SALEM HEALTH

MAGILL'S MEDICAL GUIDE

SALEM HEALTH

MAGILL'S MEDICAL GUIDE

Eighth Edition

Volume 4

Nasal polyp removal – Skin disorders

Medical Editors

Bryan C. Auday, Ph.D.
Gordon College

Michael A. Buratovich, Ph.D.
Spring Arbor University

Geraldine F. Marrocco, Ed.D., APRN, CNS, ANP-BC
Yale University School of Nursing

Paul Moglia, Ph.D.
South Nassau Communities Hospital

SALEM PRESS
A Division of EBSCO Information Services, Inc.
Ipswich, Massachusetts

GREY HOUSE PUBLISHING

Magill's Medical Guide: Health and Illness, 1995
Supplement, 1996
Magill's Medical Guide, revised edition, 1998
Second revised edition, 2002
Third revised edition, 2005
Fourth revised edition, 2008
Sixth edition, 2011
Seventh edition, 2014
Eighth edition, 2018

∞ The paper used in these volumes conforms to the American National Standard for Permanence of Paper for Printed Library Materials, Z39.48 1992 (R2009).

Note to Readers

The material presented in *Magill's Medical Guide* is intended for broad informational and educational purposes. Readers who suspect that they suffer from any of the physical or psychological disorders, diseases, or conditions described in this set should contact a physician without delay; this work should not be used as a substitute for professional medical diagnosis or treatment. This set is not to be considered definitive on the covered topics, and readers should remember that the field of health care is characterized by a diversity of medical opinions and constant expansion in knowledge and understanding.

Publisher's Cataloging-in-Publication Data
(Prepared by The Donohue Group, Inc.)

Names: Auday, Bryan C., editor.
Title: Magill's medical guide / medical editors: Bryan C. Auday, Ph.D., Gordon College [and three others].
Other Titles: Salem health (Pasadena, Calif.)
Description: Eighth Edition. | Ipswich, Massachusetts : Salem Press, a division of EBSCO Information Services, Inc. ; Amenia, NY : Grey House Publishing, 2018. | Includes bibliographical references and index. | Contents: Volume 1. Abdomen-Chronic wasting disease -- Volume 2. Chyme-Gram staining -- Volume 3. Growth-Nervous system -- Volume 4. Neuralgia, neuritis, and neuropathy-Shingles -- Volume 5. Shock-Zoonoses, Appendixes, Indexes.
Identifiers: ISBN 9781682176313 (set) | ISBN 9781682176320 (v.1) | ISBN 9781682176337 (v.2) | ISBN 9781682176344 (v.3) | ISBN 9781682176351 (v.4) | ISBN 9781682176368 (v.5)
Subjects: LCSH: Medicine--Encyclopedias.
Classification: LCC RC41 .M345 2018 | DDC 610.3--dc23

First Printing

printed in the United States of America

Complete Table of Contents

Volume 1

Volume 2

Volume 3

Volume 4

Shading indicates current volume.

Shading indicates current volume.

Shading indicates current volume.

Volume 5

SALEM HEALTH
MAGILL'S MEDICAL GUIDE

Nasal polyp removal

Procedure

Anatomy or system affected: Head, nose

Specialties and related fields: Family medicine, general surgery, otorhinolaryngology

Definition: The excision of benign growths that project from the mucous membrane lining the nasal cavity.

Indications and Procedures

Nasal polyps are swollen masses that project from the nasal wall. These benign structures are commonly found in patients with allergies. They may cause chronic nasal obstruction, which results in diminished air flow through the nasal cavity.

Once a polyp is detected, the physician may prescribe a nasal spray to reduce its size, such as the corticosteroids beclometasone or flunisolide. This treatment is usually effective for small nasal polyps that cause only minor symptoms. When pharmacological management is not successful, the polyps should be removed surgically.

Surgical removal of nasal polyps (nasal polypectomy) is typically done as an outpatient procedure. It requires either general anesthesia or local anesthesia with sedation. After the patient is asleep or sedated, the lining of the nasal cavity is injected with a combination of local anesthesia and epinephrine to control pain and bleeding. The surgeon (usually an otorhinolaryngologist) visualizes the polyps with a headlight, and the polyps are removed with specialized long surgical instruments inserted into the nasal cavity. After the polyps are removed, the nasal passages are packed with ointment-coated gauze to help control bleeding and aid in the healing of the nasal mucosa. The gauze is re-

moved in the physician's office a few days after the surgery. Once the packing is removed, the patient enjoys improved breathing through the nasal passages.

Uses and Complications

There are relatively few complications associated with nasal polyp removal. Some of the more common complications include bleeding from the surgical site, nasal and ear discomfort or anxiety as a result of the packing, and nausea from the anesthesia. The recurrence of nasal polyps after polypectomy is not unusual. Patients with cystic fibrosis have a high rate of occurrence of nasal polyps and often have recurrent problems.

—*Matthew Berria, Ph.D. and Douglas Reinhart, M.D.*

See also Allergies; Nasopharyngeal disorders; Oral and maxillofacial surgency; Otorhinolaryngology; Polyps; Sense organs; Sinusitis; Smell.

For Further Information:

Adelman, Daniel C., Thomas B. Casale, and Jonathan Corren, eds. *Manual of Allergy and Immunology*. 5th ed. Philadelphia: Wolters Kluwer Health/Lippincott Williams & Wilkins, 2012.

Benjamin, Bruce, et al. *A Colour Atlas of Otorhinolaryngology*. Edited by Michael Hawke. Philadelphia: J. B. Lippincott, 1995.

Bull, P. D. *Lecture Notes: Diseases of the Ear, Nose and Throat*. 10th ed. Malden, Mass.: Blackwell Science, 2007.

PDxMD. *PDxMD Ear, Nose, and Throat Disorders*. Philadelphia: Author, 2003.

Icon Health. *Nasal Polyps: A Medical Dictionary, Bibliography, and Annotated Research Guide to Internet References*. San Diego, Calif.: Author, 2004.

Kimball, Chad T. *Colds, Flu, and Other Common Ailments Sourcebook*. Detroit, Mich.: Omnigraphics, 2001.

Lewy, Jennifer, and Marcin Chwistek. "Nasal Polyp." *Health Library*, March 15, 2013.

Morelock, Michael, and J. B. Vap. *Your Guide to Problems of the Ear, Nose, and Throat*. Philadelphia: Lippincott Williams & Wilkins, 1985.

"Nasal Polyps." *Mayo Clinic*, February 19, 2011.

Settipane, Guy A., et al., eds. *Nasal Polyps: Epidemiology, Pathogenesis and Treatment*. Providence, R.I.: OceanSide, 1997.

Vorvick, Linda J., Seth Schwartz, and David Zieve. "Nasal Polyps." *MedlinePlus*, August 31, 2011.

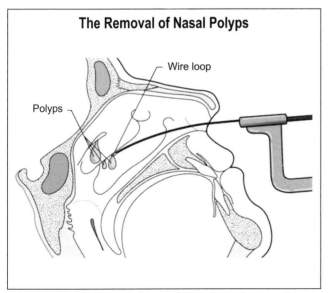

The Removal of Nasal Polyps

Wire loop

Polyps

Allergies or chronic sinus infections can lead to the development of nasal polyps, distended areas of the nasal lining. If they interfere with breathing or the sense of smell or if they cause frequent nosebleeds, the polyps may be removed with a wire loop.

Nasopharyngeal disorders

Disease/Disorder

Anatomy or system affected: Nose, respiratory system, throat

Specialties and related fields: Family medicine, occupational health, otorhinolaryngology

Definition: Disorders of the nose, nasal passages (sinuses), and pharynx (mouth, throat, and esophagus).

Key terms:

acute disease: a short and sharp disease process

chronic disease: a lingering illness

esophagus: the tube that leads from the pharynx to the stomach

larynx: the organ that produces the voice, which lies between the pharynx and the trachea; commonly called the voice box

nasopharyngeal: referring to the nose and pharynx (the upper part of the throat that leads from the mouth to the esophagus) *trachea*: a tube that leads from the throat to the lungs; commonly called the windpipe

Causes and Symptoms

Nasopharyngeal disorders are all the diseases that can be present in the nasal cavity and the pharynx. These include the common cold, pharyngitis (sore throat), laryngitis (inflammation of the larynx), epiglottitis (inflammation of the lid over the larynx), tonsillitis (inflammation of the lymph nodes at the rear of the mouth), sinusitis (inflammation of the sinus cavities that surround the nose), otitis media (earache that is often associated with nasopharyngeal infection), nosebleed, nasal obstruction, halitosis (bad breath), and various other disorders.

The common cold is one of the most prevalent diseases that afflict humankind. Pharyngitis, or sore throat, often accompanies the common cold, or it may appear by itself. Acute infections can be caused by viruses or bacteria, often by certain streptococcus strains-hence the common term for the disorder, strep throat. Acute pharyngitis can also be caused by chemicals or radiation. As a chronic disorder, pharyngitis can be caused by lingering infection in other organs such as the lungs and sinuses, or it can be attributable to constant irritation from smoking, drinking alcohol, or breathing polluted air. The usual symptoms of pharyngitis include sore throat, difficulty swallowing, and fever. The infected area appears red and swollen.

Ordinarily, pharyngitis is not serious. If certain strains of streptococcus are the cause, however, then the infection may progress to rheumatic fever. This disease appears to be the result of an immune system reaction to some streptococcus bacteria. It can have painful effects in many parts of the body, including the joints, and can do permanent damage to parts of the heart. In rare cases, rheumatic fever can be fatal.

Acute laryngitis is usually caused by a viral infection, but bacteria, outside irritants, or misuse of the voice are other causes. Ordinarily, the vocal cords produce sounds by vibrating in response to the air passing over them. When inflamed or irritated, they swell, causing distortion in the sounds produced. The affected person's voice becomes hoarse and raspy and may even diminish to a soft whisper. This distortion of sound is the main symptom of laryngitis; other possible symptoms include a sore throat and congestion that causes constant coughing. The condition generally resolves itself and requires no treatment. Chronic laryngitis has the same symptoms but does not go away spontaneously. It may be caused by an infectious agent but more likely is attributable to some irritant activity, such as constantly misusing one's voice, smoking, drinking alcohol, or breathing contaminated air.

The epiglottis is a waferlike tissue covered by a mucous membrane that sits on top of the larynx. It can become infected by such microorganisms as the bacteria *Haemophilus influenzae* type b, causing a condition called epiglottitis. Although the symptoms of epiglottitis can resemble those of pharyngitis, the infection can quickly progress to a very serious, life-threatening disor-

> ## Information on Nasopharyngeal Disorders
>
> **Causes:** May include bacterial or viral infection, nasal obstruction (polyps), environmental allergens or toxins
>
> **Symptoms:** Sore throat; inflamed lymph nodes, larynx, and sinus cavities; earache or ear infection; nosebleeds; nasal obstruction; fever; difficulty breathing or swallowing; general malaise; bad breath
>
> **Duration:** Acute to chronic
>
> **Treatments:** Antibiotics, over-the-counter medications, surgery; if severe, emergency intubation

der. Epiglottitis usually afflicts children from two to four years of age, but adults can also be affected. The infection can begin rapidly, causing the epiglottis to swell and obstruct the airway to the lungs, creating a major medical emergency. Within twelve hours of the onset of symptoms, 50 percent of patients require hospitalization and intubation (insertion of a breathing tube into the trachea). The symptoms are high fever, severe sore throat, difficulty breathing, difficulty swallowing, and general malaise. As the airway becomes more and more occluded, the patient begins to gasp for air. The lack of oxygen may cause cyanosis (blue color in the lips, fingers, and skin), exhaustion, and shock.

Another disease associated with the larynx is croup, or laryngotracheobronchitis. As the medical name indicates, croup involves the larynx, the trachea, and the bronchi (the large branches of the lung). It is usually caused by a virus, but some cases are attributable to bacterial infection. Children from three to five years of age are the usual victims. This disease causes the airways to narrow due to inflammation of the inner mucosal surfaces. Inflammation causes coughing, but the narrowed airway causes the cough to be sharp and brassy, like the barking of a seal. Croup is usually relatively benign, but sometimes it progresses to a severe disease requiring hospitalization.

Various other disorders can afflict the larynx, such as damage to the vocal cords because of infection by bacteria, fungi, or other microorganisms. The vocal cords can also be damaged by misusing one's voice, smoking, or breathing contaminated air. Polyps (masses of tissue growing on the surface), nodes (little knots of tissue), or so-called singer's nodules may develop. Sores called contact ulcers may form on the vocal cords.

Tonsillitis is an inflammation of the tonsils, two large lymph nodes located at the back of the throat. It may also involve the adenoids, lymph nodes located at the top of the throat. The function of these lymph nodes is to remove harmful pathogens (disease-causing organisms) from the nasopharyngeal cavity. At times, the load of microorganisms that they absorb becomes more than they can handle, and they become infected. The tonsils and adenoids may then become enlarged. A sore throat develops, along with a headache, fever, and chills. Glands of the neck and throat feel sore and may become enlarged. Young adults can also suffer from quinsy, or peritonsillar abscess. In this condition, one of the tonsils becomes infected and pus forms between the tonsil and the soft tissue surrounding it. Quinsy is characterized by pain in the throat or the soft palate, pain on swallowing, fever, and a tendency to lean one's head toward the affected side.

The nasal sinuses are four pairs of cavities in the bone around the nose. There are two maxillary sinuses, so called because they are found in the maxilla, or upper jaw. Slightly above and behind them are the ethmoid sinuses, and behind them are the sphenoid sinuses. Sitting over the nose in the lower part of the forehead are the two frontal sinuses. All these sinuses are lined with a mucous membrane and have small openings that lead into the nasal passages. Air moves in and out of the sinuses and allows mucus to drain into the nose. In acute sinusitis, infection builds up in the mucous membrane of any or all of the sinuses. The membrane lining the sinus swells and shuts the opening into the nasal passages. At the same time, membranes of the nose swell and become congested. Mucus and pus build up inside the sinuses, causing pain and pressure. Most often, sinusitis accompanies the common cold: the mucous membrane that lines the nose extends into the sinuses, so the infection of a cold can readily spread into the sinuses. The various viruses responsible for the common cold may be involved, as well as a wide group of bacteria. Chronic sinusitis can be caused by repeated infections that have allowed scar tissue to build up, closing the sinus openings and impeding mucus drainage, or it may be the result of allergies.

According to the Centers for Disease Control and Prevention, chronic sinusitis is the most common long-term illness in the United States, surpassing the rates for asthma, arthritis, and congestive heart disease and causing nearly fourteen million doctor's office visits per year. For reasons that are not yet understood, sinusitis sufferers are often beset with inflammation of the ducts, trapping mucus, bacteria, and viruses inside and allowing nasal polyps to develop. Researchers have been very interested in finding causes and effective treatments for sinusitis. In the late twentieth century, most chronic cases of sinusitis were treated with fiber-optic surgery that allowed access to the cramped sinus passageways. However, patients often returned within weeks or months with ongoing problems. This fact has recently prompted a reconsideration of the problem and its underlying causes as well as a struggle to redefine sinusitis. Some medical experts suspect that inflammation or the responses of the immune system are the culprit but note that additional research must be completed before any definitive answers are found.

Tissues in the nasopharyngeal cavity may be affected by conditions occurring in other parts of the body. For example, vocal cord paralysis may be caused by vascular accidents, certain cancers, tissue trauma, and other events.

Some infections in the nasopharyngeal cavity can spread to the ear through the eustachian tubes that connect the two areas. Chief among the diseases of the ear that can be asso-

ciated with nasopharyngeal disorders are the various forms of acute otitis media, an earache occurring in the central part of the ear. There are four basic types of otitis media. In the first type, serous otitis media, there is usually no infection, but fluid accumulates inside the middle ear because of the blockage of the eustachian tube or the overproduction of fluid; the condition is usually mild, with some pain and temporary loss of hearing. The second type is otitis media with effusion; with this condition comes both infection and accumulation of fluid. The third form is acute purulent otitis media, the most serious type. Pus builds up inside the middle ear, and its pressure may rupture the eardrum, allowing discharge of blood and pus. The fourth type is secretory otitis media, which usually occurs after several bouts of otitis media. Cells within the middle ear start producing a fluid that is thicker than normal and produced in greater amounts.

Chronic otitis media is bacterial in origin. It is characterized by a perforation of the eardrum and chronic pus discharge. The eardrum is a flat, pliable disk of tissue that vibrates to conduct sounds from the outside to the inner-ear structures. The perforation that occurs in chronic otitis media can be one of two types: a relatively benign perforation occurring in the central part of the eardrum or a potentially dangerous perforation occurring near the edges of the ear-

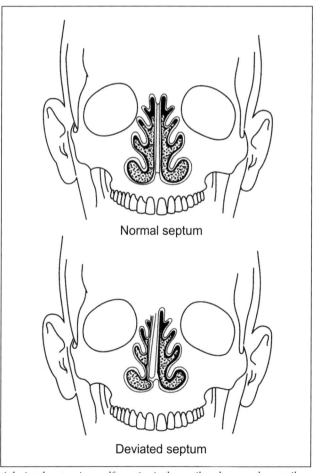

A deviated septum is a malformation in the cartilage between the nostrils, either present at birth or caused by a blow to the nose.

drum. The latter perforation can be associated with loss of hearing, increased discharge of pus and other fluids, facial paralysis, and the spread of infection to other tissues. When the perforation of chronic otitis media is near the edges of the eardrum, something called a cholesteatoma develops. This accumulation of matter grows in the inner ear and can be destructive to bone and other tissue.

The same organisms that cause otitis media can be responsible for a condition called mastoiditis. The mastoid process is a bone structure lined with a mucous membrane. Infection from otitis media can spread to this area and in severe cases can destroy the bone. Mastoiditis used to be a leading cause of death in children.

Nosebleeds are common and most often result from a blow to the nose, but they can also be caused by colds, sinusitis, and breathing dry air. The septum (the cartilaginous tissue that separates the nostrils) and the surrounding intranasal mucous membrane contain many tiny blood vessels that are easily ruptured. If an individual receives a blow to the nose, these vessels can break and bleed. They can also rupture due to irritation from a cold or other condition. Breathing very dry air sometimes causes the nasal mucous membrane to crust over, and bleeding can follow. Nosebleeds are not usually serious, but sometimes they are indicative of an underlying condition, such as hypertension (high blood pressure), a tumor, or another disease.

Nasal obstruction is common during colds and allergy attacks, but it can also be caused by a deviated septum, a malformation in the cartilage between the nostrils that can be congenital or caused by a blow to the nose. Nasal obstruction can also be attributable to nasal polyps, nasal tumors, or swollen adenoids. A common source of nasal obstruction is overuse of nasal decongestants. These agents relieve nasal congestion by reducing intranasal inflammation and swelling. If used too often or for too long, however, they can cause the very problem that they were intended to cure: intranasal blood vessels dilate, the area swells, secretions increase, and the nose becomes blocked. This is known as rebound congestion or, in medical terminology, rhinitis medicamentosa (nasal inflammation that is caused by a medication).

Halitosis, or bad breath, can be considered a nasopharyngeal disorder in the sense that it can originate in the mouth. It can be caused by diseases of the teeth or gums, but the most common causes are smoking or eating aromatic foods such as onions and garlic. Bad breath may also be a sign of disease conditions in other parts of the body, such as certain lung disorders or cancer of the esophagus. Hepatic failure, a liver dysfunction, may be accompanied by a fishy odor on the breath. Azotemia, the retention of nitrogen in the blood, may give rise to an ammonia-like odor. A sweet, fruity odor on the breath of diabetic patients may accompany ketoacidosis, a condition that occurs when there are high levels of glucose in the blood. Sometimes, young children stick foreign objects or other materials into their noses; it has been reported that these materials can fester, causing severe halitosis. Bad breath is rarely apparent to the individual who has it, however offensive it may be to others. A good way to check one's breath is to lick the back of one's hand and smell the spot; malodor, if it exists, will usually be apparent.

Treatment and Therapy

Nasopharyngeal disorders are most often mild illnesses that can be treated at home. For example, acute pharyngitis, or sore throat, is easily managed most of the time. The patient is advised to rest, gargle with warm salt water several times a day, and soothe the pain with lozenges or anesthetic gargles. If the infection is caused by a virus, it usually will clear without further treatment. If the physician suspects that the infection is bacterial in origin, throat smears may be taken so that the organism can be identified. If bacteria are discovered, antibiotic therapy will be undertaken to eradicate the pathogens. This is particularly important if the infection is caused by certain strains of streptococcus bacteria. In this case, it is vital to destroy the organism in order to avoid the development of rheumatic fever.

In cases of acute laryngitis caused by viral infection, the patient is advised to rest his or her voice, inhale steam, and drink warm liquids. If bacteria are the cause of the laryngitis, antibiotic therapy is undertaken. In treating chronic laryngitis, the physician must discover the cause and remove it. If allergy is the cause, antihistamine therapy could help. If the cause is bacterial, antibiotic therapy is used. If smoking or drinking alcohol is the problem, the patient should be counseled to stop. The simple palliative measures used for acute laryngitis-resting the voice, drinking warm liquids, and breathing steam-are also useful for chronic laryngitis.

Symptoms of epiglottitis are often similar to those of sore throat. If there is any evidence of difficulty in breathing, however, the patient should be seen by a physician quickly, as an emergency situation may be developing. If epiglottitis is obstructing the airway, the patient should be treated in an intensive care setting. Antibiotics must be given to the patient to treat the infection. It is important to make an airway for the patient, and it may be necessary to insert a tube into the trachea to allow the patient to breathe.

Before the age of antibiotics, tonsillitis was often treated surgically, with both tonsils and adenoids removed. This procedure is now rare, as the infection usually responds to antibiotic therapy. Similarly, in the case of peritonsillar abscess or quinsy, antibiotics usually clear the condition satisfactorily. In some cases, accumulations of pus may be removed surgically. If the abscesses return, it may be advisable to remove the tonsils.

As a rule, a child with croup is treated at home. Because the disease is usually caused by viruses, antibiotics are not used unless bacteria are known to be involved. Steam is often used to help liquefy mucus deposits on the interior walls of the trachea, the larynx, and the bronchi. The patient is given warm liquids to drink and is closely watched so that any signs that the condition is getting worse will be detected. The following symptoms should alert the caregiver to the possibility that an emergency situation is developing and that medical help is needed quickly: drooling, difficulty breathing or swallowing, inability to bend the neck forward, blue or dark color in the lips, high-pitched sounds when inhaling, rapid heartbeat, and loss of consciousness.

The main goals of therapy for sinusitis are to control infection, relieve the blockage of the sinus openings to permit drainage, and relieve pain. When sinusitis is known to be of bacterial origin, an appropriate antibiotic will be used to eradicate the organism. Often, however, sinusitis is attributable to viral infection, and other procedures are used to treat it. Inhaling steam is useful for thinning secretions and promoting drainage, as are mucolytic agents such as guaifenesin. Decongestant sprays and oral decongestants reduce swelling and open passages. Analgesics can be given for pain. In certain circumstances, the sinuses are drained surgically.

Acute otitis media is most often diagnosed with the aid of an otoscope, an instrument that the doctor uses to look at the eardrum and surrounding tissues. The eardrum will be a dull red color, bulging, and perhaps perforated. While a viral infection may precede otitis media, the causative microorganisms for this and related ear infections, such as mastoiditis, are usually bacteria. Antibiotics are used both to treat the infections and to prevent the spread of disease to other areas. The drugs are usually taken orally. Penicillin and its derivatives are used, as are erythromycin and sulfisoxazole. Antibiotic therapy for acute otitis media is usually continued for ten days to two weeks. Sometimes pus and other fluids and solid matter build up in the inner ear, and it may be necessary to pierce the eardrum in order to remove these deposits. To help relieve blockage of the eustachian tubes, a topical vasoconstrictor may be used in the nose to reduce the swelling of blood vessels. Antihistamines could be helpful to patients with allergies but are otherwise not indicated.

For chronic otitis media, it is necessary to clean both the outer ear canal and the middle ear thoroughly. A mild acetic acid solution with a corticosteroid is used for a week to ten days. Meanwhile, aggressive oral antibiotic therapy is undertaken to eradicate the pathogen. The perforated eardrum associated with chronic otitis media can usually be repaired surgically with little or no loss of function, and the cholesteatoma must be surgically removed.

Simple nosebleeds can be treated by pinching the nose with the fingers and breathing through the mouth for five or ten minutes to allow the blood to clot. Also, a plug of absorbent paper or cloth can be inserted into the bleeding nostril. A nosebleed that does not stop easily should be seen by a physician.

Nasal obstruction resulting from colds or allergies is treated by appropriate medications, decongestants for colds and antihistamines for allergies. A deviated septum may require surgery. The only therapy for rhinitis medicamentosa, or rebound congestion caused by overuse of nasal decongestants, is to stop the medication and endure the congestion for as long as it takes the condition to clear. Sometimes it is necessary to consult a physician.

For simple halitosis caused by smoking or food, breath fresheners (with or without "odor-fighting" chemicals) are often used, even though they usually simply replace a "bad" odor with a "good" one. Some people believe that chewing parsley or other leaves rich in chlorophyll will counteract the smell of garlic. When halitosis is attributable to tooth or gum disease, it will persist until the condition is cured. Halitosis may be of diagnostic value in certain situations where a characteristic odor could alert the physician to the possibility of a disease condition.

Perspective and Prospects

Diseases and infections of the nasal cavity and throat have always been common among human populations, as have therapies to deal with them. Until the advent of antibiotics, some of these disorders were quite serious, especially in young children, but modern medications and surgeries, where appropriate, have greatly lessened the danger. The widespread use of a vaccine against *Haemophilus influenzae* type b, the most common causative organism of epiglottitis, has made this life-threatening disease a rarity. Many over-the-counter drugs are used to combat sore throats, sinus congestion, and other nasopharyngeal symptoms of the common cold, although colds themselves remain incurable because of the hundreds or thousands of different microorganisms that may be responsible.

Despite the numerous medications that can be taken, however, more serious infections or diseases, such as chronic tonsillitis or laryngitis, require a doctor's care, with more potent prescription drugs and surgery if needed. The treatments available to physicians and patients for the symptoms of nasopharyngeal disorders are many, but the search continues for better drugs and perhaps preventive measures such as vaccinations to address the causes of these conditions.

—*C. Richard Falcon*

See also Allergies; Antihistamines; Choking; Common cold; Decongestants; Ear infections and disorders; Ears; Earwax; Esophagus; Halitosis; Hearing; Hearing loss; Laryngectomy; Laryngitis; Mouth and throat cancer; Multiple chemical sensitivity syndrome; Nasal polyp removal; Nosebleeds; Oral and maxillofacial surgery; Otorhinolaryngology; Pharyngitis; Pharynx; Plastic surgery; Respiration; Rhinitis; Rhinoplasty and submucous resection; Sinusitis; Smell; Sore throat; Strep throat; Taste; Tonsillectomy and adenoid removal; Tonsillitis; Tonsils; Voice and vocal cord disorders.

For Further Information:

Friedman, Ellen M., and James P. Barassi. *My Ear Hurts! A Complete Guide to Understanding and Treating Your Child's Ear Infections.* Darby, Pa.: Diane, 2004.

Greene, Alan R. *The Parent's Complete Guide to Ear Infections.* Allentown, Pa.: People's Medical Society, 1999.

Kimball, Chad T. *Colds, Flu, and Other Common Ailments Sourcebook.* Detroit: Omnigraphics, 2001.

Litin, Scott C., ed. *Mayo Clinic Family Health Book.* 4th ed. New York: HarperResource, 2009.

PDxMD. *PDxMD Ear, Nose, and Throat Disorders.* Philadelphia: Author, 2003.

Wagman, Richard J., ed. *The New Complete Medical and Health Encyclopedia.* 4 vols. Chicago: J. G. Ferguson, 2002.

National Cancer Institute (NCI)

Organization

Definition: A federal agency devoted to the study of cancer, as well as communication and education about this condition.

Key terms:
carcinogenesis: the biological process of the initiation, promotion, and progression of cancer
epidemiology: the study of the relationships between a host, an agent, and an environment that lead to a condition or disease

Overview

The US Department of Health and Human Services (HHS) is the federal agency responsible for public health. The HHS includes eleven divisions, one of which is the National Institutes of Health (NIH). The National Cancer Institute (NCI) is one of twenty-seven institutes and centers within the NIH. The institute was established in 1937 under the National Cancer Institute Act and in 1944 was made part of the National Institutes of Health under the Public Health Service Act. NCI is the principal federal agency for cancer research and training. Following special legislation in 1971 that amended the Public Health Service Act and created the National Cancer Act, the scope of the NCI has continued to broaden through new initiatives and legislation.

The purpose of the NCI is to eliminate cancer as far as possible and to discover treatment for those cancers which cannot be eradicated. The NCI approaches these goals by supporting research, coordinating efforts in prevention and treatment, facilitating the movement of research findings into medicine, and providing education and resources for patients and their families, health educators, and scientists. The NCI conducts research in its own laboratories and clinics in Bethesda, Maryland, but also supports and coordinates research projects conducted by universities, hospitals, research foundations, and businesses throughout the United States and many other countries.

The Organization and Focus of the NCI

The NCI is organized by the Office of the Director into nearly thirty centers, offices, and divisions. Each of the intiatives specializes in a different aspect of cancer research, although there is overlap among them. The Office of Cancer Centers, for example, supports cancer research at academic and research institutions across the United States, while the Office of Cancer Genomics specifically supports research programs that focus on the molecular components of cancer.

Another group, the Office of Cancer Nanotechnology Research, is in charge of the NCI Alliance for Nanotechnology in Cancer Program, which works to develop nanotechnology-based tools for research, detection, treatment, monitoring, and prevention. The Center to Reduce Cancer Health Disparities works through research, training, and partnerships to reduce cancer disparities among diverse populations. The Center for Global Health fosters international collaboration and sharing of research resources among government agencies, nongovernment organizations, biotechnology companies, and pharmaceu-

tical companies. In 1998, the Office of Cancer Complementary and Alternative Medicine was established to coordinate research and communication activities in the arena of complementary and alternative medicine, both within the NCI and with other agencies.

The main purpose of the NCI's basic, clinical intramural research program, the Center for Cancer Research, is to improve the lives of those affected by cancer as well as by HIV/AIDS. The NCI's other intramural initiative is the Division of Cancer Epidemiology and Genetics, whose goal is prevention. This division focuses on the factors that could lead to cancer growth, namely genetic predisposition, lifestyle factors, environmental contaminants, occupational exposures, medications, radiation, and infectious agents; the group also works on epidemiological methods development.

Research in cancer cell biology, such as carcinogenesis and cancer immunology, falls within the realm of the extramural Division of Cancer Biology. This division also examines the biological and health effects of exposures to ionizing and nonionizing radiation. The efforts of the Division of Cancer Prevention center on early detection methods and the efficacy of nutritional or lifestyle changes on cancer prevention. The results of research in this area led to the 5 a Day for Better Health program. Initiated in 1991, this program is a collaborative effort between the food industry and the NCI, which encourages Americans to eat five or more servings of vegetables and fruits each day as part of a low-fat, high-fiber diet. The goal of this type of diet is to prevent the risk of cancer, heart disease, diabetes, and stroke. The Division of Cancer Treatment and Diagnosis includes programs in biomedical imaging, cancer diagnosis, cancer therapy evaluation, developmental therapeutics, and radiation research. The Division of Cancer Control and Population Sciences supports a wide array of research in the areas of surveillance, genetics, epidemiology, and behavior.

The mission of the Coordinating Center for Clinical Trials (CCCT), established in 2006, is to facilitate the bringing of new scientific discoveries and tools to the medical clinic. Research areas supported by the CCCT include cancer genetics, cancer vaccines and immunotherapy, molecular therapeutics, experimental transplantation, and advanced technology. The clinical cancer genetics program integrates all aspects of clinical and laboratory medicine, particularly in studies of breast, colon, renal, and prostate cancer. Processes include molecular diagnostics, novel imaging techniques, and the molecular assessment of normal tissues in at-risk populations. The cancer vaccines and immunotherapy program investigates the clinical feasibility of using vaccines against known conditions associated with cancer, such as the human papillomavirus (HPV vaccines Cervarix and Gardasil) and human immunodeficiency virus (HIV), as well as with cancer-specific products, such as in melanoma and in lymphomas. The molecular therapeutics program is concerned with most clinical trial experiments. Important discoveries include the development of paclitaxel (Taxol) as an effective anticancer agent, the development of zidovudine (AZT, Retrovir) as an important anti-HIV drug, and the use of adoptive immunotherapy in the treatment of malignant melanoma. The scientific thrust of the molecular therapeutics program is the belief that the analysis of the molecular profile of individual cancers will help determine the most effective chemotherapeutic approaches. The experimental transplantation program examines bone marrow biology in order to advance transplantation techniques and the effectiveness of this approach.

Integrating many programs and divisions is the advanced technology initiative. New technology is an essential key to identifying genetic elements involved in cancer initiation and progression, as well as in drug efficacy and drug resistance. Although many drugs have been discovered that inhibit the growth of cancer cells successfully, they also affect healthy cells. This causes side effects that have a negative impact on patients' health and quality of life. New therapeutics and technology have been investigated to minimize or eliminate these side effects and enhance the effectiveness of therapy.

Another division of the NCI is the Division of Extramural Activities, which is responsible for handling all applications for funding and for monitoring research that has received funding from the NCI. Extramural activities also include the oversight of scientific communications. To enhance communication, the NCI has a number of advisory boards and groups that provide the institute with input from the public, medical, and research communities.

The NCI has helped strengthen the information base for cancer care decision making. Researchers, medical providers, and patients seek to better understand what constitutes quality cancer care. The Cancer Information Service, established in 1975, is the section of the NCI that is the link to the public, attempting to explain research findings in a clear, timely, and understandable manner. To this end, the Cancer Information Service helps develop education efforts that target minority audiences and people with limited access to health care information or services.

Perspective and Prospects

To be successful in managing this range of responsibilities and breadth of mission, the NCI has a budget in the billions of dollars. Although cancer is the second leading cause of death in the United States and is a leading cause of death worldwide, through the years, the work of the NCI has led to a decline in the number of deaths due to this disease. Creative and dedicated scientists at the NCI are committed to lowering its numbers even further.

—*Karen Chapman-Novakofski, R.D., L.D.N., Ph.D.*

See also Cancer; Chemotherapy; Clinical trials; Department of Health and Human Services; Environmental diseases; Environmental health; Epidemiology; Genetics and inheritance; National Institutes of Health (NIH); Nutrition; Oncology; Preventive medicine; Radiation therapy.

For Further Information:

"About NCI." *National Cancer Institute*, 2013.

"Cancer." *World Health Organization*, Jan. 2013.

"Cancer: Addressing the Cancer Burden at a Glance." *Centers for Disease Control and Prevention*, 30 Aug. 2012.

Hewitt, Maria Elizabeth, et al., eds. *Ensuring Quality Cancer Care*. Washington, DC: National Academy Press, 1999.

Lerner, Barron H. *The Breast Cancer Wars: Fear, Hope, and the Pursuit of a Cure in Twentieth-Century America*. New York: Oxford University Press, 2003.

National Cancer Institute. *The Cancer Information Service: A Fifteen-Year History of Service and Research*. Bethesda, Md.: Author, 1993.

National Cancer Institute. *National Cancer Institute's Research Programs: Pursuing the Central Questions of Cancer Research*. Bethesda, Md.: Author, 1999.

National Cancer Institute. *NCI Fact Book*. Bethesda, Md.: Author, 1979.

"NCI Mission Statement." National Cancer Institute, 2013.

"NCI Organization." *National Cancer Institute*, 2013.

Reuben, Suzanne H. *Assessing Progress, Advancing Change: 2005-2006 Annual Report*. Bethesda, Md.: National Institutes of Health, National Cancer Institute, 2006.

Varmus, Harold. "Professional Judgment Budget 2013." *National Cancer Institute*, 2013.

National Institutes of Health (NIH)

Organization

Definition: The National Institutes of Health (NIH), composed of more than twenty-five separate institutes, centers, and offices, is one of eight agencies constituting the U.S. Department of Health and Human Services.

Key terms:

AIDSLINE: a database that is part of the National Library of Medicine (NLM) and is devoted to the topic of research on acquired immunodeficiency syndrome (AIDS)

CATLINE: the online catalog of books and manuscripts in the NLM

grant proposals: research plans that outline scientific methods to pursue new knowledge, the required budget, and the resulting products and significance of that work

institute: a specific subagency of the NIH that has the charge of advancing scientific discovery and clinical practice in a specific area of medical science

MEDLINE: a database that is available via the Internet featuring current and historical medical literature, research articles, monographs, presentations, and abstracts

History and Mission

The National Institutes of Health (NIH) is a US federal agency that occupies a multibuilding campus in Bethesda, Maryland. It consists of a variety of offices, institutes focused on specific medical problems, research laboratories and centers, a center for scientific review, and a national medical library. Its main goal is to discover knowledge that will improve the state of public health for all persons, especially those in the United States. This goal extends to all medical conditions afflicting men, women, and children of all ethnic backgrounds. It also extends to seeking knowledge in areas of basic biological research, clinical research, and research on policy and practice in health care.

The National Institute of Health (precursor to the NIH) was formally established by the Ransdell Act of 1930, which bestowed the name on what was formerly called the Hygienic Laboratory (HL) of the Marine Hospital Service

(MHS) in New York. The Ransdell Act also allowed for the establishment of fellowships for basic medical and biological research. The very beginnings of the NIH extend back to 1887, however, when basic laboratory work into medical problems was pursued by the MHS, the founding body of the United States Public Health Service (PHS). The MHS was formed in 1798 to provide hospital care for seamen, but by the 1880s it had shifted its focus to screening ship passengers for infectious diseases capable of starting epidemics.

New European research in the 1880s suggesting that microorganisms caused such diseases spurred American interest in medical research and helped form the original HL. Work by the HL continued, with the laboratory eventually moving from the MHS to its own Washington, DC, campus. The study of microorganisms continued, extending from study of individual persons to studying the effects of bacteria on water and air pollution. Progress for such work was rewarded in 1901 with governmental money for the construction of a building (completed in 1904) to house the HL and further foster work focused on advancing the public health. Because the value of such work was not well established, however, no permanent funding was provided, leaving the organization subject to ongoing evaluation and supplemental funding.

In 1902 the MHS was reorganized and renamed the Public Health and Marine Hospital Service (PH-MHS); in 1912 it adopted the shortened name of the Public Health Service (PHS). During the intervening time, the HL continued its work and expanded to work in chemistry, pharmacology, zoology, immunology, and the regulation and production of vaccines and antitoxins. Additionally, new scientific staff were added to the staff of medical doctors already on board. Changes in the mission of the organization in 1912 also opened the door for the pursuit of research on noncontagious diseases and water pollution. This work continued during World War I in the form of examining sanitation, anthrax outbreaks, smallpox, tetanus, influenza, and other combat-related conditions. The success of the PHS's work in these areas caught the attention of legislators and resulted in the Ransdell Act of 1930, which established both the National Institute of Health and the practice of setting aside public monies for funding medical research. In 1937, the National Cancer Institute (NCI) was created. In 1944, the PHS formally designated the NCI as a component of the NIH, setting the pattern of a problem-focused structure within the NIH that continues to the present.

World War II led the NIH to focus almost exclusively on war-related problems. This involved examinations of fitness for military service and issues such as dental problems and syphilis. The effects of hazardous substances and conditions on workers in war industries; risks armed service professionals faced from lack of oxygen, cold temperatures, and blood clots while flying; burns, shock, bacterial infections, and fever; and the development of vaccines and therapies for tropical diseases such as malaria also composed much of its work during this time.

Successes established during the wars by such medical research led the PHS to take the 1944 Public Health Service Act to Congress. This act led to grant-funding mechanisms being extended from the NCI alone to the entire National Institute of Health. Additionally, an increasing public interest in health organizations caused Congress to create additional institutes for research on mental health, dental diseases, and heart disease between 1946 and 1949. In 1948, the National Heart Act allowed for the formal pluralization of the National Institutes of Health, rather than a singular institute with the NCI as a subinstitute. The Public Health Service Act of 1944 also provided funding for the Warren Grant Magnuson Clinical Center, which opened in 1953 to focus exclusively on clinical research on health.

From this point forward, each of the individual institutes now composing the NIH came into being. By 1960 there were ten institutes, and by 2013 there were twenty-seven institutes and centers. As different health interests develop and advances in medical knowledge are needed, the NIH has responded by allocating its resources to pursue goals in those areas. This has been done both by developing institutes and also by creating specialized offices to pursue contemporary medical problems.

Illness and medicine know no boundaries, however, so the NIH has also maintained an interest in global public health issues. Such interest was formally shown in 1947, when grants were first awarded to investigators abroad. Similarly, in 1968, the John E. Fogarty International Center (FIC) was created to coordinate international research efforts, involving liaisons with the World Health Organization and a variety of international research organizations. The FIC also supports language translation, documentation, and reviews of new health findings. It facilitates biomedical communications through its maintenance of the National Library of Medicine (NLM), MEDLINE, CATLINE, AIDSLINE, and numerous other databases for researchers, physicians, and the public at large. Similarly, focused consensus development conferences, where investigators and clinicians from around the world can meet to evaluate new and existing therapies, are another way in which international interests are pursued.

In keeping with its practical focus, the NIH has strived to seek out knowledge that yields new drugs, devices, and procedures that are useful not just for the government but for the public at large as well. In 1986, the Technology Transfer Act allowed for a partnership between NIH-funded research and the private sector. Encouraging researchers to examine possible commercial and practical applications of basic medical research to wide-reaching clinical or research use benefits overall scientific and health progress. Partnering with business allows private industries to take over the process of marketing and developing products in a manner more affordable to them than to the government, allowing the government to focus on development while benefiting through the use of the eventual marketed products.

Organizational Structure and Method

The NIH is organized to accomplish its goals by using its offices, institutes, and research centers. Research is conducted on the NIH campus in its own funded laboratories as well as in the labs of scientists supported by NIH funding, who are stationed in institutes of higher education, teaching hospitals, and research institutions in the United States and other countries. In addition to supporting ongoing research, the NIH also supports research infrastructure by maintaining a library and a variety of printed and electronic resources to facilitate communication among its researchers, the larger scientific community, policymakers, and the public. Scientific research also is supported through development of one of the most valuable resources known to medicine: new researchers. The NIH sponsors a variety of training programs focusing on medical training and research in order to keep a large body of high-quality scholars and investigators in development. Such programs extend from career development for postdoctoral researchers and predoctoral training, to high school level learning in the sponsoring of internships and other learning experiences for teenagers interested in medical science careers.

Funding for research and training programs outside the NIH campus and research centers is facilitated through grant proposal programs that distribute federal tax monies devoted to such endeavors. Applicants to such programs are able to submit independent proposals for work related to the goals of the NIH that they believe is demanded by the state of science and knowledge. They are also able to submit proposals in response to program announcements and calls for proposals on specific topics as outlined by the institutes and offices of the NIH. Many different grant mechanisms exist for such proposals, including grants supporting the work of individual trainees, training programs for cohorts of researchers at different stages of career development, the ongoing work of career scientists, small grants for new or experimental work, focused projects, and even centers of research excellence where many researchers focus on the same topic of study. In addition, grant support is offered to sponsor conferences and academic meetings on special topics in health research and training.

To receive this funding, those wishing to be considered must submit proposals for confidential peer review through the Center for Scientific Review (CSR), which is part of the NIH structure. Proposals are reviewed by panels of experts who evaluate the research plans, goals, staff, environment, and overall innovation and merit of the work proposed. In addition, ethical considerations about the proposed research are reviewed and considered for both animal welfare and the welfare of human research participants. Emphasis on ethical issues has been a long-standing issue for medical research. It was, however, highlighted in the 1960s, when grantees receiving NIH grant monies were required to state the ethical principles guiding their research on humans, and in 1979, when written guidelines for research on human subjects were established. Once through peer review, proposals are reviewed again by a national advisory council to determine the priority of the work in addressing the

goals of the NIH and its institutes and offices. After the proposals are approved by this council for advancement, the individual institutes (sometimes cooperating with specific NIH offices) work to fund them with the monies allotted. Unfortunately, not all proposals can be funded. It should be noted that even after funding, the work of the NIH continues so as to ensure that proper research ethics are followed through the life of the research.

Research funded by the NIH is facilitated by the various institutions and research offices that fall under its organizational umbrella, each focusing on a discrete area of health interest. Some of the institutions involved include the NCI; the National Eye Institute; the National Heart, Lung, and Blood Institute; and the National Human Genome Research Institute. Also included are the National Institutes on Aging, Alcohol Abuse and Alcoholism, Allergy and Infectious Diseases, Arthritis and Musculoskeletal and Skin Diseases, Child Health and Human Development, Deafness and Other Communication Disorders, Dental and Craniofacial Research, Diabetes and Digestive and Kidney Diseases, Drug Abuse, Environmental Health Sciences, Mental Health, Minority Health and Health Disparities, and Neurological Disorders and Stroke.

In addition to these institutes, the NIH has numerous offices focusing on specific issues or populations that need to be addressed in health research. These offices focus on contemporary issues of importance for research and include the Offices of Technology Transfer, AIDS Research, Research on Women's Health, Behavioral and Social Sciences Research, Dietary Supplements, Rare Diseases, Science Policy, Biotechnology Activities, Science Education, and Information Technology. There are also offices that focus on the management of research, specific organizational issues at the NIH, or the communication of information from the NIH to members of the public. These include the Offices of Intramural Research, Extramural Research, Evaluation, Human Resources, Financial Management, Acquisition and Logistics Management, Management Assessment, and Communications and Public Liaison as well as the NIH Legal Advisor and the Freedom of Information Act Office.

Perspective and Prospects

The NIH has been responsible for supporting some very influential research for more than one hundred years, garnering more than eighty Nobel Prizes for NIH-supported work. More vaccines against infectious diseases are available than ever before. The successful mapping of the human genome has set the stage for enhanced genetic testing and the development of gene therapies. Substantial decreases in mortality rates have been achieved for heart disease and strokes. Survival rates for individuals afflicted by cancer have increased, as have survival rates for infants with respiratory distress syndrome. Recovery from spinal cord injuries has been enhanced so as to lessen the probability of long-term disability. Advances in the pharmacological and behavioral treatment of mental health problems such as depression, anxiety, bipolar disorders, and schizophrenia have been achieved. Preventive approaches in dentistry have been highly successful in stopping and slowing dental problems.

Given such successes, billions of dollars of federal tax monies continue to be devoted to the NIH budget to foster continued scientific advances. New work focused on improving prevention, screening, assessment, diagnosis, and treatment for conditions such as AIDS, alcoholism and drug dependence, Alzheimer's disease, arthritis, blindness, communication disorders, diabetes, heart disease, kidney disease, lung cancer, lupus, mental illnesses, Parkinson's disease, stroke, and other persisting conditions continues on a daily basis. While great successes have been achieved to date, new research is needed that will focus on specialized approaches that may enhance health for women, minorities, youth, and the elderly. The combination of these needs, past successes, and governmental commitment to improving the state of the public health ensures that the NIH will continue onward with its mission for the foreseeable future.

—*Nancy A. Piotrowski, Ph.D.*

See also Childhood infectious diseases; Department of Health and Human Services; Disease; Environmental diseases; Environmental health; Epidemics and pandemics; Epidemiology; Health Canada; Immunization and vaccination; National Cancer Institute (NCI); Occupational health; World Health Organization.

For Further Information:

Desalle, Rob. *Epidemic! The World of Infectious Disease.* New York: New Press, 1999.

Eberhart-Philips, Jason. *Outbreak Alert: Responding to the Increasing Threat of Infectious Diseases.* Oakland, Calif.: New Harbinger, 2000.

Garrett, Laurie. *Betrayal of Trust: The Collapse of Global Public Health.* New York: Hyperion, 2001.

Guest, Charles, et al. Oxford Handbook of Public Health Practice. 3d ed. Oxford: Oxford University Press, 2013.

Institute of Medicine. *Scientific Opportunities and Public Needs: Improving Priority Setting and Public Input at the National Institutes of Health.* Washington, D.C.: National Academy Press, 1998.

Lee, Philip R., and Carroll L. Estes, eds. *The Nation's Health.* 7th ed. Sudbury, Mass.: Jones and Bartlett, 2003.

National Institutes of Health. "About NIH." US Department of Health and Human Services, June 6, 2013.

National Institutes of Health. "Institutes, Centers, and Offices." US Department of Health and Human Services, August 1, 2013.

Shnayerson, Michael, and Mark J. Plotkin. *The Killers Within: The Deadly Rise of Drug Resistant Bacteria.* Boston: Little, Brown, 2003.

Tulchinsky, Theodore H., and Elena A. Varavikova. *The New Public Health: An Introduction for the Twenty-first Century.* San Diego, Calif.: Academic Press, 2000.

Nausea and vomiting

Disease/Disorder

Anatomy or system affected: Brain, gastrointestinal system, nervous system, stomach

Specialties and related fields: Gastroenterology, otorhinolaryngology

Definition: Nausea is an unpleasant subjective sensation, accompanied by epigastric and duodenal discomfort, which often culminates in vomiting, the regurgitation of the contents of the stomach.

Key terms:

affect: the emotional reactions associated with experience

antiemetics: drugs that prevent or relieve the symptoms of nausea and/or vomiting

chemoreceptor trigger zone: a sensory nerve ending in the brain that is stimulated by and reacts to certain chemical stimulation localized outside the central nervous system

emesis: the act of vomiting

psychogenic: of mental origin

psychotropics: drugs that affect psychic function, behavior, or experience

Causes and Symptoms

Nausea is defined as a subjectively unpleasant sensation associated with awareness of the urge to vomit. It is usually felt in the back of the throat and epigastrium and is accompanied by the loss of gastric tone, duodenal contractions, and reflux of the intestinal contents into the stomach. Retching is defined as labored, spasmodic, rhythmic contractions of the respiratory muscles (including the diaphragm, chest wall, and abdominal wall muscles) without the expulsion of gastric contents. Vomiting, or emesis, is the forceful expulsion of gastric contents from the mouth and is brought about by the powerful sustained contraction of the abdominal muscles, the descent of the diaphragm, and the opening of the gastric cardia (the cardiac orifice of the stomach).

Nausea and vomiting are important defense mechanisms against the ingestion of toxins. The act of emesis involves a sequence of events that can be divided into three phases: preejection, ejection, and postejection. The preejection phase includes the symptoms of nausea, along with salivation, swallowing, pallor, and tachycardia (an abnormally fast heartbeat). The ejection phase comprises retching and vomiting. Retching is characterized by rhythmic, synchronous, inspiratory movements of the diaphragm, abdominal, and external intercostal muscles, while the mouth and the glottis are kept closed. As the antral (cavity) portion of the stomach contracts, the proximal (nearest the center) portion relaxes and the gastric contents oscillate between the stomach and the esophagus. During retching, the hiatal portion of the diaphragm does not relax, and intra-abdominal pressure increases are associated with a decrease in intrathoracic pressure.

In contrast, relaxation of the hiatal portion of the diaphragm (near the esophagus) permits a transfer of intra-abdominal pressure to the thorax during the act of vomiting. Contraction of the muscles of the anterior abdominal wall, relaxation of the esophageal sphincter, an increase in intrathoracic and intragastric pressure, reverse peristalsis (movement of the contents of the alimentary canal), and an open glottis and mouth result in the expulsion of gastric contents. The postejection phase consists of autonomic and visceral responses that return the body to a quiescent phase, with or without residual nausea.

The complex act of vomiting, involving coordination of the respiratory, gastrointestinal, and abdominal musculature, is controlled by what researchers label the emetic center. This center in the brain stem has access to the motor

Information on Nausea and Vomiting

Causes: May include gastrointestinal diseases, infections, intracranial disease, toxins, radiation sickness, migraines, motion sickness, pregnancy, anesthesia, psychological trauma

Symptoms: Increased salivation and swallowing, pallor, rapid heartbeat, sweating

Duration: Typically acute; can be recurrent with acute episodes

Treatments: Depends on cause; may include drug therapy, diet regulation, lifestyle change, emotional support

pathways responsible for the visceral and somatic output involved in vomiting, and stimuli from several areas within the central nervous system can affect this center. These include afferent (inward-directed) nerves from the pharynx and gastrointestinal tract, as well as afferents from the higher cortical centers (including the visual center) and the chemoreceptor trigger zone (CTZ) in the area postrema (a highly vascularized area of the brain stem). The CTZ can be activated by chemical stimuli received through the blood or the cerebrospinal fluid. Direct electrical stimulation of the CTZ, however, does not result in emesis.

Clinical assessment of nausea and vomiting usually focuses on the occurrence of vomiting, that is, the frequency and number of episodes. Nausea, however, is a subjective phenomenon unobservable by another. Few data collection instruments that measure separately the patient's experience of nausea and vomiting and his or her symptom distress have been reported in the literature. In fact, the Rhodes Index of Nausea and Vomiting (INV) Form 2 is the only available tool that measures the individual components of nausea, vomiting, and retching. This index measures the patient's perception of the duration, frequency, and distress from nausea. The frequency, amount, and distress from vomiting; and the frequency, amount, and distress from retching (dry heaves). The INV score provides a measurement of the total symptom experience of the patient.

While the causes of nausea and vomiting are numerous-they include gastrointestinal diseases, infections, intracranial disease, toxins, radiation sickness, psychological trauma, migraines, and circulatory syncope-three of the most common causes are motion sickness (air, sea, land, or space), pregnancy, and anesthesia administered during operative procedures.

The sequence of symptoms and signs that constitute motion sickness is fairly characteristic. Premonitory symptoms often include yawning or sighing, lethargy, somnolence, and a loss of enthusiasm and concern for the task at hand. Increasing malaise is directed toward the epigastrium, a sensation best described as "stomach awareness," which progresses to nausea. Diversion of the blood flow from the skin toward the muscles results in pallor. A feeling of warmth and a desire for cool air is often accompanied by sweating. Frontal headache and a sensation of disorientation, dizziness, or light-headedness may also occur. As symptoms progress, vomiting occurs early in the sequence of symptoms for some; in others, malaise is severe and prolonged and vomiting is delayed. After vomiting, there is often a temporary improvement in well-being; however, with continued provocative motion, symptoms build again and vomiting recurs. The symptoms may last for minutes, hours, or even days.

The most coherent explanation for the development of motion sickness is provided by sensory conflict theory. Motion sickness is generally thought to occur as the result of a "sensory conflict" between information arising from the semicircular canals and organs of the vestibular system, visual and other sensory input, and the input that is expected on the basis of past experience or exposure history. It is argued that conflicts between current sensory inputs are by themselves insufficient to produce motion sickness since adaptation occurs even though the conflicting inputs continue to be present. Visual input alone, however, can produce symptoms of motion sickness, such as watching motion pictures shot from a moving vehicle or looking out of the side window (as opposed to the front window) of a moving vehicle.

Nausea and/or vomiting in the early morning during pregnancy, so-called morning sickness, is so common that it is accepted as a symptom of normal pregnancy. Occurring soon after waking, it is often retching rather than actual vomiting and usually does not disturb the woman's health or her pregnancy. The symptoms nearly always cease before the fourteenth week of pregnancy. In a much smaller proportion of cases, approximately one in one thousand births, the vomiting becomes more serious and persistent, occurring throughout the day and even during the night. The term "hyperemesis gravidarum" is given to this serious form of vomiting. Theories on the etiology of morning sickness have tended to be grouped under four main areas: endocrine (caused by estrogen and progesterone levels), psychosomatic (a conscious or unconscious wish not to be pregnant), allergic (a histamine reaction), and metabolic (a lack of potassium).

Nausea and vomiting occur frequently as unpleasant side effects of the administration of anesthesia in many clinical procedures. Most postoperative vomiting is mild, and only in a few cases will the problem persist so as to cause electrolyte disturbances and dehydration. The factors affecting postoperative nausea and vomiting may be divided into two categories: by the type of patient and surgery, and by the anesthetic and preoperative and postoperative medication uses. Patients with a history of motion sickness have a predisposition to postoperative vomiting. Nearly 43 percent of patients who vomited following previous surgery vomited again, whereas slightly more than 14 percent of those who did not vomit previously had an emetic episode at their next operation. Patients undergoing their first anesthetic procedure had an incidence of vomiting of approximately 30 percent.

No direct association between vomiting and age has been found. That vomiting may be hormonally related, however, is suggested by the higher incidence of nausea and vomiting in the latter half of the menstrual cycle. Other factors that may affect nausea and vomiting associated with anesthesia include patient weight (female obese patients being particularly more vulnerable), amount of hydration, metabolic status, and psychological state.

With regard to the type of surgery performed, the highest incidence of nausea and vomiting appears to be associated with abdominal surgery, as well as ear, nose, and throat surgery, with middle-ear surgery being the major category. The length of surgery, and therefore the duration of anesthesia, also has a direct effect on nausea and vomiting. Short (thirty-minute to sixty-minute) operations using cyclopropane had an emetic incidence of 17.5 percent, while operations lasting one and a half to three and a half hours had an incidence of 46.4 percent.

Most of the causes of vomiting associated with general anesthesia are expected to be eliminated with regional or spinal anesthesia. The type of anesthesia used also has an effect on nausea and vomiting. Research indicates that cyclopropane, ether, and nitrous oxide are potent emetics.

Treatment and Therapy

Since the generation of sensory conflict underlies all motion environments that give rise to motion sickness, practical measures that reduce conflict are likely to reduce motion sickness incidence. Motion sickness can be minimized if the subject has the widest possible view of a visual reference in which the earth is stable. Passengers aboard ships are less likely to be seasick if they remain on deck at midship, where vertical motion is minimized, and view the horizon. In a car or bus, individuals should be in a position to see the road directly ahead, since the movement of this visual scene will correlate with the changes in the direction of the vehicle. While head movements in a rotating environment are known to precipitate motion sickness, there is no clear experimental evidence that they elicit nausea in mild linear oscillation. Thus, some nonpharmacologic remedies for motion sickness are restricting head movements, lying in a supine position, or closing the eyes. In addition, the use of acupressure wrist bands has proven effective in combating motion sickness.

Pharmacologically, the drug hyoscine hydrobromide (also called hyoscine or scopolamine) emerged as a valuable prophylactic drug following extensive research during World War II into the problems of motion sickness in troops transported in aircraft, ships, and landing craft. It remains one of the most effective drugs for short-duration exposures to provocative motion. Doses in excess of 0.6 milligram, however, are very likely to lead to drowsiness, and there is much experimental evidence that hyoscine impairs short-term memory. Hyoscine can be absorbed transdermally, and in order to extend the duration of action, a controlled-release patch was developed to deliver 1.2 milligrams on application and 0.01 milligram hourly thereafter. There is substantial evidence of its sustained effectiveness, but, perhaps as a result of variable absorption rates, there is an increased risk of blurred vision after more than twenty-four hours of use.

Amphetamines, ephedrine, and a number of antihistamines (such as dimenhydrinate) have been found to be clinically useful in motion sickness. Following oral administration, these drugs are generally slower than hyoscine in reaching their peak efficacy, but they have a longer duration of action.

For most susceptible subjects whose exposure to motion sickness-inducing stimuli is infrequent, prophylactic drugs offer the only useful treatment. When exposure to provocative stimuli is more frequent, as for example in professional aircraft pilots, spontaneous adaption occurs during training and an initially high incidence of motion sickness decreases with time.

In medical conditions in which the cause is relatively unknown, it is usual to find a wide variety of suggested therapies; nausea and vomiting during pregnancy and hyperemesis gravidarum (the serious, persistent form of vomiting in pregnancy) are no exception. Prior to 1968, treatments numbered approximately thirty. In subsequent years, however, suggested therapy has been mainly drugs of the antiemetic variety. Yet since the thalidomide tragedy (in which severe deformities occurred in the children of women who took this drug), there has been a reluctance to use drugs of any kind during early pregnancy. Probably the only value of drug therapy is at the stage of morning sickness, when antiemetics or mild sedatives may counter the feeling of nausea and prevent women from experiencing excessive vomiting and entering the vicious cycle of dehydration, starvation, and electrolyte imbalance. Once the patient has reached the stage of hyperemesis gravidarum, much more basic therapy is required, and the regimen calls for correction of dehydration, carbohydrate deficiency, and ionic deficiencies. This program is best managed by intravenous therapy, with or without the addition of vitamin supplements and sedative agents.

Nonpharmacologic self-care actions for morning sickness fall into the three broad categories of manipulating diet, adjusting behavior, and seeking emotional support. Some of the most effective self-care actions are getting rest, eating several small meals rather than three large ones, avoiding bad smells, avoiding greasy or fried foods, avoiding cooking, and receiving extra attention and support.

In terms of postoperative nausea and vomiting caused by anesthesia, it has been found that routine antiemetic prophylaxis of patients undergoing elective surgical procedures is not indicated, since fewer than 30 percent of patients experience postoperative nausea and vomiting. Of those who develop these symptoms, many have transient nausea or only one or two bouts of emesis and do not require antiemetic therapy. In addition, commonly used antiemetic drugs can produce significant side effects, such as sedation. Nevertheless, antiemetic prophylaxis may be justified in those patients who are at greater risk for developing postoperative nausea and/or vomiting. Such therapy is often given to patients with a history of motion sickness or to those undergoing gynecologic procedures, inner-ear procedures, oral surgery (in which the jaws are occluded by wires, causing a high risk of breathing in vomitus), and operations on the ear or eye and plastic surgery operations (in order to avoid disruption of delicate surgical work).

Many different antiemetic drugs are available for the treatment of postoperative nausea and vomiting. Researchers have found it difficult to interpret the results of antiemetic drug studies because the severity of postoperative vomiting and the response to therapeutic agents can be influenced by many variables in addition to the antiemetic drug being studied. Even with the use of the same drugs in a homogeneous population undergoing the same procedure, the severity of emesis varies from individual to individual.

Because antiemetic drugs have differing sites of action, better results can be obtained by using a multidrug approach. If a combination of drugs with a similar site of action is used, however, the incidence of side effects may be increased. There are few data regarding combination antiemetic prophylaxis or therapy for postoperative nausea and emesis. Drug combinations have been avoided in postsurgical patients because of concerns about additive central nervous system toxicity. An exception is the combination of low-dose droperidol and metoclopramide, which appears to be more effective than droperidol alone for outpatient gynecologic procedures.

Although a full stomach is best avoided before any operative procedure, with situations such as emergencies, in which danger from vomiting is acute, a rapid sequence of administering anesthesia (induction) and clearing the air passage (intubation) remains the method of choice to avoid nausea and vomiting in patients with a full stomach. After the procedure, it is recommended that the patient minimize movement in order to avoid nausea and vomiting. Also, it has been found that avoiding eating solid food for at least eight hours after a surgical procedure is helpful in preventing postoperative nausea and vomiting.

Perspective and Prospects

Though it has existed for as long as there have been human beings, the symptom of nausea has never received much attention in health care practice or research. In fact, until the early 1970s the sensation of nausea was frequently dismissed as merely a passing phenomenon. The rationale for this dismissal was most likely the understanding that nausea is self-limiting (it always passes with time), is never life-threatening in itself, is probably psychogenic in nature (at least to some degree), and, being subjective, is very difficult to measure. In addition, in the past the most predictable nausea was related to pregnancy, which may also explain the lack of attention given to nausea.

Until the late 1980s, there was still little research being conducted on the nausea associated with pregnancy, although it is a common symptom. The historical lack of interest in nausea and vomiting during pregnancy may be traced to the fact that, since the symptoms generally persist only through the first trimester, health care professionals have viewed the problem as relatively insignificant. As more pregnant women work outside the home in demanding positions, however, these women have exhibited less

tolerance for illness. Demands upon the health care industry and upon personal physicians for more research and effective treatment have become more widespread.

While it is surprising that nausea has received scant attention in the history of clinical research, it is even more astonishing that vomiting, an observable behavior, has received so little attention as well. Although vomiting is a primitive neurologic process that has remained almost unchanged in the evolution of animals, the mechanisms that regulate the behavior remain virtually unknown.

One reason for the paucity of information on the subject of nausea in particular stems from the lack of a reliable animal model. This fact has hampered research aimed at establishing the etiological basis for nausea and its relationship to vomiting. While some species of lower animals, for example rats, cannot vomit, it is not known whether rats experience the phenomenon of nausea. Thus no effective means of measuring nausea in lower animals has been devised.

Since the early 1970s, there has been a noticeable increase in research on nausea as a drug side effect because it was so frequently seen in cancer chemotherapy clinical trials sponsored by the National Cancer Institute and the American Cancer Society. As more powerful chemotherapy agents and aggressive combinations were clinically investigated, patients began to experience severe, potentially life-threatening nausea and vomiting. Older drugs such as antihistamines, phenothiazines, and benzodiazepines are still used for their antiemetic characteristics, but they are augmented by newer agents such as benzamides, neurokinin-1-receptor antagonists, and serotonin antagonists.

Aside from the pharmacological investigations of new drugs and drug combinations in the treatment of nausea and vomiting, an interesting branch of scientific investigation has begun the process of exploring alternative ways of managing these symptoms. Behavioral interventions, such as progressive muscle relaxation, biofeedback, imagery, or music therapy, have been used to alleviate postchemotherapy anxiety. These methods may also be used to treat other patients suffering from the symptoms of nausea and vomiting, such as pregnant women.

Another noninvasive, nonpharmacologic measure that has been considered in the relief of nausea and vomiting is transcutaneous electrical nerve stimulation (TENS). Several research studies indicate that TENS may be useful in alleviating chemotherapy-related nausea and vomiting, including delayed nausea and vomiting. Side effects from using TENS units are negligible, and with further study they may prove to be an acceptable, helpful relief measure.

—*Genevieve Slomski, Ph.D.*

See also Acid reflux disease; Anesthesia; Appetite loss; Botulism; Bulimia; Chemotherapy; Colitis; Crohn's disease; Diaphragm; Digestion; Eating disorders; Esophagus; Food biochemistry; Food poisoning; Gastroenteritis; Gastroenterology; Gastroenterology, pediatric; Gastrointestinal disorders; Gastrointestinal system; Heartburn; Indigestion; Influenza; Lactose intolerance; Motion sickness; Multiple chemical sensitivity syndrome; Noroviruses; Poisoning; Poisonous plants; Pregnancy and gestation; Radiation sickness; Rotavirus; Salmonella infection; Stomach, intestinal, and pancreatic cancers; Ulcer surgery; Ulcers; Vagotomy.

For Further Information:
Blum, Richard H., and W. LeRoy Heinrichs. *Nausea and Vomiting: Overview, Challenges, Practical Treatments, and New Perspectives.* Philadelphia: Whurr, 2000.

Casey, Georgina. "Treating Nausea and Vomiting." *Kai Tiaki Nursing New Zealand* 18, no. 11 (December, 2012): 20-24.

Edmundowicz, Steven A., ed. *Twenty Common Problems in Gastroenterology.* New York: McGraw-Hill, 2002.

Funk, Sandra G., et al., eds. *Key Aspects of Comfort: Management of Pain, Fatigue, and Nausea.* New York: Springer, 1989.

Hesketh, Paul J., ed. *Management of Nausea and Vomiting in Cancer and Cancer Treatment.* Sudbury, Mass.: Jones and Bartlett, 2005.

Kucharczyk, John, David J. Stewart, and Alan D. Miller, eds. *Nausea and Vomiting: Recent Research and Clinical Advances.* Boca Raton, Fla.: CRC Press, 1991.

Litin, Scott C., ed. *Mayo Clinic Family Health Book.* 4th ed. New York: HarperResource, 2009.

Palatty, Princy Lous, et al. "Ginger in the Prevention of Nausea and Vomiting." *Critical Reviews in Food Science and Nutrition* 53, no. 7 (2013): 659.

Rao, Kamakshi V., and Aimee Faso. "Chemotherapy-Induced Nausea and Vomiting: Optimizing Prevention and Management." *American Health and Drug Benefits* 5, no. 4 (July, 2012): 232-240.

Sleisenger, Marvin H., ed. *The Handbook of Nausea and Vomiting.* New York: Caduceus Medical/Parthenon, 1993.

Neck injuries and disorders. *See* Head and neck disorders.

Necrosis

Disease/Disorder
Also known as: Gangrene, mortification
Anatomy or system affected: Bones, cells
Specialties and related fields: Oncology, orthopedics
Definition: Tissue damage occurring as a result of cell death.

Causes and Symptoms

Necrosis refers to the degeneration of cells or tissues after cell death occurs for any reason, generally in localized regions of the body. Thus, necrosis is tissue degeneration, which occurs secondary to cell death from any cause. Necrosis is most commonly the result of ischemia, traumatic injury, bacterial infection, or toxins (including excessive steroids or alcohol).

In its earliest stage, there are often no symptoms of necrosis. Tissue damage begins to occur within twelve hours of cell death. When symptoms do begin to occur, they range from atrophy to decreased range of motion and pain to the development of gangrenous tissue.

Treatment and Therapy

The damage done to the tissue resulting from cell death is permanent. Any treatment of necrosis is aimed at minimizing further cell death and tissue injury. In the case of heart disease, treatment of the underlying condition to alleviate hypoxia prevents further cell death from ischemia. In the case of bacterial infection, antibiotics are used to treat the infection and prevent cell death and tissue damage. In the case of necrosis of bone tissue from decreased blood supply, the aim of treatment is to minimize further bone loss.

Information on Necrosis

Causes: Cell death leading to degeneration of tissue over time
Symptoms: Pain, tissue decay
Duration: Permanent, irreversible
Treatments: Pain relievers (NSAIDs), surgery

This type of necrosis, known as "avascular necrosis" or "osteonecrosis," is treated with nonsteroidal anti-inflammatory drugs (NSAIDs) to relieve pain, exercise to improve range of motion, electrical treatment to stimulate bone growth, or surgery to reshape or graft bone or to replace joints.

Perspective and Prospects

The term "necrosis" was used nearly two thousand years ago in ancient Greek textbooks to refer to changes within tissue, long after cell death had occurred, that were visible to the naked eye. With the advent of light microscopy, the tissue damage following cell death became visible within twelve to twenty-four hours.

In 1859, Rudolf Virchow, in his renowned text *Cellular Pathology as Based upon Physiological and Pathological Histology,* discussed degeneration, necrosis, mortification, and gangrene, using these terms more or less synonymously. It should be noted that he used the term "necrosis" to refer to an advanced stage of tissue breakdown. At this point, the breakdown had to be visible to the naked eye, since light microscopy had not yet been developed. Today, using the microscope, tissue damage resulting from cell death is obvious and often identical whether caused by ischemia, traumatic injury, bacteria, or toxins.

—*Robin Kamienny Montvilo, R.N., Ph.D.*

See also Cells; Circulation; Gangrene; Ischemia; Necrotizing fasciitis; Osteonecrosis; Pathology; Vascular medicine; Vascular system.

For Further Information:
A.D.A.M. Medical Encyclopedia. "Necrosis." *MedlinePlus*, March 23, 2013.

"Cell Death." In *Pathology: Clinicopathologic Foundations of Medicine*, edited by Raphael Rubin, David Sheldon Strayer, and Emanuel Rubin. 6th ed. Baltimore: Lippincott, 2012.

Majno, G., and I. Joris. "Apoptosis, Oncosis, and Necrosis: An Overview of Cell Death." *American Journal of Pathology* 146, no. 1 (1995): 3-15.

"Necrosis." In *Taber's Cyclopedic Medical Dictionary*, edited by Donald Venes. 21st ed. Philadelphia: F. A. Davis, 2010.

Parker, J. N., and P. M. Parker. *The Official Patient's Sourcebook on Avascular Necrosis.* San Diego, Calif.: Icon Health, 2002.

Necrotizing fasciitis

Disease/Disorder
Anatomy or system affected: Blood vessels, muscles, skin
Specialties and related fields: Bacteriology, critical care, dermatology, emergency medicine, epidemiology, histology, plastic surgery, vascular medicine
Definition: An invasive bacterial infection that occurs in the connective tissue between the skin and muscle known as

the fascia, cutting off blood flow; it must be urgently treated surgically and, even in the best circumstances, has a high mortality rate.

Causes and Symptoms

Although it had been identified in the past, in 1994 there were numerous headline newspaper reports describing a new "flesh-eating bacteria." These articles detailed the devastating effect of seemingly minor wounds infected with streptococcal bacteria. Patients quickly become very sick, with a rapidly progressive downward course, even from trauma resulting in a deep muscle bruise or muscle strain or in "minor" cuts and scrapes.

In the former nonpenetrating injuries, it is likely that the bacteria were already present in the blood and then seeded the site of damage. Most of these patients, however, did not recall any prior recent infection that may have made them susceptible. Penetrating injuries, where the normally protective barrier of the skin has been broken, were often minor and not originally treated as contaminated or infected. Other cases of necrotizing fasciitis are caused by surgical infections and bowel contamination. These cases are more rare and often found to have a mixture of bacteria, such as staphylococci or *Escherichia coli* (*E. coli*).

Information on Necrotizing Fasciitis

Causes: Bacterial infection
Symptoms: Fever, inflammation, severe pain, blistering at site of infection, tissue death
Duration: Acute
Treatments: Emergency care, extensive surgical debridement, antibiotics

---

Patients with necrotizing fasciitis have fever, inflammation, severe pain, and blistering at the site of infection. If this cellulitis is not recognized and urgently treated, the infection will quickly spread in the layers of connective tissue just under the skin known as the fascia. As the bacteria multiply, they cause blood vessels supplying the skin to form clots and thus cut off blood flow to the skin. Without nutrients, oxygen, and the ability to remove waste products, the skin dies. Once this occurs, the nerves are destroyed and the patient no longer has the excruciating pain. The skin at this point appears to be "eaten away." The possibility exists that the underlying muscle adjacent to the fascia will become infected. Thus, the potential for muscle death as well as skin death is of great concern, particularly if the infection begins in the arms, legs, abdomen, or back, as these areas have large muscle groups directly underlying the skin. In necrotizing fasciitis, the extremities and the area around the genitals and anus (perineum) are most commonly and extensively involved. Multiplication and movement of these streptococcal bacteria and their toxins into the bloodstream produces a shock-like state.

Treatment and Therapy

The patient with necrotizing fasciitis must be stabilized quickly in an intensive care unit, where fluids can be administered and heart and lung condition can be closely monitored. The only lifesaving treatment available is extensive surgical debridement to remove the necrotic (dead) tissue and slow the spread of the bacteria. Antibiotics including penicillins, clindamycin, and gentamicin are given to help eradicate the pathogen. Because the infection spreads so rapidly, death often results even with heroic surgical and drug therapy unless the condition is diagnosed and treated early. Fortunately, these infections remain relatively rare.

—*Matthew Berria, Ph.D.*

See also Antibiotics; Bacterial infections; Bacteriology; Connective tissue; Dermatology; Epidemiology; Fascia; Necrosis; Shock; Skin; Skin disorders; Streptococcal infections; Toxic shock syndrome; Wounds.

For Further Information:

Berman, Kevin. "Necrotizing Soft Tissue Infection." *MedlinePlus*, November 22, 2011.
Biddle, Wayne. *A Field Guide to Germs*. 3d ed. New York: Anchor Books, 2010.
Forbes, Betty A., Daniel F. Sahm, and Alice S. Weissfeld. *Bailey and Scott's Diagnostic Microbiology*. 12th ed. St. Louis, Mo.: Mosby/Elsevier, 2007.
MedlinePlus. "Streptococcal Infections." *MedlinePlus*, May 7, 2013.
Roemmele, Jacqueline A., and Donna Batdorff. *Surviving the Flesh-Eating Bacteria: Understanding, Preventing, Treating, and Living with the Effects of Necrotizing Fasciitis*. Garden City Park, N.Y.: Avery, 2000.
Snyder, Larry, et al. *Molecular Genetics of Bacteria*. 4th ed. Washington, D.C.: ASM Press, 2013.
Wilson, Brenda A., Abigail A. Salyers, et al. *Bacterial Pathogenesis: A Molecular Approach*. 3d ed. Washington, D.C.: ASM Press, 2011.
Wilson, Michael, Brian Henderson, and Rod McNab. *Bacterial Disease Mechanisms: An Introduction to Cellular Microbiology*. New York: Cambridge University Press, 2002.

Neonatal brachial plexus palsy

Disease/Disorder

Also known as: Erb's palsy, obstetric brachial plexus palsy, birth brachial plexus palsy
Anatomy or system affected: Arms, nerves
Specialties and related fields: Neonatology, neurology, obstetrics, organizations and programs, orthopedics, pediatrics, perinatology, physical therapy, plastic surgery, psychology, radiology
Definition: A motor disability evident early in life that manifests as weakness of the affected arm due to stretching or compression of the nerves of the brachial plexus during the perinatal period, with passive range of motion greater than active.

Key terms:

brachial plexus: complex of nerves that carry motor and sensory function to the arm
contractures: permanent shorting of muscles or joints
Erb's palsy: stereotyped clinical presentation of neonatal brachial plexus palsy resulting from injury to the C5, C6, and sometimes C7 spinal nerve roots
Horner's syndrome : ptosis (eyelid drooping), miosis (

abnormal constriction of the pupil of the eye), and anhydrosis (decreased sweating on the face)

incidence: the rate at which a certain event occurs or the number of new cases of a specific disorder occurring during a certain period in a population at risk

pan-plexopathy: a form of neonatal brachial plexus palsy comprising of injury to all of the spinal nerve roots manifesting as a flaccid arm

perinatal period: the period immediately before and after birth, commencing at 20 weeks of gestation and ending at 28 weeks after birth (140 days total)

range of motion: movement of a joint from full flexion to full extension

shoulder dystocia: diagnosed when the delivery of the fetal head is not followed by the emergence of the shoulder due to impaction of the fetus' shoulder in the birth canal

Causes and Symptoms

Children with neonatal brachial plexus palsy (NBPP) have a weak or paralyzed arm, and their passive range of motion is greater than their active range of motion. NBPP becomes evident early in life and usually results from stretching or compression of the nerves of the brachial plexus during the perinatal period. NBPP occurs with an incidence of 1.5 cases per 1000 live births, with or without shoulder dystocia at the time of both vaginal and cesarean delivery. Risk factors for NBPP include abnormal positioning of the

---

Information on Neonatal Brachial Plexus Palsy

Causes: Damage to the nerves of the brachial plexus during or after birth

Symptoms: One of the arms does not move normally

Duration: Depends on the severity; some children recover completely, others only partially, while some are permanently affected

Treatments: Physical and occupational therapy, exercises, orthopedic or neural surgery

---

fetus, labor abnormalities, artificial labor induction, large fetus, and shoulder dystocia. However, except for shoulder dystocia, none of these risk factors are statistically significant clinical predictors for the occurrence of NBPP.

Compression or stretching of the nerves of the brachial plexus can occur during development in the uterus or during the descent and emergence of the fetus from the uterus and pelvis with maternal pushing and naturally expulsive forces. Biomechanically, nerve injury can result from forces applied by clinicians, or natural physical events that move the fetus from the uterus through the birth canal and out of the mother's pelvis. No one force or factor seems to be responsible for the cause of NBPP, but the available data do suggest that the occurrence of NBPP may be a multifactorial event.

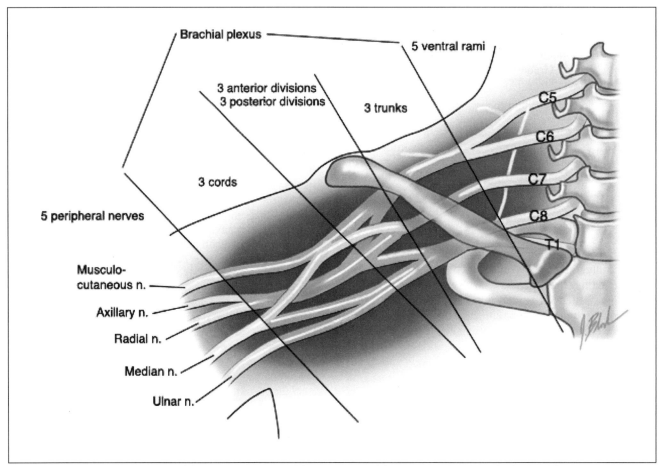

Nerves of the brachial plexus, cervical and thoracic spinal nerves and the major nerves of the upper arm. (http://www.backpain-guide.com)

The brachial plexus is a very complex structure that connects the spinal nerves in the neck to their terminal branches in the arm and is divided into 5 zones: (1) C5 through T1 spinal nerve roots; (2) upper, middle, and lower trunks; (3) anterior and posterior divisions of each trunk; (4) lateral, posterior, and medial cords; and (5) terminal branches. These nerves carry the signals necessary for the normal movement and sensation in the entire arm. The brachial plexus is analogous to a set of intersecting highways with overpasses, underpasses, and multiple merging traffic intersections, with several roads leading into (analogous to the spinal nerve roots) and out of (analogous to the terminal branches) the intersections. However, for simplicity, the nerve roots can be indexed to the muscles in the following fashion: C5-shoulder movement, C6-elbow flexion, C7-elbow extension, C8/T1-hand and finger movement.

Not all cases of NBPP are the same, and the symptoms may be radically different depending on which parts of the brachial plexus are injured. The intricate intersecting nature of the brachial plexus implies that thousands of potentially different palsies can ensue, but in reality, only a few variations actually occur. The most useful classification scheme for clinical presentation of NBPP is the Narakas Grade system that represents the extent of the spinal nerve root injury: only C5 and C6 nerve roots are injured in Grade 1, C5, C6, C7 nerve roots in Grade 2, and C5 through T1 injured in Grade 3 (without Horner's syndrome) and Grade 4 (with Horner's syndrome). When this classification system is used in 2-4 week old affected babies, it may guide the prognosis for spontaneous recovery, since up to 90 percent of the patients with Grade 1 NBPP regain functional use of the affected arm, but less than 5 percent of the patients with Grade 4 NBPP regain functional use without medical and/or surgical intervention.

Other classification systems are based on the clinical manifestations of NBPP. Erb's palsy, the most common type of NBPP, is synonymous with an "upper" plexus palsy that specifically results from damage to C5, C6, and sometimes C7 spinal nerve roots. Patients with Erb's palsy present a "waiter's tip" posture when their affected arm is pulled toward the midline of the body, an internally rotated shoulder, flexed wrist, extended fingers that result from loss of both shoulder control and elbow bending. Contrastingly, the extremely rare Klumpke's palsy is synonymous with a "lower" plexus palsy characterized by a flaccid hand attached to an otherwise active arm. Total plexus palsy or pan-plexopathy is equivalent to Narakas Grade 3 and 4 and is recognized by loss of total function of the arm.

Treatment and Therapy

Lack of normal arm movement observed during the perinatal period warrants confirmation of the diagnosis of NBPP by a specialist. Possible skeletal injuries or fractures should be confirmed by clinical and radiographic evaluation since these injuries may preclude early occupational/physical therapy. Immobilization of the arm is not recommended except in the case of skeletal injuries.

With regard to the specific motor function of the affected arm, the treating physician assesses the passive and active range of motion of the affected arm. Available assessment scales of motor function in NBPP are used to determine the extent and severity of nerve injury, to prognosticate potential functional recovery, and to guide and assess the outcomes from further treatment. Traditional scales focus only upon the affected arm, but more recently, assessment methods are focusing upon the overall function of the child. Supplementing the physical examination with electrodiagnostic / electromyographic (EMG) and radiographic (magnetic resonance imaging, MRI) findings are helpful to decide whether surgical nerve reconstruction will be beneficial.

Early referral of those babies with severe or extensive NBPP to interdisciplinary specialty clinics can improve overall functional outcomes as the baby grows. Regardless of the need for surgical intervention, rehabilitation management is critical. Occupational/physical therapy to maintain the normal passive range of motion in all upper extremity joints (especially shoulder external rotation and forearm rotation) facilitates successful functional recovery. Parents and caregivers should consider themselves to be the patient's primary therapist by performing range of motion exercises regularly, with multimedia assistance if available (e.g., during every diaper change). Reinforced use of the affected arm while constraining the normal arm (similar to patching a lazy eye) can aid the child's recognition of the arm and strengthen the arm through increased arm use during age-appropriate activities. Normal childhood developmental milestones must be encouraged, including crawling. Splinting may be used during sleep to avoid contractures or to protect floppy joints. As the child grows, recreational activities like swimming, dance, sports, and potentially therapist-designed video game platforms can help to sustain the goals of formal occupational/physical therapy.

For NBPP patients who do not recover with conservative management, surgical nerve reconstruction may be an option, usually occurring between 3-9 months of age. Although the indications and timing for nerve reconstruction have not been absolutely established, most practitioners agree that babies with the extensive total brachial plexus palsy and those with the severe Erb's palsy will benefit from nerve surgery. The goal of nerve reconstruction is not to regain a normal arm, but surgical intervention is a step towards a functional arm with adequate movement, if not power. Nerve repair using autologous nerve graft and/or nerve transfer (using a good nerve to re-innervate an injured one) constitute the primary options for reconstructing the function of the brachial plexus. As nerve repair and transfer rely upon regrowth of the normal portions of the nerve through the residual pathways after injured nerve is cleared away (Wallerian degeneration), and as this nerve regeneration is very slow, the ultimate functional outcome from nerve reconstruction surgery may not be apparent for 1-3 years.

Toddlers and older children with incomplete recovery following neurosurgical or conservative treatment may have functional limitations because of residual muscle weakness and soft tissue contractures, especially around the shoulder and elbow. MRI imaging can guide the decision to pursue orthopedic intervention. Internal rotation contracture of the shoulder is most common and can be associated with progressive shoulder joint deformity and instability. Indications for surgical intervention include persistent internal rotation contracture despite aggressive nonsurgical therapy, progressive joint deformity, and obvious joint dislocation. Surgical options include muscle lengthening combined with tendon transfers, corrective bone surgery (osteotomies), and open or arthroscopic reduction of the shoulder joint.

For children with residual elbow, forearm, and hand problems, secondary procedures by a hand surgeon may be appropriate. These procedures include soft tissue releases, joint fusions, muscle transfers, and corrective osteotomies. The usual age for secondary reconstruction of the elbow/forearm function is 4-6 years of age, and for wrist/hand function is 6-13 years of age.

For all surgical interventions, the most important factor in producing the optimal result is a cooperative child with intense investment from assertive parents/caretakers. The parents must understand the objectives of the surgical procedure and work hard with their children in postoperative rehabilitation-and maintenance of function by being their children's primary therapists. Surgery alone without subsequent rehabilitation management and therapy is unlikely to yield the desired outcome.

Perspective and Prospects

Overall, the majority of infants with NBPP have a good prognosis for recovering adequate functional use of the affected arm-with rehabilitation management and therapy, supplemented with surgical intervention when and where appropriate and desired by the patient and parents/caretakers. Early occupational/physical therapy can support the spontaneous recovery of function and minimize consequent musculoskeletal comorbidities along with more efficient recovery of function after surgery. Despite the similar incidence of NBPP to cerebral palsy, public awareness of this perinatal disorder and its lifelong implications (medical and psychosocial) for the more extensively/severely affected children are significantly lacking. Similarly, published research studies regarding NBPP number only a fraction of that regarding cerebral palsy. Therefore, current efforts exist not only to find new medical treatment techniques but also to increase awareness, to address and improve the quality of life for patients with NBPP via traditional and recent technology-assisted modalities. Early referral to an interdisciplinary specialty brachial plexus clinic can avail the patient of the most current treatment paradigms to achieve the optimal outcome.

—*Lynda J.-S. Yang, M.D., P.D., F.A.A.N.S.*

See also Neonatology; Neurology; Neurology, pediatric; Obstetrics; Occupational health; Orthopedics; Physical rehabilitation

For Further Information:
Bowerson, M., V.S. Nelson, and L.J. Yang. "Diaphragmatic Paralysis Associated with Neonatal Brachial Plexus Palsy." *Pediatric Neurology* 42, no. 3 (March 2010) 234-236. Case study of a NBPP baby whose diaphragm was also paralyzed.
Chung, Kevin C., Lynda J.-S.Yang, and John E. McGillicuddy, eds. *Practical Management of Pediatric and Adult Brachial Plexus Palsies.* London: Elsevier, 2011. Extensive overview of the medical and surgical techniques for managing disorders of the brachial plexus. Presents a multidisciplinary approach to pediatric brachial plexus palsy treatment and rehabilitation, obstetric considerations, and other timely topics in the field (includes DVD).
Mehta, S.H., and B. Gonik. "Neonatal Brachial Plexus Injury: Obstetrical Factors and Neonatal Management." *Journal of Pediatric Rehabilitation Medicine* 4, no. 2 (2011) 113-118. A review of the potential causes of and risk factors for NBPP.
Murphy, K.M., L. Rasmussen, S.L. Hervey-Jumper, D. Justice, V.S. Nelson, and L.J. Yang. "An Assessment of the Compliance and Utility of a Home Exercise DVD for Caregivers of Children and Adolescents with Brachial Plexus Palsy: A Pilot Study." *PM & R* 4, no. 3 (March 2012) 190-197. Small, initial study of the efficacy of home exercises for NBPP children.
Piatt, J.H., Jr. "Birth Injuries of the Brachial Plexus." *Clinical Perinatology* 32, no. 1 (March 2005) 39-59. Excellent summary of the classification of various types of NBPP.
Squitieri, L.. B.P. Larson, K.W. Chang, L.J. Yang, and K.C. Chung. "Medical Decision-Making among Adolescents with Neonatal Brachial Plexus Palsy and Their Families: A Qualitative Study." *Plastic and Reconstructive Surgery* 131, no. 6 (June, 2013): 880e-887e. A study that examines why patients make particular treatment choices and stresses the need for proper patient education.

Neonatology

Specialty

Anatomy or system affected: All

Specialties and related fields: Cardiology, critical care, embryology, genetics, obstetrics, pediatrics, perinatology

Definition: A subspecialty of pediatrics that involves the care of newborn infants from birth through the first month of life, especially those infants with life-threatening conditions such as prematurity, genetic defects, and serious illnesses.

Key terms:

congenital disorders: abnormalities present at birth that occurred during fetal development as a result of genetic errors, exposure to toxins and microorganisms, or maternal illness

incubator: in the nursery, a plexiglass unit that encloses the premature or sick infant to allow strict temperature regulation

intrauterine growth retardation: the condition of infants who are born significantly smaller than the standard for the number of weeks that they have spent in the uterus

neonatal intensive care unit: a hospital nursery with advanced equipment and specially trained staff to maintain the vital functions of sick newborns and to monitor their progress closely

neonatal period: the first month of life; derived from the Greek *neo* (meaning "new") and the Latin *natum* (meaning "birth")

prematurity: strictly defined, birth before a full-term pregnancy (thirty-eight weeks); more commonly associated with birth before thirty-five weeks

respirator: a machine that inflates and deflates the lungs, imitating normal breathing; connected to the patient through a tube placed into the windpipe (endotracheal tube)

respiratory distress syndrome: a life-threatening illness primarily of premature infants; immature lungs lack surfactant, a vital substance that keeps the tiny air sacs (alveoli) from collapsing upon exhalation

Science and Profession

Neonatology has grown dramatically since its beginnings in the late 1960s, and neonatologists have become an integral part of the obstetric-pediatric team at major medical centers throughout the world. In addition to being cared for by physicians who specialize in neonatology, some neonatal infants, in particular those who are critically ill or premature, are cared for by nurse practitioners with the specialty certification of neonatal nurse practitioner (NNP). In large part because of an ever-expanding technological base and marked advances in scientific research, these health care professionals have changed the outlook for premature and sick newborns.

As a subspecialty of pediatrics, neonatology is concerned with the most critical time of transition and adjustment-the first four weeks of life, or the neonatal period-whether the infant is healthy (a normal birth) or sick (as a result of genetic problems, obstetric complications, or medical illness). By the early 1970s, it became increasingly clear to health administrators that hospitals throughout the United States had varying abilities to care for medical and pediatric cases requiring the most sophisticated staff and equipment. Consequently, they developed a system that designated hospitals as either level I (small, community hospitals), level II (larger hospitals), or level III (major regional medical centers, also called tertiary care centers). It was in the last group that the most advanced neonatal care could be delivered. In these major centers, there are two types of nurseries, separating the normal healthy infant from the sick or high-risk infant: the routine nursery and the neonatal intensive care unit (NICU).

Routine nurseries are the temporary home of the vast majority of newborns. The services of the neonatologist are rarely needed here, and the general pediatrician or family practitioner observes and examines the infant for twenty-four to forty-eight hours to be sure that it has made a smooth transition from intrauterine to extrauterine life. These babies soon leave the hospital for their homes. Those neonates with minor problems arising from multiple births, difficult deliveries, mild prematurity, and minor illness are easily managed by a primary care physician in consultation with a neonatologist, perhaps at another hospital. It is in the neonatal intensive care unit, however, that the most difficult situations present themselves. Here several teams of pediatric subspecialists-surgeons, cardiologists, anesthesiologists, and highly trained nurses, along with many other health professionals-are led by a neonatologist, who coordinates the team's efforts. These newborns have life-threatening conditions, often as a result of extreme prematurity (more than six weeks earlier than the expected date of de-livery), major birth defects (genetic or developmental), severe illness (such as overwhelming infections), or being born to drug- or alcohol-addicted mothers. They require the most advanced technological and medical interventions, often to sustain life artificially until the underlying problem is corrected. It is in this setting that the most dramatic successes of neonatology are found.

After hours of being inside a forcefully contracting uterus and sustaining the stress of passing through a narrow birth canal, the newborn emerges into a dry, cold, and hostile environment. The umbilical cord, which has provided oxygen and nutrients, is clamped and cut; the fluid-filled lungs must now exchange air instead, and the respiratory center of the infant's brain begins a lifetime of spontaneous breathing, usually heralded by crying. The vast majority of neonates make this extraordinary adjustment to extrauterine life without difficulty. At one minute and again at five minutes, the newborn is evaluated and scored on five physical signs: heart rate, breathing, muscle tone, reflexes, and skin tone. The healthy infant is vigorously moving, crying, and pink regardless of race. These Apgar scores, named for neonatology pioneer Virginia Apgar, evaluate the need for immediate resuscitation. A brief physical examination follows, which can identify other life-threatening abnormalities.

It is essential to remember that the medical history of a neonate is in fact the medical and obstetric history of its mother, and seemingly normal infants may develop problems shortly after birth. Risk factors include very young or middle-aged mothers; difficult deliveries; babies with Rh-negative blood types; mothers with diabetes mellitus, kidney disease, or heart disease; and concurrent infections in either the mother or the baby. Anticipating these problems of the healthy newborn by using the Apgar scores and the results of the physical examination allows the proper assignment of the infant to the nursery or NICU.

The NICU is a daunting place containing high-tech equipment, a tangle of wires and tubes, the sounds of beeps and alarms, and tiny, fragile infants. All this technology serves two simple purposes: to monitor vital functions and to sustain malfunctioning or nonfunctioning organ systems. Looked at individually, however, the machines and attachments become much more understandable. The incubator, perhaps the most common device, maintains a warm, moist environment of constant temperature at 37 degrees Celsius (98.6 degrees Fahrenheit). Small portholes with rubber gloves allow people to touch the child safely. Generally, the infants will have small electrodes taped on their chests, connected to video monitors that record the heart and breathing rates and that will sound alarms if significant deviations occur. These monitors will also record blood pressure through an arm or thigh cuff. To ensure immediate access to the blood, for delivering medications and taking blood for testing, catheters (plastic tubes) are placed into larger arteries or veins near the umbilicus, neck, or thigh (in adults, intravenous access is found in the arms).

The remaining equipment is used for the very serious business of life support, in particular the support of the re-

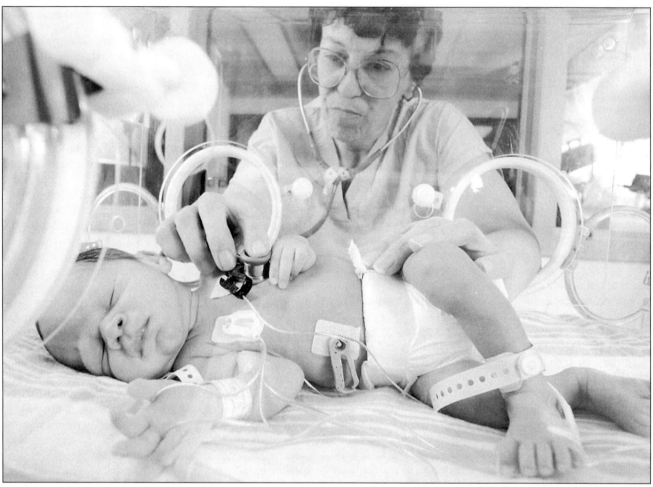

Newborns at risk may require a special environment such as an incubator. (Digital Stock)

spiratory system. Maintaining adequate oxygenation is critical and can be accomplished in several ways, depending on the baby's needs. The least stressful are tubes placed in the nostrils or a face mask, but these methods require that breathing be spontaneous although inadequate. More often, unfortunately, neonates with the types of problems that bring them to an intensive care unit cannot breathe on their own. In these cases, a tube must be connected from the artificial respirator into the windpipe (the endotracheal tube). Warm, moistened, oxygen-rich air is delivered under pressure and removed from the lungs rhythmically to simulate breathing. Tranquilizers and paralytic agents are used to calm and immobilize the infant. Sick or premature infants are also generally unable to feed or nurse naturally, by mouth. Again, several methods of feeding can be employed, depending on the problems and the length of time that such feedings will be needed. For the first few days, simple solutions of water, sugar, and protein can be given through the intravenous catheters. These lines, because of the very small, fragile blood vessels of the newborn, are seldom able to carry more complex solutions. A second method, known as gavage feeding, employs tubing that is inserted through the nose directly into the stomach. Through that tube, infant formula (water, sugar, protein, fat, vitamins, and minerals) and, if available, breast milk

can be given.

As the underlying problems are resolved, the infant is slowly weaned, first feeding orally and then breathing naturally. Next, the infant will be placed in an open crib, and gradually the tangled web of tubes and wires will clear. With approval from the neonatologist, the baby is transferred to the routine nursery, a transitional home until discharge from the hospital is advisable.

Diagnostic and Treatment Techniques

Neonatology has amassed an enormous body of knowledge about normal neonatal anatomy and physiology, disease processes, and, most important, how to manage the wide variety of complications that can occur. Specific treatment protocols have been developed that are practiced uniformly in all neonatal intensive care units. Short-term stays (twenty-four to forty-eight hours) are meant to observe and monitor the infant with respiratory distress at birth that required immediate intervention. Long-term stays, lasting from several weeks to months, are the case for the sickest newborns, most commonly those with severe prematurity and low birth weight (less than 1,500 grams), respiratory distress syndrome (also known as hyaline membrane disease), congenital defects, and drug or alcohol addictions.

Infants born prematurely make up the major proportion

of all infants at high risk for disability and death, and each passing decade has seen younger and younger babies being kept alive. While many maternal factors can lead to preterm delivery, often no explanation can be found. The main problem of prematurity lies in the functional and structural immaturity of vital organs. Weak sucking, swallowing, and coughing reflexes lead to an inability to feed and to the danger of choking. Lungs that lack surfactant, a substance that coats the millions of tiny air sacs (alveoli) in each lung to keep them from collapsing and sticking together after air is exhaled, cause severe breathing difficulty as the infant struggles to reinflate the lungs. When premature delivery is inevitable but not immediate, lung maturity can be increased by administration of steroids to the mother. An immature immune system cannot protect the newborn from the many viruses, bacteria, and other microorganisms that exist. Inadequate metabolism causes low body temperature and inadequate use of food or medications. Neurological immaturity can lead to mental retardation, blindness, and deafness.

Aggressive management of the preterm baby begins in the delivery room, with close cooperation between the obstetrician and the neonatologist. Severely preterm infants, some born after only twenty weeks of pregnancy, require immediate respiratory and cardiac support. Placement of the endotracheal tube, assisted ventilation with a handheld bag, and delicate chest compressions similar to the cardiopulmonary resuscitation (CPR) performed on adults to stimulate the heartbeat are each accomplished quickly. Once the respiratory and circulatory systems have been stabilized, excess fluid will be suctioned, while a brief physical examination is performed to note any abnormalities that require immediate attention. As soon as transport is consid-

ered safe, the newborn is sent to the NICU. If the infant has been delivered at a small community hospital, this may involve ambulance or even helicopter transport to the nearest tertiary care center.

Once in the unit, the neonate will be placed in an incubator and attached to video monitors that record heart rate, breathing, and blood pressure. The endotracheal tube can now be attached to the respirator machine, and intravenous or intra-arterial catheters will be placed to allow the fluid and medication infusions and the blood drawing for the battery of tests that the neonatologist requires. Feeding methods can be set up as soon as the infant has stabilized. Within a short time after delivery, the premature newborn has had a flurry of activity about it and is surrounded by the most sophisticated equipment and staff available. Supporting the immature organs becomes the first priority, although the ethical issues of saving very sick infants must soon be addressed as complications begin to occur. Nearly 15 percent of surviving preterm infants whose birth weights were less than 2,000 grams have serious physical and mental disabilities after discharge. The majority, however, grow to lead normal, healthy lives.

Congenital defects are common, and it is estimated that the majority of miscarriages are a direct result of congenital defects that are incompatible with life. Many infants that do survive development and delivery die shortly after birth despite the most sophisticated and heroic attempts to intervene. The causes of such defects are arbitrarily assigned to two broad categories, although a combination of these factors is the most likely explanation: genetic errors (such as breaks, doubling, and mutations) and environmental insults (such as chemicals, drugs, viruses, radiation, and malnutrition). In the United States, among the most common

Number of Infant Deaths in the United States, 2014

Cause of Death	
Congenital malformations, deformations and chromosomal abnormalities	4,746
Disorders related to short gestation and low birth weight, not elsewhere classified	4,173
Newborn affected by maternal complications of pregnancy	1,574
Sudden infant death syndrome	1,545
Accidents (unintentional injuries)	1,160
Newborn affected by complications of placenta, cord and membranes	965
Bacterial sepsis of newborn	544
Respiratory distress of newborn	460
Diseases of the circulatory system	444
Neonatal hemorrhage	441
All other causes	7,163
Total	23,215

Source: National Center for Health Statistics.

birth defects that require immediate intervention are heart problems, spina bifida (an open spine), and tracheoesophageal fistulas and esophageal atresias (wrongly connected or incomplete wind and food pipes).

The birth of a malformed infant is rarely expected, and the neonatologist's team plays a key role in its survival. Congenital heart disease is the most prevalent life-threatening defect. During development in utero, the umbilical cord supplies the necessary oxygen; it is not until birth, when that lifeline is cut, that the neonate's circulatory and respiratory systems acquire full responsibility. At delivery, all may appear normal, and the one-minute Apgar score may be high. Several minutes later, however, the pink skin color may begin to darken to a purplish blue (cyanosis), indicating that insufficient oxygen is being extracted from the air. Immediately, the infant receives rescue breathing from the bag mask. Upon admission to the neonatal unit, the source of the cyanosis must be determined. A chest x-ray may provide significant information about the anatomy of the heart and lungs, but special tests are usually needed to pinpoint the problem. Catheters that are threaded from neck or leg vessels into the heart can reveal the pressure and oxygen content of each chamber in the heart and across its four valves. Echocardiograms, video pictures similar to sonograms generated by sound waves passing through the chest, enhance the data provided by the x-rays and catheterizations, and a diagnosis is made. Based on the physical signs and symptoms of the newborn, a treatment plan is devised.

Because of the nature of congenital defects and structural abnormalities, their correction generally requires surgery. Openings between the heart's chambers (septal defects), valves that are too narrow or do not close properly, and blood vessels that leave or enter the heart incorrectly are all common defects treated by the pediatric heart surgeon. Because of the delicacy of the operation and the vulnerability of the newborn, surgery may be postponed until the baby is larger and stronger while it is provided with supplemental oxygen and nutrients. The risk of such operations is high, and depending on the degree of abnormality, several operations may be required.

Another group of infants who have benefited from advances in neonatology are those born to drug-addicted women. The lives of these infants are often complicated by congenital defects and life-threatening withdrawal symptoms. For example, heroin-addicted babies are quite small, are extremely irritable and hyperactive, and develop tremors, vomiting, diarrhea, and seizures. The newborn must be carefully monitored in the unit, and sedatives and antiseizure medications are given, sometimes for as long as six weeks. Cocaine and its derivatives frequently cause premature labor, fetal death, and maternal hemorrhaging during delivery. Infants that do survive often have serious congenital defects and suffer withdrawal symptoms. The risk of acquired immunodeficiency syndrome (AIDS) adds another dimension to an already complicated picture.

Perspective and Prospects

Throughout human history, maternal and neonatal deaths have been staggering in number. Ignorance and unsanitary conditions frequently resulted in uterine hemorrhaging and overwhelming infection, killing both mother and baby. Highly inaccurate records at the beginning of the twentieth century in New York City show maternal death averaging 2 percent; in fact, the rate was probably greater, since most births occurred at home. Neonatal deaths from respiratory failure, congenital defects, prematurity, and infection loom large in these medical records. The expansion of medical, obstetric, and pediatric knowledge and technology that began after World War II has dramatically lowered maternal and infant mortality. It should not be forgotten, however, that nonindustrialized nations, the majority in the world, remain devastated by the neonatal problems that have plagued civilization for thousands of years.

Ironically, the problems associated with neonatology in Western nations are now at the other end of the spectrum: saving and prolonging life beyond what is natural or "reasonable." As neonatology advanced scientifically and technically, saving life took precedence over ethical issues. The famous and poignant story of Baby Doe in the early 1980s illustrates the dilemmas that occur daily in neonatal intensive care units. Baby Doe was a six-pound, full-term male born with Down syndrome and severe congenital defects of the heart, trachea, and esophagus. These malformations were deemed surgically correctable, although the underlying problem of Down syndrome, a disease characterized by intellectual disabilities and particular facial and body features, would remain. The parents did not agree to any operations and requested that all treatment be withheld. Baby Doe was given only medication for sedation and died within a few days. The case was later related by the attending physician in a letter to *The New England Journal of Medicine*, sparking enormous controversy. On July 5, 1983, a law was passed in effect stating that all newborns with disabilities, no matter how seriously afflicted, should receive all possible life-sustaining treatment, unless it is unequivocally clear that imminent death is inevitable or that the risks of treatment cannot be justified by its benefit. The legislators believed that Baby Doe had been allowed to die because of his underlying condition of Down syndrome.

Since then, attorneys, ethicists, juries, and courts have used the example of Baby Doe, and the law that grew from it, to interpret many cases that have come to light. Life-and-death decisions are made on a daily basis in the neonatal care unit. They are always difficult, but they usually remain a private matter between the parents and the neonatologist. These cases become public matters, however, when the family disagrees with the medical staff. Then the question of what is in the best interest of the child is compounded by who will pay for the treatments and who will care for the baby after it is discharged.

Such ethical dilemmas will continue as expertise and technology grow. A multitude of questions, previously relegated to philosophy and religion, will arise, and the benefits of saving a life will have to be weighed against its quality and the resources necessary to maintain it.

—*Connie Rizzo, M.D., Ph.D.;*
updated by Alexander Sandra, M.D.

See also Apgar score; Birth defects; Blue baby syndrome; Bonding; Cardiology, pediatric; Cesarean section; Childbirth; Childbirth complications; Chlamydia; Circumcision, male; Cleft lip and palate; Cleft lip and palate repair; Cognitive development; Colic; Congenital disorders; Congenital heart disease; Craniosynostosis; Critical care, pediatric; Cystic fibrosis; Developmental disorders; Developmental stages; Down syndrome; Embryology; Endocrinology, pediatric; Failure to thrive; Fetal alcohol syndrome; Fetal surgery; Gastroenterology, pediatric; Genetic diseases; Genetics and inheritance; Hematology, pediatric; Hemolytic disease of the newborn; Hydrocephalus; Intraventricular hemorrhage; Jaundice, neonatal; Metabolic disorders; Motor skill development; Multiple births; Nephrology, pediatric; Neurology, pediatric; Obstetrics; Orthopedics, pediatric; Pediatrics; Perinatology; Phenylketonuria (PKU); Polydactyly and syndactyly; Premature birth; Pulmonary medicine, pediatric; Rh factor; Shunts; Sudden infant death syndrome (SIDS); Surgery, pediatric; Tay-Sachs disease; Teratogens; Toxoplasmosis; Urology, pediatric; Well-baby examinations.

For Further Information:

Behrman, Richard E., Robert M. Kliegman, and Hal B. Jenson, eds. *Nelson Textbook of Pediatrics.* 18th ed. Philadelphia: Saunders/Elsevier, 2007.

Bradford, Nikki. *Your Premature Baby: The First Five Years.* Toronto, Ont.: Firefly Books, 2003.

Crisp, Stuart, and Jo Rainbow, eds. *Emergencies in Paediatrics and Neonatology.* 2d ed. Oxford: Oxford University Press, 2013.

Cunningham, Nicholas, ed. *Columbia University College of Physicians and Surgeons: Complete Guide to Early Child Care.* New York: Crown, 1990.

Levin, Daniel L., and Frances C. Morriss, eds. *Essentials of Pediatric Intensive Care.* 2d ed. New York: Churchill Livingstone, 1997.

MacDonald, Mhairi G., Mary M. K. Seshia, and Martha D. Mullett, eds. *Avery's Neonatology: Pathophysiology and Management of the Newborn.* 6th ed. Philadelphia: Lippincott Williams & Wilkins, 2005.

Martin, Richard J., Avroy A. Fanaroff, and Michele C. Walsh, eds. *Fanaroff and Martin's Neonatal-Perinatal Medicine: Diseases of the Fetus and Infant.* 2 vols. 8th ed. Philadelphia: Mosby/Elsevier, 2006.

Meeks, Maggie, Maggie Hallsworth, and Helen Yeo, eds. *Nursing the Neonate.* 2d ed. Malden: Wiley-Blackwell, 2013.

Moore, Keith L., and T. V. N. Persaud. *The Developing Human.* 8th ed. Philadelphia: Saunders/Elsevier, 2008.

Ruhlman, Michael. *Walk on Water: Inside an Elite Pediatric Surgery Unit.* New York: Viking-Penguin, 2003.

Sadler, T. W. *Langman's Medical Embryology.* 11th ed. Philadelphia: Lippincott Williams & Wilkins, 2009.

Sinha, Sunil, Lawrence Miall, and Luke Jardine. *Essential Neonatal Medicine.* 5th ed. Malden: Wiley-Blackwell, 2012.

Woolf, Alan D., et al., eds. *The Children's Hospital Guide to Your Child's Health and Development.* Cambridge, Mass.: Perseus, 2002.

Nephrectomy

Procedure

Anatomy or system affected: Abdomen, kidneys, urinary system

Specialties and related fields: General surgery, nephrology, oncology, urology

Definition: The removal of the kidney, which may be performed to treat disorders and disease or for the purpose of transplantation.

Key terms:

adrenal gland: a small hormone-producing gland which is adjacent to the upper pole of the kidney

donor nephrectomy: a procedure in which a kidney is removed for transplantation into another patient; the kidney can be removed from a person who is brain-dead but whose heart is still beating (cadaveric donor nephrectomy) or from a relative of the recipient (a living related donor)

nephroureterectomy: a procedure similar to a radical nephrectomy, with the additional removal of the ureter and a cuff of the bladder; performed to treat transitional cell carcinomas of the ureters and the pelvis of the kidneys

radical nephrectomy: a procedure in which a kidney is removed along with the covering layers of tissue and the adjacent adrenal gland; performed with cancerous conditions

renal cell carcinoma (RCC): cancer of the small tubules of the kidney; generally known as kidney cancer

simple nephrectomy: a procedure in which a kidney is removed but the covering layers of tissue and the adjacent adrenal gland are left intact; usually performed to treat benign (noncancerous) conditions

transitional cell carcinoma (TCC): cancer arising from the lining of the urine-collecting system of the kidneys, ureters, and bladder

ureters: the tubes that drain urine from the kidneys to the bladder

Indications and Procedures

A kidney may be removed for several reasons, including congenital defects, trauma, cancer, inflammation, and transplantation. Congenital problems, or birth defects, associated with thekidneys include abnormal development, nonfunctional cysts, blockage, tumors, and cysts that leave the kidneys functional but which cause difficulty in breathing because of their large size. A kidney may be removed if the organ or its main blood vessels have been damaged beyond repair by trauma, such as a gunshot wound. Cancer is one of the most common reasons for nephrectomy; kidney cancers include renal cell carcinomas, transitional cell carcinomas, and tumors in the capsules of the kidneys or in surrounding layers of tissue. Infections or abscesses in the kidney that are beyond medical treatment and that become life-threatening may also necessitate a nephrectomy. Finally, a kidney may be removed from a donor for transplantation.

Simple nephrectomies involve removal of the kidney only, whereas radical nephrectomies include removal of the kidney and surrounding glands. Depending on the underlying disease and the surgeon's preference and experience, the kidney can be approached from the front, side, or back. The incisions used to reach the kidney are similar for simple, radical, and donor nephrectomies, but the steps that follow differ once the abdomen has been entered. For a nephroureterectomy, in which the kidney, the connecting ureter, and a part of the bladder are removed, the surgeon makes either one long, S-shaped incision starting in the flank and ending near the bladder, or two separate incisions.

Nephrectomy

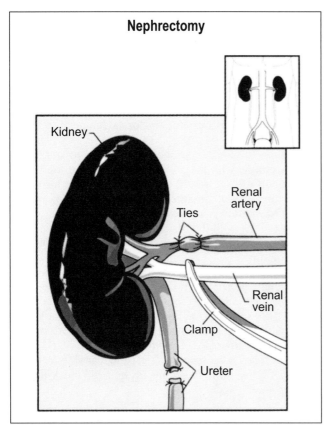

Kidney

Ties

Renal artery

Renal vein

Clamp

Ureter

The removal of a kidney may be necessary because of disease or because the kidney is intended for transplantation into another patient; the inset shows the location of the kidneys.

In the frontal approach to nephrectomy, the patient lies on his or her back and the abdomen and peritoneal cavity are opened. The intestines near the kidney are pushed to the side, and the kidney is approached from the front. The advantage of this approach includes better evaluation of the liver and the structures surrounding the kidney, better control of the blood vessels, and easy removal of clots from veins if necessary. The disadvantages of this approach are the possibility of adhesions developing in the intestines and lung complications after the surgery. The frontal approach may also be laparoscopic, in which a number of small incisions are made in the abdomen; a camera is fed through one incision, and surgical tools through another; one of the incisions is then made larger for the removal of the kidney. A laparoscopic nephrectomy takes longer to perform but has a shorter recovery period with less postoperative discomfort.

In the side approach, the patient is placed on his or her side and the incision is made through the eleventh or twelfth ribs. The kidney is approached from behind. This type of incision involves cutting into muscle and results in significant postoperative pain. The main advantage is that the peritoneal cavity is not entered.

In the back approach, known as a dorsal lumbotomy, the patient is placed face-down and a muscle-splitting incision is used. The kidney is approached from behind. This method is usually used for a simple nephrectomy. Its primary advantages are less postoperative pain and avoidance of the peritoneal cavity. Its main disadvantage is a limited view of the surgery site.

In a simple nephrectomy, after the kidney has been exposed, Gerota's fascia (the covering envelope of the kidney) is opened, and the fat around the kidney is dissected. The adjacent blood vessels and the connecting ureter are tied and cut, and the kidney is removed. In a radical nephrectomy, the adjacent adrenal gland and surrounding lymph glands are also removed in the one block. For a nephroureterectomy, the ureter is not cut close to the kidney but is removed all the way down to the bladder. A 2-centimeter cuff of bladder is cut off, the entire specimen is removed, and the hole in the bladder is closed.

The techniques used with kidney transplantation differ for cadaveric (deceased) donor nephrectomy and living related donor (LRD) nephrectomy. For cadaveric donor nephrectomy, the abdominal aorta (the main artery bringing blood to the kidney) and the inferior vena cava (the main vein taking blood away from the kidney) are isolated above and below the kidneys and cannulated with pipes to irrigate both kidneys with cold preservation fluid. Both kidneys and ureters, along with their related blood vessels, are removed. For LRD nephrectomy, the kidney is dissected along with its blood vessels and ureter. Great care is taken to obtain the maximum length of ureter and blood vessels without causing damage to the donor.

Uses and Complications

The major complications of nephrectomy during surgery are bleeding, damage to surrounding structures, and problems related to anesthesia. Therefore, there is significant evaluation of the patient before surgery. A battery of tests may be performed, including blood testing, urinalysis, electrocardiography, and x-rays. A thorough medical examination is done to determine whether the patient can be placed under anesthesia safely. The patient's blood is also typed and cross-matched in the event that a transfusion is required. Good surgical skills, the availability of blood for transfusion, and proper anesthesia techniques usually ensure that any complications that occur are not life-threatening. Nevertheless, the patient may also experience complications during the procedure that are not directly related to the surgery, such as a heart attack.

After a nephrectomy, the patient is at some risk for other problems. These complications may include bleeding, infection, intestinal obstruction, blood clots in the legs or lungs, or a heart attack.

Perspective and Prospects

Significant advances have been made in nephrectomy since the first such procedure was performed by Gustav Simmons in 1869. Thorough preoperative evaluation; improved anesthesia techniques; a greater understanding of anatomy, physiology, and pathology (including the nature of infections and microorganisms); and the discovery of antibiotics have all led to better surgical techniques. As a result, the death rate for nephrectomy operations is only 1 percent.

—Saeed Akhter, M.D.

See also Adrenalectomy; Dialysis; Hemolytic uremic syndrome; Kidney cancer; Kidney disorders; Kidney transplantation; Kidneys; Nephritis; Nephrology; Nephrology, pediatric; Transplantation.

For Further Information:
Brenner, Barry M., et al., ed. *Brenner and Rector's The Kidney.* 9th ed. Philadelphia: Saunders/Elsevier, 2012.

Danovitch, Gabriel M., ed. *Handbook of Kidney Transplantation.* 5th ed. Philadelphia: Lippincott Williams & Wilkins, 2010.

Hinman, Frank, Jr. *Atlas of Urologic Surgery.* 2d ed. Philadelphia: W. B. Saunders, 1998.

"Kidney Removal." *MedlinePlus*, October 9, 2012.

Kohnle, Diana. "Nephrectomy." *Health Library*, May 23, 2013.

Marshall, Fray F., ed. *Textbook of Operative Urology.* Philadelphia: W. B. Saunders, 1996.

"Nephrectomy (Kidney Removal)." *Mayo Clinic*, May 23, 2012.

Novick, Andrew C., and Stevan B. Streem. "Surgery of the Kidney." In *Campbell-Walsh Urology*, edited by Patrick Walsh et al. 9th ed. 4 vols. Philadelphia: Saunders/Elsevier, 2007.

Schrier, Robert W., ed. *Diseases of the Kidney and Urinary Tract.* 8th ed. Philadelphia: Wolters Kluwer Health/Lippincott Williams & Wilkins, 2007.

Nephritis
Disease/Disorder
Anatomy or system affected: Blood vessels, immune system, kidneys

Specialties and related fields: Immunology, internal medicine, nephrology

Definition: An inflammatory response of the kidneys, particularly of the glomeruli, to infectious agents or immunological challenges.

Key terms:
albuminuria: excretion in the urine of the protein albumin, usually as a result of changes occurring in the glomeruli

amyloidosis: the deposition of immunoglobulin fibrils in various tissues, including the kidneys

dialysis: the use of artificial membranes to remove metabolites from the blood when the kidneys fail; the peritoneum can also be used (peritoneal dialysis)

filtration rate: the amount of fluid passing per minute from blood across the glomerular capillaries to form glomerular fluid

glomeruli: structures consisting mainly of capillary blood vessels contained in a capsule, across whose walls water and solutes pass (filter) to form glomerular fluid

glomerulonephritis: inflammation of glomeruli

hematuria: the presence of red blood cells or red blood cell casts in the urine

immunoglobulins: proteins associated with immune responses

nephrotic syndrome: a condition involving edema, the retention of water and of sodium and chloride ions, urinary protein losses greater than 3 grams per day, and hypoalbuminemia

proteinuria: the presence of proteins, including globulins, in the urine; usually considered a sign of changes in the glomerular structures

renal blood flow: the amount of whole blood entering the renal arteries per minute; a fraction of water and solutes is removed to form urine

renal failure: severe kidney insufficiency requiring the use of dialysis or transplantation to return and maintain composition of body fluids at or near normal values

renal insufficiency: the inability of the kidneys to maintain a normal internal environment of the body and its fluids

streptococci: bacteria responsible for the development of some cases of acute glomerulonephritis, but without infection of the kidneys

tubules: hollow structures conducting glomerular fluid to the collecting ducts and the renal pelvis; they produce composition and volume changes of glomerular fluid passing through them and may reabsorb some of the protein that crosses the glomerular capillaries

Causes and Symptoms
Nephritis means any inflammatory responses of the kidney, whether the cause is infectious or immunological. Generally, it involves mainly the glomeruli, where the initial formation of urine takes place. The term is therefore equivalent in meaning to glomerulonephritis. Pathological changes may also occur in the interstitium (the extravascular, extracellular domain in which the tubules are embedded) and affect tubular functions. This condition, referred to as tubulointerstitial nephritis, is associated with localized cellular infiltrates and the accumulation of fluid.

The classic cause of acute glomerulonephritis is an infection in the throat or of the skin by a nephritogenic strain of Group A streptococci. The clinical presentation can be dramatic and can be associated not only with a sore throat but also with headaches, shortness of breath, and swelling of the ankles. Physical examination may find hypertension, rales in the lungs, peripheral pitting edema, and changes in the retinal vessels. In the chronic form, the onset is usually insidious; an infection may have been forgotten or ignored, without specific complaints except for some ankle edema, tiredness, and perhaps pallor. The physical findings for chronic glomerulonephritis are similar to but less striking than in the acute form.

The diagnosis in each type of nephritis is presumed on the basis of urinalysis, with a finding of blood (hematuria) in the acute form; proteinuria (actually mainly albuminuria, although globulins may also be present); and a decreased glomerular filtration rate. Diagnosis is established on the basis of renal biopsy with examination by both light and electron microscopy. Throat cultures and streptococcal group determination are appropriate if an infection is suspected.

Both conditions may be followed by the development of nephrotic syndrome, which is characterized by major losses of albumin in the urine, decreased serum albumin concentrations (hypoalbuminemia), the retention of water and of sodium and chloride ions, and massive edema and ascites (fluid leakage from blood vessels into the abdomen). Nephrotic syndrome may also appear without any history or evidence of a preceding episode of acute glomerulonephritis. On renal biopsy, essentially no changes or only minimal changes may be noted on inspection by light microscopy (minimal change disease), although characteristic changes are found with electron microscopy affecting particularly the foot processes (podocytes) of the glomeruli.

Information on Nephritis

Causes: Inflammation of kidney from bacterial infection (often streptococcal) or immune disorder

Symptoms: In acute form, sore throat, headache, shortness of breath, ankle swelling, hypertension, edema; in chronic form, ankle swelling, fatigue, pallor; either may lead to nephrotic syndrome (loss of albumin in urine, decreased serum albumin, water retention, sodium and chloride ion retention, massive edema and ascites)

Duration: Acute or chronic

Treatments: Usually none needed for acute form; for nonresolving or chronic form, dietary control (decreased protein and potassium), steroids, hemodialysis or peritoneal dialysis, kidney transplantation

Acute glomerulonephritis resolves spontaneously and rapidly in about 95 percent of cases, without detectable residual damage to kidney functions. Apart from control of hypertension, no specific treatment is available. The edema is rarely sufficient to warrant the use of diuretics. Antibiotics are not indicated unless there is evidence of an infection. Patients can be considered to be cured but should nonetheless be followed in the event of a reappearance of symptoms or manifestations.

In nonresolving acute glomerulonephritis and in chronic glomerulonephritis, there can be progression of damage to the glomeruli so that the number of functioning glomeruli (normally, about one million in each kidney) diminishes. This process may be gradual or may occur as a part of acute exacerbations that subside but leave the patient with diminished renal functions. As a result, glomerular filtration is decreased and the accumulation of metabolic end-products, particularly urea, occurs in the blood and tissue fluids. Abnormalities of acid-base regulation appear with decreased blood pH (acidemia), decreased serum bicarbonate concentration, and increased potassium concentration. Generally, a significant anemia exists, and renal blood flow is decreased so that the metabolic activities of the renal tubule cells are affected. Renal insufficiency is established, and dietary control is instituted, with decreased intakes of protein and potassium. Paradoxically, with decreased glomerular function, proteinuria decreases, serum albumin increases, and edema decreases or disappears.

Unfortunately, the progression of glomerular dysfunction continues, and dietary measures provide insufficient control of metabolic abnormalities. Resort is then made to hemodialysis or peritoneal dialysis to control the metabolic abnormalities and lift dietary restrictions to some degree while the patient awaits kidney transplantation. During this waiting period, stimulants of the bone marrow, such as erythropoietin, are administered in the expectation of maintaining the red cell count and the hematocrit at a satisfactory level. Transplants will require the use of immunosuppressive agents to prevent rejection unless an identical twin is the donor.

Other diseases in which glomerular damage can occur include diabetes mellitus, amyloidosis, systemic lupus erythematosus (SLE), Wegener's granulomatosis, Goodpasture's syndrome, syphilis, and human immunodeficiency virus (HIV) infection. Common problems associated with glomerular damage of any etiology are hypertension, strokes, heart failure, pulmonary edema, arteriolar vasoconstriction and sclerosis, impaired vision from exudates, pericarditis, and pericardial effusions.

Treatment and Therapy

Acute glomerulonephritis is characterized by the disappearance of signs and symptoms, or at least their marked reduction, in most patients. In 90 to 95 percent of cases, there is no progression and no recurrence. In some patients, the problems may reappear after apparent complete remission, while in others the disease progresses, often to nephrotic syndrome. This phase, too, disappears as the disease worsens, reaching the stage where hemodialysis or peritoneal dialysis becomes necessary. A renal biopsy can aid in determining the appropriate treatment. For example, if the biopsy confirms that poststreptococcal nephritis is present, then no specific treatment is available. If progressive glomerulonephritis is the diagnosis, then steroids may be indicated.

Hemodialysis depends on an arteriovenous shunt being created, usually in the forearm, so that the patient's blood can pass through a dialysis machine, which functions in a manner similar to glomeruli. Usually, several sessions, two or three times per week for several hours at a time, are required. Peritoneal dialysis involves the introduction of large amounts of fluid into the peritoneal cavity and its withdrawal after adequate exchanges with body fluids across the peritoneal surfaces have occurred. Hemodialysis requires going to a hospital or specialized facility, while pertoneal dialysis can be performed at home. Both procedures require careful and frequent monitoring of the patient's acid-base, electrolyte, and metabolic statuses.

While arrangements can usually be made for local dialysis, patients on dialysis lose a significant degree of mobility and independence. This independence can be regained to a considerable degree through kidney transplantation. Kidneys may be obtained from cadavers, unrelated living donors, and related living donors, such as identical twins. Except with the latter group, rejection phenomena may occur. Infections can occur with the use of immunosuppressive agents. Rarely, malignancies can be introduced with transplanted kidneys.

A low protein intake is recommended in the later stages of glomerulonephritis because too high a protein intake may accelerate the progression of the disease. Lack of control of water intake may lead to edema. Anemia is common in the later stages and may require the administration of erythropoietin.

In the nephrotic phase and in minimal change disease, control of edema is sought through one or more of the following measures: salt restriction, diuretics, intravenous (IV) administration of concentrated human serum albumin, corticosteroids (such as prednisone, which is more likely to be effective in minimal change disease), and other immunosuppressive agents. Nephrotic syndrome may occur in the presence of other underlying diseases, such as lupus, diabetes mellitus, HIV infection, syphilis, amyloidosis, and microvascular angiopathies. Specific treatments should be used when applicable.

Perspective and Prospects

The monograph *Reports of Medical Cases* by Richard Bright, published in 1827, marks the first clear description of nephritis through clinical findings (edema), laboratory assessment (proteinuria), and gross structural changes in the kidneys at postmortem. For many years, nephritis was referred to as Bright's disease. Apart from the measurement of blood constituents such as urea and creatinine, functional assessment was limited until the development, by Donald D. Van Slyke, of the clearance concept, defined as the amount of a given substance excreted in the urine per unit time relative to its concentration in plasma or blood. Van Slyke focused on the clearance of urea, while P. B. Rehberg in Denmark proposed that the clearance of creatinine could be used as a measure of the glomerular filtration rate. Glomerular fluid had been shown by Newton Richards to have the same composition as an ultrafiltrate of plasma. Accordingly, if creatinine was neither secreted nor reabsorbed by the tubules, then its clearance would be equivalent to the glomerular filtration rate.

The assumptions with respect to creatinine were shown to be incorrect, and inulin, a polyfructoside studied by Homer Smith, was found to be a reliable and correct indicator for measuring the glomerular filtration rate. Smith and his collaborators systematized and advanced knowledge of the kidney as a whole organ in a quantitative manner. Detailed understanding of the components of the whole organ progressed rapidly with the discovery of the significance of countercirculation in establishing the solute concentration gradient from cortex to medulla reported by H. Wirz and B. Hargitay. Functions of limited segments of the tubules (and later of individual cells) have provided additional important information on transport and metabolic processes in the kidneys.

On the clinical side, the introduction of renal biopsies and of hemodialysis (and later peritoneal dialysis) by way of an arteriovenous shunt made for more accurate diagnoses and longer life expectancies for patients with chronic renal disease. Further encouragement was provided by the development of techniques for successful renal transplants, first from identical twins, then from living donors and cadavers. Problems of rejection remain. Another major challenge is to find the means of delaying or arresting the progression of chronic renal disease before dialysis and transplants become necessary.

A study published in the *Journal of Epidemiology and Community Health* in May 2013 reported that half of over 1,100 adults treated for stroke in Boston, Massachusetts between 1999 and 2004 lived in close proximity to a major roadway. According to researchers, there is evidence that air pollution caused by traffic can cause harm to the arteries that supply blood to the kidneys.

—*Francis P. Chinard, M.D.*

See also Bacterial infection; End-stage renal disease; Hemolytic uremic syndrome; Kidney cancer; Kidney disorders; Kidneys; Nephrectomy; Nephrology; Nephrology, pediatric; Proteinuria; Pyelonephritis; Renal failure; Stone removal; Stones; Streptococcal infection; Systemic lupus erythematosus (SLE); Transplantation.

For Further Information:
Brenner, Barry M. "Retarding the Progression of Renal Disease." *Kidney International* 64 (2003): 370-378.
_____, ed. *Brenner and Rector's The Kidney.* 8th ed. Philadelphia: Saunders/Elsevier, 2008.
Cameron, J. Stewart, and Richard J. Glassock, eds. *The Nephrotic Syndrome.* New York: Marcel Dekker, 1988.
D'Amico, G., and C. Bazzi. "Pathophysiology of Proteinuria." *Kidney International* 63 (2003): 809-825.
Eddy, A. A., and J. M. Symons. "Nephrotic Syndrome in Children." *The Lancet* 362 (2003): 629-639.
Hricik, D. E., M. Chung-Park, and J. R. Sedor. "Glomerulonephritis." *New England Journal of Medicine* 339 (1998): 888-899.
Lue, Shih-Ho. "Residential Proximity to Major Roadways and Renal function."Â *Journal of Epidemiology and Community Health.* 10.1136 (2012). Print.

Nephrology

Specialty

Anatomy or system affected: Abdomen, blood, kidneys, urinary system

Specialties and related fields: Biochemistry, biotechnology, endocrinology, genetics, hematology, internal medicine, urology

Definition: The field of medicine that deals with the anatomy and physiology of the kidneys.

Key terms:

analyte: any chemical substance undergoing measurement; includes charged electrolytes found in the blood, such as sodium or potassium

creatinine: a nitrogen-containing by-product of metabolism; levels of creatinine may be indicative of kidney function

endocrine: referring to a process in which cells from an organ or gland secrete substances into the blood; these substances in turn act on cells elsewhere in the body

glomerulonephritis: inflammation of the glomeruli, the clusters of blood vessels and nerves found throughout the kidney

nephritis: any disease or pathology of the kidney that results in inflammation

nephron: the structural and functional unit of the kidney; composed of the renal corpuscle, the loop of Henle, and renal tubules

nephrotic syndrome: an abnormal condition of the kidneys characterized by a variety of conditions, including edema and proteinuria; often accompanies glomerular dysfunction and diabetes

renal: pertaining to the kidney

urea: a waste product of protein metabolism that represents the form in which nitrogen is eliminated from the body

Science and Profession

Nephrology is the branch of medicine that deals with the function of the kidneys. As a consequence, a nephrologist frequently deals with problems related to homeostasis, that is, the maintenance of the internal environment of the body. The most obvious function of the kidneys is their ability to regulate the excretion of water and minerals from the body, at the same time serving to eliminate nitrogenous wastes in the form of urea. While such waste material, produced as by-products of cell metabolism, is removed from the circulation, essential nutrients from body fluids are retained within the renal apparatus. These nutrients include proteins, carbohydrates, and electrolytes, some of which help maintain the proper acid-base balance within the blood. In addition, cells in the kidneys regulate red blood cell production through the release of the hormone erythropoietin.

The human excretory system includes two kidneys, which lie in the rear of the abdominal cavity on opposite sides of the spinal column. Urine is produced by the kidneys through a filtration network composed of 2 million nephrons, the actual functional units within each kidney. Two ureters, one for each kidney, serve to remove the collected urine and transport this liquid to the urinary bladder. The urethra drains urine from the bladder, voiding the liquid from the body.

Each adult human kidney is approximately 11 centimeters in length, with a shape resembling a bean. When the kidney is sectioned, three anatomical regions are visible: a light-colored outer cortex; a darker inner region, called the medulla; and the renal pelvis, the lowest portion of the kidney. The cortex consists primarily of a network of nephrons and associated blood capillaries. Tubules extending from each nephron pass into the medulla. The medulla, in turn, is visibly divided into about a dozen conical masses, or pyramids, with the base of the pyramid at the junction between the cortex and medulla and the apex of the pyramid extending into the renal pelvis. The loops (such as the loop of Henle) and tubules within the medulla carry out the reabsorption of nutrients and fluids that have passed through the capsular network of the nephron. The tubules extend through the medulla and return to the cortical region.

There are approximately 1 million nephrons in each kidney. Within each nephron, the actual filtration of blood is carried out within a bulb-shaped region, Bowman's capsule, which surrounds a capillary network, the glomerulus. In most individuals, a single renal artery brings the blood supply to the kidney. Since the renal artery originates from a branch of the aorta, the body's largest artery, the blood pressure within this region of the kidney is high. Consequently, hypotension, a significant lowering of blood pressure, may also result in kidney failure.

The renal artery enters the kidney through the renal pelvis, branching into progressively smaller arterioles and capillaries. The capillary network serves both to supply nutrition to the cells that make up the kidney and to collect nutrients or fluids reabsorbed from the loops and tubules of the nephrons. Renal capillaries also enter the Bowman's capsules in the form of balls or coils, the glomeruli. Since blood pressure remains high, the force filtration in a nephron pushes about 20 percent of the fluid volume of the glomerulus into the cavity portion of the capsule. Most small materials dissolved in the blood, including proteins, sugars, electrolytes, and the nitrogenous waste product urea, pass along within the fluid into the capsule. As the filtrate passes through the series of convoluted tubules extending from the Bowman's capsule, most nutrients and salts are reabsorbed and reenter the capillary network. Approximately 99 percent of the water that has passed through the capsule is also reabsorbed. The material which remains, much of it waste such as urea, is excreted from the body.

Nephrology is the branch of medicine that deals with these functions of the kidney. Loss of kidney function can quickly result in a buildup of waste material in the blood; hence kidney failure, if untreated, can result in serious illness or death. Within the purview of nephrology, however, is more than the function of the kidneys as filters for the excretion of wastes. The kidneys are also endocrine organs, structures that secrete hormones into the bloodstream to act on other, distal organs. The major endocrine functions of the kidneys involve the secretion of the hormones renin and erythropoietin.

Renin functions within the renin-angiotensin system in the regulation of blood pressure. It is produced within the juxtaglomerular complex, the region around Bowman's capsule in which the arteriole enters the structure. Cells within the tubules of the nephron closely monitor the blood pressure within the incoming arterioles. When blood pressure drops, these cells stimulate the release of renin directly into the blood circulation.

Renin does not act directly on the nephrons. Rather, it serves as a proteolytic enzyme that activates another protein, angiotensin, the precursor of which is found in the blood. The activated angiotensin, called angiotensin II, has several effects on kidney function that involve the regulation of blood pressure. First, by decreasing the glomerular filtration rate, it allows more water to be retained. Second, angiotensin II stimulates the release of the steroid hormone aldosterone from the adrenal glands, located in close association with the kidneys. Aldosterone acts to increase sodium retention and transport by cells within the tubules of the nephron, resulting in increased water reabsorption. The result of this complex series of hormone interactions within the kidney is a close monitoring of both salt retention and blood pressure and volume. In this manner, nephrology also relates to the pathophysiology of hypertension-high blood pressure.

The kidneys also regulate the production of erythrocytes, red blood cells, through the production of the hormone erythropoietin. Erythropoietin is secreted by the peritubular cells associated with regions outside the nephrons in response to lowered oxygen levels in the blood, also monitored by cells within the kidney. The hormone serves to stimulate red cell production within the bone marrow. Approximately 85 percent of the erythropoietin in blood fluids is synthesized within the kidneys, the remainder by the liver.

Since proper kidney function is related to a wide variety of body processes, from the regulation of nitrogenous waste disposal to the monitoring and control of blood pressure, nephrology may deal with a number of disparate syndromes. The kidney may represent the primary site of a disease or pathology, an example being the autoimmune phenomenon of glomerulonephritis. Renal failure may also result from the indirect action of a more general systemic syndrome, as is the case with diabetes mellitus. In many cases, the decrease in kidney function may result from any number of disorders, which poses many problems for the nephrologist.

Proper function of the kidney is central to numerous homeostatic processes within the body. Thus nephrology by necessity deals with a variety of pathophysiological disorders. Renal dysfunction may involve disorders of the organ itself or pathology associated with individual structures within the kidneys, the glomeruli or tubules. Likewise, the disorder within the body may be of a more general type, with the kidney being a secondary site of damage. This is particularly true of immune disorders such as lupus (systemic lupus erythematosus) or diabetes. Conditions that affect proper kidney function may result from infection or inflammation, the obstruction of tubules or the vascular system, or neoplastic disorders (cancers).

Immune disorders are among the more common processes that result in kidney disease. They may be of two types: glomerulonephritis or the more general nephrotic syndrome. Glomerulonephritis can result either from a direct attack on basement membrane tissue by host antibodies, such as with Goodpasture's syndrome, or indirectly through deposits of immune (antigen-antibody) complexes, such as with lupus. Nephritis may also be secondary to high blood pressure. In any of these situations, inflammation resulting from the infiltration of immune complexes and/or from the activation of the complement system may result in a decreased ability of the glomeruli to function. Treatment of such disorders often involves the use of corticosteroids or other immunosuppressive drugs to dampen the immune response. Continued recurrence of the disease may result in renal failure, requiring dialysis treatment or even kidney transplantation.

Activation of the complement system as a result of immune complex deposition along the glomeruli is a frequent source of inflammation. Complement consists of a series of some dozen serum proteins, many of which are pharmacologically active. Intermediates in the complement pathway include enzymes that activate subsequent components in a cascade fashion. The terminal proteins in the pathway form a "membrane attack complex," capable of significantly damaging a target (such as the basement membrane of a Bowman's capsule). Activation of the initial steps in the pathway begins with either the deposition of immune complexes along basement membranes or the direct binding of antibodies on glomerular surfaces. The end result can be extensive nephrotic destruction.

Nephrotic syndrome, which can also result in extensive damage to the glomeruli, is often secondary to other disease. Diabetes is a frequent primary disorder in its development; approximately one-third of insulin-dependent diabetics are at risk for significant renal failure. Other causes of nephrotic syndrome may include cancer or infectious agents and toxins.

Diagnostic and Treatment Techniques

Nephrologists can measure glomerular function using a variety of tests. These tests are based on the ability of the basement membranes associated with the glomeruli to act as filters. Blood cells and large materials such as proteins dissolved in the blood are unable to pass through these filters. Plasma, the liquid portion of the blood containing dissolved factors involved in blood-clotting mechanisms, is able to pass through the basement membrane, the driving force for filtration being the hydrostatic pressure of the blood (blood pressure).

The glomerular filtration rate (GFR) is defined as the rate by which the glomeruli filter the plasma during a fixed period of time. Generally, the rate is determined by measuring either the time of clearance of the carbohydrate inulin from the blood or the rate of clearance of creatinine, a nitrogenous by-product of metabolism. Though the rate may vary with age, it generally is about 125 to 130 milliliters of plasma filtered per minute.

Any significant decrease in the GFR is indicative of renal failure and can result in significant disruptions of acid-base or electrolyte balance in the blood. A decrease in the GFR can sometimes be observed through measurements of urine output. Healthy individuals usually excrete from 1 to 2 liters of urine per day. If the urine output drops to less than 500 milliliters (0.5 liter) per day, a condition known as oliguria, the body suffers a diminished capacity to remove metabolic waste products (urea, creatinine, or acids). Taken to an extreme, in which the filtering capacity is completely shut down and urine formation drops below 100 milliliters per day (anuria), the resulting uremia may cause death in a matter of days.

Anuria may have a variety of causes: kidney failure; hypotension, in which blood pressure is insufficient to maintain glomerular filtration; or a blockage in the urinary tract. As waste products, fluids, and electrolytes (especially sodium and potassium) build up, the person may appear puffy, be feverish, and exhibit muscle weakness. Heart arrhythmia or failure may also occur. Mediation of the problem, in addition to attempts to alleviate the reasons for kidney dysfunction, include regulation of fluid, protein, and electrolyte uptake. Medications are also used to increase the excretion of potassium and tissue fluids, assuming that the cause is not a urinary blockage.

The nephrologist or other physician may also monitor kidney function through measurements of serum analytes or through observation of certain chemicals within the urine. The levels of blood, urea, and nitrogen (BUN), nitrogenous substances in the blood, present a rough measure of kidney function. Generally, BUN levels change significantly only after glomerular filtration has been significantly disrupted. The levels are also dependent on the amount of protein intake in the diet. When changes occur as a result of renal dysfunction, BUN levels can be a useful marker for the progression of the disease. A more specific indicator of renal function can be the creatinine concentration within the blood. Serum creatinine, unlike BUN levels, is not related to the diet. In the event of renal failure, however, changes in BUN levels usually can be detected earlier than those of creatinine.

As the glomeruli lose their ability to distinguish large from small molecules during filtration, protein can begin to appear in the urine, the condition known as proteinuria. Usually, the level of protein in the urine is negligible (less than 250 milligrams per day). A transient proteinuria can result from heavy exercise or minor illness, but persistent levels of more than 1 gram per day may be indicative of renal dysfunction or even complications of hypertension. Generally, if the problem resides in the loss of tubular reabsorption, levels of protein generally are below 1 to 2 grams per day, with that amount usually consisting of small proteins. If the problem is a result of increased glomerular permeability caused by inflammation, levels may reach greater than 2 grams per day. In cases of nephrotic syndrome, excretion of protein in the urine may exceed 5 grams per day.

Measurement of urine protein is a relatively easy process. A urine sample is placed on a plastic stick with an indicator pad capable of turning colors, depending on the protein concentration. Analogous strips may be used for detection of other materials in urine, including acid, blood, or sugars. The presence of either red or white blood cells in urine can be indicative of infection or glomerulonephritis.

In addition to the filtration of blood fluids through the nephrons, the reabsorption of materials within the tubules results in increased urine concentration. A normal GFR within a healthy kidney produces a urine concentration three or four times as great as that found within serum. As kidney failure progresses, the concentration of urine begins to decrease, with the urine becoming more dilute. The kidneys compensate for the decreased concentration by increasing the amount of urine output: The frequency of urination may increase, as well as the volume excreted (polyuria). In time, if renal failure continues, the GFR will decrease, resulting in the retention of both analytes and water.

Determination of urine concentration is carried out following a brief period of dehydration: deprivation of fluids for about fifteen hours prior to the test. This dehydration will result in increased production by the hypothalamus of antidiuretic hormone (ADH), or vasopressin, a chemical that decreases the production of urine through increased renal tubule reabsorption of water. The result is a more concentrated urine. Following the dehydration period, the patient's urine is collected over a period of three hours and assessed for concentration. Significantly low values may be indicative of kidney disease.

A battery of tests in addition to those already described may be utilized in the diagnosis of kidney disease. These may include intravenous pyelography (in which a contrast medium is injected into the blood and followed as it passes through the kidneys), kidney biopsy, and ultrasound examinations. Diagnosis and course of treatment depend on an evaluation of these tests.

Perspective and Prospects

The roots of modern nephrology date from the seventeenth century. In the early decades of that century, the English physician William Harvey demonstrated the principles of blood circulation and the role of the heart in that process. Harvey's theories opened the door for more extensive analysis of organ systems, both in humans and in other animals. As a result, in 1666, Italian anatomist Marcello Malpighi, while exploring organ structure with the newly developed microscope, discovered the presence of glomeruli (what he called Malpighian corpuscles) within the kidneys. Malpighi thought that these structures were in some way connected with collecting ducts in the kidneys that had recently been found by Lorenzo Bellini. Malpighi also suspected that these structures played a role in urine formation.

Sir William Bowman, in 1832, was the first to describe the true relationship of the corpuscles discovered by Malpighi to urine secretion through the tubules. Bowman's capsule, as it is now called, is a filter that allows only the liquid of the blood, as well as dissolved salts and urea within the blood, into the tubules, from which the urine is secreted. It remained for Carl Ludwig, in 1842, to complete the story. Ludwig suggested that the corpuscles function in a passive manner, in that the filtrate is filtered by means of hydrostatic pressure through the capsule into the tubules and from there concentrated as water and solutes that are reabsorbed.

The first definitive work on urine formation, *The Secretion of the Urine*, was published by Arthur Robertson Cushny in 1917. In the monograph, Cushny offered a thorough analysis of the data published on kidney function. Though Cushny was incorrect in some of his conclusions, the work catalyzed intensive research activity on the functions of the kidney. A colleague of Cushny, E. Brice Mayrs, made the first attempt to determine the glomerular filtration rate, measuring the clearance of sulfate in rabbits. In 1926, the Danish physiologist Poul Brandt Rehberg demonstrated the superiority of creatinine as a marker for glomerular filtration; the "guinea pig" for the experiment was Rehberg himself.

A pioneer in renal physiology, Homer William Smith, began his research while serving in the United States Army during World War I. Until he retired in 1961, Smith was involved in much of the research related to renal excretion. It was Smith who developed inulin clearance as a measure of the GFR; his later years dealt with studies on mechanisms of solute excretion.

With the newer technology of the late twentieth century, more accurate methods for analysis became available. These have included ultrasound scanning, intravenous pyelography, and angiography. In addition, better understanding of immediate causes of many kidney problems has served to control or prevent some forms of renal failure.

—*Richard Adler, Ph.D.*

For Further Information:

Brenner, Barry M., ed. *Brenner and Rector's The Kidney*. 8th ed. Philadelphia: Saunders/Elsevier, 2008.

Cameron, Stewart. *Kidney Disease: The Facts*. 2d ed. New York: Oxford University Press, 1990.

Floege, Jurgen, Richard J. Johnson, and John Feehally. *Comprehensive Clinical Nephrology: Expert Consult*. St. Louis: Mosby/Elsevier, 2010.

Hricik, Donald E., R. Tyler Miller, and John R. Sedor, eds. *Nephrology Secrets*. 2d ed. Philadelphia: Hanley & Belfus, 2003.

Legrain, Marcel, et al. *Nephrology*. Trans. M. Cavaillé-Coll. New York: Masson, 1987.

Lerma, Edgar, and Allen R. Nissenson. *Nephrology Secrets*. 3d ed. Philadelphia: Elsevier Mosby, 2011.

Marieb, Elaine N. *Essentials of Human Anatomy and Physiology*. 9th ed. San Francisco: Pearson/Benjamin Cummings, 2009.

Mitchell, Rosner H, and Edgar V. Lerma. *Clinical Decisions in Nephrology, Hypertension and Kidney Transplantation*. New York: Springer, 2013.

O'Callaghan, Chris A., and Barry M. Brenner. *The Kidney at a Glance*. Boston: Blackwell Scientific, 2000.

Tanagho, Emil A., and Jack W. McAninich, eds. *Smith's General Urology*. 17th ed. New York: McGraw-Hill, 2008.

Wallace, Robert A., Gerald P. Sanders, and Robert J. Ferl. *Biology: The Science of Life*. 4th ed. New York: HarperCollins, 1996.

Whitworth, Judith A., and J. R. Lawrence, eds. *Textbook of Renal Disease*. 2d ed. New York: Churchill Livingstone, 1994.

Nervous system

Anatomy

Anatomy or system affected: Ears, nerves, spine
Specialties and related fields: Neurology
Definition: The major control system of the body, which synchronizes physiologic activity by interpreting incoming stimuli and which is responsible for memory and reasoning; it is composed of the central nervous system (the brain and spinal cord) and the peripheral nervous system (nerve processes, sensory receptors, and ganglia).

Key terms:

cerebrospinal fluid (CSF): the extracellular fluid of the central nervous system; it flows through the ventricles of the brain and the central canal of the spinal cord, circulating nutrients and providing a cushion for the brain

effector: a general term referring to skeletal, smooth, and cardiac muscles or glands that respond to impulses produced by the nervous system

glial cells: nonexcitable cells of the nervous system; they include astrocytes, microglial cells, oligodendrocytes, and Schwann cells

receptors: membrane-bound proteins with specific binding sites for neurotransmitters

synapse: a juncture between neurons or between neurons and muscle

Structure and Functions

The nervous system serves as the major control system of the human body. It is responsible for the synchronization of body parts, the integration of physiologic activity, the interpretation of incoming stimuli, and all intellectual activity, including memory and abstract reasoning. The nervous system regulates these activities by communication between various nerve cells; by controlling the actions of skeletal, smooth, and cardiac muscle; and by stimulating the secretion of products from various glands of the body.

Anatomically, the nervous system is divided into the central nervous system, which is composed of the brain and the spinal cord, and the peripheral nervous system, which includes all nervous structures outside the central nervous system-primarily nerve processes, sensory receptors, and a limited number of cells of the nervous system that are located in special structures known as ganglia. Ganglia are found at various locations throughout the body. They are the only locations of neurons outside the central nervous system. Information from incoming cells can be transmitted to the ganglion cells, which in turn can transmit that information to other locations.

Although the brain and the spinal cord contain several different types of cells that are morphologically unique, there is only one type of functional cell present, which by convention is always referred to as the neuron. The neuron is one of the few cells in the body that cannot reproduce; a fixed number of these cells develop in infancy, and the number never increases, though it can decrease in the event of injury or disease.

The neuron consists of a cell body that is similar to that of the typical animal cell familiar to most people. In addition, the neuron has extensions called processes. In the typical neuron, there are two types of processes: dendrites and axons.

Usually a neuron has many dendrites. Dendrites are very short; they receive information from nearby cells and relay that information to the cell body. Each cell has only a single axon, which may be very long, extending up and down the spinal cord or from the spinal cord to the ends of the fingers or toes. The axons conduct information from the cell bodies to the effectors-that is, the muscles and glands-or to other neurons.

Functionally, the nervous system is divided into two areas: the somatic nervous system and the autonomic nervous system. The somatic system controls posture and locomotion by stimulating the skeletal muscles. It is responsible for knowing where the body is in space and for ensuring that there is sufficient muscle contraction (tone) to maintain posture. Responses of the somatic system occur through the motor neurons.

The autonomic nervous system regulates internal activities through the innervation, or nerve stimulation, of the smooth muscles or the glands. It is anatomically different from the somatic nervous system in that the stimulation of body parts always involves two neurons. The cell body of the second neuron in the sequence is located in a ganglion outside the central nervous system.

The Nervous System

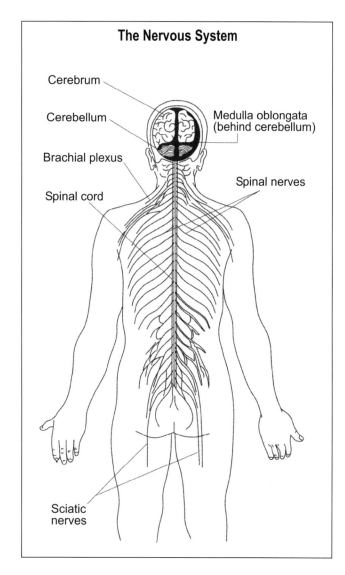

Cerebrum
Cerebellum
Medulla oblongata (behind cerebellum)
Brachial plexus
Spinal cord
Spinal nerves
Sciatic nerves

The autonomic nervous system is broken down further into two divisions: the sympathetic and the parasympathetic. The sympathetic system is also known as the "fight or flight" reaction, since it evolved from the mechanism in lower animals by which an animal would prepare to fight a predator or run from it. More commonly, it is referred to in humans as the adrenaline response, which is active during stressful situations, strenuous physical activity, public performance, or competition.

The parasympathetic system, which is responsible for the digestive functions of the body, controls stimulation of salivary gland secretions, increased blood flow to digestive organs, and movement of material through the digestive system. The sympathetic and parasympathetic systems usually function in balance; the parasympathetic system predominates after meals, and the sympathetic system predominates during periods of stress or physical activity.

Neurons communicate with other neurons or effectors through the release of chemical messengers known as neurotransmitters. At the termination of the axon, there is a widened area known as the synaptic knob, which produces and stores neurotransmitters. The effects of neurotransmitters are always localized and of short duration. There are many types of neurotransmitters, some of which are well known, such as acetylcholine and norepinephrine.

Neurotransmitters are released in response to an electrical impulse that is conducted along the axon. Once released, a neurotransmitter binds to cells that have appropriate receptors on their dendrites. Neurotransmitters may either stimulate or inhibit the activity of the second cell. If there is significant stimulation of the second cell, it will conduct the information along its axon and release a neurotransmitter from the axon terminal, which will in turn stimulate or inhibit the next neuron or effector. There must be a mechanism for the immediate removal of neurotransmitters from the synaptic cleft if the stimulation of the second neuron is to cease and if other impulses are to be conducted.

Neurotransmitters can influence only those cells that have the appropriate receptors on their surfaces. It is through the neurotransmitter-receptor complex that neurotransmitters are able to influence cells, and any alteration of the number or type of receptors on a cell membrane will lead to an alteration of cellular functioning.

The axons of some neurons are covered with multiple layers of a cell membrane known as myelin. The myelin is produced by specialized cells in the brain known as oligodendrocytes and by cells in the peripheral axons known as Schwann cells. Myelin serves as an insulator for axons and is effective in speeding up the conduction of nerve impulses. It is essential for the normal functioning of the nervous system.

The brain and spinal cord are enclosed by three membranes of dense connective tissue called the meninges, which separate the nervous system from other tissue and from the skull and spinal cord. From the outside inward, they are the dura mater, the arachnoid mater, and the pia mater. Many of the blood vessels of the brain travel through the meninges; therefore, the surface of the brain is very vascular and is subject to bleeding or clotting after trauma.

Disorders and Diseases

Diseases of the nervous system can be arranged into several general categories: infections, congenital diseases, seizure disorders, circulatory diseases, traumatic injury, demyelinating diseases, degenerative diseases, mental diseases, and neoplasms.

Infections of the nervous system are described according to the tissues infected. If the meninges are infected, the disease is known as meningitis; if the brain tissue is infected, the disease is referred to as encephalitis. The development of abscesses in the nervous tissue can also occur. The conditions described can be caused by viruses, bacteria, protozoa, or other parasites.

In most cases, the organism that causes meningitis is spread via the bloodstream. It is also possible for infections to be spread via an infected middle ear or paranasal sinus, a skull fracture, brain surgery, or a lumbar puncture. The infectious agent can usually be determined by analyzing the spinal fluid. Bacterial infections are treated with antibiotics, while viral infections receive only supportive treatment.

An abscess of nervous tissue is usually a complication resulting from an infection at some other anatomical site, particularly from middle-ear infections or sinus infections. Abscesses may also occur following penetrating injuries. The abscess can create pressure inside the skull and, if left untreated, may rupture and lead to death.

Viral encephalitis is an acute disease that is often spread to humans by arthropods from animal hosts. After a carrier insect bites a human, the virus is spread to the brain of the human via the bloodstream. The specific causative agent often goes undiagnosed. Some well-known forms of encephalitis are herpes simplex encephalitis, poliomyelitis, rabies, and cytomegalovirus encephalitis. In addition, some forms of encephalitis fall into the category of slow virus infections, which have latent periods as long as several years between the time of infection and the development of encephalitis.

Other serious infections include neurosyphilis, which occurs in the late stages of untreated syphilis infections; toxoplasmosis, a protozoan infection that is extremely dangerous to fetuses but rarely causes serious problems in adults; cerebral malaria; and African trypanosomiasis, which is also known as sleeping sickness.

Congenital diseases of the brain vary in the degree of malfunction they produce. Spina bifida is a general term for a group of disorders in which the vertebrae do not develop as they should. As a result, the spinal cord may protrude from the lower back. In some cases, the effects may be so minimal as to produce no symptoms; in other cases, however, these malformations may lead to major neurologic impairment.

Hydrocephalus is another congenital malformation, one that may lead to an increase in the size of the ventricles of the brain. It may be caused by blockage of the flow of spinal fluid in the fetus. In some cases, the spinal fluid produced by the nervous system fills the ventricles and limits the space available for the growing brain and nervous tissue. The result under these conditions is the presence of larger-than-normal ventricles and a smaller-than-normal amount of nervous tissue.

A seizure disorder is any sudden burst of excess electrical activity in the neurons of the brain. Epilepsy is a general term for seizure disorders. The condition may be mild and have only minimal effects, or it may be severe, leading to convulsions. The cause is often unknown, but epilepsy may result from infection, trauma, or neoplasms.

Cerebrovascular accident (CVA) is the term used to describe a variety of malfunctions of blood circulation in the nervous system that are not a result of trauma. More commonly, the term *stroke* is used to describe the condition. Strokes have many causes that generally fall into two categories: ischemic and hemorrhagic.

Ischemic strokes are those in which the nervous tissue is deprived of oxygen as a result of an impairment of blood flow to the area. An ischemic stroke is most commonly the result of a blood clot that blocks the blood vessels leading to the brain or the blood vessels in the brain itself. Since the cells can live for only a few minutes without oxygen, an ischemic stroke can result in neurological impairment or even death.

In hemorrhagic strokes, there is bleeding in the brain itself. It may be caused by hypertension or by the rupture of a weakened blood vessel, which is known as an aneurysm. Both ischemic and hemorrhagic strokes lead to the death of neurons in the affected area. The degree of damage to the brain is determined by the number of cells destroyed by the oxygen deprivation.

Traumatic injury to the brain can generally be classified as penetrating or nonpenetrating. Penetrating injuries produce a risk of infection as well as bleeding at the site of the wound. Since many large blood vessels are located in the meninges, even injuries that penetrate only into the meninges may be sufficient to cause serious injury. Nonpenetrating injuries may also cause bleeding of the meninges, which can limit blood flow to the nervous tissue or put excessive pressure on the tissue.

Injury to the spinal cord may result in severing the spinal cord from the brain. If this should occur, communications between the brain and any structures below the area of the injury are lost, as is all sensory and motor function in those areas. Since neurons are unable to regenerate and axon repair is limited, there is little hope for reversal of this condition, although extensive research is being conducted in this area.

Demyelinating diseases are those that result in changes in the myelin sheaths of neurons. The most common example is multiple sclerosis, which affects myelin in the central nervous system but not in the peripheral nervous system. Although there are varying degrees of severity, the condition causes limb weakness, impaired perception, and optic neuritis, among other things. Some cases present only mild symptoms, while others are degenerative and can lead to death, sometimes within months. Many patients, however, survive for more than twenty years. The cause of these diseases is not yet clear, although viral infections have been associated with some demyelinating diseases.

Degenerative diseases are those in which there is a gradual decline in nervous function. The disease may be hereditary, as in the case of Huntington's disease, or may occur without any apparent genetic basis, as in the case of Parkinson's disease. Parkinson's disease involves the death of certain neurons in the brain and a decreased concentration of neurotransmitters. As the disease progresses, there is a gradual loss of motor ability and, ultimately, a complete loss of motor function. Not much is known about neurotransmitter replacement or mechanisms to stop degenerative diseases.

Little is known about mental diseases such as schizophrenia and manic depression. They appear to involve abnormal levels of neurotransmitters or errors in the membrane receptors associated with those neurotransmitters. Success in localizing the causes of these diseases has been slow in coming; there has been much more success in the development of medications to treat them.

Cancer of the brain can be primary or metastatic. Metastatic tumors, the more common variety, can arise from any source. Of the primary neoplasms, the most common are those derived from glial cells, which are responsible for more than 65 percent of all primary neoplasms. The second most common are neoplasms resulting from transformation of cells of the meninges. Since neurons cannot divide, neuron tumors are almost nonexistent except in children.

Perspective and Prospects

When the control system of the body experiences a malfunction, the effects are wide ranging. Since the nervous system is responsible for regulating so many diverse activities, nervous-system injury or disease must be treated immediately if the patient is to survive. This problem is further complicated by the fact that the brain is a difficult organ to study, because of its location within the skull and because its cells are vital and can be studied only after they have died.

Disease or injury of the cells of the nervous system, especially the brain, creates problems that are unique to that organ for several reasons, including the fact that those cells cannot repair themselves and cannot divide. In addition, the cells of the brain are restricted to a limited area. The cells of the nervous system are unique in that they are so highly specialized that they are not capable of cell division. As a result, humans have the greatest number of neurons during early childhood. Any neural injury or disease that kills cells results in a decreased number of neurons. Furthermore, the space in the skull is tightly packed with cells and cerebrospinal fluid, leaving no room for blood that might result from an injury or fluid accumulation due to tissue infection or tumors. Any of these conditions will increase the pressure within the skull and will also increase the extent of the injury to the nervous tissue.

Although there is no mechanism for replacing cells that have died, the prognosis is not totally bleak. There are cells in the brain that can, in the event of disease or injury, assume the responsibilities of the dead cells. For example, a person who has lost the capacity to speak following a stroke may be retaught to speak using cells that previously did not perform that function.

Among the problems with which the nervous system must cope, there are many things that can go wrong at the synapse of a neuron. The cell may produce too little or too much neurotransmitter. It is possible that the neurotransmitter may not be released on cue or that, if it is released, the postsynaptic cells will not have the appropriate receptors. There also may be no mechanism for removal of the neurotransmitter from the synaptic cleft. These are only a few of the problems that can interfere with communication between different neurons or between neurons and other effectors. As science learns more about the communication system of neurons, efforts to correct these problems will intensify. Already there are many drugs available that can alter activity at the synapse. Correcting these errors can lead to methods for the treatment of mental diseases.

Someday it may be possible to transplant healthy neurons from one person to another. This procedure may permit physicians to prevent total paralysis in a person who has suffered a broken neck or total loss of motor function in an individual who suffers from Parkinson's disease. In 1990, normal neurons were grown in tissue culture for the first time. Such scientific breakthroughs will lead to more and better treatments for individuals who suffer from diseases of the nervous system.

—Annette O'Connor, Ph.D.

See also Acupressure; Acupuncture; Alzheimer's disease; Amnesia; Amputation; Anesthesia; Anesthesiology; Aneurysmectomy; Aneurysms; Anxiety; Aphasia and dysphasia; Apnea; Aromatherapy; Ataxia; Autism; Balance disorders; Behçet's disease; Bell's palsy; Biofeedback; Botox; Brain; Brain damage; Brain disorders; Brain tumors; Caffeine; Carpal tunnel syndrome; Cells; Cerebral palsy; Cluster headaches; Coma; Computed tomography (CT) scanning; Concussion; Craniotomy; Cysts; Deafness; Dementias; Disk removal; Dizziness and fainting; Dyslexia; Ear infections and disorders; Ear surgery; Ears; Electrical shock; Electroencephalography (EEG); Electromyography; Encephalitis; Epilepsy; Fetal alcohol syndrome; Fetal tissue transplantation; Ganglion removal; Guillain-Barré syndrome; Hallucinations; Head and neck disorders; Headaches; Hearing loss; Hemiplegia; Huntington's disease; Hydrocephalus; Hypothalamus; Intellectual disability; Intraventricular hemorrhage; Laminectomy and spinal fusion; Lead poisoning; Learning disabilities; Leprosy; Leukodystrophy; Lower extremities; Lumbar puncture; Memory loss; Meningitis; Migraine headaches; Motor neuron diseases; Motor skill development; Multiple sclerosis; Narcolepsy; Neuralgia, neuritis, and neuropathy; Neurofibromatosis; Neuroimaging; Neurology; Neurology, pediatric; Neurosurgery; Numbness and tingling; Paget's disease; Palsy; Paralysis; Paraplegia; Parkinson's disease; Physical rehabilitation; Poisoning; Poliomyelitis; Porphyria; Premenstrual syndrome (PMS); Quadriplegia; Rabies; Reflexes, primitive; Restless legs syndrome; Sciatica; Seizures; Sense organs; Shingles; Shock therapy; Skin; Sleep disorders; Snakebites; Spina bifida; Spinal cord disorders; Spine, vertebrae, and disks; Strokes; Sympathectomy; Systems and organs; Tetanus; Tics; Touch; Toxicology; Transient ischemic attacks (TIAs); Tremors; Unconsciousness; Upper extremities; Vagotomy; Vagus nerve.

For Further Information:

Afifi, Adel K., and Ronald A. Bergman. *Functional Neuroanatomy: Text and Atlas.* 2d ed. New York: Lange Medical Books/McGraw-Hill, 2005.

"Autonomic Nervous System Disorders." *MedlinePlus*, April 17, 2013.

Barondes, Samuel H. *Molecules and Mental Illness.* 2d ed. New York: Scientific American, 1999.

Bear, Mark F., Barry W. Connors, and Michael A. Paradiso. *Neuroscience: Exploring the Brain.* 3d ed. Philadelphia: Lippincott Williams & Wilkins, 2007.

Bloom, Floyd E., M. Flint Beal, and David J. Kupfer, eds. *The Dana Guide to Brain Health: A Practical Family Reference from Medical Experts.* New York: Dana Press, 2006.

Goldman, Steven A. "Biology of the Nervous System." *Merck Manual Home Health Handbook*, November 2007.

McCance, Kathryn L., and Sue M. Huether. *Pathophysiology: The Biologic Basis for Disease in Adults and Children.* 6th ed. St. Louis, Mo.: Mosby/Elsevier, 2010.

McLendon, Roger E., Marc K. Rosenblum, and Darell D. Bigner, eds. *Russell and Rubinstein's Pathology of Tumors of the Nervous System.* 7th ed. 2 vols. London: Hodder Arnold, 2006.

"Neurologic Diseases." *MedlinePlus*, July 4, 2013.

Nicholls, John G., et al. *From Neuron to Brain.* 5th ed. Sunderland, Mass.: Sinauer, 2012.

Underwood, J. C. E., and S. S. Cross, eds. *General and Systematic Pathology*. 5th ed. New York: Churchill Livingstone/Elsevier, 2009.

Woolsey, Thomas A., Joseph Hanaway, and Mokhtar H. Gado. *The Brain Atlas: A Visual Guide to the Human Central Nervous System*. 3d ed. Hoboken, N.J.: Wiley, 2007.

Neuralgia, neuritis, and neuropathy

Disease/Disorder

Anatomy or system affected: Nerves, nervous system, spine

Specialties and related fields: Neurology

Definition: Pathological conditions affecting the peripheral nerves of the body and interfering with the proper functioning of those nerves.

Key terms:

autonomic neuropathy: a disorder involving the nerves that work independently of conscious control, and including those nerves that go to small blood vessels, sweat glands, the urinary bladder, the gastrointestinal tract, and the genital organs

axon: the portion of a neuron that carries electrical impulses away from the nerve cell body

mononeuropathy: a neuropathy involving only one peripheral nerve

nerve: a bundle of sensory and motor neurons held together by layers of connective tissue

neuralgia: pain associated with a nerve, often caused by inflammation or injury

neuritis: inflammation of a nerve

neuron: a nerve cell that is capable of conducting electrical impulses; several different types of neurons exist, including motor neurons, sensory neurons, and interneurons

neuropathy: a disorder that causes a functional disturbance of a peripheral nerve, brought about by any cause

peripheral nervous system: the portion of the nervous system found outside the brain and spinal cord

polyneuropathy: a disease that involves a disturbance in the function of several peripheral nerves

Causes and Symptoms

Peripheral nerves, those nerves found outside the brain and spinal cord, function to carry information between the central nervous system and the other portions of the body. These peripheral nerves consist of a bundle of nerve cells, also called neurons, which are wrapped in a protective sheath of connective tissue. A nerve consisting only of neurons that carry impulses toward the central nervous system is termed a sensory nerve. Nerves that contain only neurons that carry information from the central nervous system to the periphery of the body are called motor nerves, because they usually carry information telling a particular body part to move. Most nerves, however, consist of both sensory and motor neurons and are thus called mixed nerves.

The nerves of the peripheral nervous system can be divided into two different categories, cranial nerves and spinal nerves. Cranial nerves come directly out of the brain and supply information to and about the head and neck. There are twelve pairs of cranial nerves. Spinal nerves come directly out of the spinal cord and provide information to and from the arms, legs, chest, gut, and all other parts of the body not supplied by cranial nerves. In humans, there are usually thirty-one pairs of spinal nerves. Both cranial and spinal nerves can be affected by neuropathies.

Neurons (nerve cells) are highly specialized structures designed to convey information from one part of the body to another. This information is passed along in the form of electrical impulses. Neurons consist of three main parts: a cell body, which contains the nucleus and is the control center of the entire neuron; dendrites, which are slender, fingerlike extensions that convey electrical impulses toward the cell body; and an axon, which is a slender extension that carries electrical impulses away from the cell body.

Most of the dendrites and axons of peripheral nerves are covered with a white, fatty substance called myelin. Myelin acts to protect and insulate axons and dendrites. By insulating the axons and dendrites, myelin actually speeds up the rate at which an electrical impulse can be carried along these two structures. Damage to the myelin sheath surrounding axons and dendrites can greatly impair the function of a nerve.

Often, when a nerve becomes pinched, damaged, or inflamed, the result is excessive electrical stimulation of the nerve, which will be registered as pain. The pain associated with the damaged nerve is referred to as neuralgia. One of the most common forms of neuralgia occurs upon the striking of the "funny bone." This area around the elbow is the spot where the ulnar nerve is easily accessible. The ulnar nerve runs from just under the shoulder to the little finger, and when the ulnar nerve is struck near the elbow it is compressed or pinched, leading to pain or a tingling sensation from the elbow down to the little finger.

Compression of nerves for prolonged periods can also lead to neuralgia. The most common example of compression neuralgia is carpal tunnel syndrome. In this syndrome, the median nerve becomes compressed at the wrist, usually as a result of an inflammation of the sheaths of the tendons located on either side of the median nerve. The swelling of these tendon sheaths causes the compression of the median nerve, which may initially lead to neuralgia. As this condition progresses, it can lead to a loss of feeling along the palm side of the thumb and the index and middle fingers. This condition is most common in people who use their fingers for rigorous work over prolonged periods of time, such as typing.

Sciatica is another common form of neuralgia, in which pain is associated with the sciatic nerve. The sciatic nerve is the longest nerve in the human body, running from the pelvis down the back of the thigh to the lower leg and then down to the soles of the feet. The symptoms of sciatica include sharp pains along the sciatic nerve. The pain may involve the buttocks, hip, back, posterior thigh, leg, ankle, and foot. Sciatica can result from many different causes, but the most common cause is from a ruptured intervertebral disk that puts pressure on, or causes a pinching of, the sciatic nerve.

Neuritis is defined as the inflammation of a nerve or of

**Information on
Neuralgia, Neuritis, and Neuropathy**

Causes: Wide ranging; may include toxic exposure to solvents, pesticides, or heavy metals; viral infection; certain medications; excessive alcohol use; vitamin deficiency; loss of blood to nerve; carpal tunnel syndrome; injury; disease (e.g., leprosy, shingles, diabetes)

Symptoms: Pain; inflammation; tingling, prickling, and burning sensations; inability to perceive touch, heat, cold, or pressure; localized muscle weakness

Duration: Acute to chronic

Treatments: Depends on cause; may include antibiotics, anti-inflammatory drugs, surgery

---

the connective tissue that surrounds the nerve. Many diseases can lead to the inflammation of peripheral nerves. Perhaps the most common disease leading to neuritis is shingles. Shingles are caused by the occurrence of herpes zoster, a virus that attacks the dorsal root ganglion, a place near the spinal cord that houses the cell bodies of neurons. A rash, swelling, and pain progress from the dorsal root ganglion along one or more spinal nerves. The rash along the course of the spinal nerves usually disappears within a few days to a couple of weeks, but the pain along this path can persist for months.

Leprosy is another disease that leads to the inflammation of nerves. Leprosy is a bacterial disease caused by *Mycobacterium leprae*. These bacteria invade the cells that make up the myelin sheath that surrounds the nerve. The result is a noticeable swelling of the nerves affected, primarily those that are close to the skin. Many times, this swelling will lead to neuralgia and, if left untreated, to muscle wasting.

"Neuropathy" is a general term used to describe a decrease in the function of peripheral nerves, which may be caused by many factors. The first signs of a neuropathy are usually a tingling, prickling, or burning sensation in some part of the body. This is followed by a sensory loss; the inability to perceive touch, heat, cold, or pressure; and a weakness in the muscles in the area affected. This weakness may eventually lead to a loss of muscle termed muscular atrophy. Neuropathies may affect sensory neurons, motor neurons, or both and can occur in both spinal and cranial nerves. A neuropathy may develop over a few days or many years. Neuropathies can be caused by a number of factors, including toxic exposure to solvents, pesticides, or heavy metals; viral illness; certain medications; metabolic disturbances such as diabetes mellitus; excessive use of alcohol; vitamin deficiency; loss of blood to the nerve; or cold exposure.

Neuropathies can be categorized based on the number of nerves that they affect, whether it is the myelin sheath surrounding the axon that is affected or the axon itself is destroyed, and the amount of time before symptoms of the neuropathy occur and progress. Thus, neuropathies are usually broken down into four different types:

polyneuropathy, in which more than one nerve is affected; mononeuropathy, in which only one nerve is affected; axonal neuropathy, in which the axon is affected and degenerates; and demyelinating neuropathy, in which the myelin sheath surrounding the nerve is destroyed. Each of the four categories can be further subdivided based on the time frame in which the symptoms occur. Those neuropathies that appear over days are termed acute, those that appear over weeks are termed subacute, and those neuropathies whose symptoms slowly appear over months or years are termed chronic.

Another type of neuropathy is autonomic neuropathy, a condition that affects the nerves of the autonomic nervous system. These are the peripheral nerves that go to the sweat glands, small blood vessels, gastrointestinal tract, urinary bladder, and genital organs. These nerves are referred to as autonomic since they automatically provide information between these organs and the central nervous system without the individual's conscious effort. The symptoms associated with this form of neuropathy include loss of control over urination, difficulty swallowing food, occasional stomach upset, diarrhea, impotence, and excessive sweating.

The most common cause of neuropathies in the Western world is diabetes mellitus, while leprosy is the more common cause of neuropathies elsewhere. It is estimated that at least 70 percent of all diabetics have some degree of peripheral neuropathy. In most of these cases, the neuropathy is very slight and causes the patient no noticeable symptoms. In about 10 percent of those diabetics with a neuropathy, however, the symptoms will be serious.

Treatment and Therapy

Often, the first notable feature of a neuropathy that prompts a patient to seek medical attention is a tingling, prickling, or burning sensation in a particular area of the body. The occurrence of these sensations without any external stimuli is termed paresthesias. Since diabetes is the most common cause of neuropathy in the Western world, the sensations experienced by a diabetic patient can serve as an example of the symptoms that are associated with common neuropathies. These patients may first notice the abovementioned symptoms in the balls of the feet or tips of the toes. As the neuropathy progresses, patients may lose feeling in their feet and experience a weakness in the muscles of the feet, leading to a difficulty in flexing the toes upward. This makes walking difficult, and many patients remark that they feel as if they are walking on stumps. This condition may lead to difficulties in maintaining balance. The neuropathy will begin to affect the legs above the ankles and then travel up the legs, eventually leading to atrophy of the leg muscles.

As the neuropathy worsens, it is critical that patients seek help because they can no longer feel pain. This situation is dangerous, as the patient may no longer sense the pain that can be caused by injuries from sharp objects or even a pebble in the shoe. If unnoticed, these injuries lead to ulcers that can easily become infected.

The first step in treating a neuropathy is to diagnose the type of neuropathy affecting the patient. A patient's medical history is taken to identify any recent viral or bacterial illness, any exposure to toxic substances such as pesticides or heavy metals, the patient's habits concerning alcohol use, or any other illness or injury that might have brought about a possible neuropathy. Next, a physical exam will be performed to determine if the patient's sensations regarding touch, pain, pressure, or temperature have been affected, as well as the ability of the patient to react to these stimuli. The physician may also feel the affected area to determine if the nerve or nerves are inflamed and enlarged.

If the patient's history and the physical examination point toward a neuropathy, further testing using electrodiagnostic tests will be performed. These tests measure the speed at which an electrical impulse travels down a nerve, which is called the nerve conduction velocity. Motor nerve conduction velocity is measured by stimulating the nerve with electrodes placed on the skin above the nerve. Stimulation of the nerve is typically done at two different sites. Using the arm as an example, one electrode would be placed on the inside of the arm at the elbow. The time that it takes for the impulse to reach a recording electrode on the thumb would be measured. A second site at the wrist would be tested to determine the time that it takes for the electrical impulse to reach the recording electrode on the thumb. The time that it took for the impulse to travel from the wrist to thumb would be subtracted from the amount of time that it took for the impulse to go from the inside of the arm at the elbow to the thumb. The resulting value would then be divided by the distance between the site at the wrist and the site at the elbow, giving a nerve conduction velocity value measured in meters per second.

The typical nerve conduction velocity for the motor and sensory peripheral nerves of adults is approximately 40 to 80 meters per second. If a neuropathy is the result of demyelination, the affected nerve will have a much slower nerve conduction velocity. If the neuropathy is a result of axonal damage, then the nerve conduction velocity is usually not altered from normal. Thus, electrodiagnostic testing helps to determine if the neuropathy is a demyelination neuropathy or an axonal neuropathy. Such a determination is important because the different neuropathies are caused by different diseases and are thus treated differently. Electrodiagnostic tests can also provide useful information regarding the site of the neuropathy and whether the neuropathy is affecting sensory neurons, motor neurons, or both.

The last diagnostic test to be performed, if other methods are inconclusive, is a biopsy of the affected nerve. This procedure involves the surgical removal of a portion of the afflicted nerve. The small sample of nerve will be placed under a microscope and examined for specific changes in the nerve. The nerve sample may also be subjected to various biochemical studies to determine if metabolic disturbances have occurred. Nerve biopsies are rarely performed, however, and are usually not recommended.

Once the type of neuropathy afflicting the patient has been determined, treatment can begin. Unlike axons in the central nervous system, axons in the peripheral nervous system are capable of regenerating under certain conditions. If the neuropathy is the result of exposure to toxic substances such as pesticides or heavy metals, removal of the patient from the exposure to such substances is the simple cure. If the neuropathy is the result of viral or bacterial infections, the treatment and recovery from these infections will also usually correct the neuropathy. The same principle applies to neuropathies caused by metabolic diseases and vitamin deficiencies: corrections of these problems will lead to the correction of the neuropathy.

Should the neuropathy be of the mononeuropathy type and caused by trauma, anti-inflammatory drugs such as corticosteroids may be used or surgery may be performed to repair the nerve. If the mononeuropathy is caused by compression, as in carpal tunnel syndrome, surgery may also be needed to increase the space around the nerve and thus relieve the compression. Surgery is also used to remove tumors on the nerve that might be causing a neuropathy.

The time required to recover from a neuropathy is dependent on the severity and type of neuropathy. Recovery from demyelination is typically quicker than recovery from axonal neuropathies. If only the myelin surrounding the axon is damaged, and not the axon itself, the axon can quickly replace the damaged myelin. Demyelinating neuropathies usually require three to four weeks for recovery. In contrast, recovery from axonal neuropathies may take from two months to more than a year, depending on the severity of the neuropathy.

Perspective and Prospects

Perhaps the earliest documentation of peripheral neuropathies occurred during biblical times, when the term "leprosy" was coined. It is likely, however, that this term was employed rather loosely, as it was used to describe not only the disease leprosy but also a number of skin diseases not involving neuropathies, such as psoriasis.

The actual diagnosis of neuropathies and their subsequent categorization did not occur until the advent of electrical diagnostic testing. The earliest use of electricity to study nerve function occurred in 1876 when German neurologist Wilhelm Erb noted that the electrical stimulation of a damaged peripheral nerve below the site of injury resulted in muscular contraction. In contrast, electrical stimulation at a site above the injured nerve brought about no activity in the muscle. Erb concluded that the injury blocked the flow of electrical impulses down the nerve.

The actual use of electrical diagnostic testing did not take place until the late 1940s, when electrodes and an oscilloscope, an instrument that measures electrical activity, were used to measure the rate at which an electrical impulse could travel down a nerve. This discovery allowed the testing of nerve function and would become useful in the discrimination between axonal and demyelinating neuropathies. During this period, the invention of the electron microscope and the discovery of better nerve-staining techniques enhanced the ability of scientists to study the physiological and anatomical changes that occur in nerves with the onset of neuropathies.

Neuropathies received considerable attention in 1976 when approximately five hundred cases of the neuropathy called Guillain-Barré syndrome occurred in the United States following a national vaccination program for swine flu. The reason that the swine flu vaccine caused this neuropathy has never been discovered, but this syndrome often occurs after an upper respiratory tract or gastrointestinal infection.

Those suffering from neuropathies that result from exposure to toxic substances, viral or bacterial infections, or metabolic diseases have a good prognosis of recovery if the underlying cause of the neuropathy is treated. The prognosis of recovery is not as good for those who suffer neuropathies as a result of hereditary diseases. Advances made in genetic research and continued research in gene therapy may someday greatly increase the prognosis of recovery for those suffering from hereditary neuropathies.

—*David K. Saunders, Ph.D.*

See also Batten's disease; Botox; Carpal tunnel syndrome; Cerebral palsy; Chiari malformations; Cluster headaches; Diabetes mellitus; Electromyography; Encephalitis; Epilepsy; Guillain-Barré syndrome; Hallucinations; Headaches; Hemiplegia; Huntington's disease; Lead poisoning; Leprosy; Leukodystrophy; Meningitis; Migraine headaches; Motor neuron diseases; Multiple sclerosis; Nervous system; Neuroimaging; Neurology; Neurology, pediatric; Neurosurgery; Numbness and tingling; Pain; Palsy; Paralysis; Paraplegia; Parkinson's disease; Quadriplegia; Radiculopathy; Restless legs syndrome; Sciatica; Seizures; Shingles; Sympathectomy; Tics; Vagotomy; Vagus nerve.

For Further Information:

"Conditions." *Facial Neuralgia Resources*, Jan. 31, 2007.

Kandel, Eric R., James H. Schwartz, and Thomas M. Jessell, eds. *Principles of Neural Science.* 5th ed. Norwalk, Conn.: Appleton and Lange, 2006.

"Knowledge Base." *TNA Facial Pain Association*, Apr. 18, 2013.

Margolis, Simeon, and Hamilton Moses III, eds. *The Johns Hopkins Medical Handbook: The One Hundred Major Medical Disorders of People over the Age of Fifty.* Rev. ed. Garden City, N.Y.: Random House, 1999.

Marieb, Elaine N. *Essentials of Human Anatomy and Physiology.* 10th ed. San Francisco: Pearson/Benjamin Cummings, 2012.

"NINDS Peripheral Neuropathy Information Page." *National Institute of Neurological Disorders and Stroke*, Sept. 19, 2012.

Parker, James N., and Philip M. Parker, eds. *The Official Patient's Sourcebook on Peripheral Neuropathy.* San Diego, Calif.: Icon Health, 2002.

"Peripheral Nerve Disorders." *MedlinePlus*, May 9, 2013.

Senneff, John A. *Numb Toes and Other Woes: More on Peripheral Neuropathy.* San Antonio, Tex.: MedPress, 2001.

Stahl, Rebecca J., and Rimas Lukas. "Neuropathic Pain." *Health Library*, Mar. 15, 2013.

Neuroethics

Ethics

Specialties and related fields: Bioethics, neuroscience, addiction research, social psychology

Definition: Two interrelated disciplines: the ethical, societal, and legal implications of neuroscience, and the cognitive basis for ethics and moral behavior.

Key terms:

brain-machine interface: direct communication between a living brain and a computer or other external device

neuroenhancement: drugs or therapies that improve or modify cognition

neuroimaging: a category of research techniques that produce images of brain anatomy and/or activity

psychopathy: a class of behavioral disorders characterized by a lack of remorse and empathy, antisocial behavior, and poor self-control

Science and Profession

The easiest definition of neuroethics is "the neuroscience of ethics, and the ethics of neuroscience." While this is perhaps too glib, it encapsulates the dual nature of the discipline-one that allows professionals from many disciplines to fit under the "neuroethics" umbrella. Neuroethicists range in profession from lawyers to policymakers, with concentrations in neuroscience and philosophy.

Legal teams often consult with neuroethicists about the use of neuroscience in the courtroom, especially as it pertains to personal responsibility. Some have argued that the neurological basis of morality should play a role in how offenders are prosecuted and treated. Using neuroimaging as a lie detector test has been widely debated, although it has been largely dismissed from American courts.

Neuroethicists also influence public policy about the ethical use of neuroscientific information and research, sitting on panels such as the Presidential Commission for the Study of Bioethical Issues.

Doctors and neuroscientists are frequently confronted with neuroethical questions. In the course of their research, scientists may discover unexpected health information, such as a predisposition to a progressive neurological disorder. They must then decide whether to disclose this information to the subject. Patients also regularly ask their physicians for prescriptions to drugs with off-label uses as neuroenhancers, including attention deficit hyperactivity disorder (ADHD) and narcolepsy medications.

A number of major universities now have departments exclusively dedicated to neuroethics. They generally grant masters and Ph.D.'s in the discipline. There are also two peer-reviewed neuroethics journals, Neuroethics and the American Journal of Bioethics-Neuroscience (AJOB-Neuro).

Perspective and Prospects

Both neuroscience ethics and the cognitive basis for morality have a long tradition in medicine, as well as in law and philosophy. However, neuroethics as a defined field can be traced back to a Dana Foundation meeting called "Neuroethics: Mapping the Field." The proceedings of this meeting were published in a book that has become a widely-used reference guide.

Some neuroethics topics are simply bioethical issues that are specific to neuroscience. The idea of "brain doping," sometimes called cosmetic pharmacology, taps into the wider discussion of improving performance in healthy people, although there is the added dimension of personhood and morality. Because of these additional layers, neuroethics can diverge widely from traditional biomedical ethics to include issues of the self and identity.

For instance, some neuroethicists have discussed a "morality pill," a theoretical pill that could make a person more likely to adhere to a given set of ethics (i.e., giving a psychopath a treatment for empathy). Many mental illnesses or personality disorders might be treatable with direct intervention, but potential loss of memory or personality must be weighed against the benefits.

The use of brain scans in the courtroom is often a cause for controversy. Some data shows a correlation between psychopathy and specific patterns of brain activity or anatomy, rising to a discussion of biology versus responsibility. If a person is biologically incapable of controlling their impulses, are they still legally responsible for their actions?

The growing use of brain-machine interfaces is another ripe topic for discussion. Brain implants have been used to restore vision to the blind, while gamers can don special headsets to turn brainwaves into screen action. Each use of a brain-machine interface requires a risk-benefit analysis. Is the implant safe enough? Will "mind-reading" devices violate privacy? Neuroethicists have even been called on to discuss the use of mind reading in police or military interrogations.

Future neuroethical discussions will likely focus on access to and use of new, better neuroenhancement techniques, and privacy issues arising from the use of neuroscience in marketing, law, and medical treatment.

—*Caroline Taylor Ferguson*

See also Cognitive enhancement; Concussion; Neurology; Neuroscience; Traumatic brain injury

For Further Information:

The Center for Neuroscience and Society at the University of Pennsylvania. http://neuroethics.upenn.edu/. Up-to-the-minute information on neuroethics news and events, as well as educational resources and briefs on a number of neuroethics topics.

Churchland, Patricia. *Braintrust: What Neuroscience Tells Us about Morality*. Princeton, NJ: Princeton University Press, 2011. Written for a general audience, Churchland discusses the biological basis of empathy, cooperation, and other moral behaviors.

Farah, Martha J., ed. *Neuroethics: An Introduction with Readings*. Cambridge, MA: MIT Press, 2010. A primer packed with writings from prominent neuroethicists around the world, commonly used in classroom settings.

Gazzaniga, Michael. *The Ethical Brain*. New York: Dana Press, 2005. Written by the father of cognitive neuroscience, this compulsively readable book covers the biological basis of morality, personhood, and enhancement.

Glannon, Walter. *Bioethics and the Brain*. New York: Oxford University Press, 2006. Glannon focuses on the ethical implications of modern neuroscience technologies at a graduate school-level.

Illes, Judy, and Barbara J. Sahakian, eds. *Oxford Handbook of Neuroethics*. Oxford: Oxford University Press, 2011. Features 50 chapters that cover the majority of the field so far, written by a variety of the leading experts.

The International Neuroethics Society website, http://www.neuroethicssociety.org. Includes information on the annual meeting, links to books and blogs by members, and a calendar of neuroethics-related events.

Levy, Neil. *Neuroethics: Challenges for the 21st Century*. Cambridge: Cambridge University Press, 2007. This graduate school-level book delves into the philosophy underlying neuroethical studies.

Marcus, Steven J., ed. *Neuroethics: Mapping the Field*. New York: Dana Press, 2004. Proceedings of the 2002 Dana Foundation meeting that defined neuroethics as a discipline.

Sahakian, Barbara, and Jamie N. LaBuzetta. *Bad Moves: How Decision Making Goes Wrong and the Ethics of Smart Drugs*. New York: Oxford University Press, 2013. The authors discuss what scientists know about the biological underpinnings of decision making, and how that can be altered with drugs.

Neurofibromatosis

Disease/Disorder

Also known as: Von Recklinghausen disease

Anatomy or system affected: Bones, nervous system, skin

Specialties and related fields: Dermatology, genetics, neurology, orthopedics, plastic surgery

Definition: A genetic disease affecting the nervous system, skin, and bones that produces multiple nerve tumors (neurofibromas), deeply pigmented areas of skin (café-au-lait spots), and bone deformities.

Causes and Symptoms

Most infants born with neurofibromatosis, which is also known as Von Recklinghausen disease, have few symptoms until puberty. Disease progression and signs and symptoms vary from mild (in about one-third of affected children) to moderate and severe disfigurement and organ failure. The disease causes abnormal growths of nerve tissue along the peripheral nerve tracts of the head, neck, trunk, and extremities, usually involving the brain and spinal cord (the central nervous system) later. These so-called neurofibromas appear as multiple, visible growths lying beneath the skin. Also typical are the many areas of deeply pigmented skin, known as café-au-lait (coffee-and-milk) spots. In addition, severely disfiguring bone defects of the skull and spine can be caused by neurofibromas.

Some patients lead nearly normal lives, with only cosmetic problems from the café-au-lait spots and visible neurofibromas. Most patients, however, experience serious consequences from deep growths and skeletal deformities. Depending on the size and location of these tumors, they can cause blindness, deafness, developmental disorders, seizures, pain, and paralysis. Other organs, especially the kidneys and glands, are frequently damaged as well. The

---

Information on Neurofibromatosis

Causes: Genetic factors

Symptoms: Multiple nerve tumors, deeply pigmented areas of skin (café-au-lait spots), bone deformities

Duration: Chronic

Treatments: Supportive therapy, including surgical removal of neurofibromas, reconstructive plastic surgery to correct disfigurement, counseling

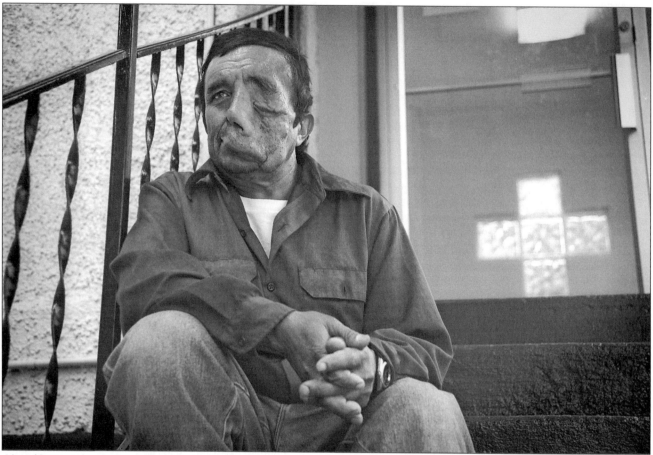

Manuel Raya was born with neurofibromatosis, a genetic disease that causes tumors to grow on nerves. (AP/Wide World Photos)

most feared complication is the transformation of these benign tumors into cancerous ones.

Treatment and Therapy

No cure exists for neurofibromatosis. Supportive therapy includes surgical removal of the neurofibromas and reconstructive plastic surgery for the sometimes severe disfigurement that can result from deep tumors and bone deformities. The skull, spine, and eye sockets are particularly affected. Social isolation and embarrassment are serious problems with neurofibromatosis, and counseling is essential. The prognosis is variable depending on the size and location of the tumors. Both cancer and organ failure can shorten the patient's life.

Because neurofibromatosis is genetic, occurring in one in three thousand births, genetic analysis of the parents is essential if there is a family history of the disease. Prenatal testing can determine if the fetus has inherited the defect. Research is now focusing on correcting the genetic error in the developing fetus.

—*Connie Rizzo, M.D., Ph.D.*

See also Bone disorders; Bones and the skeleton; Dermatology; Dermatopathology; Genetic diseases; Genetics and inheritance; Nervous system; Neuralgia, neuritis, and neuropathy; Neurology; Neurology, pediatric; Skin; Skin cancer; Skin disorders; Skin lesion removal; Tumor removal; Tumors.

For Further Information:

Ablon, Joan. *Living with Genetic Disorder: The Impact of Neurofibromatosis*. Westport, Conn.: Auburn House, 2001.

Children's Tumor Foundation. http://www.ctf.org.

Currey, John D. *Bones: Structures and Mechanics*. 2d ed. Princeton, N.J.: Princeton University Press, 2006.

Daube, Jasper R., ed. *Clinical Neurophysiology*. 3d ed. New York: Oxford University Press, 2009.

Korf, Bruce R., and Allan E. Rubenstein. *Neurofibromatosis: A Handbook for Patients, Families, and Health Care Professionals*. 2d ed. New York: Thieme Medical, 2005.

"Learning About Neurofibromatosis." *National Human Genome Research Institute*, September 16, 2012.

"Neurofibromatosis Fact Sheet." *National Institute of Neurological Disorders and Stroke*, January 13, 2012.

Nicholls, John G., A. Robert Martin, and Bruce G. Wallace. *From Neuron to Brain*. 4th ed. Sunderland, Mass.: Sinauer, 2007.

Rosenblum, Laurie. "Neurofibromatosis." *Health Library*, August 30, 2012.

Victor, Maurice, and Allan H. Ropper. *Adams and Victor's Principles of Neurology*. 9th ed. New York: McGraw-Hill, 2009.

Neuroimaging

Procedure

Also known as: Neuroradiology

Anatomy or system affected: Back, blood vessels, brain, head, neck, nerves, nervous system, spine

Specialties and related fields: All

Definition: The art and science of photographing living brain or nervous system tissue.

Key terms:

cerebral angiography: X-ray photography of blood vessels inside the skull

computed tomography (CT): originally computed axial tomography (CAT) scan; any of several techniques, with or without contrast media, for creating images of internal body structures by means of the mathematical reconstruction of a large series of parallel sectional X rays

contrast medium: any substance or chemical that is inserted, ingested, or injected into the body to improve the visibility of certain parts seen by X-ray or other medical imaging technique

echoencephalography: a technique of using reflected ultrasound to create a graphic representation of brain structures

electroencephalography (EEG): electronic measurement and graphic depiction of brain waves

magnetic resonance imaging (MRI): a technique of creating images by resonating hydrogen nuclei inside the body

magnetoencephalography (MEG): a type of MRI, designed to measure brain activity directly rather than infer it from other data

positron emission tomography (PET): a type of CT using a short-lived radioactive isotope as a contrast medium

single photon emission computed tomography (SPECT): a type of CT using a gamma camera to record the pattern of gamma rays emitted from a radioactive drug given to the patient

Indications and Procedures

Images of the living brain or other part of the central nervous system are indicated for any disorder anywhere in the body that may have neurological involvement or complications. Psychiatrists may also order neurological images for their patients whose mental disorders may have physical causes. Typical indications for neuroradiologic diagnosis include cancer, stroke, and head trauma, especially closed head injury.

Depending on what tissue is involved and what condition is suspected, the physician may order any of dozens of neuroimaging methods. The most common in the early twenty-first century are computed tomography (CT), magnetic resonance imaging (MRI), positron emission tomography (PET), single photon emission computed tomography (SPECT), and magnetoencephalography (MEG). Additional methods include electroencephalography (EEG), near infrared spectroscopy (NIRS), diffuse optical imaging (DOI), and other techniques.

Uses and Complications

Besides clinical uses in diagnosing disease in individual patients, neuroimaging is also valuable as a research tool for studying Alzheimer's disease, Parkinson's disease, multiple sclerosis, epilepsy, and other degenerative and acute conditions that affect the central nervous system. It can also increase the understanding of drug effects on the brain, natural aging processes, brain function localization, autism, psychiatric disorders, and many other kinds of physiological events. Well-funded initiatives exist for "brain mapping" to create precise, molecular-level, function-specific atlases of the human brain, as well as the brains of mice, rats, and many other animals. The Laboratory of Neuro Imaging (LONI) at the University of California, Los Angeles (UCLA) is the world leader in this kind of research.

Risks are minimal for patients undergoing brain scans. Usually the worst that can happen is that the scan may provide inadequate diagnosis. The physical dangers are generally the same as for CT or MRI scans on other parts of the body. Occasionally, CT brain scans trigger seizures, especially in children. The chance of these inadvertent seizures is much less with MRI. Another safety advantage of MRI over CT is that MRI does not use radioactive materials. On the other hand, MRIs can be harmful if there is metal inside the body, such as from bone or joint repair, or a pacemaker; doctors must be notified of this ahead of time.

Perspective and Prospects

Neuroimaging began almost immediately after German physicist Wilhelm Conrad Röntgen discovered x-rays in 1895. The limits of using plain film x-rays to diagnose nervous system diseases and other soft tissue disorders soon became apparent. Nevertheless, because of its simplicity and thanks to the pioneering work of Austrian neurologist Artur Schüller and Swedish radiologist Erik Lysholm, physicians until the early 1970s generally preferred plain film to the three other methods available for intracranial and spinal diagnosis: pneumography, radiopaque myelography, and cerebral angiography. These other three all involved using contrast media to improve the detail in the x-ray.

American physician Walter Dandy invented pneumography at Johns Hopkins University in 1918. After observing that x-rays show air as black, soft tissue as gray, and bone as white, Dandy developed techniques to inject air into the central nervous system to serve as a contrast medium. The resulting x-rays clearly highlighted abnormalities such as tumors, but the technique was very dangerous. French scientists Jean Athanase Sicard and Jacques Forestier developed radiopaque myelography, the use of contrast media in spinal x-rays, in the early 1920s.

In the 1920s, Portuguese physician António Egas Moniz developed cerebral angiography, a technique in which a rapid series of skull x-rays were taken immediately after injecting a radioactive contrast medium into both carotid arteries. This proved to be an excellent method of showing abnormalities and displacements caused by tumors, but was disfavored because of its significant danger to the patient and the ugly surgical scars left on the patient's neck.

British physicist Godfrey Newbold Hounsfield and his team of radiologists built the first practical clinical CT scanning machine in 1971. Between 1971 and 1977, several scientists developed practical MRI from facts about the magnetic properties of atomic nuclei that had been known since the 1950s. These two methods soon superseded both plain film and cerebral angiography as the preferred methods of neuroimaging. Today, there are a great variety of specialized MRI techniques geared toward different kinds of body imaging and diagnosis; an especially important one for brain imaging is functional MRI (fMRI), which can measure neural activity.

—Eric v. d. Luft, Ph.D., M.L.S.

See also Angiography; Brain; Computed tomography (CT) scanning; Echocardiography; Imaging and radiology; Magnetic resonance imaging (MRI); Mammography; Nervous system; Noninvasive tests; Nuclear medicine; Nuclear radiology; Positron emission tomography (PET) scanning; Radiation sickness; Radiation therapy; Radiopharmaceuticals; Single photon emission computed tomograph (SPECT); Ultrasonography.

For Further Information:

Cabeza, Roberto, and Alan Kingstone, eds. *Handbook of Functional Neuroimaging of Cognition.* 2d ed. Cambridge, Mass.: MIT Press, 2006.

Carter, Rita, and Christopher D. Frith. *Mapping the Mind.* Rev. ed. Berkeley: University of California Press, 2010.

Clarke, Edwin, and Kenneth Dewhurst. *An Illustrated History of Brain Function: Imaging the Brain from Antiquity to the Present.* 2d rev. ed. San Francisco: Norman, 1996.

Damasio, Hanna. *Human Brain Anatomy in Computerized Images.* 2d ed. New York: Oxford University Press, 2005.

D'Esposito, Mark. *Functional MRI: Applications in Clinical Neurology and Psychiatry.* Boca Raton, Fla.: Taylor & Francis, 2006.

Dumit, Joseph. *Picturing Personhood: Brain Scans and Biomedical Identity.* Princeton, N.J.: Princeton University Press, 2004.

Mori, Susumu, et al. *MRI Atlas of Human White Matter.* Boston: Elsevier, 2005.

"Neuroimaging and Mental Illness: A Window into the Brain." *National Institutes of Mental Health,* 2013.

"Neurological Imaging." *National Institutes of Health,* March 29, 2013.

Taveras, Juan M. "Diamond Jubilee Lecture: Neuroradiology-Past, Present, and Future." *Radiology* 175 (1990): 593-602.

Toga, Arthur W., and John C. Mazziotta, eds. *Brain Mapping: The Methods.* 2d ed. Boston: Academic Press, 2002.

Toga, Arthur W., and John C. Mazziotta, eds. *Brain Mapping: The Systems.* San Diego, Calif.: Academic Press, 2000.

Toga, Arthur W., John C. Mazziotta, and Richard S. J. Frackowiak, eds. *Brain Mapping: The Disorders.* San Diego, Calif.: Academic Press, 2000.

Van Bruggen, Nick, and Timothy P. L. Roberts, eds. *Biomedical Imaging in Experimental Neuroscience.* Boca Raton, Fla.: CRC Press, 2003.

Neurology

Specialty

Anatomy or system affected: Brain, ears, hands, head, muscles, musculoskeletal system, nerves, nervous system, psychic-emotional system, spine

Specialties and related fields: Audiology, endocrinology, genetics, physical therapy

Definition: The study of the structure and function of the nervous system.

Key terms:

axon: the cellular extension of the neuron that conducts electrical information, transmitting it to the dendrite of the next neuron through the synaptic gap between them

cellular automaton: a self-reproducing entity and mathematical model for complex systems, including animal nervous systems

dendrite: the extension of the neuron that receives electrical information from neurotransmitters moving across the synaptic gap from the axon of a preceding neuron

neuroglial cell: a supportive cell for neurons within the central nervous system of animals

neuron: the principal nervous system cell that conducts electrical information from its dendritic extensions, through its cell body, to its axonic extensions, and on to other cells

neurotransmitter: a chemical messenger or hormone that relays electrical information across a synapse from the axon of one neuron to the dendrite of another neuron

plasticity: a phenomenon of many animal nervous systems, particularly those in higher vertebrates, in which central nervous system neurons grow in patterns based upon input information

Schwann cell: a supportive cell for neurons in the peripheral nervous systems of vertebrate animals that wraps around and insulates axons using the protein myelin

synapse: the gap between the transmitting axon of one neuron and the receiving dendrite of another neuron

von Neumann machine: a cellular automaton or machine that can think and self-replicate; based on the attempts of the physicist John von Neumann to duplicate the human nervous system in computers

The Physiology of the Nervous System

Neurology is the study of the nervous system, an intricate arrangement of electrically conducting nerve cells that permeate the entire animal body. Nervous tissue, which represents a principal means of cell-to-cell communication within animals, is one of four adult tissues found within the organs of most animals. The remaining three adult tissues-epithelia, connective tissue, and muscle-rely heavily on nervous tissue for their proper functioning, particularly muscle tissue.

Nervous tissue is a primary characteristic of most animal species. Evolutionarily, nerve tissue arose from cells that primarily were endocrine in origin. Endocrine cells are hormone producers that secrete hormones for distribution through the organism via the organism's bodily fluids and circulatory systems. Hormones and closely related chemical messengers called neurotransmitters are molecules that are produced in one part of the organism (such as by an endocrine cell or gland), travel through the organism, and target cells in another part of the organism. Hormones or neurotransmitters usually are composed of proteins (long chains of amino acids, or polypeptides) or of fats such as steroids. These chemical messengers affect gene expression within their target cells. Hormones and neurotransmitters determine whether genes are active or inactive. In active genes, the deoxyribonucleic acid (DNA) of the gene encodes messenger ribonucleic acid (mRNA), which encodes protein. An inactive gene does not encode protein. All events within the target cell are influenced by the presence or absence of gene-encoded proteins.

Hormones are effective cell-to-cell communicative and control molecules within all organisms, including animals. In animals, however, hormones and neurotransmitters have become elaborated as parts of extensive nervous systems. The nervous systems of animals have developed according to the evolution of a specialized nervous cell type called a neuron.

The neuron, a specialized, electrically conducting cell, is the basic unit of the nervous system. A neuron is unlike many other cells because it can assume diverse shapes and can assume (relatively) great lengths, sometimes spanning many centimeters. A neuron consists of a cell body containing a nucleus, where the genetic information resides, and numerous organelles, including the energy-producing mitochondria and protein-synthesizing ribosomes. There may be a few or many cellular extensions of its cytoplasm and membrane that twist the neuron into a very distorted appearance. The two principal types of extensions are axons and dendrites.

A dendrite is an electrically receiving extension of a neuron; it receives electrical information from another neuron. An axon is an electrically transmitting extension of a neuron; it transmits electrical information to another neuron. An axon of one neuron transmits electrical information to the dendrite of another neuron. Yet the two neurons are not in direct contact; the axon does not touch the dendrite. A gap called a synapse separates the axon from the receiving dendrite.

Electrical information crosses the synapse via a special type of hormone called a neurotransmitter, a protein encoded by the genes and synthesized by the ribosomes of the neuron. Electrical information traveling along the axon of a neuron triggers the release of a specified quantity of neurotransmitter proteins at the synapse. The neurotransmitters diffuse across the synapse where, upon making contact with the dendritic membrane of the next neuron, they depolarize the dendrite and allow the electrical information transmission to continue unabated.

Actual electrical conduction in a neuron involves membrane depolarization and the influx of sodium ions and the efflux of potassium ions. Electrical conduction along a neuronal segment involves the depolarization of the membrane with the movement of sodium cations into the neuron. Electrical conduction for a particular neuronal segment ends with repolarization of the neuronal membrane as potassium cations move across the neuronal membrane and out of the neuron. The passing electrical action potential, which is measured in millivolts, involves simultaneous depolarization and repolarization in successive regions of the neuron. The initial depolarization is triggered by neurotransmitters contacting the dendritic membrane. Sodium and potassium ion pumps continue the successive stages of depolarization and repolarization along the dendrites, cell body, and axons of the neuron until neurotransmitters are released from a terminal axon across a synaptic gap to depolarize the membrane of the next neuron.

Within animal nervous systems, neurons are very plastic: they grow in specified patterns, much like crystals, in response to stimuli and contacts with other neurons. A neuron may have one or many axonic and dendritic extensions. A neuron with one dendrite and one axon is termed bipolar. A neuron with many dendrites and many axons is termed multipolar; such a neuron makes many contacts with other neurons for the transmission of electrical information along many different neural pathways.

Animal nervous systems usually consist of centralized, concentrated neurons that form the center of nervous control, called the central nervous system. In vertebrate animals, the central nervous system consists of the billions of neurons composing the brain and spinal cord. Additionally, peripheral neurons extend throughout the animal body, permeating virtually every cell and tissue region and thus forming the peripheral nervous system, composed of billions of dispersed neurons.

Functionally, neurons are of three principal types: sensory, motor, and internuncial neurons. Sensory neurons detect stimuli and transmit the electrical information from the stimulus toward the central nervous system. The sensory neurons are arranged one after another, transmitting the electrical action potential from axon to neurotransmitter to dendrite, and so on. The central nervous system processes this information, usually utilizing an intricate array of connected internuncial neurons and specialized neuronal regions devoted to specific bodily functions. Once the central nervous system has processed a response to the stimulus, the response is affected by motor neurons, which transmit electrical information back to the body. Motor neurons will transmit electrical information between each other in the same fashion as sensory neurons. The motor neurons, however, often will terminate at some effector tissue, usually a muscle. Neurotransmitters released from the last motor neuron will depolarize the muscle membranes and trigger the biochemical and physical contraction of muscle. The muscle responds to the stimulus.

The primary purpose of nervous systems in animals is to respond to stimuli, both internal and external. Sensory neurons detect stimuli and direct this information to the central nervous system, where internuncial neurons process the information to appropriate decision centers, which direct a response along a chain of motor neurons to a muscle or muscles that physically respond to the initial stimulus. This chain of nervous communication is called a reflex arc. Virtually every activity in the body requires reflex arcs involving central and peripheral nervous system sensory, internuncial, and motor neurons.

The neurons of vertebrate animal nervous systems are very plastic and make trillions of neuron-to-neuron interconnections for the accurate processing of information, the reception of stimuli information, and the direction of response information along reflex arcs. Within the central and peripheral nervous systems of the human body, millions of information transfer processes occur by reflex arcs every second along trillions of neuronal interconnections. The number of such electrical information transfers that must occur accurately every moment within the body is staggering, yet the human nervous system accomplishes these amazingly intricate tasks with ease. No supercomputer yet devised even comes close to the complexity and efficiency of the vertebrate animal nervous system.

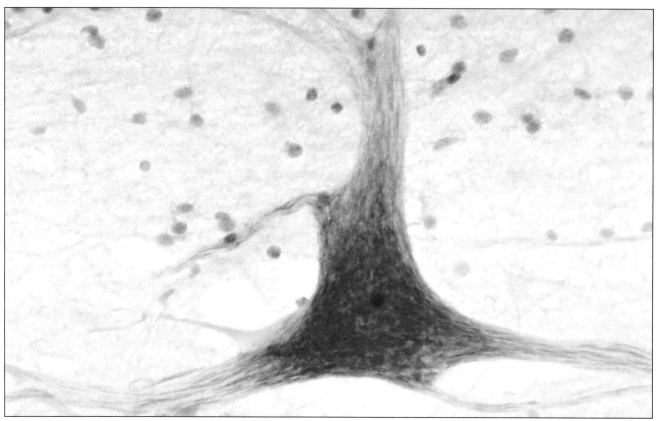

A nerve cell. (Digital Stock)

Science and Profession

Neurologists attempt to understand the structure of the nervous system, including the functioning of the neuron, neuronal plasticity, supporting nerve cells (neuroglia and Schwann cells), neurotransmitters, neuronal patterning in learning, how vision and hearing occur, nerve disorders, and the embryological development of the nervous system.

Neurons are among the most flexibly specialized cells in animal tissues. Animal nerve tissue is derived from embryonic ectodermal tissue. The ectoderm is a tissue layer of cells formed very early in animal development. Very early in development following conception, all animals undergo a blastula stage, in which the embryo is a hollow sphere of roughly five hundred cells. A region of the blastula called the blastopore folds to form a channel of cells through the blastula, thus initiating the gastrula stage.

The gastrula has three embryonic tissues: ectoderm, mesoderm, and endoderm. The ectoderm and endoderm continue to divide and differentiate into epithelial cells. Mesodermal cells multiply and differentiate into muscle and connective tissue cells. Dorsal ectodermal cells (cells that will become the back side of the organism) fold inward to form a nerve cord. The neurons of this nerve cord multiply and differentiate into central and peripheral nervous tissue.

In humans, the dorsal nerve cord becomes the billions of centralized neurons composing the spinal cord. The neurons in the anterior region of the spinal cord will fold, multiply, and differentiate into the various brain regions. The

complete, fully functional human brain has an estimated one hundred billion neurons that grow plastically and form trillions of interconnections for the accurate processing of electrical information.

The embryonic brain consists of three principal enfolded regions: the prosencephalon (forebrain), the mesencephalon (midbrain), and the rhombencephalon (hindbrain). Each of these three embryonic regions folds and differentiates further. The prosencephalon neurons multiply and differentiate to become the cerebrum, thalamus, and hypothalamus. The mesencephalon region becomes the corpora quadrigemina and cerebral peduncles, areas that connect other brain regions and coordinate sensory and motor impulses for basic reflexes. The rhombencephalon becomes the cerebellum, pons, and medulla oblongata; these are brain regions that control basic bodily processes such as coordination, prediction of movements, and maintenance of heart rate and respiration.

Furthermore, special regions of brain tissue develop into external sensory apparatuses: eyes for vision, ears for hearing and balance, and nasal and tongue chemoreceptors for smell and taste. Millions of sensory neurons flow from these special sense organs to highly complicated brain regions that analyze, interpret, learn from, and react to these sensory stimuli. Neurophysiologists attempt to decipher the mechanisms by which the brain processes information. For example, the hundreds of thousands of retinal neurons in the eye collect light images reflected from objects, convert these diverse stimuli into thousands of bits of electrical information, and combine this information along an optic nerve. The optic nerve then transmits the electrical information of vision to the posterior occipital region of the cerebrum within the brain, where millions of visual processing neurons position the inverted, reversed visual image and interpret it.

How the brain neurons process such information is not well understood and is the subject of intense study. While neurophysiologists have a fairly good understanding of nervous system structure, nervous system function represents a tremendous challenge to investigating scientists.

Structurally, neurons are supported by nerve cells called neuroglia in the central nervous system and Schwann cells in the peripheral nervous system. Neuroglia include four cell types: astrocytes, ependyma, microglia, and oligodendrocytes. Astrocytes stabilize neurons, ependyma allow cerebrospinal fluid exchange between brain ventricles and neurons, microglia clean up dead and foreign tissue, and oligodendrocytes insulate neurons by wrapping around them and secreting an electrically insulating protein called myelin. In the peripheral nervous system, Schwann cells behave much like oligodendrocytes; they wrap around axons and electrically insulate the axons with myelin for the efficient conduction of electrical information.

Specific neurological research is focused on neuronal plasticity in learning, the effects of various neurotransmitters upon neural activity, and diseases of the central nervous system. Various models of neuronal plasticity have been proposed to explain how learning occurs in higher vertebrates, including humans and other mammals. Most of these neuronal processing models involve the spatial patterning of neural bundles, which orient information in space and time. The plastic growth of these neurons in specified directions and locking patterns contributes to memory, learning, and intelligence in higher mammals such as primates (which include humans and chimpanzees) and cetaceans (dolphins and whales).

Neurotransmission can be affected by a variety of physical states and chemical influences. The extensive use and misuse of pharmaceuticals and drugs can have serious effects upon the nervous system. Furthermore, developmental errors of the nervous system and aging can contribute to various diseases and disorders.

Perspective and Prospects

The nervous system of humans and higher vertebrate animals presents a tremendous variety of exciting research possibilities. The brain, the seat of human consciousness, represents a mystery to scientists even with the intense scientific scrutiny devoted to this organ. The brain is studied to understand how humans learn and how they might accelerate this exceptional ability. The intricate connections between billions of very plastic cerebral cortical neurons enable millions of electrical information impulses to direct millions of simultaneous activities every second. Brain structure, neural pathways, and techniques of learning and cognition are studied indirectly in human subjects and more directly in other intelligent mammals such as chimpanzees, gorillas, dolphins, and whales. These studies

include analyses of the senses as well as poorly understood extrasensory perceptions that may be linked to exceptional nervous system activity.

Researchers in the field of artificial intelligence attempt to generate cellular automatons, machines that can think and self-replicate. Artificial intelligence research began with the work of the brilliant physicist and computer pioneer John von Neumann, who attempted to mimic the human nervous system within computer systems-systems that have been called von Neumann machines. Yet no true thinking machines have been developed. The best supercomputers yet devised by humans may process data far more rapidly than the human brain, but they are no match for the human brain's capacity to process millions of data items simultaneously.

While the basic physical and chemical mechanisms of neuronal function have been deciphered by neurological scientists, research into neurotransmission across synaptic gaps continues. One principal neurotransmitter at muscular junctions is acetylcholine, which triggers muscle contractions following a motor neural impulse. When acetylcholine is not needed, it is destroyed by a molecule called acetylcholinesterase. Two types of molecular poisons can affect neuromuscular activity: acetylcholine inhibitors, which compete with acetylcholine; and antiacetylcholinesterases, which inhibit acetylcholinesterase and, therefore, accelerate acetylcholine activity. Acetylcholine competitors (such as atropine, nicotine, caffeine, morphine, cocaine, and valium) block acetylcholine at neuromuscular junctions, thereby stopping muscular contractions and producing flaccid paralysis; death can result if the heart or respiratory muscles are affected. Antiacetylcholinesterases, such as the pesticides sevin and malathion, leave acetylcholine free to contract muscles endlessly, thereby causing convulsions.

Neurology also is devoted to understanding the biochemical and genetic basis for various neurological disorders, including Alzheimer's disease, parkinsonism, seizures, abnormal brain wave patterns, paralysis, and coma. Neurological research also is concerned with the nature of pain, the sense organs, and viral diseases of the nervous system, such as meningitis, encephalitis, herpes simplex virus 2, and shingles. The complexity of the human nervous system has inspired an enormous variety and quantity of research.

—David Wason Hollar, Jr., Ph.D.

See also Alzheimer's disease; Amnesia; Anesthesia; Anesthesiology; Aneurysmectomy; Aneurysms; Aphasia and dysphasia; Apnea; Ataxia; Attention-deficit disorder (ADD); Audiology; Balance disorders; Batten's disease; Behçet's disease; Bell's palsy; Biofeedback; Biophysics; Botox; Brain; Brain damage; Brain disorders; Brain tumors; Carpal tunnel syndrome; Cerebral palsy; Chiari malformations; Cluster headaches; Concussion; Craniotomy; Creutzfeldt-Jakob disease (CJD); Critical care; Critical care, pediatric; Cysts; Dementias; Disk removal; Dizziness and fainting; Dyslexia; Ear infections and disorders; Ear surgery; Ears; Electrical shock; Electroencephalography (EEG); Electromyography; Emergency medicine; Encephalitis; Epilepsy; Fetal tissue transplantation; Ganglion removal; Grafts and grafting; Guillain-Barré syndrome; Hallucinations; Head and neck disorders; Headaches; Hearing loss; Hemiplegia; Huntington's disease; Hypothalamus; Intraventricular hemorrhage; Laminectomy and spinal fusion; Learning disabilities;

Leukodystrophy; Lower extremities; Lumbar puncture; Memory loss; Ménière's disease; Meningitis; Migraine headaches; Motor neuron diseases; Motor skill development; Multiple sclerosis; Narcolepsy; Nervous system; Neuralgia, neuritis, and neuropathy; Neurofibromatosis; Neuroimaging; Neurology, pediatric; Neurosurgery; Numbness and tingling; Otorhinolaryngology; Palsy; Paralysis; Paraplegia; Parkinson's disease; Physical examination; Poliomyelitis; Porphyria; Prion diseases; Psychiatry; Psychiatry, child and adolescent; Psychiatry, geriatric; Quadriplegia; Rabies; Radiculopathy; Reflexes, primitive; Restless legs syndrome; Sciatica; Seizures; Sense organs; Shock therapy; Skin; Sleep disorders; Smell; Snakebites; Spina bifida; Spinal cord disorders; Spine, vertebrae, and disks; Strokes; Subdural hematoma; Sympathectomy; Taste; Tay-Sachs disease; Tetanus; Tics; Touch; Transient ischemic attacks (TIAs); Tremors; Unconsciousness; Upper extremities; Vagotomy; Vagus nerve.

For Further Information:
Alberts, Bruce, et al. *Molecular Biology of the Cell*. 5th ed. New York: Garland, 2008.

Bear, Mark F., Barry W. Connors, and Michael A. Paradiso. *Neuroscience: Exploring the Brain*. 3d ed. Philadelphia: Lippincott Williams & Wilkins, 2007.

Bloom, Floyd E., M. Flint Beal, and David J. Kupfer, eds. *The Dana Guide to Brain Health*. New York: Dana Press, 2006.

"Brain Basics: Know Your Brain." *National Institute of Neurological Disorders and Stroke*, 20 Mar. 2013.

Chiras, Daniel D. *Biology: The Web of Life*. St. Paul, Minn.: West, 1993.

Daube, Jasper R., ed. *Clinical Neurophysiology*. 3d ed. New York: Oxford University Press, 2009.

"Disorder Index." *National Institute of Neurological Disorders and Stroke*, 2013.

Lilly, John C. *Programming and Metaprogramming in the Human Biocomputer*. Rev. 4th ed. New York: Julian Press, 2000.

Marieb, Elaine N. *Essentials of Human Anatomy and Physiology*. 10th ed. San Francisco: Pearson/Benjamin Cummings, 2012.

Nicholls, John G., A. Robert Martin, and Bruce G. Wallace. *From Neuron to Brain*. 5th ed. Sunderland, Mass.: Sinauer, 2012.

"Neurologic Diseases." *MedlinePlus*, 13 Aug. 2013.

Snyder, Solomon H. "The Molecular Basis of Communication Between Cells." *Scientific American* 253, no. 4 (October, 1985): 132-141.

Neurology, pediatric

Specialty

Anatomy or system affected: Brain, ears, hands, head, muscles, musculoskeletal system, nerves, nervous system, psychic-emotional system, spine

Specialties and related fields: Audiology, endocrinology, genetics, neonatology, pediatrics, perinatology, physical therapy

Definition: The treatment of nervous system disorders in infants and children.

Key terms:

autonomic nervous system: the body system that regulates involuntary vital functions and is divided into sympathetic and parasympathetic divisions

brain stem: the medulla oblongata, pons, and mesencephalon portions of the brain, which perform motor, sensory, and reflex functions and contain the corticospinal and reticulospinal tracts

cerebrum: the largest and uppermost section of the brain that integrates memory, speech, writing, and emotional response

lesion: a visible local tissue abnormality such as a wound,

sore, rash, or boil, which can be benign, cancerous, gross, occult, or primary

neurologic: dealing with the nervous system and its disorders

paralysis: the loss of muscle function or sensation as a result of trauma or disease

pediatric: pertaining to neonates, infants, and children up to the age of twelve

Science and Profession

Neurologic illness and injury are principal causes of chronic disability when they occur in children because they result in the development of abnormal motor and mental behaviors and/or in the loss of previously existing capabilities, with a common problem in children being musculoskeletal dysfunction. Pediatric neurology involves the ongoing assessment of an infant's or child's neurologic function, which requires the pediatric neurologist to identify problems; set goals; use appropriate interventions, including physical therapy, teaching, and counseling; and evaluate the outcome of treatment.

The pediatric neurologist looks for certain positive or negative signs of dysfunction in the nervous system. Positive signs of neurologic dysfunction include the presence of sensory deficits; pain; involuntary motor events such as tremor, chorea, or convulsions; the display of bizarre behavior or mental confusion; and muscle weakness and difficulty controlling movement. Negative signs are those that represent loss of function, such as paralysis, imperception of external stimuli, lack of speaking ability, and/or loss of consciousness.

Neurologic disease can manifest in a variety of ways. There are disorders of motility, such as motor paralysis, abnormalities of movement and posture caused by extrapyramidal motor system dysfunction, cerebellum dysfunction, tremor, myoclonus, spasms, tics, and disorders of stance and gait. Pain and other disorders of somatic sensation, headache, and backache may occur, such as general pain and localized pain in the craniofacial area, back, neck, and extremities. There are disorders of the special senses, such as smell, taste, hearing, vision, ocular movement, and pupillary function, as well as dizziness and equilibrium disorders. Epilepsy and disorders of consciousness, such as seizures and related disorders, coma and related disorders, syncope, and sleep abnormalities also fall under the category of neurologic disease. Derangements of intellect, behavior, and language as a result of diffuse and focal cerebral disease-such as delirium and other confusional states, dementia, and Korsakoff syndrome-fall under this category as well, as do lesions in the cerebrum and disorders of speech and language. Anxiety and disorders of energy, mood, emotion, and autonomic and endocrine functions are other signs of neurological disease, such as lassitude and fatigue, nervousness, irritability, anxiety, depression, disorders of the limbic lobes and autonomic nervous system, and hypothalamus and neuroendocrine dysfunction.

Diagnostic and Treatment Techniques

The pediatric neurologist begins with a medical history of the infant or child to determine if the problem is congenital or acquired, chronic or episodic, and static or progressive. The focus of the pediatric neurologist in taking the patient's history is on genetic disorders, the medical history of family members, and perinatal events, with an emphasis on the mother's health, nutrition, and medications, as well as tobacco, alcohol, or drug use during pregnancy. Considerable information about a child's or infant's behavior or neuromuscular function can be obtained by observation of the child's alertness and curiosity, trust or apprehension, facial and eye movements, limb function, and body posture and balance during simple motor activities. If possible, the pediatric neurologist will ask the child about instances of weakness, numbness, headaches, pain, tremors, nervousness, irritability, drowsiness, loss of memory, confusion, hallucinations, and loss of consciousness. Headaches, abdominal pain, or reluctance to attend school may be associated with neurologic disturbances, with contributing factors including subtle developmental disabilities, specific learning disabilities, and depression. Disorders of movement include tics, developmental clumsiness, ataxia, chorea, myoclonus, or dystonia.

A complete neurologic examination includes an evaluation of mental status, craniospinal inspection, cranial nerve testing, sensory testing, musculature evaluation, an assessment of coordination, and autonomic function testing. Mental status evaluation involves the assessment of orientation, memory, intellect, judgment, and affect. Craniospinal inspection includes the palpation, percussion, and auscultation of the cranium and spine. Cranial nerve testing assesses the motor and sensory function of the head and neck. Sensory testing measures peripheral sensations, including responses to pinprick, light touch, vibration, and fine movement of the joints. In musculature evaluation, weakness is associated with altered tendon reflexes, indicating lower motor neuron lesions, whereas exaggerated tendon reflexes are associated with an extensor response of the big toe following plantar stimulation (Babinski reflex). In coordination assessment, smooth fine and gross motor movements demand integrated function of the pyramidal and extrapyramidal systems, whereas hyperreflexia, increased muscle stiffness, and problems with muscle coordination reflect spasticity. The evaluation of autonomic function involves bowel and bladder function, emotional state, and symmetry of reflex activity, particularly resting muscle tone and positioning of the head. Additional diagnostic aids include lumbar puncture (spinal tap), complete blood count (CBC), myelography, electroencephalography (EEG), and computed tomography (CT) scanning.

Perspective and Prospects

Pediatric neurologists have been greatly assisted in their recognition of neurologic disease in infants and children by brain-imaging techniques, such as CT scanning and magnetic resonance imaging (MRI). Event-mediated evoked potentials are also used to assess the conduction and processing of information within specific sensory pathways. These advances have enabled an accurate evaluation of the integrity of the visual, auditory, and somatosensory pathways and the uncovering of single and multiple lesions within the brain stem and cerebrum. Particularly noteworthy are CT scanning and sonographic detection of clinically silent intracranial hemorrhages in premature infants.

Late twentieth- and early twentieth-century success in assisting premature infants has produced a population of patients at risk for developing cerebral palsy, developmental disabilities, epilepsy, and various learning disorders. The higher incidence of neurologic disease in the pediatric age group likely results from the increased ability of medical science to detect nervous system disturbances and from the increased survival rate of premature infants. Neurologic patients are compromised in nearly every aspect of living and have a high incidence of psychiatric problems, and their recovery is often slow and unpredictable. Because medical advances have resulted in an increased survival rate following serious neurological insult, more individuals are in need of long-term rehabilitation. The financial cost associated with this care presents an ongoing challenge to health care systems and to researchers examining effective means to restore function.

—*Daniel G. Graetzer, Ph.D.,*
and Charles T. Leonard, Ph.D., P.T.

See also Amnesia; Anesthesia; Anesthesiology; Aphasia and dysphasia; Apnea; Ataxia; Attention-deficit disorder (ADD); Audiology; Batten's disease; Biofeedback; Biophysics; Brain; Brain damage; Brain disorders; Brain tumors; Carpal tunnel syndrome; Cerebral palsy; Chiari malformations; Cluster headaches; Concussion; Craniotomy; Creutzfeldt-Jakob disease (CJD); Critical care, pediatric; Dizziness and fainting; Dyslexia; Ear infections and disorders; Ear surgery; Ears; Electrical shock; Electroencephalography (EEG); Emergency medicine; Encephalitis; Epilepsy; Ganglion removal; Grafts and grafting; Guillain-Barré syndrome; Hallucinations; Head and neck disorders; Headaches; Hearing loss; Huntington's disease; Hydrocephalus; Intraventricular hemorrhage; Laminectomy and spinal fusion; Learning disabilities; Leukodystrophy; Lower extremities; Lumbar puncture; Memory loss; Ménière's disease; Meningitis; Migraine headaches; Motor neuron diseases; Motor skill development; Multiple sclerosis; Narcolepsy; Nervous system; Neuralgia, neuritis, and neuropathy; Neurofibromatosis; Neuroimaging; Neurology; Neurosurgery; Numbness and tingling; Otorhinolaryngology; Palsy; Paralysis; Paraplegia; Pediatrics; Physical examination; Poliomyelitis; Porphyria; Prion diseases; Psychiatry, child and adolescent; Quadriplegia; Rabies; Reflexes, primitive; Seizures; Sense organs; Skin; Sleep disorders; Smell; Snakebites; Spina bifida; Spinal cord disorders; Spine, vertebrae, and disks; Sympathectomy; Taste; Tay-Sachs disease; Tetanus; Tics; Touch; Tremors; Unconsciousness; Upper extremities.

For Further Information:

"Diseases and Conditions: Brain and Nervous System." *KidsHealth.* Nemours Foundation, 2013.

"Disorder Index." *National Institute of Neurological Disorders and Stroke,* 2013.

Fenichel, Gerald M. *Clinical Pediatric Neurology: A Signs and Symptoms Approach.* 6th ed. Philadelphia: Saunders/Elsevier, 2009.

Hay, William W., Jr., et al., eds. *Current Diagnosis and Treatment in Pediatrics.* 21st ed. New York: McGraw-Hill Medical, 2012.

"Head, Neck, and Nervous System." *HealthyChildren.org.* American Academy of Pediatrics, 2013.

Kliegman Robert, et al., eds. *Nelson Textbook of Pediatrics*. 19th ed. Philadelphia: Saunders/Elsevier, 2011.

"Neurologic Diseases." *MedlinePlus*, 13 Aug. 2013.

Victor, Maurice, et al. *Adams and Victor's Principles of Neurology*. 9th ed. New York: McGraw-Hill Medical, 2009.

Volpe, Joseph J. *Neurology of the Newborn*. 5th ed. Philadelphia: Saunders/Elsevier, 2008.

Neuropsychology

Specialty

Anatomy or system affected: Brain

Specialties and related fields: Neurology, neuroscience, pharmacology, psychiatry, psychology, rehabilitation

Definition: The scientific study of the biological underpinnings of behavior such as emotion, awareness, memory, language, and cognition.

Key terms:

amnesia: a condition exhibited by memory problems

aphasia: a condition exhibited by language problems

neuropsychological tests: standardized assessments used to evaluate a person's strengths and weaknesses of cognitive functioning

occupational therapy: the use of treatment programs to help people learn or recover skills associated with activities of daily living or work

traumatic brain injury: injury to the brain that usually results from an accident

Science and Profession

Neuropsychology is an interdisciplinary field that emerges from the study of biological mechanisms underlying psychological phenomena such as emotion, language, memory, perception, movement, and consciousness. In contrast to the discipline of cognitive psychology, which explores the conceptual and theoretical processes of the mind, neuropsychology investigates the relationship between brain function and behavior.

Most neuropsychologists have earned doctorates, with degrees coming from programs specifically in the area of neuropsychology or a general experimental program that includes postdoctoral work in neuropsychology. Neuropsychologists work in academia (colleges and universities), in private industry, for federal and state government agencies, and in private practice. They should not be confused with neurologists and psychiatrists who are physicians with medical degrees (M.D.'s). Those who study neuropsychology find that knowledge in the field opens up a variety of occupational choices, such as biomedicine, nursing, psychiatric health care, cognitive rehabilitation, occupational therapy, physical therapy, neurology, psychiatry, neuroscience, laboratory technician, and pharmacology.

Neuropsychology is typically broken down into two areas of inquiry: experimental neuropsychology (also known as cognitive neuroscience) and clinical neuropsychology (sometimes referred to as human neuropsychology). Experimental neuropsychologists most often work in university settings and conduct laboratory studies using either nonhuman animals (mice, rats, etc.) or humans who suffer from head trauma, neurological disease, or illness. A common goal of empirical research is to learn more about the basic neurological or neurophysiological mechanisms associated with specific behaviors, with an emphasis on understanding more about brain/behavior relationships. In contrast, clinical neuropsychologists usually work in health care settings (hospital, health clinic, rehabilitation center), where they assess and evaluate clinical populations such as those who suffer from traumatic brain injury, amnesia, aphasia, and other brain-based problems. More importantly, the clinical neuropsychologist wants to help patients by developing treatment protocols that will help them either improve or maintain their current level of functioning. The U.S. Department of Labor/Employment and Training Administration, which sponsors the Occupational Information Network (O*NET), lists some of the major tasks of neuropsychologists as follows:

- Conduct neuropsychological evaluations such as assessments of intelligence, academic ability, attention, concentration, sensory-motor function, language, learning, and memory.
- Write or prepare detailed clinical neuropsychological reports using data from psychological or neuropsychological tests, self-report measures, rating scales, direct observations, or interviews.
- Diagnose and treat conditions involving injury to the central nervous system such as cerebrovascular accidents, neoplasms, infectious or inflammatory diseases, degenerative diseases, head traumas, demyelinating diseases, and various forms of dementing illnesses.
- Interview patients to obtain comprehensive medical histories.
- Establish neurobehavioral baseline measures for monitoring progressive cerebral disease or recovery.
- Diagnose and treat psychiatric populations for conditions such as somatoform disorder, dementias, and psychoses.
- Distinguish between psychogenic and neurogenic syndromes, two or more suspected etiologies of cerebral dysfunction, or between disorders involving complex seizures.

One of the largest patient populations that a clinical neuropsychologist works with comprises those who suffer from a traumatic brain injury (TBI). The range of therapeutic needs for a TBI patient can vary greatly. A neuropsychologist will begin to assess cognitive and behavioral deficits by conducting a series of neuropsychological tests. Once an assessment has been completed, a treatment plan can then be developed to help the individual progress as far as they are capable. Since a brain injury can influence several systems in the body, it is common for a neuropsychologist to work in conjunction with an interdisciplinary team. A TBI patient can receive several supportive therapies such as cognitive therapy, sensory-motor therapy, occupational therapy, speech and language therapy, physical therapy, among others.

Perspective and Prospects

Neuropsychology is a subspecialty of the discipline of psychology. It is difficult to pinpoint when scientists and physicians first began to study behavior as a method to explore brain functioning; however, by the late 1800s, definite evidence supporting localization theory began to emerge. This theory hypothesized the brain was composed of separate areas that were responsible for different functions. In competition with localization theory was the concept of equipotentiality, which held the belief that mental abilities depended on the whole brain rather than just a single localized area. Thus, when those who subscribed to equipotentiality encountered a brain injury, the amount of brain damage that occurred was more important than the specific area that was compromised.

In 1861, Paul Broca, a French surgeon, treated a patient who had been unable to speak for several decades. After the patient's death, Broca performed an autopsy and discovered a lesion in the left frontal lobe near the lateral fissure that demarcates the frontal lobe from the temporal lobe of the brain. After studying several additional cases of patients with a similar language disturbance, Broca published his results in 1865. This paper supported localization theory since language processes were localized to specific brain structures. This language disturbance is now known as Broca's aphasia.

The discipline of neuropsychology continued to gain acceptance as additional brain structures that mediated specific behaviors were discovered. The development of neuropsychological tests along with the introduction of functional brain imaging technologies (e.g., functional magnetic resonance imaging, positron emission tomography) were also pivotal in the growth of neuropsychology.

—*Bryan C. Auday, Ph.D., and Elaine Hong*

See also Concussion; Glasgow coma scale; Neurology; Neuroscience; Traumatic brain injury

For Further Information:

Brain Injury Association of America: http://www.biausa.org/.

Kalat, James W. *Biological Psychology.* 11th ed. Belmont, CA: Wadsworth, 2013.

Kolb, Bryan, and Ian Q. Whishaw. *Fundamentals of Human Neuropsychology.* 6th ed. New York: Worth Publishers, 2009.

Horton Jr., Arthur MacNeill, and Danny Wedding. *The Neuropsychology Handbook.* 3rd ed. New York: Springer Publishing Company, 2008.

Lambert, Kelly G., and Craig H. Kinsley. *Clinical Neuroscience: Psychopathology and the Brain.* 2nd ed. New York: Oxford University Press, 2011.

Zillmer, Eric A., Mary V. Spiers, and William C. Culbertson. *Principles of Neuropsychology.* 2nd ed. Belmont, CA: Thomson Wadsworth, 2008.

Neurorehabilitation

Procedure

Anatomy or system affected: Brain

Specialties and related fields: Neurology, Neuroscience, Psychiatry, Psychology, Rehabilitation

Definition: The systematic use of structured activities designed to improve cognitive, emotional, and social functioning in a person recovering from an injury to the brain.

Key terms:

functional compensation: a process that allows for recovery of function by rerouting neural connections to alternate brain structures that will take over the processing demands of a damaged area

neural plasticity: the ability of the nervous system to change structurally or chemically in order to enhance its ability to adapt to environmental change

neuropsychologist: a doctoral-level professional with specialized training in brain-behavior relationships to assess and to develop treatment plans for patients who suffer from brain injury

traumatic brain injury: any wound to the brain that results from a blow to the head

Overview

Each year in the United States, approximately 1.7 million people sustain a traumatic brain injury. This does not include hundreds of thousands of people who are diagnosed with neurological diseases (e.g., stroke, Parkinson's disease, dementia) or illnesses (e.g., viral encephalitis). Any of these conditions can lead to permanent brain injury that can produce impairments in cognitive, behavioral, emotional, and psychosocial functioning. In many instances, these impairments require rehabilitation services designed to improve functional outcomes for patients.

Once a patient with a brain injury has attained a level of health where he/she does not require any immediate, life-sustaining medical treatment, a neuropsychologist, along with other rehabilitation specialists, such as physical therapists, occupational therapists, speech therapists, and sensory-motor therapists, will complete a comprehensive evaluation. This evaluation, which uses a set of standardized measures, will provide information about a patient's strengths and deficiencies in areas related to cognition, such as memory, language, and decision-making. In addition, social and emotional processing will be evaluated along with possible physical problems such as balance, gait, and other mobility issues.

After the comprehensive assessment is completed, it will be used to guide and construct a rehabilitation treatment plan that involves the implementation of therapies to address deficits caused by brain injury. Over the course of treatment, a neuropsychologist, in consultation with other specialists, will continue to assess functional outcomes in order to determine the effectiveness of the treatment plan.

Mechanisms Involved with Neurorehabilitation

Understanding how the brain is able to recover from an injury can help both patients and rehabilitation specialists. Both groups frequently need reminding that recovery tends to happen in a two-stage process. Acute recovery occurs over days and months and involves several structural and chemical processes. One of these processes includes the restabilization of neurochemical imbalances that can arise with neuropathways become damaged. Another acute recovery process involves the repairing of vascular structure in order for vital oxygen, glucose (the primary source of energy for brain cells), and nutrients to be delivered to surviving tissue. Long-term recovery occurs over years and can involve strengthening cerebral reorganization, which is a type of compensatory strategy to reinstate brain functionality. Typically, this involves rerouting connections from a damaged area to a healthy structure that then begins the task of processing neural signals that was previously performed by the damaged tissue. Another potential mechanism for recovery of function involves the regenerative sprouting or axonal regrowth of neurons that are able to create new connections with nearby healthy brain cells. This ability to create new connections among brain cells, which is referred to as synaptogenesis, can reestablish neuronal pathways that had been compromised by injury.

The various mechanisms just described allow the central nervous system to change both in terms of structure and function. This ability to change is referred to as neural plasticity. Plasticity is a central player in recovery from brain injury. Age is directly correlated with plasticity—in general, the younger the individual who suffers from brain injury, the better the long-term prognosis for recovery. In addition to age, cognitive reserve is another important factor related to neurorehabilitation. Individuals with higher levels of education are more resilient to the deleterious effects of brain injury. It is theorized that these individuals maintain more intricate neuroanatomical pathways. This affords them a redundancy of neural pathways which acts as a sort of back-up system if the primary neural networks become damaged. The additional pathways make it easier for the brain to establish functional compensation.

In general, recovery of function in the central nervous system is related to the size of the lesion and its location. Early recovery within the first week can be an excellent indicator for overall neurorehabilitation improvement.

—*Bryan C. Auday, PhD*

See also: Neurology, Neuroscience, Brain injury

For Further Information:

Ashley, Mark J. "Repairing the Injured Brain: Why Proper Rehabilitation is Essential to Recovering Function." *Cerebrum*, July, 2012.
Barisa, M.T., Dean, R.S., and Noggle, C.A. (Eds.). *Neuropsychological Rehabilitation*. New York, NY: Springer Publication Company, 2013.
Kolb, B. and I.Q. Whishaw. *Fundamentals of Human Neuropsychology*. 6th ed. New York, NY: Worth Publishers, 2009.
Lambert, K.G. and C.H Kinsley. *Clinical Neuroscience: Psychopathology and the Brain*. 2nd ed. New York, NY: Oxford University Press, 2011.

Neuroscience

Specialty

Anatomy or system affected: Brain, autonomic nervous system

Specialties and related fields: Neurology, psychiatry, pediatrics, pharmacology, geriatrics, toxicology, neuropsychology

Definition: The scientific study of nerves, the nervous system, and associated behaviors.

Key terms:

axon: the part of a neuron responsible for sending information to other neurons

dendrite: the part of a neuron responsible for receiving information from other neurons through the binding of neurotransmitters

electroencephalograph: a physiological instrument used to record electrical activity from the scalp

electrophysiology: the study of the electrical properties of cells

excitation: one consequence of the binding of neurotransmitters to the dendrite of a neuron; when the neuron receives enough excitation in its dendrite, the cell will release the neurotransmitter from its axon onto other cells

neuron: the basic cell of the nervous system; commonly referred to as a "brain cell"

neurotransmitter: any of a number of chemicals that facilitate communication between neurons

plasticity: a characteristic of brain cells that allows them to change as a result of stimulation and/or changes in activity

synapse: the space between the axon of one neuron and the dendrite of another where communication between cells takes place

Science and Profession

Neuroscience is a broad, interdisciplinary field that spans many disciplines, including medicine, psychology, biology, chemistry, physics, computer science, mathematics, economics, education, ethics, and law. The term neuroscience replaced several earlier labels for the field, including psychobiology, biopsychology, and biological psychology. Neuroscience is closely related to neurology and neurobiology, although the former focuses on clinical and medical phenomena and the latter is concerned more with biology than behavior. Most neuroscientists have earned Ph.D.'s, though some will also hold M.D.'s (to contrast, all neurologists are physicians).

There are many subdisciplines within neuroscience, such as behavioral neuroscience (which examines the relationship between the brain and behavior using animal models), cellular and molecular neuroscience (explores chemical and electrical events at the cellular level), cognitive neuroscience (uses neuroimaging to study the brain's role in thinking, feeling, and behaving in humans), computational neuroscience (uses computer modeling to understand how neurons and neuronal networks work), and developmental neuroscience (examines how the nervous system changes over the course of a lifetime).

Perspective and Prospects

Though the heart was seen as the seat of intellect in the ancient world, the Greek Hippocrates and later the Roman, Galen, theorized that it may be the brain that is responsible for complex behaviors. Despite the accuracy of these early thinkers, it would be hundreds of years before neuroscience advanced beyond the gross anatomical studies that existed during the middle ages and early Renaissance. It was only after several notable discoveries about the physics of electrical conduction that neuroscientific progress resumed, this time with advances in electrophysiology.

Around the turn of the twentieth century, the two great neuroanatomists, Camillo Golgi and Santiago Ramon y Cajal debated whether the structure of the nervous system was a "reticulum" (Golgi) or a discontinuous series of "connections" between neurons (Cajal). Though neither anatomist possessed a microscope powerful enough to determine who was correct at the time, over fifty years later Palade and Palay used electron microscopy to verify the existence of synapses and show that it was Cajal who was correct. This demonstration, along with the work of Nobel Laureates John Eccles and Bernard Katz, among others, solidified a modern understanding of the typical structure and workings of the nervous system: namely that though communication within individual neurons is electrical in nature, communication between neurons is chemical and occurs through the release of a neurotransmitter from an axon into the synapse. Once in the synapse, the neurotransmitter then binds to the dendrite of a different neuron, thus creating a change in the electrical potential within that neuron.

While neuroanatomists and neurophysiologists were unraveling where and how messages are sent in the nervous system, the Canadian psychologist, Donald Hebb, theorized about how information could be retained. In his 1949 book, On the Organization of Behavior, Hebb outlined the parameters via which the nervous system could be modified in response to activity, the phenomenon now known as "plasticity." His book, one of the most influential texts in all of neuroscience, laid the foundation for everything from development of the visual system to learning and memory.

Though prior to the 1950s, most neuroscientific research was conducted using animal models, the advent of modern neuroimaging techniques, such as functional magnetic resonance imaging, or fMRI, revolutionized the study of the brain and behavior in humans. Unlike brain wave recordings collected using an electroencephalograph (EEG), which had been used for decades, fMRI allowed neuroscientists to see exactly where within the brain activity was taking place when a human was thinking or behaving.

Continuing advances in technology now allow neuroscientists to peer into the brain with greater resolution and detail. Because of this enhanced ability to see what happens within the brain when a human engages in complex reasoning, these advances have facilitated the integration of neuroscience with seemingly unrelated fields such as economics and education.

—*Jerome L. Rekart, Ph.D.*

See also Neuropsychology; Neurology; Psychiatry

For Further Information:

Carter, Rita. *Mapping the Mind.* Berkeley, CA: University of California Press, 2010.
Gazzaniga, Michael S. *The Cognitive Neurosciences.* Cambridge, MA: MIT Press, 2009.
Gross, Charles G. *A Hole in the Head: More Tales in the History of Neuroscience.* Cambridge, MA: MIT Press, 2012.
Hebb, Donald O. *The Organization of Behavior: A Neuropsychological Theory.* New York: Wiley, 1949.
Kalat, James W. *Biological Psychology.* 11th ed. Belmont, CA: Wadsworth, 2013.
Kandel, Eric, James Schwartz, Thomas Jessell, Steven Siegelbaum, and A.J. Hudspeth. *Principles of Neural Science.* 5th ed. New York: McGraw Hill Professional, 2012.
LeDoux, Joseph. *Synaptic Self: How Our Brains Become Who We Are.* 2nd ed. London: Penguin Books, 2003.
McGill University. *The Brain from Top to Bottom.* http://thebrain.mcgill.ca.
Satel, Sally, and Scott O. Lilienfield. *Brainwashed: The Seductive Appeal of Mindless Neuroscience.* New York: Basic Books, 2013.
Society for Neuroscience. BrainFacts.org. http://www.brainfacts.org.

Neurosis

Disease/Disorder

Anatomy or system affected: Brain, nerves, nervous system, psychic-emotional system

Specialties and related fields: Ethics, family medicine, neurology, psychiatry, psychology, public health

Definition: A psychiatric disorder in which the patient continues to be rational and in touch with reality.

Key terms:

agoraphobia: the fear of being in crowds

anxiety disorder: an emotional state that ranges from mild concern to disabling fear

bipolar disorders: disorders characterized by periods of depressed and elevated mood

hysterical amnesia: a dissociative disorder in which patients, capable of reading and writing, cannot remember simple things like their names

obsessive-compulsive disorder: a condition characterized by the ritualistic performance of repetitive actions

somatization disorder: a persistent condition in which patients complain about physical problems for which no cause is apparent

Causes and Symptoms

The distinction between neurosis and psychosis is that those suffering from neuroses are in touch with reality and usually realize that they have a problem. In contrast, psychotics frequently lose touch with reality and do not recognize that they are sick and in need of immediate professional help.

The most common neurosis is depression. Those with major depression experience, for no overt reason, a persistent and overwhelming sadness coupled with an all-encompassing sense of despair. It is normal for people who suffer such ills as the death of a loved one, the loss of a job, or severe financial reverses to be depressed. In such cases, their depression is usually mitigated when the cause is removed or when they distance themselves from it. On the other hand, those who suffer from major depression cannot attribute their suffering to an immediate cause. They are frequently sad and usually do not know why. Depression is also a major component of bipolar disorders, in which episodes of major depression are followed by periods of mania, or elevated mood.

Other common forms of neurosis are obsessive-compulsive disorder (OCD), somatization disorder, hypochondria, various phobias or fears, anxiety disorders, psychosexual

Information on Neurosis

Causes: Psychological disorder
Symptoms: Distressing and unacceptable anxiety, impaired daily functioning, depression, abnormal fear
Duration: Often chronic; may involve acute episodes
Treatments: Counseling, psychoactive medications

disorders, and hysterical amnesia. All these problems occur less frequently than major depression.

An example of obsessive-compulsive disorder may be the compulsion of its victims to wash their hands thirty or forty times a day. Those who have a somatization disorder complain of largely imagined illnesses for which no physical cause can be detected. Often termed hypochondria, this disorder is more frequent in women, especially middle-aged women, than in men.

Most people suffer from one or more phobias that do not disable them. Fear of heights (acrophobia) and abnormal fear of public or open areas (agoraphobia) are quite common, as are the fear of some living things such as spiders or scorpions (arachnophobia) or the fear of closed places (claustrophobia). Many of those suffering from such phobias can usually control them by confronting them rationally, although some phobias may be so intense that they result in panic.

Hysterical amnesia, a dissociative disorder, is relatively rare. Often it is connected with anxiety disorder. Victims tend to panic to the point that they suffer temporary memory loss. Although they remain in touch with reality, they may not be able to remember their names, addresses, telephone numbers, and other obvious bits of information.

Post-traumatic stress disorder (PTSD) has become increasingly common. In extreme cases, it may result in psychotic behavior, although it is more often neurotic in its manifestation. PTSD usually occurs in people who have been subjected to combat situations or to life-threatening natural disasters such as earthquakes, hurricanes, floods, and fires.

Treatment and Therapy

The usual treatment in persistent cases of neurosis is psychotherapy rendered by a clinical psychologist or psychiatrist, frequently over an extended period. Severe cases may require meetings with a professional three or four times a week in order to be effective. Mild cases can sometimes be dealt with in only two or three visits, especially if the patient is cooperative and committed to dealing with the problem.

Neuroses usually do not require such drastic treatment as electric shock therapy or brain surgery, although such treatment was sometimes prescribed in the past. Currently, more than twenty prescription drugs exist to treat such neuroses as bipolar and somatization disorders. Often, patients need to try several of these medications before finding the one that suits them best. Patients must be cautioned, however, not to expect immediate results. When they find a

medication that works well for them, they are advised to continue taking it even after their initial symptoms disappear.

Perspective and Prospects

Substantial biochemical advances during the early years of the twenty-first century have resulted in improved understanding of the relationship between body chemistry and both neuroses and psychoses. Such advances have also been accompanied by changes in the way psychiatric therapy is delivered. Group therapy reduces the cost of treatment. In many situations, because it is so interactive, it proves superior to the one-on-one therapy that psychotherapy and psychoanalysis provide.

The public at large has become more sophisticated than past generations in dealing with neuroses. Nevertheless, the management of the most common neurosis, depression, remains challenging. Most suicides are committed by those suffering from the depths of depression, a condition that gives them a sense of hopelessness.

—*R. Baird Shuman, Ph.D.*

See also Antianxiety drugs; Anxiety; Bipolar disorders; Depression; Hypochondriasis; Midlife crisis; Obsessive-compulsive disorder; Panic attacks; Paranoia; Phobias; Postpartum depression; Post-traumatic stress disorder; Psychiatric disorders; Psychiatry; Psychiatry, child and adolescent; Psychiatry, geriatric; Psychoanalysis; Psychosis; Psychosomatic disorders; Stress.

For Further Information:

American Psychiatric Association. *Diagnostic and Statistical Manual of Mental Disorders: DSM-5.* 5th ed. Washington, D.C.: American Psychiatric Association, 2013.
Craske, Michelle G. *Origins of Phobias and Anxiety Disorders: Why More Women than Men?* New York: Elsevier, 2003.
Frankl, Victor E. *On the Theory and Therapy of Mental Disorders: An Introduction to Logotherapy and Existential Analysis.* New York: Brunner-Routledge, 2004.
Gossop, Michael. *Theories of Neurosis.* New York: Springer, 1981.
Rapee, Ronald M., and David H. Barlow, eds. *Chronic Anxiety: Generalized Anxiety Disorder and Mixed Anxiety-Depression.* New York: Guilford Press, 1991.
Russon, John. *Human Experience: Philosophy, Neurosis, and Elements of Everyday Life.* Albany: State University of New York Press, 2003.

Neurosurgery

Procedure

Anatomy or system affected: Bones, brain, glands, head, nerves, nervous system, psychic-emotional system, spine

Specialties and related fields: General surgery, neurology, psychiatry

Definition: Surgery involving the brain, spinal cord, or peripheral nerves, including craniotomy, lobotomy, laminectomy, and sympathectomy.

Key terms:

aneurysm: the swelling of a blood vessel, which occurs with the stretching of a weak place in the vessel wall

cannula: a tube or hypodermic needle implanted in the body to introduce or extract substances

commissurotomy: the severing of the corpus callosum, the fiber tract joining the two cerebral hemispheres *hematoma*: a localized collection of clotted blood in an organ or tissue as a result of internal bleeding

lesion: a wound or tumor of the brain or spinal cord

lobectomy: the removal of a lobe of the brain, or a major part of a lobe

lobotomy: the separation of either an entire lobe or a major part of a lobe from the rest of the brain

trephination: the opening of a hole in the skull with an instrument called a trephine

Indications and Procedures

Neurosurgery refers to any surgery performed on a part of the nervous system. Brain surgery may be used to remove a tumor or foreign body, relieve the pressure caused by an intracranial hemorrhage, excise an abscess, treat parkinsonism, or relieve pain. In cases of severe mental depression or untreatable epilepsy, psychosurgery (such as lobotomy) may alleviate the worst symptoms, although these procedures are now rare. Surgery may be performed on the spine to correct a defect, remove a tumor, repair a ruptured intervertebral disk, or relieve pain. Surgery may be performed on nerves to remove a tumor, relieve pain, or reconnect a severed nerve.

Most brain operations share some common procedures. Bleeding from the numerous tiny blood vessels in the brain is controlled by use of an electric needle, a finely pointed instrument that shoots a minute electric current into the vessel and seals it. (This same instrument can be used as an electric knife for bloodless cutting.) Brain tissue is kept moist by continued washing with a dilute salt solution. The brain tissue itself is handled with damp cotton pads attached to the end of forceps.

If the brain is swollen, it may be treated by intravenous injections of urea. The resulting increase in the salt concentration of the blood draws the water away from the brain. In addition to drawing off excess water, the brain's size is temporarily reduced, giving the surgeon extra room to maneuver. To help reduce bleeding within the brain, the patient's blood pressure can be lowered by half temporarily through an injection of a drug into the blood. The patient's temperature is also reduced, which lowers the brain's need for oxygen and ensures that the reduced blood flow will not be deleterious.

An operation in which a hole is cut into the skull is called a craniotomy. If only a small hole is required, the procedure is called trepanation (or trephination) and uses an instrument called a trephine, resembling a corkscrew with a short, nail-like tip and a threaded cutting disk. The size of the opening that is made ranges from 1.5 centimeters (0.6 inches) to 3.8 centimeters (1.5 inches) in diameter and, if necessary, may be enlarged with an instrument called a rongeur. This type of surgery is performed to insert needles or cannulas and to remove subdural hematomas. If too much of the bony skull has to be removed (or is fractured by accidental means), a substitute for the bone is inserted. The substitute is usually made of plastic, such as acrylic.

Brain surgery for advanced Parkinson's disease will not cure the disease but may help alleviate some of its symptoms. The major symptoms are tremor, stiffness, weakness, and slowed movements. For patients who do not respond well to medication, a form of neurosurgery called deep brain stimulation (DBS) can be used to reduce or stop the shaking, by implanting a small device called a brain pacemaker that emits electrical impulses to block abnormal activity in affected regions of the brain.

When pain becomes unbearable, such as the pain associated with cancer, the nerves carrying these pain messages can be interrupted anywhere between the brain and the cancerous region. The nerve to the affected organ can be severed, the nerve roots of the spinal cord can be cut, or the cut can be made within the spinal cord.

Hypophysectomy is the surgical removal of the pituitary gland. It is usually performed to slow the growth and spread of endocrine-dependent malignant tumors of the breast, ovary, or prostate gland. It may also be used to stop the deterioration of the retina that may come with diabetes mellitus or to remove a pituitary tumor. Hypophysectomy is considered only as a last resort when cryosurgery or radioactive implants fail to destroy the pituitary tissue. There are two ways to reach a diseased pituitary gland by surgery. One way is to go through the nose. The skull is entered through the sphenoid sinus, and the floor of the bony saddle of the middle of the skull is cut to reach the gland. The second means is by craniotomy. The skull is opened through an incision in the hairline above the forehead. A flap of bone, hinged at eyebrow level, is brought forward so that the surgeon can see the entire affected area clearly. The gland is completely excised.

Psychosurgery is now considered only as a last resort, when nothing else can possibly work. It is rarely undertaken because of the availability of so many drugs to control mental illnesses. In the cases when a lobotomy is performed, it can be done under local anesthesia through tiny holes drilled in the roof of the eyes' orbits. An instrument is then inserted to separate the lobes of the brain.

A laminectomy is performed to relieve compression of the spinal cord caused by injury (the displacement of a bone) or by the degeneration of a disk; it may also be used to find and remove a displaced intervertebral disk. A laminectomy is performed under general anesthesia. The surgeon makes an incision in the back, vertically over the tips of the vertebral bones. The large, thick muscles that lie on either side are peeled back from the surface of the bones. The lamina itself is the part of a vertebral bone that forms the back wall of the spinal canal. When the laminae are cut away, the spinal canal is opened so that the spinal cord covering can be cut. Once the cord is exposed, a particular condition can be treated. It may then be necessary to fuse the vertebrae. The removal of the laminae causes little interference with support or motion of the spine, although recovery from the surgery requires that the patient remain prone for several days to keep the spine in alignment.

Fusion of the vertebrae is the surgical joining of two or more spinal vertebrae to stabilize a segment of the spinal column following severe trauma, a herniated (ruptured) disk, or a degenerative disease. The surgery is performed under general anesthesia. The cartilage pads are removed from between the posterior portions of the affected vertebrae. Bone chips are cut from the vertebral ridges and inserted as a replacement for the removed cartilage. Postoperative motion must be limited until the articulating bones heal.

Severe pain that cannot be controlled by analgesics (painkillers) may be treated by surgery. One procedure, a cordotomy, removes a section of the spinal cord so that most of the nerve fibers that transmit pain messages to the brain are destroyed. At first, the patient does experience less pain, but after a few months, the pain can recur and become worse than before. The recurrence of pain is likely attributable to the reconstruction of some axons that carry ascending messages. Other painful conditions can be treated with surgery. Trigeminal neuralgia (or tic douloureux) is one such condition. These severe attacks of stabbing pain in the face may last a minute or more. The trigeminal nerve can be injected with a concentrated alcohol solution, which will prevent it from working for a year or two. This condition is usually treated surgically by drilling a burr hole in the temple and cutting across the lower two-thirds of the nerve trunk at the site.

Asympathectomy surgically interrupts a part of the sympathetic nerve pathways. It is used to relieve the pain of vascular disease. The surgery involves removing the sheath from around an artery. This sheath carries the sympathetic nerve fibers that control vasoconstriction. Once the sheath is removed, the vessel relaxes and expands so that more blood travels through it.

Uses and Complications

While neurosurgery offers the hope of recovery to people suffering with tumors, aneurysms, and brain injuries, it may result in complications that can bring disability, coma, or even death. Therefore, three issues must be taken into account before neurosurgery is performed. First, these surgeries involve higher risk than most other procedures. Second, diseases that necessitate neurosurgical treatment may render patients wholly or partially incompetent to understand the implications of their surgery. Third, sometimes matching the appropriate surgery to the patient's condition is an uncertain process. Even standard neurosurgical procedures have not been proven in every event.

Because the diagnosis of a brain tumor is often seen as fatal, many believe that surgery has little value as therapy, especially for malignant tumors. Others suggest, however, that the more radical the surgery, the greater the chance of survival for the patient. The problem arises when a tumor is found within the center area of the brain, where the primary sensory and motor cortices are situated. Surgical methods of the past tended to exacerbate the problems of the patient. The use of lasers and microscopy, however, may increase the chance of successful treatment. Using these tools, incisions of no longer than 2 centimeters can be made. Using the microscope, the surgeon can guide the laser to the tumor, which is gently melted and vaporized-all without disturbing the brain. This method is especially useful for reaching deep-seated tumors.

Stereotactic surgery is a means by which monitoring devices are inserted into the brain cortex. These devices can detect lesions, stimulate or record areas within the cortex, or in some other way study the brain. The two things necessary to perform this surgery are a stereotactic atlas (or map) of the brain and the instrumentation for the procedure. The atlas is a series of individual maps, each representing a slice of the brain. The stereotactic instrument consists of two parts: a head holder, which maintains the patient's head in a particular position and orientation, and an electrode holder, which holds the device that is to be inserted.

The purpose of the lesion method of stereotactic surgery is to remove, damage, or destroy a part of the brain in such a way that the behavior of the patient can be monitored to determine the functions of the affected area. Surgery to produce lesions is an extremely precise, and therefore dangerous, surgery. Structures within the brain are tiny, convoluted, and tightly packed, and any surgery performed on an area may therefore damage adjacent areas. There are four different methods of producing lesions.

Aspiration lesions are performed when the target site is in a more accessible area of the brain, where the surgeon can see it clearly and can use the proper instruments. The cortical tissue is aspirated by a handheld pipette, and then the tougher white matter layers are peeled away. Deeper lesions are created with high-frequency (radiofrequency) currents passed through carefully placed electrodes. The heat of the current destroys the tissue. The amount of tissue to be removed is regulated through control of the current's duration and intensity. In the third method, a nerve or tract to be removed can be cut with a scalpel. A tiny incision severing the nerve does not have to do damage to surrounding tissues, so the lesion is small.

The fourth method is cryogenic blockade. In this method, a coolant is pumped through the tip of an implanted cryoprobe to cool the area. When the tissue is cooled, the neurons do not fire. The temperature must remain above freezing, however, to prevent destruction of the tissue. Although the result is not a true lesion, since function returns, this cooled area acts as a lesion because the behavior that it governs is interrupted. Consequently, cryogenic blockade is said to produce a reversible lesion.

A commissurotomy, or severing the connection between the two cerebral hemispheres, may be performed in cases of severe epilepsy if no other treatment is successful. After the two halves are separated (the brain stem is left intact), each hemisphere maintains all the centers that mediate its functions, except that each cortex sees only half the world. For example, visual messages are crossed so that the opposite hemisphere is stimulated by only one eye's input. If both eyes and both hemispheres are working, however, vision should be unaffected. In fact, no real deficits should occur in these patients' behavior. They retain the same verbal intelligence, reasoning, perception, motor coordination, and personality, because of the brain's extraordinary ability to preserve unity, or oneness.

Commissurotomies were first performed in the hope of reducing the severity of convulsions and seizures associated with epilepsy. The rationale was that the severity of the convulsions would be reduced if discharges could be limited to the hemisphere from which they originated. The benefits far surpassed expectations; many patients never experience another convulsion.

Perspective and Prospects

Archaeological evidence shows that people living in the Stone Age performed trepanation. This operation was likely performed to release evil spirits or demons: There is little evidence of fractures of the skulls that have been found, and the pieces of skulls that were excised were preserved and worn as talismans. Today, surgeons in some tribal cultures perform the same surgery; in some cases, some are done for ritual purposes, while others are performed for head injuries as well as headache, dizziness, and epilepsy. Trepanation laid the groundwork for brain surgery as it is still practiced.

Perhaps the most intriguing possibility for future research is transplanting brains or brain tissue. Brain transplants have come a long way from their portrayal in science fiction. In 1971, the first real evidence that transplanted tissue could survive was found. These successful attempts were made in rats. Further studies have shown that transplants have a higher survival rate in tissue richly vascularized with sufficient room to grow. It is hoped that neurotransplant surgery can be used to treat brain damage. One approach would be to develop procedures of implantation that would stimulate the regeneration of the patient's own tissue. A second approach would be to replace damaged tissue with healthy tissue of the same type.

The major question that will have to be answered before successful regeneration is accomplished is why neurons of the peripheral nervous system (PNS) regenerate but the neurons of the central nervous system (CNS) do not. One hypothesis would be that they are too structurally different. This theory is disputed by studies that show CNS neuron regeneration in the peripheral nervous system, while PNS neurons do not regenerate in the central nervous system. Other evidence to refute the hypothesis is that peripheral sensory neurons regenerate until they reach the spinal cord, then regeneration ceases. Therefore, perhaps there is an environmental factor within the central nervous system that prohibits regeneration, such as scar tissue that forms only in the area of CNS damage. Experiments to prove or disprove this theory are inconclusive. The other possibility is that the insulating cells wrapped around CNS neurons are different enough from the Schwann cells of PNS neurons that regeneration is discouraged.

Attempts to replace damaged tissue with healthy tissue have been most useful in treating Parkinson's disease (with its rigidity, tremors, and lack of spontaneous movement). One type of tissue used for replacement is fetal neural tissue. It not only survives but also innervates adjacent tissue, releases neurotransmitters (in this case dopamine), and alleviates the symptoms of parkinsonism. A possible substitute for neural tissue is autotransplantation with some of the patient's own adrenal medulla. This tissue could be used because it too releases dopamine. Investigations thus far have been controversial, but the operation is being performed worldwide.

—*Iona C. Baldridge*

See also Aneurysmectomy; Brain; Brain damage; Brain disorders; Brain tumors; Chiari malformations; Craniotomy; Cysts; Electroencephalography (EEG); Fetal tissue transplantation; Ganglion removal; Laminectomy and spinal fusion; Laser use in surgery; Lumbar puncture; Nervous system; Neuroimaging; Neurology; Neurology, pediatric; Pain; Pain management; Parkinson's disease; Positron emission tomography (PET) scanning; Psychiatric disorders; Psychiatry; Radiculopathy; Spina bifida; Spinal cord disorders; Spine, vertebrae, and disks; Stem cells; Subdural hematoma; Tics; Tumor removal; Tumors.

For Further Information:

Bear, Mark F., Barry W. Connors, and Michael A. Paradiso. *Neuroscience: Exploring the Brain.* 3d ed. Philadelphia: Lippincott Williams & Wilkins, 2007.
Bloom, Floyd E., M. Flint Beal, and David J. Kupfer, eds. *The Dana Guide to Brain Health.* New York: Dana Press, 2006.
Daube, Jasper R., ed. *Clinical Neurophysiology.* 3d ed. New York: Oxford University Press, 2009.
Pinel, John P. J. *Biopsychology.* 8th ed. Boston: Pearson Allyn & Bacon, 2011.
Post, Kalmon, et al., eds. *Acute, Chronic, and Terminal Care in Neurosurgery.* Springfield, Ill.: Charles C. Thomas, 1987.
"What Is Neurosurgery?" *Patient Education Institute,* April 2, 2009.
Zollinger, Robert M., Jr., E. Christopher Ellison, and Robert M. Zollinger, Sr. *Zollinger's Atlas of Surgical Operations.* 9th ed. New York: McGraw-Hill, 2011.

Neutrophil

Biology

Anatomy or system affected: immune system, circulatory system

Specialties and related fields: immunology, hematology, cytology

Definition: A neutrophil is a type of white blood cell that fights infection and is the most abundant of the white blood cell types.

Key terms:

white blood cells: White blood cells function in the immune system and are made in the bone marrow. There are many types of white blood cells, including granulocytes, monocytes, and lymphocytes.

polymorphonuclear leukocytes: Polymorphonuclear leukocyte, or PMN, is another term for neutrophil, based on the irregularly-shaped multi-lobed nuclei characteristic of this cell type.

granulocytes: Granulocytes are a type of white blood cell with granules which contain enzymes released during infection or other immune responses such as allergy. The different types of granulocytes include neutrophils, eosinophils, and basophils.

phagocytosis: A phagocyte is a cell that eats, 'phago' being derived from the Greek word 'for eat'.

Structure and Functions

Neutrophils play essential roles in the immune system. They are the most abundant white blood cell type and the first cells to arrive at the site of infection or injury. Neutrophils comprise about 55-75% of a normal white blood cell count, with normal cell counts ranging from 2-7 billion cells per liter of blood. Along with eosinophils and basophils, neutrophils comprise a type of white blood cell known as granulocytes, so named because they contain small 'granules' or grain-like shapes, within their cytoplasm. These granules store microbe-fighting enzymes. Neutrophils specialize in the capture, engulfment, and killing of microorganisms.

Neutrophils are produced in the bone marrow and are short-lived with lifespans measured in hours. In the bone marrow, it takes about one week for a neutrophil to develop from a progenitor cell into a mature neutrophil. The bone marrow produces about 100 billion neutrophils every day. Once produced, neutrophils live only about 4-10 hours in the blood stream or 1-2 days if they migrate into tissue. To prevent rapid depletion of neutrophils during an infection, the bone marrow stores a large number of granulocytes that can be mobilized quickly in response to infection. Newly formed cells have a round nucleus, but as cells mature, the nucleus become more irregular and lobular, which gives the appearance of having multiple nuclei. Because of their multi-lobed nuclei, these cells are often referred to as polymorphonuclear leukocytes. Neutrophils are characterized histologically by cytoplasmic granules, nuclear features, and staining characteristics and functionally by their role in immune responses against infectious microorganisms.

When an invasion of foreign organisms is detected by the body, the cells of the body send out chemical signals that recruit cells to the site of invasion. An important feature of the role of neutrophils in immune defense is their mobility; unlike some of the other white blood cells, neutrophils aren't limited to a specific area of circulation. They can move freely through the walls of veins and into tissues of the body to immediately attack antigen. The neutrophils are the first cells to respond and travel through the bloodstream to the site of infection. Once at the site of infection, neutrophils attach themselves to walls of blood vessels and enter surrounding tissue to attack invaders and prevent more organisms from entering the blood.

A primary function of neutrophils is phagocytosis and killing of microorganisms. Although neutrophils utilize an arsenal of antimicrobial weapons to destroy their target, phagocytosis, or 'cell-devouring' is one of their primary strategies. Neutrophils surround and engulf bacteria and other microorganisms, the granules of the neutrophil, which are filled with enzymes that can digest many types of cellular material, are released to destroy the organisms. At the same time, neutrophils can also release potent forms of reactive oxygen-based molecules-such as superoxide or hydrogen peroxide-that can destroy bacteria in a process known as 'oxidative burst'. Even in dying, neutrophils have developed a method to kill their targets. Under certain conditions, a neutrophil can undergo a process called NETosis, a form of cell death that releases a mesh-like network of fibers containing antimicrobial enzymes and chemicals. Scientists have termed these neutrophil extracellular traps (NET).

Disorders and Diseases

Normally, the body regulates production of neutrophils and other white blood cells to respond to infection or injury. Abnormal neutrophil counts may be caused by infection or another condition. Too many or too few neutrophils in the blood stream can indicate blood disorders with the potential to be serious conditions. Neutrophilia, a high number of neutrophils in the blood, can result from infection or reaction to medication. Neutrophilia is generally associated with acute inflammation, although it may result from certain diseases such as chronic myelogenous leukemia, which is a type of cancer of blood-forming tissues. More common is a disorder called neutropenia, which is an abnormally low number of neutrophils in the blood. Neutropenia is most often found in cancer patients undergoing chemotherapy but can also result from inherited disorders that affect the immune system as well as by a number of acquired diseases. Neutropenia significantly increases the risk of life-threatening bacterial infection.

Perspective and Prospects

Neutrophils are critical in immune response, and are first responders to infection. In addition to direct uptake and destruction of invading pathogens, neutrophils also secrete chemicals that recruit reinforcements, including other specialized cell types, to the site of infection to assist with immune defense. Although neutrophils are the most abundant circulating leukocyte, their full spectrum of biological functions in the immune system is still emerging. Enhanced understanding of the full capabilities of neutrophils can hopefully lead to improved treatment options for diseases involving neutrophils.

—*Catherine J. Walsh, PhD*

For Further Information:

Bain, Barbara J. *Blood Cells: A Practical Guide*. 5th ed., Wiley Blackwell, 2015. A guide for identifying different blood cells and includes information on blood collection and clinical laboratory tests.

Gabrilovich, Dmitry, editor. *The Neutrophils: New Outlook for Old Cells*. 3rd ed., Imperial College P, 2013. Provides an overview of the biology of neutrophils, including role of neutrophil in cancer and ways to use neutrophils in treatment.

Territo, Mary. "Neutrophilic Leukocytosis." *Merck Manual*, www.merckmanuals.com/home/blood-disorders/white- blood-cell-disorders/neutrophilic-leukocytosis. Accessed 19 Jan. 2017. The information provided on this website focuses on neutrophilic leukocytosis, or high number of leukocytes, including possible diseases associated with the condition.

"Types of White Blood Cells." *New Health Advisor*, www.newhealthadvisor.com/Types-of-White-Blood-Cells.html. Accessed 21 Sept 2017. An informative website with general information about the types of white blood cells important in human health, including a short video explanation on white blood cell types.

"White Blood Cell Disorders." *Dana-Farber/Boston Children's Cancerand Blood Disorders Center*, www.danafarberboston childrens.org/conditions/blood-disorders/white-blood-cell-disorders.aspx. Accessed 19 Jan. 2017. A website that includes a brief description of some white blood cell disorders in children and possible treatments.

Niacin

Anatomy or Biology

Also known as: Vitamin B3; nicotinic acid

Anatomy or system affected: All

Specialties and related fields: Endocrinology; nutrition

Definition: A water-soluble vitamin that serves a key role in several body systems including the breakdown of fats, proteins, and carbohydrates into energy and the production of certain adrenal hormones.

Key terms:

adrenal: an endocrine gland located above each kidney; the inner part of each gland secretes epinephrine (adrenaline) and the outer part secretes hormones that help regulate blood pressure, blood sugar levels, and metabolism

cholesterol: a waxy substance made by the liver and also acquired through diet. High levels in the blood may increase the risk of cardiovascular disease

cirrhosis: chronic degenerative liver disease in which normal cells are replaced by fibrous tissue and normal liver function is disrupted

gout: a disease in which uric acid, a waste product that normally passes out of the body in urine, collects in the joints and the kidneys

plaque: a compound made up of fat, cholesterol, calcium, and other substances found in the blood. It can stick to the walls of arteries, partially or totally blocking blood flow

watersoluble: a compound that dissolves in water. Water-soluble vitamins are not stored in the body the way fat-soluble vitamins are, so the body needs a regular supply of water-soluble vitamins.

Background

Niacin, also known as vitamin B3 or nicotinic acid, is a water-soluble vitamin that serves a key role in metabolism. The liver makes a small amount of niacin, but not enough for human health. Most niacin must be obtained from food. Niacin occurs naturally in many foods and is added to other foods. It is also added to over-the-counter multivitamins. Niacin supplements are available in high concentrations for people who need them for health reasons, but high-dose supplements require a physician's prescription. Although niacin occurs naturally and is important to several body systems, excessive amounts of niacin can have serious, and even life-threatening, side effects.

Sources of Niacin

Good natural sources of niacin include red meat, fish, and poultry. In 1938, the United States began fortifying flour with niacin, so today most flours, cereals, bread, and pasta contain niacin. These products are labeled "fortified" or "enriched." Because of the fortification program, most Americans get enough niacin from their diet without taking a dietary supplement. In addition, the liver can manufacture small amounts of niacin from the amino acid tryptophan, which occurs in many of the foods that contain niacin, as well as seeds, tofu, dairy products, lentils, and beans.

The niacin in supplements is synthesized in a laboratory either chemically or through microbial fermentation, a process by which bacteria or other microbes digest or process one substance to produce another.

Benefits

Niacin is necessary for healthy skin and proper nerve function. It helps in digestion and metabolism, the process by which the body breaks down protein, carbohydrates, and fats to generate energy. The presence of niacin helps the adrenal glands in the production of hormones and aids the liver in processing harmful chemicals and other substances so they can be removed from the body.

The circulatory system also benefits from the presence of niacin. Prescription-strength niacin may be used to regulate cholesterol levels in the blood, although this is less common now that statin drugs are available. Studies have shown that niacin can increase high-density lipoprotein (HDL)—"good cholesterol"—by as much as 30 percent. HDL collects and transports low density lipoprotein (LDL) to the liver, where it is removed from the blood stream. LDL is considered "bad cholesterol" because it clogs arteries and leads to the formation of plaque and cardiovascular disease. Niacin is known to help with migraine headaches and dizziness, both of which can be related to circulation issues. In addition, niacin's beneficial effects on the circulatory system can help some men with erectile dysfunction.

Niacin also has been shown to help some skin disorders. Acne patients who use a topical gel containing niacin have shown improvement in their condition. Nicotinamide, a form of niacin, has been shown to help prevent some forms of skin cancer, especially in patients who already have had skin cancer.

Side Effects

Niacin is water soluble, so excessive amounts are generally excreted in the urine and not stored in the body. However, some people do experience side effects when taking niacin and can have serious problems if too much is consumed. The most notable and common side effect is known as niacin flush. Niacin flush can occur even with normal levels of the vitamin such as those found in a fortified cereal, especially if consumed close to the same time as a multivitamin or other source of the vitamin. A person experiencing niacin flush feels warmth and redness, itching, and/or tingling of the face, neck, and arms, which eventually subsides on its own. Niacin flush is not dangerous, but it can be uncomfortable or frightening, especially if the individual does not realize that it is caused by excess niacin and is not a symptom of a more serious condition. Consuming hot beverages or alcohol can worsen niacin flush and should be avoided at the time of taking a niacin supplement. For those who take prescription-strength niacin on a regular basis for a health problem, the issue of flushing may lessen with time.

Taking too much niacin for an extended period can cause liver damage, high blood glucose (sugar) levels, gout, stomach ulcers, and skin rashes. However, too little niacin can cause problems, too. Deficiencies are uncommon in developed countries but can result from alcoholism, prolonged diarrhea, and liver disorders such as cirrhosis. A deficiency can make the skin especially prone to damage from the sun.

Niacin Deficiency

The most severe result of niacin deficiency is pellagra, a disorder characterized by digestive problems including diarrhea, skin inflammations, and dementia or impairment of mental processes. Pellagra occurs often in poor populations that rely on corn as a food staple. Corn contains significant amounts of niacin but not in a form that can be absorbed through normal human digestion. The niacin does become digestible—or bioavailable—if the corn is first treated in an alkaline solution, such as the lime solution used for the preparation of corn tortillas in Mexico. The digestive issues caused by pellagra often lead to other nutritional deficits as well, and the condition can be fatal. Pellagra is treated through the administration of niacin and by supplementing nutrition to overcome other deficiencies caused by the condition.

Supplements

While niacin supplements are readily available, many physicians do not recommend taking them, especially without medical direction or supervision. As previously noted, deficiencies are uncommon in developed countries because sources of niacin are readily available through diet. Many physicians say that supplementation is not necessary and may cause uncomfortable side effects such as flushing, nausea, and stomach upset. It also can alter liver test results and lead to muscle breakdown.

—*Janine Ungvarsky;*
updated by Tish Davidson, MA

For Further Information:

Johnson, Larry. E. "Niacin." *Merck Manual-Consumer Version.* Merck Sharp & Dohme Corp. 2017. http://www.merckmanuals .com/home/disorders-of-nutrition/vitamins/niacin 25 (accessed July 31, 2017). An easy-to-understand source of information on niacin deficiency and toxicity.

Natural Standard. "Niacin." Mayo Clinic, 2017. http://www. mayoclinic.org/drugs-supplements/niacin—niacinamide/background/hrb-20059838 (accessed July 31, 2017). Comprehensive explanation of the role of niacin in human health.

"Niacin." *Linus Pauling Institute Micronutrient Information Center.* Oregon State University July 2012. http://lpi.oregonstate.edu/ mic/vitamins/niacin (accessed July 31, 2017). A somewhat technical but authoritative monograph on the function of niacin in the body.

"Vitamin B3." University of Maryland Medical Center August 6, 2015. http://www.umm.edu/health/medical/altmed/supplement/ vitamin-b3-niacin (accessed July 31, 2017). Clear, direct overview of niacin and its role in the body.

U.S. National Library of Medicine. "Niacin." MedlinePlus, February 2, 2015.https://www.nlm.nih.gov/medlineplus/ency/article/ 002409.htm (accessed July 31, 2017). Easy to understand summary of the importance of niacin in health.

Nicotine

Treatment

Anatomy or system affected: Central nervous system, lungs

Specialties and related fields: Drug dependency, rehabilitation

Definition: an active ingredient in tobacco products that stimulates the central nervous system in low doses

Today's advertising for cigarettes must carry stern warnings concerning the dangers of smoking and even secondhand smoke from those irresponsible people who have no concern for their own health. Those who have "kicked the habit" are amused to see movie stars or athletes of another day proudly displaying snuff, pipes or a chaw. It is now widely accepted that tobacco is strongly addictive and dangerous to our health. Campaigns by government offices and private foundations, sales restrictions, and high rates of taxation have reduced usage, but smoking remains a major health concern.

While smoking has been found to fill the mouth, throat, and lungs with an astounding array of unhealthy chemicals it is still true that nicotine is the cause of what is undeniably an addiction. The sole beneficial use of this poisonous chemical has been in administering progressively smaller amounts to aid in overcoming one's dependency.

Brief History

The use of nicotine has a long history. There is evidence that humans who first migrated from Asia to the Americas at least 15,000 years ago imported a strong affinity for the use of psychoactive plants. It appears that their belief system centered on a spirit world. These plants provided hallucinations and a number of species that enhanced out-of-body experiences. At least one species, *Nicotiana rustica,* was partially domesticated. While initially, ingestion was by chewing sucking, drinking, or licking, smoking became the preferred method. This observation may have been related to the smoke that suggested its relation to the spirits.

There is a large amount of evidence that the use of tobacco was very wide spread among Native Americans when European explorers and missionaries arrived. In most cases the growing of the plants, curing of the leaves, and consumption of the product was a male activity. The sailors returning to Europe in the sixteenth century brought the fad with them. The English were smoking extensively and in 1595 produced the first book devoted to tobacco. That volume contains illustrations of Europeans smoking a pipe. Soon not only Europe, but also many remote parts of the world were described as "besotted with the herb".

These observations raise the question of why the civilized world adopted so readily a habit of those usually referred to as savages. A tempting suggestion points to the fact that the medical community almost universally endorsed smoking. The evidence shows that its use was recommended as efficacious, or even as a cure, for everything from flatulence to the bubonic plague. This rapid growth occurred in spite of the strong efforts of rulers to suppress its use. Smokers might be decapitated in China and Persians were threatened with loosing parts of their body nose, lips, or ears.

Overview

There appears to be little question that nicotine has harmful effects on the human body. The ingestion of this drug causes the heart to beat faster and blood pressure to rise. There is evidence that smokers are at significant risk of strokes and heart attacks. Pregnant women are strongly advised to refrain from smoking since nicotine seems to interfere with the transfer of oxygen and nutrition to the fetus. Research on possible links between nicotine and cancer continue and thus far they do not seem to be direct. On the other hand, it does appear to promote the growth of tumors.

In spite of huge efforts by the tobacco industry to suppress evidence of nicotine's harmful effects, the courts have acted against them since the early 1990's. Among the several efforts to promote "safer" methods of using tobacco, none have shown the promise of e-cigarettes. Numerous ads have claimed that such devices afford the pleasure of smoking while eliminating the health risks.

These devices create a solution of nicotine and flavoring in glycerol or the closely related propylene glycol and vaporize it with a heated coil. The vapor created, is inhaled as in traditional smoking. It has been shown that the mist inhaled does contain chemicals known to be undesirable. It has also been found that the smoker's lungs are exposed to tiny particles of metal that likely come off the metal coil or its solder joints. These bits of matter are so small that they can travel deep into the lungs. A variety of ailments can be made worse, for example, asthma, bronchitis, and emphysema. Studies of these potential concerns are facing several problems. No one has determined how much vapor users breathe in. Each study makes different assumptions. It is also true that we have yet to determine the products produced by the vaporization of glycol or propylene glycol.

On the legal front there is still no restriction on the contents and they do not have to be specified. It is also true that, unlike tobacco products, there are no age restrictions on the purchase of e-cigarettes. They are readily available through electronic media. It appears that it will be a while before serious studies reveal just how safe vaping really is.

It has also been suggested that the use of e-cigarettes is an ideal way to quit smoking. Once again the hard, scientific evidence is not available. Until carefully conducted studies are published it is impossible to answer this question. A government bureau recommends that the smoker wishing to quit, explore the available, proven, safe, and effective methods.

—*K. Thomas Finley, PhD*

See also: Addiction, Stimulants

For Further Information:
Balfour, David J. K. *The Neurobiology and Genetics of Nicotine and Tobacco*. Cham: Springer, 2015.
Brick, John, and Carlton K. Erickson. *Drugs, the Brain, and Behavior: The Pharmacology of Drug Use Disorders*. New York: Routledge, 2013.
Di Giovanni, G. *Nicotine Addiction: Prevention, Health Effects, and Treatment Options*. Hauppauge: Nova Biomedical, 2012.
Dina, Fine Maron. "Smoke Screen: Are E-Cigarettes Safe?" *Scientific American* 310 (May 2014): 31-32.
Ferrence, Roberta, *et al. Nicotine and Public Health*. Washington DC: American Public Health Association, 2000.
Garrett, Bob. *Brain & Behavior: An Introduction to Biological Psychology*. Los Angeles: SAGE, 2015.
Kuhar, Michael J. *The Addicted Brain: Why We Abuse Drugs, Alcohol, and Nicotine*. Upper Saddle River: FT P, 2012.
Owens, Carlton L. *Nicotine Dependence, Smoking Cessation and Effects of Secondhand Smoke*. Hauppauge: Nova, 2015.
Wand, Kelly. *Tobacco and Smoking*. Detroit: Greenhaven, 2012.

Niemann-Pick disease
Disease/Disorder

Anatomy or system affected: Bones, brain, liver, lungs, nervous system, respiratory system, spleen

Specialties and related fields: Biochemistry, endocrinology, family medicine, genetics, hematology, internal medicine, neurology, pathology, pediatrics, public health

Definition: This lipid disease group, resulting from inactive sphingomyelinase and cholesterol-modifying enzymes, causes lipid buildup in the brain and other organs, mental and physical debilitation, and a short life span.

Key terms:

enzyme: a protein biocatalyst that speeds up a biochemical reaction

foam cell: a large, foamy-appearing, lipid-rich cell, usually a white blood cell

lipid: a fatlike substance

Causes and Symptoms

Niemann-Pick disease (NPD), which consists of several lipid storage diseases, is characterized by an enlarged liver and spleen and the accumulation of fatlike sphingomyelin and cholesterol. Many patients have enlarged spleens and livers soon after birth and develop severe mental damage. In others, symptoms lag; mental damage may not occur, or organ enlargement and mental damage may be postponed. The main forms, types A through C, are attributable to low levels of sphingomyelinase, which normally alters sphingomyelin for use and excretion.

Type A, or infantile NPD, is the most common type. The abdominal organs enlarge, and nervous system damage occurs in early infancy. The spleen and liver enlarge by the age of six months, motor function and intellectual capabilities are then lost, and death occurs by four years of age. Patients are emaciated, jaundiced, and have swollen abdomens and cherry-red spots in the macular region of the eye. Large histiocytes (foam cells) abound in the bone marrow, spleen, lymph nodes, adrenal glands, and lungs.

Type B, or juvenile nonneuropathic NPD, is also common. Enlarged abdominal organs develop as quickly as in type A, but no neurological impairment occurs. An enlarged spleen appears first, followed by liver enlargement. Lungs are often so damaged that frequent breathlessness occurs. Abdominal pain is caused by the huge size of the liver, and the patient is susceptible to respiratory infections. Nevertheless, patients with this type of disease reach adulthood in fair health.

Type C, a rarer chronic form, is asymptomatic for approximately two years. Symptoms then develop gradually, accompanied by lost speech and motor coordination and epilepsy. The liver and spleen are smaller than in types A and B. These patients die in their teens.

Information on Niemann-Pick Disease

Causes: Genetic enzyme deficiency
Symptoms: Liver and spleen enlargement; sometimes severe mental damage, loss of motor function, emaciation, jaundice, swollen abdomen, red spots in eyes, breathlessness
Duration: Chronic and progressive
Treatments: None; enzyme and genetic testing of prospective parents, symptom alleviation through spleen removal or antibiotics

---

Type D, a very rare form, is similar to Type C and has only been found in French Canadians in Nova Scotia.

The pathology of Niemann-Pick disease includes abundant foam cells in the spleen, bone marrow, liver, lungs, and lymph nodes. Nervous tissue may be altered similarly. Foam cells contain brown lipofuscin pigment. This and blue to blue-green stained intracellular material leads to an alternate name, sea-blue histiocytes.

The spleen of a patient with NPD is large, pale, and filled with foam cells, though few hematologic changes occur except for anemia late in the disease. The liver of a type A patient is usually about 50 percent larger than normal, while the liver of a type B patient grows so large that it deforms and causes abdominal pain. Foam cells soon fill the liver, although it usually functions adequately. They also fill the lymph nodes, spleen, lungs, and bone marrow. Their number varies with NPD type and duration. In most types, the foam cell-filled adrenal glands, gonads, thyroid, pituitary, and pancreas function adequately. However, the brains of type A and C patients drop in weight by 25 to 50 percent and are severely damaged.

The predominant lipid accumulant is sphingomyelin, made of fatty acids joined to substances called sphingosine and phosphocholine. Sphingomyelin content in the spleens of type A, B, and C patients is twenty-five, eighteen, and two to twelve times normal, respectively. A thirtyfold increase of liver sphingomyelin occurs in types A and B. Smaller increases, approximately ten times normal, occur in type C. Also, sphingomyelin levels increase threefold to sevenfold in the lymph nodes of all NPD patients. Cholesterol and other sphingolipids also increase in the tissues of NPD patients. It is believed that lipid increases are causative.

Sphingomyelinase deficiency is greatest in types A and C, in which 4 to 20 percent of normal levels occur. In type C, they are about 50 to 90 percent normal levels. The NPD defect is genetic alteration of sphingomyelinase, yielding mutant enzyme less able to break down sphingomyelin.

Treatment and Therapy

Niemann-Pick disease can be prevented only through the enzymatic and genetic testing of prospective parents. Members of at-risk ethnic groups can be tested for sphingomyelinase in their lymphocytes and muscle cells. Genetic counseling can also be used. The disease is transmitted through an autosomal recessive gene, so both parents must carry the gene to transmit disease. If both parents are carriers of a defective NPD gene, each of their children has a 25 percent chance of having the disease and a 50 percent chance of being an asymptomatic carrier.

There is no cure for Niemann-Pick disease. Therapeutic approaches include spleen removal, which diminishes abdominal pain, but it is not widely used. Patients with lung damage who experience frequent respiratory infections and pneumonia are treated with antibiotics, but long courses and high doses are required. Bone marrow transplantation has been done, with mildly encouraging results for patients with type B, but it is not a common treatment. Some children or teenagers with type C disease have been helped by low-cholesterol diets. However, the life expectancy of patients with NPD has not been prolonged much. Miglustat can help alleviate the nervous system symptoms of type C patients.

Perspective and Prospects

In 1914, Albert Niemann, a German pediatrician, reported an eighteen-month-old Jewish child with huge liver and spleen, swollen lymph glands, and jaundice. The child had poor motor control, could not suckle, and died before age two. Postmortem examination showed large lipid deposits in the liver, spleen, lymph nodes, kidneys, and adrenal glands. The overall symptoms and rapid death suggested a new illness. In the 1920s, Ludwig Pick studied other cases and named Niemann-Pick disease. NPD, seen in all ethnic groups, is most common in Ashkenazic Jews. Type B patients are often of Spanish ancestry. Type C, which is less common, occurs most in Nova Scotians.

It is believed that enzyme replacement therapy (mostly sphingomyelinase) may ease the lives of NPD victims when an effective methodology for the frequent delivery of purified enzymes is developed and the enzymes are available in sufficient amounts. Recombinant deoxyribonucleic acid (DNA) research should contribute greatly. However, such treatment of severe NPD (types A and C) will be difficult because of the need to deliver enzymes to the brain.

Another avenue is transplanting healthy livers and spleens, which is presently done to treat other diseases. The problems are scarce donated organs and difficulty placing them in debilitated NPD patients. Transplantation may prove more promising in the future. Also, researchers have identified animal models and genes that, when defective, contribute to NPD. Understanding these issues may produce successful NPD treatments.

—Sanford S. Singer, Ph.D.;
updated by LeAnna DeAngelo, Ph.D.

See also Brain damage; Enzyme therapy; Enzymes; Gaucher's disease; Genetic counseling; Genetic diseases; Glycogen storage diseases; Lipids; Metabolic disorders; Metabolism; Mucopolysaccharidosis (MPS); Screening; Tay-Sachs disease.

For Further Information:

Dugdale, David C. "Niemann-Pick Disease." *MedlinePlus*, December 7, 2012.
Lichtman, Marshall A., et al., eds. *Williams Hematology.* 8th ed. New York: McGraw-Hill, 2011.

National Institute of Neurological Disorders and Strokes. "Niemann-Pick Disease Information Page." *National Institute of Neurological Disorders and Stroke*, October 6, 2011.

National Niemann-Pick Disease Foundation. *NPD: National Niemann-Pick Disease Foundation Inc.*, May 21, 2013.

Parker, James, and Phillip Parker, eds. *Official Parent's Sourcebook on Niemann-Pick Disease*. San Diego, Calif.: Icon Health, 2007.

Raddidadi, Ali A., and Abdulazix Al Twaim. "Type A-Niemann-Pick Disease." *Journal of European Academy of Dermatology and Veneriology* 14 (July, 2000): 301-303.

Nonalcoholic steatohepatitis (NASH)

Disease/Disorder

Also known as: Fatty liver, nonalcoholic fatty liver disease (NAFLD)

Anatomy or system affected: Endocrine system, gastrointestinal system, liver

Specialties and related fields: Endocrinology, family medicine, gastroenterology, internal medicine, pediatrics

Definition: Fatty inflammation of the liver that is not caused by alcohol.

Key terms:

central obesity: excessive abdominal fat

hyperlipidemia: an excess of fat or lipids in the blood

insulin resistance syndrome: a condition characterized by the decreased sensitivity to insulin that is associated with central obesity, metabolic syndrome, and diabetes

metabolic syndrome: a condition defined by the presence of three or more of high blood pressure, abdominal obesity, high triglycerides, low high-density lipoproteins (HDL) cholesterol, and abnormal fasting blood sugar

nonsteroidal anti-inflammatory drugs (NSAIDs): a class of medications for inflammation that do not contain steroids; includes aspirin and ibuprofen

Causes and Symptoms

The liver is a complex organ located in the right upper abdomen. It plays a role in converting carbohydrates, fats, and proteins from food into usable forms for the body. It also manufactures cholesterol, stores sugar, and metabolizes certain medications and chemicals. Nonalcoholic steatohepatitis (NASH) is characterized by the storage of excess fat in the liver, with associated inflammation. The cause of this disorder is not completely understood. The accumulation of excess fat in the liver is related to the body's inability to use its own insulin, a common problem found in adults and children with central obesity. NASH is also found in individuals with other medical conditions, such as diabetes, metabolic syndrome, high blood pressure, and hyperlipidemia. Other causes of excess fat storage are certain medications, exposure to occupational toxins, and some surgical procedures. The excess fat causes damage to the cells of the liver that is similar to the damage caused by excess alcohol intake.

The majority of people with NASH have no symptoms, and the disorder is suspected from liver function tests. Studies have shown, however, that elevated liver enzymes do not always occur in individuals with NASH. If symptoms are present, then they may include fatigue or mild discomfort in the upper right side of the abdomen. The liver

---

Information on
Nonalcoholic Steatohepatitis (NASH)

Causes: Accumulation of fat in the liver; related to diabetes, metabolic syndrome, high blood pressure, hyperlipidemia

Symptoms: Often none, sometimes fatigue or mild abdominal discomfort; enlarged liver and severe liver disease may develop

Duration: Chronic

Treatments: Often none; treatment of associated conditions, liver transplantation if severe

---

may be enlarged. Fatty liver may be identified on ultrasound, but a biopsy of the liver must be performed in order to determine the extent of the disorder. A liver biopsy is a minor surgical procedure that is performed by inserting a needle into the liver through a small incision and removing cells for evaluation under the microscope. The disorder may range from inflammation of the liver to cirrhosis, a chronic, progressive disease with extensive scarring of the liver that causes destruction of liver cells. If the destruction advances, then the liver loses the ability to function. Severe liver disease occurs in approximately 20 percent of those with NASH.

Treatment and Therapy

Treatment goals include the identification and treatment of associated conditions and the reduction of insulin resistance. Adopting a healthy lifestyle is the primary treatment for NASH. Those who are overweight are encouraged to lose weight gradually and to exercise. Triglyceride and cholesterol levels should be kept within normal limits. Strict blood sugar control is indicated for diabetics with NASH. A few studies have found that daily vitamin E reduces abnormal liver enzymes. Insulin-sensitizing drugs, normally used by diabetics, have also shown promise for the treatment of NASH and its associated insulin resistance. Lipid-lowering drug studies have also shown some improvement in blood liver function tests, but not in the follow-up biopsy tests for inflammation and damage.

It is generally recommended that individuals with NASH avoid alcohol and certain medications, such as acetaminophen, that may further damage the liver. If the individual develops severe cirrhosis, then a liver transplant may be necessary to avoid death.

Perspective and Prospects

In 1958, fatty liver disease was first identified in a small group of obese individuals. In 1980, the term nonalcoholic steatohepatitis was coined to describe a small group of patients at the Mayo Clinic who had liver biopsy findings similar to those with alcoholic liver disease. Since 2000, pediatricians have reported the presence of NASH in obese children, as well as in children with other endocrine disorders. The increase in obesity and diabetes in the United States has been linked to the increasing numbers of individuals diagnosed with NASH.

Diagnosis is confirmed with a liver biopsy, or, less commonly, with a noninvasive diagnostic method. Ultrasound and abdominal computed tomography (CT) scans are sometimes used, as are newer x-ray techniques and laboratory blood analyses.

Drug therapy continues to be investigated after promising pilot studies. Further study is also needed in the area of the disease process and its potential for progression in some individuals.

—*Amy Webb Bull, D.S.N., A.P.N.*

See also Abdomen; Abdominal disorders; Alcoholism; Cholesterol; Cirrhosis; Diabetes mellitus; Gastroenterology; Gastroenterology, pediatric; Gastrointestinal disorders; Gastrointestinal system; Hypercholesterolemia; Hyperlipidemia; Inflammation; Insulin resistance syndrome; Internal medicine; Liver; Liver disorders; Liver transplantation; Metabolic syndrome; Metabolism; Obesity; Obesity, childhood; Transplantation.

For Further Information:

Adams, L. A., and P. Angulo. "Treatment of Non-alcoholic Fatty Liver Disease." *Postgraduate Medicine Journal*, 82 (May, 2006): 315-322.

Harrison, Stephen A., and Adrian M. Di Bisceglie. "Advances in the Understanding and Treatment of Nonalcoholic Fatty Liver Disease." *Drugs* 63, no. 22 (2003): 2379-2394.

Howson, Alexandra. "Nonalcoholic Fatty Liver Disease." *Health Library*, May 14, 2013.

"Liver Disease: Fat Inflames the Liver." *Harvard Health Letter* 26 (February, 2001): 4.

Nakajima, Kenichirou, et al. "Pediatric Nonalcoholic Steatohepatitis Associated with Hypopituitarism." *Journal of Gastroenterology* 40, no. 3 (March, 2005): 312-315.

"Nonalcoholic Fatty Liver Disease." *Mayo Clinic*, February 19, 2011.

Nonalcoholic Steatohepatitis." *National Digestive Diseases Information Clearinghouse*, April 30, 2012.

Porth, Carol M. "Disorders of Hepatobiliary and Exocrine Pancreas Function." In *Pathophysiology: Concepts of Altered Health States*. 8th ed. Philadelphia: Wolters Kluwer/Lippincott Williams & Wilkins, 2010.

Noninvasive tests

Procedures

Anatomy or system affected: All

Specialties and related fields: Cardiology, emergency medicine, nuclear medicine, obstetrics, pathology, preventive medicine, radiology

Definition: Diagnostic techniques that do not involve the collection of tissue or fluid samples or the introduction of any instrument into the body; most noninvasive tests involve imaging or the measurement of electrical activity.

Key terms:

computed tomography (CT) scanning: a method of producing images of cross sections of the body

diagnosis: recognition of diseases based on physical examination, the microscopic and chemical results of laboratory findings, and an analysis of imaging results

Doppler shift: the increase in frequency of sound waves as the source of the waves approaches the observer or instrument; Doppler techniques are often used to assess blood flow in body channels such as veins

echocardiogram (EC): a graph of cardiac motion and heart valve closure produced by sending sound waves to the heart and recording their deflections

electrocardiogram (EKG or ECG): a diagnostic tool used to detect disturbances in the electrical activity of the heart

magnetic resonance imaging (MRI): a procedure using magnetic fields to determine blood vessel condition, fluid flow, and tissue contours and to detect abnormal masses

signal-averaged electrocardiogram (SAECG): a sophisticated EKG which detects subtle and potentially lethal cardiac conduction defects

sonography: the use of sound waves deflected from internal body organs to find growing masses (including fetuses) and abnormal lesions; also called ultrasound

X radiology: the use of ionizing radiation of short wavelength to detect abnormalities in primarily dense portions of the body

Indications and Procedures

Noninvasive tests are used in the initial diagnosis of a disease or abnormality and for the monitoring of certain conditions and body processes. Most such tests involve imaging techniques. Primary among them are x-radiology, computed tomography (CT) scanning, magnetic resonance imaging (MRI), electrocardiography (EKG or ECG), and ultrasound.

Diagnostic x-ray examinations are often the first step in complex technological solutions to medical diagnoses and health problems. New uses for diagnostic x-rays are constantly being devised. It is common practice for hospitals to require chest x-rays for all outpatients visiting x-ray departments, and hospital inpatients are usually given chest x-rays before admission or surgery.

Computed tomography (CT) scanning, also known as computed axial tomography (CAT) scanning, uses a computer to interpret multiple x-ray images in order to reconstruct a cross-sectional image of any area of the body. The inventors of the procedure for CT scanning were awarded a Nobel Prize in 1979.

After the patient is placed in the CT scanner, an x-ray source rapidly rotates around it, taking hundreds of pictures. The pictures are electronically recorded and stored by a computer. The computer then integrates the data into cross-sectional "slices." The CT scanner can assess the composition of internal structures, which it is able to discriminate from fat, fluid, and gas. The scanner can show the shape and size of various organs and lesions and has the capability of detecting abnormal lesions as small as one or two millimeters in diameter.

Magnetic resonance imaging (MRI), unlike CT scanning (which uses x-rays), uses magnetic fields passing through the body to detect details of anatomy and physiology.

MRI equipment consists of a tunnel-like magnet that creates a magnetic field around the patient. This magnetic field causes the hydrogen atoms found in the body-water has two hydrogen atoms and one oxygen atom in the molecule-to line up. At the same time, a radio frequency signal is quickly transmitted to upset the uniformity of the formation. When the radio frequency signal is turned off, the hydrogen atoms return to their proper lineup, and a small current is generated. By detecting the speed and volume with which the atoms return, the computer can display a diagnostic image on a monitor.

MRI is noninvasive, and no pain or radiation is involved. The procedure takes from fifteen to forty-five minutes, depending on the number of views needed. Diagnostic x-rays rely on variations of density on film, and areas of soft tissue, for example, produce little or no shadow and are difficult to distinguish in any detail. MRI images, on the other hand, allow tumors, muscles, arteries, and vertebrae to be seen with great clarity.

Monitoring and providing electrical support to the heart constitute other useful noninvasive techniques. A healthy heart generates electrical impulses rhythmically and spontaneously; this activity is controlled by the sinoatrial (S-A) node, the heart's natural pacemaker. From there, the impulses pass through specialized conduction tissues in the atria and into the atrioventricular (A-V) node. Then the electrical impulses enter the ventricular conduction system, the bundle of His, and the right and left bundle branches. From the bundle branches, the impulses spread into the ventricles through the network of Purkinje fibers. The spread of electrical stimulation through the atria and the ventricles is known as depolarization. The standard electrocardiogram (ECG or EKG) records this activity from twelve different angles. The EKG records the heart's electrical activity and provides vital information concerning its rate, rhythm, and conduction system status. Detecting changes in the EKG can help to diagnose ventricular conduction problems and ventricular hypertrophy.

The signal-averaged electrocardiogram (SAECG) is another noninvasive procedure that is a promising diagnostic tool for many cardiac patients. Unlike the standard twelve-lead EKG, the SAECG can detect conduction abnormalities that often precede sustained ventricular tachycardia-which is second only to myocardial infarction (heart attack) as the leading cause of sudden death. The SAECG records the heart's electrical activity via six electrodes applied to the frontal and posterior chest walls. The SAECG can often pick up repolarization delays that occur when ischemic (damaged) tissue impedes the passage of electrical impulses through a portion of the myocardium, a condition that can lead to ventricular tachycardia.

A valuable weapon in the battle against sudden cardiac death is the temporary pacemaker, which provides support for the heart's electrical conduction system. Such devices can provide vital support when there is no time to prepare for an invasive procedure and are also used when invasive procedures are contraindicated.

Another method for diagnosing heart problems is echocardiography, a technique for recording echoes of ultrasonic waves when these waves are directed at areas of the heart. The principle is similar to that used in the sonar detection of submarines and other underwater objects. In this very simple and painless procedure, the patient lies on a table while a small, high-frequency generator (transducer) is moved across the chest. The instrument projects ultrasonic waves and receives the returning echoes. As the waves pass through the heart, their behavior differs, depending on whether there is any calcification present, whether there is a blood clot or any other mass in the cavity of the heart, whether certain heart chambers are enlarged, whether the valves within the heart open and close in the proper fashion, and whether any part of the heart is thicker than it should be.

Sonography, or ultrasound, imaging and the images produced are unique: patients can hear their blood flowing through the carotid arteries of the neck, and physicians can see a braintumor or watch a human fetus suck its thumb. This simple and inexpensive imaging technique has aided in the development of fetal medicine as a subspecialty. Sonography uses sound waves to look within the body by using a piezoelectric crystal to convert electric pulses into vibrations that penetrate the body. These sound waves are reflected back to the crystal, which reconverts them into electric signals. Many doctors foresee much growth in the use of ultrasound as a noninvasive procedure.

Uses and Complications

Historically, diagnostic x-rays have been used for the detection of metal objects, cavities in teeth, and broken bones. Films of various parts of the body, such as the abdomen, skull, and chest, have been taken ever since x-rays were first discovered in the late nineteenth century. Dentists and orthodontists use x-rays to check for jaw fractures, tooth misalignment, gum disease, tartar deposits, impacted teeth, and bone cancer. Chronic illnesses that can be detected by x-rays include arthritis, tuberculosis, osteoporosis, emphysema, ulcers, pneumonia, and urinary tract infections.

The CT scanner uses a series of narrow, pencil-like x-ray beams to scan the section of the body under investigation. CT scans allow the rapid diagnosis of brain abnormalities, cysts, tumors, and blood clots. Newly developed body scanners assist in the early detection of cancers and other diseases of the internal organs.

Magnetic resonance imaging has undergone an explosive growth in applications. In 1982, there were only six machines in operation. Hospitals often used a portable MRI device, which can be driven from place to place with a tractor-trailer truck. As the cost for MRI machines decreases, however, more hospitals are purchasing this equipment instead of sharing it.

The MRI machine is able to differentiate the brain's gray matter (nerve cells) from the brain's white matter (nerve fibers). Gray matter contains 87 percent water, and white matter contains 72 percent water. Thus, since MRI detects the protons in the hydrogen in water, a great difference in contrast between the two types of brain material is seen on the resulting scan. MRI is also useful in detecting and monitoring the progression of multiple sclerosis because the fatty tissue that normally exists around nerve fibers deteriorates, and these abnormal, fat-free areas can be clearly imaged.

MRI research seeks ways of analyzing the numerous chemical elements found in the body and aids in the study, diagnosis, treatment, and cure of a host of human diseases.

EKGs are useful in the detection of irregularities in the heart's electrical conduction system. This technology can also help in the diagnosis of ventricular hypertrophy, pulmonary emboli, and intraventricular conduction problems.

Echocardiograms, based on sound waves, are used to detect infarcts (areas of necrosis, or tissue death), valve closure between heart chambers, and abnormal thickening of myocardial muscle. Sonography is perhaps best known for its contribution to diagnostic medicine in the study of human fetal development. Determining the age of a developing embryo is now standard procedure, and clear images can be obtained at five weeks of gestation, when the embryo is only five millimeters long. Fetal weight can be determined by volume, and fetal anatomy can also be studied. Congenital heart defects can be spotted very early, and neural brain defects can be discovered as well.

The great advantage of ultrasound is that it emits no ionizing radiation and thus can be used on pregnant women without danger to the fetus. Ultrasound can also detect gallstones, kidney stones, and tumors and can monitor blood flow. Its applications have grown exponentially since its discovery.

Noninvasive tests such as x-rays, MRI, and CT scanning have become a crucial part of the detection and treatment of cancer. They are vital in determining the source and extent of the malignancy.

Mammography is a subset of x-ray imaging that is useful in detecting breast cancer. The equipment used in mammography is designed to image breast tissue, which is usually soft and of uniform density. Very small changes in density can be identified in fine detail, including small areas of calcification. Radiation doses must also be kept to a minimum. The film interpretation of mammograms is difficult, but early detection of breast cancer is often possible.

In the United States, the Public Health Service, in a memo dated June 1, 1993, delegated authority for implementing the Mammography Quality Standards Act (MQSA) of 1992 to the Food and Drug Administration (FDA). The MQSA is intended to ensure that mammography is reliable and safe. The act makes it unlawful for any facility to provide services unless it is accredited by an approved private nonprofit or state body and it has received federal certification indicating that it meets standards for quality. Each facility must also pass an annual inspection conducted by approved federal personnel. The law was enacted in response to the need for safe, early detection of breast cancer. Mammography is the most effective technique for early detection of this type of cancer.

Given a choice, most persons would prefer a noninvasive diagnostic tool. The earliest used diagnostic tool was the x-ray. X-rays were discovered in 1895 by a German professor named Wilhelm Conrad Röntgen. The first x-rays were produced in a Crookes tube, a pear-shaped glass tube in which two electrodes, the cathode (negative electrode) and anode (positive electrode), were placed at right angles to each other. The tube was then evacuated of gas. In Röntgen's first experiment, the cathode was "excited" with an electrical current, producing a beam of cathode rays, or electrons. These electrons were directed across the tube from the cathode and struck the glass, causing it to glow and, at the same time, producing x-rays, which excited a fluorescent screen. In a modern x-ray tube, the cathode ray strikes a target in the anode rather than the glass. Modern equipment also uses high-energy electricity in order to energize the tube at the high voltages necessary for producing x-rays.

Radiology has come far. From a medical discipline with a limited but vital function (that of aiding diagnosis), it has become interventional. It is a field that has moved into therapy-repairing a growing variety of abnormalities, averting surgery, and sometimes achieving results beyond the reach of surgery.

In addition to the simple x-ray, physicians now have more powerful diagnostic devices: MRI, CT scanning, and sonography. Cardiac conditions and abnormalities are quite easily analyzed via the ECG or echocardiogram. Where once the diagnosis of gallstones required a two-day x-ray test and twelve grams of diarrhea-causing pills, now ultrasound allows a diagnosis to be made painlessly and noninvasively, in ten to fifteen minutes.

The computer has been the core in the revolution in imaging. As more information becomes available and the density of information grows exponentially, larger and faster computers have been developed to assimilate this information. Computer visualization both interprets data and generates images from data in order to provide new insight into disease states through visual methods. Visualization and computation promise to play a key role in diagnostic medicine.

—*Jane A. Slezak, Ph.D.*

See also Computed tomography (CT) scanning; Diagnosis; Echocardiography; Electrocardiography (ECG or EKG); Electroencephalography (EEG); Imaging and radiology; Magnetic resonance imaging (MRI); Mammography; Neuroimaging; Physical examination; Prognosis; Radiation therapy; Screening; Single photon emission computed tomography (SPECT); Ultrasonography; Urinalysis.

For Further Information:

A.D.A.M. Medical Encyclopedia. "Imaging and Radiology." *MedlinePlus*, March 22, 2012.

Chopra, Sanjiv. *The Liver Book: A Comprehensive Guide to Diagnosis, Treatment, and Recovery.* New York: Simon & Schuster, 2002.

Crawford, Michael, ed. *Current Diagnosis and Treatment-Cardiology.* 3d ed. New York: McGraw-Hill Medical, 2009.

Galton, Lawrence. *Med Tech.* New York: Harper & Row, 1985.

Griffith, H. Winter. *Complete Guide to Symptoms, Illness, and Surgery.* Revised and updated by Stephen Moore and Kenneth Yoder. 5th ed. New York: Perigee, 2006.

MedlinePlus. "Diagnostic Imaging." *MedlinePlus*, May 24, 2013.

Merva, Jean. "SAECG: A Closer Look at the Heart." *RN* 56 (May, 1993): 51-53.

National Institute of Biomedical Imaging and Bioengineering. "Image-Guided Interventions." *National Institutes of Health*, March 29, 2013.

Pagana, Kathleen Deska, and Timothy J. Pagana. *Mosby's Diagnostic and Laboratory Test Reference.* 9th ed. St. Louis, Mo.: Mosby/Elsevier, 2009.

Sochurek, Howard. *Medicine's New Vision.* Easton, Pa.: Mack, 1988.

Solomon, Jacqueline. "Take the EKG One Step Further." *RN* 55 (May, 1992): 56-60.

Wolbarst, Anthony Brinton. *Looking Within: How X-Ray, CT, MRI, Ultrasound, and Other Medical Images Are Created.* Berkeley: University of California Press, 1999.

Non-steroidal anti-inflammatory drugs (NSAIDs)

Treatment/Pharmaceutical

Anatomy or system affected: Any area of inflammation or pain throughout the body

Specialties and related fields: Primary care, internal medicine, family medicine, orthopedic surgery, rheumatology, nurse practitioner, physician assistant

Definition: Nonsteroidal anti-inflammatory drugs (NSAIDs) are medications that are used to control pain and inflammation in the body.

Key terms:

arachidonic acid: an omega-6 unsaturated fatty acid the body requires to function properly; when broken down in the body, prostaglandins are produced

COX-1 AND COX-2: cyclooxygenase 1 and 2 (COX-1 and COX-2) are important enzymes in the function of the human body; they both convert arachidonic acid to prostaglandins, and are implicated in pain, inflammation, cell multiplication, and other key biologic responses

NSAIDs: nonsteroidal anti-inflammatory drugs (NSAIDs) are medications that are used to control pain and inflammation in the body

osteoarthritis: a progressive disorder of the joints caused by gradual loss of cartilage that can result in the development of bone spurs and cysts at the margins of joints

prostaglandins: one of a number of hormone-like substances that participate in a wide range of body functions such as the contraction and relaxation of smooth muscle, the dilation and constriction of blood vessels, control of blood pressure, and modulation of inflammation

Reye syndrome: a rare but serious disease that most often affects children ages 6 to 12 years old; can cause brain swelling and liver damage; may be related to using aspirin to treat viral infections

Indications

Enzymes known as COX-1 and COX-2 are produced by cells in the body and are responsible for the creation of substances called prostaglandins from a fatty acid called arachidonic acid. Arachidonic acid is generated by the degradation of membrane phospholipids by enzymes called phospholipases A_2, which are activated when cells are damaged in any way. Prostaglandins are responsible for many functions in the body and can foster inflammation, pain, and fever. Nonsteroidal anti-inflammatory drugs (NSAIDs) are used to inhibit the activity of the COX-1 AND COX-2 enzymes, which cause the pain and inflammation.

The most well-known NSAIDs are aspirin, ibuprofen, and naproxen, but there are many other NSAIDs including the following generic drugs: ketoprofen, sulindac, fenoprofen, diclofenac, flurbiprofen, ketorolac, piroxicam, indomethacin, mefenamic acid, meloxicam, nabumetone, oxaprozin, famotidine, meclofenamate, tolmetin, and salsalate.

NSAIDs are used to reduce fever and inflammation and for pain control. Currently, they are among the most commonly prescribed medications used for inflammation and pain control, particularly for osteoarthritis, joint pain, or muscle strain.

NSAIDs are commonly indicated for use in the following conditions: joint pain and inflammation from osteoarthritis and rheumatoid arthritis; gout (build-up of uric acid causing pain in the extremities); headaches; pain after surgery; pain from an injury such as sprains or strained muscles; and pain from kidney stones.

Many NSAIDs also have an anti-clotting effect. Preventing clotting can have an effect on reducing strokes and other cardiovascular issues, however, NSAIDs are not generally taken to prevent cardiovascular disease. A common side effect of NSAIDs is high blood pressure (hypertension), which offsets the anti-platelet action.

However, low-dose aspirin (81 mg.) is often recommended to patients who have already been diagnosed with cardiovascular disease to reduce the chances of heart attack and stroke. Many people also take low-dose aspirin as a preventative measure, but researchers are still unsure whether or not it is helpful for a healthy individual to take low-dose aspirin as a preventative treatment against heart attack or stroke.

Uses and Complications

Although NSAIDs are generally safe, it is reported that as many as 30-35% of individuals who take NSAIDs experience some side effects or adverse drug reactions. Various NSAIDs may affect individuals differently.

The most common reported side effects of NSAIDs are gastrointestinal problems. Usually, the reactions are mild, but sometimes they can result in more serious problems. The following gastrointestinal side effects may include nausea, indigestion, excess gas, vomiting, stomach ulcers or intestinal bleeding.

To lessen the chance of gastrointestinal side effects, many over-the-counter NSAIDs are produced with a special coating called an enteric coating, but to date there is no evidence that coating the medication is effective in reducing the possibility of digestive side effects.

NSAIDs carry an increased risk of cardiovascular disease. Some research implies that the occurrence of serious cardiovascular disease such as heart attacks and stroke can be twice as likely in people using NSAIDs, even if there is no pre-existing heart disease.

As mentioned in the Indications section, low-dose aspirin is an exception to this adverse reaction, and it is often used to reduce the risk of further heart attack and stroke among those who have a pre-existing condition.

Kidney problems can also be a side effect of using NSAIDs, especially when these drugs are combined with use of other drugs such as those used to treat high blood pressure. Sometimes NSAIDs can also affect the kidneys' filtering ability, leading to water retention and high blood pressure. Recent studies have suggested that routine increased use of NSAIDs by athletes, for example, ultrarunners, to decrease pain from muscle soreness or stiffness and pain, may lead to increasing the chance of them developing acute kidney injury.

If an individual using NSAIDs experiences pain in the kidneys, a reduction in the amount of urine produced, or changes in the urine color, etc., they should let their healthcare provider know immediately.

The use of NSAIDs has been linked to erectile dysfunction, but it is not understood exactly why this is the case. Men—particularly middle-aged men—regularly taking NSAIDs are up to 2.4 times more likely to suffer from erectile dysfunction.

Less common side effects of taking NSAIDs may also include an allergic skin reaction to sunlight (rash).

A positive effect of NSAIDs, however, is its use in colon cancer increased survival. A recent study at Fred Hutchinson Cancer Research Center in Seattle, Washington, concluded that the use of NSAIDs improved survival for certain colorectal cancer patients. In the study, NSAIDs were associated with about a 25 percent reduction in all-cause mortality. However, the benefit versus increased risk of cardiovascular issues needs to still be determined.

Aspirin and other NSAIDs are also thought to prevent the growth of intestinal polyps that can precede the development of colorectal cancer. Aspirin and other NSAIDs activate cell suicide pathways found in intestinal stem cells that can carry a certain mutated and dysfunctional gene known as APC and make the cells dysfunctional. NSAIDs activate the early auto-destruction of cells that could lead to precancerous polyps and tumors, according to the 2014 study at the Pittsburgh Cancer Institute (UPCI) and the School of Medicine.

Precautions

NSAIDs are not recommend to be taken during pregnancy, especially the last trimester of pregnancy. These drugs can affect the infant's developing heart and kidneys, and may also contribute to premature birth and miscarriage. Also, NSAIDs should not be used in individuals with kidney disease, congestive heart failure, or liver cirrhosis to prevent the kidneys from failing (acute renal failure).

NSAIDs should not be given to an individual who is taking an anti-clotting medication (other than low-dose aspirin if prescribed by their healthcare provider) since this may increase the risk of bleeding.

The use of aspirin for viral infections in children or teens should not be given because of the risk of Reye's syndrome.

NSAIDs are not recommended for individuals with uncontrolled diabetes, active congestive heart failure, nasal polyps, or in phenylketonuria (an inherited disorder that prevents the disposal of the amino acid phenylalanine), ulcerative colitis, and gastroesophageal reflux disease (GERD).

It is important for an individual to let their healthcare provider about any other medications that they are taking since some drug combinations should not be used with NSAIDs. When taken with some kidney and blood pressure medications, for example, NSAIDs may cause those medications to work less effectively.

The use of NSAIDs should always be discussed with an individual's healthcare provider. Usually, treatment with higher doses of NSAIDs is used to control pain and reduce inflammation, e.g., in osteoarthritis, a sprain, etc. A prescription from a healthcare provider is needed for the higher doses to be taken at regular intervals throughout the day as prescribed. For temporary conditions to relieve pain, like back pain for example, over-the-counter doses of NSAIDs are adequate.

The Federal Drug Administration (FDA) suggests individuals obtain medical attention right away if any of the following occur: chest pain, shortness of breath, trouble breathing, slurred speech, or weakness on one side or part of the body.

—*Joanne R. Gambosi, BSN, MA*

See also: Anti-inflammatory medications; Aspirin; Over-the-counter pain medications; Treatments for arthritis

For Further Information:

Doheny K. "FDA strengthens warnings on NSAIDs and heart risk." *WebMD*, July 2015.

Fred Hutchinson Cancer Research Center. "NSAIDs improve survival for certain colorectal cancer patients, study shows." *ScienceDaily*, 15 June 2017.

University of Pittsburgh Schools of the Health Sciences. "NSAIDs prevent colon cancer by inducing death of intestinal stem cells that have mutation." *ScienceDaily*, 3 November 2014.

Singh, M. "Study reveals harmful effects on kidney of Ibuprofen." *The Stanford Daily*, July 20, 2017.

U.S. Food and Drug Administration. "Health Hints: Use Caution with Pain Relievers." Accessed 4/19/2016.

Noroviruses

Disease/Disorder

Also known as: Norwalk-like viruses

Anatomy or system affected: Gastrointestinal system, immune system

Specialties and related fields: Gastroenterology, immunology, virology

Definition: A family of viruses that cause acute gastroenteritis.

Key terms:

gastroenteritis: an inflammation of the stomach and large intestines

Norwalk virus: a virus named for a 1968 outbreak of acute gastroenteritis in Norwalk, Ohio; it is the prototype strain for a group of single-stranded ribonucleic acid (RNA) viruses now called noroviruses

Causes and Symptoms

Noroviruses, also known as Norwalk-like viruses (NLV), are members of the family Caliciviridae and are the leading cause of nonbacterial acute gastroenteritis outbreaks in the United States. Noroviruses are suspected of causing over twenty million cases of acute gastroenteritis annually with an estimated 570-800 deaths, 56,000-71,000 hospitalizations, 400,000 emergency department visits, and 1.7-1.9

Information on Noroviruses

Causes: Viral infection transmitted through contaminated food or water, fecal-hand-oral contamination, direct person-to-person contact, or direct contact with contaminated surface

Symptoms: Sudden onset of nausea, vomiting, abdominal cramps, and watery diarrhea; may also include headache, fever, chills, and muscle pain

Duration: Twelve to sixty hours

Treatments: None; prevention through food safety measures (proper handing) and good hygiene (frequent hand-washing, germicides)

million outpatient visits each year. Often, norovirus-caused gastroenteritis is thought to be "stomach flu," but it is not related to influenza, a respiratory illness caused by the influenza virus. Norovirus infection is also commonly referred to as "food poisoning," although there are other numerous causes of food poisoning. Noroviruses are not related to bacteria or parasites that can cause gastroenteritis.

The illness associated with a norovirus infection lasts twelve to sixty hours and is characterized by a sudden onset of nausea, vomiting, abdominal cramps, and watery diarrhea. Vomiting is more prevalent among children, whereas adults tend to experience diarrhea. Additional symptoms, including headache, fever, chills, and myalgia (muscle pain), are also reported. Although NLV causes a self-limited acute gastroenteritis, the elderly, children, and those with severe underlying medical conditions are at increased risk for complications as a result of volume depletion, dehydration, and electrolyte disturbances. Although rare, severe dehydration caused by NLV gastroenteritis can be fatal. Hospitalization of otherwise healthy adults infected with NLV is rare.

The incubation period after exposure to a norovirus is 24 to 48 hours. The virus is transmitted by a fecal-hand-oral contamination route, directly from person to person, through contaminated food or water, or by direct contact with a contaminated surface. One of the main transmission sources is the diapers of infants with diarrhea. Aerosolized vomit has also been implicated as a transmission mode. Noroviruses are very contagious (less than 100 virus particles can establish an infection), and can spread rapidly throughout closely populated environments. Schools, hospitals, restaurants, amusement parks, fairgrounds, summer camps, and cruise ships are especially susceptible to mass infections. However, any place that food or drink is served, including the home environment, is susceptible to NLV infection. Because of high rates of infection and the persistence of noroviruses in the environment, transmission is difficult to control through routine sanitary procedures. People infected with NLV are contagious from the moment that they begin feeling symptoms to at least three days after recovery. In some cases, infected individuals have been contagious up to two weeks after recovery. Patients with compromised immune systems can shed viruses for months

following infection.

Most people infected with noroviruses recover in twenty-four to forty-eight hours, with no long-term health effects related to their infection. No evidence suggests that infected persons can become long-term carriers of the virus, but it is essential for those recovering from an infection to use good hand-washing and other hygienic practices.

Treatment and Therapy

Outbreaks of norovirus gastroenteritis can occur in multiple settings. According to the Centers for Disease Control and Prevention, between 2010 and 2011, of the 1,518 confirmed norovirus outbreaks in the United States, a total of 14 percent was contracted in restaurants or at catered events; 63 percent in nursing homes, residential institutions, and hospitals; 4 percent in schools and day care centers; 4 percent in vacation settings, including camps and cruise ships; and the rest in other settings. While person-to-person spread of the disease extends NLV outbreaks, the initial event is often the contamination of a common source such as a surface or food or water. Thus, efforts to prevent an initial contamination and subsequent transmission help to prevent the occurrence and spread of norovirus gastroenteritis outbreaks.

Food contamination by food handlers is the most frequent transmission agent. Any food item has the potential to be infected with norovirus through fecal contamination, and certain foods show a higher concentration of infections. Shellfish tend to concentrate NLVs in their tissues if they live in contaminated waters in which fecal waste is either dumped overboard from ships or released from shoreline sewage systems. Ready-to-eat foods that require handling but no subsequent cooking also pose a risk. Noroviruses are relatively resistant to environmental change and can survive temperatures as high as 140 degrees Fahrenheit (60 degrees Celsius) and chlorine levels of up to 10 parts per million, which far exceeds chlorine levels in public water systems. NLV infection can occur from the ingestion of contaminated water, including municipal water, well water, stream water, commercial ice, lake water, and swimming pools.

Noroviruses can be spread person-to-person by direct fecal-oral contact and airborne transmission. This is the most effective way that the virus spreads in populations in close proximity, such as people in nursing homes and on cruise ships. The most effective means of stopping the transmission of NLV is by frequent hand-washing with soap and hot water. Unfortunately, noroviruses are quite stable in the environment and resist temperatures up to 60°C (140°F), and freezing, and disinfection with alcohol or chlorine. Therefore, it is recommended that all surfaces be lathered with soap vigorously for ten seconds, then rinsed thoroughly under moving water. A mask should be worn by anyone cleaning areas contaminated with feces or vomitus. Soiled linen and clothes should be handled carefully and with a minimum of agitation. Soiled surfaces should be cleaned with a germicidal product containing at least 10 percent bleach.

Neither a specific antiviral treatment nor a vaccine has

been developed for noroviruses, although the development of a vaccine is underway. NLV infection cannot be treated with antibiotics because it is not caused by bacteria. Because there are many different strains of norovirus, developing an individual long-lasting immunity is difficult. Consequently, NLV infections can recur throughout a person's lifetime. Because of genetic factors, some people are more likely than others to be infected and to develop severe symptoms.

—Randall L. Milstein, PhD;
updated by Michael A. Buratovich, PhD

See also: Childhood infectious diseases; Common cold; Diarrhea and dysentery; Epidemics and pandemics; Epidemiology; Fever; Food poisoning; Gastroenteritis; Gastroenterology; Gastroenterology, pediatric; Gastrointestinal disorders; Influenza; Nausea and vomiting; Rotavirus; Viral infections.

For Further Information:

Barclay, Leslie, et al. "Notes from the Field: Emergence of New Norovirus Strain GII.4 Sydney-United States." *Morbidity and Mortality Weekly Report* 62,03. (January 25, 2013): 55.

Centers for Disease Control and Prevention. "Outbreaks of Gastroenteritis Associated with Noroviruses on Cruise Ships-United States, 2002." *Morbidity and Mortality Weekly Report* 51 (2002): 1112-1115.

"'Cruise Ship Virus' Also Sickens One Million US Kids Yearly." *MedlinePlus/HealthDay*, March 20, 2013.

Dolan, Raphael. "Noroviruses-Challenges to Control." *New England Journal of Medicine* 357. (2007): 1072-1073.

Fankhauser, R. L., S. S. Monroe, J. S. Noel, et al. "Epidemiologic and Molecular Trends of 'Norwalk-Like Viruses" Associated with Outbreaks of Gastroenteritis in the United States." *Journal of Infectious Disease* 186. (2002): 1-7.

Hall, Aron J. et al. "Updated Norovirus Outbreak Management and Disease Prevention Guidelines." *Morbidity and Mortality Weekly Report* 60, RR03. (March 4, 2011): 1-15.

Meyers, H. "Norwalk Virus, Noroviruses, and Viral Gastroenteritis." *Public Health Bulletin, County of Orange Health Care Agency* 52, 2. (2003): 1-8.

"Norovirus Infection." *Mayo Clinic*, April 5, 2011. "Norovirus is Now the Leading Cause of Severe Gastroenteritis in US Children." *Centers for Disease Control and Prevention*, March 21, 2013.

Umesh, D. P., E. S.Wuiroz, A.W. Mounts, et al. "Norwalk-Like Viruses: Public Health Consequences and Outbreak Management." *Morbidity and Mortality Weekly Report* 50, RR-9. (2001): 1-13.

Nuclear medicine

Specialty

Anatomy or system affected: Bones, brain, gallbladder, glands, kidneys, heart, and musculoskeletal system

Specialties and related fields: Cardiology, endocrinology, internal medicine, nephrology, neurology, oncology, radiology, urology

Definition: The field of medicine that employs radioactivity for both diagnostic and therapeutic purposes; the former involves imaging techniques, while the latter uses large amounts of radioactive material to destroy cells.

Key terms:

cathode-ray tube: a display device used for the presentation of nuclear medicine data; it displays images in real time

collimator: a device used for restricting and directing gamma rays by passing them through a grid made of metal, which absorbs the rays

gamma radiation: electromagnetic radiation of a short wavelength that is emitted by the nucleus of a radionuclide during radioactive decay

half-life: a unique characteristic of a radionuclide defined by the time during which its initial activity is reduced by one-half; this period varies among radionucleotides from less than one-millionth of a second to millions of years

pharmacological stresstesting: a procedure wherein a pharmacological agent is administered to a patient to increase blood flow to the heart, thereby enabling coronary artery disease, if present, to manifest itself

radionuclide: a species of atom (of natural or artificial origin) that exhibits radioactivity

radiopharmaceutical: a sterile, radioactively tagged compound that is administered to a patient for diagnostic or therapeutic purposes

scintillation: the production of flashes emitted by luminescent substances when excited by high-energy radiation

tomography: the term that describes all types of body-section imaging techniques, in which a visual representation is restricted to a specified section or "cut" of tissue within an organ

tracer: a radioactive substance introduced into the body, the progress of which may be followed by means of an external radioactivity detector; it must not affect the process that it is used to measure

Science and Profession

Nuclear medicine is the branch of medicine that uses radioactive substances in the diagnosis and treatment of diseases. A discussion of such technology requires an understanding of the nature of radioactivity and the tools employed by specialists in this medical field.

Radioactivity is the spontaneous emission of particles from the nucleus of an atom. Several kinds of emissions are possible. Gamma-ray emission is the type with which nuclear medicine imaging is concerned. The activity of radionuclides is measured in terms of the number of atoms disintegrating per unit time. The basic unit of measurement is the curie. Radiopharmaceuticals that are administered are in the microcurie or millicurie range of activity. Most radionuclides used in nuclear medicine are produced from accelerators, reactors, or generators. Accelerators are devices that accelerate charged particles (ions) to bombard a target. Cyclotron-produced radionuclides that are used frequently in nuclear medicine include gallium 67, thallium 201, and indium 111. The core of a nuclear reactor consists of material undergoing nuclear fission. Nuclides of interest in nuclear medicine that are formed from reactors include molybdenum 99, iodine 131, and xenon 133.

In generator systems, a "parent" isotope decays spontaneously to a "daughter" isotope in which the half-life of the parent is longer than that of the daughter. The parent is used to generate a continuous supply of the relatively short-lived daughter radionuclides and is therefore called a generator. The most commonly used generator system is molybdenum 99 (with a half-life of sixty-seven hours) and technetium 99m (with a half-life of six hours). The daughter, technetium 99m, is the most widely used radioisotope in nuclear medicine. It is obtained from the generator in a physiologic sodium chloride solution as the pertechnetate ion. It can be used alone to image the thyroid, salivary glands, or gastric mucosa, or it can be labeled to a wide variety of complexes that are picked up physiologically by various organ systems.

The scintillation camera, or Anger camera (named for its inventor, Hal O. Anger), is the most commonly used static imaging device in nuclear medicine. The scintillation camera produces a picture on a cathode-ray tube of the distribution of an administered radionuclide within the target organ of a patient. It uses the gamma rays emitted by the nuclide and a collimator to create the image as a series of light flashes on a disk-shaped sodium iodide crystal. The system determines the location of each scintillation and then produces a finely focused dot of light on the face of the cathode-ray tube in a corresponding position. The complete picture is then produced on photographic film. The camera normally contains two parts, the head and the computer console. The head serves as the gamma-ray detector. It absorbs incoming gamma rays and generates electrical signals that correspond to the positions where the absorptions took place. These signals are sent to a computer to be processed and to produce a picture that can be displayed on film or stored on disk for video display.

The collimator normally consists of a large piece of lead with many small holes in it. There are many types of collimators; the most common being parallel-hole types. The holes are of equal, constant cross section, and their axes form a set of closely spaced, vertical, parallel lines. The materials between the holes are called septa. Once a radioisotope is injected or ingested, it travels to the target organ. Gamma-rays from the target organ are emitted in all directions. The collimator allows only those gamma rays traveling in a direction essentially parallel to the axis of its holes to pass through to the crystal. The crystal is made of sodium iodide, with a small amount of thallium impurity. The thallium is transparent and emits light photons whenever it absorbs a gamma ray. This action by the collimator causes the light flashes in the crystal to form an image of the nuclide distribution located below it. This image will preserve gray-scale information, since the number of gamma rays received by any given region of the crystal will be directly proportional to the amount of nuclide located directly below that region.

Single-photon emission computed tomography (SPECT) is a tomographic imaging technique employing scintillation cameras to display the information at a given depth in sharp focus, while blurring information above and below that depth. There are two distinct methods of SPECT, each based on the type of images produced. The first, longitudinal section tomography, provides images of planes parallel to the long axis of the body. The second method, transverse section tomography, is perpendicular to the long axis of the body. Transverse section tomography with a rotating gamma camera has received wide clinical acceptance, partly because of the information that it provides and its multiple-use capability, since these systems can perform routine planar imaging as well as SPECT imaging. In this system, the gamma camera is a device mounted to a gantry and capable of rotating 360 degrees around the patient. These systems must be interfaced with a computer. The orbit around the patient is circular, and from 32 to 180 equiangular images are acquired over a 360-degree arc. Image acquisition is by computer. The images are stored digitally, and image reconstruction is achieved by filtering each projection, with geometric correction for photon attenuation. Noise reduction is generally accomplished by the application of filters. The efficiency of rotating systems can be improved by incorporating additional detectors (most often two or three), which rotate around the patient. Virtually any organ in the body for which an appropriate radiopharmaceutical exists can be studied with SPECT techniques.

Positron emission tomography (PET) scanning utilizes positron-emitting radionuclides, such as carbon 11, nitrogen 13, oxygen 15, and fluorine 8 (a bioisosteric substitution for hydrogen), which are isotopes of elements that occur naturally in organic compounds. These tracers enter into the biochemical processes in the body so that blood flow; oxygen, glucose, and free fatty acid metabolism; amino acid transport; pH; and neuroreceptor densities can be measured. A positron is an antimatter electron. This positron-emitting radiopharmaceutical is distributed in a patient's system. As a positron is emitted, it travels several millimeters in tissue until it meets a free electron and annihilation occurs. Two gamma rays appear and are emitted 180 degrees apart from each other. A scintillation camera could be used to detect these gamma rays, but a collimator is not needed. Instead, the patient is surrounded by a ring of detectors. By electronically coupling opposing detectors to identify the pair of gamma rays simultaneously, the location where the annihilation event must have occurred (the coincidence) can be determined. The raw PET scan consists of a number of coincidence lines. Reconstruction could simply be the drawing of these lines as they would cross and superimpose wherever there is activity in the patient. In practice, the data set is reorganized into projections.

Diagnostic and Treatment Techniques

Nuclear medicine is widely used in the diagnosis and prognosis of coronary artery disease, especially in conjunction with either physical stress testing (treadmill or bicycle exercise) or pharmacological stress testing. The patient is instructed to exercise on the treadmill until his or her heart rate has significantly increased. At peak exercise, a radioisotope, usually thallium 201 or technetium 99m, is injected into a vein. Stress images are obtained. Because the injected tracer corresponds to the blood flow through the arteries that supply oxygen to the heart muscle, those vessels that have a blockage exhibit decreased flow, or decreased tracer delivered to that area of the heart. Rest images are also obtained. Rest and stress images are

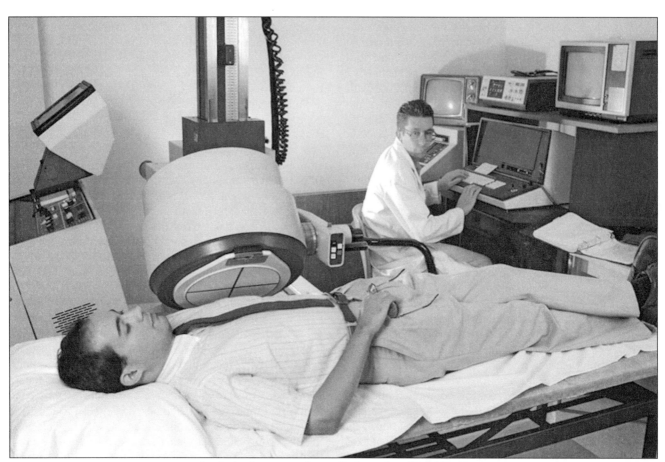

A patient undergoes a nuclear medical procedure. (Digital Stock)

compared, and differences in the intensity of the tracer, analyzed by a computer, help to identify blocked arteries and the extent of the blockage. This technique is also used in follow-up of patients who have undergone bypass surgery or angioplasty to determine if blockage has recurred. Nuclear cardiology is also used to measure the ejection fraction (the amount of blood ejected by the left ventricle to all parts of the body) and motion of the heart. Patients with cardiomyopathy, coronary artery disease, or congenital heart disease often have decreased function of the heart. Certain medications used in cancer therapy can also damage the heart muscle. These patients are followed closely to determine if they are developing toxicity from their drug therapy. In these studies, commonly called MUGA scans, a small portion of the patient's blood is extracted. A radioactive tracer is tagged to this blood, which is then reinjected. The gamma camera takes motion pictures of the beating heart and, through the aid of computers, calculates the ejection fraction.

Nuclear medicine can be very helpful in locating primary or metastatic tumors throughout the body, and it is unique in its ability to assess the viability of a known lesion and its response to radiation or chemotherapy. Breast cancer, lymphomas (especially low-grade), differentiated thyroid cancer, and most sarcomas (both bone and soft tissue) are tumors that will metabolize the appropriate injected radiopharmaceutical. The resulting images will show in-

creased localization in an active tumor but none in those masses that have been destroyed by treatment. By injecting a radioisotope that has been tagged by bone-seeking agents, doctors can view images of an entire skeleton. Multiple fractures, metastatic disease, osteomyelitis, osteoporosis, and Paget disease are but a few of the diseases that can be identified quickly and with minimal exposure of the patient to radiation.

Functional as well as anatomical information can be obtained by using nuclear medicine techniques to image the genitourinary tract, especially the kidneys. A perfusion study may be performed as the first phase of structural imaging. This study is done primarily to evaluate the vascularity (amount of blood vessels) of renal (kidney) masses. Cystic lesions and abscesses are usually avascular (having few or no blood vessels), and tumors are usually moderately or highly vascular. Uncommonly occurring arteriovenous (A-V) malformations show high vascularity. An evaluation of blood flow may also be important in patients who have received a kidney transplant. Anatomical renal imaging is performed to evaluate the position, size, and shape of the kidneys. Renal function studies have proven to be very sensitive in the diagnosis of both bilateral and unilateral kidney disease. By following specific tracers through the kidneys, doctors are able to evaluate the filtration by the glomeruli (capillary tufts) and the function of the tubules. Radionuclide cystography (imaging of the bladder), although not performed routinely, is extremely useful in diagnosing vesicoureteral reflux (urine reflux from the bladder back to the ureters), a relatively common problem in children.

Radionuclide imaging plays a significant role in the diagnosis of disease involving the gastrointestinal tract. Swallowing function, esophageal transit, gastroesophageal reflux, gastric emptying, gallbladder function, pulmonary aspiration of liver disease, and gastrointestinal bleeding can all be evaluated with nuclear medicine. The application of radioactive materials in the endocrine system provides historical benchmarks in the field of nuclear medicine with the use of radioiodine to assess the dynamic function of the thyroid gland. Radioiodine uptake testing is important and useful in the diagnosis of thyroid disease, specifically hyperthyroidism and hypothyroidism, thyroiditis, and goiters. Thyroid imaging is employed for the detection and functional evaluation of solitary or multiple thyroid nodules and the evaluation of aberrant thyroid tissue, metastases of thyroid cancer, and other tumors containing thyroid tissue. The therapeutic value of nuclear medicine is best demonstrated in its role in the treatment of Graves' disease, toxic adenoma, toxic multinodular goiter, and metastatic thyroid carcinoma. The purpose of the therapeutic application of radioiodine to hyperthyroidism (an overactive thyroid) is to control the disease and return the patient to a normal state. The accumulation and retention of radioiodine, with the subsequent radiation effects upon the thyroid cells, underlie the basic principle behind radionuclide therapy. The treatment of thyroid carcinoma with radioiodine is directed toward the control of metastatic foci and palliation of patients with thyroid carcinoma. Not all thyroid tumors localize radioiodine; therefore, care must be taken for proper patient selection by assuring a tumor's response to iodine.

Monoclonal antibody imaging has become important not only diagnostically but also therapeutically. Antibodies with perfect specificity for antigens of interest—in this case, malignancies—are produced. These antibodies are labeled with a large dose of radioactivity and injected into the patient. This "magic bullet" is then directed only to the antigen-producing areas. As in thyroid treatment, the radiation effect destroys only those cells to which the radioactivity is attached, leaving the noncancerous cells undamaged. Although this treatment is primarily a research protocol, the future role of radioactive monoclonal antibodies in the treatment of malignant disorders could be significant.

Clinical applications of PET scanning have focused on three areas: cardiology, oncology, and neurology/psychiatry. The principal clinical utility of PET in cardiology lies primarily in accurately differentiating infarcted, scarred tissue from myocardium, which is viable but not contracting because of a reduced blood supply. PET offers a noninvasive procedure to distinguish tissue viability, which allows more accurate patient selection for surgery and angioplasty than conventional approaches. In cancer cases, PET can determine cellular viability and the growth of tumor tissue and can directly measure the effectiveness of a given radiation or chemotherapy regimen on the metabolic process within the tumor. PET can differentiate tumor regrowth from radiation necrosis. Because of the unique ability of PET scanning to assess metabolic function, it can aid in the diagnosis of dementia and other psychoses as well as offer possible effective treatment of these disorders. PET is also helpful in detecting the origin of seizures in patients with complex epilepsy and can be used to locate the lesion prior to surgical intervention. PET can determine the viability of brain tissue after a stroke (one of the most common causes of death in the United States), permitting the clinician to select the most effective (and least invasive and expensive) form of treatment.

Nuclear imaging techniques are quite safe. Allergic reactions to isotopes are essentially nonexistent. In fact, the few that have been reported can be traced back to a contaminant in the injected dose. The radiation burden is far less than that of fluoroscopic radiographic examination and is equal to that of one chest x-ray, regardless of the picture produced.

Having said that, health concerns surround repeated CT scans of children. Epidemiological studies have established that children are significantly more sensitive to radiation than adults. Furthermore, children have a longer life expectancy than adults, which increases their opportunities to acquire and express radiation damage. Despite the advances in CT scanning technology that provide higher-quality images at lower doses of radiation, the settings of the CT machine must take into account the child's smaller size or the child will receive too much radiation. Also, multiple CT scans should be avoided in children when necessary.

Perspective and Prospects

Natural radioactivity was discovered in the late nineteenth century. The first medical success with a radioisotope was Robert Abbe's treatment of an exophthalmic goiter with radon in 1904. In 1934, the Joliot-Curies produced artificial radioisotopes, specifically phosphorus 32. In 1938, Glenn T. Seaborg synthesized iodine 131. Phosphorus 32 was used to treat chronic leukemia and iodine 131 to treat thyroid cancer. Both treatments fell victim to radiation hysteria fueled by the aftermath of World War II. For a decade, nuclear medicine was equated with the "atomic cocktail" and was used only sporadically as a therapeutic modality. In 1949, the first gamma camera was introduced by Benjamin Cassen. It was called a tap scanner because as it measured radioactivity, it would tap ink on a piece of paper. The intensity of the ink mark was directly proportional to the radioactivity that was being scanned. The first nuclear medicine image was that of a thyroid gland.

Although discovered in the late 1930s, the imaging properties of the short-lived technetium 99m were not understood until the early 1960s. Its six-hour half-life and its chemical properties were ideally suited to imaging with the scintillation camera newly introduced in 1965. From that time on, nuclear medicine grew in its role as a diagnostic tool, with technetium agents becoming the primary radiopharmaceuticals employed in the detection of disease.

With the addition of computers and array processors to the technology, tomographic imaging became increasingly useful in the localization and quantification of disease states. Improved body attenuation correction and computerized three dimensional imaging enable physicians to quantify the size and extent of abnormalities quite accurately. When one examines the relative role and costs of transmission computed tomography (CT) scanning versus SPECT, a number of factors must be kept in mind. On the side of advantage of SPECT are the low costs compared to CT scanning. Additionally, no contrast is required in the SPECT study, which lessens the chance of adverse patient reaction. CT scanning is still primarily an anatomic diagnostic tool, while SPECT, by employing physiological radiopharmaceuticals, demonstrates the functional features of organs. By repeated imaging during the course of treatment, minute changes in the physiologic biochemical process can be detected and appropriately addressed.

Because of the physiologic nature of nuclear medicine, the development of radiopharmaceuticals to detect other disease states is essential for further growth in this field. It is interesting that much activity in this area is now centered on the treatment of diseases, primarily malignant ones. As PET scanning becomes more frequently used, new positron radiopharmaceuticals will be introduced. Theoretically, all biochemical reactions in the body can be imaged, if the proper radiopharmaceutical is produced.

—Lynne T. Roy;
updated by Michael A. Buratovich, PhD

See also: Biophysics; Imaging and radiology; Invasive tests; Magnetic resonance imaging (MRI); Noninvasive tests; Nuclear radiology; Positron emission tomography (PET) scanning; Radiation therapy; Radiopharmaceuticals; Single photon emission computed tomography (SPECT).

For Further Information:

Brown, G. I. *Invisible Rays: A History of Radioactivity*. Stroud, England: Sutton, 2002.

Brucer, Marshall. *A Chronology of Nuclear Medicine, 1600-1989*. St. Louis, Mo.: Heritage, 1990.

Christian, Paul E., Donald Bernier, and James K. Langan, eds. *Nuclear Medicine and PET: Technology and Techniques*. 5th ed. St. Louis, Mo.: Mosby, 2004.

Gupta, Tapan K. *Radiation, Ionization, and Detection in Nuclear Medicine*. London: Springer, 2013.

Iskandrian, Ami E., and Mario S. Verani, eds. *Nuclear Cardiac Imaging: Principles and Applications*. 4th ed. New York: Oxford University Press, 2008.

Iturralde, Mario P. *Dictionary and Handbook of Nuclear Medicine and Clinical Imaging*. 2d ed. Boca Raton, FL: CRC Press, 2002.

National CancerInstitute, "Radiation Risks and Pediatric Computed Tomography (CT): A Guide for Health Care Providers." https://www.cancer.gov/about-cancer/causes-prevention/risk/radiation/pediatric-ct-scans, June 7, 2012.

Powsner, Rachel A., Matthew R. Palmer, and Edward R. Powsner. *Essentials of Nuclear Medicine Physics and Instrumentation*. 3d ed. Malden: Wiley-Blackwell, 2013.

Taylor, Andrew, David M. Schuster, and Naomi P. Alazraki. *A Clinician's Guide to Nuclear Medicine*. 2d ed. Reston, Va.: Society of Nuclear Medicine, 2006.

Ziessman, Harvey, Janis O'Malley, and James Thrall. *Nuclear Medicine: The Requisites*. 4th ed. Philadelphia: Elsevier, 2014.

Nuclear radiology

Procedure

Also known as: Nuclear medicine

Anatomy or system affected: Bones, brain, glands, kidneys, musculoskeletal system, nervous system

Specialties and related fields: Nuclear medicine, radiology

Definition: The use of radiopharmaceuticals for the diagnosis of disease and the assessment of organ function.

Key terms:

collimator: a device that directs photons into a crystal for their detection

gamma camera: a system composed of a cesium-iodide crystal, collimator, and computer which is used to detect radioactivity and create an image of its distribution

radioisotope: a radioactive atom

radiopharmaceutical: the combined form of a pharmaceutical labeled with a radioisotope

Indications and Procedures

Nuclear radiology, also known as nuclear medicine, is similar to conventionalradiology in that radiation is used to look inside the patient's body. Unlike conventional radiology, however, nuclear radiology looks not only at the anatomy of the patient but also at the functioning of the organ of interest. In conventional radiology (X-rays), the radiation or X-ray photon is produced by accelerating electrons, elemental negative charges, up to 50,000 to 125,000 volts and then ramming them into a metal anode. The physical act of stopping the electrons causes about 0.2 percent of the electrons to give off the accelerating energy as packets of energy called photons. This radiation is then directed by the lead housing of the X-ray tube toward the patient. The radiation transmitted through the patient is then recorded on either film or an image-intensifying tube.

Nuclear radiology differs from conventional radiology because there is no X-ray tube generating the radiation. The radiation comes from the pharmaceuticals injected into the patient. The source of the radiation is from a radioactive atom attached to a pharmaceutical (therapeutic drug). The physiological action and distribution of the pharmaceutical determines the diagnostic ability of the radiation given to the patient. The radiation can be emitted in any direction from the atom. The radiation, which travels in the direction of a piece of cesium-iodine crystal and through a collimator, or set of lead holes, is detected. The cesium-iodine crystal with the accompanying computer is known as a gamma camera.

The radioactive atom used in most nuclear radiology departments is an isotope of technetium. The isotope is in a semistable state known as a metastable state. When it becomes unstable and decays, it emits a single photon with the energy equivalent of an electron accelerated in a 140,000 volt potential (140 keV). After the emission of this single photon, the technetium atom is nonradioactive. The number of photons given off is dependent on the number of technetium atoms present in the metastable state. The time required for half of those present to emit the photons is called its half-life. The half-life of technetium is 6.02

hours. Because of its ease of production and reasonable half-life, technetium is used in many pharmaceuticals.

Specialty isotopes are also used. A gaseous isotope of xenon 133 is used for some lung studies. Xenon has a more complicated decay than does technetium. Xenon decays by the release of an energetic electron to unstable states of cesium 133. Cesium 133 gives off six gamma rays, with the predominant one being 80.9 keV. The half-life of xenon is 5.31 days. Xenon, being a noble gas, is chemically inert.

An isotope that can be used without being attached to a pharmaceutical is thallium 201. Thallium can be used in cardiac studies since it is readily taken up in the cardiac tissue. When thallium 201 decays, it becomes mercury 201. As mercury 201 becomes stable, it gives off high-energy X-rays and gamma rays with the predominant energy being between 68.8 and 80 keV. Iodine is another isotope that does not necessarily need to be attached to a pharmaceutical. The three isotopes of iodine used are iodine 123, 125, or 131. All give off gamma rays that can be detected, predominant being 159.1, 35.4, and 364.4 keV, respectively. Iodine 131 also gives off energetic electrons when it decays and as such is used when energetic electrons are desired for therapy purposes. The emission of energetic electrons can damage surrounding tissues. Iodine 123 and iodine 125 decay by absorbing an electron from the atom and only emit gamma rays. The use of one over the other depends on the cost, with iodine 123 more costly because of its thirteen-hour half-life. Iodine 125 has a half-life of 60.2 days. Iodine 131 has a half-life of 8.06 days. Other isotopes are used for specialty purposes, such as chromium 51, which can be used to attach to red blood cells. Chromium has a half-life of 27.7 days, with a predominant gamma emission of 320 keV.

A collimator is employed to force only the radiation from the front of the crystal through a known path to be detected. A collimator can consist of a piece of metal, usually lead, with one or multiple holes. The size and length of the hole determine the number of photons that will reach the crystal. The collimator works because it absorbs the photons that are not directed along the axis of the hole. The higher the energy of the photon being directed, the thicker the sides of the holes, known as septa, must be. The smaller the hole, the better the spatial resolution and ease of detecting small concentrations of the isotope of interest. The longer the hole, the better defined the path will be from the crystal face out through the hole to the patient. The limitations of the size and length are dictated by the need to detect a sufficient number of photons to give a diagnostic result. Unlike conventional radiology, in which the films are acquired in a short time (usually a fraction of a second), nuclear radiology can require fifteen to thirty minutes or more to acquire enough photons for a clinician to make a diagnostic determination.

Perspective and Prospects

The main structures that nuclear medicine studies are blood, brain, heart, thyroid gland, parathyroid glands, liver, kidneys, lungs, and bones. Blood studies use several different pharmaceuticals and radioisotopes depending on what is being measured. These studies involve the measurement of the blood volume or blood filtration. Brain studies use technetium with several different pharmaceuticals. Some pharmaceuticals will not pass the blood-brain barrier and can be used to detect bleeding in the cranial compartment. Others pass easily through the blood-brain barrier and can be used to detect sections of the brain that are either hyperactive or hypoactive. Heart studies are involved in determining the health of the cardiac muscles. By the use of thallium and new, additional technetium-labeled pharmaceuticals, the viability of heart tissue after a heart attack can be assessed, along with the thickness of cardiac structures such as the septa between the right and left ventricles. Other properties such as the filling and ejection fractions can be determined in this study. Thyroid studies look at the size and location and are easiest to use with iodine isotopes. A different thallium-labeled radiopharmaceutical can be used to look at the same properties of the parathyroid glands. Liver studies involve the determination of areas that are not functioning and that are revealed as voids on a scan. These pharmaceuticals use technetium as the labeled isotope. Kidney studies, which determine whether the kidneys are filtering the blood properly and in sufficient quantities, use technetium as the labeled isotope. Lung studies determine if all the lobes of the lungs are filling properly by using an inhalation isotope of xenon or aerosol compounds labeled with technetium. The health of the alveoli can be determined by the introduction of a radiopharmaceutical that congregates in the alveolar space. Bone studies are involved in determining whether new bone is being formed.

—*Anthony J. Wagner, Ph.D.*

See also Biophysics; Imaging and radiology; Invasive tests; Magnetic resonance imaging (MRI); Nuclear medicine; Positron emission tomography (PET) scanning; Radiation therapy; Radiopharmaceuticals.

For Further Information:

Bontrager, Kenneth, and John P. Lampignano. *Textbook of Radiographic Positioning and Related Anatomy.* 8th ed. St. Louis, Mo.: Mosby/Elsevier, 2013.

Cherry, Simon R., James A. Sorenson, and Michael E. Phelps. *Physics in Nuclear Medicine.* 4th ed. Philadelphia: W. B. Saunders, 2012.

"Children's (Pediatric) Nuclear Medicine." *RadiologyInfo.org.* American College of Radiology and Radiological Society of North America, Mar. 7, 2013.

"General Nuclear Medicine." *RadiologyInfo.org.* American College of Radiology and Radiological Society of North America, May 9, 2013.

Saha, Gopal B. *Physics and Radiobiology of Nuclear Medicine.* 4th ed. New York: Springer, 2013.

Sandler, Martin P., R. Edward Coleman, and James A. Patton, eds. *Diagnostic Nuclear Medicine.* 4th ed. Philadelphia: Lippincott Williams & Wilkins, 2003.

"What Is Nuclear Medicine?" *Society of Nuclear Medicine,* n.d.

Numbness and tingling

Disease/Disorder

Also known as: Paresthesias, dysesthesias, hypesthesias

Anatomy or system affected: Legs, muscles,

musculoskeletal system, nerves, nervous system, skin
Specialties and related fields: Neurology, physical therapy
Definition: Abnormalities of sensation that are attributable to nerve damage or disorders.

Symptoms. Patients commonly report various sensory aberrations that are often described as "pins and needles," tingling, prickling, burning of varying severity, or sensations resembling electric shock. The accepted term for these symptoms is *paresthesias* or *dysesthesias*. When severe enough to be painful, they can be referred to as painful paresthesias.

The other major sensory symptom is a reduction or loss of feeling in an area of skin. Most patients use the relatively unambiguous term *numbness*; however, the more formal medical term is *hypesthesia*. Paresthesias and hypesthesias are usually restricted to a part rather than all of the cutaneous territory of a damaged root or nerve.

The distribution of nonparesthetic pain is seldom as anatomically specific as the paresthesias themselves. Patients with carpal tunnel syndrome, for example, often have arm and shoulder pain that suggests compression of a cervical root rather than of the distal median nerve (a combined motor and sensory nerve). The paresthesias, by contrast, are usually localized to the tips of the fingers innervated by the median nerve. Similarly, in patients with cervical or lumbosacral radiculopathies (any diseased condition of the roots of spinal nerves), the distribution of pain in the upper or lower limbs often correlates poorly with the root involved. The paresthesias, however, are felt usually either along the entire area or, more commonly, in the distal part of the skin area innervated by the damaged root (the dermatome).

Examination. In attempting to localize the site of a lesion, the physician innervates major muscles from the spinal nerve roots (myotomes) through the plexuses, the individual peripheral nerves and their branches, and also the cutaneous areas supplied by each of these components of the peripheral nervous system. Traditionally, the site of the lesion can be deduced from which muscles and nerves are involved and from where the various branches of the peripheral nerves arise.

In motor examination, the muscles and tendon reflexes are examined first because weakness and reflex changes are often easier to elicit than are sensory signs. The muscles are first examined for atrophy. Since muscles become atrophic when denervated, the focal atrophy can sometimes identify accurately a nerve lesion. The lack of atrophy in a weak muscle either indicates an upper motor neuron lesion or raises the suspicion of spurious weakness. A systematic examination of individual muscles is then performed.

In sensory examination, the patient describes the area of sensory abnormality, which often tells as much as a formal examination. Testing light touch with the examiner's finger is frequently all that is required for confirmation. If this reveals no abnormality, retesting with a pin may disclose an area of sensory deficit. Pinpricks in normal and abnormal areas are compared.

It is important to examine the entire course of an affected nerve for bone, joint, or other abnormalities that may be

---

Information on Numbness and Tingling

Causes: May include neurological damage or disease, exposure to environmental toxins, infection, carpal tunnel syndrome, injury or trauma, metabolic disturbances

Symptoms: Prickling or burning sensations; pain and inflammation; impaired mobility

Duration: Acute to chronic

Treatments: Varies; may include physical therapy, use of ergonomic or corrective devices, surgery, drug therapy

---

causing the nerve damage. Local tenderness of the nerve and/or a positive Tinel's sign (paresthesias produced in the area of the nerve when the nerve is tapped or palpated) may also help to identify the site. Many normal persons experience mild tingling when nerves such as the ulnar at the elbow or the median at the wrist are tapped lightly, so this finding is significant only when the nerve is very sensitive to light percussion. Conversely, a badly damaged nerve may be totally insensitive to percussion or palpation.

Nerve conduction studies and the electromyographic examination of muscles evaluate the function of large-diameter, rapidly conducting motor and sensory nerve fibers. These two complementary techniques are valuable tools in the accurate assessment of focal peripheral neuropathies, helping in the localization of the nerve lesion and the assessment of its severity.

Diagnosis. Peripheral nerves causing sensory symptoms may be damaged anywhere along their course from the spinal cord to the muscles and skin that they innervate. The site of a focal neuropathy (the focus of neurologic disease) may therefore be in the nerve roots, the spinal nerves, the ventral or dorsal rami (branches), the plexuses (network of nerves), the major nerve trunks, or their individual branches. The character, site, mode of onset, spread, and temporal profile of sensory symptoms must be established and precipitating or relieving factors identified. These features-and the presence of any associated symptoms-help identify the origin of sensory disturbances, as do the physical signs. Sensory symptoms or signs may conform to the territory of individual peripheral nerves or nerve roots. Involvement of one side of the body, or of one limb in its entirety, suggests a central lesion. Distal involvement of all four extremities suggests polyneuropathy (several neurologic disorders), a cervical cord or brain-stem lesion, or, when symptoms are transient, a metabolic disturbance such as hyperventilation syndrome. Short-lived sensory complaints may be indicative of sensory seizures or cerebral ischemic phenomena (local and temporal deficiency of blood supply caused by obstruction of the circulation to a part) as well as metabolic disturbances. In patients with cord lesions, there may be a transverse sensory level. Dissociated sensory loss is characterized by the loss of some sensory modalities and the preservation of others. Such findings may be encountered in patients with either peripheral or central disease and must therefore be interpreted in the clinical context in which they are found.

The absence of sensory signs in patients with sensory symptoms does not mean that symptoms have a nonorganic basis. Symptoms are often troublesome before signs of sensory dysfunction have had time to develop.

—*Genevieve Slomski, Ph.D.*

See also Carpal tunnel syndrome; Nervous system; Neuralgia, neuritis, and neuropathy; Neurology; Neurology, pediatric; Pain; Sense organs; Spinal cord disorders; Spine, vertebrae, and disks.

For Further Information:

Heller, Jacob L. "Numbness and Tingling." *MedlinePlus*, April 3, 2011.

Herkowitz, Harry N., et al. *Rothman-Simeone The Spine.* 5th ed. Philadelphia: Saunders/Elsevier, 2006.

Mathers, Lawrence H., Jr. *The Peripheral Nervous System: Structure, Function, and Clinical Correlations.* Menlo Park, Calif.: Addison-Wesley, 1985.

National Institute of Neurological Disorders and Stroke. "NINDS Paresthesia Information Page." *National Institute of Neurological Disorders and Stroke*, May 6, 2010.

Rosenbaum, Richard B., and José L. Ochoa. *Carpal Tunnel Syndrome and Other Disorders of the Median Nerve.* 2d ed. Boston: Butterworth-Heinemann, 2002.

Senneff, John A. *Numb Toes and Other Woes: More on Peripheral Neuropathy.* San Antonio, Tex.: MedPress, 2001.

Sutton, Amy L., ed. *Back and Neck Disorders Sourcebook.* 2d ed. Detroit, Mich.: Omnigraphics, 2004.

Nursing

Specialty

Anatomy or system affected: All

Specialties and related fields: Critical care, emergency medicine, geriatrics and gerontology, neonatology, nutrition, oncology, occupational, primary care, informatics, midwifery, pediatrics, perinatology, preventive medicine, research, public health

Definition: A helping profession that focuses on the care of the sick and disabled and on the maintenance of the health and well-being of all individuals.

Key terms:

assessment: the systematic process of collecting, validating, and communicating patient data; these data will include information gathered from the patient's history and from physical examination and laboratory test results

healing: the restoration to a normal physical, mental, or spiritual condition

health: a condition in which all functions of the body, mind, and spirit are normally active

holistic: the philosophy that individuals function as complete units or integrated systems and are not understood merely through their parts

illness: the condition of being sick or diseased

nurture: the act or process of raising or promoting development and well-being

service: work done or duty performed for another or others

treatment: any specific procedure used for the cure or improvement of a disease or pathological condition

The Role of Nursing

It is difficult at times to distinguish nursing from medicine, since there are so many ways in which they interrelate. Whereas some people think that nursing began with Florence Nightingale (1820-1910), nursing is as old as medicine itself. Throughout history, there have been periods when the two fields functioned interdependently and times when they were practiced separately from each other. It seems likely that the role of the mother-nurse would have preceded the magician-priest or medicine-man. Even the seeds of medical knowledge were sown by the natural remedies used by the mother. Over the course of human history, the words *nurse* and *nursing* have had many meanings, and the connotations have changed as tribes became highly developed and sophisticated nations. The word *nurse* comes from the Latin *nutrix*, which means "nursing mother." The word *nursing* originated from the Latin *nutrire*, meaning "to nourish." The word *nurse* as a noun was first used in the English language in the thirteenth century, being spelled "norrice," then evolving to "nurice" or "nourice," and finally to the present "nurse." The word *nurse* as a verb meant to suckle and to nourish. The meanings of both the noun and the verb have expanded to include more and more functions related to the care of all human beings. In the sixteenth century, the meaning of the noun included "a person, but usually a woman, who waits upon or tends the sick." By the nineteenth century, the meaning of the verb included "the training of those who tend the sick and the carrying out of such duties under the supervision of a physician." With the origin of nursing as mother care came the idea that nursing was a woman's role. Suckling and nurturing were associated with maternal instincts. Ill or helpless children were also cared for by their mothers. The image of the nurse as a loving and caring mother remains popular. The true spirit of nursing, however, has no gender barriers. History has seen both men and women respond to the needs of the sick. The role of the nurse has certainly expanded from that of the mother in the home, nourishing infants and caring for young children. Care of the sick, infirm, helpless, elderly, and handicapped and the promotion of health have become vital aspects of nursing as a whole. In history, the role of nursing developed with the culture and society of a given age. Tribal women practiced nursing as they cared for the members of their own tribes. As tribes developed into civilizations, nursing began to be practiced outside the home. As cultures developed, nursing care became more complex, and qualities other than a nurturing instinct were needed to do the work of a nurse. Members of religious orders, primarily those composed of women, responded by devoting their lives to study, service, and self-sacrifice in caring for the needs of the sick. These individuals were among the educated people of their time, and they helped set the stage for nursing to become an art and a science.

It was not until the nineteenth century that the basis of nursing as a profession was established. The beliefs and examples of Florence Nightingale laid that foundation. Nightingale was born in Italy in 1820, but she grew up in England. Unlike many of the children of her time, she was educated by governesses and by her father. Against the wishes of her family, she trained to be a nurse at the age of

Types of Nursing

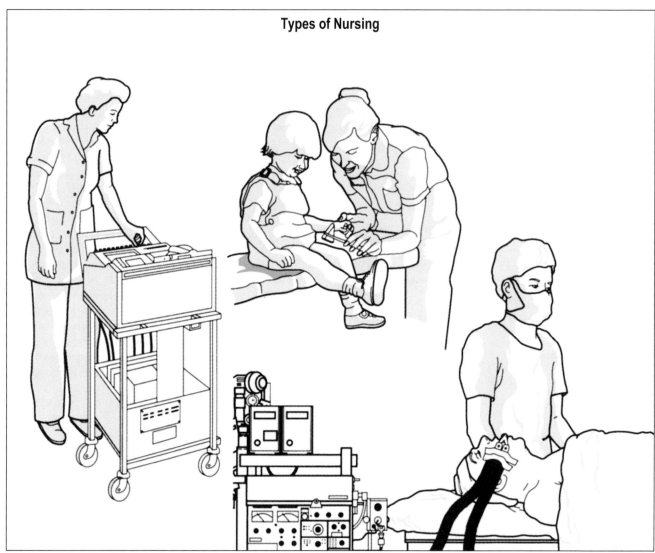

Nurses may become involved in many areas of health care, including the administration of diagnostic tests, the performance of physical examinations, and assistance during surgical procedures.

thirty-one. Amid enormous difficulties and prejudices, she organized and managed the nursing care for a military hospital in Turkey during the Crimean War. She returned to England after the war, where she established a school, the Nightingale Training School for Nurses, to train nurses. Again, she encountered great opposition, as nurses were considered little more than housemaids by the physicians of the time. Because of her efforts, the status of nurses was raised to a respected occupation, and the basis for professional nursing in general was established.

Nightingale's contributions are noteworthy. She recognized that nutrition is an important part of nursing care. She instituted occupational and recreational therapy for the sick and identified the personal needs of the patient and the role of the nurse in meeting those needs. Nightingale established standards for hospital management and a system of nursing education, making nursing a respected occupation for women. She recognized the two components of nursing: promoting health and treating illness. Nightingale believed that nursing is separate and distinct from medicine as

a profession.

Nightingale's methods and the response of nursing to American Civil War casualties in the 1860s pointed out the need for nursing education in the United States. Schools of nursing were established, based on the values of Nightingale, but they operated more like apprenticeships than educational programs. The schools were also controlled by hospital administrators and physicians.

In 1896, nurses in the United States banded together to seek standardization of educational programs, to establish laws to ensure the competency of nurses, and to promote the general welfare of nurses. The outcome of their efforts was the American Nurses Association. In 1900, the first nursing journal, the *American Journal of Nursing*, was founded. The effects of World War II also made clear the need to base schools of nursing on educational objectives. Many women had responded to the need for nurses during the war. A great expansion in medical knowledge and technology had taken place, and the roles of nurses were expanding as well. Nursing programs developed in colleges and universities and offered degrees in nursing to both women and men. While there were impressive changes in the expectations and styles with which nursing care has been delivered from ancient times into the twenty-first century, the role and function of the nurse have been and continue to be diverse. The nurse is a caregiver, providing care to patients based on knowledge and skill. Consideration is given to physical, emotional, psychological, socioeconomic, and spiritual needs. The role of the nurse-caregiver is holistic and integrated into all other roles that the nurse fulfills, thus maintaining and promoting health and well-being.

The nurse is a communicator. Using effective and therapeutic communication skills, the nurse strives to establish relationships to assist patients of all ages to manage and become responsible for their own health needs. In this way, the nurse is also a teacher who assists patients and families to meet their learning needs. Individualized teaching plans are developed and used to accomplish set goals.

The nurse is a leader. Based on the self-confidence gained from a nursing education and experience, the nurse is able to be assertive in meeting the needs of patients. The nurse facilitates change to improve care for patients, whether individually or in general. The nurse is also an advocate. Based on the belief that patients have a right to make their own decisions about health and life, the nurse strives to protect their human and legal rights in making those choices.

The nurse is a counselor. By effectively using communication skills, the nurse provides information, listens, facilitates problem-solving and decision-making abilities, and makes appropriate referrals for patients.

Finally, the nurse is a planner, a task that calls forth qualities far beyond nurturing and caring. In an age confronted with controversial topics such as abortion, organ transplants, the allocation of limited resources, and medical research, the role of nurses will continue to expand to meet these challenges in the spirit that allowed nursing to evolve and become a respected profession.

Science and Profession

While the nurse-mother of ancient times functioned within a very limited framework, the modern nurse has the choice of many careers within the nursing role. The knowledge explosion of the last century created many job specialties from which nurses can choose a career. The clinical nurse specialist is a nurse with experience, education, or an advanced degree in a specialized area of nursing. Some examples are enterostomal therapy, geriatrics, infection control, oncology, orthopedics, emergency room care, operating room care, intensive and coronary care, quality assurance, and community health. Nurses who function in such specialties carry out direct patient care; teach patients, families, and staff members; act as consultants; and sometimes conduct research to improve methods of care.

The nurse practitioner is a nurse with an advanced degree who is certified to work in a specific aspect of patient care. Nurse practitioners work in a variety of settings or in

independent practice. They perform health assessments and give primary care to their patients.

The nurse anesthetist is a nurse who has also successfully completed a course of study in anesthesia. Nurse anesthetists make preoperative visits and assess patients prior to surgery, administer and monitor anesthesia during surgery, and evaluate the postoperative condition of patients.

The nurse midwife is a nurse who has successfully completed a midwifery program. The nurse midwife provides prenatal care to expectant mothers, delivers babies, and provides postnatal care after the birth.

The nurse administrator functions at various levels of management in the health care field. Depending on the position held, advanced education may be in business or hospital administration. The administrator is directly responsible for the operation and management of resources and is indirectly responsible for the personnel who give patient care. The nurse educator is a nurse, with a master's or doctoral degree, who teaches or instructs in clinical or educational settings. This nurse can teach both theory and clinical skills.

The nurse researcher usually has an advanced degree and conducts special studies that involve the collection and evaluation of data in order to report on and promote the improvement of nursing care and education.

Duties and Procedures

Creativity and education are the keys to keeping pace with continued changes and progress in the nursing profession. Nurses are expected to play many roles, function in a variety of settings, and strive for excellence in the performance of their duties. A service must be provided that contributes to the health and well-being of people. The following examples of nursing-an operating room nurse and a home health nurse-provide a limited portrait of how nurses function and what roles they play in health care.

Operating room nurses function both directly and indirectly in patient care and render services in a number of ways. Operating room nurses, usually known as circulating nurses, briefly interview patients upon their arrival at the operating room. They accompany patients to specific surgery rooms and assist in preparing them for surgical procedures. They are responsible for seeing that surgeons correctly identify patients prior to anesthesia. They are also directly attentive to patients when anesthesia is first administered.

Circulating nurses perform the presurgical scrub, which is a cleansing of the skin with a specified solution for a given number of minutes. It is their overall responsibility to monitor aseptic (sterile) techniques in certain areas of the operating room and to deal with the situation immediately if aseptic techniques are broken. They count the surgical sponges with surgical technologists before the first incision is made, throughout the procedure as necessary, and again before the incision is closed. They secure needed items requested by surgical technologists, surgeons, or anesthesia personnel: medications, blood, additional sterile instruments, or more sponges. At times, they prepare and assist with the operation of equipment used for surgeries, such as lasers, insufflators (used for laparoscopic surgery), and blood saver and reinfuser machines. They arrange for the transportation of specimens to the laboratory. They may also be instrumental in sending communications to waiting family members when the surgery takes longer than anticipated. When the surgery is completed, they accompany patients to the recovery room with the anesthesia personnel.

Home health nurses, on the other hand, function in a very different manner. This type of nurse usually works for a private home health services agency, or as part of an outreach program for home services through a hospital. Referrals come to the agency or program via the physician, through the physician's office, by way of the social services department in a hospital, or by an individual requesting skilled services through the physician.

The following scenario is an example of a patient whom a home health nurse may be requested to see: a seventy-six year-old man who was hospitalized with a recent diagnosis of diabetes mellitus, for which he is now insulin-dependent. He also has an open wound on his right ankle. The number of days allowed for hospitalization for his diagnosis has expired, but he still needs help using a glucometer to take his blood sugar readings and assistance with drawing up his insulin. He still has questions about how to manage his diabetes, especially the dietary parameters. He is unable to manage the wound care on his right ankle. His wife is willing to assist him, but she has no knowledge about diabetes or wound care. The home health nurse performs the following assessments on the initial visit: general physical condition, the patient's level of knowledge and understanding and his ability to manage his diabetic condition, all medications used, and the patient's understanding of the actions, side effects, and interactions of these medications. An assessment is made of the home setting in general: the patient's safety, the support system, and any special needs, such as assistive devices. If services such as physical therapy, occupational therapy, or speech therapy are needed, the nurse makes these referrals. If the patient requires additional in-home services, a referral to a medical social worker is made. Wound care is performed, and the nurse will then set up a plan of care, with the patient's input, for follow-up visits. Guidelines requested by the physician, as well as approval needed by health insurance companies covering the cost for home health services, will be taken into consideration when planning ongoing visits. If the home health agency has a nurse who is a diabetic specialist, the nurse can either consult with that specialist about the care of this patient or have the diabetic specialist make a home visit.

Perspective and Prospects

From the beginning of time, nursing and the role of the nurse have been defined by the people and the society of a particular age. Nursing as it is known today is still influenced by what occurred over the centuries.

In primitive times, people believed that illness was su-

pernatural, caused by evil gods. The roles of the physician and the nurse were separate and unrelated. The physician was a medicine man, sometimes called a shaman or a witch doctor, who treated disease by ritualistic chants, by fear or shock techniques, or by boring holes into a person's skull with a sharp stone to allow the evil spirit or demon an escape. The nurse, on the other hand, was usually the mother who tended to family members and provided for their physical needs, using herbal remedies when they were ill.

As tribes evolved, the centers for medical care were temples. Some tribes believed that illness was caused by sin and the displeasure of gods. The physician of this age was a priest and was held in high regard. The nurse was a woman, seen as a slave, who performed menial tasks ordered by the priest/physician. Living in the same era were Hebrew tribes who used the Ten Commandments and the Mosaic Health Code to develop standards for ethical human relationships, mental health treatment, and disease control. Nurses visited the sick in their homes, practiced as midwives, and provided for the physical and spiritual needs of family members who cared for the ill.

These nurses provided a family-centered approach to care. With the advent of Christianity, the value of the individual was emphasized, and the responsibility for recognizing the needs of each individual emerged. Nursing gained an elevated position in society. A spiritual foundation for nursing was established as well. The first organized visiting of the sick was done by deaconesses and Christian Roman matrons of the time. Members of male religious orders also cared for the sick and buried the dead.

During the time of the Crusades, there were both male and female nursing orders, and nursing at this time was a respected vocation. Men usually belonged to military nursing orders, who cared for the sick, on one hand, and defended the hospital when it was under attack, on the other. In medieval times, hospitals became a place to keep, not cure, patients. There were no methods of infection control. Nursing care was largely custodial, and the practice of accepting individuals of low character to supplement inadequate nursing staffs became common.

The worst era in nursing history was probably from 1500 to 1860. Nursing at this time was not a respected profession. Women who had committed a crime were sent into nursing as an alternative to serving a jail term. Nurses received poor wages and worked long hours under deplorable conditions. Changes in the Reformation and the Renaissance did little or nothing to improve the care of the sick. The attitude prevailed that nursing was a religious and not an intellectual occupation. Charles Dickens quite aptly portrayed the nurse and nursing conditions of the time through his caricatures of Sairey Gamp and Betsey Prig in *Martin Chuzzlewit* (1843-1844).

It was not until the middle of the nineteenth century that this situation began to change. Through Nightingale's efforts, nursing became a respected occupation once more. The quality of nursing care improved tremendously, and the foundation was laid for modern nursing education. As innovations in health care have an impact on nursing, nurses' roles will continue to expand in the future. Nursing can also be a background from which both men and women begin to bridge gaps of service where other affiliations are needed: computer science, medical-legal issues, health insurance agencies, and bioethics, to name a few. The words of Florence Nightingale still echo as a challenge to the nursing profession:

> *May the methods by which every infant, every human being will have the best chance of health, the methods by which every sick person will have the best chance of recovery, be learned and practiced! Hospitals are only an intermediate state of civilization never intended, at all events, to take in the whole sick population.*

Nursing will continue to meet this challenge to improve the quality of health care around the world.

—Karen A. Mattern and Mary Dietmann,
EdD, APRN, CNS;
updated by Geraldine Marrocco

See also: Aging: Extended care; Allied health; Anesthesiology; Cardiac rehabilitation; Critical care; Critical care, pediatric; Emergency medicine; Geriatrics*and gerontology; Holisticmedicine; Hospitals; Immunizationand vaccination; Intensive care unit(ICU); Neonatology; Nutrition; Pediatrics; Physical examination; Physician assistants; Preventive medicine; Surgical procedures; Surgical technologists; Terminally ill: Extended care.*

For Further Information:

American Nurses Association. *NursingWorld*, 2013. Delaune, Sue C., and Patricia K. Ladner, eds. *Fundamentals of Nursing: Standards and Practices*. 4th ed. Albany, N.Y.: Delmar Thomson Learning, 2011.

Dolan, Josephine A., M. Louise Fitzpatrick, and Eleanor K. Herrmann. *Nursingin Society: A Historical Perspective*. 15th ed. Philadelphia: W. B. Saunders, 1983.

Donahue, M. Patricia. *Nursing: The Finest Art*. 3d ed. Maryland Heights: Mosby Elsevier, 2011.

Kozier, Barbara, et al. *Fundamentals of Nursing: Concepts, Process, and Practice*. 2d ed. Harlow, England; NewYork: Pearson, 2012.

MedlinePlus. "Health Occupations." *MedlinePlus*, August 29, 2013.

Park, Melissa, et al. "Nurse Practitioners, Certified Nurse Midwives, and Physician Assistants in Physician Offices." *Centers for Disease Control and Prevention:NCHSDatabrief*, August 17, 2011.

United States Department of Labor. "Licensed Practical and Licensed Vocational Nurses." *Bureau of LaborStatistics: OccupationalOutlook Handbook*, March 29, 2012.

United States Department of Labor. "Registered Nurses." *Bureau of LaborStatistics: OccupationalOutlook Handbook*, March 29, 2012.

Vorvick, Linda J. "Types of Health Care Providers." *MedlinePlus*, August 14, 2012.

Nutrition

Biology
Anatomy or system affected: All
Specialties and related fields: Biochemistry, preventive medicine, public health
Definition: The science of food and beverage analysis, metabolism, physical needs for health and disease prevention.

Key terms:

calorie: a measure of the energy in food or of the energy used by the body

carbohydrate: one of three macronutrients; foods that provide carbohydrates are starches, sugars, fruit, vegetables, and milk products

fat: one of three macronutrients; foods that provide fat are oils, margarine, butter, meat, and dairy

macronutrient: carbohydrate, protein, or fat

minerals: inorganic substances that are essential for body processes; the major minerals include calcium, phosphorus, magnesium, sodium, chloride, and potassium

protein: one of three macronutrients; foods that provide protein are meat and dairy, with smaller amounts of protein found in starches

vitamins: organic (carbon-containing) substances found in plants and animals that are essential for body processes; examples include vitamins A, C, and D and the B vitamins

Structure and Functions

Nutrients are necessary for all aspects of living, including cellular metabolism, individual organ function, and multiple organ systems function. Breathing, moving, thinking, playing, and working all rely on the availability of nutrients. The study of nutrition has revolved around either healthy growth and development or nutrition in relation to the prevention and treatment of disease. Periods of noticeable growth, such as pregnancy, infancy, childhood, and adolescence, are particular areas of study in nutrition because nutrient needs change during these periods.

The amount of calories required to maintain a healthy weight during each stage of the life cycle depends upon the amount of energy expended. Higher caloric requirements are found when body mass is relatively large and energy output is relatively high, as seen in later adolescence and young adulthood. Because men generally have a larger body mass than women, they usually have a larger caloric requirement.

Macronutrients. Carbohydrates are an important source of energy. The recommended range of intake is 45 to 65 percent of the total caloric intake. Each gram of carbohydrate contributes 4 calories to the diet. Carbohydrates are found in starchy foods such as potatoes or corn, in vegetables and fruits, and in milk and yogurt. Carbohydrates are not found in meats or fats unless the food is a mixed dish, such as a hamburger casserole or a candy bar. Simple carbohydrates are those that require little digestion, such as sucrose or sugar. Complex carbohydrates include those that require more digestion, such as starches and fiber. General dietary guidelines suggest an increase in the higher fiber foods. The recommendation is to consume 25 to 35 grams of fiber each day; Americans generally consume 5 to 10 grams. In addition to fruits and vegetables, nuts and seeds, whole wheat bread, and cereal are higher fiber foods.

Dietary protein is required to supply essential amino acids so that the body can synthesize new proteins such as enzymes or hormones, or structural proteins to build muscle. Meats (including pork, beef, chicken, or turkey), fish, eggs, and nuts contain substantial amounts of protein. Protein is also found in dairy products such as milk, cheese, and yogurt. Some protein can be found in most foods, including starches and vegetables, the exception being those foods that are all fat, such as oil, or all simple carbohydrates, such as sugar. Each gram of protein contributes 4 calories to the diet. Protein requirements are closely related to caloric intake. With adequate or excess calories, protein is pared, meaning that less can be consumed while still meeting all body demands for protein. In these cases, protein does not need to be used for energy. With inadequate caloric intake, however, higher levels of protein are required to meet the body's needs because some protein will also be converted to calories for energy needs. The recommended intake assumes that adequate calorie needs are consumed. Protein requirements may be higher than the recommend levels in cases of stress. Although both psychological and physical stress can increase protein requirements, physical stress (including surgery and burns) usually causes a more substantial increase in requirements.

Dietary fat is a risk factor in the development of atherosclerosis or heart disease. Because of this, dietary fat intake recommendations are restricted both in total intake and type of fat ingested. Saturated fat is solid at room temperature and is derived from animals. Lard, shortening, and bacon fat are examples. Unsaturated fat can either have many unsaturated bonds (polyunsaturated) in the structure or one (monounsaturated). Polyunsaturated fat is liquid at room temperature and derived from plants such as corn or soybeans. Monounsaturated fat is derived from plants such as canola or olive oil. Whereas recommendations had previously specified levels of intake for both polyunsaturated and monounsaturated fats, current recommendations reflect only a limited total fat intake with a restriction on transfats in particular. Transfat is an unsaturated fat that has been partially hydrogenated. This process causes a liquid fat to become more solid and is sometimes desirable in baked products. Transfats are linked to cardiovascular disease and should be limited. Foods that have higher values of transfat should be labeled as such and are most often processed baked goods, such as cookies, cakes, or pies, or snack foods, such as chips. Regardless of the type of fat, each gram of fat contributes 9 calories to the diet.

Minerals. The major minerals include calcium, phosphorus, magnesium, sodium, chloride, and potassium. These minerals are at times referred to as electrolytes, meaning that they can have a negative or positive charge, thus conducting electricity. In the body, these anions (negatively charged) and cations (positively charged) are important for the action potentials of cells, nerve conduction, and the excitation of muscles. The trace minerals are so called because only very small amounts are needed on a daily basis. One of the most common trace minerals is iron. The amounts of minerals in a particular food often vary depending on the soil in which a plant is grown or the feed that an animal consumes. Minerals are inorganic and cannot be destroyed with cooking or processing.

Calcium is required for normal growth and development of bone as well as nervous and muscular activity, enzyme regulation, and blood clotting. Food labels may designate a food as an excellent source (at least 200 milligrams of calcium) or a good source (100 to 199 milligrams of calcium). Poor intake of calcium is associated with the development of porous bones, or osteoporosis.

Most phosphorus is in bone as hydroxyapatite, although phosphorus also occurs as phospholipids in most cell membranes and is a component of nucleic acids. Phosphorus functions as an acid-base buffer, in enzymatic reactions, and in energy transfer. Phosphorus is found in nearly all foods, but good sources include meat, milk products, eggs, grains and legumes, and soft drinks.

About half of the body magnesium is found in bone, but magnesium is essential for hundreds of enzymatic reactions as well as muscle contraction. Green leafy vegetables, fruits, grains, and nuts as well as milk, meat, shellfish, and eggs are good sources of magnesium.

Potassium is found in many foods, including milk, meat, fruit, and vegetables. Together with sodium, potassium is involved with maintaining fluid balance. A diet high in sodium and low in potassium may be involved in the development of high blood pressure, or hypertension. The major source of sodium in the diet is salt, which is sodium chloride. Foods high in sodium include any food with visible salt (such as crackers and snack foods), pickled foods, processed foods such as lunch meat, canned soup, canned meat, and cured foods such as bacon and ham. A diet high in potassium and calcium and low in sodium is recommended to prevent hypertension.

Most of the body's iron is found in hemoglobin in red blood cells, where its function is to transport oxygen in the blood. Food sources of iron are either heme (from meat) or nonheme (from plant sources or iron-fortified foods). Very little iron is excreted from the body, with most of the iron from degraded hemoglobin being reabsorbed in the gastrointestinal tract. A deficiency of iron occurs gradually with chronic poor intake of iron-rich foods. Other causes of iron deficiency include excess blood loss and malabsorption. Chronic iron deficiency will cause anemia.

Vitamins. Vitamin A food sources include both animal sources (retinoids) and plant sources (carotenoids). Good animal food sources of vitamin A include liver, egg yolks, milk fat, and fish oils. Carotenoids can be converted to retinol in the intestinal mucosa and will then have the same metabolic role as retinoids from animal sources. The most common of these is beta carotene, but there are more than five hundred carotenoids. Vitamin A is required for optimal vision, with most of its effects found in the maintenance of night vision. Vitamin A also has a role in maintaining epithelial tissues, mucus production, and bone health. Vitamin A appears to have a role in fertility and in maintaining immune function as well.

Vitamin C is an important antioxidant with the biochemical ability to neutralize free radicals. Free radicals are metabolites of oxygen used in the cell and are believed to promote aging and several chronic diseases. Good sources of vitamin C include citrus fruits, broccoli, kiwi, potatoes, strawberries, and tomatoes, as well as most other fruits and vegetables. Heat, alkalinity, and exposure to air will destroy vitamin C. Therefore, certain cooking, processing, and storage practices can greatly reduce the vitamin C content of food.

Another antioxidant is vitamin E. Vitamin E is really a group of compounds, the most common of which is α-tocopherol. Good sources of vitamin E include vegetable oils, margarines, and nuts. Vitamin E is not destroyed by exposure to air, primarily because it is protected in dietary fat. Vitamin E can be destroyed by high temperatures such as in frying.

Vitamin D food sources are very limited. While milk is fortified with vitamin D, other dairy products, such as cheese and yogurt, generally are not. Some new products are being fortified with both calcium and vitamin D, such as yogurt, margarine, and juice. Exposure of the skin to sunlight converts a pre-vitamin D compounds to vitamin D_3 (cholecalciferol). Cholecalciferol will be hydroxylated in the liver and the kidney before it becomes active vitamin D. Vitamin D is required for calcium regulation and bone health, but emerging areas of research suggest that vitamin D may have a role in autoimmune diseases as well.

The B vitamins are water soluble and include thiamin, niacin, riboflavin, pantothenic acid, vitamin B_6, biotin, folate, and vitamin B_{12}. As a group, the B vitamins are essential for the metabolism of macronutrients, as well as cell growth and division and all organ functions. The B vitamins are found in a variety of foods, although vitamin B_{12} is primarily found in animal products. Once a concern for vegetarians, vitamin B_{12} is now fortified in many cereals and nonmeat breakfast foods.

Disorders and Diseases

Most chronic diseases result as a complex interaction between genetics and environmental factors. Diet is an important environmental factor that is potentially modifiable, and it has received much attention in the prevention of chronic disease. Most chronic disease prevention or treatment includes a nutritional component. The most prevalent chronic diseases in the United States are cancer, cardiovascular disease, diabetes, obesity, and osteoporosis.

Cancer. Although overall rates are declining in the United States, cancer continues to be a major cause of mortality. In general, cancer involves three phases: initiation, promotion, and progression. During the initiation step, there is a genetic alteration that may remain quiescent or continue though the second step of promotion. During promotion, cellular proliferation is stimulated and the abnormal cells begin to grow without regulation. The third phase is progression, when the neoplastic cells become invasive and spread or metastasize to other parts of the body. Dietary components may be involved in the initiation and promotion of certain cancers as well as their inhibition. The dietary components that have been linked to the development of cancer include dietary fat, total calories, and alcohol, as well as salted, cured foods and molds that may grow in certain foods.

Antioxidants have been investigated as inhibitors of cancer. Fruits and vegetables are rich sources of antioxidants, and high fruit and vegetable intake has been linked to a lower incidence of certain cancers. The results of many studies, however, are inconclusive. Although high intake of dietary fat and red meat has been associated with an increased risk of colon cancer, lower fat diets have not proved to be an effective intervention in decreasing colon cancer incidence. Nevertheless, a diet high in fruits and vegetables, at least five servings each day, and lower in fat and alcohol is recommended as a preventive measure against cancer. Some of the benefit of high fruit and vegetable intake may be attributable to the fiber content of these foods. Higher fiber diets increase fecal bulk, thereby diluting any carcinogens that enter the gastrointestinal tract. By increasing intestinal motility, fiber also decreases the amount of time that fecal material is in the gastrointestinal tract, thereby limiting exposure of the mucosa to potential toxins.

Cardiovascular disease. Cardiovascular diseases are the leading cause of death in the United States. They include arrhythmias, congestive heart failure, and valvular diseases, but most of the morbidity and mortality is related to coronary heart disease, or atherosclerosis. Hyperlipidemia is a risk factor for atherosclerosis, and dietary fat has influence on the level of blood lipids. According to the Center for Disease Control (CDC), the recommended intake of fat is 25 to 35 percent of total calories per day. Of that dietary fat, less than 7 percent of total calories should be saturated fat and less than 1 percent should be transfat. Lower fat meats and dairy are recommended, as well as replacement of some meat with vegetable alternatives. Sources of transfat should be limited. The effects of various levels of polyunsaturated and monounsaturated fats are debated. While limited intake of cholesterol is recommended, cholesterol intake has had less of an effect on blood lipids than total fat and transfat.

Eating fish, especially oily fish, is recommended as a source of omega-3 fatty acids, which are long-chain polyunsaturated fatty acids associated with a decreased risk of certain heart diseases. The two omega-3 fatty acids are eicosapentaenoic acid (EPA) and docosahexaenoic acid (DHA). Although fish may contain contaminants known to be hazardous to health, the benefits of eating it are believed to outweigh the risks for adults. Restricted intake may be recommended for children and pregnant women. Supplements of DHA and EPA are not recommended for the prevention of heart disease, although they may be prescribed as treatment under a physician's supervision.

Higher intakes of fruits, vegetables, and whole grains are recommended to prevent heart disease. In addition to fiber, these foods may contain antioxidants or other bioactive compounds that are beneficial to health. In addition, these foods may displace other, higher calorie foods from the diet, thus promoting a healthy weight. Limiting foods high in added sugars is recommended because of the association of these foods with weight gain and obesity. Obesity is a significant risk factor for cardiovascular disease, and achieving a healthy weight through diet and physical activity is important.

A healthy weight is also significant in the maintenance of optimal blood pressure. Because sodium intake is associated with increases in blood pressure on average, limiting sodium intake is also recommended for heart health. Limited amounts of alcohol, if alcohol is consumed at all, is also included as a healthy lifestyle measure for the prevention of heart disease. Moderate alcohol intake is generally considered to be two drinks for men and one drink for women each day.

Foods that are being investigated concerning their role in the prevention of cardiovascular disease include soy and plant stanols. Supplements of antioxidants and fish oils for their DHA and EPA are generally not recommended, but foods containing these compounds may be beneficial.

Diabetes. The incidence of diabetes continues to grow in parallel to the incidence of obesity. Diabetes mellitus has been categorized as either insulin-dependent diabetes mellitus (IDDM), which is also called type 1 diabetes, and non-insulin-dependent diabetes mellitus (NIDDM), also known as type 2 diabetes. Nutrition is an important component of both the prevention and treatment of diabetes, regardless of type.

Obesity enhances insulin resistance. Therefore, a main goal in type 2 diabetes is to prevent or reduce obesity. Weight loss in obese persons with type 2 diabetes improves glycemic control and blood lipid profile. Because carbohydrates are the main determinant of postprandial plasma glucose, the amount of carbohydrates and timing of foods eaten may need to be regulated. The total amount of carbohydrates in the diet or meal is more important than the type of carbohydrate, with certain exceptions. Liquid carbohydrates are more easily digested and absorbed than those from solid foods. Beverages such as milk and orange juice may cause a more rapid rise in blood glucose. Sucrose and sucrose-containing foods do not need to be eliminated, but these foods do need to be included in the total carbohydrates and calories consumed for meal planning and coverage with medication. Restriction of sucrose and sucrose-containing foods usually relates to the restriction of total calories. The glycemic response to carbohydrates depends on many components, including the type of carbohydrate, the cooking or processing, prior food intake, other macronutrients in the food, and glycemic control of the individual. Because dietary modifications need to be individualized, people with diabetes should receive individualized medical nutrition therapy, preferably by a registered dietitian or certified diabetes educator.

Obesity. Obesity occurs when caloric intake exceeds the needs of the individual and is therefore stored in adipose tissue. Although normal weight varies with age, gender, and height, for each group there are indicators of obesity. Usual indicators of obesity are based on the assumption that variations in weight at various heights are attributable to body fat and are often calculated as the body mass index (BMI). According to the CDC, a BMI of between 25 and 30 is considered overweight, and above 30 is considered obese. The optimal macronutrient distribution to facilitate weight loss is not known. Higher and lower amounts of protein, fat, and carbohydrates have been investigated, without clear conclusions. Consuming fewer calories while increasing the amount of calories used through physical activity remains the cornerstone of obesity prevention and treatment.

Osteoporosis. As with other chronic diseases, the incidence of osteoporosis continues to rise. Osteoporosis is asymptomatic until the condition produces deformity or contributes to fractures. While genetics play an important role in the development of osteoporosis, modifying risk factors include diet and physical activity. Optimal levels of calcium have been shown to be beneficial in maintaining high bone mineral density, which is critical in preventing osteoporosis. Most calcium is obtained from dairy products, although increasingly grain-based foods and juices are being fortified with calcium. Vitamin D plays a critical role in regulating calcium balance. Therefore, adequate vitamin D status is important in preventing osteoporosis. Vitamin D deficiency can be a contributing factor to osteoporosis in older individuals secondary to poor skin synthesis, lower hydroxylation of vitamin D in the kidneys, and inadequate nutritional intake. As with calcium, more food products are being fortified with vitamin D with an increasing awareness of osteoporosis.

Perspective and Prospects

Although the science of nutrition began as a branch of biochemistry, early discoveries of the health properties of food date to the eighteenth century and the discovery that limes could prevent the painful bleeding disorder scurvy. Since then, the knowledge of nutrition has progressed beyond identifying deficiency diseases toward an understanding and appreciation of the complexity of nutrition in optimal health. In addition to further investigations into macronutrients, vitamins, and minerals, many bioactive substances in foods are being identified, such as bioflavinoids and probiotics. The interactions of these and more traditional nutrients are being investigated as potential modifiers of chronic disease and promoters of longevity.

—*Karen Chapman-Novakofski, R.D., L.D.N., Ph.D.*

See also Acid reflux disease; Aging: Extended care; Anorexia nervosa; Antioxidants; Appetite loss; Arteriosclerosis; Beriberi; Breast-feeding; Bulimia; Caffeine; Cancer; Carbohydrates; Carcinogens; Cholesterol; Diabetes mellitus; Dietary reference intakes (DRIs); Digestion; Eating disorders; Enzyme therapy; Enzymes; Failure to thrive; Fiber; Food biochemistry; Food Guide Pyramid; Gastroenterology; Gastroenterology, pediatric; Gastrointestinal system; Gastrostomy; Geriatrics and gerontology; Heart disease; Hirschsprung's disease; Hypercholesterolemia; Hyperlipidemia; Kwashiorkor; Lactose intolerance; Lipids; Macronutrients; Malabsorption; Malnutrition; Mercury poisoning; Metabolic disorders; Metabolism; Obesity; Obesity, childhood; Osteoporosis; Phenylketonuria (PKU); Phytochemicals; Pinworms; Protein; Roundworms; Scurvy; Sports medicine; Supplements; Tapeworms; Taste; Tropical medicine; Vitamins and minerals; Weaning; Weight loss and gain; Weight loss medications; Worms.

For Further Information:

American Diabetes Association. *American Diabetes Association Complete Guide to Diabetes.* 4th rev. ed. New York: Bantam Books, 2006.

"Defining Overweight and Obesity." *Centers for Disease Control..* July 17, 2013.

Duyff, Roberta Larson. *American Dietetic Association Complete Food and Nutrition Guide.* 3d ed. Hoboken, N.J.: John Wiley & Sons, 2007.

Lichtenstein, Alice H., et al. "Diet and Lifestyle Recommendations Revision 2006: A Scientific Statement from the American Heart Association Nutrition Committee." *Circulation* 114, no. 1 (July 4, 2006): 82-96.

"Nutrition for Everyone: Dietary Fat." *Center for Disease Control.* July 17, 2013.

"Nutrition for Everyone: Vitamins and Minerals." *Center for Disease Control.* July 17, 2013.

U.S. Department of Health and Human Services and U.S. Department of Agriculture. *Dietary Guidelines for Americans 2005.* 6th ed. Washington, D.C.: Government Printing Office, 2005.

Obesity
Disease/Disorder

Anatomy or system affected: Abdomen, blood vessels, circulatory system, endocrine system, gastrointestinal system, heart, intestines, joints, psychic-emotional system, respiratory system, stomach

Specialties and related fields: Endocrinology, family medicine, internal medicine, nutrition, psychiatry, psychology, public health

Definition: A condition in which the body carries abnormal or unhealthy amounts of fat tissue, leading the individual to weigh in excess of 20 percent more than his or her ideal weight.

Key terms:

adipose tissue: fat; a soft tissue of the body composed of cells (adipocytes) that contain triglyceride, a compound consisting of glycerol and fatty acids; in obesity, there may be increased numbers of adipocytes, and the cells may contain an increased amount of triglyceride

basal metabolic rate(BMR): the minimal energy expended for maintenance of the vegetative functions of the body (respiration, heat production, and so on), expressed as calories per hour per square meter of body surface

body mass index(BMI): weight in kilograms divided by height in meters, squared (kg/m2); since this value is relatively independent of height and sex, the same standard values can be used for all adults.

calorie: 1 kilocalorie, which is the amount of heat (energy) needed to raise the temperature of 1 kilogram of water by 1 degree Celsius

metabolism: the sum of the physical and chemical processes by which living matter is produced, maintained, and transformed

resting metabolic rate(RMR): similar to the BMR, but more easily measured (the subject is resting rather than in a truly basal state)

Causes and Symptoms

Obesity is a condition in which the body accumulates an abnormally large amount of adipose tissue, or fat. It is a multifactorial, chronic disease that is rapidly increasing and having devastating effects on health, especially in the United States. The disease has social, cultural, genetic, metabolic, behavioral, and psychological components. People who are obese also face stigma and discrimination in work and social settings. Obesity is the second leading cause of preventable deaths in the United States, resulting in an estimated 300,000 deaths each year.

Because it is not practical to measure body fat content directly but it is easy to measure weight and height, the body mass index (BMI), is the most widespread method to identify and quantify obesity. BMI also closely correlates with body fat Being overweight and being obese are not the same condition. A BMI of 25 to 29.9 is considered to be overweight, a BMI of 30 or more is obese, and a BMI of 40 or more is severely obese. In 2012 the National Center for Health Statistics reported that in 2009 to 2010 35.7 percent of adults in the United States were obese. In 2006, it was estimated that 64.5 percent of adults in the United States were overweight, 30.5 percent were obese, and 4.7 percent were

Information on Obesity

Causes: May include endocrine disorders, poor diet, lack of exercise, psychic-emotional disorders, genetic factors

Symptoms: Excessive weight possibly leading to such health problems as strain on weight-bearing body parts leading to arthritis, hypertension, arteriosclerosis, difficulty breathing, sleepiness from inadequate oxygen delivery to tissues

Duration: Often chronic

Treatments: Diet and lifestyle regulation, medications, surgery

severely obese. This latter figure increased from only 2.9 percent in a 1994 survey done by the National Health and Nutrition Examination Survey, which also found that 46.6 percent of adults were overweight and 14.4 percent were obese.

The Centers for Disease Control and Prevention cites a 2009 report in *Health Affairs*, which estimated that the annual cost of obesity in the United States was $147 billion in 2008 dollars. The National Institutes of Health funded approximately $836 million in obesity research for fiscal year 2012, and set funding estimates for fiscal year 2014 at about $843 million. The Patient Protection and Affordable Care Act of 2010 listed obesity screening and counseling among the preventative services that all new group health plans and individual market plans under the act are required to provide without patient cost sharing.

An important function of adipose tissue is to store energy. If the intake of energy in the form of food calories is greater than the expenditure of energy, then the excess calories are stored, mainly in the adipose tissue, with a resulting gain in weight. Expenditure of energy depends largely on the resting metabolic rate or resting energy expenditure, defined as the calories used each day to maintain normal body metabolism. Additional calories are expended by exercise or other activity, by the digestion and metabolism of food, and by other metabolic processes. Because of this simple relationship between energy intake, energy utilization, and energy storage, weight gain can occur only when there is increased caloric intake, decreased caloric expenditure, or both.

Genetic factors appear to be very important in determining the presence or absence of obesity. Body weight tends to be similar in close relatives, especially in identical twins, who share the same genetic makeup. The extent to which genetic factors affect food intake, activity level, or metabolic processes is not known.

One theory holds that each individual has a "set point" that determines body weight. When food intake is decreased, experiments have shown less weight loss than predicted by the caloric deficit, suggesting that the body has slowed its metabolic rate, thus minimizing the deviation from the original set point.

Many believe that physiologic regulation of body weight, which tends to maintain a preferred weight for each individual, explains some of the difficulty in treating obesity. The discovery and role of leptin in regulating weight helps to explain this apparent set point of weight for each individual. There are other causes of obesity as well. Lesions in the hypothalamus, a part of the brain, can make animals eat excessively and become obese, and rare cases of obesity in humans are attributable to disease of the hypothalamus. In hypothyroidism, a condition in which the thyroid gland produces too little thyroid hormone, the metabolic rate is slowed, which may cause a mild gain in weight. In Cushing's syndrome, which is caused by excessive amounts of the adrenal hormone cortisol or by drugs that act like cortisol, there is an accumulation of excessive fat in the face and trunk, which disappears when the disease is cured or the drug is stopped. Weight gain has also occurred with the use of other drugs, including some antidepressants and tranquilizers.

While most physicians and the public assume that the main factor causing obesity is excessive food intake in relation to physical activity, it has not been possible to prove that overweight people eat more than slender people do. This may be the case because it is very difficult to measure food intake under normal conditions, or perhaps because obese individuals tend to underestimate their food intake when dietary histories are taken. Some experts believe, however, that differences in metabolic efficiency and the physiologic set point for body weight are the principal causes of obesity in some people, rather than excessive food intake. The basal metabolic rate (BMR) varies fairly widely among persons of the same age, sex, and body size, and studies have shown large differences in the daily caloric intake needed to maintain a constant body weight in normal people; these observations support the possibility that metabolic differences could contribute to obesity.

Many health problems are associated with obesity. The majority of people who develop non-insulin-dependent diabetes mellitus are overweight, and manifestations of the disease commonly improve or disappear if the individual succeeds in losing weight. Hypertension (high blood pressure) is more common with obesity, and weight loss may lower the blood pressure enough to lessen or avoid the need for medication. Arteriosclerosis, or "hardening of the arteries," is more prevalent in obese persons and causes an increased risk for heart attacks and strokes. Certain forms of cancer are more prevalent with obesity: cancer of the colon, rectum, and prostate in men and cancer of the uterus, gallbladder, ovary, and breast in women. Severe obesity can cause difficulties in breathing, namely obstructive sleep apnea, with sleepiness resulting from inadequate oxygen delivery to the tissues and sometimes from interruption of sleep at night. In addition, conditions such as arthritis may be worsened by the additional strain that obesity places on weight-bearing parts of the body.

The distribution of excess adipose tissue differs among individuals. Two main patterns have been described: android obesity (more commonly affecting men), in which fat accumulates mainly in the abdomen and upper body; and gynoid obesity (more common in women), in which fat ac-

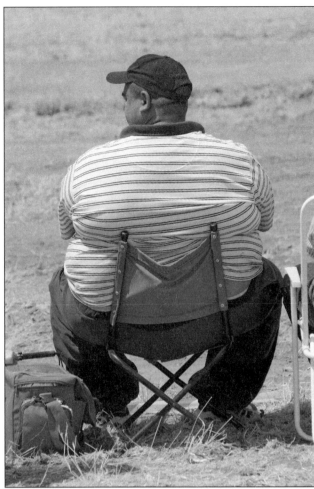

The rates of severe obesity are increasing in the United States. (© Armand Upton/Dreamstime.com)

cumulates mainly in the hips, thighs, and lower body. This distinction has received much attention because persons with android obesity are more likely to suffer from diabetes, hypertension, and cardiovascular disease. The closest association with these diseases is seen when sensitive measurements of abdominal visceral fat mass are made with computed tomography (CT) scanning. A simple measurement of the waist circumference compared with the hip circumference—the waist-to-hip ratio—can also be used to identify those obese individuals at greater risk for diabetes and cardiovascular disease.

Treatment and Therapy

Many obese people are highly motivated to lose weight because of the common perception that a slim body build is more attractive than an obese one. Many other overweight individuals desire to lose weight because of health problems related to obesity. As a result, the human and financial resources devoted to weight loss efforts are extensive. Unfortunately, the long-term results of the treatment of obesity are successful in only a minority of cases. The only measures useful in the treatment of obesity are those that decrease the intake or absorption of calories or those that increase the expenditure of calories. The basis for any long-term weight reduction program is a low-calorie diet. The average daily calorie requirement in the United States is approximately 1,600 calories for women and 2,300 calories for men; decreasing an individual's intake, usually to between 800 and 1,500 calories, will result in weight loss, provided that energy expenditure does not decrease. A balanced diet, with 20 percent to 30 percent of the calories derived from fat (considerably less fat than is found in the typical American diet) is usually recommended. Many unbalanced diets, or "fad diets," have enjoyed periods of popularity. Rice diets, low carbohydrate diets, vegetable diets, and other special diets may produce rapid weight loss, but long-term persistence with an unbalanced diet is rare and the lost weight is often regained.

Many patients fail to lose weight with low-calorie diets. More severe calorie restriction can be achieved with very low-calorie diets that provide only 400 to 800 calories daily. This level of caloric restriction is unsafe unless a very high proportion of the diet consists of high-quality protein, with correct amounts of other nutrients such as vitamins and minerals. These requirements can be met with special formula diets under careful medical supervision. Such a program is recommended for severely obese patients who are otherwise healthy enough to tolerate this degree of caloric restriction. Because most people find it difficult to lower their calorie intake, behavioral management programs may be combined with dietary restrictions. Dieters can be taught techniques for self-monitoring of food intake, such as keeping a daily log of meals and exercise, which will increase the awareness of eating behavior as well as point out ways in which that behavior can be modified. There are techniques for reducing exposure to food and the stimuli associated with eating, such as keeping food out of sight, keeping food handling and preparation to a minimum, and eliminating the occasions when food is eaten out of habit or as part of a social routine. Ways can be sought to increase the social support of friends and family for weight-losing behavior and for reinforcement of compliance with dietary restrictions. Interestingly, the "diet merry-go round" which many mildly obese individuals experience—restricting their caloric intake until a weight goal is achieved, ending the diet only to resume overeating and regain the weight lost—often results in higher weight. Over time, such a pattern can "cycle" the individual to a dangerously high weight. Such individuals tend to experience more success if they can adjust their long-range eating behavior to moderate, rather than restrictive, intake of food. Many physicians would prefer to see their obese patients remain relatively stable in weight, reducing slowly over time, to avoid physical stress and ensure success. When establishing dietary weight loss programs, it is crucial to set realistic goals such as an initial goal of 5-7% of body weight loss. The Mediterranean diet, which involves high consumption of fruits, vegetables, grains, and legumes with limited dairy and meat intake, has been shown to have numerous health benefits including diabetes prevention and reduced risk of cardiovascular disease.

Because obesity is caused by an excess of calorie intake over calorie expenditure, another approach to weight loss is to increase energy utilization by increasing physical activity. Some studies have shown that overweight individuals are less active than their non-obese counterparts. This fact could contribute to their obesity, since less energy utilization results in more energy available for storage as fat. Decreased activity could also be a result of obesity, since a heavier person must do more work, by carrying more pounds, than a non-obese person who walks or climbs the same distance. Each pound of fat contains energy equal to about four thousand calories. If an obese person expends four hundred extra calories each day by walking briskly for one hour, it will take ten days for this activity to result in the loss of one pound. In a year, this increased calorie expenditure would result in a thirty-six-pound weight loss. More vigorous exercise, such as running, swimming, or calisthenics, would lead to more rapid weight loss, but might not be advisable for every person because of the increased prevalence of certain health problems in obese individuals, such as heart disease, hypertension, and musculoskeletal disorders. For this reason, any exercise program that involves vigorous physical activity should be undertaken with medical supervision.

Exercise as part of a weight-loss program has additional benefits. The function of the cardiovascular system may be improved, and muscles may be strengthened. Exercise will lead to loss of adipose tissue and gain in lean body mass as weight is lost, a change in body composition that is beneficial to overall health. Although some fear that physical activity will lead to an increase in appetite, studies show that any increase in food intake that occurs after exercise is usually not great enough to match the calories expended by the exercise. Medications that decrease appetite are occasionally used to help people comply with a low-calorie diet. Some appetite suppressants act like adrenaline and may cause such side effects as nervousness, irritability, and increased heart rate and blood pressure. Other drugs may stimulate serotonin, a chemical transmitter in the central nervous system that decreases appetite, and may cause drowsiness as a side effect. The use of these medications is controversial because of their side effects and their limited effectiveness in promoting weight loss. Several surgical procedures, collectively referred to as bariatric surgery, have been used to treat severe obesity that has impaired the patient's health and has resisted other treatment. There are stringent criteria for being a surgical candidate. Typically a patient has to have a BMI>40 or have a BMI between 35.0 to 39.9 with at least one serious comorbidity, which can include type 2 diabetes, hypertension, asthma or sleep apnea. Pre-operative counseling as well as psychological and cognitive assessments often takes place to ensure patients are realistic about goals post-surgery and are prepared to make serious lifestyle modifications.

Bariatric surgical procedures lead to weight loss through two basic mechanisms: malabsorption and restriction. Malabsorptive procedures decrease nutrient absorption through the removal of a portion of intestine. Restrictive procedures decrease caloric intake through restriction of stomach capacity anatomically. The most commonly performed bariatric procedures done today include the following:

Roux-en-Y gastricbypass: a combined restrictive and malabsorptive procedure wherein the stomach is divided and a new, smaller gastric pouch is created, and the small intestine is also divided with a limb created and connected to the gastric pouch to bypass the initial portion of the intestine

Sleeve gastrectomy: a restrictive procedure in which the majority of the stomach is removed. This is the most commonly performed procedure both globally and in the U.S.

Laparoscopic adjustable gastricbanding: a restrictive procedure where an adjustable band is placed around the entrance to the stomach. This procedure is being performed less in light of the aforementioned procedures which cause increased weight loss and improved comorbidity resolution.

Liposuction is not a suggested weight loss strategy as studies indicate it does not actually cause improvements in insulin sensitivity or cardiovascular risk factors.

Perspective and Prospects

Fat has several important functions in the human body. It serves as a cushion for the body frame and internal organs, it provides insulation against heat loss, and it is a storage site for energy. Fat stores energy very efficiently since it contains approximately nine calories per gram, compared with approximately four calories per gram in protein and carbohydrate. The presence of reserve stores of energy in the form of fat is particularly important when regular food intake is interrupted and the body becomes dependent on its fat deposits to maintain a source of fuel for daily metabolism and physical activity. In affluent, culturally advanced societies, however, where food is abundant and modern conveniences greatly reduce the need for physical exertion, many people tend to accumulate excessive amounts of fat, since energy that is taken in but not utilized is stored in the adipose tissue. In the early twenty-first century, health officials were concerned by findings that showed one in every fifty Americans were "extremely obese," meaning their BMI measured at least 50 and they were at least one hundred pounds overweight. This number had quadrupled since the 1980s. Obesity is a critical public health problem because it increases the risk of diabetes, hypertension, cardiovascular disease, and other illnesses. Also, many overweight men and women are distressed by the effects of their weight on their social interactions and self-image, and, despite laws, face discrimination in workplace settings. Therefore, many obese individuals desire to lose weight. Childhood and adolescent obesity is also becoming a growing problem, with the prevalence of severe obesity increasing. Childhood obesity is more common among American Indian, Mexican-American and black children and is also more prevalent among lower-income communities. Childhood obesity increases the risk for comorbidities later in life including diabetes, hypertension, and heart disease.

Unfortunately, the results of weight-loss programs and countless individual efforts at dieting to achieve this goal have often been disappointing. Short-term weight loss can often be achieved; programs utilizing low-calorie diets, behavior modification, exercise, and sometimes appetite-suppressing drugs usually lead to a weight loss of ten to thirty pounds or more over a period of several weeks or months. The problem is that after a year or more, the great majority of these dieters have regained the lost weight. It appears that the maintenance of a low-calorie diet and an increase in physical activity require a degree of commitment and willingness to endure inconvenience, self-deprivation, and sometimes even physical discomfort that most people can accept for short periods of time but not indefinitely. There are exceptions—some people do succeed in maintaining long-term weight loss—but more commonly dieters return to or surpass their original weight. It is as if the body's set point can be overcome temporarily by intense effort, but not permanently. Because of the poor prognosis for long-term weight loss, some experts now question the extent to which efforts should be devoted to the treatment of obesity. Nevertheless, because one cannot predict which obese individuals will succeed in achieving long-term weight reduction and because of the important health benefits of maintaining a normal body weight, most physicians agree that serious efforts should be made to treat obesity. Overweight individuals should identify the modifications in their diet and lifestyle that would be most beneficial and should attempt, with medical supervision, to initiate and maintain the behavior needed to bring about permanent weight loss.

Bariatric surgery has been enjoying increasing popularity as a weight loss strategy. According to the American Society of Metabolic and Bariatric Surgery, there were 196,000 bariatric surgery procedures done in 2015, compared to 158,000 in 2011. With the advent of laparoscopic, minimally-invasive surgery, patients now have improved recovery and diminished morbidity compared to open surgery. Expected weight loss at 2 years post surgery is 60% for sleeve gastrectomy and 70% for Roux-en-Y gastric bypass. Because of the rapid weight loss that takes place, patients often are counseled that they may have excess loose skin that will require plastic surgery for removal.

In 2006, in an effort to reduce the incidence rate of obesity in the United States, the Alliance for a Healthier Generation, the William J. Clinton Foundation, and the American Heart Association announced an agreement to fight childhood obesity. Five leading food manufacturers vowed to reformulate their products in order to provide more nutritious choices for children in schools. In 2010 President Barack Obama and First Lady Michelle Obama each announced initiatives to help prevent childhood obesity.

—E. Victor Adlin, MD and Karen E. Kalumuck, PhD;
updated by LeAnna DeAngelo, PhD
and Ananya Anand, MSc

See also: Arteriosclerosis; Bariatric surgery; Cholesterol; Cushing's syndrome; Diabetes mellitus; Eating disorders; Endocrine disorders; Endocrinology; Exercise physiology; Glands; Heart disease; Hormones; Hyperadiposis; Hypercholesterolemia; Hyperlipidemia; Hypertension; Malnutrition; Metabolic syndrome; Metabolism; Nutrition; Obesity, childhood; Prader-Willi syndrome; Sleep apnea; Thyroid disorders; Weight loss and gain; Weight loss medications.

For Further Information:

American Academy of Pediatrics. *A Parent's Guide to Childhood Obesity: A Roadmap to Health.* Edited by Sandra G. Hassink. Elk Grove Village, Ill.: Author, 2006.

American Obesity Treatment Association. *American Obesity,* n.d.

Björntorp, Per, ed. *International Textbook of Obesity.* Chichester: Wiley, 2002.

Brownell, Kelly D., and Katherine Battle Horgen. *Food Fight: The Inside Story of America's ObesityCrisis and What We Can Do About It.* New York: McGraw-Hill, 2004.

Carson-DeWitt, Rosalyn. "Overweight in Adults." *Health Library,* June 24, 2013.

Centers for Disease Control and Prevention. "Overweight and Obesity." *Centers for Disease Control and Prevention,* April 27, 2012.

Finkelstein, Eric A., et al. "Annual Medical Spending Attributable to Obesity: Payer- and Service-Specific Estimates." *Health Affairs* 28, no. 5 (2009): w822-w831.

Koplan, Jeffrey P., Catharyn T. Liverman, and Vivica I. Kraak, eds. *Preventing Childhood Obesity: Health in the Balance.* Washington, D.C.: National Academies Press, 2005.

MedlinePlus. "Obesity." *MedlinePlus,* August 29, 2013.

National Heart, Lung, and Blood Institute. "What Are Overweight and Obesity?" *National Heart* Obesity Society. *Obesity.org,* 2010.

Ogden, C. L., et al. "Prevalence of Obesity in the United States, 2009-2010." *NCHS Data Brief* no. 82 (January, 2012).

Wadden, Thomas A., and Albert J. Stunkard, eds. *Handbook of ObesityTreatment.* Rev. ed. New York: Guilford Press, 2004.

Obesity, childhood

Disease/Disorder

Anatomy or system affected: Abdomen, blood vessels, circulatory system, endocrine system, gastrointestinal system, heart, intestines, joints, psychic-emotional system, respiratory system, stomach

Specialties and related fields: Endocrinology, family medicine, internal medicine, nutrition, pediatrics, psychiatry, psychology, public health

Definition: Having a body mass index (BMI) at or above the 95th percentile for children of the same age and sex. Rapid changes from infancy through adolescence are part of normal and expected development, and the norm used to identify childhood obesity must be correct for that child's age and sex.

Key terms:

adipose tissue: a type of fat storage cell constellation that is also involved in energy regulation and hormone release

body mass index (BMI): a formula that estimates the percentage of body fat compared to overall weight; usually expressed in metrics, a person's weight in kilograms divided by height in meters, squared (kg/m^2)

hormones: chemical signaling substances in the bloodstream that foster communication between individual organs and the rest of the body

metabolic syndrome: a cluster of traits that can include obesity, high blood pressure, abnormal lipid levels, and high insulin levels in blood; their presence often marks the first phase of more serious diseases

Causes and Symptoms

A chronic or recurrent imbalance between energy expended (how active one is) and energy ingested (how much one eats and drinks) will promote ill health. When ingestion regularly exceeds expenditure, the unused energy is

Information on Childhood Obesity

Causes: May include poor diet, lack of exercise, genetic factors

Symptoms: Excessive weight relative to age and height, possibly leading to health problems and adult obesity

Duration: Often chronic

Treatments: Improved diet and increased activity

stored in adipose tissue, or body fat. Animal species that developed the capacity to store fat had a better chance of surviving times of scarcity. Chronic storage of excessive energy, as commonly occurs when high levels of physical activity are less and less necessary for survival, produces its own physical pathology. Almost every person who eats and drinks more than he or she uses in energy (usually calculated in calories) will produce adipose tissue to store the excess energy.

Peptide hormones such as leptin and adiponectin regulate and balance energy expended with energy ingested. When leptin is absent (leptin deficiency), massive obesity is present; this condition improves when people are given leptin. Adiponectin, the most abundant hormone in fat cells, is also an insulin sensitizer and an anti-inflammatory signaler. Leptin and adiponectin, along with other peptide hormones, initiate a series of signaling processes that eventually lead to signaling hormones that turn on the food-seeking abilities of organs and muscles.

The formal definition of obesity in children is a BMI greater than or equal to the 95th percentile. Children between the 85th and 95th percentiles are at risk for obesity; those less than the 85th percentile are generally considered to have normal weight when correlated with their height.

Childhood obesity has many detrimental effects and comorbidities (other diseases and disorders) that often extend into adolescence and adulthood. It is simplistic to say that obese children will become obese adults. Still, childhood obesity often produces a metabolic syndrome that children easily bring into adolescence and adulthood. This syndrome has serious implications for quality of life and life expectancy. Metabolic syndrome is a combination of high insulin levels (hyperinsulinemia), obesity, high blood pressure (hypertension), and abnormal lipid levels (dyslipidemia). Metabolic syndrome initiates a process that leads to an excess of insulin production that, in turn, promotes high blood pressure and dyslipidemia. Together, these produce aortic and coronary atherosclerosis (hardening of the arteries) and clogging of the arteries by fatty deposits in the blood.

Genetic factors play a fundamental role in childhood obesity, as genetically obese families illustrate. People cannot exchange the genes that they have inherited, but environmental factors are also important, as they are the only ones where management is possible.

The psychosocial impact of childhood obesity is no less serious than physical syndromes, leading to poor body image, low self-confidence, social isolation, recurrent anger, early forms of eating disorders, clinical depression, and

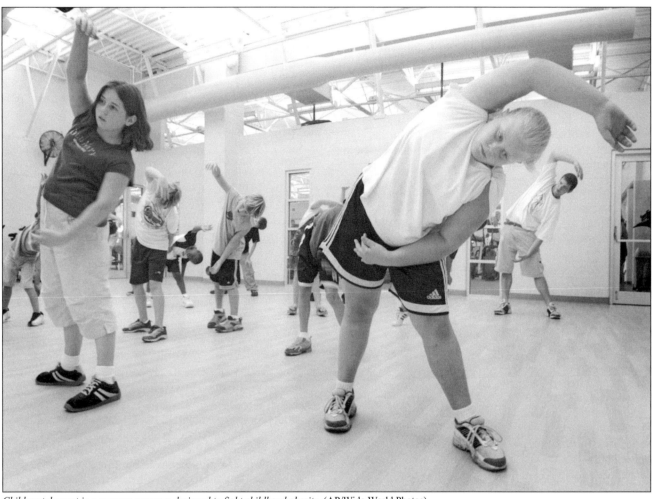

Children take part in a summer program designed to fight childhood obesity. (AP/Wide World Photos)

negatively acting-out in school and other social settings. Obese children are more likely to become underachievers who are underactive, less popular, and unhappy. Promoting physical activity is an important intervention to lessen the psychological harm of obesity as much as is controlling the amount and type of food and drink.

Treatment and Therapy

The most effective treatment for child obesity is prevention, and it can begin shortly after birth. Research shows that breast-fed children have significantly lower rates of obesity in later years. All children must gain weight as they grow, and having an adequate amount of fat cells during early antenatal development is critically important for maximal growth of key organs. Baby fat is important; its absence is problematic. As infants become toddlers and toddlers become children, the difference between healthy weight gains and weight gains that suggest the onset of obesity often require the expert eye of a pediatrician or family physician. A healthy five-pound weight gain in one five-year-old child may not be healthy in another child of the same age.

It is not until adolescence that children play a significant role in choosing and purchasing food. Until then, whatever children eat is most likely what adults have purchased or provided. Preventing obesity and correcting it when it occurs requires thoughtful selection of food and beverage items at home and school. Fast and take-out foods are always an easy solution to busy, hectic family schedules, but they are almost always obesity-promoting. Junk food snacks, also a quick solution to the transient hunger pangs of youth, are similarly harmful.

Prevention and treatment are almost one and the same in dealing with child obesity. Parents control the food world of children, and making available a variety of healthy choices becomes an important part of achieving and maintaining healthy bodies that have modest amounts of adipose tissue, as children with a BMI of less than 20 are also unhealthy. Obesity is much less likely to occur in families and schools that support healthy lifestyles: balanced nutritional consumption, physical activity and exercise, and sufficient sleep. (As a group, children who consistently get less sleep than they need are more likely to be obese than are children who sleep enough. The specific number of hours any child might need is a function of several factors, including age.)

Successful school-based interventions in the management of obesity include a prioritization of physical education classes, healthy choices on the student menu and in vending machines, proportional servings, encouraging water as the main beverage, and the ready availability of after-school activities that involve physical activity, such as intramural sports. When these elements are not present, effective obesity management for school-age children is difficult.

The key to successful long-term obesity prevention and treatment involves awareness of and respect for the individual child's personal preferences and enjoyments-nothing will enhance motivation more. Decreasing sitting time and the active encouragement of free play is far more effective than mandates to exercise or reduce food intake. Even in families where genetics play a major role in obesity, a healthy lifestyle will decrease the negative impact that obesity can have on the children's overall health.

Perspective and Prospects

In 2010, the Centers for Disease Control and Prevention (CDC) reported that data from the 2007-8 National Health and Nutrition Examination Survey showed that about 17 percent of US children and adolescents from ages two to nineteen are obese. Although a national study by the CDC showed that obesity among low-income preschoolers declined in nineteen states between 2008 and 2011, childhood obesity remains anepidemicthat has achieved the status of a public health crisis. Obesity has profound impacts on children's long-term physical and psychological health and, more often than not, leads to serious comorbidities in adulthood that are costly to treat and difficult to control. Focused strategies on modifying behavior and the slow but steady acquisition of healthy habits are the only ways that children will reliably manage the balance between calories consumed and calories burned. Adult habits, good and bad, are usually fostered during childhood. They reflect the level of care, attention, and perseverance of caregivers. Childhood obesity can be a problem of adults' mismanagement much more than it is a problem of children's choices. Parents and teachers make a major contribution to children when they provide a health-oriented environment in which children are more likely to acquire the habits that promote wellness throughout their lives.

In 2006, in an effort to reduce the incidence rate of obesity in the United States, the Alliance for a Healthier Generation, the William J. Clinton Foundation, and the American Heart Association announced an agreement to fight childhood obesity. The five leading food manufacturers-Campbell's Soup, Dannon, Kraft, Mars, and PepsiCo-vowed to reformulate their products in order to provide more nutritious choices for children in schools. On February 9, 2010 President Barack Obama created the Task Force on Childhood Obesity, which was charged with reviewing existing programs and formulating a national plan of action, and First Lady Michelle Obama announced the start of her own campaign to end childhood obesity, Let's Move.

—*Paul Moglia, Ph.D., and Kenneth Dill, M.D.*

See also Bariatric surgery; Cholesterol; Diabetes mellitus; Eating

disorders; Endocrine disorders; Endocrinology; Exercise physiology; Glands; Heart disease; Hormones; Hyperadiposis; Hypercholesterolemia; Hyperlipidemia; Hypertension; Malnutrition; Metabolic syndrome; Metabolism; Nutrition; Obesity; Thyroid disorders; Weight loss and gain; Weight loss medications.

For Further Information:

Berg, Frances. *Underage and Overweight: America's Childhood Obesity Epidemic-What Every Parent Needs to Know.* New York: Random House, 2005.

Centers for Disease Control and Prevention. "Childhood Overweight and Obesity." *Centers for Disease Control and Prevention*, August 5, 2013.

Centers for Disease Control and Prevention. "Obesity Among Low-Income Preschoolers Declines in Many States." *CDC Newsroom*, August 6, 2013.

Jones, Pamela. "Obesity-Children and Teens." *Health Library*, March 18, 2013.

MedlinePlus. "Obesity in Children." *MedlinePlus*, August 22, 2013.

Ogden, Cynthia, and Margaret Carroll. "NCHS Health E-Stat: Prevalence of Obesity among Children and Adolescents: United States Trends 1963-1965 through 2007-2008." *Centers for Disease Control and Prevention*, June 4, 2010.

Okie, Susan. *Fed Up! Winning the War Against Childhood Obesity.* Washington, D.C.: National Academies Press, 2005.

Sothern, Melinda S., Heidi Schumacher, & T. Kristian von Almen. *Trim Kids: The Proven 12-Week Plan that has Helped Thousands of Children Achieve a Healthier Weight.* New York: HarperCollins, 2003.

Obsessive-compulsive disorder

Disease/Disorder

Anatomy or system affected: Psychic-emotional system

Specialties and related fields: Psychiatry, psychology

Definition: An anxiety disorder characterized by intrusive and unwanted but uncontrollable thoughts, by the need to perform ritualized behavior patterns, or both; the obsessions and/or compulsions cause severe stress, consume an excessive amount of time, and greatly interfere with a person's normal routine, activities, or relationships.

Key terms:

anal stage: the stage of psychosexual development in which a child derives pleasure from activities associated with elimination

anxiety: an unpleasant feeling of fear and apprehension

biogenic model: the theory that every mental disorder is based on a physical or physiological problem

major affective disorder: a personality disorder characterized by mood disturbances

monoamine oxidase inhibitors: antidepressant compounds used to restore the balance of normal neurotransmitters in the brain

phobia: a strong, persistent, and unwarranted fear of a specific object or situation

selective serotonin reuptake inhibitors (SSRIs): primary medications used for obsessive-compulsive disorder

Tourette's syndrome: a childhood disorder characterized by several motor and verbal tics that may develop into the compulsion to shout obscenities

tricyclics: medications used to relieve the symptoms of depression

Causes and Symptoms

Obsessive-compulsive disorder (OCD) is an anxiety disorder characterized by intrusive and uncontrollable thoughts and/or by the need to perform specific acts repeatedly. Obsessive-compulsive behavior is highly distressing because one's behavior or thoughts are no longer voluntarily controlled. The more frequently these uncontrolled alien and perhaps unacceptable thoughts or actions are performed, the more distress is induced. A disturbed individual may have either obsessions (which are thought-related) or compulsions (which are action-related), or both. At various stages of the disorder, one of the symptoms may replace the other.

OCD affects 1 to 2 percent of the population; most of those afflicted begin suffering from the disorder in early adulthood, and it is often preceded by a particularly stressful event such as pregnancy, childbirth, or family conflict. It may be closely associated with depression, with the disorder developing soon after a bout of depression or the depression developing as a result of the disorder. OCD affects men and women equally.

Obsessions generally fall into one of five recognized categories. Obsessive doubts are persistent doubts that a task has been completed; the individual is unwilling to accept and believe that the work is done satisfactorily. Obsessive thinking is an almost infinite chain of thought, targeting future events. Obsessive impulses are very strong urges to perform certain actions, whether they be trivial or serious, that would likely be harmful to the obsessive person or someone else and that are socially unacceptable. Obsessive fears are thoughts that the person has lost control and will act in some way that will cause public embarrassment. Obsessive images are continued visual pictures of either a real or an imagined event.

Four factors are commonly associated with obsessive characteristics, not only in people with OCD but in the general population as well. First, obsessive individuals are unable to control their mental processes completely. Practically, this means the loss of control over thinking processes, such as intrusive thoughts of a loved one dying or worries about hurting someone unintentionally. Second, there may be thoughts and worries over the potential loss of motor control, perhaps causing impulses such as shouting obscenities in church or school or performing inappropriate sexual acts. Third, many obsessive individuals may be afraid of contamination and suffer irrational fear and worry over exposure to germs, dirt, or diseases. The last factor is checking behavior, or backtracking previous actions to ensure that the behavior was done properly, such as checking that doors and windows are shut, faucets are turned off, and so on. Some common obsessions are fear of having decaying teeth or food particles between the teeth, worry about whether the sufferer has touched germs, and fear of contracting a sexually transmitted disease.

Compulsions may be either mild or severe and debilitating. Mild compulsions might be superstitions, such as refusing to walk under a ladder or throwing salt over one's shoulder. Severe compulsions become fixed, unvaried ritu-

Information on Obsessive-Compulsive Disorder

Causes: Psychological factors; may involve physical defects, genetics, or biochemical disorders

Symptoms: Excessive repetitive behavior, anxiety, depression, intrusive and uncontrollable thoughts, irrational fears, checking behavior

Duration: Often chronic with acute episodes

Treatments: Psychotherapy, drug therapy

alized behaviors; if they are not practiced precisely in a particular manner or a prescribed number of times, then intense anxiety may result. These strange behaviors may be rooted in superstition; many of those suffering from the disorder believe that performing the behavior may ward off danger. Compulsive acts are not ends in themselves but are "necessary" to produce or prevent a future event from occurring. Although the enactment of the ritual may assuage tension, the act does not give the compulsive pleasure.

Several kinds of rituals are typically enacted. A common ritual is repeating; these sufferers must do everything by numbers. Checking is another compulsive act; a compulsive checker believes that it is necessary to check and recheck that everything is in order. Cleaning is a behavior in which many compulsives must engage; they may wash and scrub repeatedly, especially if they think that they have touched something dirty. A fourth common compulsive action is avoidance; for certain superstitious or magical reasons, certain objects must be avoided. Some individuals with compulsions experience compelling urges for perfection in even the most trivial of tasks; often the task is repeated to ensure that it has been done correctly. Some determine that objects must be in a particular arrangement; these individuals are considered "meticulous." A few sufferers are hoarders; they are unable to throw away trash or rubbish. All these individuals have a constant need for reassurance; for example, they want to be told repeatedly that they have not been contaminated.

No single cause for OCD has been isolated. Several theories provide some examples of attempts to explain the basis of OCD psychologically. They involve guilt, anxiety, and superstition. Sigmund Freud first proposed that obsessive thoughts are a replacement for more disturbing thoughts or actions that induce guilt in the sufferer. These thoughts or behaviors, according to Freud, are usually sexual in nature. Freud based his ideas on the cases of some of his young patients. In the case of a teenage girl, for example, he determined that she exchanged obsessive thoughts of stealing for the act of masturbation. The thoughts of stealing produced far fewer guilt feelings than masturbation did. Replacing guilt feelings with less threatening thoughts prevents one's personal defenses from being overwhelmed. Other defense mechanisms may be parlayed into OCD. Undoing, one of these behaviors, is obliterating guilt-producing urges by undergoing repetitive rituals, such as handwashing. Since the forbidden urges continue to recur, the behavior to replace those urges must continue. These behaviors are then negatively reinforced because anxiety decreases when the behavior is performed, thereby maintaining the behavior. Another mechanism is reaction formation. When an unacceptable thought or urge is present, the sufferer replaces it with an exactly opposite behavior. Many theorists believe that both obsessive and compulsive behaviors arise as a consequence of overly harsh toilet training. Thus the person is fixated at the anal stage and, by reaction formation, resists the urge to soil by becoming overly neat and clean. A third mechanism is isolation, the separation of a thought or action from its effect. Detachment or aloofness may isolate an individual from aggressive or sexual thoughts.

The superstition hypothesis proposes a connection between a chance association and a reinforcer that induces a continuation of the behavior. Many theorists believe that the same sequence is involved in the formation of many superstitions. A particular obsessive-compulsive ritual may be reinforced when a positive outcome follows the behavior; anxiety results when the ritual is interrupted. An example would be a student who only uses one special pencil or pen to take exams, based on a previous good grade. In actuality, there is seldom a real relationship between the behavior and the outcome. This hypothesis, too, fails to explain the development of obsessions.

Another theory is accepted by those who believe that mental disorders are the result of something physically or physiologically amiss in the sufferer, employing data from brain structure studies, genetics, and biochemistry. Indeed, brain activity is altered in those suffering from OCD, and they experience increased metabolic activity. Whether the activity is a cause or an effect, however, is unclear. Studies of genetics in families, at least in twins, reinforce the idea that genetics may play a small role in OCD because there appears to be a higher incidence of the disorder in identical twins than in other siblings. Yet these results may be misleading: Because all the studies were carried out on twins who were reared together, environment must also be considered as a contributing cause. It should be noted, however, that relatives of OCD sufferers are twice as likely as unrelated individuals to develop the same disorder, indicating that the tendency for the behavior could be heritable.

Treatment and Therapy

Obsessional symptoms are not uncommon in the general population. While many people have been diagnosed with OCD, others are too horrified to admit to their symptoms, or they do not realize that their behavior is abnormal and do not seek treatment.

Diagnostic techniques evaluating OCD usually involve psychological evaluation. It is important to determine whether an individual is actually suffering from OCD or other potential problems such as schizophrenia or a mood disorder. Additionally, it is important to determine whether more than one disorder is present. OCD may occur in conjunction with other disorders, such as substance use disorders, eating disorders, and mood disorders. When this occurs, treatment must be adjusted. For example, when

depression is also noted, both disorders must be treated.

In cases when differentiation is required between OCD and schizophrenia, the concern is to understand the nature of the dysfunctional thoughts and behaviors. For instance, a distinction can be made by determining the motive behind the ritualized behavior. Stereotyped behaviors are symptomatic of both disorders. In the person with schizophrenia, however, the behavior is triggered by delusions rather than by true compulsions. People suffering from true delusions cannot be shaken from them. They do not resist the ideas inundating their minds, and ritualized behavior does not necessarily decrease the feelings associated with the intrusive ideas. On the other hand, obsessive people usually experience decreases in anxiety when they perform their rituals and may be absolutely certain of the need to perform their rituals, though other aspects of their thinking and logic are perfectly clear. They generally resist the ideas that enter their minds and realize the absurdity or abnormality of the thoughts to some extent. As thoughts and images intrude into the obsessive person's mind, the person may sometimes appear to have symptoms that mimic schizophrenia.

Other problems having symptoms in common with OCD are Tourette syndrome and stimulant use. What seems to separate the symptoms of these disorders from those experienced with OCD is that the former are organically induced. Thus, the actions of a sufferer from Tourette syndrome may be mechanical since they are not intellectually dictated or purposely enacted. In the case of the stimulant user, the acts may bring pleasure and are not resisted, but reinforced by the drug effects.

"Normal" people also have obsessive thoughts; in fact, the obsessions of normal individuals are not significantly different from the obsessions of those with OCD. The major difference is that those with the disorder have longer-lasting, more intense, and less easily dismissed obsessive thoughts. The importance of this overlap is that mere symptoms are not a reliable tool to diagnose OCD, since some of the same symptoms are experienced by the general population.

Assessment of OCD separates the obsessive from the compulsive components so that each can be examined. Obsession assessment should determine the triggering fears of the disorder, both internal and external, including thoughts of unpleasant consequences. The amount of anxiety that these obsessions produce should be monitored. The compulsive behaviors then should be examined in the same light.

The greatest chance for successful treatment occurs with individuals who experience mild symptoms that are usually obsessive but not compulsive in nature, who seek help soon after the onset of symptoms, and who had few problems before the disorder began. While OCD can be challenging to treat, many valuable and successful treatment strategies are available. Types of treatment fall into four categories: psychotherapy, behavioral therapy, drug therapy, and psychosurgery. The treatments of choice tend to be behavioral and drug therapies.

When psychotherapy is attempted, it usually begins with some type of analysis. The degree of dysfunction, the stressor triggering the symptoms, and the psychological makeup of the individual often determine whether the analysis will be successful. The major goal of a more psychoanalytical approach is to find and then remove an assumed repression so that the individual can deal with whatever they fear in an open and honest fashion. Some analysts believe that focusing on the present is most beneficial, since delving into the past may strengthen the defensive mechanism (the compulsive behavior). If the patient attempts to "return" to the mitigating event, then the analyst usually intervenes directly and actively and brings the individual back to the present by encouraging, pressuring, and guiding him or her.

The most effective treatment for controlling OCD is the behavioral approach. Behavioral therapy focuses on breaking the connection between the stimulus (what induces the compulsion or obsession) and the compulsions and obsessions. Response prevention involves two stages. First, the individual is subject to flooding, the act of exposing the individual to the real and/or imagined stimuli that cause anxiety. This process begins with brief exposure to the stressors while the therapist assesses the individuals's thoughts, feelings, and behaviors during the stimulus period. In the second stage, the individual is flooded with the stimuli but restrained from acting on those stressors. Although flooding may produce intense discomfort at first, patients are gradually desensitized to the stimuli, causing the resulting anxiety to decrease. The therapist must expend considerable time preventing the response, discussing the anxiety as it appears, and supporting the person as the anxiety abates. To be more effective, treatment may also occur in the home with the guidance and support of family members who have been informed about how best to interact with the person needing treatment. Therapists may also help the person break the connection between triggers and responses by aiding the individual in replacing the symptoms of the obsession or compulsion with healthier preventive or replacement actions. Similarly, aversive methods may be used to break the chain of behavior. They might include a nonvocal, internal shout of "Stop!" The action of snapping a rubber band on the wrist when the obsessive thoughts enter the mind or physically restraining oneself if the compulsive action begins may also be helpful. This latter approach may be so uncomfortable and disconcerting to the patient that it may work only under the supervision supplied by a hospital. With any of these approaches, however, if the individual is also depressed or has other complicating conditions, then successful treatment will require additional steps.

Drugs commonly used to treat OCD that have met with some success include selective serotonin reuptake inhibitors (SSRIs), antidepressants, tricyclics, monoamine oxidase inhibitors, LSD, and tryptophan. SSRIs often have remarkable effects on OCD, helping individuals to experience a change in their thinking and behavior, as well as relief. They are usually the first line of treatment in addressing OCD through drug therapy. Psychiatrists also may prescribe tranquilizers to reduce the client's anxiety; however, these drugs are usually not adequate to depress the frequent obsessive thoughts or compulsive actions and so are not a treatment of choice. More general antidepressants may benefit those suffering from depression as well as OCD. It has also been observed that as depression lifts, some of the compulsive behavior may also decrease. Monoamine oxidase inhibitors (MAOIs), another form of antidepressants, are used in treating

OCD associated with panic attacks, phobias, and severe anxiety. When medication is halted, however, the patient often relapses into the previous obsessive-compulsive state, so these too are not necessarily a treatment of choice. Drugs such as tryptophan may provide some relief through its affects on melatonin. Similarly, LSD and other hallucinogenic drugs have been tested as potential treatments for this condition because of their effects on serotonin receptors; however, their status as illicit drugs and the significant side effects from other aspects of the actions of these substances do not make them practically useful.

Some psychosurgeons may resort to psychosurgery to relieve a patient's symptoms. The improvement noted after surgery may simply be attributable to the loss of emotion and dulling of behavioral patterns found in any patient who has undergone a lobotomy. Because such surgery may result in a change in the patient's intellect and emotional response, it should be considered only in extreme, debilitating cases. Newer surgical techniques do not destroy as much of the cerebral cortex. These procedures separate the frontal cortex from lower brain areas in only an 8-centimeter square area.

Perspective and Prospects

Descriptions of OCD-like behavior go back to medieval times; a young man who could not control his urge to stick out his tongue or blurt out obscenities during prayer was reported in the fifteenth century. Medical accounts of the disorder and the term "obsessive-compulsive" originated in the mid-nineteenth century. At that time, obsessions were believed to occur when mental energy ran low. Later, Freud stated that OCD is accompanied by stubbornness, stinginess, and tidiness. He attributed the characteristics to a regression to early childhood, when there are perhaps strong urges to be violent and/or to dirty and mess one's surroundings. To avoid acting on these tendencies, he theorized, an avoidance mechanism is employed, and the symptoms of obsession and/or compulsion appear. Other features related to this regression are ambivalence, magical thinking, and a harsh, punitive conscience.

An unpleasant consequence of OCD behavior is the effect that the behavior has on the people who interact with the sufferer. The relationships with an obsessive person's family, schoolmates, or coworkers all suffer when a person with OCD takes up time with uncontrollable and lengthy rituals. These people may feel not only a justifiable concern but also resentment. Some may feel guilt over the resentful feelings because they know the obsessive-compulsive cannot control these actions. An obsessive-compulsive observing these conflicting feelings in others may respond by developing depression or other anxious feelings, which may cause further alienation.

Although not totally disabling, OCD behaviors can be strongly incapacitating. A famous figure who suffered from OCD was millionaire and aviator Howard Hughes (1905-1976). A recluse after 1950, he became so withdrawn from the public that he communicated only via telephone and intermediaries. His obsession-compulsion was the irrational fear of germs and contamination. It began with his refusal to shake hands with people. If he had to hold a glass or open a door, he covered his hand with a tissue. He would not abide any of his aides eating foods that gave them bad breath. He disallowed air conditioners, believing that they collected germs. Because Hughes acted on his obsessions, they became compulsions.

Most parents will agree that children commonly have rituals to which they must adhere or compulsive actions they carry out. A particular bedtime story may be read every night for months on end, and children's games involve counting or checking rituals. It is also not atypical for adults without psychiatric disorders to experience some mild obsessive thoughts or compulsive actions, as seen in an overly tidy person or in group rituals performed in some religious sects. Excessively stressful events may trigger obsessions as well.

Further research into the biopsychosocial causes of OCD will be important in developing future treatment approaches. Such causes and treatment may also be useful for understanding other behaviors that have compulsive features, such as problems related to substance use, gambling, eating, and sexual behavior.

—Iona C. Baldridge;
updated by Nancy A. Piotrowski, Ph.D.

See also Addiction; Anorexia nervosa; Antianxiety drugs; Anxiety; Bipolar disorders; Bulimia; Depression; Eating disorders; Grief and guilt; Neurosis; Panic attacks; Paranoia; Phobias; Post-traumatic stress disorder; Psychiatric disorders; Psychiatry; Psychiatry, child and adolescent; Psychiatry, geriatric; Psychoanalysis; Schizophrenia; Stress; Tics.

For Further Information:

American Psychiatric Association. *Diagnostic and Statistical Manual of Mental Disorders: DSM-5.* 5th ed. Arlington, Va.: Author, 2013.

Barlow, David H. *Anxiety and Its Disorders.* 2d ed. New York: Guilford Press, 2004.

Barlow, David H., ed. *Clinical Handbook of Psychological Disorders.* 4th ed. New York: Guilford Press, 2008.

Kring, Ann M., et al. *Abnormal Psychology.* 12th ed. Hoboken, N.J.: John Wiley & Sons, 2012.

McCoy, Krisha, and Michael Woods. "Obsessive-Compulsive Personality Disorder." *Health Library*, Sept. 30, 2012.

Menzies, Ross, and Padmal de Silva, eds. *Obsessive Compulsive Disorder: Theory, Research, and Treatment.* New York: Wiley, 2003.

"Obsessive-Compulsive Disorder." *MedlinePlus*, Apr. 11, 2013.

"Obsessive-Compulsive Disorder: When Unwanted Thoughts Take Over." *National Institute of Mental Health*, 2010.

Oltmanns, Thomas F., et al. *Case Studies in Abnormal Psychology.* 9th ed. Hoboken, N.J.: John Wiley & Sons, 2012.

Scholten, Amy, and Brian Randall. "Obsessive-Compulsive Disorder." *Health Library*, Sept. 10, 2012.

"What You Need to Know about Obsessive-Compulsive Disorder." *International OCD Foundation*, 2012.

Obstetrics

Specialty

Anatomy or system affected: Reproductive system, uterus

Specialties and related fields: Embryology, genetics, gynecology, neonatology, perinatology

Definition: The medical science dealing with pregnancy and childbirth, including the health of both mother and unborn infant and the delivery of the child and the placenta at the time of birth.

Key terms:

amniocentesis: a technique by which a fine needle is inserted through a pregnant woman's abdomen and into the uterus and amniotic sac in order to collect fetal amniotic cells for biochemical and genetic analysis

birth defect: a genetic or developmental abnormality which occurs in utero that leads to anatomic or functional problems after birth; the defect can be serious, with potentially significant consequences for the fetus or mother, or the defect can be minor

cesarean section: a surgical procedure whereby the infant is delivered through an incision on the mother's abdomen

forceps: curved metal blades that are carefully placed around the fetal head through the vagina to facilitate delivery

gestation: the period from conception to birth, in which the fetus reaches full development in order to survive outside the mother's body

placenta: an organ in the uterus through which the fetus receives its oxygen and nutrients and removes its waste products; it serves as a blood barrier between the mother's circulatory system and the fetal circulatory system

Rh0(D) immune globulin: also known as RhoGAM; a type of gamma globulin protein injected into Rh-negative mothers who may have an Rh-positive fetus to protect the fetus from an immune reaction called isoimmunization

trimester: one of three periods of time in pregnancy, each period lasting three months; the first trimester is zero to twelve weeks of gestational age, the second trimester is thirteen to twenty-four weeks of gestational age, and the third trimester is twenty-five to thirty-seven weeks of gestational age

ultrasonography: an imaging modality in which sound waves penetrate bodily tissues in order to generate an image; in obstetrics, this technique is commonly used to assess the fetus, amniotic fluid, and uterus and ovaries

vacuum: a device with a suction cup that is applied to the fetal head through the vagina to assist in delivery of the infant

Science and Profession

Obstetrics is the branch of medical science dealing with pregnancy and childbirth in women. Once conception has occurred and a woman is pregnant, major physiological changes occur within her body as well as within the body of the developing embryo or fetus. Obstetrics deals with these changes leading up to and including childbirth. As such, obstetrics is a critical branch of medicine, for it involves the complex physiological events by which every person comes into existence.

The professional obstetrician is a licensed medical doctor whose area of expertise is pregnancy and childbirth. Often, the obstetrician is also a specialist in the closely related science of gynecology, the study of diseases and conditions that specifically affect women, particularly nonpregnant women. The obstetrician is especially knowledgeable in female anatomy and physiology, including the major bodily changes that occur during and following pregnancies. Obstetricians also have a detailed understanding of the necessary diagnostic procedures for monitoring fetal and maternal health, and they are educated in the latest technologies for facilitating a successful pregnancy and childbirth with minimal complications. Obstetrical care is also provided by certified nurse midwives (CNMs) and by nurse practitioners, particularly those with certification in women's health (women's health care nurse practitioners).

Broadly, the diseases and conditions managed by the clinicians in this field include preconception counseling, normal prenatal care, and the management of pregnancy-specific problems such as preeclampsia, gestational diabetes, premature labor, premature rupture of membranes, multiple gestations, fetal growth problems, and isoimmunization. In addition, obstetricians manage medical problems that can occur in any woman but that take on special importance in pregnancy, such as thyroid disorders or infections. Obstetricians make assessments and decisions regarding when a baby is best delivered, particularly if there are in utero conditions that make it safer for the baby to be born immediately, even if prematurely. Obstetricians manage both normal and abnormal labors. They are able to assess the progress and position of the infant as it makes its way down the birth canal. They are knowledge-

able about pain control options during labor and make decisions regarding when a cesarean section is indicated. Obstetricians assist with normal vaginal deliveries, either spontaneous or induced, and sometimes use special instruments such as forceps or vacuum-suction devices. They also perform cesarean sections. Obstetricians are trained in appropriate postpartum care for the mother and infant.

In natural, spontaneous fertilization, pregnancy begins with the fertilization of a woman's egg by a man's sperm following sexual intercourse, the chances of which are highest if intercourse takes place during a two-day period following ovulation. Ovulation is the release of an unfertilized egg from the woman's ovarian follicle, which occurs roughly halfway between successive periods during her menstrual cycle. Fertilization usually occurs in the upper one-third of one of the woman's fallopian tubes connecting the ovary to the uterus; upon entering the woman's vagina, sperm must travel through her cervix to the uterus and up the fallopian tubes, only one of which contains a released egg following ovulation.

Once fertilization has occurred, the first cell of the new individual, called a zygote, is slowly pushed by cilia down the fallopian tube and into the uterus. Along the way, the zygote undergoes several mitotic cellular divisions to begin the newly formed embryo, which at this point is a bundle of undifferentiated cells. Upon reaching the uterus, the embryo implants in the lining of the uterus. Hormonal changes occur in the woman's body to maintain the pregnancy. One of these hormones is human chorionic gonadotropin, which is the chemical detected by most pregnancy tests. Failure of the embryo to be implanted in the endometrium and subsequent lack of hormone production (specifically the hormone progesterone) will cause release of the endometrium as a bloody discharge; the woman will menstruate, and there will be no pregnancy. Therefore, menstrual cycles do not occur during a pregnancy.

The embryo will grow and develop over the next nine to ten months of gestation. The heart forms and begins beating at roughly five and one-half weeks following conception. Over the next several weeks and months, major organ systems begin to organize and develop. By the end of the first three months of the pregnancy, the developing human is considered to be a fetus. All the major organ systems have formed, although not all systems can function yet. The fetus is surrounded by a watery amniotic fluid within an amniotic sac. The fetus receives oxygen and nutrients from the mother and excretes waste products into the maternal circulation through the placenta. The fetus is connected to the placenta via the umbilical cord. During the second and third trimesters, full organ system development; massive cell divisions of certain tissues such as nervous, circulatory, and skeletal tissue; and preparation of the fetus for survival as an independent organism occur. The fetus

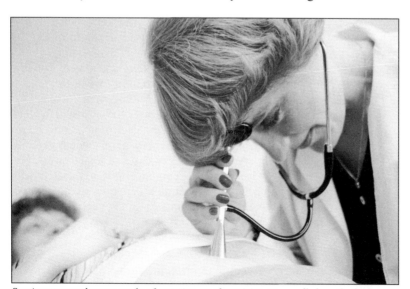

Starting at around twenty weeks of gestation, an obstetrician can usually hear the fetal heartbeat using a special stethoscope called a fetoscope. (PhotoDisc)

cannot survive outside the mother's body, however, until the third trimester.

Changes also occur in the mother. Increased levels of the female steroid hormone estrogen create increased skin vascularization (that is, more blood vessels near the skin) and the deposition of fat throughout her body, especially in the breasts and the buttocks. The growing fetus and stretching uterus press on surrounding abdominal muscles, often creating abdominal and back discomfort. Reasonable exercise is important for the mother to stay healthy and to deliver the baby with relative ease. A balanced diet also is important for the nourishment of her body and that of the fetus.

Late in the pregnancy, the protein hormones prolactin and oxytocin will be produced by the woman's pituitary gland. Prolactin activates milk production in the breasts. Oxytocin causes muscular contractions, particularly in the breasts and in the uterus during labor. Near the time of birth, drastically elevated levels of the hormones estrogen and oxytocin will cause progressively stronger contractions (labor pains) until the baby is forced through the vagina and out of the woman's body to begin its independent physical existence. The placenta, or afterbirth, is discharged shortly thereafter.

Diagnostic and Treatment Techniques

The role of the obstetrician is to monitor the health of the mother and unborn fetus during the course of the pregnancy and to deliver the baby successfully at the time of birth. Once the fact of the pregnancy is established, the obstetrician is trained to identify specific developmental changes in the fetus over time in order to ensure that the pregnancy is proceeding smoothly.

The mainstay of diagnosis is the physical examination during prenatal visits. Early in the pregnancy, prenatal visits occur monthly, but they become more frequent as the pregnancy progresses. During these visits, the woman may receive counseling regarding a balanced diet, folic acid and iron supplementation, and substances or foods to avoid that may pose a risk to the pregnancy. The woman's growing uterus is measured to confirm proper growth, and, if indicated, a vaginal or cervical examination may be performed. After ten weeks of gestational age, fetal heart tones are also assessed at every prenatal visit using a simplified ultrasonic technique, to ensure that they are within the normal number of beats per minute. Fetal heart tones that are abnormally slow may indicate a fetus in jeopardy.

The other main component of diagnosis is through laboratory tests. Early in the pregnancy, the woman will receive a Pap test to screen for cervical cancer. Blood tests will be ordered to determine whether the mother is a carrier of the human immunodeficiency virus (HIV) or hepatitis B or C viruses, which can be transmitted to the fetus. In addition, the mother is checked for anemia, and the blood type of the mother is assessed. If the mother's blood type indicates that she is Rh negative, she will receive RhoGAM in the third trimester to prevent the development of a disease called isoimmunization, a condition that could be fatal to the fe-

tus. An additional diagnostic test performed routinely during pregnancy is a screening test for diabetes, which pregnant women are at increased risk for.

Another important method of diagnosis in obstetrics is ultrasonography. Ultrasonography early in pregnancy can determine the gestational age of a pregnancy in cases in which a woman's last menstrual period is unverified. The correct development of the fetus and the presence of any birth defects can be assessed using this procedure. Ultrasound can also determine whether the placenta is growing in a safe location and whether the proper amount of amniotic fluid is found in the amniotic sac. Toward the end of pregnancy, ultrasound is an invaluable diagnostic tool for determining fetal well-being and the position of the infant in the uterus in preparation for delivery. Ultrasound is also a useful tool in guiding diagnostic procedures. For instance, amniocentesis can be extremely safe when performed under ultrasound guidance. Finally, one of the main methods of diagnosis in the third trimester is fetal heart monitoring. This technique involves following the heartbeat of the infant while in utero.

The heart rate of the infant is typically followed for twenty to thirty minutes. Any concerning dips in the heart rate may be indicative of a poor fetal state and a cause for increased monitoring or, in extreme cases, delivery of the infant.

Obstetricians have at their disposal a variety of treatment modalities. They are trained to turn manually fetuses that are in a breech (feet-first) position, a procedure called external cephalic version. In cases where the artificial induction of labor is desirable, the obstetrician may employ mechanical or hormonal means of cervical dilation, followed by infusions of a hormone called pitocin to stimulate contractions or the artificial rupture of the amniotic sac to promote natural contractions. When immediate delivery of the infant is needed and the chances of it emerging via the vaginal route are remote, then the obstetrician may perform a cesarean section. Common indications for cesarean section include fetal distress and lack of progress in labor.

Other treatments commonly used by obstetricians include the use of medications such as magnesium to relax the uterus in cases of premature labor and maternal steroid injections to induce fetal lung maturity when the fetus is premature but delivery is anticipated. When a woman experiences difficulty in the final stages of labor and the fetal head has descended almost to the vaginal opening, the obstetrician may employ forceps or vacuum devices to facilitate the delivery, particularly in cases of fetal distress. Obstetricians also treat the complications associated with childbirth, including postsurgical care after a cesarean section and repair of any lacerations of the vagina, cervix, or rectum after vaginal delivery.

Perspective and Prospects

Obstetrics is central to medicine because it deals with the very process by which all humans come to exist. The health of the fetus and its mother in pregnancy is of primary concern to these doctors. The field of obstetrics has blossomed as a sophisticated specialty, more likely to be practiced by obstetricians, certified nurse midwives, and specially trained and certified nurse practitioners, rather than the general practitioners who used to provide this care.

Advances in medical technology have enabled more precise analysis and monitoring of the fetus inside the mother's uterus, and obstetrics has therefore become a complex specialty in its own right. Technology such as ultrasonography and fetal heart rate monitoring, among other techniques, allows the obstetrician to collect a much larger supply of fetal data than was available to the general practitioner of the 1960s. Increased data availability enables the obstetrician to monitor the pregnancy closely and to identify any problems earlier.

New advances in product development continue to improve the diagnostic ability of obstetricians. One example is the development of a test for fetal fibronection, which enables obstetricians to predict which patients are at low risk of premature delivery. This test involves a simple swab of the upper vagina. When negative, this test is highly reliable and allows the pregnant patient to leave the hospital and avoid prolonged and unnecessary hospitalization.

Advances in prenatal diagnosis and basic science have made it possible for parents to obtain information about their fetuses down to the molecular level. Through techniques such as amniocentesis and chorionic villus sampling (in which a small sample of placental cells is obtained early in pregnancy), genetic analysis has enabled the detection of chromosomal defects responsible for mental retardation and single-gene defects responsible for inherited diseases (such as cystic fibrosis). Amniocentesis has also made it possible to detect biochemical changes that may be indicative of major structural defects in the fetus, as well as to assess the developmental maturity of organs such as the lungs.

Advances in medical practice have dramatically decreased the morbidity and mortality of premature birth. For instance, with the introduction and widespread use of maternal steroid injections, the severity of serious diseases of prematurity, such as respiratory distress syndrome, has been dramatically reduced. The development of drugs against HIV has prevented the transmission of the virus from mother to infant in many cases.

The medical science of obstetrics continues to advance. There is ongoing research into the physiology and basic science of preeclampsia and eclampsia, common and potentially dangerous diseases peculiar to pregnancy. Fetal surgery programs at academic centers open the possibility that serious birth defects may be correctable while the fetus is in utero. Although many controversies currently exist in the field of obstetrics, an increased push toward medical practice grounded in scientific evidence promises many exciting advances in the future. It is hoped that many of these advances will result in improved outcomes and quality of life for patients.

—*David Wason Hollar, Jr., Ph.D.;*
updated by Anne Lynn S. Chang, M.D.

See also Amniocentesis; Assisted reproductive technologies; Birth defects; Breast-feeding; Breasts, female; Cesarean section; Child-birth; Childbirth complications; Chorionic villus sampling; Conception; Congenital disorders; Critical care; Down syndrome; Ectopic pregnancy; Embryology; Emergency medicine; Episiotomy; Family medicine; Fetal alcohol syndrome; Fetal surgery; Gamete intrafallopian transfer (GIFT); Genetic counseling; Genetic diseases; Genital disorders, female; Gestational diabetes; Gonorrhea; Growth; Gynecology; In vitro fertilization; Incontinence; Miscarriage; Multiple births; Neonatology; Ovaries; Pap test; Perinatology; Placenta; Postpartum depression; Preeclampsia and eclampsia; Pregnancy and gestation; Premature birth; Reproductive system; Rh factor; Rubella; Spina bifida; Stillbirth; Teratogens; Toxoplasmosis; Ultrasonography; Urology; Uterus; Women's health.

For Further Information:

American College of Obstetricians and Gynecologists. *American College of Obstetricians and Gynecologists*, 2013.

Cohen, Barbara J. *Memmler's The Human Body in Health and Disease*. 11th ed. Philadelphia: Wolters Kluwer Health/Lippincott Williams & Wilkins, 2009.

Doyle, Kathryn. "Midwife-Led Care Linked to Fewer Premature Births." Reuters Health Information. *MedlinePlus*, August 28, 2013.

Gabbe, Steven G., Jennifer R. Niebyl, and Joe Leigh Simpson, eds. *Obstetrics: Normal and Problem Pregnancies*. 6th ed. Philadelphia: Saunders, 2012.

Gaudin, Anthony J., and Kenneth C. Jones. *Human Anatomy and Physiology*. New York: Harcourt Brace Jovanovich, 1997.

Harkness, Gail, ed. *Medical-Surgical Nursing: Total Patient Care*. 10th ed. St. Louis, Mo.: Mosby, 1999.

Limmer, Daniel, et al. *Emergency Care*. 12th ed. Boston: Brady, 2012.

MedlinePlus. "Childbirth." *MedlinePlus*, August 13, 2013.

MedlinePlus. "Pregnancy." *MedlinePlus*, August 29, 2013.

Vorvick, Linda J. "Certified Nurse-Midwife." *MedlinePlus*, September 12, 2011.

Vorvick, Linda J. "Choosing the Right Health Care Provider for Pregnancy and Childbirth." *MedlinePlus*, August 23, 2012.

Wallace, Robert A., Gerald P. Sanders, and Robert J. Ferl. *Biology: The Science of Life*. 4th ed. New York: HarperCollins, 1996.

Occupational health

Specialty

Anatomy or system affected: All

Specialties and related fields: Environmental health, epidemiology, internal medicine, preventive medicine, psychology, public health, pulmonary medicine, toxicology

Definition: The application of health care that focuses on injury and illness prevention and the treatment of injuries that can occur in the workplace or that result from a person's employment.

Science and Profession

The discovery that eighteenth-century chimney sweeps were prone to developing testicular cancer is often cited as the first example of an acknowledged occupational illness. In fact, physicians and other health care professionals had been aware for many centuries that certain jobs were linked to particular medical disorders: millers developed coughs, and hatmakers became mentally unbalanced. Textbooks urged physicians to consider a patient's occupation both in diagnosing and in treating illness. The emergence of occupational health as a distinct specialty within the medical professions is, however, a relatively recent phenomenon.

The Industrial Revolution brought with it not only the separation of one's home life from one's work life but also an increased risk of injury from factory machinery. Spinning jennies, power looms, mill wheels and belts, and early assembly line processes all carried the risk of accidental amputations, mangled limbs, and other permanently crippling injuries. Not surprisingly, much of the early emphasis of occupational health focused on safety. While company doctors treated the injured workers, engineers sought ways to reduce the job hazards.

By the twentieth century, several different but related specialties had evolved that focused on different aspects of occupational health. Industrial hygienists combine training in engineering and public health and attempt to improve safety in the workplace by providing education and training for workers and by redesigning the work area to eliminate hazards. Doctors of occupational medicine are employed by both government and industry to diagnose and to treat occupational illnesses and work-related disabilities. In addition to diagnosing and treating work-related injuries and illnesses, occupational health care providers may provide preemployment physical examinations, health screenings, and health promotion education and risk management programs based on occupational hazards and outcomes of trends of injuries or risks identified in the workplace. Public awareness of occupational health issues has led to the passage of legislation creating such agencies as the United States Occupational Safety and Health Administration (OSHA). All occupational health specialists in the United States must work within guidelines established by OSHA. There is a high cost to society from such disabilities as the black lung disease suffered by coal miners and the toxic or radioactive exposure experienced by workers ranging from hospital laboratory technicians to pipefitters and welders. As a result, occupational health has become an ever-expanding, complex, and important medical specialty.

Diagnostic and Treatment Techniques

Because occupational health problems can affect any part of the human anatomy, their diagnostic and treatment techniques are drawn from all areas of medical science. If a worker is injured on the job or suffers from an easily recognizable problem, such as a repetitive motion disorder, diagnosis and treatment can be quite straightforward. In the case of repetitive motion, problems such as carpal tunnel syndrome, which is sometimes experienced by word processing operators, might be treated by advising patients to change their work posture, providing them with splints to align the wrists and hands properly, employing corrective surgery to alleviate pain, and redesigning the work site to prevent future problems. The treatment for many on-the-job injuries will also include an extensive course of physical and rehabilitative therapy to allow the worker to return to work eventually, either at the old job or at a new one.

Many occupational health problems, however, are not as readily diagnosed as carpal tunnel syndrome. The industrial hygienist and the doctor of occupational medicine often must rely on the expertise of epidemiologists and toxicologists to determine the substances to which occupational exposure may be responsible for a worker's ill health. In cases in which workers complain of vague symptoms such as chronic fatigue, nausea, or neuropathy (loss of nerve function), an accurate diagnosis can prove elusive. The medical literature contains numerous examples of occupational illnesses that mimicked other common disorders. For example, doctors misdiagnosed a cosmetologist as suffering from multiple sclerosis (a degenerative disease of the central nervous system) when she was actually experiencing nerve damage caused by many years of exposure to the chemical solvents used to apply and remove artificial fingernails. Because many occupational illnesses can take years or even decades to appear, in some cases an accurate diagnosis may never be achieved. Once a diagnosis is made, treatment for an occupational illness caused by exposure to chemicals, for example, can be as simple as assigning the worker to tasks that eliminate exposure or as technologically sophisticated as using dialysis or chemical chelation to remove toxins from a patient's blood.

Perspective and Prospects

Occupational health is one of the most challenging specialties in modern medicine. Practitioners must combine skills and knowledge gleaned from a wide spectrum of related skills. The proliferation of technologically complex methods and materials in the workplace has resulted in occupational exposures and illnesses that were unknown until the twentieth century. At the time that occupational health first emerged as a distinct concern in the medical community, industrial hygiene focused almost exclusively on safety in the workplace. If the factory could be designed so that workers did not risk losing a limb whenever they operated machinery, the hygienist could feel a sense of accomplishment.

Workplace safety remains a concern in occupational health, but obvious hazards such as poorly lit work areas or exposed moving parts on machines have been joined by a host of subtler threats to workers' well-being. Epidemiologists and toxicologists have linked on-the-job exposure to dust, heavy metals, radiation, solvents and other chemicals, and even blood-borne pathogens to a host of cancers, disabling diseases, reproductive problems, and other concerns. Yet, not only must the industrial hygienist and doctor of occupational medicine worry about protecting workers from these physical hazards, but the modern occupational health specialist must also be concerned with the long-term effects of repetitive motions, noise exposures, and even emotional stress. As the influence of workers' jobs on those workers' health and on the health of their families is recognized as a major factor in a family's overall well-being, the importance of the occupational health specialist becomes increasingly obvious within modern society. Occupational health specialists employed in government, industry, and private practice, each approaching the question of worker wellness from a slightly different perspective, all fill a vital and expanding niche in modern medical practice.

The regulatory agency OSHA was created by Congress

in 1970 to ensure safe work environments free of hazards that could cause death or serious physical harm to employees. It has the authority to fine or charge employers who do not follow safety regulations. The National Institute of Occupational Safety and Health (NIOSH), also created in 1970, conducts research and advise OSHA on issues related to hazards in the workplace.

—Nancy Farm Mannikko, Ph.D.; updated by
Sharon W. Stark, R.N., A.P.R.N., D.N.Sc.

See also Allied health; Altitude sickness; Asbestos exposure; Asphyxiation; Biofeedback; Carcinogens; Cardiac rehabilitation; Carpal tunnel syndrome; Chronic obstructive pulmonary disease (COPD); Environmental diseases; Environmental health; Hearing loss; Interstitial pulmonary fibrosis (IPF); Law and medicine; Lead poisoning; Lung cancer; Lungs; Mesothelioma; Multiple chemical sensitivity syndrome; Nasopharyngeal disorders; Preventive medicine; Pulmonary diseases; Pulmonary medicine; Pulmonary medicine, pediatric; Radiation sickness; Skin disorders; Stress; Stress reduction; Tendon disorders; Tendon repair; Teratogens; Toxicology.

For Further Information:

Caplan, Robert D., et al. *Job Demands and Worker Health: Main Effects and Occupational Differences.* Ann Arbor: University of Michigan Press, 1980.

Cralley, Lester V., and Patrick R. Atkins, eds. *Industrial Environmental Health: The Worker and the Community.* 2d ed. New York: Academic Press, 1975.

Gatchel, Robert J., and Izabela Z. Schultz. *Handbook of Occupational Health and Wellness.* New York: Springer, 2012.

Guzik, Arlene. *Essentials for Occupational Health Nursing.* Malden: Wiley-Blackwell, 2013.

Koren, Herman. *Illustrated Dictionary and Resource Directory of Environmental and Occupational Health.* 2d ed. Boca Raton, Fla.: CRC Press, 2005.

Levy, Barry S., et al., eds. *Occupational Health: Recognizing and Preventing Disease and Injury.* 5th ed. Philadelphia: Lippincott Williams & Wilkins, 2006.

Morgan, Monroe T. *Environmental Health.* 3d ed. Belmont, Calif.: Thomson/Wadsworth, 2003.

Sadhra, Steven S., and Krishna G. Rampal, eds. *Occupational Health: Risk Assessment and Management.* Malden, Mass.: Blackwell Scientific, 1999.

Sellers, Christopher C. *Hazards of the Job: From Industrial Disease to Environmental Health Science.* Chapel Hill: University of North Carolina Press, 1999..

Smedley, Julia, et al., eds. *Oxford Handbook of Occupational Health.* 2d ed. Oxford: Oxford University Press, 2012.

World Health Organization. "Occupational Health." http://www.who.int/occupational_health/en.

Oncology

Specialty

Anatomy or system affected: All

Specialties and related fields: Critical care, cytology, general surgery, genetics, immunology, pathology, pharmacology, radiology

Definition: The study of cancer-its causes, its possible spread throughout and destruction of the body, and its medical treatment.

Key terms:

cancer: a tumorous growth of abnormal cells that invade other tissues, choke off available resources, and eventually destroy major organs and the organism

carcinogen: a chemical or radiation mutagen that causes changes in genes, leading to the cancerous state in a cell

cellular transformation: the process in which a cell becomes cancerous, which begins with abnormal changes in gene expression and cell differentiation

hormone: a chemical messenger, usually composed of protein or steroid, that controls the gene expression within target cells and thereby affects cellular development

mutagen: a chemical or an ionizing radiation that causes a change in the nucleotide sequence of the DNA of a gene, possibly affecting the gene's normal expression

mutation: a change in the nucleotide sequence of the DNA (that is, the genetic information) of a gene

oncogene: a gene within the chromosomes of all the cells of an individual organism that triggers cancerous cellular transformation when it is expressed incorrectly

protein kinase: an enzyme type that often is encoded by oncogenes; this enzyme attaches phosphate molecules to certain amino acids on specifically targeted proteins

tumor: an uncontrollable growth of cells within a tissue region that may be benign (noninvasive) or malignant (invasive cancer)

virus: an obligate intracellular parasite, composed of nucleic acid protected by a protein capsid, which reproduces inside cells

Science and Profession

Oncology is the scientific study and treatment of cancers, tumors, and other abnormal tissue growths. This field is an important part of medical science because of the prevalence of cancer within the human population, particularly in the progressively older populations of Western societies, in which people enjoy life-prolonging medical advances. Cancer ranks second only to heart disease as a killer of people in Western nations. Its victims number in the hundreds of thousands each year.

The study of cancer and its various physiological manifestations involves an understanding of several diverse biological disciplines, including genetics, developmental biology, embryology, neurology, endocrinology, and general physiology. The oncologist must synthesize information from these scientific fields in diagnosing, monitoring, and treating the disease. The oncologist works closely with the cancer patient's physician, surgeons, laboratory technicians, radiation therapists and chemotherapists, and pharmacists in treating cancerous tumors.

A tumor is an abnormal growth of cells within a specific tissue or organ beyond that tissue or organ's normal developmental pattern. Tumors may be either benign or malignant. Benign tumors are noninvasive; benign tumor cells multiply more rapidly than normal cells within a single, localized region that grows larger and larger. A benign tumor does not spread to other body regions. A malignant tumor, however, is invasive; it grows rapidly and uncontrollably. A malignant tumor is a cancer that consists of grotesquely aberrant cells that break off and are carried through the affected individual's bloodstream to other body regions, where they lodge and overcrowd or outcompete normal body cells.

Cells function normally as a result of the hormonal control of thousands of protein-encoding genes located on twenty-three pairs of chromosomes. The order of nucleotide nitrogen bases on a gene's deoxyribonucleic acid (DNA) polynucleotide chain serves as the genetic code. A change in the nucleotide sequence of DNA is called a mutation. A substance causing a mutation, which is called a mutagen, may be ionizing radiation (for example, ultraviolet light, x-rays, or gamma radiation) or a chemical. The DNA of a gene encodes ribonucleic acid (RNA), which encodes protein. Thus, an alteration in the nucleotide sequence of DNA, such as the replacement of a cytosine by an adenine nitrogen base, affects the messenger RNA nucleotide information sequence and, subsequently, the protein amino acid sequence. Proteins serve important structural, enzymatic, and hormonal roles within and between cells. A mutation within the DNA nucleotide sequence of a particular cellular gene affects the resulting protein encoded by that gene. Consequently, a variety of cellular functions are affected in sequence. In some cases, the cell is transformed into a cancerous state.

Mutagens that alter certain genes and then trigger cellular transformation into a cancerous state are called carcinogens. Only certain mutagens are carcinogens. An altered gene encodes a protein that has an incorrect amino acid sequence, thereby altering the normal functioning of the protein. An aberrant protein enzymatically or hormonally alters the functioning of other molecules within the cell, thereby directing the cell into the cancerous state.

The precise genes and proteins that are affected in transformed cells have not been identified completely. It appears that certain cancer-causing genes called oncogenes are involved, as well as certain oncogene-encoded enzymes called protein kinases. Protein kinases attach phosphate molecules to certain amino acids on certain cellular proteins, thereby altering the functioning of the proteins and triggering developmental changes within the cell. Certain viruses can also trigger these changes by activating oncogenes and protein kinases. The cell becomes cancerous as a result of these influences.

Diagnostic and Treatment Techniques

Oncologists must confront a variety of cancers that affect many different tissues. Common cancers affecting women include breast, colon, lung, uterine, ovarian, and lymphatic cancers, while common cancers affecting men include prostate, lung, colon, bladder, and lymphatic cancers. Oncologists must identify and treat these tumors as rapidly and as efficiently as possible.

The successful treatment of cancer begins with its early detection. The classic seven warning signs of cancer are a sore that does not heal, a lump on the body, a persistent cough, difficulty in swallowing, unusual bleeding, a change in a wart or mole, and a change in bladder or bowel movements. The presence of cancer in a patient can be identified by an oncologist by means of several techniques, including cytological (cellular) analysis, biopsy, and direct observation. Cytological techniques employ the microscopic examination of discarded cells from the suspected cancerous region. Biopsy involves the surgical removal of suspected cancerous tissue from an individual and the subsequent chemical and microscopic analysis of the removed tissue cells. Cancer cells are morphologically and chemically distinct from normal body cells.

Cancerous cell masses can be directly observed within the body by means of probing tubes that contain fiber-optic imaging devices and that can be inserted into body cavities. Such medical technology can visualize directly the trachea, bronchi, and larger bronchioles of the lungs; the esophagus and stomach; the colon and rectum; and the reproductive organ passageways, such as the vagina and cervix. Cancerous tumors also can be located via more elaborate techniques, such as computed tomography, magnetic resonance imaging, mammography, radioactive isotopes, x-rays, and ultrasound.

Computed tomography (CT) scanning is an enhanced x-ray survey of selected regions of the patient's body. The patient lies within the device, which rotates and x-rays around the patient, thereby generating a three-dimensional, computer-enhanced image of the tumor. Conventional x-rays can identify many tumors; however, computed tomography can penetrate deeper tissues with greater sensitivity. Mammography is an example of a regular x-ray treatment that utilizes low-energy x-rays beamed at a woman's breasts. Mammography is recommended every two years for women of age fifty or older with an average risk for breast cancer.

Similarly, the ingestion of certain radioactive isotopes such as iodine can be used to localize tumors. Certain elemental isotopes concentrate in specific body tissues and organs. The radioactive isotope concentrates in a particular tissue, the tissue is imaged, and any abnormal growths can be detected. Magnetic resonance imaging and ultrasound use magnetic fields and sound waves, respectively, to image interior tissues and abnormalities in tissue growth.

Once the presence of cancer and the type of cancer have been established, prompt treatment must ensue. The oncologist must determine the appropriate course of treatment. Surgical removal of the tumor may be possible. Radiotherapy and chemotherapy can be used in conjunction with, or instead of, surgery. Radiotherapy, or radiation therapy, involves the killing of the cancerous tumor through the use of a concentrated beam of ionizing radiation such as x-rays or gamma rays or an ingested radioactive isotope (such as cobalt 60) that will concentrate in the target cancerous tissue. Chemotherapy involves the internal administration of cytotoxic (cell-killing) chemicals to the patient; cancer cells are particularly susceptible to these chemicals.

Treatment for all forms of cancer involves combinations of chemotherapy and radiation therapy. Cancer cells are more sensitive to these treatments than are normal body cells, and they are killed more easily as a result. Early detection of cancer is critical to the success of such treatments. Accessible cancers, such as skin cancers, can be removed surgically or frozen.

Common chemicals used in cancer chemotherapy include alkylating agents, antimetabolites, antibiotics, plant alkaloids, human and synthetic hormones, and enzymes.

All these chemicals kill cells, especially cancer cells. Examples of alkylating agents are cisplatin for the treatment of testicular and ovarian cancers, cyclophosphamide for the treatment of breast and lymphatic cancers, and mechlorethamine for the treatment of Hodgkin's disease. A typical antimetabolite is 5-fluorouracil, which is used for the treatment of breast and colon cancer. Examples of antibiotics are mitomycin-C and actinomycin-D. Vincristine is a plant alkaloid that is used to treat leukemia. The human male hormone testosterone and the female hormone progesterone are both used to treat breast cancer, while the female hormone estrogen is used to treat prostate cancer.

Radiation therapies include concentrated beams of x-rays or gamma rays aimed at target cancerous tissues or the ingestion of specific radioactive isotopes that concentrate in target cancerous tissues. Both radiation and chemical therapies for cancer have numerous side effects, because normal cells are damaged as well as cancerous cells in both treatments. Such side effects include nausea, weakness, vomiting, diarrhea, loss of hair, and anemia.

In cases of certain tissue tumors and cancers, such as leukemia and bone cancer, tissue transplants from carefully matched individuals have been very effective in saving the lives of these cancer patients. The advent of molecular cloning and the use of tissue-specific viral gene vectors provide another avenue by which the oncologist will treat cancer in the future.

The oncologist's goals are to remove or kill the cancerous growth and to arrest its spread (metastasis) to other body tissues. The prevention of metastatic spreading is of critical importance, because the establishment of tumors in multiple body regions makes treatment much more difficult and patient death much more likely. Also, the oncologist must help the patient to cope psychologically with the disease and the possibility of dying.

Oncological research and the treatment of neoplastic (cancerous) tissues represent formidable tasks for medical science. Cancer is the number-two killer of Americans, and tumors are responsible for countless other ailments and millions of dollars of medical expenses. The use of surgery, cytotoxic chemical agents, and radiation to destroy or remove cancers has proven to be effective in saving thousands of lives.

Perspective and Prospects

Cancer is an increasing problem in Western societies, where medical science is increasing longevity and where industry and business place extraordinary levels of stress upon individuals. Most theories of aging maintain that accumulated genetic mutations in somatic cells during organismal development contribute to the breakdown of body systems, particularly the immune system. Aging is contained for much of an individual's life. Aging accelerates, however, following the end of an individual's period of reproduction. Although cancer can occur at any age, its probability of occurrence accelerates with aging.

Cancer cells are present in the bodies of all humans. Out of approximately 1,000 trillion cells within the human body, it is inevitable that mistakes will occur frequently within the gene regulation mechanisms of certain cells. Humans and other life-forms are exposed continuously to radiation and carcinogenic chemicals of varying types. A critical gene within a critical cell eventually will mutate so that the cell follows a cancerous pathway.

A healthy person with a strong immune system, however, quickly will destroy these mutated, transformed cancers. Individuals having weakened immune systems as a result of stress, aging, illness, and so forth are more susceptible to cancer because the mutated cells have the opportunity to multiply and spread rapidly throughout the body before the person's immune system can respond. Many scientists are beginning to identify aging and stress as diseases, and cancer as a symptom of these diseases.

As the body ages, more and more mutations accumulate, thereby increasing the probability that cancer cells will develop, survive, and multiply. At the same time, the aging immune system cannot respond to abnormal cells and infections as rapidly. Consequently, cancer cells elude the victim's immune system and spread to other body regions.

Evidence is implicating stress as a contributor to incidences of disease, illness, cancer, aging, and premature death in the human population. Stress causes abnormal elevations in nerve and endocrine (hormonal) systems that affect a tremendous variety of cellular and tissue-specific processes within the human body. Elevated levels of hormones for prolonged periods of time can permanently alter the gene expression of certain body tissues, causing these tissues to develop abnormally. Stress is a major problem in fast-paced, technological societies, and it is probably no coincidence that heart disease and cancer are the two principal killers of people in such societies.

Additionally, certain cancers may be infectious. In 1910, Peyton Rous determined that the Rous sarcoma virus, which infects chickens, can trigger cancerous tumors. Subsequent investigators corroborated Rous's findings, and nearly two dozen viruses have been identified that are capable of initiating cellular transformation in animals. Such oncogenic viruses either carry an oncogene or activate oncogenes in their host cells when they infect cells. All viruses must infect cells in order to reproduce. Some viruses can insert their genetic material into the host cell's DNA, thereby affecting the expression of host-cell genes at the viral insertion point; this may be one method of oncogenic viral cellular transformation into cancer. Among the oncogenic viruses that infect humans are hepatitis B; the papillomavirus, which also causes warts; and the Epstein-Barr virus. The Epstein-Barr virus usually causes infectious mononucleosis. In a region of western central Africa, however, humans develop a deadly lymph node cancer called Burkitt lymphoma when exposed to the virus-a phenomenon that has baffled oncologists.

Genetic damage caused by chemicals and radiation to which humans are exposed has a substantial effect upon the incidences of tumors and cancer. The link between ionizing radiation (for example, ultraviolet light or gamma radiation) and cancer has been established. The links between various chemicals and cancer are more difficult to sustain, however, often leading to controversies over the banning of certain substances and the health risks associated with contact with such substances (for example, saccharin or motor oil). The Ames test for chemical mutagens is a very effective assessment of whether a chemical is mutagenic; it was developed by biochemist Bruce Ames and his colleagues at the University of California, Berkeley, in the 1970s.

The problems posed by cancer are immense and will require decades of intense medical research. Advances in oncological research are saving many lives each year. Understanding gene regulation within living cells and developing more effective diagnostic techniques and cancer-inhibiting treatments are important steps in conquering this disease.

—David Wason Hollar, Jr., Ph.D.

See also Amputation; Anal cancer; Biopsy; Bladder cancer; Bladder removal; Blood testing; Bone cancer; Bone grafting; Bone marrow transplantation; Breast biopsy; Breast cancer; Breasts, female; Burkitt's lymphoma; Cancer; Carcinogens; Carcinoma; Cells; Cervical, ovarian, and uterine cancers; Chemotherapy; Colorectal cancer; Colorectal polyp removal; Cytology; Cytopathology; Dermatology; Dermatopathology; Endometrial biopsy; Gallbladder cancer; Gene therapy; Genital disorders, female; Genital disorders, male; Gynecology; Hematology; Histology; Hodgkin's disease; Hysterectomy; Imaging and radiology; Immunology; Immunopathology; Kaposi's sarcoma; Kidney cancer; Laboratory tests; Laryngectomy; Liver cancer; Lung cancer; Lymphadenopathy and lymphoma; Malignancy and metastasis; Mammography; Mastectomy and lumpectomy; Melanoma; Mouth and throat cancer; National Cancer Institute (NCI); Nephrectomy; Parathyroidectomy; Pathology; Plastic surgery; Proctology; Prostate cancer; Prostate gland removal; Radiation therapy; Sarcoma; Screening; Serology; Skin cancer; Skin lesion removal; Stomach, intestinal, and pancreatic cancers; Stress; Terminally ill: Extended care; Testicular cancer; Thyroidectomy; Tumor removal; Tumors.

For Further Information:
Alberts, Bruce, et al. *Molecular Biology of the Cell.* 5th ed. New York: Garland, 2008.

Berger, Ann, et al., eds. *Principles and Practice of Palliative Care and Supportive Oncology.* 4th ed. Philadelphia: Lippincott Williams & Wilkins, 2012.

Dark, Graham G. *Oncology at a Glance.* Malden: Wiley-Blackwell, 2013.

DeVita, Vincent T., et al., eds. *Cancer: Principles and Practice of Oncology.* Philadelphia: Lippincott Williams & Wilkins, 2011.

Dollinger, Malin, et al. *Everyone's Guide to Cancer Therapy.* 5th ed. Kansas City, Mo.: Andrews McMeel, 2008.

Eyre, Harmon J., Dianne Partie Lange, and Lois B. Morris. *Informed Decisions: The Complete Book of Cancer Diagnosis, Treatment, and Recovery.* 2d ed. Atlanta: American Cancer Society, 2002.

Harnett, Paul, John Cartmill, and Paul Glare, eds. *Oncology: A Case-Based Manual.* New York: Oxford University Press, 1999.

Joesten, Melvin D., Mary E. Castellion, and John L. Hogg. *The World of Chemistry: Essentials.* 4th ed. New York: Brooks Cole, 2007.

Jorde, Lynn B., et al. *Medical Genetics.* 3d ed. St. Louis, Mo.: Mosby/Elsevier, 2006.

Ophthalmology

Specialty
Anatomy or system affected: Eyes
Specialties and related fields: General surgery, optometry
Definition: The study of the anatomy and physiology of the eye, as well as treatment of vision problems or diseases, ranging from corrective lenses to delicate surgery.

Key terms:
ciliary body: a ring of tissue that surrounds the eye; the uveal portion of this tissue contains the ciliary muscle that adjusts the degree of curvature of the lens
cornea: the transparent portion of the first layer of the eye
keratitis: a state of inflammation of the cornea that may cause partial or total opacity, leading to loss of vision
retina: the key sensory element located in the eye's inner layer
sclera: the opaque portion of the outer layer of the eye; commonly referred to as the "white of the eye"

Science and Profession
Among the sense organs and functions in the body, probably the most complex are the eye and the process of vision that it supports. Ophthalmologists study both the anatomy and the physiology of the eye in order to understand and treat common and rare eye diseases.

The principal anatomical element of vision is the eyeball, or eye globe, located in the right and left orbital openings of the skull. It is embedded in a complex system of tissues surrounded by ocular muscles that control its movement. Adjacent to the eye and also within the bony orbit is the lacrimal gland, which is responsible for keeping the eye moist. Only the front third of the globe is exposed. This exposed area is made up of the central transparent portion, the cornea, and a surrounding white portion, which is only part of the sclera, the main component mass of the globe itself. The sclera is a very dense collagenous (protein-rich) structure which has two large openings (the anterior and posterior scleral foramina) and a number of smaller apertures that allow for the passage of nerves and blood vessels into the eye. It is through the posterior scleral foramen that three main components sustaining the eye's functions pass: the optic nerve, the central retinal vein, and the central retinal artery.

The eye has three main layers, within which are further specialized divisions. The outer layer consists essentially of the transparent cornea and opaque sclera. The middle layer, called the uvea, is made up of the choroid, which is the outer coating of the layer; the ciliary body, which contains key eye muscles that affect the degree of curvature in the lens; and the iris, which, with the lens located immediately behind it, separates the anterior from the posterior chambers of the eye. This iris itself has two layers, the stroma and the epithelium. The latter is immediately recognizable to the layperson, since its cells are markedly pigmented, giving to each individual a characteristic eye color.

It is the opening in the iris, called the pupil, that allows the passage of light into the inner layer of the eye, which contains the key sensory portion of the organ, the retina. Before light reaches the inner layer and the retina, it passes through the lens of the eye, located immediately behind the iris (which it supports), and through the largest area of open space within the eye, the vitreous cavity. This posterior cavity, like the smaller forward cavity of the eye, is filled with a transparent hydrogel called aqueous humor, made up mainly of water (about 95 percent of its total mass) in a collagenous framework within which the main component is hyaluronic acid. The aqueous humor is very similar to plasma but lacks its protein concentration. The pupil of the eye serves a purpose similar to the diaphragm (or f-stop) on a camera; it opens wider (dilates) or closes (contracts) according to the intensity of light striking the eye. (This reaction explains why, after a few minutes in an apparently totally dark room, the eye adjusts at least in part to the lower intensity of light.) For purposes of examining the internal structures of the eye, ophthalmologists sometimes place special drops in the eye to cause the pupil to dilate.

The lens of the eye, which is held in place behind the pupil by zonular fibers, consists of onionlike lens fibers. These are the product of epithelial cells that "migrate" from their place of origin in a germinative zone next to the edges of the lens to the anterior portion of the concentric structure of the lens. The central or internal layers of lens fibers, called the embryonic nucleus, represent the earliest cell specialization processes before birth. By contrast, the anterior and posterior lens fibers are constantly renewed at the surface.

As light passes through the transparent lens fibers, the phenomenon of refraction results, in the simplest possible explanation, both from the concentric shape of the lens itself and from a differential in the index of refraction occurring in the "younger" outside layers of lens fibers and that of the "older" central layers; the latter have a greater index of refraction than the former. Another phenomenon that increases the refractive power of the lens occurs when the zonular fibers that hold it in place relax under the influence of the ciliary muscle, making the lens more spherical in shape. The resultant increase in refractive power is called accommodation.

It is the retina, located in the last layer of the eye, that receives the light images passing through the lens and transmits them to the brain via the optic nerve. Physiologists consider the nerve-related function of the retina to be comparable in many details with all other sensory phenomena in the body, including touch and smell. The retina itself consists of a very thin outer layer, called the retinal pigment epithelium, and an inner layer, the sensory retina. On the surface of the retina, one finds a layer of photoreceptor cells. Once affected by the absorption of light rays reaching them from the lens, these cells form synapses with an intermediate layer of modulator cells. A synaptic relationship may be defined as an excitatory functional contact between two nerve cells, causing either a chemical or an electrical response. The modulator cells-referred to as neurons when their function is to receive synaptic transmissions from receptor cells-in turn pass the "message" of light to ganglion cells forming the innermost cellular layer of the retina. These cells transmit electrical discharges through the optic nerve to the brain, where they are registered as images.

Diagnostic and Treatment Techniques

Ophthalmologists must deal with a wide variety of problems affecting the eyes, ranging from injuries to the diagnosis of vision problems that can be corrected with eyeglasses or contact lenses. Perhaps the most important area of applied ophthalmology, however, involves treating the diseases that may occur in several areas of the eye.

An entire category of diseases can appear in the conjunctiva, the thin mucous membrane that lines the inner portion of the eyelid and covers the exterior of the sclera. Conjunctivitis refers to inflammatory conditions that may attack this membrane. Some conditions cause mere irritation, while others may lead to serious infections. In acute catarrhal, or mucopurulent, conjunctivitis, the conjunctival blood vessels become congested with mucus and then with pus, which accumulates on the margins of the eyelids. If untreated, this form of contagious, easily transmitted infection begins to affect the cornea, by causing prismatic distortions and eventually abrasions that may infect the cornea itself. A more serious form of conjunctivitis is referred to as purulent conjunctivitis; it is sometimes associated with complications of the sexually transmitted disease gonorrhea.

Inflammation of the cornea, or keratitis, usually comes from the passage of virulent organisms from the conjunctival sac, which, although exposed to the external environment, may not itself react to the presence of bacteria. There are many different types of keratitis. Individuals may be vulnerable to infections in the cornea as a result of abrasions (one of the main reasons that all ophthalmologists recommend against rubbing the eye to remove irritating particles) or because of abnormal conditions affecting the surface of the cornea. Among the latter, ophthalmologists list excessive dryness in the eye and the side effects of malnutrition leading to a condition called keratomalacia, which is common in underdeveloped countries.

Bacteria such as pneumococci (the primary contributor to pneumonia in the lungs) may cause infections that result in corneal ulceration, the most common form of keratitis. In such cases, the area affected by the ulceration may increase considerably as epithelial tissue in the cornea attaches itself to the ulcer. Corneal ulcers may be removed by surgery, although the effect of remaining scar tissue may reduce the level of vision. The prospect of success in corneal transplant operations has not eliminated the need for ulcer removal surgery, since transplants depend on the availability of "fresh" cornea donors.

Another form of corneal infection, herpes zoster (a form of skin rash also called shingles), is caused by the virus that causes chickenpox; it is common among aged patients whose cellular immunity systems suffer from decreased efficiency. In herpes zoster ophthalmicus, an infection that begins in the eye spreads via the nasociliary branch of the ophthalmic nerves and appears as red blotches on the surface of the skin (usually near the eye orbits on the side of the infection only). Zoster attacks are accompanied by rather severe pain. Ophthalmologists use several key drugs to treat this condition, including Distalgesic, Fortral, or Pethidine. Resultant depression in the patient may be relieved by prescribing amitriptyline.

Inflammation and possible infection of other regions of the eye also occur. Some zones, such as the sclera, tend to be more resistant to invasion because of the density of their fibrous tissues. Superficial inflammation of the sclera, called episcleritis, may be transitory but recurrent. Ophthalmologists will prescribe the anti-inflammatory drug Tandearil in the form of drops. More serious but much less common is the condition called scleritis, which extends much deeper into the tissue of the sclera and may affect the cornea and the uveal tract in the middle layer of the eye. Treatment of scleritis involves the use of steroid therapy, such as the corticosteroid drug prednisolone, often supplemented with Tandearil.

Uveitis is a term that applies to inflammations that occur in the uveal tract. The name suggests that such complications are not limited to one or another of the parts of the uveal zone (the iris or the ciliary body): All are affected and must be treated simultaneously.

The most common vision problem is myopia (nearsightedness). While most people still choose to correct nearsightedness with contact lenses or glasses, laser techniques such as photorefractive keratectomy (PRK) and laser in situ keratomileusis (LASIK) have shown some promise in treating myopia. Early enthusiasm for radial keratotomy has waned because of erratic results.

The most widely known eye disorders are probably glaucoma and cataracts. Glaucoma occurs when pressure caused by an excessive amount of aqueous humor increases inside the eyeball, specifically in the area of the retina. Impairment of vision may be slight, occurring at first in the peripheral area of sight. Further deterioration, however, may lead to blindness in the eye. Regular treatment with drugs that reduce the production of aqueous humor is necessary in patients suffering from chronic glaucoma. Acute glaucoma, which is very sudden, represents only about one-tenth of recorded cases. It must be treated within less than a week to avert permanent blindness.

Cataracts occur when there is a loss of full transparency in the lens of the eye. Cataracts occurring among children are congenital or hereditary in origin. Cataract-like damage to the lens of the eye may also result from exposure to the sun's rays (which is especially dangerous when one views the sun without protection during eclipses), extreme heat, x-rays, or nuclear radiation. Most characteristically, however, cataracts (from slight to advanced stages) are associated with the aging process. Formerly, cataract surgery was difficult and the recovery period slow, so patients were advised to wait as long as possible to have cataracts removed. Improvements in surgical techniques and materials mean that patients no longer need to wait until their vision is severely impaired to have this surgery. Most cataract extractions are combined with implantation of an intraocular lens, so that patients do not need to wear specially prescribed contact lenses or thick glasses following surgery.

Ophthalmologists make use of laser surgery for an increasing number of eye disorders. Lasers are used to treat eye problems caused by diabetes and hypertension, to treat or prevent some types of glaucoma, and to treat other, rarer eye conditions. Macular degeneration, an important cause of decreased central vision, may be arrested by laser therapy, but the technique does not repair existing damage.

Microsurgical techniques have further revolutionized eye care and have led to more effective management of conditions (such as retinal detachment) that formerly caused blindness.

Perspective and Prospects

Knowledge of the anatomy and physiology of the eye evolved gradually through history and then spectacularly in the latter half of the twentieth century. The most extraordinary advances in the later period were made in the field of eye surgery. For an understanding of how vision itself worked, it took centuries for surprisingly unscientific views to cede to the first modern theories and then, with the advance of anatomical dissection, the practical possibility of examining both normal and abnormal conditions of the organ in the laboratory.

An early but not widespread theory of how the eye sees, held into the Middle Ages, depended on what now seems to be the fantastic conception of *eidola*, or "skins." Those who believed this theory held (in part correctly) that something must be leaving the objects that one perceives through the eyes. This "something" was thought to be a skinlike picture that, once detached from the object in question, actually entered the eye (after an unexplainable physical contraction) through the pupil, the aperture in the eye that is visible in many different animals. Another widespread theory was a prescientific version not of light rays but of "visual rays" that were thought to leave the interior of the eye, returning to record the colors and shapes of objects encountered.

Historians generally agree that the tenth-century Arab scientist Ibn al-Haytham, known in the West as Alhazen, was the first to suggest that rays of light entered the eye to stimulate what he called the "sensorium." Although Alhazen's theory predated a scientific explanation of the nature of light itself, he based his views on the phenomenon of the lingering image on the eye's "sensorium" of strong light, particularly that of the sun, even after the eyelids closed out the object emitting light. He even proposed a basic theory of refraction of light inside the eye. According to his theory, the sensorium recorded images according to an exact formula that reconstituted both the "shape" and the "order" in which rays are received by the eye, depending on the angle at which they strike the spherical surface of the cornea. Alhazen even warned that although the eye's sensorium always duplicated this formula exactly, the observer (actually, the observer's brain) could be "tricked" by the reproduction of certain ray patterns that might resemble something that was not "real"-the optical illusion.

Alhazen's views would be examined and extended during the late sixteenth and mid-seventeenth centuries in the West by the scientific pioneers of optics, specifically the Italian Francesco Maurolico (died 1575) and the famous German astronomer Johannes Kepler (1571-1630). Kepler's best-known work complemented that of his Italian contemporary Galileo Galilei (1564-1642), marking a breakthrough in the science of optics and the use of lenses to make telescopes in order to explore the skies. Only in later generations, however, did the ophthalmological relevance of some of his findings concerning the measurement of light reflected off the objects "seen" by a lens become clear.

As specialized interest in the eye progressed along with the constant advance of science in the eighteenth and nineteenth centuries, exact observation of the internal features of the organ of vision hinged on both the historical progress of anatomical dissection and the development of instruments to look into the living eye. One of the principal figures who contributed to the latter field was the Swedish ophthalmologist Allvar Gullstrand (1862-1930). Gullstrand received the Nobel Prize in Physiology or Medicine in 1911 for his application of physical mathematics to the study of refraction of light in the eye. He gained additional worldwide attention for his research on astigmatism (the failure of rays to be focused by the lens accurately on a single central point) and for devising the so-called slit lamp for viewing the interior of the eye through the use of an intense beam of light.

In the area of eye surgery, a major landmark was achieved in the 1960s when the Spanish ophthalmologist Ramón Castroviejo began to develop a method for surgical transplant of fully transparent corneas from deceased donors to replace damaged corneas in eye patients.

—*Byron D. Cannon, Ph.D.;*
updated by Rebecca Lovell Scott, Ph.D., PA-C

See also Aging: Extended care; Albinos; Astigmatism; Biophysics; Blindness; Blurred vision; Cataract surgery; Cataracts; Color blindness; Conjunctivitis; Corneal transplantation; Eye infections and disorders; Eye surgery; Eyes; Geriatrics and gerontology; Glaucoma; Keratitis; Laser use in surgery; Macular degeneration; Microscopy, slitlamp; Myopia; Optometry; Sense organs; Trachoma; Vision; Vision disorders.

For Further Information:

Buettner, Helmut, ed. *Mayo Clinic on Vision and Eye Health: Practical Answers on Glaucoma, Cataracts, Macular Degeneration, and Other Conditions.* Rochester, Minn.: Mayo Foundation for Medical Education and Research, 2002.

Kaufman, Paul L., and Albert Alm. *Adler's Physiology of the Eye: Clinical Application.* 10th ed. St. Louis, Mo.: Mosby, 2003.

Museum of Vision. "Healthy Eyes, Healthy Body." *Foundation of the American Academy of Ophthalmology,* 2011.

Newell, Frank W. *Ophthalmology.* 8th ed. St. Louis, Mo.: Mosby, 1996.

Palay, David A., and Jay H. Krachmer, eds. *Primary Care Ophthalmology.* 2d ed. Philadelphia: Mosby/Elsevier, 2006.

Remington, Lee Ann. *Clinical Anatomy of the Visual System.* New York: Butterworth-Heinemann/Elsevier, 2012.

Riordan-Eva, Paul, and John P. Whitcher. *Vaughan and Asbury's General Ophthalmology.* 17th ed. New York: Lange Medical Books/McGraw-Hill, 2007.

Ronchi, Vasco. *Optics: The Science of Vision.* Translated and revised by Edward Rosen. Rev. ed. New York: Dover, 1991.

Spalton, David J., Roger A. Hitchings, and Paul A. Hunter, eds. *Atlas of Clinical Ophthalmology.* 3d ed. Oxford: Mosby/Elsevier, 2013.

Sutton, Amy L., ed. *Eye Care Sourcebook: Basic Consumer Health Information About Eye Care and Eye Disorders.* 3d ed. Detroit, Mich.: Omnigraphics, 2008..

Yanoff, Myron, and Jay S. Duker, eds. *Ophthalmology.* 3d ed. St. Louis, Mo.: Mosby/Elsevier, 2009.

Opportunistic infections

Disease/Disorder

Anatomy or system affected: All

Specialties and related fields: Bacteriology, immunology, internal medicine, microbiology, virology

Definition: Potentially life-threatening diseases occurring in people with weakened immune systems by microorganisms that typically do not cause severe illnesses in otherwise healthy people.

Key terms:

CD4: a type of white blood cell (specifically a type of T cell) that is affected by the human immunodeficiency virus (HIV)

encephalitis: inflammation of the brain

immunocompromised: the state of having a weakened immune system

lumbar puncture: also known as a spinal tap; a procedure that involves insertion of a needle into the lumbar spinal column

pneumonia: infection of the lung

prophylaxis: a method of preventing a disease

Causes and Symptoms

Opportunistic infections can be caused by various microorganisms, including viruses, bacteria, fungi, and protozoa. While they are capable of infecting healthy persons, the infection is either without symptoms or the disease is mild. It is in those who lack a healthy immune system that these organisms cause disastrous infections. Acquired immunodeficiency syndrome (AIDS), resulting from human immunodeficiency virus (HIV), is a widely known disease that weakens the immune system. There are other situations, however, in which the immune system can be compromised and become susceptible to opportunistic infections, such as being on chronic glucocorticoid therapy, taking immunosuppressive medications after organ transplantation, undergoing chemotherapy for cancer, being malnourished, or having a genetic predisposition.

Pneumocystis jirovecii is a fungus capable of causing life-threatening pneumonia in the immunocompromised. In those with HIV, the majority of *Pneumocystis* pneumonia develops in those with a very low CD4 cell count. Common symptoms include fever, cough, progressive difficulty breathing (especially with exertion), fatigue, chills, chest pain, and weight loss.

Toxoplasmosis is a ubiquitous infection caused by the intracellular protozoan parasite *Toxoplasma gondii*, which makes cats their hosts. Transmission is via ingestion of contaminated soil or undercooked meats that contain the protozoan oocyte. Infection in the healthy person is usually asymptomatic, but the organism can remain dormant in the host indefinitely. In immunocompromised patients such as those with very low CD4 cells, the organism reactivates and causes active infection. The central nervous system is the principal site of involvement. *T. gondii* can cause encephalitis and masses within the brain. Symptoms may in-

---

Information on Opportunistic Infections

Causes: Viruses, bacteria, fungi, protozoa
Symptoms: Fever, weakness, lack of appetite, rash, cough, difficulty breathing, confusion, headache, blurry vision, chest pain, weight loss, night sweats
Duration: Acute to chronic
Treatments: Antibiotics, antiviral medications, antifungal medications, antiprotozoan medications

---

clude confusion, fever, seizures, and headache. *T. gondii* can also cause pneumonia accompanied by difficulty breathing, fever, and cough. Other organs such as the intestines, liver, bone marrow, bladder, spinal cord, testes, pancreas, eyes, heart, and liver can be infected, although this is less common. Pregnant women who have an active infection can pass it to their offspring, leading to infantile neurological deficits, mental retardation, and eye infections.

Mycobacterium avium complex (MAC) usually causes widespread disease in the immunocompromised and is due to two nontuberculous species, *M. avium* or *M. intracellulare*. These organisms are ubiquitous in the environment such as in soil, with transmission typically through inhalation or ingestion. Acquisition of infection typically takes place when the CD4 count is extreme low. Symptoms include fever, night sweats, abdominal pain, diarrhea, weight loss, weakness, and wasting.

Cytomegalovirus (CMV) is a herpes virus found worldwide. It is commonly transmitted via feces, saliva, breast milk, urine, and genital secretions. In immunocompetent individuals, the virus remains latent and usually does not cause any severe disease. In the immunocompromised, however, the dormant virus reactivates and infection occurs. Symptoms generally include fever, night sweats, chills, fatigue, and muscle and joint aches. Other symptoms depend on the organ system affected: Gastrointestinal involvement typically produces symptoms of colitis (inflammation of the colon), such as abdominal pain and bloody diarrhea; lung involvement produces a pneumonitis (inflammation of the lung) with cough and difficulty breathing; and eye involvement (retinitis) can lead to blindness. The adrenal gland and the nervous system can also be affected.

Another opportunistic fungus associated with immunocompromised hosts is *Cryptococcus neoformans*, which causes cryptococcosis. The organism is normally found in soil contaminated with pigeon droppings, and transmission is usually through inhalation. The initial site of infection is in the lungs where it subsequently spreads to the brain, causing what is known as meningoencephalitis (inflammation of the brain and its surrounding protective tissues). Meningoencephalitis is the most common clinical syndrome in immunocompromised patients, developing slowly over one to two weeks with fever, malaise, headache, stiff neck, photophobia (aversion to bright lights), and vomiting. Disseminated rash is another symptom occurring in those with a weakened immune system.

There are many other causes of opportunistic infections, including the viruses *Varicella* and herpes simplex; the bacteria *Nocardia*, *Listeria*, and the less common *Mycobacterium* species; the protozoans *Cryptosporidium*, *Isospora*, *Microsporidia*, and *Cyclospora*; and the fungi *Coccidioides*, *Candida*, *Histoplasma*, and *Aspergillus*. While all these organisms are capable of causing disease in the healthy, their impact on the immunocompromised is much more severe.

Treatment and Therapy

Treatment of specific infections is important in addressing the disease, but what is more important is to correct the underlying deficit, which is the weakened immune system. In some cases, this may not be possible, such as in those who require immunosuppressive therapy after organ transplantation or those undergoing chemotherapy for cancer. However, advances in HIV therapy with the implementation of highly active antiretroviral therapy (HAART) as well as institution of prophylaxis against opportunistic infections have dramatically decreased the mortality rate in these patients.

Treatment of *Pneumocystis* pneumonia requires the demonstration of organisms from respiratory specimens. Treatment is with anti-Pneumocystis regimens typically for twenty-one days, with or without corticosteroids. The latter is used in severe cases when oxygenation becomes problematic. Symptoms typically worsen after two to three days of therapy as a result of increased inflammation in response to dying microorganisms. After initial therapy, prophylactic therapy against future infections is instituted.

Treatment of toxoplasmosis requires antiprotozoan medications for at least six weeks. Prophylaxis against future infection is also required, which is the same medication as that used for *Pneumocystis* prophylaxis. In high-risk persons, as a means of prevention it is important to avoid undercooked meats and cat litter boxes. Treatment of MAC involves combination antibiotics for at least twelve months, with subsequent prophylaxis.

CMV infection is treated with antiviral agents. Immunoglobulin may be used to reduce the risk of infection in certain transplant recipients. If the eye is involved, then a pellet that releases an antiviral agent may be implanted into the eye with surgery. While not curative, this treatment may hinder the progression of the eye disease.

The treatment of cryptococcosis is with antifungal agents, initially with combination medications for what is known as induction therapy, followed by consolidation therapy, and finally maintenance therapy. Because the disease can also cause an increased pressure surrounding the brain, frequent lumbar punctures are sometimes required to relieve this pressure, or if severe enough, a drain placed in the spinal cord may be necessary to continuously relieve the pressure.

While prophylactic therapy is needed when the CD4 cell count is low, it may be withdrawn when the CD4 cells improve.

Perspective and Prospects

Pneumocystis was originally identified by the Brazilian physician Carlos Chagas in 1909. Chagas was also the discoverer of the protozoan *Trypanosoma cruzi*, the organism that causes trypanosomiasis, or Chagas' disease. Initially, he mistakenly thought that the *Pneumocystis* cysts from the lungs of rats were part of the *Trypanosoma* life cycle. It was in 1910 that the Italian physician Antonio Carini discovered that these cysts were also present in lungs without *T. cruzi* infection, and he thus concluded that these cysts were a different type of infection. In 1912, Pierre and Marie Delanoe at the Pasteur Institute also confirmed that these cysts were present in the absence of *T. cruzi* infection, and they subsequently named these cystlike organisms *Pneumocystis carinii*, after Carini. Because these infections appeared to affect only rats, however, the organism did not become a major issue at that time.

It was not until the 1940s that *P. carinii* was found to cause pneumonia in human infants and adults. However, these patients all had some type of immune system compromise, such as malnutrition, genetic immune deficiency, or immunosuppressive medications. Before the AIDS epidemic, there were fewer than one hundred confirmed cases per year in the United States. It was later determined that there were several species of *Pneumocystis*, one of which causes disease in rats and another in humans. It was in 1999 when the term *P. jirovecii* (named after the Czech parasitologist Otto Jiroveci) was officially coined to refer to the disease occurring in humans. *P. carinii* still refers to the disease in rats. It was also in 1999 that *Pneumocystis* was recognized as a fungus rather than a protozoan, as previously thought.

In late 1980 to early 1981, the Centers for Disease Control and Prevention (CDC) described a cluster of five cases of *Pneumocystis* pneumonia in young gay men. Since then, the cases of *Pneumocystis* pneumonia increased, as did the cases of Kaposi's sarcoma (rare HIV-related skin cancer). It was soon realized that both of these illnesses were not exclusive to gay males; they also affected heterosexuals, intravenous drug users, and others who were immunocompromised. In 1982, the CDC officially coined the term "acquired immunodeficiency syndrome," or AIDS, for this syndrome. In 1983, Luc Montagnier and his team from the Pasteur Institute isolated a virus that was thought to be the causative agent of AIDS, which they termed lymphadenopathy-associated virus. In 1984, Robert Gallo and his team from the United States also isolated a virus presumptive to cause

AIDS; they named it human T lymphotropic virus type III (HTLV-III). Later, it was recognized that both viruses were the same, and the virus was officially termed human immunodeficiency virus (HIV) in 1986.

In the beginning of the AIDS epidemic, death was certain. Treatment of HIV did not begin until 1986, when the Food and Drug Administration (FDA) approved the first antiviral agent, zidovudine, a nucleoside reverse transcriptase inhibitor (NRTI)-an agent that inhibits viral replication. However, single agent therapy did not prove to be as effective due to drug resistance. In 1995, newer classes of antiviral medications were approved-non-nucleoside reverse transcriptase inhibitor (NNRTI) and protease inhibitors (PI)-and began the trend of combination therapy of what is now known as highly active antiretroviral therapy (HAART). The thought behind combination therapy is that if the virus develops a genetic mutation and becomes resistant to one drug, the other two would still be active against it. However, while successful, even this powerful combination of drugs is still not adequate enough to achieve a complete cure since the virus is capable of remaining dormant inside cells and becoming resistant to medications even after a brief episode of missed doses.

In 2007, the FDA approved two new classes of antiretroviral therapy, integrase inhibitors and CCR5 co-receptor antagonists, which are used for advanced stages of HIV infection.

As of 2013, there are currently no available vaccines effective against HIV, although there are vaccines in various stages of clinical trial. A report in 2009 of a study of healthy volunteers with an experimental HIV vaccine in Thailand showed only a modest success rate (about 31 percent) in the prevention of HIV. In 2013, however, a two-year-old child was declared "functionally cured" of HIV infection, but further research will be conducted to determine if the results can be replicated in clinical trials involving other HIV-infected children.

While there are still obstacles to conquer in the fight against HIV, the battle against opportunistic infections has made great strides with the introduction of HAART and prophylactic medications.

—*Andrew Ren, M.D.*

See also Acquired immunodeficiency syndrome (AIDS); Bacterial infections; Fungal infections; Human immunodeficiency virus (HIV); Immune system; Immunodeficiency disorders; Immunology; Kaposi's sarcoma; Protozoan diseases; Terminally ill: Extended care; Viral infections.

For Further Information:

Fauci, Anthony, eds. *Harrison's Principles of Internal Medicine.* 17th ed. New York: McGraw-Hill, 2008.
Mandell, Gerald, et al., eds. *Mandell, Douglas, and Bennett's Principles and Practice of Infectious Diseases.* 7th ed. Philadelphia: Churchill Livingstone/Elsevier, 2010.
Mathis, Diane J., and Alexander Y. Rudensky, eds. *Immune Tolerance.* Cold Spring Harbor, N.Y.: Cold Spring Harbor Laboratory Press, 2013.
"Opportunistic Infections and Their Relationship to HIV/AIDS." *AIDS.gov,* November 16, 2011.
Rubin, Robert, eds. *Clinical Approach to Infection in the Compromised Host.* 4th ed. New York: Kluwer Academic, 2002.
St. Georgiev, Vassil. *Opportunistic Infections: Treatment and Prophylaxis.* Totowa, N.J.: Humana Press, 2003.
Stine, Gerald James. *AIDS Update 2013: An Annual Overview of Acquired Immune Deficiency Syndrome.* New York: McGraw-Hill, 2013.
"Surveillance for Norovirus Outbreaks." *Centers for Disease Control and Prevention,* January 28, 2013.
"Toddler 'Functionally Cured' of HIV Infection, NIH-Supported Investigators Report." *National Institutes of Health,* March 4, 2013.

Optometry

Specialty
Anatomy or system affected: Eyes
Specialties and related fields: Ophthalmology
Definition: A field involving the provision of eye exams, the prescription of corrective lenses, and the diagnosis and treatment of eye disease, but not eye surgery.

Key terms:

clinical refraction: the determination of appropriate optical powers and related parameters to promote optimal visual acuity

contact lens: a small, shell-like glass or plastic lens that rests directly on the external surface of the eye to serve as a new anterior surface and thus correct refractive error as an alternative to spectacles, to protect the eye, or to serve as a prosthetic device promoting a more normal appearance of a disfigured eye

ophthalmologist: a physician who specializes in the comprehensive care of the eyes and the visual system; ophthalmologists provide visual, medical, and surgical eye care and diagnose general diseases of the body

prism: an optical element or component that, by virtue of two nonparallel plane faces, deviates the path of a beam of light

spectacles: a pair of ophthalmic lenses held together with a frame or mounting; also called glasses

Science and Profession

Optometry has been defined as "the art and science of vision care" by Monroe J. Hirsch and Ralph E. Wick in *The Optometric Profession* (1968). The American Optometric Association has stated that "Doctors of Optometry are independent primary health care providers who specialize in the examination, diagnosis, treatment and management of diseases and disorders of the visual system." Optometrists examine eyes and the visual system. They prescribe spectacles and contact lenses, optimize binocularity (the manner in which the two eyes work together), and improve visual function. Optometrists are trained to detect, treat, and manage disorders and diseases of the eyes and related structures.

Optometry is one of the youngest of the learned professions, which were originally restricted to law, medicine, and theology. Following the earlier lead of organized medicine, optometrists successfully organized and passed the first optometry practice law in 1901. Optometrists today complete a university education and then spend four additional years in a specialized school or college of optometry to receive the OD (doctor of optometry) degree. Many optometrists spend an additional year training in special-interest residency programs after graduation. Optometrists practice independently in private offices, although increasing numbers of optometrists also work in groups, the military, public health agencies, and university and hospital environments.

Distinctions are made between optometrists, ophthalmologists, and opticians. Ophthalmologists are physicians who diagnose and treat eye diseases and who perform eye surgery. They complete a premedical university education, four years of medical school, one year of internship, and three or more years of specialized training in ophthalmology. Many ophthalmologists also complete one or more years of fellowship subspecialty training. Opticians are technicians trained in the manufacture and dispensing of optical aids.

Diagnostic and Treatment Techniques

A portion of the eye examination performed by optometrists is called clinical refraction. To the physicist, refraction is the bending of light as it passes through an interface separating two differing media (such as water and air). Refraction, however, has also come to mean the clinical evaluation of the human visual system. Clinical refraction generally results in a spectacle prescription; such a prescription will contain the spherical optical power, and the astigmatic optical power and its axis when appropriate, that are necessary to provide optimally focused light on the retina for each eye.

A clinical refraction also includes an assessment of binocularity, which is the way in which both eyes are used simultaneously such that each retinal image contributes to the final visual percept. (The retina is the inner nerve layer of the eye upon which the optics of the eye focuses the image of the outside world.) Much effort is made, during a refraction, to attain maximum visual comfort by optimizing binocularity. Occasionally, it is necessary to utilize a prismatic element in the spectacle prescription as well as optical powers to this end. In other cases, the clinician may suggest a course of eye exercises to assist the patient in achieving improved binocularity without, or in supplement to, spectacles. Some patients may be found to suffer from severe binocular dysfunction and are referred for surgical consideration.

Near vision is tested during a refraction, especially for those people more than forty years of age who might require optical assistance for near work. The cornea is the clear, circular "window" in the front of the eye through which the colored iris is seen. Behind the iris is a crystalline lens. The cornea and the lens act together to focus light on the retina. The cornea provides most of the refractive power of the eye, and the lens serves to fine-tune the image in a process called accommodation. As one ages, however, the ability to accommodate deteriorates. Some form of near correction, either with two pairs of spectacles or with some form of bifocal, is then necessary. Only minimal optical power is needed at first, but as the aging process continues, the need for stronger near correction increases.

For a given patient, an analysis of binocularity, the determination of near vision requirements, and a consideration of additional occupational or avocational tasks (such as sports) make up his or her "functional vision." For some patients, the data gleaned in a standard refraction will provide the optometrist with all the information necessary to recommend comfortable visual correction for all tasks. For other patients, some additional thought and consideration may be required. For example, a very tall, fifty-year-old patient may not require as strong a reading correction as another shorter individual of the same age because the former has longer arms and is more used to holding reading material at a greater distance than the latter. In addition, providing visual care to patients using computers and video display terminals has become a rapidly growing subarea in functional vision.

No clinical refraction would be complete without an assessment of ocular health. This examination consists of observation of the eyes and related structures, as well as a testing of function. Good visual acuity, in and of itself, is fairly good evidence that the function of the eye is normal. Some ocular diseases, however, may occur and-at least initially-leave central vision intact. The structures of the eye are inspected with the assistance of instruments such as a clinical biomicroscope, or slitlamp microscope, to examine the outer ocular structures, and an ophthalmoscope, which allows inspection of the structures of the inner eye. Pupillary dilation with pharmaceutical agents in the form of drops allows inspection of the peripheral retina. The pressure in the eye should be tested, a process called tonometry, and the field of vision evaluated. Many optometrists also bear the responsibility for the treatment of certain ocular diseases.

As is true for all professionals, when the management of a specific problem is beyond one doctor's training, interest, or licensure, referral is made to another, more appropriate, doctor. For example, a patient with an age-related cataract (clouding of the crystalline lens) may be referred to an ophthalmologist for surgery, and an optometrist who suspects multiple sclerosis will refer the patient to a neurologist.

There are subspecialty areas in optometry, such as the prescription of appropriate visual aids for patients with particularly poor vision, known as low vision rehabilitation. Other subspecialty areas include industrial vision, developmental vision and vision therapy, and ocular disease. Contact lens care has become a large subspecialty in optometry. In fitting contact lenses, the curvature of the cornea, the quality of the patient's tears, and the health of the ocular surface and associated structures (such as eyelids) are all important considerations. Contact lenses are usually intended as devices to provide vision as an alternative to spectacles (although there are occasions when contact lenses may be used as prosthetics, to cover a damaged eye, or as therapy for a specific disease). The clinician must modify the original refractive findings to adjust for the placement of the lens because it will rest directly on the ocular surface instead of being attached to a frame half an inch from the eye. The contact lens must be designed so that the surface of the eye is not compromised by its presence. The proper contact lens care system is vitally important for the initial and continued success of a contact lens fitting. Continuing professional supervision is essential in maintaining optimal vision and safe contact lens wear.

Perspective and Prospects

Evidence suggests that spectacles were first used to assist human vision in Europe at about the end of the thirteenth century. Organizations of spectacle makers were formed in Europe in the fourteenth and fifteenth centuries. These guilds policed the quality of spectacles and the working conditions under which their manufacture occurred. Spectacles were sold to the public in stores and by peddlers. Individuals self-selected the lens or lenses that seemed most appropriate to them for their visual tasks. Retailers selling spectacles eventually began to assist their clientele in making an informed selection. Over time, spectacle vendors evolved into opticians. Some "refracting" opticians tested vision to provide what they believed to be the most appropriate correcting lenses for a particular person. Physicians at that time did not recommend or examine the eyes for spectacles, preferring the use of medication for eye difficulties.

The impetus for optometry's modern development and legal recognition in the United States began with a confrontation between optometry and ophthalmology. A New York refracting optician named Charles Prentice referred a patient to Henry D. Noyes, an ophthalmologist, in 1892. Noyes wrote Prentice a thank-you note for the referral but suggested that Prentice should not have charged a fee (of three dollars) for his services-such being the right reserved

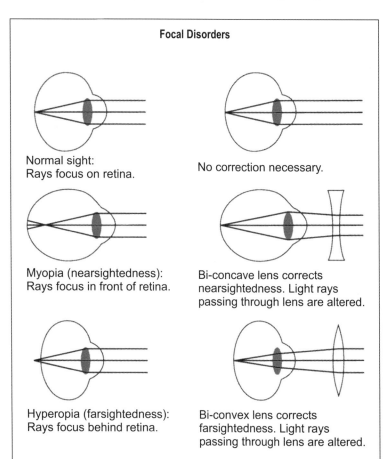

Focal Disorders

Normal sight:
Rays focus on retina.

No correction necessary.

Myopia (nearsightedness):
Rays focus in front of retina.

Bi-concave lens corrects nearsightedness. Light rays passing through lens are altered.

Hyperopia (farsightedness):
Rays focus behind retina.

Bi-convex lens corrects farsightedness. Light rays passing through lens are altered.

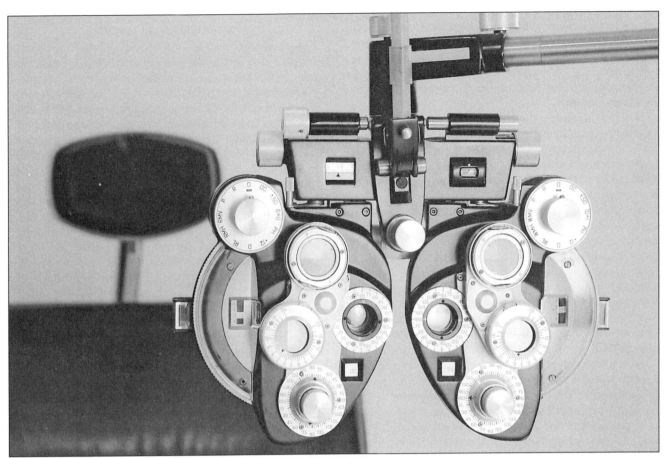

A device called a phoropter, which is used to evaluate a patient's vision. (Digital Stock)

to professionals such as physicians. Prentice responded, defending his practice of charging for his services. Noyes sent Prentice's letters to another ophthalmologist, D. B. St. John Roosa, who expressed his opinion that Prentice was in violation of the law by charging a fee for his services. By 1895, Roosa had announced that he would seek legislation to prevent opticians from practicing, and Prentice responded by organizing the Optical Society of the State of New York. This society eventually introduced a bill to the New York legislature to regulate the "practice of optometry." Optometry was defined as refraction, dispensing (that is, selling) spectacles, and related services.

This bill was quite controversial and never came to a vote. Later, however, another New York optometrist, Andrew J. Cross, while visiting Minnesota to teach a program in optics, scoffed at the notion that Minnesota could pass an optometry practice act before New York. Thus inspired, the Minnesotans passed their law, which included a regulatory board, in 1901. Arguing that optometry was separate and distinct from medicine, optometrists proceeded to obtain practice acts in all the states over the next twenty-three years.

Optometrists sought to be professionals rather than businesspeople and developed an agenda that included the formation of organizations: both the American Optometric Association (AOA) and the American Academy of Optometry were established early in the twentieth century. Efforts were made both to reduce the commercial aspects of practice and to improve educational standards. A code of ethics and stringent rules of conduct were adopted by the AOA.

The first American optometric schools were extensions of apprenticeships and offered short courses (one to two weeks) in refraction. Eventually, private schools were established to train both physicians and nonphysicians. Academic programs developed from these independent schools, such as the Southern California College of Optometry and the Illinois College of Optometry. A milestone two-year optometry course began at Columbia University in New York in 1910; Cross and Prentice were instrumental in preparing the curriculum. Ohio State University began a four-year program in 1915, and the University of California, Berkeley, established an optometry course in 1923. By the late twentieth century, seventeen schools and colleges of optometry trained optometrists in the United States; many of the university programs also provided academic postgraduate studies. Similar programs were created in England, Australia, Canada, Europe, Asia, Africa, and South America.

Optometrist and lawyer John G. Classe credits the major change in the way optometry developed in the latter half of the twentieth century to contact lenses and modern tonometry. Prior to technical improvements in contact lenses and tonometry, the practice of optometry was limited and nonmedical. The commercial success of contact lenses brought about research in physiology, which in turn expanded biological knowledge and improved contact lenses. The ability to use a tonometer without drops to test for increased intraocular pressure (a condition called glaucoma) gave optometrists additional responsibility in ocular disease management. Unfortunately, the subsequent changes in practice placed optometry in even greater direct conflict with ophthalmology.

In a meeting held in January 1968, many of the leaders of the schools and colleges of optometry, the chair of the AOA's Council on Optometric Education, and the editor of the *Journal of the American Optometric Association* unofficially discussed the future of the profession. Court decisions had ruled that optometrists had the legal responsibility to detect, diagnose, and refer ocular disease, and many optometrists were frustrated by the limited scope of their practice. This group believed that optometry should discard its original concept of being a drugless profession dedicated solely to ocular function. They argued that optometric education should be expanded in the fields of ocular pharmacology, anatomy, physiology, and pathology so that optometrists would become primary entry points into the health care system for patients. Finally, it was concluded that the state laws that govern the practice of optometry should be updated to allow the optometrist to practice what he or she was taught, including the appropriate use of pharmaceutical agents.

In 1971, Rhode Island became the first state to amend its optometry law to permit the use of diagnostic pharmaceutical drugs. Despite continued opposition from ophthalmology, all fifty states followed over the next twenty years. In 1976, West Virginia became the first state to permit the use of therapeutic drugs, and thirty-two states had enacted similar laws by 1993.

—*Barry A. Weissman, O.D., Ph.D.*

See also Aging: Extended care; Astigmatism; Biophysics; Blurred vision; Cataracts; Eye infections and disorders; Eyes; Geriatrics and gerontology; Glaucoma; Myopia; Ophthalmology; Optometry, pediatric; Sense organs; Strabismus; Trachoma; Vision; Vision disorders.

For Further Information:

Buettner, Helmut, ed. *Mayo Clinic on Vision and Eye Health: Practical Answers on Glaucoma, Cataracts, Macular Degeneration, and Other Conditions*. Rochester, Minn.: Mayo Foundation for Medical Education and Research, 2002.

Classe, John G. "Optometry: A Legal History." *Journal of the American Optometric Association* 59, no. 8 (1988): 641-50.

Eger, Milton J. "Now It Can and Should Be Told." *Journal of the American Optometric Association* 60, no. 4 (1989): 323-26.

Gregg, James R. *History of the American Academy of Optometry*. Washington, D.C.: American Academy of Optometry, 1987.

Millodot, Michel. *Dictionary of Optometry and Visual Science*. 7th ed. New York: Butterworth-Heinemann/Elsevier, 2009.

Museum of Vision. "Healthy Eyes, Healthy Body." *Foundation of the American Academy of Ophthalmology*, 2011.

Remington, Lee Ann. *Clinical Anatomy of the Visual System*. New York: Butterworth-Heinemann/Elsevier, 2012.

Sutton, Amy L., ed. *Eye Care Sourcebook: Basic Consumer Health Information About Eye Care and Eye Disorders*. 3d ed. Detroit, Mich.: Omnigraphics, 2008.

"What Is a Doctor of Optometry?" *American Optometric Association*, June 2012.

Oral and maxillofacial surgery

Specialty

Anatomy or system affected: Gums, head, mouth, teeth

Specialties and related fields: Anesthesiology, dentistry, oncology, otorhinolaryngology, plastic surgery

Definition: A specialty of dentistry that deals with the diagnosis and management of diseases or conditions of the mouth, teeth, jaws, and face.

Key terms:

mandible: the lower bone of the jaw

maxilla: two fused bones that make up the upper jaw and the mid-portion of the facial skeleton

nitrous oxide: a chemical compound that at room temperature forms a colorless gas, also known as laughing gas, used to produce anesthesia and analgesia during surgery

obstructive sleep apnea: periods of interrupted breathing during sleep caused by airway obstruction in the nose or throat

orthgnathic surgery: surgical procedures of the jaws to correct structural deformity caused by congenital or growth defects

temporomandibular joint: the hinged joint that attaches the head of the mandible to the skull

Science and Profession

The specialist in oral and maxillofacial surgery deals with the anatomical region of the head that includes the oral cavity and the hard and soft tissues that compose that part of the facial skeleton formed by the mandible and the maxilla. The mandible is the bone that forms the lower jaw, and the maxilla is the fusion of the two bones that form the middle part of the face, or the upper jaw.

The maxilla forms the roof of the mouth, the lateral walls and floor of the nose, and the floor of the eye cavities. The maxilla contains the maxillary sinuses and holds the upper teeth. The mandible holds the lower teeth and attaches to the temporal bone of the skull at the temporomandibular joint (TMJ).

The diseases and conditions treated by oral and maxillofacial surgeons are numerous and diverse. They may include extraction of impacted teeth, dental implants, benign and malignant lesions of the oral cavity, TMJ disorders, management of facial pain syndromes, facial fractures, obstructive sleep apnea, and surgical correction of congenital deformities. Oral and maxillofacial surgeons will treat infections of the jaws, oral cavities, and salivary glands and may perform facial cosmetic procedures.

Most oral and maxillofacial surgeons begin their training after dental school. Increasingly, medical doctors are being integrated into the specialty through additional dentistry training and subsequent entry into an oral and maxillofacial training program. The oral and maxillofacial surgical residency includes general surgery, plastic surgery, medicine, and anesthesia. A four-year residency program grants a degree that makes these surgeons board eligible in oral and maxillofacial surgery. Some American oral and maxillofacial surgeons complete a six-year residency program that grants a medical degree as well. Graduates of the residency program may elect to pursue additional fellowship training in head and neck cancer, cosmetic facial surgery, pediatric maxillofacial surgery, or maxillofacial trauma.

Oral and maxillofacial surgery is recognized as a dental specialty. The American Board of Oral and Maxillofacial Surgery is responsible for certifying oral and maxillofacial surgeons in the United States. The board is recognized and approved by the Council on Dental Education of the American Dental Association. In order to become board certified, a typical applicant will have completed four years of undergraduate studies and four years of dental school, followed by an approved training program. Candidates must present letters of recommendation from board-certified oral and maxillofacial surgeons and then pass a written and oral examination. After completion of these qualifications, applicants are granted the title of diplomat of the American Board of Oral and Maxillofacial Surgery. The board requires that its diplomats be recertified every ten years.

Diagnostic and Treatment Techniques

Oral and maxillofacial surgeons take careful and detailed histories of present and past medical conditions, including family history, medication history, and allergy history. Examination of the oral and maxillofacial area includes a complete examination of the oral cavity and the use of radiologic techniques to visualize the soft tissues and bone structure of the jaw and the mid-face. Many oral and maxillofacial surgeons perform conventional radiographs (x-rays) and panoramic radiographs of the upper and lower jaw in their office. The diagnosis of oral and maxillofacial conditions is further aided by the use of diagnostic images from computed tomography (CT) scans and magnetic resonance imaging (MRI).

Oral and maxillofacial surgeons perform surgical procedures both at the hospital and in the office. Because many biopsies and dental procedures are done in the office, these specialists must be proficient in administering oral sedation, local anesthetics, nitrous oxide, intravenous sedation, and general anesthesia. Patients who come to oral and maxillofacial surgeons come from all age groups. They may have multiple medical conditions and require a broad range of medical and surgical care. The oral and maxillofacial surgeon must be part medical doctor, part general surgeon, and part dentist.

Some of the more common treatment techniques in oral and maxillofacial surgery include dental procedures for removal of impacted teeth or teeth that cannot be restored. These surgeons may work along with restorative dentists to reconstruct bone for placement of dental implants. In the event of facial trauma, oral and maxillofacial surgeons may be called upon to repair routine and complex fractures, repair lacerations, and reconstruct damaged nerves and blood vessels. Oral and maxillofacial surgeons may diagnose and treat benign cysts and growths in the oral cavity, including cysts that form in the salivary glands. Head and neck cancer diagnosis and treatment may include malignant lesions of the jaws, lips, or oral cavity.

A major component of the specialty involves reconstructive and orthognathic surgery to correct congenital deformities such as facial asymmetry, bite deformities, and cleft lip or palate. Obstructive sleep apnea is being increasingly recognized; severe cases may be life threatening and may be an indication for surgical intervention by an oral and maxillofacial specialist. Maxillomandibular advancement surgery may be performed in selected cases. The procedure involves moving the upper and lower jaws forward. The bones are surgically separated and advanced to increase the opening of the airway. The procedure is done in the hospital under general anesthesia and may take three to four hours to complete. In cases of severe obstructive sleep apnea that do not respond to conservative treatments, this type of orthognatic surgery may be the treatment of choice.

Chronic facial pain disorders that oral and maxillofacial surgeons deal with include TMJ disease and neurogenic pain syndromes. TMJ disorders may cause pain in the ear, headache, or pain when moving the jaw. The oral and maxillofacial surgeon may treat this condition conservatively with medication or splint therapy. In more severe cases, open or arthroscopic joint surgery may be indicated. The most common craniofacial pain syndrome is trigeminal neuralgia. If medications are not effective, then the oral and maxillofacial surgeon may treat this condition with local nerve block, surgical destruction of the nerve, or microvascular decompression of the trigeminal nerve root.

Because of their surgical training, their familiarity with the soft tissue and structural anatomy of the face, and their experience with office-based surgery and anesthesia, oral maxillofacial surgeons are uniquely qualified and positioned to take advantage of recent developments in facial cosmetic surgery. Facial cosmetic surgery may be indicated for birth defects, deformity resulting from injury, or aging process reversal. Facial plastic surgery that may be performed by the oral and maxillofacial surgeon includes cheekbone implants, chin augmentation, facial and neck liposuction, lip enhancement, and face lift surgery. These specialists may also use the surgical laser to remove outer layers of damaged skin, inject collagen to fill wrinkles, and use Botox injections to reduce muscle activity that causes wrinkles.

Perspective and Prospects

Hesy-Re, an Egyptian scribe who lived around 2600 BCE, is credited as the first dentist. The Greek physician Hippocrates, who lived between 500 and 300 BCE, described treatments of diseased teeth and gums, including the use of forceps to extract teeth and wires to stabilize fractured jaws. During the early part of the Middle Ages, most oral surgery was performed by monks; after the popes forbade monks from practicing medicine, barbers became responsible for extracting teeth and draining dental abscesses. In 1723, the French surgeon Pierre Fauchard described the practice of dentistry, including oral anatomy and operative and restorative procedures; he is credited with being the founder of modern dentistry. The American Revolutionary War figure Paul Revere advertised himself as a dentist, in addition to being a fine silversmith. The first dental school was established in 1840 as the Baltimore College of Dental

Surgery, and in 1867 the Harvard Dental School became the first university-affiliated dental school. In 1844, the Connecticut dentist Horace Wells performed the first dental extractions done using nitrous oxide as an anesthetic.

Simon P. Hullihen of Wheeling, West Virginia, both a medical doctor and a dentist, is considered to be the founder of oral surgery. He specialized in operations on defects of the mouth and head and performed hundreds of operations for cleft lip, cleft palate, and other abnormalities of the mouth and jaw.

Another contributing factor to the development of the specialty of oral and maxillofacial surgery was the devastating injuries suffered by soldiers during the great wars of the twentieth century. It became clear to battlefield surgeons that dentists were needed to help align dental occlusion in facial injuries and fractured jaws. Dentists became valued members of the surgical team, and today dentistry is still the field from which most oral and maxillofacial surgeons come.

In 1945, a committee was authorized to establish an American Board of Oral Surgery (ABOS). In 1947, the ABOS was approved by the American Dental Association. The name of the board was changed to the American Board of Oral and Maxillofacial Surgery in 1978 to reflect the complete scope of the specialty.

Advancements in cosmetic and reconstructive surgery put the oral and maxillofacial surgery specialist at the cutting edge of medical innovation. An example is the French oral and maxillofacial surgeon Bernard Devauchelle, who along with his colleagues at the University Hospital Center of Amiens, France, performed the first human face transplant. In November 2005, Devauchelle and his team transplanted the central and lower face of a thirty-eight-year-old woman whose nose, lips, and chin had been lost as a result of a dog bite. Their success was reported around the world and hailed as a milestone in surgical history. Today, the specialty of oral maxillofacial surgery is a dynamic field that attracts both medical and dental school graduates. Although the residency program is long and arduous, the rewards of the specialty are great.

—*Chris Iliades, M.D.*

See also Anesthesia; Anesthesiology; Birth defects; Cleft lip and palate; Cleft lip and palate repair; Dental diseases; Dentistry; Dentistry, pediatric; Facial transplantation; Fracture repair; Head and neck disorders; Jaw wiring; Orthodontics; Periodontal surgery; Periodontitis; Plastic surgery; Root canal treatment; Surgery, general; Teeth; Temporomandibular joint (TMJ) syndrome; Tooth extraction; Toothache; Wisdom teeth.

For Further Information:

Coulthard, Paul, et al. *Oral and Maxillofacial Surgery, Radiology, Pathology, and Oral Medicine.* 3d ed. London: Elsevier, 2013.

Ellis, Edward, et al. *Contemporary Oral and Maxillofacial Surgery.* 6th ed. St. Louis: Mosby/Elsevier, 2013.

Meneghini, Fabio, and Paolo Biondi. *Clinical Facial Analysis: Elements, Principles, and Techniques.* London: Springer, 2012.

Miloro, Michael, et al. *Peterson's Principles of Oral and Maxillofacial Surgery.* 2d ed. Philadelphia: BC Decker, 2004.

Mitchell, David A. *An Introduction to Oral and Maxillofacial Surgery.* New York: Oxford University Press, 2006.

White, R. L. "Oral and Maxillofacial Surgery: Defining Our Present, Shaping Our Future." *Journal of the American College of Dentistry* 76, no. 1. (Spring, 2009): 36-39.

Orchiectomy

Procedure

Anatomy or system affected: Reproductive system

Specialties and related fields: Urology

Also known as: Testicle removal

Definition: Excision of a testicle, usually performed as part of cancer therapy.

Key terms:

electrocautery: a needle charged with electricity that is heated and placed on the tissue; often used to remove warts and polyps

lymphadenectomy: the removal of lymph nodes, one or more in a group

seminoma: the most common cancer of the testes

Indications and Procedures

Orchiectomy is usually performed for benign or malignant conditions. For metastatic carcinoma of the prostate, bilateral orchiectomy (removal of both testicles) is often utilized. For primary tumors of the testes that are malignant, radical orchiectomy is performed for the best result.

During simple orchiectomy, the patient's genitalia are prepared in a sterile manner. An incision is made in the scrotum, and the testis is withdrawn from its sac. The spermatic cord is clamped during the procedure, and then cut.

When it comes to radical orchiectomy, the genitalia and the inguinal region (the upper groin and lower lateral abdominal region) are prepared in a sterile manner, and an inguinal skin incision is made. Then the spermatic cord is freed and clamped Next, the testis is pulled up from the scrotum. A radical orchiectomy would typically be necessary in the case of suspected testicular cancer. Once the tumor is verified, either by gross analysis or by a frozen section, the cord is doubly clamped and then cut.

It is important for patients undergoing an orchiectomy to have blood drawn and a urine sample collected and to stop any aspirins that they may be taking a week before the procedure. Also, all nonsteroidal anti-inflammatory drugs (NSAIDs) should be discontinued two days before the procedure.

Orchiectomy can also be a part of gender reassignment surgery and is mostly done in clinics that specialize in it. It is considered genital reconstruction. Prior to the genital reconstruction, patients usually undergo hormone therapy for several months or as long as a year before going through the surgery. The patient must be sure that he wants to live life as a woman with real-life experiences as a female with all the social implications.

Uses and Complications

Orchiectomy can be used to treat testicular cancer. Seminoma is a type of testicular cancer that, if the tumors are localized, in 98 percent of the patients is curable with orchiectomy and low doses of adjuvant radiotherapy.

Advanced cancer at stage II is curable with orchiectomy and radiation therapy to the involved areas for 85 to 90 percent of patients. In metastatic diseases, stage III or localized advanced disease is primarily curable in 90 percent of the patients if combined with chemotherapy. Nonseminoma germ cell tumors (NSGCTs) seem to resist radiation therapy and are more likely to travel to the lungs, brain, bones, and liver.

Both seminoma and nonseminoma are highly curable if caught early enough, even if the cancer has spread beyond the testes to other body parts and tissues, as compared to other cancers. When it comes to relapse of the disease, the risk is lowered with retroperitoneal lymphadenectomy followed by chemotherapy, but this protocol does not improve survival. It is also possible that removing the lymph nodes may cause infertility.

Patients who have undergone orchiectomy may go to work the next day, if they desire. However, some patients may need a day or two before they feel ready. It is important to drink fluids and to abstain from alcoholic beverages. Sometimes, the patient may feel nauseated if the procedure was performed because of cancer. Some pain and swelling may develop, which is normal, and the physician may prescribe medications to counteract them.

One of the major risks of orchiectomy is a sudden hormone change, and side effects may occur, such as loss of muscle mass, brittle bones, weight gain, fatigue, erection problems, loss of sexual desire, hot flashes, enlargement and tenderness in the breasts, and sterility.

Undergoing orchiectomy for male-to-female genital reconstruction requires a diagnosis from a psychiatrist, as well as letters from mental health counselors in support of this procedure.

Perspective and Prospects

In 1941, orchiectomy was first used on a patient suffering from advanced prostate cancer. Indications from this therapy showed no apparent improvement of survival from it. In 1967, the Veterans Administration Cooperative Urological Research Group or (VACURG), presented information on more than two thousand patients who had received different types of therapies, including orchiectomy.

From 1984 through 1993, a study was performed on seventy-two patients with stage C and stage D prostate cancer whereby forty-four out of sixty-one patients had a partial response, and a good response on the tumor markers.

—*Marvin Morris, L.Ac., M.P.A.*

See also Genital disorders, male; Glands; Hydroceles; Men's health; Orchitis; Reproductive system; Surgery, general; Testicles, undescended; Testicular cancer; Testicular surgery; Testicular torsion; Urology; Urology, pediatric; Vascular system.

For Further Information:

Dawson, C. "Testicular Cancer: Seek Advice Early." *Journal of Family Health Care* 12 (2002): 3.
Geldart, T. R., P. D. Simmonds, and G. M. Mead. "Orchiectomy After Chemotherapy for Patients with Metastatic Testicular Germ Cell Cancer." *BJU International* 90 (September, 2002): 451-455.
Incrocci, L., et al. " Treatment Outcome, Body Image, and Sexual Functioning After Orchiectomy and Radiotherapy for Stage I-II Testicular Seminoma." *International Journal of Radiation Oncology, Biology, Physics* 53 (August 1, 2002): 1165-1173.
Khatri, Vijay P., and Juan A. Asensio. *Khatri: Operative Surgery Manual*. Philadelphia: Saunders, 2003.
Neff, Deanna M. "Orchiectomy." *Health Library*, September 26, 2012.
"Testicular Cancer Treatments: The Inguinal Orchiectomy." *Testicular Cancer Resource Center*, December 9, 2012.

Orchitis

Disease/Disorder
Also known as: Epididymoorchitis
Anatomy or system affected: Genitals, reproductive system
Specialties and related fields: Family medicine, virology
Definition: An inflammation of one or both testicles.

Causes and Symptoms

Orchitis is usually a consequence of epididymitis, an inflammation of the tube that connects the vas deferens and the testicles. It can also result from prostate infections. The source of inflammation can be either bacterial or viral organisms. The disease is typically caused by a generalized infection, such as mumps, scarlet fever, or typhoid fever. Chronic cases of orchitis can be produced by syphilis, gonorrhea, chlamydia, tuberculosis, and parasitic infections. In most cases of orchitis, only one testis is infected.

The most frequent cause of orchitis is the mumps, a viral infection. About one-third of males with the mumps develop orchitis at some stage of the illness, usually within four to six days after it begins. In prepubertal boys, about 20 percent develop mumps-induced orchitis. It is much rarer for males who are past puberty.

Symptoms of orchitis include nausea, fever, fatigue, and tenderness and significant swelling of the affected testis. Other effects may include groin pain, pain during urination, discharge from the penis, pain associated with intercourse and ejaculation, and blood in the semen.

Treatment and Therapy

If orchitis is produced by a bacterial infection, then antibiotics are the most effective treatment. Anti-inflammatory drugs are also commonly prescribed. If the source of infection is viral, then orchitis can be treated only with proper bed rest, elevation and support of the testes, and pain-relieving drugs. The application of ice packs periodically to the infected area helps reduce the pain. If acute pain occurs in the scrotum or testicles, then immediate medical attention is necessary.

When orchitis is properly treated and the cause is bacterial, normal function of the testis is typically preserved. If mumps is the source of orchitis, then shrinking of the testicles often occurs. Sterility may also occur, though it is very rare in cases of unilateral (one-sided) orchitis. Immunization against mumps is the best preventive treatment to avoid the possible complications of orchitis, although there have been a few cases of mumps-induced orchitis developing subsequent to a mumps-measles-rubella (MMR) vac-

Information on Orchitis

Causes: Bacterial or viral infection of epididymis or prostate from mumps, scarlet fever, typhoid fever; chronic cases may result from STDs (syphilis, gonorrhea, chlamydia), tuberculosis, parasitic infections

Symptoms: Tenderness and swelling of affected testis; nausea; fever; fatigue; groin pain; pain during urination, intercourse, or ejaculation; penile discharge; blood in semen

Duration: Acute, with possible sterility

Treatments: Depends on cause; may include antibiotics, anti-inflammatory drugs, bed rest, elevation and support of testes, pain medications, ice packs

cine. Spread of bacteria associated with sexually transmitted diseases (STDs) that can cause epididymo-orchitis in sexually active men can be minimized through monogamy and the use of condoms.

Perspective and Prospects

The first recorded description of orchitis goes back to Hippocrates in the fifth century BCE. Physical examination often reveals a tender, enlarged testicle on the affected side. Tender, enlarged lymph nodes in the groin area may also indicate the presence of orchitis.

Doppler ultrasound of the groin area can be used to confirm a diagnosis of orchitis by showing increased blood flow to the affected region, as well as tissue textures that are associated with infection. This test can also reveal any presence of scrotal abscesses. Nuclear magnetic resonance (NMR) imaging may also be used to help diagnose the presence of orchitis.

—*Alvin K. Benson, Ph.D.*

See also Antibiotics; Bacterial infections; Chlamydia; Gonorrhea; Men's health; Mumps; Parasitic diseases; Prostate gland; Reproductive system; Scarlet fever; Sexually transmitted diseases (STDs); Syphilis; Testicles, undescended; Testicular cancer; Testicular surgery; Testicular torsion; Typhoid fever; Tuberculosis; Viral infections.

For Further Information:

Kliegman, Robert M., et al., eds. *Nelson Textbook of Pediatrics*. 19th ed. Philadelphia: Elsevier/Saunders, 2011.

"Orchitis." *Mayo Clinic*, October 7, 2011.

Rosenfeld, Isadore. *Symptoms*. New York: Bantam Books, 1994.

Standring, Susan, et al., eds. *Gray's Anatomy: The Anatomical Basis of Clinical Practice*. 40th ed. New York: Churchill Livingstone/Elsevier, 2008.

Taguchi, Yosh. *Private Parts: An Owner's Guide to the Male Anatomy*, edited by Merrily Weisbord. 3d ed. Toronto: McClelland & Stewart, 2003.

Van De Graaff, Kent M. *Human Anatomy*. 6th ed. New York: McGraw-Hill, 2002.

Vorvick, Linda J., Louis S. Liou, and David Zieve. "Orchitis." *MedlinePlus*, October 9, 2012.

Organs. *See* **Systems and organs.**

Orthodontics

Specialty

Anatomy or system affected: Gums, mouth, teeth

Specialties and related fields: Dentistry

Definition: A dental specialty in which the teeth are straightened and moved into positions in the jaws that yield a correct and attractive arrangement.

Key terms:

analgesic: a medication (such as aspirin) that reduces or eliminates pain

dental arch: the arched bony part of the upper and lower jaws, in which the teeth are found

lingual: related to the tongue; in orthodontics, the inner sides or faces of the teeth

malocclusion: an incorrect fit of the upper and lower teeth when they are brought together

mastication: the act of chewing food

occlusion: the fit of the upper and lower teeth when they are brought together

Science and Profession

The term "orthodontics" comes from the Greek words meaning "straight teeth." It is practiced by a dental specialist called an orthodontist. Orthodontists graduate from dental school and then specialize in orthodontics. To explore orthodontics as a field, one must first consider teeth and the mouth. Ideally, thirty-two human teeth are arranged in appropriate orientations in the dental arches of each jaw. Four incisors are located in the center of each arch; on either side of them are a cuspid or canine tooth, followed by two bicuspids (premolars) and three molars.

The first molar on the side of each jaw is viewed as particularly important to orthodontics. Appropriate tooth development within the jaw and correct tooth eruption enable proper dental health, which keeps teeth in the mouth for most of an individual's life. They also ensure appropriate mastication of food and good digestive health, as well as self-confidence with an attractive smile.

Teeth are rarely optimally placed in the jaws. One important reason for this is heredity. This facet of orthodontics relates to the teeth and to jaws. The genes that control the size and shape of human teeth and jaws vary considerably. In addition, the genes for teeth and jaws are highly individualized and often poorly related to one another. Hence, it is likely that orthodontic problems caused by tooth-jaw mismatch will occur.

Other aspects of the development of irregular tooth positioning arise from living. In some cases, teeth are damaged by decay, oral diseases, or injury. In others, poor oral habits such as thumb sucking move them out of appropriate positions. In many cases, minor problems may be handled by restorative dentistry, such as filling dental caries (cavities) or placing crowns. Most treatment of poorly positioned teeth, however, is carried out by orthodontists on nearly 5 million Americans per year. The majority of these patients are children, but many adults are presently undergoing orthodontic treatment.

There are several main goals of orthodontic treatment involving the bones of the jaws and the teeth. First, occlusion

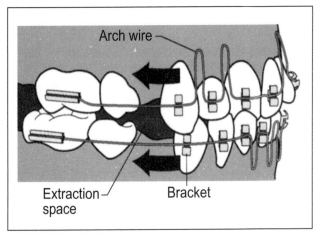

The most common orthodontic appliances are braces, which can be used to realign crooked teeth or correct malocclusion (such as underbite or overbite). In cases of tooth overcrowding, some teeth may be extracted, and the remaining teeth may be repositioned to fill the extraction space (shown here).

is improved so that all teeth engage one another properly for chewing and swallowing. Speech patterns are also improved, because almost twenty letter sounds involve interactions between tooth, tongue, and jaw movements. Another goal is increased resistance to decay and periodontal disease, which cause havoc in mouths where teeth are too close together or misaligned in other ways. The final orthodontic goal is improved appearance, which is for many individuals the primary reason for undergoing treatment.

Most orthodontic problems are termed malocclusions and are caused by defects of teeth and/or the jaws. Malocclusions are often classified according to the system developed by Edward H. Angle, the originator of modern orthodontics. He developed three classes of occlusion, defined by relationships between the upper and lower first molars.

In normal occlusion (class I), the lower first molars are seen slightly farther forward than their upper counterparts when the mouth is closed. This relationship positions the rest of the teeth for optimum chewing. When the arch length of either jaw is too small for all the teeth to be in appropriate positions, they become crowded. Also, in some individuals bimaxillary protrusion occurs, in which the front teeth of the jaws flare outward. These occurrences are unattractive and lead both to tooth decay and to periodontal disease.

Classes II and III are malocclusions that can be considered together. They are caused by improper positioning in the closed mouth of the lower first molars, either very far back or very far forward. In the first case (class II), the position of the first molars produces buck teeth because of the protrusion of the upper jaw in the closed mouth. The resulting problems are uncosmetic appearance and the ease with which buck teeth can be knocked out. Class II malocclusion is most often attributable to a hereditary size mismatch of the jawbones. Class III malocclusion is often termed crossbite. It causes the lower jaw to be positioned so that the lower front incisors are in front of the upper ones. In

some cases, this problem is treated by orthodontics; in others, surgery is required.

The Angle classification system does not include faulty vertical relationships of the jaws, which produce other problems. Examples are overbite, which hides the lower teeth entirely in the closed jaw, and open bite, which leaves a gap between the upper and lower front teeth in the closed mouth. These situations may be asymmetric and make closures lopsided.

Functional malocclusions are also caused by thumb sucking, chewing of the lower lip, or tongue thrusting. With thumb sucking, class II malocclusion may result or be enhanced, or open bite may occur. Chewing the lower lip will cause the upper front teeth to flare outward, and tongue thrusting (often a consequence of mouth breathing because of asthma) may cause open bite, crossbite, or class II malocclusion.

Defects of the teeth themselves occur as well. They are caused by overretention or underretention of the baby teeth and missing or lost permanent teeth. These conditions cause the remaining teeth to drift in the mouth and should be corrected as soon as possible in order to preclude occlusion problems.

Diagnostic and Treatment Techniques

The first stage of orthodontic treatment is an extensive diagnostic procedure that requires several office visits. First, the orthodontist compiles a complete dental and medical history. Then, the patient's mouth and teeth are examined thoroughly. This effort, accomplished in one visit, leads to a preliminary treatment plan. During the next visit, complete x-rays of the jaws are taken to show their relationship to each other, dental impressions of the teeth and jaws are made, and color photographs of the face and mouth are taken.

On the third visit, the patient is given a comprehensive diagnosis, and a treatment plan is described. At this point, the patient is informed about the problems to be treated, the probable consequences if they are left untreated, the steps to be used and their duration, the results that are expected, and any possible treatment complications. The overall cost of the treatment is also discussed. After agreement is reached, treatment begins and may require up to several years of visits at varied intervals. The process begins with the use of orthodontic appliances worn to move the teeth to new positions. After this, a simpler appliance called a retainer is worn until the bone of the tooth sockets, remodeled by the earlier treatment, is able to maintain the new dental arrangement.

Patient compliance with treatment instructions is crucial. Short-term noncompliance can lengthen the treatment period greatly; extreme noncompliance may completely destroy the endeavor. Most aspects of modern orthodontic treatment are relatively painless. If soreness occurs, it may usually be relieved quickly by combining saltwater gargles, temporary soft diets, and mild analgesics. Soreness caused by the rubbing of metal appliance parts against the inside of the cheeks or lips may be prevented by application of a wax supplied by the orthodontist. Pain that lasts for more than several days should be reported; it can usually be alleviated by an office visit where the orthodontist adjusts the offending portion of the appliance.

Throughout the course of orthodontic treatment, it is recommended that patients keep careful written records of orthodontic instructions and a complete daily record of use of the orthodontic appliance prescribed. The orthodontic appliances also need to be kept clean, stored carefully if removable, and guarded carefully during sports or other physical activities. The teeth must also be kept clean to prevent tooth decay. In addition, hard or sticky foods must be avoided.

The mechanical devices used by orthodontists vary widely. Their purposes are to direct jaw growth, to move selected teeth, to alter the behavior of the jaw muscles, and to maintain the position of the teeth once they have been moved. These appliances operate on two main principles. First, bone growth slows when pressure is applied against it and accelerates when the bone is kept in traction. This is how desired facial bone growth is attained. Second, when pressure is applied to the bone in tooth sockets, bone growth slows on the side to which the pressure is applied. Conversely, the growth of bone is stimulated on the other side of the tooth. This is the principle that generates tooth movement in the mouth. Applied properly, the combination of jaw and tooth treatment achieves results that can be fine-tuned over the treatment period. A lengthy treatment period ensures the minimum amount of pain while this movement occurs.

There are two main categories among the many orthodontic appliances used: fixed and removable appliances. Each category has numerous subcategories, and there are variants within each subcategory. Fixed appliances are firmly affixed in the mouth for the duration of treatment. They are made of metal cylinders shaped to fit snugly around individual teeth and cemented in position. The main fixed appliance types are bracketed appliances, lingual arch wires, habit control appliances, and space retainers.

Bracketed appliances, usually called braces, move teeth and direct growth of bone in the dental arches. Although braces are often disliked by patients on aesthetic grounds, orthodontists view them as an unrivaled means to cause precise tooth movement and directed bone growth. They are made up of several components. First, bands (metal cylinders) are applied around chosen anchor teeth. Then, metal or sturdy synthetic polymer brackets are cemented to each tooth in positions that determine the direction of the force to be applied to it. Next, arch wires are passed across each bracket to the anchor teeth, where they are attached to the bands. Elastic or wire ligatures keep the arch wires in the brackets at all times.

Much of the pressure that engenders tooth movement comes from the shape of the arch wires and their composition. Elastic bands are also used to provide special treatment to a given tooth or tooth group. These bands must be removed before eating and replaced daily. When necessary, external headgear is used to apply pressure to teeth and/or jaws, either pulling them forward or pushing them backward.

Lingual bracketed appliances, a newer device often called "invisible braces," are fixed appliances attached to the teeth on the inside of the dental arch. They are not externally visible except for the bands on the anchor teeth. Thus, they are advantageous aesthetically. They do not function as well as standard braces, however, and often interfere with normal speech. Other fixed appliances include lingual arch wires, habit control devices, and space retainers.

A wide variety of removable appliances may also be used. They are either entirely or partly removable by wearers. Removable appliances are most effective when worn constantly, but they can be removed at meals and on special occasions. Their use gives much less precise results than fixed appliances, however, and requires the continuous, unflagging cooperation of patients. Active, partly removable appliances put pressure on teeth and jaws. Functional appliances, which are completely removable, alter the pressure created by the muscles of the mouth and so act on the teeth and bones (for example, lip bumpers, which keep lips away from teeth).

Removable habit control appliances and space retainers are used, respectively, to prevent activities such as thumb sucking and to maintain desired spaces between teeth until the new dental arrangements have stabilized. They are specially designed bands, acrylic plates, and/or combinations. Space retainers exert enough pressure on teeth to keep them in place but not to move them. Special headgear may also be used as an auxiliary to in-the-mouth appliances. In some cases, diseased or extra teeth must be extracted as part of the treatment regimen.

Perspective and Prospects

Orthodontics has changed markedly since its inception. The changes include efforts at making braces more appealing and a changing clientele, evolving from one in which most patients were children to a population having many adult customers. The new direction in producing more cosmetic bracketed appliances arises from several factors.

First is the development of stronger and better synthetic polymer and ceramic replacements for metals, allowing the creation of materials that are less visible and that still produce the unrivaled therapeutic capabilities of bracketed appliances. A second factor is the interest of adults in orthodontic treatment. This discriminating population wishes to appear as attractive as possible, even in braces, and has both the independence of judgment and the monetary power to drive trends toward the use of such materials.

The adult move toward orthodontics in the United States is founded partly on the funding of orthodontic work by entities as diverse as Medicaid for welfare recipients and third-party group dental insurance plans. In addition, the adult public is being made more aware that it is not necessary to live out life with an unattractive smile simply because orthodontic treatment was not attempted in childhood or adolescence.

Considerable research has been carried out in the treatment of problems associated with orthodontics, including the root tip resorption that often halts such treatment. It is hoped that a combination of these endeavors and factors will continue to improve orthodontics.

—*Sanford S. Singer, Ph.D.*

See also Bones and the skeleton; Braces, orthodontic; Dentistry; Jaw wiring; Orthodontics; Periodontal surgery; Teeth; Tooth extraction.

For Further Information:

Doundoulakis, James, and Warren Strugatch. *The Perfect Smile: The Complete Guide to Cosmetic Dentistry.* Long Island, N.Y.: Hatherleigh Press, 2003.

Gluck, George M., and Warren M. Morganstein, eds. *Jong's Community Dental Health.* 5th ed. St. Louis, Mo.: Mosby, 2003.

Houston, W. J. B., C. D. Stephens, and W. J. Tulley. *A Textbook of Orthodontics.* 2d ed. Boston: Wright, 1992.

Klatell, Jack, Andrew Kaplan, and Gray Williams, Jr., eds. *The Mount Sinai Medical Center Family Guide to Dental Health.* New York: Macmillan, 1991.

"Malocclusion of Teeth." *MedlinePlus*, February 22, 2012.

Mitchell, Laura. *An Introduction to Orthodontics.* 4th ed. New York: Oxford University Press, 2013.

"Orthodontics: Braces and More." *Columbia University College of Dental Medicine*, May 5, 2010.

Smith, Rebecca W. *The Columbia University School of Dental and Oral Surgery's Guide to Family Dental Care.* New York: W. W. Norton, 1997.

Orthopedic braces. *See* Braces, orthopedic.

Orthopedic surgery

Procedure

Anatomy or system affected: Bones, feet, hands, hips, joints, knees, legs, ligaments, muscles, musculoskeletal system, nervous system, spine, tendons

Specialties and related fields: General surgery, orthopedics, physical therapy, podiatry, rheumatology, sports medicine

Definition: Surgical procedures involving the bones or joints.

Key terms:

polymethylmethacrylate: a material used in the fixation of bones

valgus: a musculoskeletal deformity in which a limb is twisted outward from the body

varus: a musculoskeletal deformity in which a limb is twisted toward the body

Indications and Procedures

Orthopedic surgery encompasses a number of different procedures carried out to repair injuries affecting the skeletal system and joints or to repair tissues associated with these structures. Such surgery may also attempt to correct associated neurological injury. In addition, orthopedic surgery is used to correct musculoskeletal problems that may be congenital in origin.

Among the congenital conditions for which orthopedic surgery may be warranted are bowlegs (valgus knees) and knock-knees (varus knees). In the case of bowlegs caused by a congenital malformation, one or both legs are bent outward at the knee. In knock-knees caused by congenital con-

ditions, the knees are curved inward, causing the lower legs to twist away from the body.

Treatment begins with a thorough evaluation of the problem. Based on x-ray analysis, an orthopedic surgeon may make a decision as to whether surgery can be used in the correction of the problem. During the surgical procedure itself, the affected limbs are properly aligned; they are splinted upon completion of the surgery. The chances of success are greatest in younger children. In an analogous situation, if a limb is twisted during fetal development, the child may exhibit misalignment of the structure following birth. Since bone at this stage of life is only beginning its growth, maintaining the limb in a splint may correct the problem. If necessary, the surgeon may decide to realign the limb at the joint through orthopedic surgery.

Tumors that originate in bone are uncommon. If they occur, such growths must be removed as quickly as possible because of the speed with which they spread to adjacent and distant structures in the body if the tumor is cancerous. The first signs of bone cancer include pain and swelling in the affected region. Spontaneous fractures may occur. X-ray and biopsy analyses are necessary to confirm the diagnosis of cancer. If the tumor is benign, it may be removed through surgery. Osteomas, which are tumors that arise from connective tissue within the bone, may require radiation or chemotherapy in addition to surgical removal.

Commonly, orthopedic surgery is used to correct fractures or dislocations. As with any procedure, a thorough evaluation is necessary prior to a final decision. This evaluation often includes x-ray and computed tomography (CT) analyses. If the injury involves the spine, treatment must both correct the problem and prevent secondary injury to the spinal cord. Fractures to the vertebral column may produce fragments that pose a threat to the spinal cord. Under these conditions, orthopedic surgery is used to immobilize or straighten the spinal column; this may involve external braces or an internal brace such as a Harrington distraction rod. The patient may be immobilized for weeks to months, depending on the extent of the injury and the course of treatment.

Uses and Complications

One of the most common applications of orthopedic surgery is the repair of trauma or fractures to bones. For example, a blow to the face, either intentional or accidental, may result in fractures to the nose or facial bones. Injuries to other skeletal structures, including the spine, may also result from the incident. This is particularly true if the source of the injury was an automobile accident. Upon clinical examination by a physician, it may be apparent that facial bones have been fractured. X-ray analysis may be used to confirm the initial diagnosis. Proper repair and restoration of features will be the primary concern of the orthopedic surgeon, assuming that the injuries are not life-threatening. In the event of facial injuries, damage to teeth and other periodontal regions will also be a consideration. In many cases, wire fixation may be a sufficient course of treatment. If more severe, the fracture may require screw-plate fixation, particularly in complicated fractures.

If uneventful or uncomplicated, the healing of such injuries usually requires about six weeks of immobilization. The procedure and immobilization, however, are inherently uncomfortable. If a muscle tear is severe or significant, resulting in a pull to the bone or joint, an associated fracture may heal improperly because of the dislocation of tissue. Proper evaluation of surgical options, including the use of metallic plates, can limit any such complications.

Although cancers originating in bone tissue are uncommon, they nevertheless present problems for the orthopedic surgeon. Fractures related to tumor development are generally treated in much the same way as uncomplicated breaks. If damage to the bone, either through the tumor itself or as a result of therapy, is severe, even surgical repair may not be sufficient to heal the structure and allow mobility or normal function. If the fracture is near the joint, the bone may require realignment or resection, resulting in a shortening of the structure. In some cases, internal fixation with polymethylmethacrylate bone cement may be used to augment repair.

Perspective and Prospects

The introduction of computed tomography (CT) scanning technology in the 1970s allowed for much more detailed evaluation of bone and joint injuries. Much of the technology is best applicable in a post-traumatic situation, evaluating the result of injury rather than its cause. Magnetic resonance imaging (MRI) is based on different technology but produces results that are similar to CT scans.

The destruction of bone as a function of aging or of disease is not well understood. Degenerative bone disease as a result of arthritis is among the most common of arthritic conditions, affecting nearly half of middle-aged adults in some manner. Such conditions, particularly among the elderly, remain to be fully addressed.

The ability to carry out bone transplants, developed extensively in the latter half of the twentieth century, allowed for at least partial replacement of damaged bone. Replacement structures may come from the patient's own body or from a cadaver. In addition, orthopedic technology has resulted in prostheses for the replacement of most joints in the body.

Joint replacements are dramatic. Individuals with crippling deformities can have nearly normal function restored through replaced joints. The most commonly replaced joints include hips and knees. Other joints can also be replaced. Individuals who have their hips and knees replaced usually start walking on the replaced joint in the first or second postoperative day. Complete rehabilitation requires several months.

—*Richard Adler, Ph.D.; updated by*
L. Fleming Fallon, Jr., M.D., Ph.D., M.P.H.

See also Amputation; Arthroplasty; Arthroscopy; Bone grafting; Bowlegs; Bunions; Casts and splints; Disk removal; Fracture repair; Hammertoe correction; Hammertoes; Heel spur removal; Hip fracture repair; Hip replacement; Jaw wiring; Joints; Kneecap removal; Knock-knees; Laminectomy and spinal fusion; Orthopedics; Orthopedics, pediatric; Physical rehabilitation; Prostheses; Rotator cuff surgery.

For Further Information:

Bentley, George, and Robert B. Greer, eds. *Orthopaedics*. 4th ed. Oxford, England: Linacre House, 1993.

Brotzman, S. Brent, and Kevin E. Wilk. *Clinical Orthopaedic Rehabilitation*. 2d ed. Philadelphia: Mosby, 2003.

Callaghan, John J., Aaron Rosenberg, and Harry E. Rubash, eds. *The Adult Hip*. 2d ed. Philadelphia: Lippincott Williams & Wilkins, 2007.

Doherty, Gerard M., and Lawrence W. Way, eds. *Current Surgical Diagnosis and Treatment*. 13th ed. New York: Lange Medical Books/McGraw-Hill, 2010.

Griffith, H. Winter. *Complete Guide to Symptoms, Illness, and Surgery*. 6th ed. New York: Perigee, 2012.

Mulholland, Michael W., et al., eds. *Greenfield's Surgery: Scientific Principles and Practice*. 5th ed. Philadelphia: Lippincott Williams & Wilkins, 2011.

Tapley, Donald F., et al., eds. *The Columbia University College of Physicians and Surgeons Complete Home Medical Guide*. Rev. 3d ed. New York: Crown, 1995.

McPhee, Stephen J., and Maxine A. Papadakis, eds. *Current Medical Diagnosis and Treatment*. Los Altos, Calif.: Lange Medical, 2011.

Zollinger, Robert M., Jr., E. Christopher Ellison, and Robert M. Zollinger, Sr. *Zollinger's Atlas of Surgical Operations*. 9th ed. New York: McGraw-Hill, 2011.

Orthopedics

Specialty

Anatomy or system affected: Bones, feet, hands, hips, joints, knees, legs, ligaments, muscles, musculoskeletal system, nervous system, spine, tendons

Specialties and related fields: Physical therapy, podiatry, rheumatology, sports medicine

Definition: The field of medicine concerned with the prevention and treatment of disorders, either developmental or caused by injury or disease, that are associated with the skeleton, joints, muscles, and connective tissues.

Key terms:

articulation: a joint between two bones of the skeleton; also called an arthrosis

bursa: a connective tissue sac filled with fluid that reduces friction at joints

collagen: a fibrous protein found in skin, bone, ligaments, tendons, and cartilage

inflammation: the reaction of tissue to injury, with its corresponding redness, heat, swelling, and pain

ligament: a structure of tough connective tissue that attaches one bone to another bone

synovial: referring to the lubricating fluid in the joints or the membrane surrounding the joints

tendon: a structure of tough connective tissue that attaches a muscle to a bone

Science and Profession

Orthopedics is the branch of medicine primarily concerned with the movement of the human body and its parts, as well as disorders that affect its function. Such activities as maintaining posture, walking, doing manual work, and exercising involve a complex relationship between the nervous system, muscular system, and skeletal system. While orthopedists must be familiar with the nervous system, they focus primarily on the prevention and treatment of disorders of the skeleton and muscles. They also have expertise in the proper development of these systems in childhood and the changes that occur as a result of aging.

When a person decides to make a movement, the brain sends signals to the muscles. The muscles contract and, by pulling on the bones to which they are attached, cause that part of the body to move. The anchor point for the muscle is the origin, and the attachment point to the bone that is being moved is the insertion. Muscles work in groups to perform a movement. The principal muscle involved is the prime mover, or agonist. The muscles that help the prime mover are called synergists. When a prime mover contracts, the muscle on the opposite side of the bone, termed the antagonist, must relax. An illustration of this would be the muscle and bone interaction involved in the flexing of the arm. The biceps muscle, anchored to bone in the shoulder, contracts, pulling on the bone in the lower arm to which it is attached by a tendon. Its synergist, the brachialis, also contracts. On the back of the upper arm, its antagonist, the triceps muscle, relaxes to allow the arm to bend. When the arm is extended, the triceps becomes the prime mover for that action, and the biceps is the antagonist.

The skeletal system is made of bone and cartilage. Bone cells, called osteocytes, take in nutrients from the blood and constantly renew the bony matrix. The chemical composition of bone includes calcium and phosphorus salts, which provide stiffness. The fibrous protein collagen gives bones some flexibility. Cartilage cells, called chondrocytes, manufacture cartilage, which is a mass of collagen and elastic fibers embedded in a gelatin-like substance. The nature of this structure gives cartilage more flexibility than bone, which makes it an ideal substitute for bone in certain areas. The ribs, for example, are attached by cartilage to the sternum, or breastbone. This arrangement allows for the expansion of the chest during breathing.

Tendons, ligaments, and bursas are also part of the skeletal and muscular systems. Tendons attach muscles to bones. They are made of fibrous tissue so strong that, under stress, the muscle will tear or the bone will break before the tendon will be damaged. Ligaments, which are also made of fibrous tissue, attach bones to other bones and provide stability at the joints. Bursas are fluid-filled connective tissue sacs that lie between muscle and bone, tendon and bone, or other areas around joints. They reduce the damage that occurs to the softer tissue as it rubs against bone with each movement. Because of their close interdependence, the skeleton, attached muscles, and other associated structures are often referred to as the musculoskeletal system.

The health of the musculoskeletal system during childhood is of primary importance to an individual in attaining full growth and physical function as an adult. In the early developmental stages of the embryo and fetus, a skeleton of cartilage is formed. This structure is replaced with bone in a process called ossification that continues for years after birth. Good nutrition is vital to this process. In particular, the body requires adequate amounts of protein, calcium, and vitamin D. The ends of a long bone are separated from the shaft of the bone by cartilage until the child reaches full growth. Care should be taken when participating in sports, since damage to these areas could affect the growth of that limb. Hormonal production influences the development of the skeleton. Adequate amounts of growth hormone are needed to ensure that proper growth is attained. At puberty, sex hormones, especially testosterone, stimulate the final growth spurts and completion of the adult skeleton.

Young adults have attained their full growth, but the skeleton must renew itself continually to remain strong and maintain its ability to repair injury. A woman of childbearing age must eat a healthy diet if she is to nourish a fetus that, in turn, is developing its own skeleton. Both men and women must take care to exercise, since the stress of activity not only builds muscle but also sends messages to the bone to maintain its strength. Calcium and vitamin D intake must continue, or the bones may begin to dissolve some of their calcium matrix. Automobile accidents, work injuries, and sports injuries are more likely to occur at this stage of life.

As adults age, metabolic and other cellular processes become less efficient, and care must be taken to maintain functions and prevent further losses. At one time, disorders such as osteoarthritis and osteoporosis were considered an inevitable part of the aging process. While heredity is certainly a risk factor in these conditions, a substantial body of evidence has been accumulated showing that some degenerative processes can be traced to lifestyle and diet. Osteoarthritis is the type of joint tissue degeneration that is associated with wear and tear on the joints. A person who is obese puts excessive pressure on the skeletal system, especially the hips, knees, and ankles. This pressure increases the damage to the joints. A person who fails to exercise begins to lose flexibility in the joints, and muscles become weaker.

Osteoporosis occurs as bones become porous and brittle. As osteocytes age, they become less efficient at calcium absorption and renewal of the bony matrix. At a time in life when more calcium is needed to make up for this inefficiency, most people consume fewer dairy products, either because of lactose intolerance or because of the ingestion of other beverages. Older women are at particular risk because their bones are lighter than those of men. After the menopause, women lose some of the protection that estrogen provided by stimulating the absorption of calcium and thus bone renewal. If older people lose the ability to move as surely as before and their reflexes slow down, then injuries are more likely to occur as a result of falls. These injuries are much more serious if the bones are brittle. Even if osteoporosis is not a factor, fractures and other injuries in an older individual do not heal as quickly as they would in a younger person.

Because of their knowledge of developmental processes, orthopedists, as well as pediatricians, are able to advise parents concerned about their growing children and the appropriate precautions for sports activities. Recommendations are made by orthopedists with regard to the design and utilization of safety equipment to prevent or reduce injury. Advice on nutrition and exercise for adults may also be given by physicians in an effort to reduce the incidence of problems as a person ages, allowing continuation of an active, independent life.

Diagnostic and Treatment Techniques

In nonemergency situations, patients with some pain or disorder of the muscles, bones, or joints are usually referred to an orthopedic surgeon. The first office visit begins with a review of the condition, during which the physician will take a general medical history and obtain a history of the current complaint. This history will include the time frame from onset, any action that may have initiated the condition, and a description of any difficulty in movement that the patient is having. A physician will then perform a physical examination to determine the specific areas affected and observe range-of-motion exercises to determine if function has been lost.

X-rays or other imaging methods are ordered to see whether any structural defect can be seen. Blood tests may be ordered if a disease process is suspected. Once a diagnosis has been made, a physician may prescribe medication, order physical therapy or home exercises, schedule surgery, or take other therapeutic measures to correct the condition. The types of abnormalities treated by orthopedists generally fall into one of three categories: injuries caused by accidents, repetitive motion disorders, and diseases affecting the skeleton, skeletal muscles, or joints.

The most common situation in which a patient sees an orthopedist is after an accidental injury. If the injury is severe, the patient may be transported to a hospital emergency room, with care taken to keep the injury site immobilized until a physician can see the patient. The type of treatment needed will be determined by the type and severity of the injury. In a closed or simple fracture, the skin is unbroken; the bones are manipulated back in line and then immobilized with a plaster cast or brace. An open or compound fracture occurs when the ends or fragments of the bone protrude through the skin. In this case, or if surgery is needed to align the bones properly, there is a higher risk of infection. In some cases, pins or wires must be used to hold the bone in position. Fractures of the skull or vertebrae are of special concern because of the possibility of permanent damage to the brain or spinal cord; a neurologist (a physician with specialty training in the nervous system) is usually called to assist an orthopedic surgeon.

Because of twisting movements, injuries that affect one or more joints are common. A dislocation occurs when the bones at a joint are separated. An orthopedist must realign the bones as closely as possible to the original positions and immobilize the joint to allow healing to occur. A sprain results from severe twisting of a joint without dislocation. The severity of joint injury and recovery time depend on the extent of the damage to surrounding ligaments, tendons, cartilage, and other tissues. A special procedure called arthroscopy may be scheduled since damage to soft tissue may not be revealed in an x-ray. An orthopedic surgeon inserts a flexible tube, called an arthroscope, into the injury site. This tube, combined with lights and a camera, allows the surgeon to view the joint cavity to see if any abnormality is present, and, if possible, to repair it.

Some damage to the musculoskeletal system is not the result of a single accident but of actions that are repeated

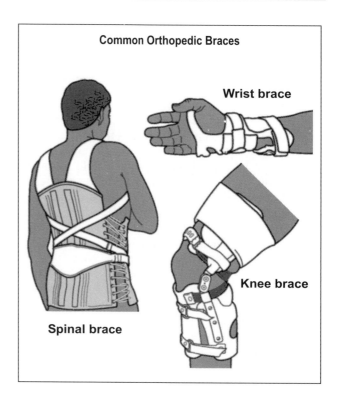

Common Orthopedic Braces

Wrist brace

Knee brace

Spinal brace

over a long period of time as a part of work duties or recreational activities. These are termed repetitive motion disorders. For example, bursitis, or inflammation of the bursas, may arise in a baseball pitcher's shoulder or a tennis player's elbow. Because the same motion is repeated over and over, the rub of the bursa and other soft tissue over bone causes irritation and inflammation, resulting in pain each time the movement is attempted. Treatment consists of reducing the inflammation by using cortisone or other similar drugs, usually by injection at the affected site, coupled with rest. Resumption of the activity may occur following recommendations from an orthopedist or therapist on a change in technique aimed at reducing the trauma. In some cases, the condition becomes chronic, and the patient may have to discontinue the activity altogether.

Many occupations arising in the mid-twentieth century involved relatively small movements of the hands and wrists. A worker on an assembly line who installs a specific part and an employee who uses a computer keyboard all day are examples of people at high risk for repetitive motion disorders. An understanding of the structure of the wrist leads to better understanding of the problem involved. The median nerve leads from the spinal cord through a tunnel in the carpal bones of the wrist and then branches out to the fingers. It is encircled, together with tendons leading to the fingers, by the transverse carpal ligament. When constant friction causes swelling of the tendons and tissues adjacent to the nerve, the nerve is pinched, resulting in pain, tingling, and weakness in the hand and fingers. This condition is termed carpal tunnel syndrome. Therapy may include changing work positions, wearing a splint to hold the wrist straight, using medications to reduce inflammation, and injecting cortisone at the injury site. If the problem continues, surgery may be needed. In this procedure, the orthopedic surgeon makes an incision in the wrist and cuts the transverse carpal ligament, thus releasing the pressure on the nerve and tendons. If the motion or activity that initially caused carpal tunnel syndrome is not stopped, the condition is likely to recur.

Diseases can affect the bones and joints. Congenital defects and inheritance may result in deformities that can be treated by orthopedic devices or surgery. Hormone therapy may be used by a physician to help a child attain full growth. Nutritional disorders, such as rickets, may cause the softening of the bones, with the corresponding bowed-leg deformity. Caused by a vitamin D deficiency, rickets must be treated not only with vitamin therapy but also with braces to keep the legs straight while the bones harden. Multiple myeloma is a form of cancer that invades the bone and bone marrow and must be treated with chemotherapy as well as surgery to remove the tumor. Infections such as gangrene affect the limbs and, if not treated in time, may necessitate amputation by the orthopedic surgeon.

Of all the diseases of the musculoskeletal system, arthritis and related disorders are the most common. "Arthritis" is a general term referring to inflammation of a joint. Osteoarthritis is a degenerative disease that results to some extent from the aging process, although it can be exacerbated by obesity, lifestyle, or injury. Arthritis can also be caused by infection or by deposits of uric acid crystals, a condition called gout. The most serious form of joint disease is rheumatoid arthritis, a term that is sometimes used to encompass a group of related disorders. These diseases are classified as autoimmune conditions because the body is making antibodies against itself-in this case, against the tissues associated with the joints. The disease process itself is often treated by a specialist called a rheumatologist, who tries various medications to alleviate the condition. An orthopedic surgeon may be called upon to help correct the deformities resulting from the disease or to replace defective joints with artificial ones. Special care must be taken in cases of juvenile rheumatoid arthritis, since the growth process may also be affected. Systemic lupus erythematosus (SLE), ankylosing spondylitis, and scleroderma are some of the other autoimmune diseases that affect the musculoskeletal system.

Perspective and Prospects

In the study of prehistoric humans, a major source of information is their skeletal remains. Archaeologists have found evidence of broken bones that were set and healed, indicating some rudimentary attempts at the treatment of injuries. Examination of hieroglyphs shows that ancient Egyptians set bones and used wooden splints held in place by the same gum and bandages that were used to wrap mummies. There were no medical specialties, and the treatment of wounds and fractures was part of the duties of any medical practitioner.

The branch of medicine known as orthopedics had its start in the eighteenth century. A physician named Jean André Venel (1740-91) opened an institute in Switzerland with the purpose of correcting skeletal deformities in children. The term "orthopedics" is actually a combination of two Greek words: *orthos*, meaning "straight" or "correct," and *pais*, meaning "child." Treatment of congenital deformities such as clubfoot and defects caused by rickets or injury was the primary function of this type of clinic.

In the nineteenth century, the development of quick-setting plaster for casts aided physicians in the immobilization of broken bones after they were set. The development of anesthesia and antiseptic techniques to prevent infection allowed the practice of orthopedic surgery to expand. Research using the microscope added to the understanding of the structure and function of bone as a living tissue.

In 1895, Wilhelm Conrad Röntgen (1845-1923) discovered that radiation from a cathode-ray tube would produce a photographic image of the bones of his hand. By the early twentieth century, the medical x-ray came into widespread use, providing an invaluable diagnostic tool for orthopedists. In the 1940s and 1950s, better understanding of radioactive phenomena allowed the development of safer x-ray equipment and techniques. In the 1970s and 1980s, other imaging techniques, such as computed tomography (CT) scanning and magnetic resonance imaging (MRI), increased the ability of orthopedic surgeons to diagnose and treat musculoskeletal disorders.

One of the greatest orthopedic surgical advances has been in the ability to treat badly damaged limbs. At one time, the best the orthopedic surgeon could do for some patients was to amputate the limb to prevent the spread of infection and the development of gangrene, then help the patient cope with the amputations by use of artificial limbs. More sophisticated techniques, incorporating the use of the microscope with computer-directed surgical instruments, allow the reattachment of limbs in many cases by enabling the surgeon to connect even the smallest blood vessels and nerves.

If amputation is necessary, artificial limbs, or prostheses, have also become more sophisticated. Artificial hands have become functional as a result of computer technology that enables the patient to direct the movement of the fingers by contracting and relaxing arm muscles. New plastics and other materials are being developed and used for synthetic joint replacements which increase the mobility of, and decrease the pain for, arthritic patients.

Joints are now routinely replaced. The most common replacements are hip and knee joints, although techniques have been developed to replace other joints in the body. The surgery is performed in a hospital. Recipients are encouraged to begin to use their replaced joints within twenty-four to forty-eight hours after surgery. Complete rehabilitation requires several months of increasingly intense physical activity and exercise. Contemporary materials have an expected useful life of twenty or more years.

A better understanding of the natural healing process at the cellular level has also allowed advances in the treatment of fractures. It has been found that attaching a device that generates a weak electric current can increase the rate of healing in some patients. This current stimulates the multiplication of osteocytes and the growth of new bone in the area.

As the understanding of disease and of degenerative processes increases, better treatments can also be devised. Osteoporosis, for example, is known to be a preventable condition when a correct diet and sufficient physical exercise are maintained throughout life. After the menopause in women, treatment with estrogen replacement therapy gives further protection against osteoporosis. New imaging devices allow osteoporosis to be detected at an earlier stage and more aggressive treatment measures to be applied. The genetic factor in diseases and conditions that trigger autoimmune disorders are other areas of research that are being pursued. While accidents will always occur, orthopedic research into the injury process can help devise methods of prevention, as well as new treatments for the orthopedic problems that do arise.

—*Edith K. Wallace, Ph.D.; updated by*
L. Fleming Fallon, Jr., M.D., Ph.D., M.P.H.

See also Amputation; Arthritis; Arthroplasty; Arthroscopy; Bone cancer; Bone disorders; Bone grafting; Bones and the skeleton; Bowlegs; Bunions; Bursitis; Cancer; Cartilage; Casts and splints; Chiropractic; Collagen; Craniosynostosis; Disk removal; Dwarfism; Ewing's sarcoma; Feet; Flat feet; Foot disorders; Fracture and dislocation; Fracture repair; Geriatrics and gerontology; Growth; Hammertoe correction; Hammertoes; Heel spur removal; Hip fracture repair; Hip replacement; Jaw wiring; Joints; Kinesiology; Kneecap removal; Knock-knees; Laminectomy and spinal fusion; Ligaments; Lower extremities; Muscle sprains, spasms, and disorders; Muscles; Neurofibromatosis; Orthopedic surgery; Orthopedics, pediatric; Osgood-Schlatter disease; Osteoarthritis; Osteochondritis juvenilis; Osteogenesis imperfecta; Osteomyelitis; Osteonecrosis; Osteopathic medicine; Osteoporosis; Paget's disease; Physical examination; Physical rehabilitation; Pigeon toes; Podiatry; Prostheses; Rheumatoid arthritis; Rheumatology; Rickets; Rotator cuff surgery; Scleroderma; Scoliosis; Slipped disk; Spina bifida; Spinal cord disorders; Spine, vertebrae, and disks; Spondylitis; Sports medicine; Systemic lupus erythematosus (SLE); Tendon disorders; Tendon repair; Upper extremities.

For Further Information:

American Academy of Orthopaedic Surgeons. http://www.aaos.org.
Cash, Mel. *Pocket Atlas of the Moving Body*. New York: Crown, 2000.
Currey, John D. *Bones: Structures and Mechanics*. 2d ed. Princeton, N.J.: Princeton University Press, 2006.
Delforge, Gary. *Musculoskeletal Trauma: Implications for Sport Injury Management*. Champaign, Ill.: Human Kinetics, 2002.
Marcus, Robert, David Feldman, and Jennifer Kelsey, eds. *Osteoporosis*. 3d ed. Boston: Academic Press/Elsevier, 2008.
Marieb, Elaine N., and Katja Hoehn. *Human Anatomy and Physiology*. 9th ed. San Francisco: Pearson/Benjamin Cummings, 2013.
"Orthopedic Services." *MedlinePlus*, March 1, 2012.
Rosen, Clifford J., Julie Glowacki, and John P. Bilezikian. *The Aging Skeleton*. San Diego, Calif.: Academic Press, 1999.
Salter, Robert Bruce. *Textbook of Disorders and Injuries of the Musculoskeletal System*. 3d ed. Baltimore: Williams & Wilkins, 1999.
Tortora, Gerard J., and Bryan Derrickson. *Principles of Anatomy and Physiology*. 13th ed. Hoboken, N.J.: John Wiley & Sons, 2012.

Orthorexia nervosa

Disease/Disorder

Anatomy or system affected: All
Specialties and related fields: Nutrition, health

Definition: Orthorexia nervosa is an obsession focused on the optimal healthfulness of an individual's diet and an obsession with eating "clean" or "pure" food.

Key terms:

cognitive behavioral therapy: a type of psychotherapy in which people learn to recognize and change negative and self-defeating patterns of thinking and behavior

Diagnostic and Statistical Manual of Mental Disorders: the handbook the American Psychiatric Society uses to categorize and diagnose mental disorders

Background

As more information about nutritional research is released to the public, it generally results in a healthier population. However, some individuals take this information as absolute fact, without understanding that research is a work in progress. They develop an unhealthy obsession with applying the knowledge at a level that most in the population do not. This obsession is most commonly focused on types of foods purported to be best for perfect health, how they should be prepared, and when and how much should be eaten.

The term orthorexia nervosa was coined by Steven Bratman, an American physician, in 1997. The term means "correct diet," and denotes an unhealthy fixation with eating food that is optimally healthy, "clean," "pure," and "correct." This obsession goes well beyond the desire to eat a healthy diet and extends to rituals involving eating the exact amount of "correctly" prepared food at the specific times during the day or allowing certain foods to be eaten only during certain seasons. This obsession can interfere with social relationships (e.g., the refusal to eat at friends' houses or in restaurants) and may result in nutritional deficits.

Orthorexia nervosa is not considered an official psychiatric disorder like anorexia nervosa or bulimia. It does not have an official diagnosis in the *Diagnostic and Statistical Manual of Mental Disorders*; however, it shares many characteristics with obsessive-compulsive disorders and anorexia nervosa. Ursula Philpot, chair of the British Dietetic Association, stated that individuals who have this condition are only concerned about the quality of food they consume, and only eat what they perceive to be "pure" food. When these individuals experience intense feelings of hunger and cravings, they punish themselves for being weak. The deprivation can be so severe that it results in death.

Physicians and eating disorder specialists often fail to distinguish between orthorexia nervosa and anorexia nervosa. It is important to understand the difference; anorexia nervosa is an eating disorder that results from the fear of being overweight, whereas in orthorexia nervosa, the goal is to achieve perfect health by controlling diet, not necessarily to lose weight. Still, both disorders can lead to malnutrition and health problems.

Even though increased attention is being given to better understanding the risk factors, behavior, and outcomes of therapy, there remains much to be learned. As of 2015, only one study has addressed the overlap of orthorexia, or other obsessive-compulsive disorders, with another type of eating disorder, including bulimia and anorexia. It appears that the longer a person is preoccupied with healthy eating, the higher the likelihood that he or she will develop a clinical eating disorder (up to 53 percent three years after diagnosis). Orthorexia can also develop in an individual recovering from another eating disorder.

Overview

Individuals with orthorexia nervosa are preoccupied with eating healthy foods, and avoid those high in fat, preservatives, animal products, or pesticides. Many of these individuals become malnourished because they avoid sources of necessary nutrition in favor of a small number of "safe" foods. One example of dietary restriction is the raw food diet. Individuals who follow this and similarly restrictive diets (i.e., veganism or fruitarianism) have an elevated risk of becoming emaciated, and can develop nutritional deficiencies if they do not sufficiently vary their diet to ensure adequate intake of vitamins, minerals, proteins, fiber, and other nutritional requirements found in food.

Orthorexia disorders are similar to and potentially overlap other psychiatric disorders such as obsessive-compulsive disorders, somatic symptom disorder, hypochondria, and psychotic spectrum disorders. One interesting overlap between orthorexia and other eating disorders is the displeasure with eating and the trading of control over one's life for control over diet.

It is not clear what demographic group is more susceptible to developing the disorder. In one 2008 study in Germany, nutrition students were investigated for developing the disorder because of their in-depth knowledge of nutrition and how to achieve optimal health. It was found that nutrition students did not have higher orthorexic tendencies than non-nutrition students. In a similar study in Portugal, it was found that orthorexic tendencies measured by a diagnostic questionnaire decreased as a nutrition student progressed through their education. The orthorexia questionnaire measured eating behaviors and attitudes toward nutrition. The students did have higher scores in regard to having more restrictive eating behaviors than non-nutrition students, but this is unsurprising given their education about healthy eating; however, it did not indicate that these students had unhealthy attitudes towards eating.

Symptoms of orthorexia nervosa include obsessive concern about one's diet, spending excessive amounts of time analyzing the source of a food for pesticides, worrying about whether milk or meat contains growth hormones or antibiotics, worrying about the safety of genetically modified foods (GMOs), overcooking food (thus losing nutrition) or eating only raw food, and avoiding packaged food. These individuals spend a lot of time planning menus, measuring portions, and obsessing about health and diet. Orthorexic individuals develop nutritional deficiencies because they tend to omit entire food groups. Nutritional deficiencies can lead to medical complications such as anemia, osteopenia, and metabolic, hormonal, and blood deficiencies.

Diagnosis of orthorexia nervosa is performed using a fif-teen-point questionnaire, called ORTO-15. This questionnaire assesses the beliefs of patients about their perception of eating healthy, food selection attitudes, food consumption habits, and the extent that food concerns affect daily life. Responses are scored using a four-point scale; a score below 40 is considered diagnostic of orthorexia whereas a score higher than 40 indicates a healthy view of eating. In addition, blood samples are drawn to assess for nutritional deficiencies.

Treatment for orthorexia nervosa has not been standardized. After a diagnosis has been made, the patient is referred to psychotherapists and dietitians, and sometimes prescribed medication (often antidepressants) and behavioral therapy. Psychotherapists focus their therapy according to the patient's needs. Among the varied approaches, patients undergo cognitive behavioral therapy to restructure their thoughts and reprogram their minds to avoid obsessive behavior and attitudes toward their diet. It appears that patients who undergo these therapies have some success in changing their attitudes towards food, with correct education about nutrition.

—Mandy M. McBroom, MPH;
updated by Tish Davidson, MA

See also: Anorexia nervosa, Nutrition

For Further Information:

Bratman, Steven. "The Authorized Orthorexia Self-Test." http://www.orthorexia.com (accessed August 1, 2017). An extensive description of orthorexia and how to determine if one has it by the doctor who coined the term.

Brytek-Matera, Anna, et al. "Predictors of Orthorexic Behaviours in Patients with Eating Disorders: A Preliminary Study." *BMC Psychiatry* 15. (2015): 1-8. https://bmcpsychiatry.biomedcentral.com/articles/10.1186/s12888-015-0628-1 (accessed August 1, 2017). A scholarly article examining the traits that predict orthorexia.

Kratina, Karin. "Orthorexia Nervosa." National Eating Disorders Association. https://www.nationaleatingdisorders.org/orthorexia-nervosa (accessed August 1, 2017). Easy-to-understand discussion about where orthorexia nervosa fits into the general picture of eating disorders.

Reddy, Sumathi. "When Healthy Eating Calls for Treatment." *Wall Street Journal - Eastern Edition* 11 Nov. 2014: D1+. https://www.wsj.com/articles/when-healthy-eating-calls-for-treatment-1415654737 (accessed August 1, 2017). Newspaper article discussing whether and when orthorexia rises to the level of needing to be treated.

Osgood-Schlatter disease
Disease/Disorder
Anatomy or system affected: Knees, musculoskeletal system, tendons
Specialties and related fields: Orthopedics, pediatrics
Definition: Pain caused by the patellar (kneecap) tendon pulling away from the tibia (shin bone).

Causes and Symptoms

Osgood-Schlatter disease is most frequently found in young athletes during their years of rapid growth. It is more common in boys, who are typically affected between the ages of thirteen and fourteen. Girls usually are affected at younger ages, ten to eleven. However, children are at risk between the

Globus, S. "Osgood-Schlatter: More than Growing Pains." *Current Health 2* 28, no. 4 (2002): 20.

Kaneshiro, Neil K. "Osgood-Schlatter Disease." *MedlinePlus*, November 12, 2012.

Lackey, E., and R. Sutton. "Rest Is Best for Common Knee Swelling." *GP: General Practitioner* 1c (2003): 75.

Parker, James N., and Philip M. Parker, eds. *The Official Patient's Sourcebook on Osgood-Schlatter Disease*. San Diego, Calif.: Icon Health, 2002.

Woodward, A. H. "Osgood-Schlatter Disease." *Pediatrics for Parents* 11, no. 1 (1990): 11.

Information on Osgood-Schlatter Disease

Causes: Rapid skeletal growth, repetitive motion associated with sports

Symptoms: Pain below kneecap; swollen, bony bump

Duration: Chronic during childhood

Treatments: Usually self-resolving; alleviation of symptoms with rest, ice, elastic bandages, leg elevation, pain medications, brace or cast in severe cases

---

ages of ten and eighteen, especially during their rapid skeletal growth years. Children who play sports that involve running or repetitive jumping have the highest risk.

The most common symptom of Osgood-Schlatter disease is pain below the kneecap. There is usually a swollen, bony bump in that area. Pain is often felt when the bump is touched or when the knee is bent or fully extended in activities such as running, jumping, kneeling, squatting, or lifting weights. As the child matures, Osgood-Schlatter disease will usually go away. When children stop growing, the patellar tendon is stronger and the pain and swelling disappear. Very seldom does the disease continue after rapid growth stops.

If the pain persists, then the child should see a pediatrician or orthopedist. The physician will examine the knee area and the location of pain in order to make a diagnosis. If the source of the pain is unclear, then an x-ray will be taken of the knee to verify Osgood-Schlatter disease.

Treatment and Therapy

The best treatment for Osgood-Schlatter disease is simply rest. Depending on the severity of the condition, the child may have to decrease activity levels or stop playing sports for several months. Deep knee bending and jumping should be minimized, and running may need to be limited. To treat the pain, the knee should get more rest, and ice should be applied for twenty minutes three times per day. Elastic bandages should be used to compress the knee area, and the leg should be elevated when possible. Over-the-counter pain relievers can be taken. In extreme cases, a brace or cast may be used.

After recovery from the pain, the child can slowly return to previous activity levels. Additionally, a physical therapist can prescribe exercises that will help strengthen the leg muscles around the knee to minimize the chances of a recurrence.

There is no surgical procedure for Osgood-Schlatter disease unless the patellar tendon is fully torn from the tibia. This should not happen if the patient gets proper rest, in which case Osgood-Schlatter disease will resolve itself.

—Bradley R. A. Wilson, Ph.D.

See also Bone disorders; Bones and the skeleton; Growth; Orthopedic surgery; Orthopedics; Orthopedics, pediatric; Physical rehabilitation; Sports medicine; Tendon disorders; Tendon repair.

For Further Information:

Dunn, J. F., Jr. "Osgood-Schlatter Disease." *American Family Physician* 41, no. 4 (1990): 173.

Osteoarthritis

Disease/Disorder

Anatomy or system affected: Joints, musculoskeletal system

Specialties and related fields: Exercise physiology, orthopedics

Definition: A degenerative joint disease that results from the wearing away of the cartilage of bones, causing inflammation, swelling, and pain in affected joints and eventually causing joint stiffness and limitation of movement, misalignment, and knoblike bone growths in the hands.

Key terms:

Bouchard's nodes: osteophytes or bony spurs that develop as a result of destruction of joint cartilage in proximal interphalangeal joints

cartilage: a smooth material covering the ends of bone joints that cushions the bone, allowing the joint to move easily

collagen: a fibrous protein substance in connective tissue, bone, tendons, and cartilage

crepitus: the scraping or grinding sound heard or felt when bone rubs over bone in joint spaces

degenerative: marked by progression to a state below what is considered normal or desirable

distal: away from the point of origin

distal interphalangeal joints: the distal joints of the fingers

Herberden's nodes: osteophytes or bony spurs that develop as a result of destruction of joint cartilage in distal interphalangeal joints

inflammatory: irritation that causes swelling, heat, and discomfort

joints: the junctions at the ends of bones that allow for movement

proximal: toward the point of origin

proximal interphalangeal joints: the proximal joints in the fingers

synovial fluid: fluid contained in the synovium of joint margins that reduces friction during movement of the joints

synovium: fluid-filled sacs in joint margins

Causes and Symptoms

There are several causes of osteoarthritis (OA), including traumatic injuries, joint overuse or repetitive movement of a joint, obesity, and genetic or metabolic diseases. The most commonly affected joints are in the hands, hips, knees, and spine. An inherited genetic defect in the production of collagen leads to defective cartilage and to more rapid joint deterioration. OA in the hands or hips may be hereditary. OA in the knees is linked to excess weight. X rays

Information on Osteoarthritis

Causes: Traumatic injuries, joint overuse, obesity, genetic or metabolic diseases

Symptoms: Joint pain (commonly in hands, hips, knees, spine); stiffness in morning or after long periods of immobility; development of nodes

Duration: Chronic and progressive

Treatments: Occupational therapy; physical therapy; moderate exercise; heat therapy (warm soaks, paraffin, mud treatments); pain medications such as topical analgesic ointments, acetaminophen, NSAIDs (ibuprofen, naproxyn); COX-2 inhibitors; glucosamine; chondroitin; injections of cortisone or hyaluronic acid; surgery in severe cases

of more than half the population over sixty-five would show evidence of osteoarthritis in at least one joint.

Cartilage containing synovial fluid and elastic tissue reduces friction as joints move. Osteoarthritis develops when the cartilage wears away and bone rubs against bone. The most prominent symptom of osteoarthritis is joint pain. Other symptoms include morning stiffness or stiffness after long periods of immobility. Early in the disease, individuals may experience joint pain after strenuous exercise. As the disease progresses, joints stiffen and diminished joint mobility is experienced even with slight activity. As joint mobility decreases, the muscles surrounding the joint weaken, thereby increasing the likelihood of further injury to the joint. As the cartilage wears away, crepitus can often be heard as bone moves against bone. The development of Herberden's nodes on the distal interphalangeal joints and Bouchard's nodes on the proximal interphalangeal joints of the hands is not uncommon.

Confirmation of osteoarthritis is based on a history of joint pain and physical findings that indicate arthritic changes in the joints. An x-ray shows a loss of joint space, osteophytes, bone cysts, and sclerosis of subchondral bone. Sometimes, a computed tomography (CT) scan or magnetic resonance imaging (MRI) may be helpful in confirming the presence of osteoarthritis.

Treatment and Therapy

The goal of treatment for OA is to preserve physical function and reduce pain. Education, physical therapy, and occupational therapy are instrumental in maintaining independence and improving muscle strength around affected joints. Pacing activities to avoid overexertion of the affected joints is an effective means to prevent further pain and injury. Heat therapies such as warm soaks, paraffin, and mud treatments may help to lessen the discomfort in tender joints. Moderate exercise such as walking, swimming, strength training, and stretching all may help to maintain mobility in arthritic joints and to improve posture and balance. Relaxation techniques, stress reduction activities, and biofeedback may also be helpful.

Topical analgesic ointments may help to reduce joint swelling and pain. Acetaminophen is very effective for controlling OA pain. However, persons who take blood-thinning medicines, have liver disease, or consume large amounts of alcohol should use acetaminophen with caution. Nonsteroidal anti-inflammatory drugs (NSAIDs) such as ibuprofen and naproxen are also effective for pain relief, but they may cause gastrointestinal bleeding. COX-2 selective inhibitors are the most recently introduced NSAIDs. This class of drugs selectively blocks the enzyme COX-2, thus controlling the production of prostaglandins, natural chemicals that contribute to body inflammation and cause the pain and swelling of arthritis. Since they do not block the COX-1 enzyme cyclooxygenase-1, which is present in the stomach and inflammation sites, the natural mucous linings of the stomach and intestine are protected, thereby reducing the incidence of upset, ulceration, or bleeding. This feature of blocking COX-2 but not COX-1 makes these drugs unique among traditional NSAIDs. COX-2 selective inhibitors include Celebrex (celecoxib), Vioxx (rofecoxib), and Bextra (valdecoxib); the latter two are no longer on the market, however. Other COX-2 inhibitors sold outside the United States include Prexige (lumiracoxib) and Arcoxia (etoricoxib). Any medication used to treat OA should be taken under the direction of a health care provider.

Glucosamine and chondroitin naturally occur in the body. Both have been promoted for the treatment of OA. Glucosamine may promote the formation and repair of cartilage, while chondroitin may promote water retention and elasticity in cartilage and prevent cartilage breakdown. However, recent studies indicate that taking glucosamine for arthritis may increase a patient's risk of developing glaucoma.

When interventions to relieve symptoms of OA no longer work, an orthopedic surgeon may inject cortisone or hyaluronic acid into joint spaces such as the knee. Hyaluronic acid is used to replace the synovial fluid that a

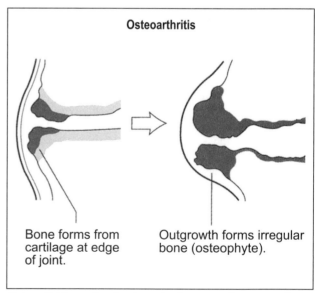

Osteoarthritis

Bone forms from cartilage at edge of joint.

Outgrowth forms irregular bone (osteophyte).

Osteoarthritis results when irregular bone growth occurs at the edge of a joint, causing impaired movement of the joint and pressure on nerves in the area.

joint has lost in order to maintain knee movement without pain. Cortisone may be injected into affected joint spaces to provide temporary relief of joint pain. Surgical intervention to trim torn and damaged cartilage from joint spaces, to partially or totally replace severely damaged joints in the knees and hips, or to fuse bones together are effective treatments in the most severe, debilitating stages of OA. Realignment of a joint (osteotomy) is another possible procedure.

Perspective and Prospects

Arthritis comprises more than one hundred diseases and conditions and is the major cause of disability in the United States. The incidence of OA increases with age, but it can affect individuals as young as eighteen. Almost 27 million people in the United States have OA, and it is the most common form of arthritis. OA is three times more common among women, although before forty-five years of age, it is more common in men. Costs for treatment of arthritis in the United States exceed $128 billion annually. There is no cure for OA, but a healthy diet, regular exercise, and weight control are measures that can slow its progress.

—*Sharon W. Stark, R.N., A.P.R.N., D.N.Sc.;*
updated by Victoria Price, Ph.D.

See also Arthritis; Bursitis; Cartilage; Collagen; Gout; Joints; Juvenile rheumatoid arthritis; Obesity; Rheumatoid arthritis; Rheumatology.

For Further Information:
Ali, Naheed. *Arthritis and You: A Comprehensive Digest for Patients and Caregivers*. Lanham, Md.: Rowman and Littlefield, 2013.
Brower, Anne C. *Arthritis in Black and White*. Philadelphia: Elsevier Saunders, 2012.
Foltz-Gray, Dorothy. *The Arthritis Foundation's Guide to Good Living with Osteoarthritis*. 2d ed. Atlanta: Arthritis Foundation, 2004.
Lane, Nancy E., and Daniel J. Wallace. *All About Osteoarthritis: The Definitive Resource for Arthritis Patients and Their Families*. New York: Oxford University Press, 2002.
Nelson, Miriam E., et al. *Strong Women and Men Beat Arthritis*. New York: G. P. Putnam's Sons, 2002.
Sayce, Valerie, and Ian Fraser. *Exercise Beats Arthritis: An Easy to Follow Program of Exercises*. Palo Alto, Calif.: Bull, 1998.
Sutton, Amy L., ed. *Arthritis Sourcebook: Basic Consumer Health Information About Osteoarthritis, Rheumatoid Arthritis, Other Rheumatic Disorders, Infectious Forms of Arthritis, and Diseases with Symptoms Linked to Arthritis*. 2d ed. Detroit, Mich.: Omnigraphics, 2004.
Yelin, E. "The Economics of Osteoarthritis." In *Osteoarthritis*, edited by K. Brandt, M. Doherty, and L. Lohmander. New York: Oxford University Press, 1998.

Osteochondritis juvenilis

Disease/Disorder

Also known as: Legg-Calvé-Perthes disease, coxa plana, pseudocoxalgia

Anatomy or system affected: Bones, circulatory system, hips, joints, musculoskeletal system

Specialties and related fields: Orthopedics, vascular medicine

Definition: The disturbance of the blood supply to the tops of the thigh bones, resulting in their destruction.

Information on Osteochondritis Juvenilis

Causes: Trauma and damage to blood vessels that serve thigh bone
Symptoms: In early stages, tenderness in hip joint, limping, pain in thigh or knee, limited leg movement
Duration: Chronic
Treatments: Physical therapy, braces and crutches, bed rest with traction

---

Causes and Symptoms

Osteochondritis juvenilis may be the result of trauma and damage to the blood vessels that serve the thigh bone (femur) in children, aged approximately two to twelve years. The patient, who in the majority of cases is male, usually experiences tenderness in the hip joint area during the early stages of the disease, accompanied by limping, pain in the thigh or knee, and limited movement of the leg. Usually it is difficult to rotate the leg or move it sideways. In 90 percent of cases, only one leg is affected. In such cases, one leg may be shorter than the other, and the child favors the affected leg. If the disease is not treated, atrophy of the thigh muscle results.

Treatment and Therapy

Most cases of osteochondritis juvenilis do not require treatment beyond observation, particularly with children under the age of six who have a small amount of damage. For children over six with most of the joint affected, a more aggressive therapy is needed, and older children with the disease are at greater risk for osteoarthritis later in live.

Physical therapy, coupled with braces and crutches or bed rest with traction, is used in the most severe cases. For most children, a Scottish Rite brace is used. Such a brace is belted around the waist and wrapped around the thighs, with a bar holding the knees apart so that the legs are held at a slight angle away from the body. The child wears the brace until the bone heals, usually in about six months.

If the child is more than eight years old, if the brace is too restrictive for an active child, or if the brace must be worn more than six months, surgical correction may be recommended. In these cases, the end of the affected bone is reshaped and the tip of the femur placed back into its socket. Occasionally, the hip socket must be reshaped instead.

—*Rose Secrest*

See also Blood vessels; Bone disorders; Bones and the skeleton; Braces; Circulation; Joints; Lower extremities; Orthopedics; Orthopedics, pediatric; Osteonecrosis; Vascular system.

For Further Information:
Currey, John D. *Bones: Structures and Mechanics*. 2d ed. Princeton, N.J.: Princeton University Press, 2006.
Kellicker, Patricia Griffin. "Legg-Calve-Perthes Disease." *Health Library*, May 7, 2013.
Kliegman, Robert M., and Waldo E. Nelson, eds. *Nelson Textbook of Pediatrics*. 19th ed. Philadelphia: Saunders/Elsevier, 2011.
Perthes Association. http://www.perthes.org.uk/.
Shapiro, Frederic. *Pediatric Orthopedic Deformities: Basic Science, Diagnosis, and Treatment*. San Diego, Calif.: Academic Press, 2001.

Staheli, Lynn T. *Fundamentals of Pediatric Orthopedics*. 4th ed. Philadelphia: Wolters Kluwer/Lippincott Williams & Wilkins, 2008.

Wenger, Dennis R., and Mercer Rang. *The Art and Practice of Children's Orthopaedics*. New York: Raven Press, 1993.

Osteoclast

Biology

Anatomy or system affected: Bone marrow, bones, cells

Specialties and related fields: Endocrinology, geriatrics, hematology/oncology, orthopedics, pathology, pediatrics

Definition: Large, specialized multinucleated cells that breaks down extracellular bone matrix and reabsorbs its tissue components

Key terms:

acidity: condition of having a low pH, or more than the normal number of protons (H^+s), which can destroy adjacent tissue

apoptosis: controlled process by which cells systematically shrink and self-destruct in response to a particular signal, in a programmed cell suicide

hydrolysis: the process of breaking down a compound, such as a protein or other complex structure, by inserting an H_2O molecule to break a covalent bond

lacuna: the small pit, or 'lake,' that an osteoclast forms over a section of bone about to be resorbed

macrophage: the general term for the large polymorphonuclear immune cells, found in numerous locations in the body, that work primarily by phagocytosing, or 'eating,' extracellular tissues

osteoblast: specialized mononucleate cell that produces the extracellular component of bone

osteoid: the extracellular substance that makes up about half the volume and mass of bone and becomes mature bone once mineralized, primarily with calcium and phosphate

protease: an enzyme that catalyzes the breakdown of proteins

Structure and Functions

Like all the dynamic, non-static tissues in the body, bone is a living substance that must be continuously broken down and resynthesized in order to function. Bone turnover happens at the cellular level and is controlled primarily by two cell types: osteoblasts and osteoclasts. Whereas osteoblasts are anabolic cells that synthesize new bone, making complex proteins from amino acids, sugars, and minerals, osteoclasts are catabolic cells that break down these materials—particularly type 1 collagen—into their basic components, such as calcium, phosphate, collagen, and water. Normal osteoclast function is necessary for ongoing remodeling of bone throughout the human lifespan, and either overactivity or underactivity of osteoclasts can lead to disease, such as osteoporosis, osteopetrosis, Paget's disease of bone, or nonunion of a fracture. Osteoclastic activity is also necessary for dissolving small bone fragments that get broken down and reabsorbed after a fracture, and for helping bones in children to remodel into their adult size and shape. The word *osteoclast* comes from the Greek for "bone," *osteon,* and "broken," *klastos*.

Bone is a type of connective tissue and, as such, is derived from mesoderm, the middle layer of the developing human embryo. In a healthy adult, bone marrow is responsible for producing most of the blood cells in the body, including platelets, red blood cells, and white blood cells. Macrophages, a destructive type of white blood cell, are the most numerous cell type in the body, and they have different names and specialized functions depending on their location in the body. For example, Kupffer cells are macrophages that reside in the liver; microglia are macrophages that migrate to the brain and spinal cord; histiocytes are activated macrophages in the lymph system; and epithelioid cells are activated macrophages involved in a foreign body reaction. Osteoclast is the name for the specialized macrophages that resorb mature bone. Unlike the aforementioned types, however, these macrophage derivatives return from the bloodstream into bones after differentiating, then fusing together to form giant, multinucleate cells. Osteoclasts may have anywhere from 5 to 200 nuclei.

Most types of macrophages destroy tissues through phagocytosis, in which they reach out multiple projections and 'eat,' or phagocytose, foreign cells or substances. Since extracellular bone forms a highly reinforced, intricate structure, osteoclasts must adopt a different strategy in order to break it down. After receiving its activation signal, an osteoclast forms a sealed pit, also called a lacuna, over a section of mature bone. *Lacuna* is actually Latin for "lake," and they are so called because when viewed under a microscope, they appear to form small lakes within the areas of bone being resorbed. Because it is sealed at its edges, the use of a pit protects nearby bone from incidental destruction by the catalytic chemical processes generated by the osteoclast.

After forming a lacuna, an osteoclast degrades bone matrix through several different methods. The most important of these are acidity, enzymatic reactions, and reactive oxygen species. Acidity refers to the generation of a low pH, which directly damages the extracellular bone matrix in the same way that acidity of the stomach breaks down food. Osteoclasts achieve this through ion channels, which pump charged hydrogen atoms, i.e. protons, directly into the sealed pit they have created. Enzymatic reactions destroy bone tissue through catalysis, in which special enzymes such as proteases break down proteins. Hydrolysis is the most notable way that proteases achieve this. Finally, osteoclasts also degrade bone matrix through the generation of reactive oxygen species. Reactive oxygen species refer to any oxygen-containing molecule in which an oxygen atom has an unpaired electron, also known as a free radical. Free radicals are highly chemically unstable and contribute significantly to the breakdown of molecules both in the setting of osteoclasts and also elsewhere in the body.

Type 1 collagen is the primary structural component of extracellular bone. After breakdown by osteoclasts, it reverts to individual amino acids and short chains of amino acids, namely lysine, proline, and especially glycine, which makes up more than a third of collagen. Other components of extracellular bone include minerals such as calcium and phosphate, and a large amount of water. After reabsorption, building blocks can then diffuse to other tissues in the body or remain in the bone for reuse by osteoblasts.

Numerous hormonal signals are known to influence osteoclasts. Chief among these is parathyroid hormone, also called PTH, which is made by the four small parathyroid glands in the neck and primarily regulates the concentration of calcium in the bloodstream. Parathyroid hormone release is triggered by a drop in blood calcium levels. In response, one of its actions is to indirectly stimulate osteoclasts, which will then increase the amount of bone they resorb in order to release calcium from mature bone and make it available for use in the bloodstream. Of note, low-level, pulsed increases in parathyroid hormone have actually been observed to have the opposite effect, stimulating osteoblasts and inhibiting osteoclasts. Thus, a synthetic form of parathyroid hormone called teriparatide has actually been approved as a last-resort treatment for osteoporosis. Estrogen is the other major hormone known to act on osteoclasts, which has an opposite effect in that it induces apoptosis, or programmed cell-death, of osteoclasts, and thereby decreases bone resorption.

Disorders and Diseases

Osteoclast dysfunction occurs primarily in one of two ways: overactivity, resulting in excess resorption of bone, or underactivity, resulting in pathologic hardening and stiffening of bone. Bone remodeling is homeostatic and requires an equal balance between formation by osteoblasts and turnover by osteoclasts. Disease can therefore occur anytime there is continued imbalance between these two forces.

Osteoporosis is an example of bone thinning and decreased density due to imbalance between osteoblasts and osteoclasts. Although its specific biochemical mechanisms are still under research, it is hypothesized to occur both from under stimulation of osteoblasts and from overstimulation of osteoclasts. Osteoporosis is a chronic process, however, and does not result in increased blood calcium and phosphate levels, unlike osteoclast stimulation by high levels of parathyroid hormone. Osteopetrosis represents the opposite end of the spectrum and is a disorder of osteoclast dysfunction. It occurs from loss of function mutations in the enzymes that generate the acidity in the resorption pit, such as carbonic anhydrase II.

Paget's disease of bone, so-called to distinguish it from Paget's disease of breast, is also known as osteitis deformans and represents a more complex example of osteoclast pathology. Paget disease is a dynamic disorder seen primarily in adults that proceeds through four phases, called the lytic, mixed, sclerotic, and quiescent phases. In the lytic phase, osteoclast overactivity predominates, and affected bones subsequently become thinner and weaker. In the mixed phase, osteoclasts and osteoblasts are both overactive and result in a disordered destruction and formation of bone. In the sclerotic phase, the osteoclast activity declines, and osteoblasts cause affected bones to be-

come dense and brittle. Finally, in the quiescent phase, both cell types decline in activity, leaving behind an overly dense, poorly formed bone mass. It can be treated with bisphosphonates such as alendronate, arrest the disease in the early stages by inhibiting osteoclast activity.

Osteoclast dysfunction is also associated with masses and tumors. *Osteitis fibrosa cystica* is Latin for "disease process of the bone consisting of fibers and fluid-filled sacs" and is one such disease process involving osteoclasts. Although its root cause is typically due to primary hyperparathyroidism, it results in cystic masses of osteoclasts. Young adults can also develop tumors of osteoclasts, which are called giant cell tumors or osteoclastomas and usually seen at the ends of the long bones of the leg, i.e. the tibia or femur.

Perspective and Prospects

Teriparatide is a relatively novel therapy for osteoporosis that was approved for use in the U.S. in 2002. Although parathyroid hormone is typically thought of as decreasing bone mass through its indirect action on osteoclasts, the pathway for stimulation osteoclasts begins with a signal upstream, from osteoblasts. Thus, in the same way that pulsating gonadotropic hormone causes normal gonad physiology, but continuous high-dose gonadotropic hormone suppresses gonadal activity, teriparatide, as a recombinant parathyroid hormone analog, stimulates osteoblasts without triggering osteoclasts if given in pulsating low doses daily.

Pharmaceutical treatment with bisophosphonates is the mainstay for osteopetrosis, which is primarily a disease of osteoclasts. But bisphosphonates are not curative, and thus can only forestall progression of this disease. Since osteoclasts are derived from bone marrow macrophages, bone marrow transplant can offer a more definitive treatment for osteopetrosis. However, bone marrow transplant for osteopetrosis may cause a pathologic increase in blood calcium levels as a side effect, which carries the risk of significant cardiac dysfunction.

—*Walter Klyce, BA and Derek T. Nhan, BS*

See also: Anabolism; Bone Marrow; Bones; Calcium; Catabolism; Enzyme; Macrophage; Osteoblast; Osteopetrosis; Osteoporosis; Paget's disease of bone; Parathyroid gland; Parathyroid hormone; Phosphate; Tumor; Vitamin D

For Further Information:

"Bone Cells." ASBMR Bone Curriculum, https://depts.washington.edu/bonebio/ASBMRed/cells.html.

"Major Progress in Understanding Osteoclast Function." Mayo Clinic, http://www.mayoclinic.org/medical-professionals/clinical-updates/endocrinology/research-explores-mechanisms-regulate-bone-resorption-formation.

"Skeleton: Bone Growth." BBC. http://www.bbc.co.uk/science/humanbody/body/factfiles/bonegrowth/femur.shtml.

"Your Bones." KidsHealth, The Nemours Foundation, http://kidshealth.org/en/kids/bones.html.

Osteogenesis imperfecta

Disease/Disorder

Also known as: Brittle bone disease

Anatomy or system affected: Auditory, cardiovascular, dental, musculoskeletal, pulmonary, visual

Specialties and related fields: Cardiology, dentistry, ophthalmology, orthopedics, otolaryngology

Definition: A

type 1 collagen defect leading to increased bony fragility and reduced bone mass, causing increased risk for fracture and extremity deformities. Also manifests systemically with heart valve abnormalities, pulmonary compromise, hearing loss, and dental abnormalities due to altered quantity or quality of collagen.

Key terms:

osteoblasts: cells responsible for the production of bone

osteoclasts: macrophage-like cells in bone marrow that degrade bone to recycle, remodel, and heal it.

type 1 collagen: a connective tissue protein involved in the structure of bone, tendons, and ligaments

Causes and Symptoms

Osteogenesis imperfecta (OI) is an inherited bone disease characterized by an overall low bone mass and increased skeletal fragility, leading to an increased risk for fractures and growth impairment. The disorder is transmitted autosomally—meaning on the 22 non-sex chromosomes—and, depending on the subtype, inherited in an either autosomal dominant or recessive pattern. It has an overall incidence of about 1 case for every 15,000 to 20,000 children.

The defect in OI occurs in the synthesis pathway for collagen, a vital structural component of connective tissue, and more specifically in the type 1 complex, which is the building block that provides the strength and stiffness for bones, tendons, and ligaments. Collagen is composed of a sequence of amino acids, the basic element of proteins, which combine to form subunits that are wound around one another to create a triple helix. These helices pack together in an organized fashion to form the fibrils capable of withstanding the significant forces necessary in bone. In OI, mutations occur in the structural genes that code for collagen synthesis (specifically COL1A1 and COL1A2), causing osteoblasts either to secrete severely abnormal collagen or an inadequate amount of collagen. Alternatively, OI is also caused by mutations in genes that cause: (1) defects in collagen modification (*CRTAP, LEPRE1, PPIB, TMEM38B*); (2) abnormalities in collagen folding and cross-linking (*SERPINH1, FKBP10, PLOD2*); (3) ossification or mineralization defects (*IFITM5, SERPINF1*); and (4) defects in osteoblast development combined with collagen insufficiencies (*WNT1, CREB3L1, SP7*).

Weakened bony architecture causes patients with OI to be particularly susceptible to skeletal deformities and ulti-

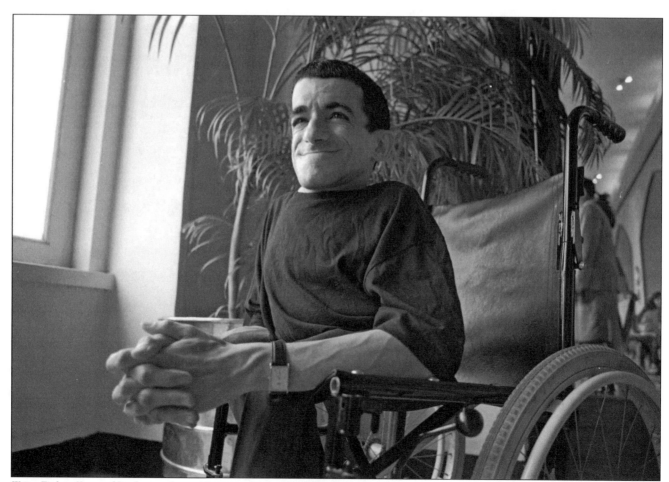

Writer Firdaus Kanga of Bombay was born with osteogenesis imperfecta. (AP/Wide World Photos)

mately fractures without obvious trauma. Fractures can occur anywhere in the body, but are most commonly seen in the ribs and long bones such as arms and legs. Many patients with OI will present immediately at birth with numerous broken bones because of trauma endured during the birthing process. Others may present during childhood, at which point OI can sometimes be difficult to distinguish from non-accidental sources of trauma, such as child abuse.

While the hallmark of OI involves increased bony fragility, contributing to various orthopedic manifestations such as fractures, scoliosis, and long-bone deformities, type 1 collagen is prevalent in numerous tissues, and, thus, can affect nearly every system in the body. Hearing loss is present in more than 50% of patients and typically develops between ages 20-40. This occurs because of the thinning and fracture of the bones in the ear, which are necessary for transmission of sound. Patients with OI also frequently have dental abnormalities because of the abnormal collagen in dentin, the substantive component of teeth. Defective tooth collagen causes a condition called *dentinogenesis imperfecta* characterized by abnormal pulp and a grey-to-yellow discoloration of the teeth. Other involvements in OI include thinning of the sclerae in the eye, which causes a blue color due to visualization of the underlying veins. However, of these extra-skeletal features, the most severe are the involvements in the cardiovascular and pulmonary systems. Cardiac involvement includes increased stiffness of the heart valves leading to poor pump function of the heart. The pulmonary complications such as respiratory distress and pneumonias are typically the most devastating for patients with OI and usually occur in combination with scoliosis and rib fractures.

Given the wide spectrum of clinical features, David Sillence, an Australian physician, developed a classification scheme based originally on 4 distinct groups of OI. Types 1 and 4 have autosomal dominant inheritance, while types 2 and 3 are inherited recessively. Type 1 is considered the mildest variant and describes a triad of hearing loss, blue sclera, and fractures that occur primarily in childhood and decrease after puberty. Patients with type 2 are typically stillborn or die within the first few weeks of life secondary to fractures of the thoracic cavity that lead to respiratory failure and frequent lung infections. Types 3 and 4 are in the spectrum between types 1 and 2. Type 3 is characterized as the most severe, non-lethal form with a large multitude of fractures that continue beyond puberty with severe scoliosis. Type 4 is associated with a moderate set of symptoms between types 1 and 3. Since the original classi-fication, four additional discrete categories have been identified, creating a total of 8 distinct groups.

Treatment and Therapy

Given that a cure has not yet been developed for OI, treatment is largely symptomatic. From a musculoskeletal perspective, treatment is focused on a combination of physical therapy, orthopedic surgery, and medications. Patients with OI have been shown to benefit from exercise programs that help to improve muscle strength and stretching for mobility. These therapies are started from the infant stage in collaboration with the parent, to teach them how to manage an unusually fragile baby. Surgery is frequently the primary modality for management of the high fracture potential in OI. The major procedures are insertion of rods described as "telescoping" which elongate as the patient grows are usually paired with osteotomies to cut and realign a misshapen bone. For OI scoliosis, bracing has been shown to have limited potential due to the fragility of the ribs. As a result, patients with OI frequently undergo fusion procedures of the spine to provide corrective alignment. Pharmacologically, bisphosphonates are the mainstay, with the idea that reducing the breakdown of bone by osteoclasts helps to increase the bony matrix to be more resistant to fractures. The improvement expected with bisphosphonates usually peaks within 2-4 years. Patients are also typically started on calcium and vitamin D, if their diet is not sufficiently fortified. Growth hormone is another medication usually started not because of abnormalities in the hormonal axis, but to improve overall bone remodeling by recruiting osteoblasts to increase bone formation and limiting bone resorption by osteoclasts.

Extra-skeletal screening is also an important adjunct to therapy for OI, specifically regular hearing screens and dental check-ups. In addition, evaluation with echocardiography is essential to evaluate for cardiac abnormalities, especially in the setting of an audible murmur or in patients with scoliosis or a history of rib fractures. Ultimately, a multidisciplinary team is vital for providing coordinated care to help patients with OI improve their mobility and daily functioning while keeping the comorbidities at bay.

Perspective and Prospects

Although the molecular basis for OI has been identified for 40 years, research is still in the early stages of developing a targeted gene-based therapy to selectively increase or correct the mutation in type 1 collagen synthesis. Preliminary studies have focused on harnessing the potential of mesenchymal stem cells from bone marrow or fetal liver that can differentiate into osteoblasts as a potential mechanism for improving the bony structure in patients afflicted with OI. Several clinical trials have shown that such stem cell treatments are safe, and that implanted stem cells engraft into bone and improve bone density and quality. Patients in these trials were still required to take prescribed bisphosphonates. Thus, management involves a multimodal approach to effectively treat the manifestations of OI.

—Derek T. Nhan, BS and Walter Klyce, BA

For Further Information:
Chan, Jerry, K. Y., and Cecilia Götherström. "Prenatal transplantation of mesenchymal stem cells to treat osteogenesis imperfecta." *Frontiers in Pharmacology* 2014; 5: 223.
"Osteogenesis Imperfecta Facts." *FastFacts — OsteogenesisImperfecta Foundation | OIF.org*, Osteogenesis Imperfecta Foundation, 2015.
"Osteogenesis Imperfecta - Genetics Home Reference." *U.S. National Library of Medicine*, National Institutes of Health, 5 Sept. 2017.
"Osteogenesis Imperfecta." *NORD (National Organization for Rare Disorders)*, National Organization for Rare Disorders, 2017.

Osteomyelitis

Disease/Disorder
Anatomy or system affected: Bones, joints, musculoskeletal system
Specialties and related fields: Bacteriology, orthopedics
Definition: A secondary bacterial infection of the bone and bone marrow.

Causes and Symptoms

After a cut, open bone fracture, or puncture wound becomes infected, a secondary infection, caused 80 percent of the time by the bacterium *Staphylococcus aureus*, can take place. In children, the bacterium usually enters the body via an infection of the mucous membranes in the throat or an infected sore on the body. In the case of a heel puncture, a bacterium that breeds in old athletic shoes, *Pseudomonas aeruginosa*, can be the culprit. In children, osteomyelitis tends to be located at the growing ends of the long bones in the legs or arms.

Osteomyelitis is generally accompanied by fever, drowsiness, dehydration, bone pain, and swelling and redness in the affected region. When a joint near the infected area is flexed, severe pain and tenderness can result. With a heel puncture, the heel tends to hurt and swell, but there is often no fever. Over time, the bacteria form pus.

Treatment and Therapy

If osteomyelitis is discovered within seven to ten days from the onset of the infection, large doses of antibiotics can be administered with success. Oral antibiotics are not recommended because compliance is hard to achieve. The recommended daily dose of the antibiotic must be ingested over four to six weeks and can cause severe side effects. Usually, patients are hospitalized and given intravenous antibiotics, which may also be administered at home. During this time, the affected bones should not be exposed to undue stress until easy, pain-free movement is achieved. The injured area may be immobilized. Risks during the time of treatment include broken bones and the onset of severe osteoporosis.

In severe cases or in cases in which the infection was not discovered early, surgery that removes the infected bone or bone marrow is necessary. If the osteomyelitis is not treated, the infection enters the bloodstream and the disease becomes chronic. Extensive bone damage, arthritis, and extrusion of pus will follow. Treatment may involve occasional removal of pus and pieces of dead bone or, in extreme cases, amputation.

For patients with difficult cases of osteomyelitis, hyperbaric oxygen therapy may be administered to deliver more oxygen to the affected bone and thereby speed healing.

—Rose Secrest

See also Antibiotics; Arthritis; Bacterial infections; Bone disorders; Bone marrow transplantation; Bones and the skeleton; Joints; Orthopedics; Orthopedics, pediatric; Osteonecrosis.

For Further Information:
A.D.A.M. Medical Encyclopedia. "Osteomyelitis." *MedlinePlus*, May 30, 2012.
Badash, Michelle, and Rosalyn Carson-DeWitt. "Osteomyelitis." *Health Library*, September, 2011.
Biddle, Wayne. *A Field Guide to Germs*. 3d ed. New York: Anchor Books, 2010.
Currey, John D. *Bones: Structures and Mechanics*. 2d ed. Princeton, N.J.: Princeton University Press, 2006.
"Osteomyelitis." *Mayo Foundation for Medical Education and Research,* November 20, 2012.
Osteomyelitis: A Medical Dictionary, Bibliography, and Annotated Research Guide to Internet References. San Diego, Calif.: Icon Health, 2004.
Norden, Carl W., ed. *Osteomyelitis*. Philadelphia: W. B. Saunders, 1990.
Wilson, Michael, Brian Henderson, and Rod McNab. *Bacterial Disease Mechanisms: An Introduction to Cellular Microbiology*. New York: Cambridge University Press, 2002.

Information on Osteomyelitis

Causes: Bacterial infection
Symptoms: Fever, drowsiness, dehydration, bone pain, localized swelling and redness
Duration: Several days to weeks
Treatments: Hospitalization, intravenous antibiotics, surgery

---

Osteonecrosis

Disease/Disorder
Also known as: Aseptic necrosis, avascular necrosis, ischemic necrosis
Anatomy or system affected: Bones, hips, joints, knees, musculoskeletal system
Specialties and related fields: Orthopedics, rheumatology
Definition: A disorder that occurs when the blood supply to bone is cut off, causing the death of bone tissue and leading to the collapse of joints in the affected areas.

Causes and Symptoms

Osteonecrosis-from *osteo*, meaning "bone," and *necro*, meaning "death"-may be either posttraumatic or nontraumatic, in some cases with risk factors identified and in others with no known cause (idiopathic). Approximately twenty thousand new cases are diagnosed each year in the United States, most commonly between the ages of twenty and fifty, with the average age of onset at thirty-eight. Osteonecrosis is of equal prevalence in men and women.

Some risk factors seem to predispose people to osteonecrosis, including the use of corticosteroids (to treat

---

Information on Osteonecrosis

Causes: Interruption of blood supply to bone; may result from trauma, corticosteroid use, excessive alcohol consumption, bone disorders, cancer treatment
Symptoms: Joint pain and loss, death of bone tissue
Duration: Chronic and progressive
Treatments: Nonsteroidal anti-inflammatory drugs (NSAIDs), anticoagulants, statins, exercises, electrical stimulation, surgery (core decompression, bone grafting, osteotomy, joint replacement)

---

inflammatory conditions) as well as excessive alcohol ingestion. Both steroid and alcohol use may lead to a buildup of lipids in the blood vessels, decreasing blood flow to bones. Injury to a bone or joint (such as a fracture) may damage the blood vessels, decreasing the blood supply and causing bone death. Medical conditions which affect the bone (gout, osteoarthritis, osteoporosis) may predispose someone to osteonecrosis. Cancer treatments (radiation and chemotherapy) and organ transplantation also increase the risk of osteonecrosis, as do other medical conditions including sickle cell disease and acquired immunodeficiency syndrome (AIDS). The medication Fosamax, a bisphosphenate used to treat osteoporosis, has been linked to osteonecrosis of the jaw.

Often, few symptoms occur in early stages of the disease. Preliminary symptoms include pain in the affected joint, followed by collapse of joint surfaces and increased pain. Pain occurs initially only when the joint is in use and later even at rest. The bones most commonly affected are the ends of the femur, the upper arm bone, and the knees, shoulders, and ankles. Within months to two years from the onset of symptoms, individuals may lose range of motion and suffer severe disability. Appropriate treatment must be undertaken to prevent the breakdown of joints, Therefore, immediate diagnosis is important. X-rays, magnetic resonance imaging (MRI), computed tomography (CT) scan, and bone scans serve as diagnostic tools when an individual is symptomatic.

Treatment and Therapy

Once the condition has been diagnosed, treatment should begin immediately. To decide on most effective treatments, physicians consider the age of the patient, the progression of the disease, the location of the bones involved, and the underlying cause. Treatment can be either medical or surgical. Medical treatments include the use of nonsteroidal anti-inflammatory drugs (NSAIDs) to decrease pain, anticoagulants (blood thinners) to improve blood supply to bone, and statins (cholesterol-lowering medications) to decrease lipid buildup in blood vessels, allowing improved blood flow to bone. Other medical treatments involve range of motion exercises, electrical stimulation to induce bone growth, and decreased weight-bearing on affected joints.

Surgical techniques used to treat osteonecrosis include core decompression, bone grafting, osteotomy, and joint replacement. In core decompression, the inner core of the bone is removed, thus reducing pressure within the bone. Core decompression is often followed by bone grafting to the decompressed area to support the joint. Osteotomy is a surgical reshaping of the bone to decrease stress on affected areas. Joint replacement is the surgical treatment of choice in advanced cases. Treatment may be an ongoing process that continues for years, as the disease progresses. Adequate treatment allows afflicted individuals to continue to live reasonably normal lives.

—Robin Kamienny Montvilo, R.N., Ph.D.

See also Alcoholism; Arthritis; Bone disorders; Bones and the skeleton; Circulation; Corticosteroids; Gout; Grafts and grafting; Joints; Necrosis; Orthopedics; Osteoarthritis, Osteoporosis; Steroids; Vascular medicine; Vascular system.

For Further Information:

Bianchi, Giancarlo I., and Pascual C. Giordano. *Osteonecrosis: Diagnosis, Treatment, and Management.* New York: Nova Science, 2013.

Icon Health. *Osteonecrosis: A Medical Dictionary, Bibliography, and Annotated Research Guide to Internet References.* San Diego, Calif.: Author, 2004.

Mont, Michael A., et al. *Osteonecrosis of the Hip.* New York: Springer, 2010.

National Institute of Arthritis and Musculoskeletal and Skin Diseases. *Osteonecrosis: Questions and Answers About Osteonecrosis (Avascular Necrosis).* Bethesda, Md.: US Department of Health and Human Services, 2011.

National Osteonecrosis Foundation. http://www.nonf.org.

Soucacos, Panayotis N., and James R. Urbaniak, eds. *Osteonecrosis of the Human Skeleton.* Philadelphia: W. B. Saunders, 2004.

Urbaniak, James R., and John Paul Jones, eds. *Osteonecrosis: Etiology, Diagnosis, and Treatment.* Rosemont, Ill.: American Academy of Orthopaedic Surgeons, 1997.

Osteopathic medicine

Specialty

Anatomy or system affected: Bones, muscles, musculoskeletal system

Specialties and related fields: Critical care, emergency medicine, family medicine, geriatrics and gerontology, internal medicine, physical therapy, preventive medicine, public health

Definition: The practice of medicine as dictated by the philosophy of treating the individual instead of merely the disease, by the belief that the musculoskeletal system is crucial to the health of the entire body, and by an emphasis on the interrelatedness of all bodily systems.

Key terms:

allopathic medicine: the traditional course of study leading to a doctorate in medicine; most practicing physicians are allopathic physicians

family medicine: the practice of medicine in which the physician cares for the basic needs of the family and emphasizes preventive health care, as well as the importance of the patient's environment

immune system: the system of the body that is responsible for the maintenance of health; includes the spleen, the thymus, bone marrow, and the lymphatic system

Medical College Admission Test (MCAT): a test of problem-solving skills taken by all candidates for medical school in the United States; used to predict which students will be successful

musculoskeletal system: the system of the body consisting of the muscles and skeleton particularly in relation to their role in the maintenance of health

obstetrics/gynecology: the practice of medicine which deals with the health of the female reproductive system; includes care of the pregnant woman and delivery of her baby, as well as care for infertile couples who need assistance in becoming pregnant

osteopathy: philosophy of medicine which emphasizes the treatment of the whole person, rather than only the disease; from the Greek *osteo*, meaning bone, and *pathos*, meaning to suffer or be in sympathy with

The History of Osteopathy

Osteopathy is a medical philosophy that treats disease in the context of the whole person, taking into consideration the functions and interrelationships of all body systems as well as such factors as nutrition, environment, and psychology. The first college of osteopathic medicine was founded in Kirksville, Missouri, in 1892, by Andrew Taylor Still (1828-1917), a frontier physician and Civil War surgeon. By the opening decades of the twenty-first century, there were more than thirty colleges of osteopathic medicine across the United States.

Still was the son of the Reverend Abraham Still, a doctor as well as a minister. As a youth, Andrew often accompanied his father on house calls, where he helped with basic medical procedures. His study of medicine led to a doctorate of medicine (MD), and he was licensed in the state of Missouri.

During the Civil War and in his practice as a frontier doctor, Still became frustrated by his inability to cure patients using the available techniques. The suffering of his patients was difficult for him to tolerate. The lack of knowledge about diseases and their treatment drove him to reconsider ways to improve the lot of the ill and injured. He also suffered a great personal loss when an epidemic of spinal meningitis spread through Kansas. Three of his children died of the disease, and three others died shortly after they were born. These tragedies nearly caused Still to abandon his career, but, in spite of the fact that the practice of modern medicine was in its infancy, he was determined to find the answers that would help him conquer disease and improve the health of his patients.

After the war ended, Still spent his life studying, observing, comparing, and experimenting in the treatment of disease. His observations closely paralleled the theories that the Greek physician Hippocrates proposed two thousand years earlier. Both Still and Hippocrates encouraged the physician to concentrate on the patient, not the disease.

Still wanted to establish the first school of osteopathy at Baker University in Baldwin, Kansas. He was refused permission to do so, however, because his philosophy of medicine did not conform to the accepted medical practice of the day. He was ostracized in Kansas, and in 1874, he moved to Missouri, where he was still licensed as a doctor and was legally able to practice medicine. As an itinerant doctor, he gained fame throughout the area and was affectionately known as the "bonesetter." It was during this time that he perfected his practice of osteopathy. Still's reputation and popularity spread, and he soon required assistance in treating the patients who sought him out. He established the first school of osteopathic medicine in Kirksville, Missouri, as the American School of Osteopathy under the law governing scientific institutions in 1892.

In 1894, he received a new charter from the state of Missouri for an educational institution. By the authority of the charter, the school could have awarded an MD degree, but Still wanted his degree to be different and chose to award a doctor of osteopathy (DO) degree instead. During the next few years, osteopathic colleges became a trend, and at one time, thirty-seven of them existed, many of which were correspondence or diploma schools.

The American School of Osteopathy taught the art of manipulative therapy. Still and his followers believed that if they could regulate and correct malfunctions of musculoskeletal function, they could return the body to a healthful state. When possible, they also eliminated the use of drugs to treat disease. Although this approach now sounds extreme, at that time few, if any, drugs were on the market, and most had severe side effects.

At the time that Still was establishing the roots of osteopathy, many significant advances were made in medical knowledge and techniques, including germ theory, the development of antiseptic surgery, the development of anesthesia, and the reorganization of medical education. The emphasis of Still on the treatment of the entire person has taken on more importance in modern times with the development of the fields of holistic medicine and preventive care.

Science and Profession

The philosophy of osteopathic medicine suggests that a human being is an ecologically and biologically unified whole. Among its tenets are that the various body systems are joined through the nervous, endocrine, and circulatory systems and that if one region of the body is diseased, the entire body is diseased.

There are five basic premises of osteopathy. First, the unity of all body parts is a benefit that assists in the maintenance of health and the resistance to disease. Second, when the body is properly nourished and structural relationships are normal, the body is able to adapt to physiological changes that might otherwise put the body out of balance. Third, a healthy body depends on a healthy circulatory system and a nervous system that is able to conduct information to all areas of the body. Fourth, the musculoskeletal system does more than simply provide a framework for the body, and its normal function is critical to a healthy body. Fifth, it is not in the patient's best interest for the physician to treat only one aspect of the disease; the physician must treat the entire body and mind if the patient is to be cured. In modern times, the osteopathic physician uses manipulative therapy-in which rhythmic stretching and thrusting movements are used to realign joints and muscles properly-as one of many tools to cure the patient.

Osteopathic physicians and allopathic physicians have much in common. Both are members of the health care community who are fully trained physicians, who have taken a prescribed amount of undergraduate work, and who have received four years of training in a medical school. After completing medical school, osteopathic physicians take a one-year rotating internship in hospitals with approved intern training programs. They may then enter a medical specialty program which may require a three- to four-year residency program.

Both allopathic and osteopathic medical programs use scientifically accepted methods of diagnosis and treatment. In the United States, the graduates of these programs are licensed by the same state medical boards and can practice in all phases of medicine in all states.

Admission to a college of osteopathic medicine in the United States requires a minimum of three years of preprofessional education in an accredited college or university. Virtually all students in osteopathic school, however, have been awarded undergraduate degrees. Many osteopathic students were science majors in undergraduate school, but all areas of study are represented. Most schools require a minimum of two semesters of study in biology, physics, and inorganic and organic chemistry. Students are also required to take the Medical College Admission Test (MCAT), submit letters of recommendation, and demonstrate an understanding of osteopathic medicine.

During the first two years in a college of osteopathic medicine, students receive basic science and preclinical instruction in a classroom or laboratory environment. Students are required to take courses in anatomy, biochemistry, physiology, pharmacology, pathology, and microbiology.

Schools are organized along one of two lines. They teach either by discipline or by system. In a discipline curriculum, the student concentrates on one subject at a time, such as biochemistry or physiology. In those programs with a curriculum that is organized by system, the student will study one organ system from the perspective of various basic science disciplines. For example, when studying the circulatory system, the student would concentrate on the anatomy, biochemistry, physiology, and pathology of the blood vessels and heart before moving on to another system.

Most students of osteopathy are required to take the first part of an examination prepared by the National Board of Osteopathic Medical Examiners near the end of their second year. At the end of the second year or in the third year, the student concentrates on clinical instruction. Students of osteopathy may do clinical rotations in teaching hospitals, community hospitals, or physicians' offices in both urban and rural areas. Clinical instruction is designed to give the student experience in the diagnosis and treatment of a patient's symptoms. Students also attend seminars and conferences that are more specialized and that emphasize the disease process and the healing process.

The second part of the national boards is taken during the last year, and the third part is taken after the student has received the DO degree. After completion of the degree, the student participates in a one-year rotating internship in an approved hospital prior to selection of a residency program. Approximately 70 percent of all doctors of osteopathy enter one of the primary care specialties, including general practice, general internal medicine, obstetrics/gynecology, and pediatrics.

Diagnostic and Treatment Techniques

Osteopathic medicine stresses the interdependence of structure and function. The application of manipulative therapy, and in particular joint mobilization, has been a hallmark of osteopathic medicine since its inception. Osteopathic physicians recognize human beings as complex biomechanical, biophysical, and biochemical organisms. They believe that structural disturbances can have wide-ranging effects that may spread to interconnecting systems. The biologic foundations of osteopathic medicine are based in the concepts of holism, homeostasis, unity of the body, environmental influences, and health-versus-disease.

Holism suggests that humans are whole beings that are not resolvable into component parts and that each "whole" is more than the sum of its parts. This premise can also be extended to mean that people are not isolated units-they are a part of their surroundings and thus are a part of their environment and the universe. The increased tendency toward specialization in health care would seem to be in conflict with this principle. Osteopathic medicine suggests a need to increase the number of generalists or primary care physicians to ensure adequate care of the whole person. It further requires time to know and understand the patient as a person in his or her own environment.

The concept of body unity suggests that the normal healthy body contains all the elements necessary to maintain optimum function. Osteopathic physicians would argue that when disease alters body function, there is adequate flexibility within the system to compensate for change and to return the body to a state of wellness. This concept is similar to the principle of general physiology known as homeostasis.

Homeostasis recognizes the fact that essential body functions such as acidity of the blood, body temperature, and blood pressure are maintained within relatively narrow limits. It is not unusual for these parameters to drift slightly from the norm, but they must be quickly and efficiently returned to normal if the body is to survive. Deviations that cannot be readjusted quickly lead to poor body function and even death. Therefore, the body expends much time and energy in maintaining homeostasis, which prevents changes in the environment from having a significant effect on body function.

The philosophy of osteopathic medicine presents the position that musculoskeletal function is important in the maintenance of homeostasis. If this system is "out of line" or in any way unhealthy, the body will have a more difficult time maintaining homeostasis. It further argues that a healthy musculoskeletal system is necessary for a healthy immune system and that an unhealthy immune system can interfere with homeostasis.

The osteopathic physician emphasizes the role of the environment in health. There is general agreement that a healthy environment contributes to a healthy body. However, a healthy environment here refers not only to the working and living environment of the patient, but also to all associates and family members who are directly involved with the patient.

The concept of health-versus-disease is central to the philosophy of osteopathic medicine. The osteopathic physician is not as concerned with the treatment of the disease as with the cause of the disease and the methods that can be used to prevent its continuation or recurrence. The concept of health implies that all components of the body are functioning as a unit and that all are contributing to the maintenance of homeostasis. Consequently, properly functioning circulatory, nervous, and endocrine systems are required. Disease, on the other hand, is present when cells do not receive appropriate circulation and/or nervous or endocrine regulation, causing a breakdown in the immune system or impairment of the adaptive mechanisms.

Although there are many similarities between allopathic and osteopathic physicians, some distinctions can be made. While the allopathic physician's philosophy emphasizes the value of the type of intervention used, the osteopathic physician stresses the importance of the body's ability to heal itself. Osteopathic medicine recognizes the musculoskeletal system as an important factor in the body's efforts to resist and overcome illness and disease. The major factor that separates osteopathic medicine from allopathic medicine is manipulative treatment, which is often called biomechanics. Osteopathic manipulative treatment is used in conjunction with other practices to provide the body with the means to cure itself.

Perspective and Prospects

In 1894, when Andrew Taylor Still opened the first osteopathic medical school in Kirksville, Missouri, the medical community was skeptical of the methods of the osteopathic physician. Although Missouri was the first state to recognize an osteopathic medical school, there was resistance to licensing the graduates. In 1896, Vermont was the first state to enact legislation legalizing the licensing of osteopathy. Licensing in Missouri followed in 1897. By 1924, thirty-eight states had legally recognized osteopathy. In 1897, the American Osteopathic Association was formed to establish professional standards of practice. Its objectives were to promote the public health and to maintain high standards of medical education in osteopathic colleges.

Members of the American Medical Association (AMA) were not as accepting of osteopathic physicians as was the general public. When World War I broke out, some allopathic physicians claimed that the osteopaths were insufficiently trained for military service. Although there was widespread disagreement across the country, these allopathic physicians were successful, and the osteopathic physicians were kept at home. This situation ultimately proved to be to the benefit of osteopathy: While allopaths were serving in foreign countries, health care in the United States was left to osteopaths.

In 1923, the AMA continued its efforts to limit the practice of osteopathic physicians by declaring that it was unethical for MDs to consult with DOs. In 1938, MDs were forbidden to engage in any professional relationship with DOs.

Acceptance of osteopathic physicians finally came in 1967, when the AMA voted to negotiate for the merger of the two professions. The American Osteopathic Association was not interested in such a merger, but allopaths and osteopaths were allowed to work side by side in hospitals, community health clinics, and offices throughout the United States.

In the United States in 2012, there were more than 82,000 osteopathic physicians across the nation, constituting almost 10 percent of practicing physicians. The education of osteopathic physicians is expected to have an increasingly important role in the United States as people continue to emphasize preventive and family medicine. In efforts to cut costs and to improve the availability of health care, the government and health care insurance providers have stressed the need for primary care-an area that has always been important to the osteopathic physician.

Two monthly journals are available in libraries throughout the United States: the *Journal of the American Osteopathic Association* and *The DO* These journals contain research studies from osteopathic physicians as well as articles regarding the profession and the education of its students.

—*Annette O'Connor, Ph.D.*

See also Alternative medicine; Bones and the skeleton; Exercise physiology; Family medicine; Holistic medicine; Massage; Muscle sprains, spasms, and disorders; Muscles; Nutrition; Physical rehabilitation; Preventive medicine.

For Further Information:

American Association of Colleges of Osteopathic Medicine. *The Education of the Osteopathic Physician*. Rev. ed. Rockville, Md.: Author, 1990.

"About Osteopathic Medicine." *American Osteopathic Association*, 2013.

Chila, Anthony G., ed. *Foundations of Osteopathic Medicine*. 3d ed. Philadelphia: Wolters Kluwer Health, 2011.

Lederman, Eyal. *Fundamentals of Manual Therapy: Physiology, Neurology, and Psychology*. New York: Churchill Livingstone, 1997.

McKone, Walter Llewellyn. *Osteopathic Medicine: Philosophy, Principles and Practice*. Malden, Mass.: Blackwell Scientific, 2001.

Nicholas, Alexander S., and Evan A. Nichols. *Atlas of Osteopathic Techniques*. 2d ed. Philadelphia: Wolters Kluwer Health, 2012.

Still, Andrew T. *Philosophy of Osteopathy*. Kirksville, Mo.: Author, 1899.

Osteopetrosis

Disease/Disorder

Also known as: Marble bone disease, Albers-Schonberg disease

Anatomy or system affected: Hematologic, immunologic, musculoskeletal, neurologic, visual

Specialties and related fields: Hematology/oncology, neurology, neurosurgery, ophthalmology, orthopaedics

Definition: Defect in osteoclast function leading to impaired bone resorption, with increased density of bone but overall weaker bony structure and reduced bone marrow volume. Patients are thus more susceptible to fractures, bony deformities, and cranial nerve compression.

Key terms:

osteoblasts: Cells responsible for the synthesis of bony matrix

osteoclasts: Cells responsible for the resorption and digestion of the bony matrix

hematopoietic stem cells: Precursor cells for the production of various blood cell components, including red blood cells and white blood cells

Causes and Symptoms

Osteopetrosis describes a group of three inherited bone disorders that cause thickening and hardening of bone due to a defect in a type of cell called an osteoclast. The incidence of this condition ranges from 1 in 20,000 for the autosomal dominant inherited form, to 1 in every 250,000 live births, for the recessive subtype.

The bony architecture is dynamic and occurs via interactions between two cells—osteoblasts and osteoclasts, which both arise from bone marrow stem cells. Osteoblasts are responsible for synthesizing and secreting the bony matrix, laying the foundation for the ultimate development of bony structure. On the other hand, osteoclasts serve as their counterpart, working to remodel bone and calcified cartilage via reabsorption of bony tissue. This process of resorption occurs via the secretion of acidic compounds that break down the matrix and allow for the creation of various bony shapes as an individual grows.

Osteopetrosis occurs when mutations develop in the pathway for secreting these acidic molecules, thereby leading to unopposed action of osteoblasts, proliferation of the bony matrix, and increased density of bone. However, the primary bone matrix and calcified cartilage, which are not resorbed in osteopetrosis, are weaker than normal bone and thereby more fragile and susceptible to fractures.

Classification of osteopetrosis is based primarily on the severity of its clinical features and occurrence at different ages. In increasing severity, the three types include benign, intermediate, and malignant/infantile types. The benign or autosomal dominant variant, also known as osteopetrosis tarda, typically manifests in adulthood and is associated with increased fractures, scoliosis, hip osteoarthritis, and long bone deformities due to stress applied on the weaker bone. In addition, thickening of the skull can lead to narrowing around the cranial nerves including the optic nerve causing blindness. The other two subtypes—the intermediate and malignant variants—are inherited in an autosomal recessive fashion and are regarded as more severe.

The intermediate form usually appears within the first few years of life with an increased frequency of fractures and compression of the cranial nerves. Of the three types, these patients are most commonly affected by osteomyelitis, or an infection of bone, within the jaw.

The malignant, or infantile, form usually occurs within months of birth. It is the rarest type of osteopetrosis, but also the most severe. Its lethal nature occurs due to the bony overgrowth that narrows the bone marrow located at the center of bones. Marrow normally houses the stem cells vital for proliferation of blood cells, but it can be severely reduced in the malignant form of osteopetrosis, causing anemia and increased susceptibility to infections. Most infants with this type of osteopetrosis generally do not survive past the age of two and succumb as a result of severe bleeding or infection.

Treatment and Therapy

Various modalities are implemented, both surgical and non-surgical, to control the deficient resorption of bone that is central to osteopetrosis. Inteferon-gamma is an immune system modulator frequently prescribed because of its ability to increase the breakdown of bone, similar to osteoclasts. Other medications that have shown benefit include the steroid prednisone, which reduces the clearance of red and white blood cells. This both prevents anemia and reduces the risk of infection. In addition, a medication called Calcitriol—the precursor to the active form of Vitamin D—can help increase osteoclast production, and it has been shown to help reduce the frequency of fractures in osteopetrosis.

Surgical options may also be implemented for osteopetrosis. One option involves preventatively inserting nails into the medullary cavity of bones to fortify their structure in the setting of the increased fracture risk. However, caution must be taken, given that osteopetrotic bones are already weaker than normal bones and thus more likely to be damaged by an intramedullary nail than healthy bone would be. For patients with end-stage osteoarthritis, total hip and knee replacements have also been shown to be beneficial, since they allow for improved mobility.

Perspective and Prospects

While 70% of cases of osteopetrosis fall into one of the three forms described above, the genetic underpinnings behind the remaining 30% have yet to be explained. Whole exome sequencing will likely play a role in this process to identify the key mutations in the osteoclast function that lead to this disorder. Further research into the mechanism of acid production by osteoclasts and the pathway for resorption of bone will also aid in the development of targeted interventions for treatment of osteopetrosis.

—*Derek T. Nhan, BS and Walter Klyce, BA*

For Further Information:

"Osteopetrosis - Genetics Home Reference." *U.S. National Library of Medicine*, National Institutes of Health, 2017.

Favus MJ, ed. Primer on the Metabolic Bone Diseases and Disorders of Mineral Metabolism, 3rd. ed. Lippincott-Raven; 1996:363-6.

"Osteopetrosis." *NORD (National Organization for Rare Disorders)*, NORD, 2015.

Osteoporosis

Disease/Disorder

Anatomy or system affected: Bones

Specialties and related fields: Endocrinology, geriatrics, nutrition, orthopedics

Definition: Decreased bone density caused by an imbalance of bone resorption relative to new bone formation, which decreases the number of interconnections in the bone and increases risk of fracture

Key terms:

osteoblasts: specialized mononucleated cells that work together to synthesize bone matrix

osteoclast: specialized multinucleated cell that breaks down bone matrix

trabeculae: small struts that form crosslinks and give bones their stability

vertebra: any of the 33 bones that form the spinal column

Causes and Symptoms

Normal bone is made up of two layers: cortical, or compact bone, which forms the hardened exterior one sees, and trabecular bone, aka cancellous or spongy bone, which forms the softer, more compliant tissue in the interior of the bone. In a healthy person, both these tissue types maintain their structure through the numerous small trabeculae that intersect at right angles and give bones their strength. In osteoporosis, the number of trabeculae is reduced, and as a result, both types of bone are much weaker and less dense. As more and more physiologic stress is placed on an osteoporotic bone, its few remaining trabeculae are less and less able to maintain its shape, which can lead either to gradual compression fractures of the bone, such as in a spinal vertebra, or to 'fragility' fractures, such as a femoral neck fracture. The word *osteoporosis* hints at this pathophysiology, given that *osteo-* means "of or relating to bone," and *porosis* is related to the English word *porous* and means "the condition of having holes."

Only a handful of tissues in the body are permanent and do not generate new cells in adulthood, such as nerves, muscles, and tooth enamel. Bones, unlike these, are a type of connective tissue, and as such they must undergo constant remodeling from stem cells throughout the human lifespan, more like hair follicles and gut epithelium. This is a homeostatic activity that is regulated primarily by the push and pull of osteoblasts and osteoclasts. Osteoblasts are most numerous in the periosteum, the thin membrane that covers bones, and are responsible for secreting the extracellular tissue of bone. This tissue is initially called osteoid and is composed mostly of type I collagen. Osteoclasts are a type of macrophage found inside bones that cause the resorption of osteoid by generating a local small area of acidity. In healthy adults, the amount of mature bone is stable, in the short term, because the generation of new bone by osteoblasts and destruction by osteoclasts are relatively equal. Osteoporosis occurs when the turnover of bone by osteoclasts overtakes its formation by osteoblasts. As the bone thins, the space originally taken up by extracellular bone matrix is slowly replaced by fat cells.

The most common cause of osteoporosis is estrogen deficiency, as estrogen inhibits osteoclasts and thereby prevents bone resorption. Since postmenopausal women are by definition estrogen deficient, they are the population

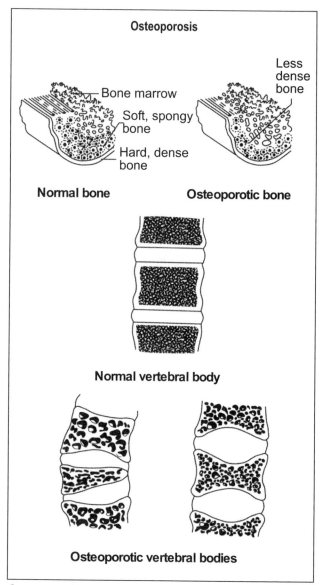

Information on Osteoporosis

Causes: Aging, disease (e.g., hyperparathyroidism, multiple myeloma), amenorrhea, anorexia nervosa, physical inactivity

Symptoms: Increased bone fractures, severe and localized back pain, reduced height

Duration: Chronic

Treatments: Hormonal therapy (estrogens, calcitonin); drug therapy (bisphosphonates, teriparatide, slow-release sodium fluoride, calcitriol, raloxifene), calcium supplements

Osteoporosis leads to bone that is less dense, more brittle, more easily broken, and degenerative.

most at risk for osteoporosis and osteoporotic fractures. However, estrogen deficiency can also be seen in premature ovarian failure, steroid use, pituitary prolactinomas, and anorexia. With regard to anorexia, the combination of an eating disorder, lack of menses, and osteoporosis has been called the Female Athlete Triad.

Certain medical conditions can also cause osteoporosis, such as diabetes, some cancers, or the production of excess thyroid hormone or steroid hormone. Other known risk factors for osteoporosis include excess alcohol use, smoking, malnutrition, some anti-seizure and acid reflux medications, and a sedentary lifestyle. Of note, race has been found to be one of the few known protective factors for women, with African-American ancestry resulting in a higher average bone mass density throughout life. Asian women, conversely, may be the population most at risk for osteoporosis, since lactose intolerance is most common in this population and can lead to decreased calcium and Vitamin D levels.

The most telling symptom of baseline osteoporosis is a vertebral compression fracture, as individual vertebrae lose their shape and slowly collapse on themselves. This process results in a kyphotic, or forward-bending, deformity of the spine, which is sometimes called a "dowager's hump" since it is most often seen in older women. Osteoporosis is also diagnosed in men, usually after the age of 65. People with osteoporosis will also have a loss of vertical height, as the vertebrae are increasingly squashed into each other. The more alarming symptom of osteoporosis is a fragility fracture, sometimes called a nontraumatic fracture, which refers to any fracture that occurs with a fall from standing height or less. The most common type of fragility fracture is snapping of the neck of the femur, often called a broken hip. Although femoral neck fractures are becoming increasingly commonplace, as the average age of the population creeps upward, they can pose a significant risk if not treated quickly, since the head of the femur has a tenuous blood supply and may quickly become oxygen-deficient if blood flow is occluded by a fracture.

Diagnosis and Treatment

Osteoporosis cannot be diagnosed by laboratory examination, as typical osteoporosis has normal values for calcium, phosphate, alkaline phosphatase, and parathyroid hormone. Imaging is the more reliable way to evaluate it. Vertebral compression fractures will show vertebral bodies that appear sunken and concave on x-ray, rather than the smooth, rectangular shape of a healthy vertebral body. Osteoporotic bones will also appear less opaque on x-ray, particularly in the outer part of the bone where the cortical bone is. However, this finding will be seen only once 40% or more of the bone mass has been lost. Only a specialized type of x-ray can be used to screen for osteoporosis preventatively. Dual-energy X-ray absorptiometry, or DEXA, can directly measure bone density, and it is recommended for all women over 65 and anyone else in whom osteoporosis is suspected. DEXA works by measuring the amount of x-ray radiation that gets trapped within the bone and calculating from that what the density of the bone is.

Surgery is the usual treatment for most fragility fractures, such as a hip fracture or forearm fracture. Vertebral compression fractures, however, typically cannot be reversed. Rather, osteoporosis is treated through early identification, preventative measures, and slowing of the disease once it occurs. This treatment can involve dietary supplements, such as calcium or vitamin D, or medications, such as bisphosphonates, which directly inhibit osteoclasts, or raloxifene, which is similar to estrogen. An active lifestyle, particularly strength training and weight exercises, has also been shown to increase bone density.

Perspective and Prospects

Hormonal replacement therapy with estrogen-like medications was recommended for most postmenopausal women in the latter half of the twentieth century, as it not only helped prevent osteoporosis, but also treated some other perimenopausal symptoms. More recently, however, estrogen replacement was found to have a number of negative side effects. Raloxifene has been shown to cause blood clots, and tamoxifen, another estrogen analog, was found to increase the risk not only of clotting but also uterine cancer. Both are still used to treat osteoporosis, but they are now used more selectively, particularly tamoxifen.

Although inactivity, such as being bedbound, is a known risk for osteoporosis, the effect of obesity on osteoporosis is still controversial. The high stress obesity places on bones is thought to be protective against osteoporosis; additionally, it is known that fat cells can produce estrogen, even after the ovaries fail. But recent research has shown that obesity increases the level of general inflammation in the body, which would seem to increase the rate of osteoporosis. This is further complicated by the fact the pathology of osteoporosis involves the replacement of bone osteoid by fat cells themselves, implying a further potential adverse role for fat cells in the pathogenesis of osteoporosis.

—*Walter Klyce, BA and Derek T. Nhan, BS*

See also: Aging; Aging: Extended care; Amenorrhea; Anorexia nervosa; Bone disorders; Bones*and the skeleton; Eating disorders; Exercisephysiology; Fracture and dislocation; Fracture repair; Hip fracture repair; Hormonetherapy; Hormones; Malnutrition; Menopause; Nutrition; Orthopedic surgery; Orthopedics; Preventive medicine; Spinal corddisorders; Spine, vertebrae, and disks; Sports medicine; Supplements; Vitaminsand minerals.*

For Further Information:

Ensrud KE, Crandall CJ. "Osteoporosis." *Ann Intern Med.* 2017;167(3):ITC17-ITC31.

Misiorowski W. "Osteoporosis in men." *MenopauseRev.* 2017;16(2):70-73.

Batur P, Rice S, Barrios P, Sikon A. "Osteoporosis Management." *J Women's Heal.* 2017;26(8):918-921.

Gambacciani M, Levancini M. "Hormone replacement therapy and the prevention of postmenopausal osteoporosis." *MenopauseRev.* 2014;13(4):213-220.

Martin M. *Exercisefor Better Bones: The Complete Guide to Safe Effective Exercises for Osteoporosis.* Kamajojo Press, 2015.

Otoplasty

Procedure

Anatomy or system affected: Ears, skin

Specialties and related fields: Audiology, family medicine, general surgery, pediatrics, plastic surgery

Definition: Cosmetic or reconstructive surgery performed on the outer ear.

Indications and Procedures

Otoplasty is performed to improve the appearance of the outer ear, typically to flatten protruding ears or to repair or reconstruct a missing or badly damaged ear. Since the ears have reached 90 percent of their adult size by the time a child reaches age five, the surgery can be performed either at this early age or later.

The first step in flattening protruding ears is to remove a flap of skin from the back of each ear. The underlying cartilage is then remolded, and the two edges of the wound are stitched together, bringing the ear closer to the head. Dressings are applied to the ears and left for a few days, when they are replaced by a headband that is worn for several weeks. The stitches are removed approximately one week after the surgery.

The reconstruction of a missing or badly damaged ear is a complex procedure that typically involves more than one operation, and long healing intervals are necessary between operations. The first step is to remove a piece of cartilage from a rib and sculpt it to resemble a normal ear. The cartilage is then transferred to a fold of skin where the ear will be located. A skin graft may be necessary. Dressings are applied to the ear for up to two weeks, and the stitches are then removed. In many cases, hearing in the reconstructed ear may not be normal. As long as hearing is normal in the other ear, however, no attempt is usually made to improve hearing in the reconstructed ear.

Uses and Complications

Possible complications associated with otoplasty operations include sensitivity of the ear to cold weather, especially during the first year after surgery, and skin graft failure. On rare occasions, excessive bleeding or infection of the surgical wounds may arise. For minor pain, the patient can take acetaminophen or ibuprofen. As the ear heals, a hard ridge usually forms along the incision, but it will gradually recede. The scar will be hidden in the crease between the scalp and the ear.

—*Alvin K. Benson, Ph.D.*

See also Ear infections and disorders; Ears; Hearing loss; Plastic surgery; Surgery, pediatric.

For Further Information:

Converse, J. M. *Reconstructive Plastic Surgery.* 2d ed. Philadelphia: W. B. Saunders, 1977.

Davis, Jack. *Otoplasty: Aesthetic and Reconstructive Techniques.* 2d ed. New York: Springer, 1997.

"Otoplasty." *Mayo Clinic,* August 23, 2012.

Stedman, Thomas Lathrop. *Stedman's Plastic Surgery/ENT/Dentistry Words.* 5th ed. Philadelphia: Wolters Kluwer Health/Lippincott Williams & Wilkins, 2008.

Townsend, Courtney M., Jr., et al., eds. *Sabiston Textbook of Surgery.* 19th ed. Philadelphia: Saunders/Elsevier, 2012.

Otorhinolaryngology

Specialty

Anatomy or system affected: Ears, nose, respiratory system, throat

Specialties and related fields: Audiology, neurology, pediatrics, plastic surgery

Definition: The study of the diseases and disorders of the ears, nose, and throat.

Key terms:

audiometer: an electronic device, often used in combination with a computer, that measures a patient's range of hearing

fenestration: the surgical opening of a passage in a closed or narrowing ear canal through which sound can pass

mastoidectomy: the surgical removal of the temporal or mastoid bone, which is located behind the ear

maxillofacial surgery: surgery of the face and neck, a form of cosmetic and reconstructive surgery

otologist: a medical doctor who specializes in diseases and disorders of the ear

stapedectomy: the surgical removal of all or part of the stapes or innermost ossicle of the ear

tomography: an X ray used in combination with sophisticated computers to create an image of a specific organ, blotting out everything in front or behind

Science and Profession

Otorhinolaryngology-whose practitioners are often referred to simply as otolaryngologists or ear, nose, and throat (ENT) doctors-is a medical specialty that requires a doctor of medicine degree followed by a hospital or medical center residency ranging from four to five years, depending on the institution in which it is served. Many physicians in this field develop subspecialties, for which additional training is requisite. Among the most common subspecialties are oncology of the head and neck, ear surgery, pediatric otolaryngology, and maxillofacial surgery.

The scope of the otorhinolaryngologist's job is broad and overlaps several other medical specialties, notably general surgery, neurosurgery, plastic surgery, pediatrics, ophthalmology, and oncology. The otorhinolaryngologist treats all diseases and lesions that occur above the clavicle or collarbone except for those belonging to two categories: diseases and disorders of the eyes, which fall into the province of ophthalmology, and brain lesions, which are usually treated by neurosurgeons.

Otorhinolaryngology has existed as a specialty since the late nineteenth century. The need for it was great because ear, nose, and throat problems had, through the centuries, been among the most persistent killers of human beings. The areas affected have much to do with the ability to take in food and air. They also are directly connected with speech, smell, taste, hearing, and balance. Dysfunction of the ears, nose, or throat can profoundly affect a person's well-being physically, emotionally, and socially.

Among the medical conditions and diseases that most frequently come under the purview of otorhinolaryngology are the following: cleft lip and palate deformities (which are often treated as well by plastic surgeons); thyroid tumors (which are also treated by oncological surgeons); skin cancers (which also fall within the practices of plastic surgeons and oncological surgeons); face lifts, the treatment of facial lacerations, and other reconstructive surgery (which plastic surgeons also handle); lumps on the salivary glands (which are sometimes treated by oncological surgeons); and jaw injuries, including fractures (which are treated by maxillofacial surgeons, many of them board-certified in otorhinolaryngology).

Some of the surgery once done by otorhinolaryngologists is now virtually unnecessary because of the development of antibiotics. For example, drugs can combat effectively the kinds of infections that used to result in mastoiditis (inflammation of the mastoid bone), which frequently required a mastoidectomy. The flexible fiber-optic endoscope permits doctors to look into areas that previously could be exposed only through surgery. Advances in research have revealed that nasal polyps, which had a high rate of recurrence and were removed on a continuous basis, can usually be treated effectively with antibiotics, making such surgery unnecessary.

Until the mid-twentieth century, the most serious operation performed by otorhinolaryngologists was the laryngectomy (removal of the larynx, or voice box). By the end of the century, however, many practitioners in this specialty were routinely performing surgeries on tongue cancers and thyroid tumors because otorhinolaryngologists are often the ones who initially discover these conditions during head and neck examinations.

Because otorhinolaryngologists have long dealt with the grafting of bone and skin and the surgical management of skin flaps, much reconstructive and cosmetic surgery now falls into their specialty. Removal of tumors from the base of the skull, the interior ear canal, or the posterior cranial depression by means of modified craniotomies can be done by otorhinolaryngologists, who sometimes work in tandem with neurosurgeons in such cases.

Diagnostic and Treatment Techniques

The illnesses treated by otorhinolaryngologists have plagued the human race throughout history but could not be treated effectively until technology was developed that enabled physicians to look into the crowded crevices deep inside the body that were the source of many illnesses. In 1854, Manuel Garcia invented a concave mirror with a hole in its center through which doctors, attaching the implement to their heads, could peer as light from the mirror illuminated a patient's ears, nose, and throat. Doctors discovered that, using the reflecting head mirror in combination with an angled mirror held as far back as possible in the throat, they could illuminate the laryngeal area and the pharynx as well as the area behind the nose, all previously unavailable for visual inspection. Eventually, rather than examining affected areas with the bare eye, physicians had available to them, imbedded in the eyepiece of a hollow instrument with a light at the end, a magnifying telescope through which they could examine remote cavities with considerable ease and in great detail.

Modern otorhinolaryngologists can also examine patients under mild local anesthetic with sophisticated endoscopes, flexible devices that can easily be inserted into the nose, mouth, or ear of the patient. Such procedures are usually carried out in the doctor's office or in a hospital on an outpatient basis. These endoscopes, originally lighted with bulbs that heated up and burned out quickly, now carry light through light-bearing fiber-optic strands. In combination with small magnifying devices and cameras designed for this purpose, physicians can examine almost any area of the ears, nose, and throat and create color images, which can be invaluable in determining the presence of disease and in making an accurate diagnosis.

Modern technology has also made available to otorhinolaryngologists laser scalpels that permit extremely intricate surgery and accurate electronic audiometers. Audiometers eliminate the subjectivity of past tests of hearing acuity: In the nineteenth century, doctors either whispered into patients' ears, increasing the volume until their whispers could be heard, or used tuning forks to determine how much their patients could hear.

Treatment of disorders and diseases of the ear, nose, and throat have changed rapidly with the introduction of increasingly sophisticated surgical equipment and with the development of new drugs to control many conditions that

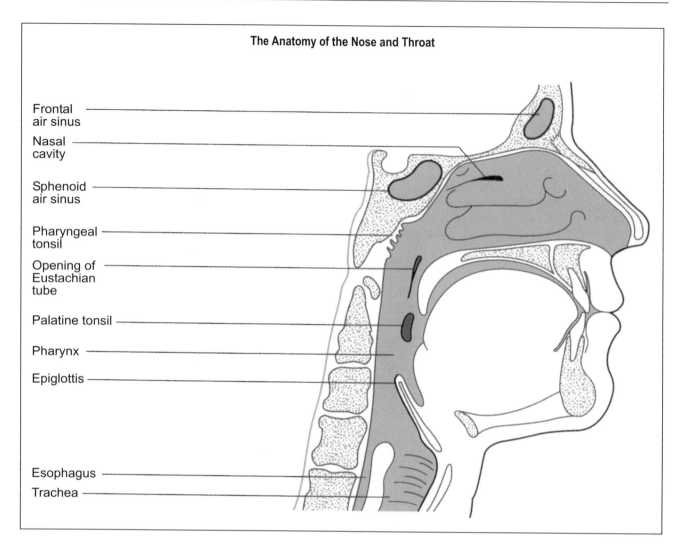

The Anatomy of the Nose and Throat

Frontal air sinus

Nasal cavity

Sphenoid air sinus

Pharyngeal tonsil

Opening of Eustachian tube

Palatine tonsil

Pharynx

Epiglottis

Esophagus

Trachea

once could be managed only by surgery. Computers have also been a valuable tool in diagnosing many of the problems that fall within this specialty.

All the anatomical areas with which otorhinolaryngologists must deal are interconnected; therefore a disease that begins in the ears can affect the nose and the throat, and vice versa. The most common diseases of the ears include deafness and Ménière's disease, an illness caused by an accumulation of fluid in the ear's labyrinth that results in loss of balance. Both of these disorders are most common among people over fifty, although they can afflict people at any age. One out of every ten thousand babies born in the United States has some hearing deficit, and many-particularly those whose mothers contracted rubella (German measles) during pregnancy-are almost totally deaf.

Otologists (physicians who treat diseases and disorders of the ear) have made considerable headway in treating some forms of deafness, particularly conductive deafness, which results from a narrowing of the ear canal to the point of closure. Shortly before 1920, it was discovered that considerable hearing can be restored through fenestration-that is, through making a small surgical opening in the eardrum through which sound can pass. The complications associated with this procedure have been largely overcome with

stapedectomy (the removal of all or part of the stapes, one of the bones of the middle ear) and the insertion of a prosthetic device, which is made of wire or Teflon and used in combination with a gelatin sponge or the patient's own veins, connective tissue, and fat. Although fenestration is highly successful in cases in which deafness is conductive, it does not alleviate deafness whose cause is sensorineural, so-called nerve deafness, which is often treated palliatively with hearing aids. These devices are constantly improving, however, as they are decreasing in size and increasing in effectiveness.

Tumors of the inner ear can now be successfully removed through a translabyrinthine approach. The ear canal is entered with tiny, well-illuminated laser instruments to which magnifying devices are attached. Such surgery is often performed by otologists, although many undertake it collaboratively with a neurologist. Pituitary tumors, once the responsibility almost solely of neurosurgeons who performed craniotomies to reach the diseased area of the brain, are often treated by otorhinolaryngologists, who approach the tumor through the nose. Thus the tumor can be removed without the need for debilitating surgery.

From the earliest beginnings of otorhinolaryngology, the larynx has been among the parts of the anatomy most often treated by its practitioners. The laryngectomy, with its radical side effect of rendering the patient unable to speak, was once the treatment of choice for malignant laryngeal tumors. Such tumors can now be treated successfully with radiation, obviating the need for more drastic treatment. Teflon injections have been used to treat patients whose vocal cords have been compromised by surgery or by radiation. Because the larynx is in the area of the thyroid glands, otorhinolaryngologists also possess expert knowledge of thyroid disorders and may perform a thyroidectomy (removal of the thyroid), a procedure that is now emphasized in their residencies.

Two of the most frequent surgical procedures of the field in the mid-twentieth century were the removal of the tonsils (tonsillectomy) and of the adenoids, the masses of lymphoid tissue in the lining at the back of the tongue that produce white blood cells, which fight disease. Tonsils and adenoids were once removed routinely if children suffered from frequent colds. Now this surgery is discouraged because it has been discovered that the tonsils and adenoids help children develop a resistance to infection. When these tissues become inflamed, they can be treated conservatively and successfully through medication.

Otorhinolaryngologists regularly work in concert with physicians in other specialties, particularly neurosurgery. An internist treating a patient who suffers from loss of balance usually refers that patient to an otologist, who orders diagnostic tests to check for fluid in the inner ear, which would suggest Ménière's disease. If such tests fail to reveal a buildup of fluid in the inner ear, the otologist usually refers the patient to a neurologist or neurosurgeon to check for other causes, including a tumor or a disorder in the central nervous system.

Otologists sometimes perform plastic surgery on ears that are abnormally protrusive. This reduction is a form of cosmetic surgery. By the end of the twentieth century in the United States, it was common for otorhinolaryngologists to perform most cosmetic and reconstructive surgeries related to these areas of the body. Consequently, residencies in this specialty offer considerable training in plastic surgery, especially in the procedures that otorhinolaryngologists have come to perform routinely in connection with thyroid, nasal, and other surgeries. They are often the physicians of choice in cases of cleft lip and cleft palate, the treatment of which normally falls largely within the province of reconstructive surgery. Because much cosmetic and reconstructive surgery involves the face, maxillofacial surgeons are often otorhinolaryngologists.

The common cold, although usually treated by an internist or family doctor if it is referred to a physician at all, sometimes involves complications such as bronchitis, pneumonia, or ancillary infections of the ears and sinuses. In such cases, an otorhinolaryngologist may be consulted for treatment. Dealing with the common cold is merely a waiting game: colds generally go away after a week or ten days. Colds afflict the average adult about four times a year and the average child twice that often (because young children have not yet built up the immunity that prevents infection).

Perspective and Prospects

Many of the illnesses that fall within the purview of otorhinolaryngology became more threatening and more frequent when the Industrial Revolution of the eighteenth century caused the relocation of large numbers of people from rural to urban settings. Cities grew as factories opened. Living conditions were often deplorable and, at best, overcrowded. Added to this situation was the pollution of the air by the waste products expelled by smokestack industries. Wherever pollution is prevalent, diseases of the upper respiratory tract are endemic.

The eighteenth century spawned conditions that compromised the environment and severely affected humans, but until physicians had a way of examining the body's more remote crevices, the diagnosis and treatment of ear, nose, and throat problems were difficult. Such treatments as bleeding frequently killed rather than cured patients. Surgery was a treatment of last resort because the major anesthetic was whiskey. Patients sometimes died of shock from the unbearable pain that they suffered during surgical procedures.

Once physicians had reliable means of seeing into the body by using such equipment as reflective mirrors, endoscopes, x-rays, tomography, and ultrasonography, they could treat many illnesses nonsurgically. It is hoped that in the future even less invasive surgery will be done in all fields of medicine, including otorhinolaryngology.

Even when surgery is indicated, in the field of otorhinolaryngology it can often be performed without an incision by entering the body through the ear canal, nose, or throat. Advanced technology has produced surgical instruments that, in combination with computer imaging, work precisely and with less trauma. In cases where incisions are necessary, the opening is often so small that it is almost undetectable a year after the procedure.

—*R. Baird Shuman, Ph.D.*

See also Antihistamines; Aromatherapy; Audiology; Cleft lip and palate; Cleft lip and palate repair; Common cold; Deafness; Decongestants; Ear infections and disorders; Ear surgery; Ears; Earwax; Esophagus; Epiglottitis; Halitosis; Hearing; Hearing loss; Hearing tests; Laryngectomy; Laryngitis; Ménière's disease; Motion sickness; Mouth and throat cancer; Myringotomy; Nasal polyp removal; Nasopharyngeal disorders; Nosebleeds; Otoplasty; Pharyngitis; Pharynx; Plastic surgery; Quinsy; Rhinoplasty and submucous resection; Sense organs; Sinusitis; Sjögren's syndrome; Smell; Sneezing; Sore throat; Strep throat; Taste; Tonsillectomy and adenoid removal; Tonsillitis; Tonsils; Voice and vocal cord disorders.

For Further Information:

American Academy of Otolaryngology-Head and Neck Surgery. "What Is an Otolaryngologist?" *American Academy of Otolaryngology-Head and Neck Surgery*, January, 2011.

Benjamin, Bruce, et al. *A Color Atlas of Otorhino- laryngology.* Edited by Michael Hawke. Philadelphia: J. B. Lippincott, 1995.

Chasnoff, Ira J., Jeffrey W. Ellis, and Zachary S. Fainman, eds. Rev. ed. *The New Illustrated Family Medical and Health Guide.* Lincolnwood, Ill.: Publications International, 1994.

Crumley, Roger L. "Otolaryngology-Head and Neck Surgery." In *Planning Your Medical Career: Traditional and Alternative Opportunities*, edited by T. Donald Rucker and Martin D. Keller et al. Garrett Park, Md.: Garrett Park Press, 1986.

Ferrari, Mario. *PDxMD Ear, Nose, and Throat Disorders.* Philadelphia: PDxMD, 2003.

Gulya, Aina J., and William R. Wilson. *An Atlas of Ear, Nose, and Throat Diagnosis and Treatment*. New York: Parthenon, 1999.

Kennedy, David W., and Marilyn Olsen. *Living with Chronic Sinusitis: A Patient's Guide to Sinusitis, Nasal Allergies, Polyps, and Their Treatment Options*. Long Island, N.Y.: Hatherleigh Press, 2007.

Vorvick, Linda J. "Types of Health Care Providers." *MedlinePlus*, August 14, 2012.

Woodson, Gayle E. *Ear, Nose, and Throat Disorders in Primary Care*. Philadelphia: W. B. Saunders, 2001.

Ovarian cancer. *See* Cervical, ovarian, and uterine cancers.

Ovarian cysts

Disease/Disorder
Anatomy or system affected: Reproductive system
Specialties and related fields: Gynecology
Definition: Benign growths that develop in the ovaries.

Causes and Symptoms

Ovarian cysts may occur at any age, individually or in numbers, on one or both ovaries. The cyst consists of a thin, transparent outer wall enclosing one or more chambers filled with clear fluids or old blood that presents as thick brownish or jellylike material; in some cases tissue material may be present as well. Such cysts range in size from that of a raisin to that of a large orange. The normal ovary measures 3 centimeters by 2 centimeters; the cystic ovary requiring investigation is one which is enlarged to more than twice its normal size. Large cysts may cause a feeling of fullness in the abdominal area, cramping pain with various levels of severity, or pain during vaginal intercourse. Often, however, there are no apparent symptoms, and the cyst is discovered only during a routine gynecologic examination when the clinician, on bimanual examination, discovers that one ovary is considerably enlarged. At this point, it is important to rule out malignancy, because ovarian cancers in their early stages also have no warning symptoms and can occur at any age.

Polycystic ovaries (ovaries containing multiple cysts) causing significant enlargement occur in a variety of conditions. For example, polycystic ovaries can result from an enzyme deficiency in the ovaries that interferes with the normal biosynthesis of hormones, resulting in the release of an abnormal amount of androgen (a substance producing or stimulating the development of male characteristics).

More than half of all ovarian cysts are functional; that is, they arise out of the normal functions of the ovary during the menstrual cycle. These cysts are relatively common. A cyst can form when a follicle (a small, spherical, secretory structure in the ovary) has grown in preparation for ovulation but fails to rupture and release an egg; this type is called a follicular cyst. Sometimes the structure formed from the follicle after ovulation, the corpus luteum, fails to shrink and forms a cyst; this is called a corpus luteum cyst.

Another type of ovarian cyst, most often found in younger women, is the dermoid cyst, which contains particles of teeth, hair, or calcium-containing tissue that are thought to

be an embryologic (developmental) remnant; such cysts usually do not cause menstrual irregularity and are very common. Dermoids are bilateral in 25 percent of cases, making careful examination of both ovaries mandatory. The cyst has a thickened, white, opaque wall and is more buoyant than other types of cysts.

Ovarian cysts cause problems when they become very large, when they rupture and cause severe internal bleeding, or when a cyst's pedicle (a tail-like appendage) suddenly twists and cuts off its blood supply, creating severe pain and possibly gangrene. Rupture of a cyst is followed by the acute onset of severe lower abdominal pain radiating to the vagina and lower back. The most severe symptoms of pain and collapse are associated with rupture of a dermoid cyst, as the cyst contents are extremely irritating.

Torsion (twisting) of a cyst may occur at any age but most often in the twenties; it may be associated with pregnancy. A

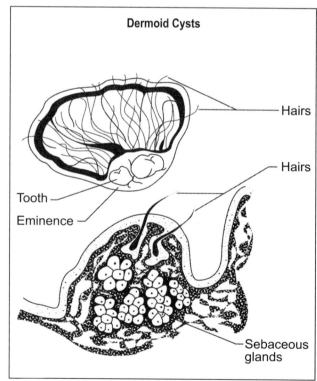

Dermoid cysts are a relatively common form of ovarian cyst often found in younger women.

twisted dermoid cyst is the most common, probably because of its increased weight. The onset of pain often occurs in the umbilical region and radiates to one or the other side of the pelvis. Pain on the right is frequently confused with appendicitis. Hemorrhage may sometimes occur from a vessel in the wall of the cyst or within the capsule.

Treatment and Therapy

The diagnosis of an ovarian cyst is made with consideration of the patient's age, medical and family history, symptoms, and the size of the enlarged ovary. In women under the age of thirty, clinicians, after a manual examination, will usually wait to see if the ovary will return to its normal size. If it does not, and pregnancy has been ruled out, a pelvic X-ray or a sonogram (the use of sound to produce an image or photograph of an organ or tissue), or both, can determine the exact size of the ovaries and distinguish between a cyst and a solid tumor. In women age forty and older, X-rays and sonograms may be done sooner. If uncertainty still exists, the physician may recommend laparoscopy, the visual examination of the abdominal cavity using a device consisting of a tube and optical system inserted through a small incision. The physician may also suggest the option of a larger incision and a biopsy.

In the case of the functional ovarian cyst, if no severe pain or swelling is present, the clinician may adopt "watchful waiting" for one or two more menstrual cycles, during the course of which this type of cyst frequently disappears on its own accord. Sometimes this process is hastened by administering oral contraceptives for several months, which establishes a regular menstrual cycle. Women already taking oral contraceptives rarely develop ovarian cysts.

In the case of torsion or rupture, surgical treatment is indicated, preferably the removal of the cyst only and preservation of as much of the normal ovarian tissue as possible. Sometimes, with a very large cyst, the ovary cannot be saved and must be removed, a procedure called oophorectomy or ovariectomy.

—*Genevieve Slomski, Ph.D.*

See also Biopsy; Cyst removal; Cysts; Genital disorders, female; Infertility, female; Laparoscopy; Ovaries; Polycystic ovary syndrome; Women's health.

For Further Information:

Altcheck, Albert, Liane Deligdisch, and Nathan Kase, eds. *Diagnosis and Management of Ovarian Disorders*. 2d ed. San Diego, Calif.: Academic Press, 2003.

Ammer, Christine, et al. *The New A to Z of Women's Health: A Concise Encyclopedia*. 6th ed. New York: Checkmark Books, 2009.

Berek, Jonathan S., ed. *Berek and Novak's Gynecology*. 14th ed. Philadelphia: Lippincott Williams & Wilkins, 2007.

Kovacs, Gabor T., and Robert Norman, eds. *Polycystic Ovary Syndrome*. 2d ed. New York: Cambridge University Press, 2012.

Leung, Peter C. K., and Eli Y. Adashi, eds. *The Ovary*. 2d ed. San Diego, Calif.: Academic Press, 2004.

Mahajan, Damodar K., ed. *Polycystic Ovarian Disease*. Philadelphia: W. B. Saunders, 1988.

"Ovarian Cyst." *Family Doctor*, August 2010.

Rosenblum, Laurie. "Ovarian Cyst." *Health Library*, September 10, 2012.

Vorvick, Linda J., Susan Storck, and David Zieve. "Ovarian Cysts." *Medline Plus*, February 26, 2012.

Ovaries

Anatomy

Anatomy or system affected: All

Specialties and related fields: Biochemistry, embryology, endocrinology, genetics, gynecology, obstetrics

Definition: The ovaries produce eggs and sex hormones in females.

Key terms:

atresia: the programmed process of cell death

corpus luteum: the structure that develops from an emptied ovarian follicle after ovulation

Fallopian tubes or oviducts: tubular structures attached at their lower ends to the uterus; the passageways for ova following ovulation

follicle: a structure composed of an oocyte and surrounding granulosa cells

hormone: a chemical messenger secreted by one cell type and acting on another to cause a predictable response

oocyte: a female germ cell that differentiates to become a mature ova

ovum (pl. ova): an egg cell

Structure and Functions

Ovaries develop from undifferentiated gonadal tissue in the absence of a Y chromosome. They are ductless glands located in the female pelvis, attached on either side of the uterus by the ovarian ligaments. Each is a flattened lumpy oval about 5 centimeters (cm) in length, 2.5 cm wide, and less than 1 cm in thickness. They are often described as being about the size and shape of an almond. There are three regions to each ovary: An outer cortex contains the developing oocytes, an inner medulla produces steroid hormones, and the hilum serves as the point of attachment and entry of blood vessels and nerves.

A principal function of the ovaries is gametogenesis, the production of ova through meiosis. This process begins during fetal life, and about 1 to 2 million immature oocytes are present in the cortex of the ovaries at birth. By puberty, this number has been reduced to about 300,000 through the process of atresia, and only about 400 mature ova are actually ovulated during life. The number of lifetime ovulated oocytes are reduced if oral contraceptives are used.

Recent research has found that it may be possible to increase oocyte numbers during life through the implantation of stem cells that are capable of mitosis. These stem cells can be isolated from the ovaries of reproductive age women. Studies done on mice have isolated germline stem cells from ovaries that can actively divide and produce oocytes when implanted in a human body.

Within the mature ovarian cortex are many follicles, each containing an oocyte. At any given time, there are oocytes in all stages of development, and only a small percentage of available oocytes ever undergo ovulation; the rest undergo atresia and are recycled by the body. This occurs because groups of oocytes are activated during ovulation, and only one makes it to the luteal stage, while the others undergo atresia.

Immature oocytes remain dormant until puberty. During this time, the hypothalamus region of the brain releases a surge of hormone, the Ganadotropin-releasing hormone, that initiates the release of hormones from the pituitary, which will drive the process of ovulation. During puberty, eggs mature successively, and one breaks through the ovarian wall each cycle in the process of ovulation. This continues until menopause, or cessation of reproductive functioning in the female. After release from the ovary, the ovum passes through the Fallopian tube and into the uterus. If the ovum is fertilized, then pregnancy ensues and the ovum (now a blastocyst) implants in the uterine lining.

Following ovulation, the empty follicle left in the ovary becomes the corpus luteum. It appears as a yellow body (because of lipid droplets in the cells) on the surface of the ovary and secretes progesterone to prepare the uterine lining for implantation. The corpus luteum deteriorates after ten to twelve days if conception does not occur, and the decrease in progesterone allows deterioration of the uterine lining, and thus, menstruation begins.

The ovarian medulla is also responsible for hormonogenesis. The primary steroids produced here are estradiol (estrogen) and progesterone. Androgens (particularly androstenedione and testosterone) are also secreted, but most of them are converted to estradiol within the ovary. Estrogens are essential for the development of ova and female body characteristics (including breasts, body shape, fat deposition, and body hair distribution) and for implantation and pregnancy maintenance. They also initiate mammary gland maturation and contribute to bone mineralization. Progesterone prepares the uterine lining for implantation and pregnancy, regulates the release of luteinizing hormone (LH) from the pituitary, and contributes to the maturation of mammary gland alveoli.

In addition to the steroid hormones, peptide hormones are produced by the ovaries. Relaxin is secreted from the corpus luteum and induces relaxation of the pelvic bones and ligaments, inhibits myometrial motility, softens the cervix, and induces uterine growth. Activins stimulate the release of follicle stimulating hormone (FSH) from the pituitary, and inhibin causes decreasing FSH output, although the mechanism is not yet understood. The ovary has been found to produce a variety of neuropeptides such as b-endorphin, adrenocorticotropin, α-melanocyte-stimulating hormone, vasopressin, and oxytocin. The physiologic roles that these peptides may play in the ovary are uncertain.

Human ovaries display a regular cycle in reproductively mature females. This cycle, known as menstruation, includes a follicular phase, during which FSH promotes growth and maturation of the granulosa cells, partial maturation of oocytes, synthesis of proteins, and estrogen secretion. Next is the ovulatory phase, during which one mature oocyte and the surrounding cells are discharged. Lastly is the luteal phase, in which progesterone is secreted. The average ovarian cycle is twenty-eight days, with a normal range between twenty-four and thirty-two days in length.

Disorders and Diseases

Polycystic ovary syndrome (PCOS), or Stein-Leventhal syndrome, is the most common ovarian disorder, affecting 6 to 10 percent of all women. The ovarian stroma becomes enlarged and produces excessive amounts of androgens. Atretic follicles accumulate and large numbers of cysts (fluid-filled sacs) may form; most are harmless and require no treatment. Ovarian follicle development is incomplete, and menstrual cycles are usually irregular. Symptoms can be alleviated with combination contraceptives and antiandrogens. Ovulation can sometimes be induced by clomiphene.

Ovulatory dysfunction is one of the causes of infertility. Most often this is hormonal in nature, and many cases of infertility can be overcome by hormone treatments.

Ovarian cancer is a major cause of death in females and comes in a variety of forms. The lifetime risk is about 1.6 percent, but it increases with age and in women with relatives who have had reproductive cancers. In women with an altered BRCA1 or BRCA2 gene, the risk is 25 to 60 percent, depending on the specific mutation. Pregnancy decreases the overall risk, as do oral contraceptives. Surgery is the treatment of choice, often followed by chemotherapy. Prognosis is poor overall, mostly due to the lack of clear symptoms that would lead to early diagnosis.

Perspective and Prospects

The human ovary was first described by Renier De Graaf in 1672. In 1701, the first surgery to remove an ovarian tumor was performed by Robert Houston, and in 1809 the first known ovary removal (ovariectomy or oophorectomy) was performed by Ephraim McDowell. Throughout the nineteenth and early twentieth centuries, study of the ovaries centered on their anatomy and physiology, while during the latter part of the twentieth century studies turned to their endocrine functions.

Many postulated ovarian hormones are still being searched and studied for their effects. They include transforming growth factor beta (TGF-β), anti-Mullerian hormone (AMH), folliculostatins, and many other peptides involved in the control of growth and differentiation. Gonadotropin surge attenuating factor (GnSAF) has also been hypothesized to be physiologically involved in the control of LH secretion during the menstrual cycle.

—Kerry L. Cheesman, Ph.D.;
updated by Catherine Avelar

See also Amenorrhea; Assisted reproductive technologies; Cervical, ovarian, and uterine cancers; Contraception; Endometrial biopsy; Endometriosis; Gamete intrafallopian transfer (GIFT); Genital disorders, female; Gynecology; Hormone therapy; Hormones; Hot flashes; Hysterectomy; In vitro fertilization; Infertility, female; Menopause; Menorrhagia; Menstruation; Obstetrics; Ovarian cysts; Pap test; Pelvic inflammatory disease (PID); Polycystic ovary syndrome; Pregnancy and gestation; Premenstrual syndrome (PMS); Puberty and adolescence; Reproductive system; Sterilization; Tubuligation; Uterus; Women's health

For Further Information:
Futterweit, Walter, and George Ryan. *A Patient's Guide to PCOS: Understanding-and Reversing-Polycystic Ovary Syndrome*. New York: Holt, 2006.

Johnson, J., J. Canning, T. Kaneko, J.K. Pru, and J.L. Tilly. "Germline Stem Cells and Follicular Renewal in the Postnatal Mammalian Ovary." *Nature* 428, no. 6979 (2004): 145-150.

Kaipia, Antti, and Aaron Hsueh. "Regulation of Ovarian Follicle Atresia." *Annual Review of Physiology* 59 (1997): 349-363.

Moore, K.L., T.V.N. Persaud, M.G. Torchia, and T.V.N. Persaud. *The Developing Human: Clinically Oriented Embryology.* Philadelphia: Saunders/Elsevier, 2008.

Plourde, Elizabeth. *Your Guide to Hysterectomy, Ovary Removal, and Hormone Replacement: What All Women Need to Know.* Ashland, OH: New Voice/ Atlas Books, 2002.

Over-the-counter medications

Treatment

Anatomy or system affected: All

Specialties and related fields: Family medicine, pharmacology, preventive medicine

Definition: Pills, capsules, tablets, or syrups that can be purchased without prescription for the self-treatment of common illnesses, such as colds, fever, and headache.

Key terms:

brand name: the name under which a drug is marketed by a pharmaceutical company

excipients: fillers, coloring, or coatings added to pills, tablets, capsules, or syrups

generic name: the unique name of a drug, typically the active chemical ingredient; a drug may be marketed under the generic name or the brand name

self-diagnosis: a determination of medical condition or illness without the benefit of a physician's input

self-prescription: the selection of over-the-counter medications without consulting a physician

self-treatment: the self-administration of one or more over-the-counter medications

Indications and Procedures

Drugs or medications that can be purchased directly, without a prescription, are called over-the-counter (OTC) medications or drugs. These medications may be suggested by physicians or simply purchased for consumption as a result of self-diagnosis and self-prescription. Most of the common OTC medications are used to treat common ailments such as cold and fever symptoms, headache, coughs, and similar complaints. Such self-treatment may be initiated at will and discontinued at any time.

Dozens of pharmaceutical companies produce and market hundreds of drugs for sale as over-the-counter medications, but they fall into only a few categories. The basic types of OTC medications, along with some brand examples, include analgesics (Advil, Tylenol), antacids (Milk of Magnesia), antidiarrheal medications (Imodium), antifungal agents (Tinactin), antihistamines (Benadryl), antiacne treatments (Clearasil), anti-inflammatory drugs (Motrin), decongestants (Sudafed), motion sickness (Meclizine), laxatives (Metamucil, Dulcolax), dandruff treatments (Selsun Blue), expectorants (Robitussin), hair growth formulas (Rogaine), and sleep aids (L-Tryptophan).

The most frequently used category of OTC medications is analgesics, which are more popularly known as painkillers. Analgesics include a diverse group of drugs that are used to relieve soreness, general body pain, and headaches. Probably the most common analgesic is aspirin, which is part of a group of medications termed nonsteroidal anti-inflammatory drugs (NSAIDs) that chemically affect the central and possibly the peripheral nervous system by leading to a decrease in prostaglandin production. Many analgesics are used in combination with other drugs such as vasoconstriction drugs that contain pseudoephedrine, which is especially important for the relief of sinus congestion, and in combination with antihistamine drugs, which relieve the worst symptoms of allergy.

Decongestants must certainly rank as the second most common category of OTC medications. Generally, decongestants are taken to relieve nasal congestion and allied symptoms of colds and flu by acting to reduce swelling of the mucous membranes of the nasal passageways. A recurring problem with most nasal decongestants is that they increase hypertension, but this effect is lessened by including one or more antihistamines in the preparation. The brand name drug Dimetapp, for example, is both an antihistamine and a decongestant, while various Tylenol products may contain drugs that collectively work to soothe sore throat, relieve nasal congestion, or suppress coughing.

Despite the fact that over-the-counter drugs are available to everyone, their marketing and use is restricted by the Food and Drug Administration (FDA) in the United States and similar agencies with regulatory powers in many other countries. The FDA mandates ingredients and labeling of OTC drugs and specifies rigid testing and safety standards that must be met prior to marketing. Pharmaceutical companies must apply to the New Drug Agency (NDA) for the approval of drugs. The NDA specifies testing requirements prior to issuing a license for the sales and marketing of the proposed new drug. Following approval, the FDA regularly reviews and maintains the right to remove or restrict marketing and sales of OTC drugs that create adverse side affects or are potentially addictive.

Following discovery, testing, and FDA approval of a new drug, it is given a unique trade name or brand name. The pharmaceutical company is awarded an exclusive patent to manufacture and market the drug for a specified period of time, usually seventeen years in the United States but of variable length in other countries. At the end of this time, the company no longer has proprietary rights to the drug, which may then be manufactured and marketed by other pharmaceutical companies. These drug companies may choose to market the drug under a new brand name of their choosing but not under the original label, which may still be manufactured by the original pharmaceutical company that designed and patented the drug. Spin-off products of these companies must still pass rigid FDA quality control standards which demonstrate that their product contains sufficient amounts of the active ingredients to promote bioequivalency before it can be marketed as an OTC medication-that is, the new drug has to be the therapeutic equal of the original drug.

Drugs manufactured by other pharmaceutical companies following patent expiration are typically called generic drugs and are strictly regulated by the U.S. Drug Price Competition and Patent Term Restoration Act (also known as the Hatch-Waxman Act), which was enacted in 1984. Tylenol, for example, is the exclusive brand name of an analgesic over-the-counter medication that contains the active chemical ingredient acetaminophen. Following the release of its patent, many other pharmaceutical companies started marketing pain relief drugs containing products for pain relief under the their own trade name or brand name. These copies are considered generic drugs and provide the consumer with a wide choice of the most popular drugs, usually at greatly reduced cost.

Manufacture and marketing of a generic drug by new companies usually means that their product costs considerably less, partly because of competition but mostly because the new drug companies did not bear the initial costs of development, marketing, and promotion that were part of the original financial investment of the parent company. Furthermore, manufacturers of generic drugs enjoy all the benefits of prior marketing, public acceptance, and possibly dependence on the most popular OTC medications. Generally, however, the parent company enjoys a certain competitive advantage of brand name recognition that promotes continued use of their marketed product, thereby reducing the impact of cheaper competition.

Over-the-counter medications may take the form of packets, tablets, capsules, pills, drops or droplets, ointments, inhalants, lotions, creams, suppositories, or syrups. Except for creams and topical ointments, OTC medications are administered orally, in contrast to drugs that are taken by injection. This mode of delivery places natural limits on their therapeutic effectiveness in several ways.

After being swallowed, OTC medications pass down the esophagus, through the stomach, and into the small intestine, where they are digested and absorbed. This mode of delivery requires a certain time interval between oral intake of the drug and its arrival in the bloodstream that transports it to target cells, tissues, and organs, thus delaying the effects of the drug. Tablets or capsules sometimes get stuck in the back of the mouth or on the lining of the esophagus, where they start to dissolve. When this happens, the ingredients may cause irritation, nausea, and sometimes vomiting, and the therapeutic value is lost. Furthermore, a certain amount of each key ingredient will be destroyed by the digestive enzymes of the gastrointestinal system, may be metabolized by cells of the intestinal epithelia, or may simply pass through the gut without being absorbed. Even following absorption into the blood, a certain amount of the drug may be lost because liver and other body cells set about removing foreign substances in the blood almost as soon as they are detected, generally by metabolizing the ingredient into a harmless chemical that will be excreted into the bile or be removed by the kidneys. This process explains why all drugs, including OTC medications, must be taken in repeated doses at regularly prescribed intervals in order to obtain maximum therapeutic value.

A final factor complicating delivery efficiency and thus the therapeutic value of OTC medications involves their packaging. Capsules, tablets, and pills in particular all contain substances in addition to the chemical ingredient, such as coatings, fillers, stabilizers, and often color additives. These substances, called excipients, do not contribute to the actual working of the drug itself, but they often modify both the rate and the extent of dissolution of the drug as it travels the gastrointestinal tract. While most excipients ultimately reduce the overall degree of delivery, some have important functions of permitting them to transit through the stomach, which has limited absorption ability, and into the small intestine, where chemical dissolution and absorption occurs at an optimum rate. For some drugs, the natural limits placed on delivery efficiency by gastrointestinal processes and excipient components can be sharply reduced by placing the capsule or tablet directly under the tongue, thus entirely bypassing the alimentary tract.

Uses and Complications

Primarily because of liability issues, all OTC medications include labels that are sometimes extensive. Label components typically consist of a list of one or more symptoms addressed by the medication, active ingredients contained in the drug, warnings, directions for use, and the date after which the medication should be discarded. For example, the label on a common OTC medication used to treat severe colds notes that it is to be used to relieve symptoms of nasal congestion, cough, sore throat, runny nose, headache and body ache, and fever. Directions for use are specific as to number of times a day, hours between use, and factors involving taking the medication, such as with or without glasses of water prior to or following administration and limits regarding food intake.

Most labels also carry prominent warnings regarding use with respect to age, alcohol consumption, sedatives or tranquilizers, and combinations of medications. Most over-the-counter medications also state that use should be continued only for a specified time and that, if symptoms persist, the user should stop taking the medication and consult a physician. Finally, the user is usually cautioned to stop taking the OTC medication immediately if headache, rash, nausea, or similar symptoms appear. Despite these warnings, even commonly used OTC medications pose certain health hazards, and the user is advised to take these medications with full recognition of potential problems.

In the United States, while the FDA periodically issues warnings regarding OTC medications, their actual use by consumers normally is not regulated, documented, or monitored. This has led to a number of concerns regarding real and potential overuse of OTC drugs, particularly for reasons unrelated to their medicinal intent. It has also led directly to the modification of certain OTC medications to engineer drugs that are highly addictive.

Because their use is unregulated-or, more correctly, cannot be regulated-over-the-counter medications can be deliberately abused. Overdosing with certain types of painkillers, for example, has become a frequent method of suicide attempt. The use of Tylenol in suicide attempts is increasing. Tylenol overdosing causes the destruction of liver cells that synthesize blood coagulants. Loss of these blood coagulants results in uncontrolled bleeding, most evidently through the eyes, nose, and mouth but also internally. Internal bleeding continues until death occurs, usually within a few days following onset.

Perhaps the most egregious misuse of OTC medications is to induce or achieve temporary "highs" that parallel those obtained by use of street or hard drugs. Cough suppressants that contain the drug dextromethorphan, for example, affect the central nervous system and can be used as mood-altering drugs that cause brain damage and even death at high doses. An even more serious abuse is the cooking of common drugs to obtain the highly addictive drug methamphetamine, popularly called meth. Also known as ice or speed, meth is a highly addictive drug that is often devastating and sometimes deadly. In some regions of the United States, it ranks with heroin and cocaine as the popular drug of choice. Record growth in use and the ability to cook meth from readily obtained OTC drugs has led to the creation of National Methamphetamine Awareness Day to draw attention at all levels to this problem.

This cooking process involves the conversion of certain OTC medications into meth. Some other sources for cooking meth include diet aids, tincture of iodine or other iodine solutions, and household cleaning solutions. In response to the widespread home manufacture of meth, a national federal law was enacted to require pharmacies to check photo identification and keep records of over-the-counter sales of cold medications that contain pseudoephedrine and ephedrine, which are the two popular ingredients in many cold medications. By-products of in-home meth cooking labs are garbage cans filled with Sudafed packages and a distinct odor of cat urine. The cooking process itself releases potentially harmful toxic chemicals that can pose serious health hazards to lungs and the respiratory system and also poses the risk of fire.

Perspective and Prospects

Originally, OTC medications were available for purchase only at pharmacies, along with physician-prescribed drugs. Today, a varied selection of OTC medications is available at many retail outlets, including supermarkets, food stores, and even convenience stores, although pharmacies still continue to offer the greatest selection. This can lead to a confusion of terms, as such medications or drugs are often no longer sold "over the counter" but instead can be found on shelves alongside other items for sale.

To complicate matters, certain drugs are offered as OTC medications at low dosages but must be obtained by prescription at higher dosages. For example, the popular analgesic ibuprofen (Advil, Motrin) can be purchased as an OTC medication at dosages of less than 200 milligrams, but higher dosages can be obtained only via prescription. Similarly, the antidiarrheal medication Imodium, an opiate, is available as an OTC medication in liquid form, while tablets of Imodium are available only by prescription.

The status of over-the-counter medications may change over time, depending on effectiveness and safety issues.

While some OTC drugs are removed from the general market following various concerns regarding safety, other drugs are transferred from prescription drugs to OTC medications. Examples include the antihistamine drug Benadryl, which is used to relieve symptoms of allergy and guard against allergic reactions, and the painkiller ibuprofen, both of which were, until recently, sold as prescription drugs only but are now available as OTC medications.

While the distribution and sale of over-the-counter medications is strictly regulated by state and federal laws in the United States, certain drugs that are deemed harmless may be offered for sale as medical cures for many ailments and thereby compete with OTC medications. These so-called miracle drugs have become increasingly popular because of the Web, which opens the door to purchases without prescription. Media promotions also sometimes offer these medications, complete with testimonials that dramatically describe their success as a cure-all for ailments. These types of medications are often labeled "quack" drugs. They pose a threat to users of prescription and OTC medications in several ways. First, they are generally useless, offering a nonexistent cure for health problems. Second, they are manufactured without regard to quality control measures that legitimate drug manufacturers must follow. Third, time may be lost in using the quack drug, especially if the condition is chronic and the symptoms need to be treated immediately. Finally, while some may be harmless, other quack drugs contain chemical ingredients that are potentially dangerous when used in combination with genuine over-the-counter medications.

—*Dwight G. Smith, Ph.D.*

See also Aging: Extended care; Antihistamines; Anti-inflammatory drugs; Aphrodisiacs; Clinical trials; Decongestants; Digestion; Food and Drug Administration (FDA); Herbal medicine; Homeopathy; Metabolism; Pain management; Pharmacology; Pharmacy; Polypharmacy; Sports medicine; Veterinary medicine.

For Further Information:

"Careful: Acetaminophen in pain relief medicines can cause liver damage." *fda.gov*, January 13, 2011.

Griffith, H. Winter, and Stephen Moore. *Complete Guide to Prescription and Non-Prescription Drugs*. Rev. ed. New York: Penguin Group, 2010.

Litin, Scott C., ed. *Mayo Clinic Family Health Book*. 4th ed. New York: HarperResource, 2009.

"Over-the-Counter Medicines." *MedlinePlus*, June 24, 2013.

Prescription and Over-the-Counter Drugs. Rev. ed. Pleasant View, N.Y.: Reader's Digest, 2001.

Sanberg, Paul, and Richard M. T. Krema. *Over-the-Counter Drugs: Harmless or Hazardous?* New York: Chelsea House, 1986.

"Use Caution with Over-the-Counter Creams, Ointments." *fda.gov*, April 1, 2008.

Overtraining syndrome

Disease/Disorder

Anatomy or system affected: Endocrine system, lymphatic system, muscles, nervous system, psychic-emotional system

Specialties and related fields: Exercise physiology, psychology, sports medicine

Definition: Perceptible and lasting decrease in athletic performance, often coupled with mood changes, which does not quickly resolve following a normal period of rest.

Causes and Symptoms

To achieve peak athletic performance, increased effort in training, sometimes to the point of overexertion, is required. Initial periods of overexertion followed by a brief decrease in performance are often referred to as overreaching, which is distinguishable from overtraining syndrome by the desired increase in performance following a brief period of rest. Overtraining syndrome appears to develop from an overload of training, psychosocial stressors, and performance without adequate recovery or rest periods.

Diagnosing this syndrome can be complicated because a single diagnostic test or tool has yet to be developed. Symptoms may vary depending on the individual athlete or the sport, so other possible causes for a long-term decrease in performance, such as diet or disease, should be ruled out first. More than eighty-four symptoms or markers have been attributed to overtraining syndrome. Most often noted in diagnosis are impaired performance, variations in heart rate, variations in blood pressure, loss of coordination, elevated basal metabolic rate, decreased body fat, weight loss, chronic fatigue, sleep disturbances, increased thirst, headaches, nausea, elevated C-reactive protein (CRP), hormone changes, excessive production of cytokines, mood changes, depression, increased susceptibility to colds, difficulty concentrating, restlessness, increased aches and pains, and muscle soreness. Sport-specific stress tests conducted to the point of exhaustion may aid in the diagnosis.

Treatment and Therapy

Rest from training, performance, and/or competition is needed. The recovery period may take anywhere from several weeks to years. As the rest period needed to fully recover from overtraining syndrome may vary greatly from one athlete to the next, prevention is seen as the better option. To reduce the risk of developing this condition, a training schedule that alternates high and low training intensities with at least one day of rest is suggested. Other possible preventive measures include managing stress and maintaining a log to track training intensities, diet, and sleep.

Information on Overtraining Syndrome

Causes: Training overload, stress, inadequate recovery or rest periods

Symptoms: Impaired performance, loss of coordination, elevated metabolism, body fat loss, chronic fatigue, sleep disturbances, increased thirst, headaches, nausea, depression, muscle soreness

Duration: Chronic

Treatments: None; prevention through rest periods, stress management

---

Perspective and Prospects

Research on the characteristics of overtraining syndrome, such as how it affects men and women differently or athletes from various sports, continues to offer new insight. More research, especially longitudinal research, is needed to better understand the condition including its diagnosis, prevention, and treatment. A number of physiological tests to aid in detecting overtraining syndrome, including hormone levels, enzyme levels, and blood plasma changes, have been implemented, but none thus far have proved to be a valid measure for diagnosing this condition.

—*Susan E. Thomas, M.L.S.*

See also Ergogenic aids; Exercise physiology; Fatigue; Kinesiology; Metabolism; Muscle sprains, spasms, and disorders; Muscles; Nutrition; Physical rehabilitation; Physiology; Preventive medicine; Sports medicine; Stress; Stress reduction.

For Further Information:

Brooks, K. A., and J. G. Carter. "Overtraining, Exercise, and Adrenal Insufficiency." *Journal of Novel Physiotherapies* 3,125. (2013).

Hausswirth, Christophe. *Recovery for Performance in Sport.* Champaign, Ill.: 2013.

Kerksick, Chad M. *Nutrient Timing: Metabolic Optimization for Health, Performance, and Recovery.* Boca Raton, Fla.: 2012

Kreider, Richard B., Andrew C. Fry, and Mary L. O'Toole, eds. *Overtraining in Sport.* Champaign, Ill.: Human Kinetics, 1998.

McDuff, David R. Sports Psychiatry: Strategies for Life Balance and Peak Performance. Arlington, Va.: American Psychiatric Publishing, 2012.

Romain, Meeusen, et al. "Prevention, Diagnosis, and Treatment of the Overtraining Syndrome." *European Journal of Sport Science* 6, 1. (2006): 1-14.

Urhausen, Axel, and Wilfried Kindermann. "Diagnosis of Overtraining: What Tools Do We Have?" *Sports Medicine* 32, 2. (2002): 95-102.

Wyatt, Frank B., Alissa Donaldson, and Elise Brown. "The Overtraining Syndrome: A Meta-Analytic Review." *Journal of Exercise Physiology* 16, 2. (April 2013): 12-23.

Oxygen therapy

Treatment

Anatomy or system affected: Chest, circulatory system, heart, lungs, respiratory system

Specialties and related fields: Anesthesiology, cardiology, critical care, emergency medicine, preventive medicine, pulmonary medicine

Definition: Giving air enhanced by added oxygen to persons suffering from hypoxia, lack of sufficient oxygen in the tissues.

Indications and Procedures

The major indication for oxygen therapy is cyanosis, in which the skin assumes a bluish tint as a result of hypoxia, a reduced arterial saturation of oxygen to the tissues. In cases of extreme breathlessness, which may be caused by extreme physical exertion, hypoxia may occur, but the condition in most cases reverses itself within minutes if the affected person rests.

In older people whose circulatory systems have been compromised by such conditions as arteriosclerosis (narrowing of the arteries), hypoxia may be chronic. Asthmatics often require immediate oxygen therapy during severe attacks. People suffering from influenza or pneumonia may have accumulated secretions in their airways that limit the amount of oxygen that can reach their tissues. Such people are usually given oxygen administered through either a nasal catheter or a face mask.

In instances where respiratory difficulties persist, as in emphysema or chronic bronchitis, patients often receive prescriptions for oxygen cylinders for home use. They may also benefit from the home installation of an oxygen concentrator, a machine that removes oxygen from the atmosphere and remixes it in high concentrations with air. Such machines can supply oxygen-enhanced air to various rooms within a house so that ambulatory patients can breathe it for prolonged periods without being confined to one location. Some patients must breathe oxygen-enhanced air for up to fifteen hours a day.

Uses and Complications

Oxygen therapy is routinely used by anesthesiologists during many surgical procedures, but very high oxygen concentrations are usually avoided. Warm, humidified oxygen is preferred in surgical situations to prevent condensation and inordinate cooling, which can lead to complications. Such therapy is often administered through a catheter and used postoperatively for up to five days to prevent hypoxemia (reduced oxygen in the blood). In emergency rooms, pure oxygen is frequently given to patients in acute distress.

In some situations, physicians must use medications such as naftidrofuryl to reduce the brain's requirement for oxygen where hypoxemia is present, and brain damage may result if this complication is not addressed immediately. A thrombus (blood clot) may reduce blood flow substantially and reduce to dangerous levels the supply of oxygen to the brain and tissues. In such situations, anticoagulants such as heparin or warfarin often reduce or eliminate the thrombus and restore the body's circulation of oxygen.

—*R. Baird Shuman, Ph.D.*

See also Alternative medicine; Altitude sickness; Asbestos exposure; Asthma; Brain damage; Bronchitis; Chronic obstructive pulmonary disease (COPD); Circulation; Drowning; Ergogenic aids; Exercise physiology; Hyperbaric oxygen therapy; Hypoxia; Influenza; Lungs; Pneumonia; Pulmonary diseases; Pulmonary hypertension; Pulmonary medicine; Pulmonary medicine, pediatric; Respiration; Sports medicine; Thrombosis and thrombus; Vascular medicine; Vascular system; Wheezing.

For Further Information:

Perry, Anne Griffin, and Patricia A. Potter, eds. *Clinical Nursing Skills and Techniques*. 6th ed. St. Louis, Mo.: Mosby/Elsevier, 2006.

Rosdahl, Caroline Bunker, and Mary Kowalski, eds. *Textbook of Basic Nursing*. 9th ed. Philadelphia: Lippincott Williams & Wilkins, 2008.

Sheldon, Lisa Kennedy. *Oxygenation*. 2d ed. Sudbury, Mass.: Jones and Bartlett, 2008.

Tallis, Raymond C., and Howard M. Fillit, eds. *Brocklehurst's Textbook of Geriatric Medicine and Gerontology*. 7th ed. Philadelphia: Saunders/Elsevier, 2010.

Oxytocin

Biology

Anatomy or system affected: reproductive

Specialties and related fields: endocrinology, gynecology

Definition: a peptide hormone primarily synthesized by the hypothalamus and stored in the pituitary that stimulates uterine contractions during childbirth and milk ejection during breast feeding

Key terms:

autismspectrum disorders: a group of developmental disorders that includes autism, and Asperger syndrome among other disorders

placenta: an organ that develops during pregnancy that allows for an exchange of gases, nutrients and wastes between the mother and developing fetus

hypothalamus: the part of the brain the synthesizes oxytocin and vasopressin, links the nervous system with the endocrine system and has a myriad of physiological effects

milkejection/letdown effect: the process by which upon stimulation of the nipple, oxytocin is released and stimulates the contraction of alveoli of the mammary glands expelling milk towards the nipple

Structure and Function

Oxytocin is a nine amino acid peptide hormone primarily synthesized by the hypothalamus and stored in the pituitary until released. Oxytocin is released late in pregnancy when the uterus and cervix become stretched. Oxytocin causes contractions of the uterus facilitating birth. The name oxytocin is derived from Greek and means "quick birth," a reference to the fact that the body produces increased amounts of oxytocin causing uterine contractions during childbirth. Oxytocin is often administered to induce labor. Oxytocin is also involved with breast feeding by playing a role in the milk ejection/letdown effect, which occurs when an infant sucks at the mother's nipple, producing nerve impulses that are communicated to the hypothalamus in the mother's brain, which then causes the pituitary gland to begin producing oxytocin. The oxytocin stimulates the contractions of the mammary sinuses expelling milk towards the nipple. Oxytocin may also be responsible for bonding enhancement that encourages the mother to continue nursing for as long as the infant is hungry, a clear evolutionary advantage, as it avoids the problem of undernourished babies of mothers who might otherwise curtail nursing. It is also thought that the oxytocin produced during nursing stimulates contractions of the uterus that help the mother heal the location at which the placenta was attached during pregnancy.

In popular culture it has gained recognition under a variety of monikers: "the social hormone," "the romantic hormone," "the intimacy drug," and so on. This is because one of oxytocin's effects appears to be the enhancement of empathy and of deep emotional bonds and the development of trust or romantic affiliation between adults. The evolutionary advantages that social bonding, affection, and love may offer are believed to support larger populations, which are more likely to survive. A number of studies have also suggested that oxytocin may play a significant role in human sexual arousal, orgasm, and fertilization. Oxytocin has been shown to be released during hugging and sexual intercourse where it may stimulate contraction for the uterus aiding the transport of sperm Since males do not give birth or breast feed, the role of oxytocin in males is not completely understood. Males and females respond somewhat differently to oxytocin.

Perspective and Prospects

Scientists have been studying oxytocin since the early part of the twentieth century. The neuropeptide was discovered in 1906 by Henry Hallett Dale, an English physiologist. Research, distinct from that involving childbirth and nursing, has to do with oxytocin's ability to assist the body in recovering from injuries. Folk wisdom has asserted that people are better able to overcome sickness and injury when they are attended by people with whom they share an affectional bond. This can even extend to animals, as indicated by the frequent use of "therapy dogs" to help patients cope with their illnesses by offering comfort and companionship. Scientists now believe there is evidence to support the observation that some types of wounds appear to heal more quickly and more completely when oxytocin is produced by the patient. This suggests a direct connection between the presence of supportive social bonds and improved patient outcomes, because having loved ones nearby during treatment causes the patient's body to produce greater amounts of oxytocin, which in turn augment the body's ability to heal itself.

A growing number of physicians believe that oxytocin may offer a number of profoundly important benefits to public health. One such benefit might be realized by those suffering from autism spectrum disorders. One aspect of autism common to many of those afflicted with the syndrome is a difficulty making connections with other people, or an impaired ability to understand or even take notice of the emotional states of others. This can give rise to the social awkwardness that is often associated with autism spectrum disorders. Those with such disorders frequently fail to respond appropriately to social cues because they are either unaware of the cues and their meaning, or they fail to notice them altogether. Some research has established a relationship between autism and the oxytocin gene. Research in progress seeks to determine whether those with autism spectrum disorders might experience a greater ability to empathize with others if they were to receive increased doses of oxytocin. The hope is that whatever mechanisms underlie oxytocin's ability to increase empathy and interpersonal bonding are the same mechanisms operating in autistic persons at an impaired level. If this research bears fruit, then there may be a host of related disorders such as social anxiety disorder and related anxiety-based syndromes worth exploring for treatment with oxytocin. The main challenge scientists face is to discover ways in which people can benefit from oxytocin in a more controlled, deliberate way, while finding ways to prevent the cynical and unethical misuse of the drug's properties.

—*Scott Zimmer, MLS, MS;*
updated by Charles L. Vigue, PhD

See also: Reproductive system

For Further Information:

Baron-Cohen, Simon, Helen Tager-Flusberg, and Michael V. Lombardo. *Understanding Other Minds: Perspectives from Developmental Social Neuroscience*. Oxford: Oxford UP, 2013.

Breuning, Loretta G. *Habits of a Happy Brain: Retrain Your Brain to Boost Your Serotonin, Dopamine, Oxytocin, &... Endorphin Levels*. Fort Collins: Adams, 2015.

Choleris, Elena, Donald W. Pfaff, and Martin Kavaliers. *Oxytocin, Vasopressin, and Related Peptides in the Regulation of Behavior*. Cambridge: Cambridge UP, 2013.

MacGill, Markus. Oxytocin: The love hormone? Medical News Today. September 4, 2017. http://www.medicalnewstoday.com/articles/275795.php

Mikulincer, Mario, and Phillip R. Shaver. *Mechanisms of Social Connection: From Brain to Group*. Washington, DC : American Psychological Assoc., 2014.

Moberg, Kerstin U. *The Hormoneof Closeness: The Role of Oxytocinin Relationships*. London: Pinter, 2013.

Stoller, K. P. *Oxytocin: The Hormoneof Healingand Hope*. Santa Fe: Dream Treader, 2012.

Takahashi, Toku, Irena Gribovskaja-Rupp, and Reji Babygirija. *Physiologyof Love: Role of Oxytocinin Human Relationships, StressResponse and Health*. New York: Nova, 2013.

Pacemaker implantation

Procedure

Anatomy or system affected: Chest, circulatory system, heart

Specialties and related fields: Biotechnology, cardiology

Definition: The introduction into the heart of a permanent instrument that uses electrical pulses to regulate its rhythm.

Key terms:

atrium: one of the two upper chambers of the heart; the right atrium receives blood returning through the veins; the left atrium receives oxygenated blood from the lungs

catheter: a thin tube that can be inserted into blood vessels, such as a vein leading into the heart, to carry electrical wires or optical fibers

circus movement: electrical impulses in the heart that continue firing instead of reaching a normal resting phase, causing heart flutter and fibrillation

electrocardiogram (ECG or EKG): a recording of electrical signals generated by the heart that are detected by electrodes placed on the chest, arms, and legs; used to diagnose heart abnormalities

fibrillations: rapid and chaotic contractions of the heart muscle that are usually fatal when they occur in the ventricles because of insufficient blood flow

heart block: a delay or blockage of the electrical signal traveling through the heart muscle, which upsets the synchronization between contractions of the upper and lower chambers

sinoatrial (S-A) node: a cluster of cells above the right atrium that emit electrical signals which initiate contractions of the heart; also called natural pacemaker cells

ventricles: the two lower chambers of the heart; the right ventricle pumps blood to the lungs, and the left ventricle pumps oxygenated blood to the body

Indications and Procedures

The first human-made pacemaker, which used electronic pulses to stimulate a regular heart rhythm, was built in the 1950s. Since then, the device has evolved into a sophisticated and reliable instrument. It was miniaturized so that it could be implanted under the skin of the patient. Tiny batteries that would last from five to fifteen years were developed. A microprocessor that can sense the need for different heart rates during sleep or strenuous exercise has become a standard component. Most recently, a small automatic defibrillator has been incorporated into some pacemakers to supply several large jolts of electrical energy in case of heart stoppage or other emergencies.

The normal rhythm of a healthy heart is regulated by natural pacemaker cells. These unique cells are located at the sinoatrial (S-A) node near the top interior of the heart, where blood empties from the veins into the right atrium. Electrical impulses originating at the S-A node travel to the atrioventricular (A-V) node, which is located where the four chambers of the heart come together. From there, the signal is relayed to the ventricles, causing the muscle fibers to contract. This pumping action forces blood to flow from the two ventricles to the lungs and the body arteries.

If the natural pacemaker cells or the nerve pathways in the heart do not function properly, the heart may beat too rapidly, too slowly, irregularly, or not at all. For example, the condition calledheart block interrupts or delays the electrical signal at the A-V node. It can happen that only every second or third pacemaker signal triggers a contraction. Sometimes, the ventricles will start a contraction on their own, but it will not be synchronized with the blood flow from the atrium. An artificial electronic pacemaker can be used to overcome heart block.

The electrical activity of the heart is observed in an electrocardiogram (ECG or EKG). Metal electrodes are placed in contact with a patient's left arm, right arm, left leg, and sometimes chest. After suitable amplification, the signal can be displayed on a video screen or recorded by an ink pen on moving paper.

For a healthy heart, the normal ECG pattern starts with a small pulse (the P wave), which is followed by a group of three closely spaced pulses (the QRS complex) and a final small pulse (the T wave). This pattern is repeated approximately seventy-two times per minute for a person sitting at rest.

In brief, the P wave indicates contraction of the atrium, the QRS complex shows contraction of the ventricles, and the T wave represents the muscles' return to the resting state. If the heart "skips a beat" because of a heart block at the A-V node, the ECG will show a missing or delayed pulsation in the otherwise regular pattern. If this happens in a sustained fashion, electronic stimulation is needed.

Two other serious malfunctions of the heart's electrical system are flutter and fibrillation. Flutter is a very rapid but still constant rhythm that may produce 200 to 300 beats per minute. Fibrillations are much more serious, causing chaotic, random contractions that can occur as often as 500 times per minute. There is insufficient time between contractions for blood to fill the ventricles. Pumping action becomes very inefficient, and death is likely to occur if the fibrillations continue.

To restore normal heart rhythm, a defibrillator is used to send a strong electric shock through the ventricular muscle fibers, which deactivates the heart's electrical system for several seconds. An electronic pacemaker may then replace the natural pacemaker cells to prevent the recurrence of fibrillations.

The cause of flutter and fibrillation is a process called "circus movement." Suppose the electrical impulses are diverted from their normal pathway by thickened or dead heart tissue. In such a case, the timing may be thrown off so that the ventricles are restimulated to contract again without waiting for the pacemaker's signal. Therefore, the heart is unable to reach its resting state.

In the ECG pattern, flutter shows up as a rapid pulsation with an indistinct QRS complex. Fibrillation is indicated by irregularly spaced pulses of random size that have no pattern at all. It is something like electrical noise coming from the heart, with no synchronization. Heart cells at many locations fire at random, producing ripples similar to those made by a handful of pebbles thrown into a lake.

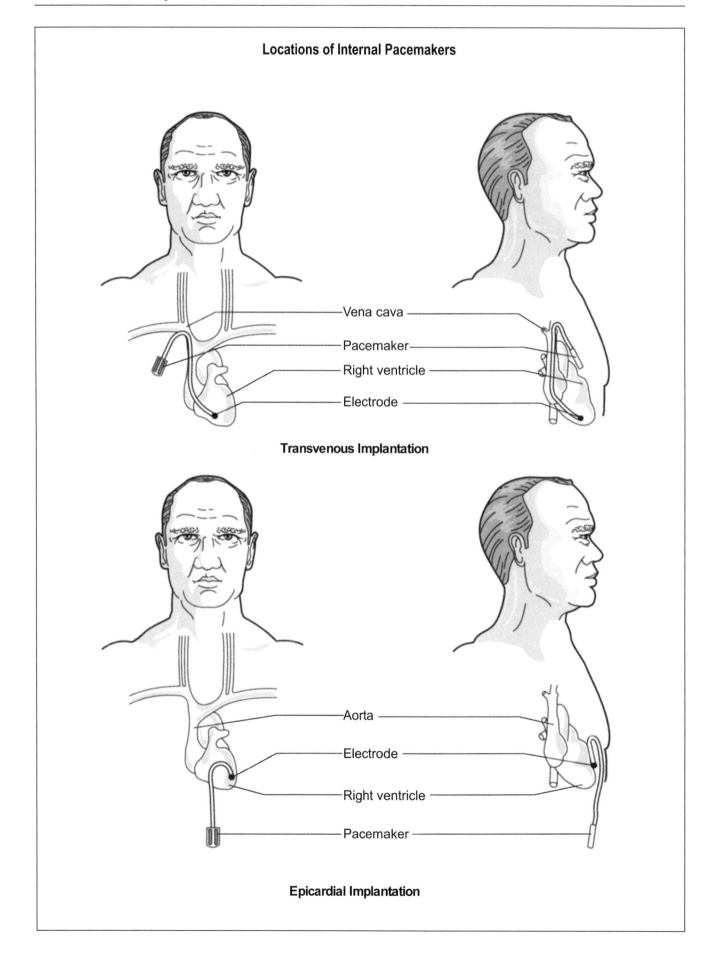

Locations of Internal Pacemakers

Vena cava

Pacemaker

Right ventricle

Electrode

Transvenous Implantation

Aorta

Electrode

Right ventricle

Pacemaker

Epicardial Implantation

The first artificial pacemaker was developed by Paul Zoll in 1952. When a patient suffering from heart block went into heart failure during surgery, Zoll inserted a needle electrode into the man's chest and applied regular voltage pulses from an external circuit. After two days, the man's heart resumed beating on its own, and the circuit was disconnected.

A portable artificial pacemaker was developed in 1957 by C. W. Lillehei and Earl Bakken. The electrode was inserted directly against the outer surface of the heart, and a battery pack and timer circuit were worn around the patient's waist. Three years later, the pacemaker was miniaturized sufficiently to be implanted under the skin of the patient's chest. This had the advantage of reducing the risk of infection.

The next major improvement was to redesign the fixed-rate pacemaker so that it could respond to variable demand during exercise or sleep. The demand pacemaker has a built-in sensor that monitors the heart's electrical system. An electronic microprocessor is programmed to recognize abnormal ECG pulses. Generally, the demand pacemaker is set to deliver a trigger pulse only when the heart rate falls below a certain point.

For people with a potential for unpredictable heart stoppage or fibrillation, a device called an implantable cardioverter defibrillator (ICD) has been developed. This unit, which is comparable to the external defibrillators used by emergency medical technicians but much smaller, can deliver several large jolts directly to the heart. Since implanted batteries are quite small, the circuit requires some time to recharge between shocks. The circuit is quite similar to the flash attachment of a camera, with its "slow charge, fast discharge" process.

Uses and Complications

The implantation of a pacemaker may become necessary as a result of a coronary artery disease, in which a buildup of plaque leads to irregularities in the heart's rhythm. Coronary artery disease is the main form of heart disease, which is the leading cause of death in the United States. Heart disease claimed nearly 600,000 American lives in 2010; it afflicts 11 percent of the US population. It is primarily a disease of modern, industrial society and is less frequently found in more rural, underdeveloped countries. In the United States, the death rate from heart attacks increased sharply after 1920, reached a peak in the mid-1960s, and has declined substantially since then.

A heart attack is usually caused by an oxygen deficiency in the heart muscle. The attack may come suddenly and without warning, but most often there is previous tissue damage that has weakened the heart over a period of time. A buildup of plaque in the arteries, called atherosclerosis, can reduce the rate of blood flow to a dangerously low level. The heart muscle tries to compensate for its reduced pumping power and may develop rhythmic irregularities, or arrhythmia. Eventually, heart block or ventricular fibrillations can ensue, leading to heart failure and death.

The famous Framingham Heart Study, initiated in 1948 in Framingham, Massachusetts, has been following the medical histories of approximately 5,000 men and women in order to identify the most important risk factors for heart disease. For example, the rate of heart disease among male smokers in this study was three times as high as that among nonsmokers. (This result is in addition to the much higher rate of lung cancer among smokers.) Other risk factors are excessive alcohol consumption, lack of exercise, high blood cholesterol, emotional or physical stress, and excess weight. Some unalterable risk factors are age, sex, and a family history of heart disease. The decline in heart attack deaths in recent years has been attributed to widespread changes of lifestyle to reduce the risk factors, as well as to improvements in medical diagnosis and treatment.

Modern pacemakers are remarkably reliable and safe. One of the few precautions for pacemaker wearers is to avoid standing near high-level microwave sources (although household microwave ovens are harmless). The problem is that the metal wire going into the heart acts like an antenna; it can pick up stray microwave radiation, which can disrupt the electronics in the sensitive pacemaker circuit. Also, the battery in a pacemaker must be changed at five- to ten-year intervals to ensure proper operation.

Thousands of people receive implanted pacemakers each year. The procedure has become so routine that even small community hospitals are equipped to handle it. Many patients with heart block and irregular rhythm, especially elderly patients, have benefited greatly from this technological development.

Perspective and Prospects

The creation of effective electronic pacemakers depends on an understanding of the structure and function of the human heart. Also, instruments such as x-ray machines and electrocardiographs are indispensable for monitoring an individual patient's response. This section will review the progress of the medical ideas and instruments that were the essential prerequisites for modern pacemakers. Good starting points are the pioneering studies of human anatomy made by Leonardo da Vinci (1452-1519) and Andreas Vesalius (1514-1564).

Leonardo dissected and studied the human body and made anatomical sketches in his notebooks. He recognized that the heart had four chambers, and he also drew the heart valves in detail. His interest in anatomy was that of an artist rather than that of a physician.

Vesalius was a professor of medicine at the University of Padua, in Italy. He taught anatomy and wrote a famous seven-volume treatise on the structure of the human body that had many excellent illustrations. His knowledge of anatomy came from the dissection of animals and of human cadavers obtained at night from paupers' graves. Some of his anatomical investigations contradicted traditional medical doctrine and brought him into conflict with the Catholic Church. Like Galileo, he believed that experimental information was superior to ancient textbooks.

William Harvey, a British physician, received his medical degree from the University of Padua in 1602. He is known for formulating the first accurate description of the circulation of the blood through the body. He showed that the volume of blood is fairly constant, so the function of the heart is to act as a recirculating pump. He had a clear understanding of the way in which the right ventricle pushes blood through the lungs and the left one circulates it to the rest of the body. There was, however, one missing link in Harvey's theory: How did the blood get from the arteries to the veins for its return flow? The invention of the microscope in the 1670s made it possible to see the tiny, previously invisible capillaries, thus providing final confirmation of the circulation process.

The scientific investigation of electricity began in the eighteenth century. Benjamin Franklin studied lightning rods, and scientists learned how to build a friction machine that produced electricity in the laboratory. Taking an electric shock became an amusing, although somewhat dangerous, entertainment at parties.

About 1790, the Italian anatomist Luigi Galvani made an important, though accidental, discovery. A metal scalpel lying near an electrostatic machine came into contact with the leg of a recently dissected frog, causing a sudden twitching of the muscle. Evidently, there was a connection between the electric shock and the muscle contraction.

The modern pacemaker that stimulates the heart muscle works in the same way that Galvani's scalpel worked; however, a major evolution in physiological knowledge and medical practice had to take place before the pacemaker could be developed.

Wilhelm Conrad Röntgen was experimenting with high voltages in his laboratory in 1896 when he observed a mysterious new type of radiation, which he called x-rays. Unlike light, x-rays were able to pass through black paper, wood, and even thin metal sheets. They could cause certain paints to glow in the dark and could expose photographic film that was still in its light-tight box. For the medical profession, the discovery of x-rays was a major breakthrough.

X-ray technology has been improved in recent years. Electronic image intensifiers were developed in the 1950s in order to brighten the dim pictures on a fluorescent screen. A major breakthrough in the 1970s was the invention of computed tomography (CT) scanning. Instead of using film or a fluoroscope, a computer generates images of the heart and other internal organs on a video screen. For pacemaker implantation, x-ray apparatus is indispensable in order to observe the electrode's precise placement into the interior of the heart.

The electrodes of most pacemakers are installed with a catheter that is inserted through a vein, through the right atrium, through the valve, and finally touches the inside of the right ventricle. The first human heart catheterization is credited to Werner Forssmann in 1929, when he was a young intern at a hospital in Berlin, Germany. He requested permission to try the procedure on a patient, but his supervisor refused. Forssmann then decided to try it on himself. He anesthetized his left elbow, opened a vein, and inserted the catheter tube. As he pushed it up the arm, he watched its progress on an x-ray fluoroscope, which he had to view by reflection in a mirror held by a nurse. When the catheter had gone in 65 centimeters, Forssmann asked an x-ray technician to record it on film to prove that it had entered his heart. During the next two years, he repeated the procedure several times, but criticism by his medical colleagues forced him to discontinue it. He became a small-town doctor and was amazed to learn in 1956 that he had been awarded the Nobel Prize for Medicine.

Accumulated knowledge about the structure of the heart, improvements in surgery, the development of new drugs, and the availability of modern instrumentation have all contributed to a substantial improvement in the medical treatment of heart ailments in modern times. The development of artificial heart valves, the heart-lung machine, the success of heart bypass surgery, the use of laser beams for surgery, and the use of drugs to control high blood pressure are recent developments.

An important contribution from the field of electronics was the development of the transistor in the early 1950s. It made possible the whole technology of miniaturized electronics, replacing the bulky vacuum tubes that were used in old radio circuits. Implantable pacemakers and microprocessor sensors would not have been possible without transistors.

Human ingenuity no doubt will continue to develop new instruments for cardiac diagnosis and rehabilitation, building on the accomplishments of the innovators of the past.

—*Hans G. Graetzer, Ph.D.*

See also Arrhythmias; Cardiac arrest; Cardiac rehabilitation; Cardiac surgery; Cardiology; Cardiology, pediatric; Cardiopulmonary resuscitation (CPR); Circulation; Echocardiography; Electrocardiography (ECG or EKG); Exercise physiology; Heart; Heart attack; Heart disease; Heart valve replacement; Vascular medicine; Vascular system.

For Further Information:

Corona, Gyl Garren. "Pacemakers: Keeping the Beat Today." *RN* 62, no. 12 (December, 1999): 50-52.

Crawford, Michael, ed. *Current Diagnosis and Treatment: Cardiology*. 3d ed. New York: McGraw-Hill Medical, 2009.

Davis, Goode P., Jr., and Edwards Park. *The Heart: The Living Pump*. Washington, D.C.: U.S. News Books, 1981.

Eagle, Kim A., and Ragavendra R. Baliga, eds. *Practical Cardiology: Evaluation and Treatment of Common Cardiovascular Disorders*. 2d ed. Philadelphia: Lippincott Williams & Wilkins, 2008.

Gersh, Bernard J., ed. *The Mayo Clinic Heart Book*. 2d ed. New York: William Morrow, 2000.

Jeffrey, Kirk. *Machines in Our Hearts: The Cardiac Pacemaker, the Implantable Defibrillator, and American Health Care*. Baltimore: Johns Hopkins University Press, 2001.

"Pacemaker." *Mayo Clinic*, April 17, 2013.

"Pacemaker Insertion." *Health Library*, November 26, 2012.

Sonnenberg, David, Michael Birnbaum, and Emil A. Naclerio. *Understanding Pacemakers*. New York: Michael Kesend, 1982.

Urone, Paul Peter. *Physics with Health Science Applications*. New York: John Wiley & Sons, 1986.

"What Is a Pacemaker?" *National Heart, Lung, and Blood Institute*, February 28, 2012.

Paget's disease

Disease/Disorder

Also known as: Osteitis deformans, Paget's disease of bone

Anatomy or system affected: Bones, head, hips, legs, musculoskeletal system, spine

Specialties and related fields: Genetics, orthopedics, rheumatology, virology

Definition: A chronic disorder resulting in enlarged and deformed bones.

Causes and Symptoms

Paget's disease of bone is a disorder characterized by excessive and abnormal formation of bone, most commonly in the spine, skull, pelvis, thighs, and lower legs. (Paget's disease of the nipple is a different disorder related to breast cancer.) The cause of this disease is under investigation. Genetic factors are a major component. Between 15 and 40 percent of all patients with Paget's disease have a positive family history of the disease, and the risk of developing Paget's disease is seven to ten times higher in relatives of those who have Paget's disease compared with relatives of those who do not have this disease. Several genes are known to regulate the cells that remodel bone, and mutations in some of these genes seem to be the main cause of Paget's disease in some patients.

Information on Paget's Disease

Causes: Unknown; possibly viral infection and genetic factors

Symptoms: Excessive and abnormal formation of bone (commonly in spine, skull, pelvis, thighs, lower legs); increased risk of fractures; curving of spine or legs; bone and joint pain

Duration: Chronic and progressive

Treatments: Bisphosphonates (pamidronate, alendronate, risedronate, tiludronate); pain medications (acetaminophen, NSAIDs); exercise; adequate intake of calcium and vitamin D; surgery

---

In adult, nongrowing bone, the structure of bone is the result of the interplay between two types of cells-one that deposits bone, the osteoblast, and another that resorbs bone, a multinucleate cell called the osteoclast. A signaling system called the RANK-RANKL-OPG system regulates osteoclast recruitment. RANK is a receptor on the surface of osteoclast precursor cells. RANKL is the ligand, or molecule, that binds to RANK to activate it. RANKL is secreted by bone marrow cells; when RANKL binds to the RANK molecules on the surface of osteoclast precursor cells, it activates an internal protein called p62. The activation of p62 pushes osteoclast precursor cells toward becoming mature, bone-resorbing osteoclasts. Osteoblasts, however, also secrete OPG, a soluble receptor that competitively binds RANKL and prevents osteoclast recruitment (see figure on page 2244). Mutations in the genes that encode RANK, OPG, or p62 cause various inherited forms of Paget's disease with varying severities and times when the disease manifests itself. Not all individuals who harbor these mutations, however, suffer from full-blown Paget's disease.

Paget's disease might also result from viral infections. Experimental infection of mouse osteoblasts with measles virus can cause Paget's disease in mice. Furthermore, osteoblasts from human patients with Paget's disease sometimes harbor measles virus or other closely related viruses. It is possible that the presence of mutations in genes that increase osteoclast activity in combination with chronic infection of osteoclasts by measles virus or similar viruses create an environment that nurtures the development of clinical Paget's disease.

Paget's disease is more common in people over the age of forty. The disease usually starts without any symptoms. It is often diagnosed when a person has radiographs taken for other reasons or has a higher-than-normal level of alkaline phosphatase in the blood. As the disease progresses, the patient may develop an enlarging skull, sometimes accompanied by headaches; increased risk of fractures; curving of the spine or legs; and bone and joint pain. Rarely, Paget's disease may lead to kidney stones, loose teeth when bones of the face are involved, and loss of hearing and vision when the enlarging skull compresses nerves to the eye and ear. People with severe Paget's disease may have heart problems such as congestive heart failure or abnormal heart

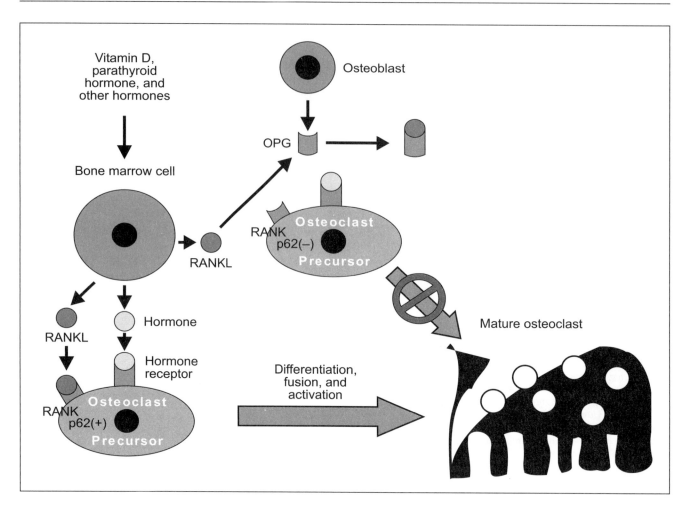

rhythms. Less than 1 percent of people with Paget's disease will develop bone cancer.

Treatment and Therapy

Bisphosphonates (such as etidronate, pamidronate, alendronate, risedronate, or tiludronate) are the main treatment for Paget's disease. Subcutaneous injections of salmon calcitonin successfully reverse the symptoms of Paget's disease, but 50 percent of all patients who receive this treatment develop an immune response against calcitonin and 10 to 20 percent of all patients become resistant to it. In patients with severe symptoms who do not respond to these more typical treatments, the antibiotic mithramycin has been used successfully, but the toxicity of this drug militates against its use for anything but worst-case scenarios.

Treatment is given when patients experience pain, deformities, nerve compression, or other symptoms or to prevent the risk of future complications when the skull, spine, legs, and/or pelvis are involved. Therapy is given until the levels of alkaline phosphatase in the blood return to normal, and it may need to be repeated if that level increases again. Acetaminophen or nonsteroidal anti-inflammatory drugs (NSAIDs) may be used to treat pain. Exercise and adequate intake of calcium and vitamin D are also recommended. Surgery may be needed to stabilize fractures, replace joints affected with severe pain from arthritis, or decompress nerves.

Perspective and Prospects

Paget's disease likely has been around for many centuries, as it has been observed in a grossly thickened Egyptian skull dating from about 1000 BCE. The disorder is named after a British surgeon, Sir James Paget, who was the first to describe this condition in 1876. He noted five patients with thickened bones that were prone to fracture and deformity. Paget thought that the disorder resulted from chronic inflammation and named it osteitis deformans. Subsequently, researchers have shown that Paget's disease of bone arises from the overproduction of poor-quality bone, rather than from chronic inflammation.

Identification of mutations in candidate genes in patients who have active Paget's disease, coupled with the expression of these mutant genes in transgenic mice in which the endogenous copy of the same gene has been eliminated (so-called knockout mice), represents one of the most powerful techniques for studying the cause and pathology of Paget's disease. Combining Paget's disease-specific mutations in transgenic mice whose osteoblasts have been chronically infected with measles virus or respiratory syncytial virus has also greatly elucidated the nongenetic causes of this disease.

—Meika A. Fang, M.D.;
updated by Michael A. Buratovich, Ph.D.

See also Bone disorders; Bones and the skeleton; Fracture and dislocation; Orthopedic surgery; Orthopedics; Orthopedics, pediatric.

For Further Information:
Daroszewska, Anna, and Stuart H. Ralston. "Genetics of Paget's Disease of Bone." *Clinical Science* 109, 3. (September, 2005): 257-263.

DeGroot, Leslie J., J. Larry Jameson, et al. *Endocrinology: Adult and Pediatric.* Philadelphia: Saunders/Elsevier, 2010.

Delmas, Pierre D., and P. J. Meunier. "Drug Therapy: The Management of Paget's Disease of Bone." *New England Journal of Medicine* 336, 8. (February 20, 1997): 558-566.

Kanis, John A. *Pathophysiology and Treatment of Paget's Disease of Bone.* 2d ed. London: Martin Dunitz, 1998.

Klippel, John H., ed. *Primer on the Rheumatic Diseases.* 13th ed. New York: Springer, 2008.

Litin, Scott C., ed. *Mayo Clinic Family Health Book.* 4th ed. New York: HarperResource, 2009.

McDermott, Michael T. *Endocrine Secrets.* Philadelphia: Elsevier, 2013.

"Paget's Disease of Bone." *MedlinePlus*, May 9, 2013.

Ralston, Stuart H. "Paget's Disease of Bone." *New England Journal of Medicine* 368.7. (2013): 644-650.

Roodman, David G., and Jolene J. Windle. "Paget Disease of Bone." *Journal of Clinical Investigation* 115, 2 (February, 2005): 200-208.

Pain

Disease/Disorder

Anatomy or system affected: All

Specialties and related fields: Most, especially anesthesiology, general surgery, genetics, internal medicine, neurology, oncology, physical therapy, psychiatry, rheumatology, sports medicine

Definition: An unpleasant, subjective experience of physical or mental suffering, a symptom of a real or potential underlying cause, condition, or injury.

Key terms:

acute pain: sudden, extreme pain that is short-term; serves as a warning of damage or disease

analgesic: a drug or medication that alleviates pain by blocking pain receptors

chronic pain: a deeper, aching pain that comes on slowly and lasts longer than the normal course for a specific injury or condition; may be constant or intermittent

cutaneous pain: caused by injuries to the skin or superficial tissues; brief and localized

endorphins: brain chemicals released by the body that act as natural painkillers

nociception: the process of transmitting pain messages to the brain through the spinal cord by sensitive nerve endings in skin and tissues

referred pain: pain experienced at a site other than the site of origin

substance P: a peptide found in nerve cells in the body, which serves as a chemical messenger (neurotransmitter) that carries pain messages along pathways to the brain

visceral pain: throbbing or aching pain that originates in the deeper body tissues and organs; of longer duration than cutaneous pain

Causes and Symptoms

Not all causes of pain are known or understood, but some basic causes of the most commonly reported pain include inflammation, as in arthritis, rheumatism, and infection; work-related and sports-related injuries; stress and tension; nerve pain, as from shingles, diabetic neuropathy, and sciatica; and pain related to such diseases as osteoporosis and cancer.

People have similar pain thresholds but different levels of pain tolerance, or how much pain they can bear. One congenital anomaly actually inhibits or eliminates the perception of pain. Pain tolerance is therefore subjective and can be influenced by socioeconomic status, cultural background, and socialization, with disparities noted in who suffers pain, what type of pain a person suffers, and how pain is perceived by the individual.

The most commonly reported types of pain are associated with the lower back, with severe or migraine headache, and with joint pain, particularly in the knees. Physiological pain is a response of the body associated with tissue damage or inflammation, or as a warning system to alert the body to potential physical harm. Although pain may be produced without a defined stimulus, such as with emotional or psychological pain, physiological pain is transmitted through stimulation of nerve pathways, a process called nociception. Nociceptors are free, sensitive nerve endings located outside the spinal column; they are found in skin and on internal surfaces, such as on the joints. Nociceptors, when stimulated, send signals through sensory neurons to the posterior horn of the spinal cord that are then transmitted to other nerve fibers, which travel upward through the brain stem to the thalamus, the gateway to conscious action in the brain. There, information is coordinated and localized and then sent to the cerebral cortex, where a conscious reaction to the stimulus is produced.

Pain is said to be referred when it is experienced at a location other than its site of origin. This occurs when nerve fibers carrying pain messages enter the spinal cord at the same place as other nerve fibers from other parts of the body using the same pathways. The other nerve fibers may become stimulated and result in painful perceptions in healthy areas of the body, such as referred pain from the heart to the neck, arm, and stomach.

Among theories of pain transmission, the gate control theory of Ronald Malzack and Patrick Wall helps to explain the differing degrees of pain that people may suffer. It is related to the amount of substance P, a peptide found in nerve cells throughout the body, that actually reaches the brain. The transmission of neurons is generally very rapid, as when touching a hot stove produces immediate action to protect the body from damage. Messages carried by substance P, however, travel more slowly, since they must pass through a special gateway in the spinal cord. At the same time, pain signals are also prompting the brain to release chemical endorphins, the body's natural painkillers, which must also pass downward through the same gate. Thus, there is some competition for passage, and the fewer receptors for substance P that actually arrive in the brain and at-

---

Information on Pain

Causes: Infection, trauma, disease
Symptoms: Sensation may range from mild to severe
Duration: Acute to chronic
Treatments: Wide ranging; may include drug therapy, surgery, physical therapy, alternative medicine

---

tach to nerve cells there, the lower the pain perception. With healing, the gate closes, but when chronic pain occurs, it remains open even after healing or without an identified underlying cause.

The two basic types of pain are chronic and acute. Acute pain comes on suddenly and, although extreme, is generally brief in duration. Acute pain is a warning to the body about damage or disease, is localized, and is more easily treated. Chronic pain, however, occurs daily and lasts longer than would be common for a specific injury. It no longer serves to warn, and it is much more difficult to treat, although most sufferers can be helped. Chronic pain may last beyond resolution of an underlying cause, or it may grow out of an acute condition. In this case, it may become a learned response that no longer has a purpose but continues to hurt. Chronic pain may also occur without any apparent cause, creating disability, depression, and suffering.

Pain may be medically classified as either superficial or deep. Superficial pain, also called fast or cutaneous pain, is carried by nerve fibers on the skin and outer linings of the organs. These nerve fibers are plentiful in the intestines, cornea, and nose, for example, and pain messages are quickly delivered to the brain, such as when one is cut or burned. Also termed somatic pain, it is experienced as intense, or burning. Kidney stones or acid reflux from the stomach may create waves of this burning pain. Deep pain, on the other hand, also referred to as slow or visceral pain, comes from nerve fibers located in muscles, bones, and tissues of the internal organs, and it travels more slowly, taking longer to reach the brain. It may be experienced as dull aching or throbbing pain. The two types of pain may also occur at the same time.

Treatment and Therapy

The major treatment for pain in the United States has been analgesic medications, or drug therapy, with sufferers spending over an estimated $18 billion a year for relief in the form of both prescription and over-the-counter medications. There are no standard guidelines for the use of analgesics, since the degree of relief varies from one patient to another. These medications are classified as narcotic, such as morphine or opium-based addictive drugs, and nonnarcotic, such as aspirin, ibuprofen, and acetaminophen. Since patients respond differently, and many of the analgesics can carry significant side effects with cardiovascular, renal, and gastrointestinal toxicity, the lowest dose of the preferred medication is usually recommended to start. Painkillers must also often be administered with other medications directed to the underlying cause of the pain and must therefore be compatible.

One subcategory of nonnarcotic analgesics is made up of nonsteroidal anti-inflammatory drugs (NSAIDs). Another alternative, acetaminophen, addresses pain but has no effect on inflammation. Another nonnarcotic class of drugs, known as COX-2 inhibitors, suppress the COX-2 enzyme, which triggers inflammation. Although these drugs are seemingly well tolerated and effective, it was found that many of them endanger the heart, and several were withdrawn from the market.

Narcotic analgesics are the most effective, but long-term use can create dependency, and these drugs are stringently protected in the United States by state and federal laws. Doctors have therefore been hesitant to use them for severe chronic pain, even in patients dying from cancer or other painful diseases, when other medications are not working. This situation appears to be changing.

Nondrug therapies include such techniques as transcutaneous electrical nerve stimulation (TENS), massage therapy, neurosurgery, physical therapy and exercise, and mind-body therapies such as guided imagery, meditation, relaxation, and hypnosis. These therapies attempt to alleviate chronic pain in various ways by stimulating blood circulation, blocking nerve pain messengers, and enlisting the help of the brain, where pain messages are processed.

A combination of biomedical and nonbiomedical therapies also utilizes a number of alternative therapies for pain. Acupuncture and acupressure, the foundation of Chinese medicine, are thought to stimulate blood circulation and possibly the autonomic nervous system through insertion of very fine needles at crucial points in the body. Herbal medicine uses substances that are derived from plants with therapeutic or pharmacologic properties and benefits. Many of today's medicines have ingredients that originated in plants and can be synthesized in the laboratory. Guided imagery, aromatherapy, creative arts therapy, magnet therapy, and therapeutic touch are often used as adjuncts to dealing with pain, but most have not been proven. Like analgesics, these therapies address the control and management of pain rather than offering a cure.

Although many of these complementary therapies are not biomedically sanctioned or recognized, many sufferers of chronic pain try some form of complementary medicine. Little or no research has been done on many of these therapies, but their popularity relates to the fact that chronic pain is closely connected with the brain, affecting emotions, attitudes, and psychological stability, which are not addressed by conventional medicine and treatment. Some of these therapies may work through the placebo effect-meaning that if one expects the therapy to alleviate pain, then it will. Some approaches are backed by positive evidence, while others may have been shown to have no effect. Very little evidence exists about how or why many of these therapies are successful, but combination therapies are vital in alleviating pain, however they may work.

Perspective and Prospects

The development of pain medicine and pain clinics

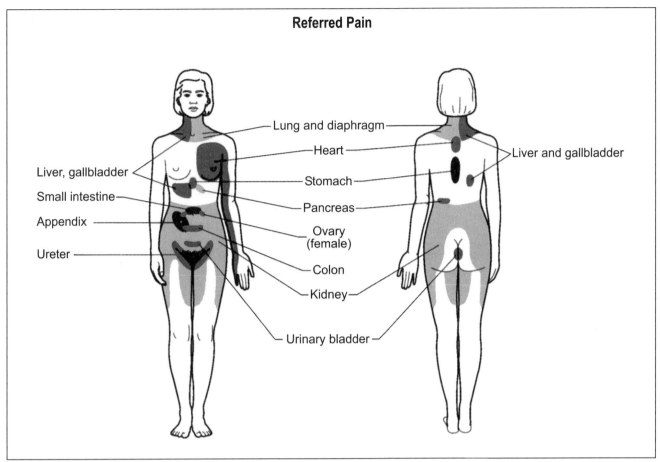

Referred Pain

Liver, gallbladder

Small intestine

Appendix

Ureter

Lung and diaphragm

Heart

Stomach

Pancreas

Ovary (female)

Colon

Kidney

Urinary bladder

Liver and gallbladder

Internal organs do not have the same type of neural sensors found in surface tissues; as a result, damage to internal organs may manifest itself in areas of the body away from the organ's location.

devoted solely to the study and alleviation of pain is a fairly recent occurrence. Since pain was traditionally seen as a symptom rather than as a disease or condition in itself, the medical profession has generally focused on treating the cause, considering pain to be purely a diagnostic tool. The discovery and development of anesthetics for surgical procedures in the latter nineteenth century, however, was a huge advance in medical care and treatment and was a precondition for the later development of pain medicine. Anesthesiologists not only had to address traumatic and postoperative pain but also worked to refine techniques and developed expertise in management relating to other types of pain.

Anesthesiology progressed rapidly during World War II, with improved use of nerve blocking and analgesics. Anesthesiologist John Bonica contributed significantly to this development of pain medicine. He was faced with extreme, intractable, complex, and phantom limb pain (the sensation of pain felt in a limb no longer there) in the injured during wartime and lacked knowledge or methods to treat them. As pain persisted and when physiological causes could not be identified, it became necessary to look elsewhere for the source of the pain. It became obvious that numerous specialists, including psychologists and psychiatrists, needed to consult and discuss their varied findings and opinions.

Practitioners of pain medicine mostly come from other medical fields most closely related to pain, such as neurology, anesthesiology, and rehabilitation. As defined by the American Academy of Pain Medicine, the specialty is concerned with the study, prevention, evaluation, treatment, and rehabilitation of people in pain. Many are certified as pain specialists through the American Board of Anesthesiology. While some pain clinics focus on specific types of pain, such as bone and joint, others address a broader spectrum of suffering and tend to use a variety of methods and treatments, including alternative therapies, to find whatever works. Some pain cannot be eliminated but can be minimized or controlled to allow the patient to function.

The need to study and understand the causes and alleviation of pain have become more urgent. According to the National Center for Health Statistics, one in four adults in the United States reported suffering pain lasting for at least twenty-four hours during the previous month, and one in ten reported pain lasting a year or more. Pain is usually seen as a result of another physical condition, but considering the costs that accompany pain and resulting disability in terms of dollars and loss of individual function reflected in absenteeism in the workplace, pain places an increasing burden on the American health care system. The general cost of pain and pain-related items is estimated to top $100 billion each year.

Research is being conducted into the origins and mechanics of pain in an attempt to identify new and more effective therapies. A study funded by the National Institutes of Health found that the perception of pain (the extent to which one feels pain) is inherited through a gene with a specific variant. This gene variant affects sensitivity to acute pain as well as the risk of developing chronic pain. Other genes may also play a role. This study opens up pathways for developing new treatments and approaches to pain.

Such professional organizations as the American Academy of Pain Medicine, the American Pain Foundation, the American Pain Society, and the International Association for the Study of Pain represent only a few of the growing number of resources for the study of pain and pain management. Alternative approaches are represented through organizations for specific therapies and the National Center for Complementary and Alternative Medicine.

—*Martha Oehmke Loustaunau, Ph.D.*

See also Acupressure; Acupuncture; Alternative medicine; Amputation; Anesthesia; Anesthesiology; Arthritis; Back pain; Bruises; Burns and scalds; Cancer; Fibromyalgia; Headaches; Healing; Hypnosis; Local anesthesia; Massage; Meditation; Narcotics; Nervous system; Neuralgia, neuritis, and neuropathy; Neurology; Over-the-counter medications; Pain management; Physical rehabilitation; Prescription drug abuse; Self-medication; Skin; Stress; Stress reduction; Substance abuse; Toothache; Touch; Wounds.

For Further Information:

Baszanger, Isabelle. *Inventing Pain Medicine: From the Laboratory to the Clinic*. New Brunswick, N.J.: Rutgers University Press, 1998.

Bellenir, Karen, ed. *Pain Sourcebook: Basic Consumer Health Information About Specific Forms of Acute and Chronic Pain*. 2d ed. Detroit, Mich.: Omnigraphics, 2002.

Coakley, Sarah, and Kay Kaufman Shelemay, eds. *Pain and Its Transformations: The Interface of Biology and Culture*. Cambridge, Mass.: Harvard University Press, 2008..

Fishman, Scott M. *Bonica's Management of Pain*. 4th ed. Philadelphia: Lippincott Williams & Wilkins, 2012.

Vertosick, Frank T., Jr. *Why We Hurt: The Natural History of Pain*. New York: Harcourt, 2000.

Waldman, Steven D. *Atlas of Uncommon Pain Syndromes*. Philadelphia: Elsevier, 2014.

Wall, Patrick David. *Pain: The Science of Suffering*. New York: Columbia University Press, 2013.

Pain management

Treatment

Anatomy or system affected: All

Specialties and related fields: Alternative medicine, anesthesiology, critical care, emergency medicine, geriatrics and gerontology, oncology, pharmacology, physical therapy, psychiatry, psychology

Definition: Any treatment or management technique to lessen or eliminate pain or make it more tolerable.

Indications and Procedures

Pain is experienced as an unpleasant reaction to either an external stimulus (such as a burn) or an internal process (such as a disease). The initial evaluation of pain is aimed at determining the cause. A good description by the patient aids diagnosis. The person experiencing the pain must be able to communicate the intensity, location, pattern (such as throbbing, steady, intermittent) and type (crushing, burning, sharp, or dull). In addition, factors that make the pain better or worse must be known and communicated. Duration is important; recent onset is termed "acute" pain while long-standing pain or pain that returns periodically is termed "chronic."

Generally, the best way to treat pain is to prevent its occurrence. Failing that, a number of different interventions should be used together. Whatever treatment is used, the therapy must be tailored both to the patient and to the nature and severity of the pain. When medications are used, review of some important principles is essential, such as the pharmacology, duration of effectiveness, and optimal dose of a certain medication. Even the route of administration must be considered in every case.

Treatment may include combinations of simple analgesics, narcotics, and other treatments. Combinations take advantage of the additive pain relief while sparing the patient potential side effects. When choosing pain medications, a stepwise approach is often used. It starts with the simple analgesics: aspirin, acetaminophen, and nonsteroidal anti-inflammatory drugs (NSAIDs). These medications are generally well tolerated, although aspirin and NSAIDs can produce gastrointestinal distress ranging from mild heartburn to bleeding ulcers. Additionally, adjuncts to these types of medications might be icing or heat, depending on the nature of the problem.

For more severe pain, the second step often includes a narcotic analgesic with or without the simple analgesics. Narcotics are very potent and have a potential for addiction. Furthermore, they may produce problems such as confusion, nausea and vomiting, constipation, and drowsiness. If the pain has a significant inflammation component that does not resolve easily with milder analgesic approaches or with narcotics, then corticosteroids may be used to alleviate the pain. This approach does not lend itself well to longer-term pain management, however, because of side effects such as fluid retention, stomach irritation, thrush, muscle weakness, weight gain, bone loss, suppressed adrenal function, and increased risk of infections, among others.

The third step in pain control involves alternative methods of pain control. Treatments here include physical therapy, nerve-blocking injections, transcutaneous electrical nerve stimulation (TENS), and behavioral approaches. The latter method seeks to identify the causes of preventable pain (physical or mental) and takes steps to minimize pain.

Medical research is leading to interesting discoveries about the management of pain. In 2002, researchers announced that they had identified a key protein that controls severe pain, a discovery that could lead to better pain management for patients who suffer from chronic pain or pain associated with terminal cancer. The protein, known by the acronym DREAM, protects the neural reflex critical to survival, allowing individuals to feel pain and quickly pull away from its source, but over time, DREAM seems to help sharp pain fade as the protein becomes disabled. Moreover, while there are many types of pain, disabling the DREAM

In the News:
FDA Panel Recommends Percocet, Vicodin Ban

In June, 2009, a Food and Drug Administration (FDA) advisory committee convened to discuss the use of acetaminophen (Tylenol) in combination drugs, the risk of acetaminophen-associated liver damage, and possible interventions to reduce the incidence of liver injury. The issue with the combination drugs Percocet (oxycodone/acetaminophen) and Vicodin (hydrocodone/acetaminophen) is their potential for severe liver damage as a result of an overdose of acetaminophen. Acetaminophen is a key drug in the treatment of pain and fever. When it is used according to directions, the risk of developing liver injury is very low. However, many people are unaware that acetaminophen overdose can cause serious liver damage. Between 1998 and 2003, acetaminophen-related liver damage was the leading cause of acute liver failure in the United States, with 48 percent of cases associated with accidental overdose. It is noteworthy that there is only a small difference between the maximum recommended daily dose and a potentially damaging dose of acetaminophen, and some people may be more susceptible to liver damage than others, such as those who use alcohol. Additionally, a multitude of over-the-counter and prescription acetaminophen products are available with a range of doses indicated for a variety of different conditions, and it may not be obvious that acetaminophen is an ingredient in some prescription drugs—for example, the label on pharmacy-dispensed containers are often identified as containing APAP.

The FDA panel voted twenty to seventeen in favor of banning Percocet and Vicodin, as well as seven other drugs that combine a narcotic with acetaminophen. Though the FDA is not required to follow the recommendations of its advisory committees, it frequently does. However, if prescription acetaminophen combination products continue to be marketed, the panel recommends implementing additional safety measures by requiring "unit-of-use" packaging and/or requiring an additional boxed warning for prescription acetaminophen combination products. "Unit-of-use" would require packaging by the manufacturer for sale in a pharmacy, with no need for repackaging at the pharmacy. Standardized information would be displayed on the prescription package (for example, prominent display of "ACETAMINOPHEN" as an active ingredient and a warning about potential liver damage). Regardless of a ban on these combination drugs, acetaminophen would continue to be available as an over-the-counter medication and opioids would be available as single-ingredient painkillers.

—*Anita P. Kuan, Ph.D.*

protein appears to reduce the severity of all of them. The next step in research will be to examine ways to disable the protein, a task that scientists deem difficult because of its location deep within individual cells. Additional research in this area recognizes that pain has different causes and that it may be more productive to examine mechanisms of pain rather than taking a disease-based approach.

—*Charles C. Marsh, Pharm.D.;*
updated by Nancy A. Piotrowski, Ph.D.

See also Acupressure; Acupuncture; Alternative medicine; Anesthesia; Anesthesiology; Biofeedback; Chiropractic; Hypnosis; Local anesthesia; Marijuana; Meditation; Narcotics; Over-the-counter medications; Pain; Palliative medicine; Pharmacology; Prescription

drug abuse; Self-medication; Substance abuse.

For Further Information:
Cousins, Michael J., and P. O. Bridenbaugh, eds. *Cousins and Bridenbaugh's Neural Blockade in Clinical Anesthesia and Management of Pain*. 4th ed. Philadelphia: Lippincott Williams & Wilkins, 2009.
Dillard, James M. *The Chronic Pain Solution: The Comprehensive, Step-by-Step Guide to Choosing the Best of Alternative and Conventional Medicine*. New York: Bantam Books, 2002.
Ferrari, Lynne R., ed. *Anesthesia and Pain Management for the Pediatrician*. Baltimore: Johns Hopkins University Press, 1999.
Ferrer-Brechner, Theresa. *Common Problems in Pain Management*. Chicago: Year Book Medical, 1990.
"DREAM Repression & Dynorphin Expression." *qiagen.com*, 2013.
Fishman, Scott, with Lisa Berger. *The War on Pain: How Breakthroughs in the New Field of Pain Medicine Are Turning the Tide Against Suffering*. New York: HarperCollins, 2001.
Loeser, John D., ed. *Bonica's Management of Pain*. 4th ed. Philadelphia: Lippincott Williams & Wilkins, 2010.
"Pain Management Facts." *lls.org*, May 2013.
"Pain Management." *nih.gov*, March 29, 2013.
"Pain Management Programs." *theacpa.org*, 2009.
Raj, Prithvi, and Lee Ann Paradise, eds. *Pain Medicine: A Comprehensive Review*. 2d ed. St. Louis, Mo.: Mosby, 2003.
Rosenfeld, Arthur. *The Truth About Chronic Pain: Patients and Professionals on How to Face It, Understand It, Overcome It*. Rev. ed. New York: Basic Books, 2005.

Palliative care

Specialty
Anatomy or system affected: All
Specialties and related fields: Most, especially critical care, internal medicine, geriatrics, oncology, pain medicine, cardiology, pulmonary, hematology, nephrology, psychology, radiology, nursing and ethics
Definition: Palliative care is a medical specialty which aims to maximize quality of life in people with life-threatening illnesses. Palliative care focuses on symptom control, pain management, and psychosocial support for patients and their families.

Key terms:
multidisciplinary care: A comprehensive care provided by professionals from different disciplines, including doctors, nurses, pharmacists, social workers, and many others.
pain management: A treatment to control pain and reduce suffering using pharmacological and/or non-pharmacological methods. The goal is to improve quality of life.
hospice: End-of-life medical care for people who are terminally ill. Similar to palliative care, the focuses are also symptom control, pain management and psychosocial support.

Overview

Palliative care is a multidisciplinary medical care approach for people with serious or life-threatening illnesses. These patients often suffer from severe pain, shortness of breath, fatigue, difficulty sleeping, or other distressing physical symptoms. They and their families may also experience stress or even depression while trying to cope with the patients' illnesses. The goal of palliative care is to maximize quality of life through pain management, symptom control

Palliative Care versus Hospice			
		Palliative Care	**Hospice**
Similarities		• Improve quality of life for people with severe illness—pain management, symptom control, psychosocial support • Patient and family-centered care • Team approach	
Differences	Timing	• During any stage of illness, doesn't need to be terminal	• Terminal stage of illness or with limited life expectancy (generally < 6 months, varies by different hospice programs)
	Location	• Hospital • Extended care facility • Nursing home • Home	• Home • Extended care facility • Nursing home
	Curative or life-prolonging treatment	• Continue	• Usually stopped
	Insurance coverage	• Medicare • Medicaid • Most private insurance	• Medicare • Medicaid • Most private insurance

as well as psychosocial support. Receiving palliative care does not mean that the patient has to stop the primary curative treatment. Instead, palliative care is like another layer of support on top of the original medical treatment plan. Palliative program not only cares for the patient, but also his or her family. It designs individualized plan of care taking into consideration the patient and the family's needs, values, beliefs, and goals.

Palliative care should not be confused with hospice, which focuses on end-of-life care and comfort. Patients in hospice programs usually have stopped the curative treatments; instead, emphasis is on pain and symptom relief and how to make the most out of the last days or months of life.

Individuals who may consider palliative care includes anyone who has severe illnesses and suffers from uncontrolled pain or other distressing physical or psychological symptoms. Examples of some devastating diseases include cancer, heart disease, lung disease, kidney failure, Human immunodeficiency virus infection / acquired immunodeficiency syndrome (HIV/AIDS). Lupus, Alzheimer's, and many others. People do not need to wait until the terminal stage of his or her illness to receive palliative care. It can be started during any stage of the illness to enhance quality of life. Applying for palliative care is not difficult. Patients and families with potential needs should talk to their doctors and ask for a referral for palliative care. Palliative care often starts in the hospital, but can be provided in various nursing facilities, outpatient clinics, hospices, or even at patients' home.

Treatment and Therapy

Palliative care is all about making the life more comfortable and meaningful for the patient and his or her loved ones. It is accomplished using a team approach. A palliative care team consists of professionals from different disciplines, including doctors, nurses, pharmacists, social workers, chaplains, nutritionists, counselors, and others. The team closely works with the patient and the family to assess their needs, values, beliefs, and goals. Patient education and counseling are also provided to help the patient better understand his or her health condition and how to more effectively cope with it. The palliative care team also works collaboratively with patient's primary health care providers to design a comprehensive and individualized treatment plan to maximize physical and emotional comfort.

The length of palliative care depends on the individual's health condition and family goals and needs. The financial aspect of the care is almost always a concern for patients and their families. The good news is that Medicare, Medicaid, and most private insurance covers all or part of palliative treatment. In instances when palliative care is not fully covered by Medicare, Medicaid, or private insurance, there may be funds available within the community or through the state to subsidize the cost.

—*Zhongqi Weng*

See also Hospice, death and dying, end of life, euthanasia, oncology, pain , psychiatry, terminally ill, ethics

For Further Information:

Mayo Clinic. (2013). *Palliative Care: Symptom Relief During Illness.* Retrieved October 12, 2013, from http://www.mayoclinic.com/health/palliative-care/ MY01051.

National Caregivers Library. (2013). *Hospice vs. Palliative Care.* Retrieved October 13, 2013, from http://www.caregiverslibrary.org/caregivers-resources/grp-end-of-life-issues/hsgrp-hospice/hospice-vs-palliative-care-article.aspx.

National Hospice and Palliative Care Organization. (2013). *Palliative Care.* Retrieved October 12, 2013, from http://www.nhpco.org/palliative-care-0.

National Institute of Health, National Institute of Nursing Research. (2009). *Palliative Care.* Retrieved October 12, 2013, from https://www.ninr.nih.gov/newsandinformation/ publications/palliative-care-brochure.

Palliative medicine

Specialty
Anatomy or system affected: All
Specialties and related fields: Anesthesiology, emergency medicine, family medicine, internal medicine, obstetrics and gynecology, pediatrics, physical medicine and rehabilitation, psychiatry and neurology, radiology and surgery
Definition: The World Health Organization (WHO) defines palliative care as: An approach that improves the quality of life of patients and their families facing the problem associated with life-threatening illness, through the prevention and relief of suffering by means of early identification and impeccable assessment and treatment of pain and other problems, physical, psychosocial, and spiritual.
Key terms:
multidisciplinary: involving several medical specialties, requiring health care practitioners from various perspectives to work closely together to meet the needs of the patient
opioid medications: pain medications derived from opiates, such as morphine, oxycodone, codeine, and fentanyl; intended to control severe pain

Science and Profession

While in the United States, The National Hospice and Palliative Care Organization (NHPCO) defines palliative care as: Treatment that enhances comfort and improves the quality of an individual's life during the last phase of life. No specific therapy is excluded from consideration. The test of palliative care lies in the agreement between the individual, physician(s), primary caregiver, and the hospice team that the expected outcome is relief from distressing symptoms, the easing of pain, and/or enhancing the quality of life. The decision to intervene with active palliative care is based on an ability to meet stated goals rather than affect the underlying disease. An individual's needs must continue to be assessed and all treatment options explored and evaluated in the context of the individual's values and symptoms. The individual's choices and decisions regarding care are paramount and must be followed.

Palliative medicine is a specialty that spans disciplines. The goal is to comfort and support patients as they face life-threatening illnesses, not only relieving their suffering but also addressing their emotional and spiritual needs. Although palliative medicine is typically associated with the final stages of life-threatening conditions, patients may also benefit from specialized care while they are still undergoing active treatment. In that case, symptom relief and other interventions to improve their quality of life help improve their strength and stamina to endure additional cycles of therapy.

Palliative care may be provided in a long-term care facility, a hospital, or the patient's home. Care is provided by a team consisting of primary care physicians, specialists in the patient's condition (for example, oncologists, cardiologists, or pulmonologists), palliative medicine specialist, nurses, social workers, mental health specialists (psychologists, psychiatrists, or counselors), nutritionists, and clergy. The level and type of care provided are guided by the wishes and needs of the patient. Pain management is often the greatest need, but the patient may also require relief of other symptoms associated with the condition or its treatment, such as nausea, vomiting, decreased appetite, inability to eat, dehydration, constipation or diarrhea, shortness of breath, malaise, fatigue, anxiety, depression, and altered consciousness.

Palliative medicine is recognized as a basic human right in the International Bill of Human Rights of the United Nations. The document declares that all people have the right to adequate health and medical care, and further states that patients with chronic and terminal illnesses have the right to avoid pain and die with dignity. Following these principles, Canada decreed that every citizen has the right to palliative care. The European Committee of Ministers and the South African Department of Health declared that palliative care is a right of all citizens. Palliative medicine is formally recognized as a specialty in Australia, France, Germany, Hong Kong, Ireland, New Zealand, Poland, Romania, Slovakia, Taiwan, the United States, and the United Kingdom.

Palliative medicine is an essential component of care for patients suffering from any chronic, life-threatening illness, but the specialty has taken on an added significance in the field of oncology. In the United States, the Institute of Medicine stated in 1997 that any comprehensive cancer care plan should include palliative care. A 2005 resolution of the 58th World Health Assembly to improve cancer care placed palliative medicine on equal footing with surgery, radiation, and medical oncology.

Although recognized as a medical specialty, palliative medicine relies on the unique contributions of numerous disciplines. Education in palliative techniques begins at the undergraduate level and is incorporated into the training of a number of medical specialties, such as oncology and gerontology. Continuing education programs focus on educating health care professionals in quality palliative care techniques. Other projects build on these efforts, using other health care professionals, such as nurse practitioners and physician assistants, to develop quality palliative medicine programs in their institutions.

The American Society for Clinical Oncology (ASCO) actively promotes continuing education in palliative medicine. Palliative care is incorporated into educational materials and programs developed by ASCO. The society published an educational curriculum for continuing medical education on palliative medicine, and it has a study program devoted to supportive care. Palliative medicine is included in the training for internists, as adopted by the American Board of Internal Medicine.

The National Consensus Project for Quality Palliative Care issued guidelines for palliative care to establish continuity of care across institutions. The clinical practice guidelines have been incorporated into the hospital accreditation standards of The Joint Commission (formerly the Joint Commission for the Accreditation of Hospitals). Institutions are assessed on the eight domains of palliative care: structure and process, physical aspects, psychological and psychiatric aspects, spiritual and religious aspects, cultural aspects, care of the imminently dying patient, the ethical aspects of care, and the legal aspects of care. Additionally, the Center for the Advancement of Palliative Care developed the State-by-State Report Card on Access to Palliative Care in Our Nation's Hospitals. The report card measures patient access to palliative care and to palliative medicine specialists, access of medical students to training in palliative care, and access of physicians to specialty training in palliative care. The report card emphasizes the importance of a multidisciplinary approach to palliative medicine.

Diagnostic and Treatment Techniques

Patient care is traditionally disease-oriented. Specialists in particular tend to focus narrowly on a specific organ or body system. Palliative care, however, takes a holistic, patient-centered approach. The emphasis is on communicating with the patient and family to assess the patient's specific needs and desires.

Palliative care can be divided into primary and secondary teams. The primary team, as defined by Medicare, is comprised by four core members (physician, nurse, social worker and spiritual counselor) and is responsible for assessing and managing symptoms, providing expertise regarding psychosocial services as well as communicating with the patient and family while involving the shared decision making model of care If, however, the patient's condition worsens and the primary team can no longer manage the symptoms, a palliative medicine specialist in the patient's condition is called. The palliative medicine specialist may be consulted on specific issues as needed or become a core member until the patient's death.

The whole-patient assessment begins with the patient's description of symptoms and level of function. Diagnostic tests may be used to evaluate symptom severity, but diagnosis is not the purpose. The emphasis is always on symptom relief.

Pain is a significant issue that must be managed properly. Inadequately controlled pain may reduce the effectiveness of treatment and wear the patient down psychologically. Proper pain management involves communication with and education of the patient and family members as well as continuous assessment of the effectiveness of pain medications. The World Health Organization (WHO) has developed an approach to pain for cancer patients, beginning with nonsteroidal anti-inflammatory drugs (NSAIDs), such as ibuprofen, and progressing through acetaminophen combined with an opioid medication, such as acetaminophen with codeine, and lastly to opioid medications such as morphine or oxycodone. The goal is to relieve pain while keeping the patient alert and in control.

The effect of the condition on the emotions and cognitive functioning of the patient is an important aspect of the palliative medicine assessment. Patients are facing serious issues while they battle their illnesses. They must cope with imminent death and the grief of their loved ones along with the fear of loss of control and dignity. Patients must be evaluated for depression and anxiety. Practical needs, such as relationship issues, legal affairs, and financial management, also need attention. The patient's spiritual needs should also be addressed. Spiritual counseling can be traditional religious advisement from a clergyperson or an informal discussion of personal beliefs, according to the desires of the patient.

Depression and anxiety are common among patients coping with life-threatening conditions. Feelings of sadness and depression are to be expected and should be managed appropriately even when they are not expected to be permanent. The members of the primary team who are in closest contact with the patient need to be alert for symptoms of depression that surpass the normal grieving process. Signs of major depression include persistent feelings of worthlessness, hopelessness, helplessness, and loss of self-esteem. Physical symptoms may include weight loss or changes in sleep habits, although these symptoms may also be attributed to the patient's underlying condition. Thoughts of suicide or requests by the patient to hasten death are not part of the coping process and are a sign of major depression. If the signs of depression fail to resolve after a few weeks, then the mental health specialists on the team are consulted and the depression should be treated.

Similarly, anxiety is an understandable and natural emotion as patients juggle financial concerns, family issues, medical concerns, and preparations for their own death. Anxiety may be managed through counseling or, if it is severe, with antianxiety medications.

The role of the palliative care team is not limited to the patient. The team assists family members in accepting the patient's condition, managing financial and insurance matters, and coping with grief. The health care team can advise family members on what to expect as the patient's condition deteriorates. Breathing difficulties, delirium or dementia, wasting, and incontinence can be upsetting for family members to experience if they are not properly prepared. After the patient's death, the palliative care team assists family members through the grieving process. The team follows up with the family through phone calls and home visits, providing grief counseling or referral to caregiver support groups or other mental health professionals when needed. Bereavement services often last for several months to a year after the patient's death.

Perspective and Prospects

In the span of two decades, palliative medicine progressed from haphazard training through chance experiences to a recognized specialty. A 1998 member survey by ASCO revealed 90 percent of the oncologists who responded had no formal training in palliative medicine. Rather, they indicated they learned through "trial and error." Alarmingly, more than one-third claimed that their education in palliative medicine was from a "traumatic experience" with a patient. Most had little training in how to discuss a poor prognosis with patients and their families, and only 10 percent had completed clinical training in palliative care.

Since that survey, ASCO and other professional societies have incorporated palliative medicine into their continuing education curricula. More important, national and international groups have formally recognized the importance of palliative medicine in preserving the dignity and well-being of patients nearing the end of their lives. In recent years, palliative medicine has been incorporated as a routine part of comprehensive cancer care plans in the United States.

Despite these advances, much work remains. The need for palliative medicine is increasing. The population is growing older while the prevalence of cancer is rising. Cancer treatments are becoming more effective. Although cancer death rates are declining, more people are living longer with the disease, resulting in growing numbers of people who will benefit from palliative medicine.

To meet the growing need, health care practitioners must be educated in palliative medicine. Fellowships in palliative medicine (currently 93 in the United States), continuing education, and readily available educational resources are needed now more than ever. Formal certifications and national guidelines and standards of practice have been adopted to ensure consistency in the quality of palliative medicine across states and individual institutions. The concept of palliative medicine continues to be incorporated into care plans across medical disciplines. In 2006 the American Board of Medical Specialties approved the creation of Hospice and Palliative Medicine as a subspecialty to 10 medical disciplines, and after 2013, only those who have completed an accredited fellowship program will be able to be certified and practice this discipline.

Improving end-of-life care requires more than educational and quality control initiatives; it also requires political will. Unless palliative medicine is viewed as a priority by administrators and policy makers, quality care cannot be ensured.

Pain management is an integral piece of palliative medicine. Unfortunately, misconceptions remain among health care practitioners as well as the general public regarding the use of opioid medications. The fear of addiction frequently results in less than optimal pain control and patient suffering. The need for higher doses of pain medications does not indicate addiction; it is more likely a sign the pain is inadequately controlled or the condition is progressing. The United Nations elevated effective pain control to a fundamental human right. In a formal statement, the UN equated inadequate pain control with "cruel, inhuman, and degrading treatment" and called for nations to supply adequate pain medications to patients.

Collectively, the United Nations, individual countries, and medical societies are striving to ensure that all patients suffering from terminal illnesses receive compassionate and comprehensive care. The strength of palliative medicine is in considering the patient as a whole rather than focusing exclusively on a particular diagnosis. Palliative medicine breaks from traditional medical practice and creates a multidisciplinary team to care for the patient. The direction of care is dictated by the wishes of the patient and encompasses physical, emotional, and the spiritual needs of the patient and their families.

—Cheryl Pokalo Jones;
updated by Felix Rivera, M.D.

See also Aging; Cancer; Death and dying; Depression; Ethics; Euthanasia; Grief and guilt; Hospice; Narcotics; Pain; Pain management; Phobias; Psychiatry; Psychiatry, child and adolescent; Psychiatry, geriatric; Stress; Suicide; Terminally ill: Extended care

For Further Information:

Chochinov, Harvey M., and William Breitbart. *Handbook of Psychiatry in Palliative Medicine.* New York: Oxford University Press, 2000. Discussion of the role of psychiatry in palliative medicine.

Doyle, Derek, et al., eds. *Oxford Textbook of Palliative Medicine.* New York: Oxford University Press, 2005. Comprehensive text on palliative medicine, including the role of different medical specialties in patient care.

Field, Marilyn J., and Cathleen K. Cassel, eds. *Approaching Death: Improving Care at the End of Life.* Washington, DC: National Academies Press, 1997. The documents from the Institute of Medicine establishing the role of palliative medicine in comprehensive cancer care.

National Hospice and Palliative Care Organization website: http://www.nhpco.org.

Woodruff, Roger. *Palliative Medicine: Evidence-Based Symptomatic and Supportive Care for Patients with Advanced Cancer.* 4th ed. New York: Oxford University Press, 2004. Review of recent research in the principles of palliative medicine and related ethical issues.

World Health Organization website on palliative care: http://www.who.int/cancer/palliative/en

Palpitations

Disease/Disorder
Also known as: Skipping beats, irregular heartbeat
Anatomy or system affected: Chest, circulatory system, heart, muscles
Specialties and related fields: Cardiology
Definition: A perceived irregularity of the normal heartbeat.

Causes and Symptoms

Individuals experiencing palpitations often describe a slight discomfort and uneasiness accompanied by a flutter or sudden change in heart rate. Palpitations are often a symptom of an abnormal heart rhythm known as an arrhythmia. Arrhythmias involve a change in the electrical activity of the heart resulting in a chaotic or irregular contraction of the heart muscle. The location of these arrhythmias within the heart muscle determines the type, duration, and intensity of the palpitations.

Palpitations are common among many people, regardless of age or gender. They are often diagnosed by cardiologists using several techniques aimed at measuring the electrical activity of the heart. Such tests include electrocardiograms (ECGs), Holter monitoring, and stress tests. Most palpitations do not indicate the presence of a serious cardiac problem. Instead, they are often the result of one cause or a combination of several causes. Several underlying causes of heart palpitations include a high caffeine intake, alcohol and tobacco use, fatigue, extreme physical exertion, stress and anxiety, and a poor diet.

Palpitations have not been shown to cause any damage to

Information on Palpitations

Causes: Abnormal heart rhythm, high caffeine intake, alcohol or tobacco use, fatigue, extreme physical exertion, stress and anxiety, poor diet

Symptoms: Flutter or sudden change in heart rate, slight discomfort and uneasiness; in severe cases, decreased blood flow leading to dizziness, loss of consciousness, chest pain, shortness of breath

Duration: Brief, sometimes recurrent

Treatments: Removal of underlying cause; in severe cases, medications (beta-blockers, calcium-channel blockers), surgery (implantable defibrillator)

the heart muscle. Extended palpitations, however, may lead to decreased blood flow to areas of the brain, heart, or other parts of the body. This decreased blood flow can create oxygen deficits in these areas, leading to dizziness, loss of consciousness, chest pain, or shortness of breath. Palpitations accompanied by such symptoms may be a sign of other structural problems of the heart muscle or surrounding blood vessels and may be diagnosed with the use of an echocardiogram (an ultrasound technique) or invasive catheterization.

Treatment and Therapy

Most palpitations are treated by removing the underlying causes. Decreasing intake of caffeine, alcohol, and tobacco products often succeeds in lowering the frequency and severity of palpitations. Reducing levels of physical and emotional stress while maintaining proper diet and sleep patterns has also been successful in treating palpitations. Medications such as beta-blockers or calcium-channel blockers or other methods such as surgery or implantable defibrillators may be used to treat palpitations in more severe cases.

Perspective and Prospects

Advances in medical technology have shown heart palpitations to be much more common than once thought. Today, heartbeat irregularities perceived as palpitations are rarely considered to be a sign of serious disease and are often easily treated or prevented.

—*Paul J. Frisch*

See also Addiction; Alcoholism; Anxiety; Arrhythmias; Caffeine; Cardiology; Cardiology, pediatric; Echocardiography; Electrocardiography (ECG or EKG); Exercise physiology; Heart; Nicotine; Panic attacks; Smoking; Stress; Stress reduction.

For Further Information:

American Medical Association. *American Medical Association Family Medical Guide.* 4th rev. ed. Hoboken, N.J.: John Wiley & Sons, 2004.
Berne, Robert M., and Matthew N. Levy. *Cardiovascular Physiology.* 8th ed. St. Louis, Mo.: Mosby, 2001.
Everett, Russell J., Mary N. Sheppard, and David C. Lefroy. "Chest Pain and Palpitations Taking a Closer Look." *Circulation* 128, no. 3 (September, 2013): 271-277. Print.
Icon Health. *Heart Palpitations: A Medical Dictionary, Bibliography, and Annotated Research Guide to Internet References.* San Diego, Calif.: Author, 2004.
Jonsb, Egil, et al. "Illness Perception Among Patients with Chest Pain and Palpitations Before and After Negative Cardiac Evaluation." *BioPsychoSocial Medicine* 6, no. 1 (2012): 19-26.
Larson, Lyle W. "Grad Students with Palpitations." *Clinicial Reviews* 23, no. 7 (July, 2013): 18-48.
Litin, Scott C., ed. *Mayo Clinic Family Health Book.* 4th ed. New York: HarperResource, 2009.
Zaret, Barry L., Marvin Moser, and Lawrence S. Cohen, eds. *Yale University School of Medicine Heart Book.* New York: William Morrow, 1992.

Palsy

Disease/Disorder

Anatomy or system affected: Muscles, musculoskeletal system, nerves, nervous system

Specialties and related fields: Neurology, physical therapy

Definition: A paralysis or partial paralysis that is usually accompanied or followed by muscle weakness and muscle wasting over the affected area; in some cases, there may be residual electrical activity present, but the amount is usually small and the activity cannot be controlled.

Key terms:

Bell's palsy: paralysis of the seventh cranial nerve (facial nerve)

cerebral palsy: a palsy arising prenatally, at birth, or early in life within the central nervous system, affecting large portions of the cerebral hemispheres, with extensive paralysis of many major muscles

hemiplegia: paralysis involving an arm and a leg on the same side of the body

palsy: a paralysis or partial paralysis involving loss of motor control, usually accompanied or followed by muscle weakness and muscle wasting over the affected area

Parkinson's disease: also called shaking palsy; a degenerative paralysis resulting from destruction of certain cells in the substantia nigra, a structure near the base of the cerebral hemispheres

quadriplegia: paralysis involving all four extremities more or less equally

spastic: characterized by uncontrollable spasms

substantia nigra: a clump of cells located near the base of the cerebral hemispheres that secrete the neurotransmitter dopamine

Causes and Symptoms

In general, the term "palsy" describes any type of dysfunction of the motor nerves that impairs or reduces the conscious control of muscles. The paralysis or loss of motor control is usually accompanied or followed by weakness and wasting of the muscles in the affected area.

The most common type of palsy is Bell's palsy, a paralysis of the seventh cranial nerve, or facial nerve, often accompanied by pain over part or all of the affected area. The number of muscles involved varies. The paralysis usually occurs on one side of the face at a time, with the result that the undamaged muscles of the opposite side pull the facial skin to that side. Typically, the eye on the affected side remains open all the time because the muscles that close it have been affected; attempts by the patient to close the eye merely result in the eyeball rotating upward. The rest of the face on the affected side generally droops but remains flat; the brow fails to wrinkle, and the cheeks never thicken. Smiles and other facial expressions are asymmetrically contorted.

Thorough neurological testing is needed to assess how much damage has been done and which branches of the facial nerve have been affected. If the damage affects either hearing or taste, this finding indicates that the damage is closer to the root of the facial nerve, and the patient's chances for recovery are correspondingly much lower. If only a few muscles are involved, it indicates that the damage is farther from the root of the nerve, which usually forecasts a better chance of recovery. In most cases, Bell's palsy is thought to arise from a reduced blood supply to the affected nerves. Viral infection by herpes simplex or herpes zoster (shingles) is also a frequent cause; the viral infections are believed to cause demyelination (deterioration of the myelin sheath that insulates nerves) of the affected parts of the facial nerve. Other causes include injuries to the area just below or in front of the external ear resulting from blows to the head, surgery in this region, or other types of trauma.

Another common type of palsy is cerebral palsy, an impairment of movement and posture caused in most cases by injury, malformation, or other damage to the immature brain. Cerebral palsy is actually a group of paralytic disorders that begin during intrauterine development, at birth, or in early infancy. The extent of the paralysis may vary, often involving large groups of muscles while sparing others. Those muscles that are not totally paralyzed are often uncoordinated in their movements or poorly controlled; this is especially true of large muscle movements such as those of the limbs. In many cases, the patient exhibits a "scissors gait" in which the lower limbs are crossed and the one behind must be swung sideways before it is placed in front of the other limb. In addition to the lack of muscular control of the limbs, other symptoms variously include spasms, athetoid (slow, rhythmic, and wormlike) movements, or muscular rigidity. Speech is in many cases difficult or unclear if the muscles used in speaking are affected.

Mental deterioration may occur in some cases but not in others: Some patients with cerebral palsy are intellectually disabled, while others have managed to display brilliant artistic or literary talents with the use of whatever muscles still function in their bodies. Some cerebral palsy patients also suffer from seizure disorders such as epilepsy. Almost all cases of cerebral palsy are accompanied by some other type of neurological impairment, the nature of which varies greatly. In general, cerebral palsy is a nonprogressive type of disease; that is, it does not continually worsen. Afflicted individuals generally experience a normal life span, though with impaired motor functions.

The most common types of cerebral palsy are those that occur in infancy or earlier. Of this group, injuries received at birth (during forceps delivery, for example) form one of the largest and most well defined groups. Cerebral hemor-

Information on Palsy

Causes: May include genetic and environmental factors, birth defects, trauma during childbirth, reduced blood flow to affected nerves, viral infection, injury in front of ear (trauma, surgery)

Symptoms: May include paralysis (partial or complete); muscle weakness, wasting, or rigidity; awkward gait; impaired facial movement; impaired speech; mental impairment; seizure disorders

Duration: Acute to chronic

Treatments: Drug therapy (vasodilators drugs such as cortisone, antiviral drugs such as acyclovir); surgery; application of warmth and avoidance of cold drafts

rhage, a cause of many cerebral palsies, may occur either during intrauterine life or at birth. Cerebral palsy may also result from embryonic malformations, from injuries received during intrauterine life, or from injuries or other damage during the first two years of life. In addition to birth trauma, many other factors may contribute to a risk of cerebral palsy: premature delivery, breech delivery, toxemia of pregnancy, impairment of the baby's oxygen supply, maternal infection (especially rubella, also called German measles), premature detachment of the placenta during the birth process, and incompatibility between the Rh blood types of mother and child. Brain injuries caused by low oxygen levels (anoxia or hypoxia) can arise before, during, or after birth and can result from damage to the blood vessels, birth trauma, or infectious diseases such as meningitis or encephalitis.

Cerebral palsies are classified into two general types: pyramidal (or spastic) and extrapyramidal (or nonspastic). The pyramidal or spastic types show muscular spasms and other symptoms that persist with age and hardly vary with changes in emotion, tension, movement, or sleep. The pyramidal tracts of the brain stem are damaged in these forms of cerebral palsy. The extrapyramidal or nonspastic types are more variable and are subdivided into several subtypes according to the types of movement exhibited: none (rigid type), weak (dystonic type), rhythmic and wormlike (athetoid type), or uncoordinated shaking (ataxic type). The extrapyramidal tracts of the brain stem are damaged in all these forms of the disease. Most forms of cerebral palsy can also be described as hemiplegia (involving both extremities on one side of the body only), diplegia (involving both legs more than the arms), bilateral hemiplegia (involving the arms more than the legs), or quadriplegia (involving all four extremities more or less equally). Attempts to group the various forms of cerebral palsy by their causes have generally resulted in a lack of agreement among experts. One scheme divides the causes into subependymal hemorrhage among premature infants, damage from oxygen deprivation to the growing brain (the vast majority of cases), and developmental abnormalities of the nervous system.

The most common form of cerebral palsy is infantile spastic hemiplegia, which accounts for about one-third of all cerebral palsies. Most cases of spastic hemiplegia (about 65 percent) are thought to result from birth trauma, either from forceps delivery or from the difficult passage of a very large head through the mother's pelvic girdle. Another 30 percent arise after birth, during the first year of life, either from head injury or from infections such as meningitis and encephalitis. Only 5 percent of spastic hemiplegias arise before birth from embryonic malformations or from toxemia of pregnancy. The rate at which cerebral palsy occurs is higher for babies born prematurely than for those born at term. It is also higher for large babies that may suffer injury during a difficult passage through the birth canal. In the United States, there is a somewhat higher incidence rate among Caucasians than among African Americans.

Parkinson's disease (also called paralysis agitans or shaking palsy) is a progressive or degenerative type of palsy. The disease usually produces a tremor that includes a distinctive "pill-rolling" movement of the thumb and forefinger; this tremor usually stops if a voluntary movement of some other kind is begun. Muscle weakness, stiffness, and muscular rigidity are common but with intermittent symptoms that come and go; movements generally become slow and difficult. The muscles involved in chewing and swallowing are often affected in Parkinson's disease, so patients are often advised to eat high-calorie, semisoft foods that require no chewing and are more easily swallowed than liquids. Involvement of the muscles of facial expression results in a masklike expression that does not alter with changes in emotion. Patients suffering from Parkinson's disease often have difficulty in initiating voluntary movements; this difficulty is often described by patients as a feeling of "being frozen in place."

The walking gait of Parkinson's disease patients is also very characteristic: The body above the waist leans forward, the head and shoulders droop, the feet shuffle slowly (and are barely lifted from the ground), and the arms are generally held slightly flexed and motionless rather than swinging. Many patients break into a trot or a run when they attempt to walk; as a result, patients often fall, most often forward. To prevent such falls, they frequently shuffle forward in very small steps. The shuffling gait is believed to result from a partial paralysis of the extrapyramidal motor system of neurons, which is generally responsible for controlling posture and coordinating motor activities.

Parkinson's disease is known to result from a disorder in the production of dopamine, a neurotransmitter chemical normally secreted by certain parts of the brain. The affected parts of the brain are the basal ganglia deep within the cerebral hemispheres, and especially the substantia nigra, a deeper structure that sends dopamine-secreting nerve fibers to the basal ganglia. In patients with Parkinson's disease, cells of the substantia nigra are often degenerate and pale from the loss of normal pigments, but this may be a result, rather than a cause, of the primary defect: an impairment of the brain's ability to convert dopa (dihydroxyphenylalanine) into the neurotransmitter dopamine.

The chemical n-methyyl-4-phenyl-1,2,3,4-tetrahydro-pyridine has been found to produce in experimental animals a disease very similar to Parkinson's disease. For this reason, many researchers suspect that the disease has an environmental cause that leads to the production of a related toxic chemical, one that presumably interferes with the production of dopamine.

Parkinson's disease is uncommon before the age of forty, but it becomes so common in people over sixty that it is the leading neurological disorder in this age group. In the United States, the incidence rate is about 130 per 100,000 in the general population and is roughly the same in all races and ethnic groups. About 10 to 15 percent of patients show mental deterioration (dementia) as the disease progresses. Patients often experience depression, social withdrawal, and generalized apathy.

Other, less common palsies include brachial birth palsy, Erb's palsy, Klumpke's palsy, true or progressive bulbar palsy, pseudobulbar palsy, Féréol-Graux palsy, posticus palsy, lead palsy, scrivener's palsy, pressure palsy, compression palsy, and creeping or wasting palsy.

Brachial birth palsy is a paralysis of the infant's arm resulting from an injury received at birth, involving the whole arm, the upper arm only (Erb's palsy), or the lower arm only (Klumpke's palsy). Erb's palsy, a brachial birth palsy of the upper arm, is caused by an injury at birth to the brachial plexus or the posterior roots of the fifth and sixth cervical nerves; the muscles involved generally include the deltoideus, biceps brachii, and brachialis, impairing the raising of the upper arm, flexion of the elbow, or supination movements involving the forearm. In Klumpke's palsy, which results from an injury at birth, the muscles of the forearm and the small muscles of the hand undergo atrophy; this form is often accompanied by paralysis of the cervical sympathetic nerves.

True or progressive bulbar palsy, a palsy and progressive atrophy of the muscles of the tongue, lips, palate, pharynx, and larynx, often occurs late in life and is caused by degeneration of the motor neurons leading to these muscles. Twitching or atrophy of the tongue and other affected muscles causes drooling, difficulties in swallowing, and ultimately a respiratory paralysis that results in death. Many experts consider true bulbar palsy to be a manifestation of the same disease that causes amyotrophic lateral sclerosis (ALS), which is popularly known as Lou Gehrig's disease.

Pseudobulbar palsy ("laughing sickness") is a paralysis of the lips and tongue that mimics true or progressive bulbar palsy, but it arises in the brain itself and is accompanied by difficulties in swallowing and by spasmodic laughter at inappropriate times. Féréol-Graux palsy, a one-sided (unilateral) paralysis of the motor nucleus of the lateral rectus muscle of one eye and the medial rectus muscle of the other eye, results from damage to the medial longitudinal fasciculus and impairs the ability to direct either eye toward the affected side. Posticus palsy is a paralysis of the posterior cricoarytenoideus muscle (cricoarytenoideus posticus), resulting in the vocal cords being held close to the midline.

Lead palsy is a paralysis of the extensor muscles of the

wrist resulting from lead poisoning, while scrivener's palsy ("writer's cramp") is a repetitive motion disorder resulting in damage to the nerve controlling the small muscles of the hand. Pressure palsy is a paralysis caused by repeated or persistent compression of a nerve or nerve trunk. Compression palsy results from nerve compression, especially of the arm, caused by pressure from the use of a crutch (crutch palsy) or from compression of a nerve during sleep. Creeping palsy and wasting palsy are general terms for progressive muscle atrophy, such as that associated with ALS.

Treatment and Therapy

Bell's palsy is treated by various methods, including the application of warmth, the avoidance of cold drafts, or the administration of vasodilating drugs such as cortisone or antiviral drugs such as acyclovir. In unusual cases, surgery is performed to enlarge the passages through which the facial nerve passes, thus relieving compression on the nerve. In past generations, physicians often recommended treating eyes that could not be closed by taping them shut, especially in sleep. This treatment is no longer recommended. Instead, physicians usually advise patients who cannot close an affected eye to wear dark glasses during the day.

Many patients with Bell's palsy recover spontaneously on their own. The chances that a particular individual will spontaneously recover depend on the location of the damage and the extent of muscle involvement; the cases with the most favorable outcomes are those in which the damage is more peripheral and fewer muscles are involved. Frequent, repeated testing of each small group of facial muscles is needed to assess the extent of damage and the extent of any recovery.

Diagnosis of cerebral palsy is best made by a trained neurologist through observation of the patient's spontaneous motor movements and reflex actions. Infants who exhibit any reflex that persists beyond its appropriate age range, or any voluntary motor pattern that fails to develop at the appropriate age, should be examined more carefully for signs of nerve damage. For example, most babies can lift their heads by one month of age and their chests by two months. By three months of age, most babies can raise themselves up on their elbows, and by four months on their wrists. Newborn babies exhibit reflexes such as the Moro reflex, a flexion and "embracing" reflex in reaction to a sudden noise or other sudden stimulus or "startle"; however, the persistence of this reflex beyond six months of age (or its asymmetrical performance) may be indicative of some form of cerebral palsy. Another reflex often used in diagnosis is the "fencer" reflex, or asymmetric tonic neck reflex: Turning the baby's head toward one side usually causes extension movements in both the arm and leg on the side toward which the chin faces, while flexion movements usually take place on the opposite side of the body. This reflex is present at birth and disappears in a few months; its persistence after six months of age should be considered suspicious.

There is no cure for cerebral palsy. Treatment generally consists of physical rehabilitation and training the patient to use whatever muscles are still capable of being con-

sciously controlled. This is a difficult form of therapy that must be tailored to the needs of each patient because individuals experience unique combinations of motor abilities and disabilities. Few patients with cerebral palsy are capable of walking on their own. Depending on the extent of impairment of muscle movements, some patients may require crutches or braces, while others use motorized wheelchairs. In cases in which there is speech impairment, speech therapy may also be needed to teach the patient to speak more clearly. Most types of cerebral palsy are already present during infancy; therapy for these types is always rather difficult because the patient is learning the necessary motor skills (such as walking or speaking) for the first time. Palsies that arise during adolescence or adulthood respond differently to therapy because the patient is relearning skills that had already been mastered.

Treatment for Parkinson's disease includes the administration of a number of drugs that are chemically related to dopamine, the missing neurotransmitter. The drug most often used is levodopa, or L-dopa, a derivative of a naturally occurring amino acid in the brain. The drug carbidopa is also given to help deliver most of the levodopa into the brain. Dopamine agonists (enhancers) such as bromocriptine and pergolide are frequently given. The antiviral drug amantadine has also been shown to have effects that counter the disease.

Perspective and Prospects

The various palsies were identified in the nineteenth century. Bell's palsy was first described by Sir Charles Bell (1774-1842), a renowned Scottish anatomist. Parkinsonism was first described by James Parkinson (1755-1824), who called it "shaking palsy"; the understanding of the neurotransmitter dopamine and the use of L-dopa in the treatment of Parkinson's disease were development of the late twentieth century. Cerebral palsy was first described in 1861 by a London physician, William J. Little; the famous psychoanalyst Sigmund Freud (1856-1939) published an account of this disease in 1883. The most thorough early work on this disease was published in 1889 by the distinguished Canadian physician Sir William Osler (1849-1919), who coined the term "cerebral palsies" to describe the several types of the disease.

Several types of cerebral palsy that were more common in the early twentieth century, such as those caused by the use of obstetrical forceps during delivery, have decreased in incidence as a result of improved medical procedures. For larger babies that formerly faced a greater risk of cerebral hemorrhage and other brain injury from passage through the mother's pelvic girdle at birth, the increased frequency of cesarean sections has greatly reduced the rates of cerebral palsy arising at birth.

—*Eli C. Minkoff, Ph.D.*

See also Amyotrophic lateral sclerosis; Bell's palsy; Cerebral palsy; Hemiplegia; Herpes; Motor neuron diseases; Nervous system; Neuralgia, neuritis, and neuropathy; Neurology; Neurology, pediatric; Paralysis; Paraplegia; Parkinson's disease; Physical rehabilitation; Quadriplegia; Shingles; Tremors.

For Further Information:

Bloom, Floyd E., M. Flint Beal, and David J. Kupfer, eds. *The Dana Guide to Brain Health*. New York: Dana Press, 2006.

Carson-DeWitt, Rosalyn. "Parkinson's Disease." *Health Library*, September 10, 2012.

Chipps, Esther, Norma J. Clanin, and Victor G. Campbell. *Neurologic Disorders*. St. Louis, Mo.: Mosby Year Book, 1992.

Daube, Jasper R., ed. *Clinical Neurophysiology*. 3d ed. New York: Oxford University Press, 2009.

Kliegman, Robert M., and Waldo E. Nelson, eds. *Nelson Textbook of Pediatrics*. 19th ed. Philadelphia: Saunders/Elsevier, 2011.

Iansek, Robert, and Meg. E. Morris, eds. *Rehabilitation in Movement Disorders*. Cambridge: Cambridge University Press, 2013.

Stanley, Fiona J., Eva Alberman, and Eva Blair. *Cerebral Palsies: Epidemiology and Causal Pathways*. New York: Cambridge University Press, 2000.

Stanton, Marion. *The Cerebral Palsy Handbook*. London: Vermilion, 2002.

United Cerebral Palsy. http://www.ucp.org.

Victor, Maurice, and Allan H. Ropper. *Adams and Victor's Principles of Neurology*. 9th ed. New York: McGraw-Hill, 2009.

Waxman, Stephen G. *Correlative Neuroanatomy*. 25th ed. New York: Lange Medical Books/McGraw-Hill, 2002.

Weiner, William J., Lisa M. Shulman, and Anthony E. Lang. *Parkinson's Disease: A Complete Guide for Patients and Families*, 3d ed. Baltimore, Md.: Johns Hopkins University Press, 2013.

Pancreas

Anatomy

Anatomy or system affected: Abdomen, endocrine system, gastrointestinal system, glands, immune system

Specialties and related fields: Endocrinology, gastroenterology, immunology, internal medicine

Definition: A vital organ that produces enzymes used in the digestive process and hormones such as insulin, which regulates blood sugar levels.

Key terms:

autoimmunity: a disorder in which the immune system starts to attack the body's cells as foreign matter

autosomal recessive disease: a disease caused by a gene (other than the X or Y chromosome) that must be on both chromosomes to be expressed

concordance: the inheritance of the same trait by both twins

duodenum: the initial part of the small intestine, where most of the digestion of food occurs

endocrine glands: ductless glands that secrete hormones directly into the bloodstream; these glands help to maintain homeostasis

exocrine glands: glands that excrete their products into tubes or ducts

Structure and Functions

The pancreas is an organ about 15 to 18 centimeters long and weighing 100 grams that is located in the abdominal cavity. The head of the organ is situated in the loop of the small intestine that forms at the site where the small intestine joins the stomach. The pancreas is enclosed in a thin connective tissue capsule. As an accessory gland of the digestive system, the pancreas is an exocrine gland. Scattered within the tissue of this exocrine gland, however, are small distinct regions known as the islets of Langerhans, which are a part of the endocrine system. The exocrine portion composes by far the greatest mass of tissue. In the guinea pig, for example, about 82 percent of pancreatic cells are exocrine cells, while the endocrine portion is about 2 percent. The remaining cells are associated with the duct system and the blood vessels.

The exocrine pancreas is an arrangement of tubules that continue to branch until they form very fine ducts called the intercalated ducts. Along the edges of the intercalated ducts are the acinar cells. These cells produce the pancreatic juices that aid in the digestion of food in the small intestine and help neutralize the contents of the small intestine. The products drain from the ducts into the main collecting duct, which joins the common bile duct and empties into the duodenum.

The islets of Langerhans, as is the case with all endocrine glands, have a well-developed blood supply. The hormones produced by these endocrine cells are emptied into the surrounding capillaries. The hormones flow into the general circulation where they are distributed to target cells throughout the body. Since the two portions of the pancreas are anatomically as well as functionally different, they will be considered independently.

The exocrine portion of the pancreas produces about 1 liter of aqueous fluid per day that is delivered directly to the duodenum. The two major components of the pancreatic juices are ions, which are used to neutralize the stomach contents as they enter the small intestine, and enzymes, which metabolize intestinal contents for absorption.

The various ions that are secreted include sodium, potassium, chloride, and bicarbonate ions. The sodium, potassium, and chloride are present in concentrations similar to their concentrations in the bloodstream. The bicarbonate ions act as the major buffer of the body. With only a few exceptions, the bloodstream and the contents of the body must be maintained at a pH of 7.4. Bicarbonate ions ensure that there is no change in pH.

The stomach is one of the areas of the body in which the pH varies. It may be as low as pH 1, which is highly acidic. The contents of the stomach empty directly into the duodenum, and while the cells of the stomach are capable of withstanding an acid environment, the cells of the small intestine are not. The acid must be rapidly neutralized in order to protect these cells. In addition, the enzymes that help to digest the food reaching the small intestine work optimally at about pH 7. If the pH varies significantly, the food will not be properly digested and vital nutrients will not be absorbed by the intestinal cells.

The production of bicarbonate by the duct cells is controlled by a hormone called secretin. The contents of the small intestine become acidic as food moves into the area from the stomach. When the pH is lowered, the cells of the small intestine release secretin, which in turn stimulates the pancreas to produce more bicarbonate. As bicarbonate enters the small intestine, it neutralizes the acid, and the stimulus to produce secretin is removed.

The pancreas also produces a variety of enzymes that digest proteins, sugars, lipids, and nucleic acids. In order for protein to be absorbed by the cells of the small intestine, it must be broken down into its building blocks, amino acids. This breakdown is an enzymatic process that occurs only when the appropriate enzymes are present and at a pH near neutrality. The enzymes that digest proteins include trypsin, chymotrypsin, and carboxypeptidase. Like protein, sugars, nucleic acids, and lipids must be digested to their subunits if they are to be absorbed. Sugars are metabolized by amylase, nucleic acids by either ribonuclease or deoxyribonuclease, and fats by lipase, phospholipase, or cholesterol esterase.

The secretion of enzymes by the pancreas is controlled by the hormone cholecystokinin. As the content of protein and fat increases in the lumen of the duodenum, the duodenal cells release cholecystokinin, which acts on the acinar cells of the pancreas to release the enzymes. As the food is digested, the level of cholecystokinin decreases and the release of enzymes from the pancreas also decreases.

The islets of Langerhans have four different cell types and produce four different hormones. The alpha and beta cells produce glucagon and insulin, respectively. The delta cells produce somatostatin, which inhibits the secretion of hormones by the alpha and beta cells. The F cells produce pancreatic polypeptide, the function of which is not yet understood.

Insulin secretion is stimulated or inhibited by a large number of factors. Blood glucose levels are the most important factor in the release of insulin from the beta cells. If blood glucose increases, insulin is released until glucose levels return to normal. When insulin is released into the bloodstream, it stimulates the uptake of glucose by target cells. Although insulin is best known for its action on glucose, it also stimulates the uptake of amino acids and fatty acids from the bloodstream during periods of adequate nutrition. Glucagon is an antagonist of insulin. It is released in response to low levels of glucose and acts on cells to release glucose, amino acids, and fatty acids into the circulatory system.

Disorders and Diseases

Diseases of the pancreas can be divided into two basic categories: diseases of the exocrine cells of the organ and those diseases that effect the function of the endocrine portion, the islets of Langerhans. The exocrine cells of the pancreas can be affected by various conditions, including acute pancreatitis, chronic pancreatitis, cystic fibrosis, and carcinoma of the pancreas. Also, because the pancreas is a gland and glandular organs typically have a large blood supply, it is at risk of injury any time that circulation is impaired. The islets of Langerhans may be affected by diabetes mellitus.

Inflammation of the pancreas (pancreatitis) can be either acute or chronic. While some cases are mild, it is considered a serious disease and has a high mortality rate. Although the acute form is more serious, patients with

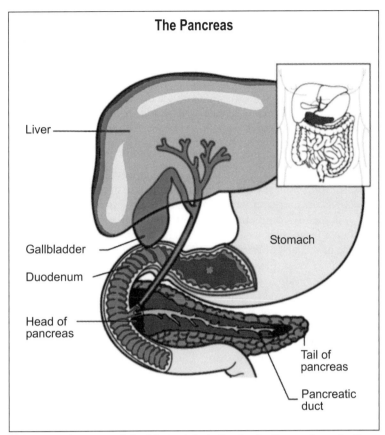

The Pancreas

The pancreas is an unusual gland that contains both endocrine tissue and exocrine tissue; the inset shows the location of the pancreas within the gastrointestinal system.

chronic pancreatitis may suffer from acute episodes.

Acute pancreatitis may result from obstruction of the pancreatic duct (possibly by gallstones from the gallbladder or by mucous plugs, as in cystic fibrosis), bile reflux, acute intoxication by alcohol, shock, infection by the mumps virus, hypothermia, or trauma. The diagnosis, pathology, and prognosis are the same regardless of the cause.

The onset of the disease is usually quite sudden, with severe pain in the abdomen, nausea, and vomiting. Diagnosis is made by the presence of amylase in the blood serum. Amylase is an enzyme produced by the pancreas that is used to digest carbohydrates in the small intestine. The presence of elevated levels of the enzyme is an indication that it is not reaching the small intestine and is spilling over into the bloodstream.

The powerful enzymes produced by the pancreas are used to digest proteins, carbohydrates, and fats. If for any reason these substances are not released from the pancreas, they will digest the cells of the pancreas and destroy them. As pancreatitis progresses, it will cause tissue inflammation and will lead to swelling of the organ. In addition, the enzymes may start to digest the cells of the blood vessels in the immediate area, causing bleeding into the tissue. The inflammation, combined with the bleeding, may lead to greater swelling and further inflammation.

Acute pancreatitis can lead to complications in other tissue as well, such as fat necrosis leading to the release of fatty acids from adipose tissue. The fatty acids bind to circulating calcium and may cause tetanus of the skeletal muscle as a result of calcium deficiency. If the enzymes released from the exocrine cells destroy the endocrine cells, the resulting loss of hormone production will lead to hyperglycemia and the complications that stem from it. Cysts or abscesses may also result from acute pancreatitis. Although this disease is usually self-limiting, in many cases it will lead to death.

Chronic pancreatitis is a recurring disease that may also demonstrate acute episodes. It has generally been associated with chronic alcoholism, which seems to be the major cause. Chronic pancreatitis is primarily a disease of middle age and occurs more frequently in men than in women. The patient generally complains of abdominal or back pain, often after a large meal or excessive alcohol consumption. Because of the lack of enzymes for lipid digestion, patients often excrete large quantities of undigested lipids. Without fat absorption, many fat-soluble substances such as vitamins A, D, E, and K will not be absorbed.

Because the patient with chronic pancreatitis is often malnourished from inadequate digestion and absorption of food and from vitamin deficiencies, there is associated weight loss and muscular wasting. The exocrine portion of the pancreas is gradually replaced by scar tissue, but the endocrine cells remain unaffected.

Disease of the pancreas can also be caused by cystic fibrosis. Cystic fibrosis, also known as mucoviscidosis, is an autosomal recessive disease of the exocrine glands. It occurs in about 1 in 2,500 live births of Caucasians but rarely occurs in African Americans or Asians. Cystic fibrosis affects the mucus-secreting glands in the body and leads to the production of abnormally thick mucus. About 80 percent of these patients have involvement of the pancreas. The onset and severity of the disease vary widely, but most infants born with cystic fibrosis have a pancreas that appears to be normal. As the abnormal mucus is produced, however, it may block the ducts of the exocrine glands and lead to the destruction of the exocrine tissue. The glandular tissue is progressively replaced by fibrous or adipose tissue or by cysts. The loss of pancreatic activity may lead to malabsorption of nutrients and vitamins. Although the islets of Langerhans are not affected by the disease in its early stages, eventually they also may be destroyed.

Tumors of the pancreas are primary tumors; there is almost no incidence of tumors metastasizing to the pancreas from other locations in the body. The exocrine tumors are generally adenocarcinomas, a type of cancer that is increasing in frequency throughout the world. An association with cigarette smoking and diabetes mellitus has been established. The tumors most commonly occur in the area of the gland where the major ducts leave the pancreas. As the tumors enlarge, they may put excessive pressure on the common bile duct, which is located in the same region. This pressure leads to the backup of bile in the liver known as obstructive jaundice; this is one of the earliest signs of pathology. Tumors located at other sites will not be detected until much later because they do not produce symptoms. Metastases of these tumors may be to the liver or surrounding lymph nodes. Because diagnosis is usually after the disease has progressed, the prognosis is poor even in operable cases.

The most common disease of the endocrine portion of the pancreas is diabetes mellitus. In 2009, over 68,000 individuals died of diabetes in the United States. Diabetes is a chronic disorder affecting carbohydrate, fat, and protein metabolism. It may be further classified as insulin-dependent or juvenile diabetes (type 1), non-insulin-dependent or adult-onset diabetes (type 2), or secondary diabetes. All forms of diabetes have a common pattern in which insulin is present in insufficient quantities, is absent, or does not function normally-all of which lead to hyperglycemia. Both type 1 and type 2 diabetes are inherited. In identical twins, there is a 50 percent concordance rate for type 1 and a 90 percent concordance for type 2. The latter figure indicates that heredity plays a more important role in type 2 diabetes.

Patients with type 1 diabetes are insulin-dependent. The disease starts at an early age and is sometimes referred to as juvenile diabetes. The decrease in insulin supply is caused by a decrease in functional beta cells in the islets of Langerhans. Evidence indicates that the beta cells are damaged or destroyed by an autoimmune reaction, which may follow a viral infection. Type 1 diabetics often have other endocrine disorders that are a result of autoimmunity. Type 2 diabetics produce some insulin, but not sufficient quantities. It appears that the tissues of these patients are resistant to insulin. The symptoms are less severe than those associated with type 1. Secondary diabetes is a result of some other disease that causes injury or destruction of beta cells. Diseases such as chronic pancreatitis or carcinoma of the pancreas can interfere with insulin production. The severity of the three forms of the disease varies widely, as does the treatment. The type 1 diabetic requires insulin for survival, while in many type 2 diabetics the disease may be controlled by diet and exercise.

Although the presence of insulin has several effects on the body, the lack of insulin has the most pronounced effect on serum glucose levels. If insulin supply is diminished or if the cells do not respond to the insulin produced, there is a rise in blood glucose levels exceeding the amount that the kidney can retain. As a result, glucose is excreted in the urine along with large quantities of water. The loss of glucose and water may lead to hypoglycemia and dehydration. The problem is further complicated if there is inadequate glucose available, which causes the cells to metabolize fats. One of the by-products of fat metabolism is the production of chemicals known as ketones, which are acids. Thus the dehydration may be accompanied by a more acidic serum.

The symptoms described above are acute and demand immediate attention. In addition to these symptoms, many abnormalities may appear in patients who have diabetes for ten or more years. The cardiovascular system is highly vulnerable to the disease, and the cause of death in about 80 percent of diabetics is a cardiovascular abnormality.

Perspective and Prospects

Since the pancreas is a vital organ, any disease or injury to it will have serious consequences. Problems with the pancreas may be magnified because the diseases associated with the exocrine portion of the gland are not easily detected. In acute cases of pancreatitis, the onset is sudden and requires immediate treatment to control the extent of the disease. Even when the disease is treated early, many patients die. Surgery is complicated by the inflammation and hemorrhaging that may have previously occurred.

Chronic pancreatitis and cancer of the pancreas are even more difficult to diagnose since many of the symptoms are common to other ailments and may not even be present until the disease has progressed to an acute stage. The chronic condition is complicated because the body cannot absorb nutrients and vitamins. By the time that the diagnosis has occurred, the patient is weakened by the loss of weight and muscular wasting from malnutrition.

Diabetes presents its own unique set of problems. In type 1 diabetes, the patient is often unable to follow the prescribed diet and must continually monitor his or her glucose levels to ensure that the insulin doses are appropriate. Assuming that the patient is able to follow the diet and takes the medication as prescribed, there will still be complications-particularly of the cardiovascular system-that may include renal damage.

Pancreas transplants provide type 1 diabetics with hope when all other standard treatments have failed and they are faced with serious and often life-threatening complications. Pancreatic transplants are often performed in conjunction with a kidney transplant since the majority of patients are in the end states of renal failure, but the procedure is rarely performed on individuals suffering from pancreatic cancer because that form of cancer is highly malignant and the probability of it returning and attacking the new pancreas is very high.

Pancreatic transplants usually involve implanting a healthy (and insulin producing) organ into a patient while leaving the original pancreas in place since it is still able to produce essential digestive enzymes. Following surgery, many patients are able to maintain normal blood glucose levels, and diabetes-related nerve damage is often stabilized and sometimes repaired following transplantation. The risks involved in the surgery, however, are significant and should be taken into consideration: In addition to the potential for blood clots, infection, and inflammation of the new pancreas, rejection of the new organ is of great concern and can occur immediately following the surgery or at any time during the recipient's life. Because of this threat, the patient must take powerful immunosuppressive drugs for the remainder of his or her life, and these drugs come with their own set of potential side effects such as thinning of the bones, high cholesterol and blood pressure, weight gain, and acne and excessive hair growth over the body.

New procedures have been employed that involve the transplantation of only the beta cells of the islets of Langerhans rather than of the entire organ. Similar side effects and risks, such as blood clots and the necessity of immunosuppressive drugs, are also associated with this procedure.

It is likely that there will be significant progress with the treatment of diabetes as more becomes known about somatic gene therapy, cell transplants, immunosuppression, and the control of insulin receptors.

—*Annette O'Connor, Ph.D.*

See also Abdomen; Abscess drainage; Abscesses; Diabetes mellitus; Digestion; Endocrine glands; Endocrinology; Endocrinology, pediatric; Enzymes; Fetal tissue transplantation; Food biochemistry; Gastroenterology; Gastroenterology, pediatric; Gastrointestinal disorders; Gastrointestinal system; Glands; Hormones; Internal medicine; Metabolic syndrome; Metabolism; Pancreatitis; Stomach, intestinal, and pancreatic cancers; Systems and organs; Transplantation.

For Further Information:

Calvagna, Mary. "Pancreatitis." *HealthLibrary*, October 31, 2012.

Goodman, H. Maurice. *Basic Medical Endocrinology.* 4th ed. Boston: Academic Press/Elsevier, 2009.

Howard, John M., and Walter Hess. *History of the Pancreas: Mysteries of a Hidden Organ.* New York: Kluwer Academic, 2002.

Marieb, Elaine N. *Essentials of Human Anatomy and Physiology.* 10th ed. San Francisco: Benjamin Cummings, 2010.

O'Reilly, Eileen, and Joanne Frankel Kelvin. *One Hundred Questions and Answers About Pancreatic Cancer.* 2d ed. Sudbury, Mass.: Jones and Bartlett Publishers, 2010.

"Pancreas Transplantation." *American Diabetes Association*, July 25, 2013.

"Pancreatic Islet Transplantation." *National Diabetes Information Clearinghouse*, August 1, 2012.

Pizer, H. F. *Organ Transplants: A Patient's Guide.* Cambridge, Mass.: Harvard University Press, 1991.

Valenzuela, Jorge E., Howard A. Reber, and André Ribet, eds. *Medical and Surgical Diseases of the Pancreas.* New York: Igaku-Shoin Medical, 1991.

Pancreatic cancer. *See* Stomach, intestinal, and pancreatic cancers.

Pancreatitis

Disease/Disorder

Anatomy or system affected: Abdomen, endocrine system, gastrointestinal system, pancreas

Specialties and related fields: Endocrinology, gastroenterology, internal medicine

Definition: Inflammation of the pancreas, which may be acute or chronic.

Causes and Symptoms

Linked to the small intestines by the pancreatic duct, the pancreas contributes enzymes necessary to digestion. When the pancreas is damaged or its duct is blocked, the enzymes may begin to digest the pancreatic tissue itself, a process called autodigestion. Inflammation ensues, resulting in acute pancreatitis. Although there may be complications, most cases are self-correcting once the damaging agent is eliminated, and the pancreatitis does not recur. With continuing damage to the pancreas, however, the disease may become self-perpetuating and either break out periodically in attacks that mimic the acute form or cause few symptoms until much of the pancreas has been destroyed, a

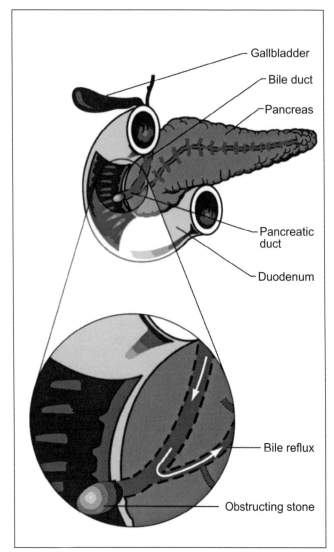

- Gallbladder
- Bile duct
- Pancreas
- Pancreatic duct
- Duodenum
- Bile reflux
- Obstructing stone

The pancreas, showing the pancreatic duct; when this duct is blocked, bile may reflux, leading to "autodigestion" of the pancreas.

Information on Pancreatitis

Causes: Sometimes unknown; often alcoholism and biliary tract disease; possibly trauma, certain medications, viral infections, hyperlipidemia, structural abnormalities in pancreas, hereditary disease
Symptoms: Pain, inflammation
Duration: Acute or chronic
Treatments: Pain medications, intravenous hydration, antibiotics, surgery, intensive care

tion, it seldom leads to chronic pancreatitis. Other, rarer causes include traumatic injury (especially the damage done by the steering wheel or seat belt during an automobile accident), damage incurred during abdominal surgery or endoscopic procedures in the small intestine, reactions to some medicines, viral infections, very high levels of fats in the blood (hyperlipidemia), structural abnormalities in the pancreas, or hereditary disease.

Despite the variety in causes, patients present a fairly limited set of symptoms, at least during an acute episode. Usually (but not always), they initially complain of steady pain in the upper abdomen that in severe cases seems to bore into them and radiate to the back. They may also have an enlarged abdomen, run a fever, experience nausea, and vomit. The physician is likely to find the abdomen distended, while the patient feels tenderness when it is touched. In severe cases, the patient may develop signs of shock, unstoppable hiccuping, jaundice, discoloration around the navel, fluid buildup in the peritoneal cavity, and impaired bowel function. While abdominal pain is a prominent feature of chronic pancreatitis as well, the most common associated symptoms are diarrhea, fatty stool, weight loss from poor digestion, and the development of diabetes mellitus.

Because none of these symptoms belongs exclusively to pancreatitis, physicians must conduct tests to establish the diagnosis; however, no single test is conclusive. Only by carefully showing that other possible diseases, such as pancreatic cancer, are not responsible for the symptoms can doctors be sure that pancreatitis is the culprit. Blood tests that detect elevated levels of amylase and lipase (pancreatic digestive enzymes) support the diagnosis. X-rays, ultrasonography, computed tomography (CT) scanning, and endoscopic inspection of the pancreas and common bile duct can identify both causes and complications of pancreatitis.

Treatment and Therapy

The treatment for pancreatitis depends on its cause. If the problem is abuse of alcohol or other drugs, physicians usually let an attack of acute pancreatitis run its course while the patient abstains from the offending substance. Nevertheless, even mild attacks frequently require hospitalization, because painkillers and intravenous hydration therapy are needed. If gallstones are thought to be the problem, plans are made to remove them by surgery. Patients with

chronic form of pancreatitis that is difficult to treat. Either form can be fatal. Acute pancreatitis causes death in less than 5 percent of cases and generally does so because of complications, such as extensive tissue destruction and hemorrhage or infection. Complications from chronic pancreatitis can be fatal in as many as 50 percent of cases.

Although a variety of damaging agents are known to lead to pancreatitis, in as much as 15 percent of cases no clear cause is detectable; doctors call these cases idiopathic pancreatitis. Of detectable causes, alcoholism and biliary tract disease account for about 80 percent of both acute and chronic cases in the United States and Europe (the percentages vary widely in other parts of the world). Alcohol is the most common toxic agent causing pancreatitis, although susceptibility varies and only a minority of heavy drinkers develop acute pancreatitis; however, a long history of steady drinking is by far the most common cause of chronic pancreatitis. Gallstones in the common bile duct, or any other stricture or obstruction that backs up bile into the pancreatic duct, can trigger acute pancreatitis. Because surgeons can correct this problem by removing the obstruc-

severe acute pancreatitis are sent to the hospital's intensive care unit, since they urgently need supportive treatment to stay alive. There, doctors insert a tube through the patient's nose and into the stomach to suck out excess gastric fluids and relieve pressure on the pancreas. They may give antibiotics if there is evidence of infection. Extra oxygen or mechanical assistance may be needed to support breathing. Occasionally, surgery may be called for even in pancreatitis not caused by gallstones, in order to cut away dead, infected tissue or drain fluid accumulations known as pseudocysts. Following an attack and treatment, a patient may require intravenous nourishment for weeks before the pancreas is ready to resume its full function.

Continued alcohol abuse will generally spur recurrent bouts of pancreatitis. Sometimes, however, the alcohol (or, rarely, slowly developing biliary tract disease) causes more subtle, gradual impairment of pancreatic function with few symptoms; in fact, some patients do not go to the doctor until the damage has become extensive and permanently disabling. Others have intense, continual upper abdominal pain that painkillers cannot reduce easily. (In fact, drug addiction from high dosages of painkillers often becomes a problem.) The doctor's first step is to stop the patient's alcohol intake. If gallstones or other obstructions are present, clearing the bile duct with surgery or an endoscopic procedure will decrease pain. Sometimes, high doses of pancreatic enzymes may be helpful in relieving pain.

In cases of uncontrollable pain, however, surgery may be needed to block the sympathetic nerves or even to remove all or part of the pancreas. If pancreatic function is sufficiently impaired by this procedure, or by the progress of the disease, chronic pancreatitis patients will digest food poorly and may require enzyme supplements to avoid continued weight loss. Since insulin is made in the pancreas, such patients may also develop diabetes. All chronic pancreatitis patients will need professional advice about appropriate diet and lifestyle changes.

—*Roger Smith, Ph.D.*

See also Alcoholism; Diabetes mellitus; Endocrine disorders; Endocrinology; Endocrinology, pediatric; Enzymes; Gallbladders; Gallbladder diseases; Hypoglycemia; Obstruction; Pancreas; Stomach, intestinal, and pancreatic cancers; Stone removal; Stones.

For Further Information:

Büchler, M. W., et al., eds. *Acute Pancreatitis: Novel Concepts in Biology and Therapy*. Boston: Blackwell Science, 1999.

Calvagna, Mary. "Pancreatitis." *Health Library*, October 31, 2012.

Feldman, Mark, Lawrence S. Friedman, and Lawrence J. Brandt, eds. *Sleisenger and Fordtran's Gastrointestinal and Liver Disease: Pathophysiology, Diagnosis, Management*. 2 vols. Philadelphia: Saunders/Elsevier, 2010.

Levine, Joel S., ed. *Decision Making in Gastroenterology*. 2d ed. Philadelphia: B. C. Decker, 1992.

Melmed, Schlomo, et al., eds. *Williams Textbook of Endocrinology*. 12th ed. Philadelphia: Saunders/Elsevier, 2011.

Munoz, Abilio, and David A. Katerndahl. "Diagnosis and Management of Acute Pancreatitis." *American Family Physician* 62, no. 1 (July 1, 2000): 164-174.

"Pancreatitis." *Mayo Clinic*, January 15, 2011.

"Pancreatitis." *National Digestive Diseases Information Clearinghouse*, August 16, 2012.

Pancreatitis Supporters' Network. http://www.pancreatitis.org.uk.

Parker, James N., and Philip M. Parker, eds. *The Official Patient's Sourcebook on Pancreatitis*. San Diego, Calif.: Icon Health, 2002.

Panic attacks. *See* Anxiety.

Pap test

Procedure

Also known as: Pap sampling, Pap smear

Anatomy or system affected: Genitals, reproductive system, uterus

Specialties and related fields: Gynecology, oncology

Definition: A sampling of cells from the cervix or vagina used to screen for dysplasia (precancer) and cancer.

Indications and Procedures

Pap testing guidelines have recently changed. Formerly, the procedure was recommended for all women over the age of eighteen or for women who are sexually active. Revised guidelines have been issued by the American Cancer Society, the American College of Obstetricians and Gynecologists, and the Preventive Services Task Force, part of the US Department of Health and Human Services. These updated guidelines all stipulate that Pap tests should begin in women aged twenty-one and older. Updated guidelines have been issued as well for human papillomavirus (HPV) testing, which frequently accompanies the procedure; it is now recommended that HPV testing be done in women aged thirty and older because HPV in younger women is usually a transient infection that will clear without need for intervention.

The guidelines also recommend less frequent Pap testing for women who have had three consecutive negative tests; the guidelines also call for a cutoff to Pap testing in older women without abnormalities. Pap testing guidelines for women who have had a hysterectomy (with sampling of the vaginal cuff) vary depending on whether the hysterectomy was done for benign or malignant causes. The guidelines recommend that only women who have had malignant disease continue Pap testing.

A Pap test is performed easily in an office visit. Generally, the patient lies on her back with legs flexed and knees apart, although alternative positions can be utilized for women with limited mobility or with disabilities. A speculum is then carefully inserted into the vagina, and the cervix is visualized. A spatula is used to gently scrape off cells from the transition zone of the cervix. A cytobrush samples cells from the cervical canal. These cells are then placed in a preservative and sent to a pathology laboratory for analysis. The term "Pap smear" derives from the fact that before the advent of liquid preservative methods of collecting samples, samples were "smeared" on a glass slide and then sent to a laboratory for analysis.

Uses and Complications

The main use of Pap testing is to identify asymptomatic cases of dysplasia (abnormal growth) of the cervix and vagina. With early treatment of dysplasia, the incidence of and number of deaths from cervical cancer have decreased dramatically. Although cancer screening is the primary purpose and use of Pap testing, incidental findings may include vaginal infections of bacteria, fungi, or parasites. In rare cases, Pap tests may also detect abnormal cells shed from the endometrium.

There are no serious risks from the procedure. Women may see a small amount of spotting after the procedure as a result of abrasions from the spatula or cytobrush.

Perspective and Prospects

The Pap test was introduced in 1943 by George N. Papanicolaou and Herbert F. Traut. Since then, the incidence of invasive cervical cancer has dramatically, although cervical cancer remains the second most prevalent malignancy among women worldwide, according to the World Health Organization.

A screening test analogous to cervical Pap sampling, called the anal cytology, or "anal Pap test," has been developed to screen for anal dysplasia and cancer. It has been used primarily on high-risk patients, such as those with human immunodeficiency virus (HIV), women who have had cervical or vulvar cancer, and HIV-negative men who have sex with men.

—*Clair Kaplan, A.P.R.N./M.S.N.;*
additional material by Anne Lynn S. Chang, M.D.

See also Biopsy; Cervical, ovarian, and uterine cancers; Cervical procedures; Genital disorders, female; Gynecology; Reproductive system; Screening; Women's health.

For Further Information:

A.D.A.M. Medical Encyclopedia. "Pap Smear." *MedlinePlus*, February 26, 2012.

"Cervical Cancer Screening." *Centers for Disease Control and Prevention*, June 13, 2013.

Kumar, Vinay, et al., eds. *Robbins Basic Pathology*. 9th ed. Philadelphia: Saunders/Elsevier, 2013.

Lentz, Gretchen M., et al. *Comprehensive Gynecology*. 6th ed. Philadelphia: Mosby/Elsevier, 2012.

National Cancer Institute. "Cervical Cancer Screening." *National Institutes of Health, US Department of Health and Human Services*, July 19, 2012.

"Pap Test." *Health Library*, March 15, 2013.

Wright, Thomas C., Jr., et al. "2001 Consensus Guidelines for the Management of Women with Cervical Cytological Abnormalities." *Journal of the American Medical Association* 287, no. 16 (April, 2002): 2120-2129.

Paralysis

Disease/Disorder

Anatomy or system affected: Legs, muscles, musculoskeletal system, neck, nerves, nervous system, spine

Specialties and related fields: Neurology, physical therapy

Definition: Pronounced weakness or the inability to produce movement in a part of the body resulting from a variety of causes.

Key terms:

brain cortex: the outer layer of the brain, or gray matter; divided into many areas, each with a different function, such as motion (the motor cortex) or sensation (the sensory cortex)

central nervous system: a system consisting of the brain, the brain stem, the cerebellum, and the spinal cord

hemiplegia: paralysis of one side of the body

motor: referring to parts of the nervous system having to do with movement production

nerve cell: the type of cells that make up the brain, spinal cord, and all the nerves; some initiate nerve impulses, some transmit impulses from one nerve cell to another, some transmit impulses from nerve cells to muscle cells, and some function to regulate other impulses

nerve impulse: a weak, localized electrical current generated by the movement of charged particles across and along a nerve cell membrane

nerves: bands of nervous tissue that carry both motor and sensory nerve impulses between the central nervous system and the rest of the body

neurotransmitters: chemical substances, such as acetylcholine, that are released by nerve cells into synapses when the nerve is stimulated; they stimulate the next nerve cell to fire in turn, thus passing the impulse from cell to cell

paraplegia: paralysis of the legs and lower trunk

peripheral nervous system: a system consisting of the nerves not located in the central nervous system; these nerves carry impulses from the central nervous system to the target muscles and relay sensory impulses from the rest of the body to the central nervous system

quadriplegia: paralysis of all four limbs

spinal cord: a large collection of nerve cells that relay impulses between the brain and the rest of the body; sometimes the spinal cord initiates nerve impulses of its own, such as reflexes

Nervous System Functions

To understand the causes of paralysis-weakness or the inability to move a part of the body-it is necessary to review briefly the motor nervous system and muscles. Following an action from initiation to completion through the motor nervous system may clarify this process. One may begin, for example, with a voluntary movement. An alarm clock rings early one morning. A sleeper hears the noise and decides to hit the snooze button. This decision is made in the cerebral cortex, which sends impulses to the nerves in the arm via the spinal cord.

The actual microscopic actions that result in a nerve impulse traveling from the motor cortex all the way to individual muscles will be briefly reviewed. An individual nerve cell, or neuron, comprises three parts: the dendrites, the cell body, and the axon. The cell body conducts the metabolism for the cell and otherwise keeps things in running order, but it has little direct involvement with the transmission of nerve impulses.

Dendrites are similar in appearance to the roots of plants. They are numerous and relatively short. Their function is to pick up impulses received either from sensory organs or from other cells. They do this when the receptors on their surface become activated by certain chemical signals released by neighboring nerve cells. Once these receptors are activated, they initiate a process known as depolarization.

Information on Paralysis

Causes: May include injury; infection, exposure to toxins, stroke, central nervous system disorders

Symptoms: Range from muscle weakness to complete immobility

Duration: Acute or chronic, depending on cause

Treatments: Depend on cause; may include surgery, physical therapy, spinal alignment and stabilization, drug therapy, toxin removal, hormonal therapy

In the most basic description, depolarization refers to the generation of a minute electrical charge on nerve cell membranes. It occurs through the motion of charged molecules, or ions, across the cell membrane. The specific ions involved include potassium, sodium, and calcium. Depolarization progresses down the length of the nerve cell. It passes through the dendrite to the cell body of the nerve cell and then to the axon. The axon is long and thin, some axons reaching lengths of three or more feet. Depending on its type and function, the axon may split into small filaments that go to several nerve or muscle cells, or it may remain single.

The sending axons do not touch the receiving cells when passing an impulse. Instead, they come close to the receiving cell's dendrites but leave a small gap (the synapse). Once a nerve impulse reaches the end of an axon, the axon releases chemical compounds called neurotransmitters.

Synthesized by the nerve cell, the neurotransmitter is collected and stored in small packets resting at the end of the axon. In response to depolarization, the small packets of neurotransmitter are released into the synapse, and the original electrical nerve impulse is converted into a chemical impulse. When the neurotransmitter is released, it diffuses across the gap and contacts specific receptors on the dendrite of the receiving nerve cell. The receiving nerve cell's receptors then depolarize the receiving nerve cell, converting the chemical impulse back into an electrical one.

The receiving nerve cell is forced to continue depolarizing until the neurotransmitter is no longer in contact with the receptor, or until the nerve cell itself becomes exhausted and cannot depolarize again. To allow the receiving nerve cell to stop firing and to prepare itself for another signal, the neurotransmitter must be removed rather quickly from the receptor. This can be done by the axon of the sending cell, which takes it back in, or by enzymes located within the synapse that actually destroy the neurotransmitter. The most common neurotransmitter is acetylcholine, and the most frequently encountered form of enzyme that destroys neurotransmitters is called acetylcholinesterase.

The transmission of the nerve impulses signaling the hand to press the alarm clock's snooze button involves passing the impulses through several nerves. The impulses form synapses on nerve cells in the spinal cord before those cells pass the impulse down the spinal cord toward the arm to cause the desired action.

The spinal cord is protected inside the vertebral column, a hollow column of bone. This column is made up of a stack of vertebrae supported by solid bone in the front and a hollow ring of thinner bone in the back through which the spinal cord runs. The vertebrae are anchored to one another by bony connections; the facets and vertebral spines; fibrous ligaments to the front, back, and side; and the intervertebral disks. Disks are made up of soft, gelatinous material surrounded by fibrous tissue. The disks and joints in the vertebral column allow the spine to flex and turn, while the bony column surrounding the spinal cord provides protection.

When the nerve leaves the spinal cord, it travels in what is called the motor ramus, or "root." The ramus passes through an opening in the vertebral column called a foramen. While passing through the foramen, the ramus passes near the intervertebral disk. The motor nerve fibers (and consequently the nerve impulses sent out to turn off the alarm clock) in the motor ramus join with the sensory nerve fibers in the sensory ramus just outside the vertebral column, and together they form the spinal nerves. These spinal nerves regroup to form peripheral nerves.

A peripheral nerve is the part of the nervous system that finally contacts the muscles that turn off the alarm clock. Peripheral nerves carry both sensory and motor information in the same nerve. They are the only locations in which sensory and motor nerve fibers are so completely joined. Peripheral nerves must sometimes pass through relatively tight or exposed locations. An example of an exposed nerve is the "funny bone," the ulnar nerve, which causes an unpleasant sensation when struck. Nerves that pass through tight spaces may suffer entrapment syndromes. A common nerve entrapment syndrome is carpal tunnel syndrome, in which the median nerve is squeezed in the fibrous band around the wrist.

Finally, the arm muscles themselves become involved in the process of turning off the alarm. The muscles are made up of numerous muscle fibers, and each muscle fiber is made up of numerous muscle cells. Inside each muscle cell are two active protein filaments, actin and myosin, which pull together when activated, causing the muscle cell to shorten. When the majority of muscle cells "fire" at once, the whole muscle contracts. The signal from nerve to muscle cell is transmitted across a synapse. The snooze button is pushed, and the alarm ends. Finally, the signals to the arm end, and the filaments slide back to their initial positions, relaxing the muscle cells.

For actin and myosin to move well, there must be adequate blood flow and adequate concentrations of substances such as oxygen, glucose, potassium, sodium, and calcium. Many other substances are needed indirectly to keep muscle cells functioning optimally, including thyroid hormone and cortisone.

Types of Paralysis

True paralysis is the inability to produce movement of a part of the body. Paralysis may result from problems at many locations in the body, such as the motor cortex of the brain, the spinal cord, the nerves in the arms or legs, the blood, or the muscle cells themselves. Doctors must determine the specific cause of paralysis or weakness since the treatment of each disease is different. The first task is to determine whether the weakness or paralysis is caused by a disease of the nervous system, the muscle cells, or one of the substances that interferes with nerve conduction or muscular contraction. Some characteristics of specific problems are helpful in this diagnosis.

Disease of the nervous system is most often associated with complete paralysis. Diseases affecting the muscle cells or the factors controlling them are usually associated with a partial rather than complete paralysis-there is weakness rather than a lack of movement. When weakness is severe, however, it may be mistaken for complete paralysis. The fact that diseases of the nervous system cause paralysis of one side of the body (hemiplegia) or one part of the body is helpful in diagnosis. Paralyzing conditions that affect muscle cells tend to result in whole-body weakness, although some muscles may be more severely affected than others. Another aid in differentiation is that neurologic diseases are almost always associated with some degree of impairment in sensation, while muscular causes are never associated with sensory loss.

Damage to the central nervous system and to the peripheral nervous system can be differentiated by features of the dysfunction. Central nervous system problems affect either half of the body or one region of the body, while peripheral damage affects only the muscles controlled by the damaged nerve or nerves. Central nervous system damage leaves pronounced reflexes, while damage to peripheral nerves results in an affected area without any reflexes. There is some muscle wasting with either type of paralysis, but the wasting seen after a peripheral nerve disease appears more quickly and more severely. When central nervous system damage occurs, the muscles involved are generally tight (spastic paralysis). Conversely, in patients with peripheral nervous system damage, muscles are usually loose. Through attention to these differentiating features, the source of paralysis can usually be discovered.

In adults, the most common cause of paralysis is stroke. A stroke results from interruption of the blood supply to a part of the brain. After being cut off from blood flow, the affected area dies. Brain tumors may also cause paralysis. Unlike strokes, however, which cause most of their damage as soon as the blood supply is interrupted, the damage produced by tumors tends to increase slowly as the tumor grows. An interesting feature of brain tumors is that they are surrounded by an area of swelling called edema. The edema, not the tumor itself, causes most of the neurologic changes. This distinction is important because edema is usually responsive to medical treatment.

Subdural hematomas are collections of blood that are outside the brain but inside the skull. They are seen most frequently in older people and alcoholics. To form a subdural hematoma, a small blood vessel becomes injured in such a way that blood slowly oozes from it, accumulates, and clots. Interestingly, the trauma may be so slight as to not be remembered by the patient. This clot may cause

pressure on the motor cortex that results in paralysis. Generally, subdural hematomas are slow in onset.

Multiple sclerosis, a disease affecting the nervous system, causes scattered, multiple small areas of destruction virtually anywhere in the brain or spinal cord. The extent of paralysis depends on the sites and extent of the damaged areas. Patients often have impairments in vision, speaking, sensation, and coordination.

If the spinal cord is the cause, the extent and location of the paralysis and numbness depend on the size, location, and level of the lesion. Spinal cord paralysis may result from trauma, tumors, interruption of blood flow, blood clots, or infections such as abscesses. These disorders are similar, except for location, in most respects to the previously described conditions in the brain. One of the conditions, however-trauma of the spinal cord-is very different from trauma of the brain.

Significant trauma may result in fracture of the vertebral column. Spinal fractures may be classified as stable or unstable. Unstable fractures, unlike stable ones, are often associated with paralysis because unstable fractures allow subluxation to occur. Subluxation is a dislocation of the vertebral column that compresses the spinal cord. If it occurs in the neck, quadriplegia (paralysis of all four limbs) results. If it occurs lower down the spine, paraplegia (paralysis of both lower limbs) is seen. On occasion, through inadvertent or excessive movement, overenthusiastic rescuers cause permanent paralysis by converting a nonsubluxated fracture to a subluxated one during rescue attempts.

Another unique type of spinal cord trauma is the rupture of an intervertebral disk, which allows the gelatinous material to press on the spinal cord or on the rami leaving the spinal cord. In addition to causing severe pain, an intervertebral disk rupture may cause weakness or paralysis. It usually affects only one or two rami and spares the spinal cord itself. Trauma to the spinal cord is particularly dangerous to individuals with conditions that weaken the bony spine. These conditions include osteoporosis of all types and rheumatoid arthritis.

Peripheral nerve damage can occur through a number of conditions that may result in nerve degeneration, including diabetes mellitus, vitamin deficiencies, use or abuse of certain medications, and poisoning by toxins such as alcohol and lead. Sometimes, a temporary nerve degeneration called Guillain-Barré syndrome follows upper respiratory tract infections and may be quite serious if the respiratory muscles are affected. A peripheral nerves may also be damaged by direct trauma, or by pressure as it passes through a narrow compartment, as happens in carpal tunnel syndrome. Peripheral nerve conditions are accompanied by numbness, tingling, and weakness or paralysis of only the area served by the affected nerve.

Paralysis may complicate diseases affecting muscles, although in these cases the patients usually demonstrate weakness rather than paralysis. In muscular diseases, the paralysis (or weakness) tends to affect all the muscles of the body, although some may be more affected than others. The most frequent causes of paralysis in children are inherited diseases such as muscular dystrophy. In adults, muscular diseases are mainly attributable to hormonal imbalances caused by problems such as an underactive thyroid gland or an overactive adrenal gland.

Paralysis may result if the concentration of certain substances in the body is significantly altered, although weakness is a much more common occurrence. The concentration of potassium, sodium, calcium, glucose, and specific hormones may dramatically affect muscle strength. A specific, though uncommon, disease of this type is periodic hypokalemic paralysis, a condition that runs in families. In this disorder, the amount of potassium in the blood can be dramatically reduced for short periods of time, resulting in brief periods of severe weakness or paralysis. These episodes rarely have serious consequences.

Weakness or paralysis may result if the body is unable to produce adequate amounts of acetylcholine, or if this neurotransmitter is destroyed in the synapse before it can pass on its message. Myasthenia gravis is the most common example of this type of disorder. Affected patients initially have adequate strength, but they develop weakness and paralysis in muscles during periods of use because acetylcholine stores become depleted. The weakness in this condition tends to become more prominent as the day wears on. The most frequently used muscles are the most affected. This type of paralysis temporarily improves after rest or medication.

Another unique type of paralysis, called Todd's paralysis, may follow a generalized epileptic seizure. It happens only when the seizure has been so extensive and prolonged that the nerve cells in the brain are literally exhausted and no longer able to initiate the nerve impulses needed to generate movements. This paralysis is temporary.

Paralysis may be caused by a variety of psychiatric disorders, including hysteria, catatonic psychosis, conversion disorder, factitious disorder, and somatization disorder. In psychological paralysis, the patient's inability to move parts of the body is psychological. This paralysis is particularly common during periods of high stress such as combat. Psychological paralysis should be differentiated from malingering. In a psychological paralysis, the patients genuinely believe that they are paralyzed, whereas malingerers, though they deny it, know that they are not paralyzed. Malingering is usually seen when some benefit resulting from the paralysis is anticipated.

Perspective and Prospects

Once a nerve cell has been destroyed, it cannot be repaired. This is the main reason that the outlook is quite poor when most types of paralysis occur. The only thing that doctors can do is to try to limit the extent of the paralysis. Improvements can be made only by training the neighboring cells to take over the functions of the lost cells.

After suffering a paralyzing event, a patient begins rehabilitation using a number of exercises. These activities are usually carried out with the help of physical therapists, occupational therapists, or kinesiotherapists. Unfortunately, progress is rather limited, and most patients are not able to resume their old lifestyle after suffering extensive paralysis.

It is very important to take seriously paralysis or weakness that is localized to a single muscle or single group of muscles. Doctors need to find out the cause of this weakness as soon as possible and take steps to minimize or reverse the damage prior to complete destruction of the nerve cells. Initial and subsequent stroke prevention, tumor treatments, hematoma evacuation, spinal alignment and stabilization, intervertebral disk surgery, toxin removal, hormonal manipulation, and ion correction are all currently available methods of dealing with paralysis.

Because of the poor prognosis for overcoming paralysis, research has focused on understanding how nerve cells grow. Some lower animals possess an ability to regenerate nerve cells when they are damaged. It is well known that a lobster which has lost one of its claws can regenerate that claw, as well as the nerves that control the claw's functioning. A lower animal nerve growth factor has been identified and is being examined by a number of researchers. It is likely that drugs which could aid regeneration of damaged nerve cells in higher animals will be discovered. Once available, these drugs will improve the outlook for recovery of patients with paralysis. These medications may also help with other conditions associated with nerve cell damage, such as Alzheimer's disease and Parkinson's disease.

Progress in medical treatment and an increased health awareness by the public will reduce the incidence of diseases such as diabetes mellitus and the intake of toxins, such as alcohol, that may cause paralysis. Seat belt laws and motorcycle helmet laws may reduce the incidence of paralysis by reducing the severity of injuries in motor vehicle accidents.

Progress in neurosurgery should also improve a patient's hope for recovery in trauma cases. Although dead nerve cells cannot regenerate, cut nerve filaments may be able to regenerate and reattach, which is why surgeons have been able to reattach severed limbs. With progressively finer techniques and equipment, the success rate should improve further. Future progress in neurosurgery may also benefit patients whose paralysis is attributable to causes other than trauma. Progress in genetic research may allow scientists to isolate the genes responsible for diseases causing paralysis. Diseases such as myasthenia gravis and muscular dystrophy could respond to treatment if genetic therapies are found.

—*Ronald C. Hamdy, M.D., Mark R. Doman, M.D., and Katherine Hoffman Doman*

See also Amyotrophic lateral sclerosis; Ataxia; Bell's palsy; Botox; Brain; Brain damage; Brain disorders; Brain tumors; Cerebral palsy; Epilepsy; Fracture and dislocation; Guillain-Barré syndrome; Hemiplegia; Motor neuron diseases; Multiple sclerosis; Muscular dystrophy; Nervous system; Neuralgia, neuritis, and neuropathy; Neuroimaging; Neurology; Neurology, pediatric; Neurosurgery; Numbness and tingling; Palsy; Paraplegia; Parkinson's disease; Quadriplegia; Seizures; Spinal cord disorders; Spine, vertebrae, and disks; Strokes.

For Further Information:

Bear, Mark F., Barry W. Connors, and Michael A. Paradiso. *Neuroscience: Exploring the Brain*. 3d ed. Philadelphia: Lippincott Williams & Wilkins, 2009.

Christopher and Dana Reeve Foundation, Paralysis Resource Center. http://www.christopherreeve.org.

Cure Paralysis Now. http://www.cureparalysisnow.org.

Goroll, Allan H., and Albert G. Mulley, eds. *Primary Care Medicine*. 5th ed. Philadelphia: Lippincott Williams & Wilkins, 2006.

Kandel, Eric R., James H. Schwartz, and Thomas M. Jessell. *Principles of Neural Science*. 5th ed. New York: McGraw-Hill Medical, 2013.

Lukas, Rimas. "Quadriplegia and Paraplegia." *Health Library*, March 15, 2013.

MedlinePlus. "Paralysis." *MedlinePlus*, August 9, 2013.

Nicholls, John G., A. Robert Martin, and Bruce G. Wallace. *From Neuron to Brain*. 5th ed. Sunderland, Mass.: Sinauer Associates, 2012.

"Progress for the Paralyzed." *MedlinePlus Magazine* 8, no. 1 (Spring, 2013): 10.

Tortora, Gerard J. *Principles of Anatomy and Physiology*. 14th ed. [S.I.]: John Wiley & Sons, 2013.

Paramedics

Specialty

Anatomy or system affected: All

Specialties and related fields: Cardiology, critical care, emergency medicine, geriatrics and gerontology, pulmonary medicine

Definition: Trained professional emergency medical technicians (EMTs) who provide sophisticated advanced life support in the field, especially intravenous therapy, cardiac monitoring, drug administration, cardiac defibrillation, and advanced airway management.

Key terms:

advanced life support (ALS): procedures such as intravenous therapy, pharmacology, cardiac monitoring, and defibrillation

basic life support (BLS): simple emergency lifesaving procedures that can aid a person in respiratory or circulatory failure

cardiopulmonary resuscitation (CPR): the artificial establishment of circulation of the blood and movement of air into and out of the lungs in a pulseless, nonbreathing patient

certification: the formal notice of certain privileges and abilities after completion of specified training and testing

defibrillation: the termination of atrial or ventricular fibrillation (irregular heart muscle contractions), with restoration of the normal rhythm

emergency medical services (EMS): the combined efforts of several professionals and agencies to provide prehospital emergency care to the sick and injured

intravenous therapy: the introduction of medication into a vein with a special needle

intubation: the introduction of a tube into a body cavity, as into the larynx

Science and Profession

Emergency medical technician-paramedics (EMT-Ps) provide hospital emergency care in the field under medical command authority to acutely ill and/or injured patients and then transport those patients to the hospital by ambulance or other appropriate vehicle. The clinical knowledge possessed by the EMT-P includes the following systems and areas: the cardiovascular system, including the recognition of arrhythmias, myocardial ischemia, and congestive heart failure; the respiratory system, including acute airway obstruction, pneumothorax, chronic obstructive pulmonary disease (COPD), and respiratory distress; trauma to the head, neck, chest, spine, abdomen, pelvis, and extremities; medical emergencies, including acute abdominal infections, diabetes mellitus, and allergic reactions; the central nervous system, including strokes, seizures, and alterations in levels of consciousness; obstetrical emergencies such as eclampsia; pediatric cases, including croup, epiglottitis, dehydration, child abuse, and care of the newborn; psychiatric emergencies, including problems with individuals who are suicidal, assaultive, destructive, resistant, anxious, confused, amnesiac, or paranoid; drug-related problems, including alcoholism, drug addiction, or overdoses; sexual assault and abuse; and various special situations, such as carbon monoxide and other noxious inhalations, poisoning, near drownings, overexposure to heat and cold, electrocution, burns, and exposure to hazardous materials.

The EMT-P must be able to fulfill many roles. First, paramedics must recognize a medical emergency, assess the situation, manage emergency care, and, if needed, extricate the patient. They must also coordinate their efforts with those of other agencies that may be involved in the care and transport of the patient. Paramedics should establish a good rapport with patients and their significant others in order to decrease their state of anxiety.

The next step is to assign priorities to emergency treatment data for the designated medical control authority. Emergency treatment priorities must be assigned in cases where the medical direction is interrupted by communication failure or in cases of immediate, life-threatening conditions. Paramedics must record and communicate pertinent information to the designated medical command authority.

Meanwhile, they must initiate and continue emergency medical care under medical control, including the recognition of presenting conditions and the initiation of appropriate treatments. Such conditions include traumatic and medical emergencies, airway and ventilation problems, cardiac arrhythmias or standstill, and psychological crises. Paramedics must also assess the response of patients to treatment, modifying the medical therapy as directed by the medical control authority. EMT-Ps exercise personal judgment; provide such emergency medical care as has been specifically authorized in advance; direct and coordinate the transport of the patient by selecting the best available methods in concert with the medical command authority; record, in writing, the details related to the patient's emergency care and the incident; and direct the maintenance and preparation of emergency care equipment and supplies.

EMT-Ps must have a good working knowledge of human anatomy and must be familiar with its topographical language. Even though paramedics are not expected to diagnose every injury or illness, they can aid emergency department personnel by conveying correct information using medical terminology. Such information is gathered after examination of a patient at the scene of an accident or sudden illness.

The most important functions of the paramedic are to identify and treat any life-threatening conditions first and then to assess the patient carefully for other complaints or findings that may require emergency treatment or transportation to a hospital setting. Paramedics must distinguish between signs (measured information such as pulse, respiration, and temperature) and symptoms (patient complaints). They must be able to take complete patient histories, document all medications, and transfer this information to medical control.

The vital role of the respiratory system is stressed in all paramedical training courses. The function of the respiratory system is to provide the body with oxygen and to eliminate carbon dioxide. Paramedics must fully understand the breathing process, including gas exchange and the role and anatomic position of the air passages and lungs. They must understand the mechanics of breathing-how the diaphragm and intercostal muscles contract and relax during inspiration and expiration-and must realize that breathing is controlled by the brain's response to levels of carbon dioxide and oxygen present in the arterial blood. Of special concern

to the paramedic is the patient with COPD, who needs specialized oxygen support and careful watching.

Basic life support (BLS), formerly called cardiopulmonary resuscitation (CPR), is a series of emergency lifesaving procedures that are carried out in order to treat respiratory arrest, cardiac arrest, or both. CPR is a method of providing artificial ventilation and circulation. Its effectiveness depends on the prompt recognition of respiratory and/or cardiac arrest and the immediate start of treatment. Very often, the paramedic is able to defibrillate the patient immediately after cardiac arrest and restart the heart. Knowledge of how to provide BLS to the laryngectomy patient is part of paramedic education; in such cases, ventilation is often given via a stoma (opening) in the neck of the patient. Basic life support procedures must be modified for infants and children, since their respiration and pulse rates are higher than those of adults and require more rapid delivery of ventilatory and cardiac assistance.

Although breathing and heart rate are the primary interests of the paramedic, serious bleeding can also be life-threatening. Hence, paramedics must be well versed in blood circulation routes, control of bleeding, and the pressure points that can help in the control of serious hemorrhage. Serious bleeding often brings on a type of shock that is termed hypovolemic (meaning low blood volume). Paramedics must be alert to signs of impending shock and deal

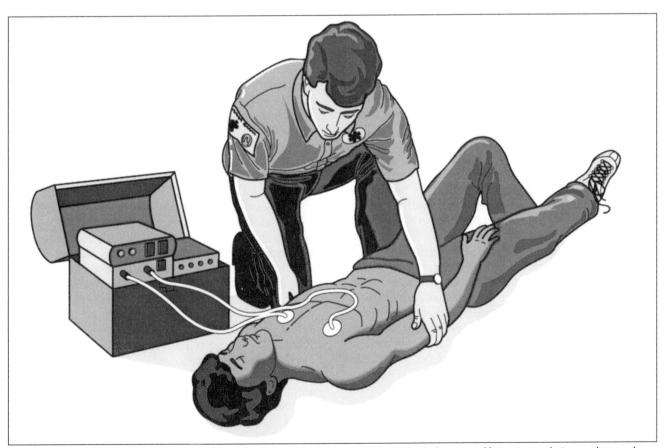

Paramedics administer emergency care in the field to sick or injured patients; among their primary tools are portable monitoring devices, such as an electrocardiograph (ECG or EKG) machine to check the electrical activity of the heart.

with this condition as soon as possible. Medical antishock trousers (MAST) are often used by paramedics to autotransfuse volumes of blood from the patient's lower extremities to the heart, lungs, and brain. These trousers are also used to control severe hemorrhage or the complications of pelvic fractures. The paramedic must be aware of the contraindications to the use of these devices as well; for example, persons with head injuries should not have the MAST device applied to them.

Paramedics need to identify the many types of shock. Anaphylactic shock is caused by an unusual or exaggerated allergic reaction of a person to a foreign protein. Psychogenic shock (fainting) is often self-correcting. Septic shock is caused by severe bacterial infections, while metabolic shock may arise from severe, untreated illnesses. Cardiogenic shock arises from an underlying cardiac condition and inefficient blood flow. In each case, the paramedic must be alert to the signs of each type of shock and be prepared to treat it, either with drugs delivered under medical control or with equipment present on the paramedic ambulance.

The more common types of injuries encountered by the paramedic are soft tissue injuries, caused by falls or accidents. The skin is the largest single organ of the body. It protects the body from the environment, regulates the body temperature, and transmits information from the environment to the brain. Soft tissue injuries can cause breaks in the skin, leaving the body vulnerable to infection and bleeding. Paramedic training includes treatment for massive traumatic wounds, such as gunshot or knife wounds.

Dealing with fractures is another part of paramedic training. While most fractures are not life-threatening, they can be painful and bring on patient shock; hence, paramedics need to deal with them quickly. Knowledge of the body's musculoskeletal system is vital to the performance of a paramedic.

Head injuries are a very challenging part of paramedic treatment, since the scalp contains many blood vessels and bleeding from head injuries is often profuse. The more serious head injury is often bloodless externally, but internal bleeding brings on pressure buildup in the skull and sudden coma. Such injuries are life-threatening and often require rapid treatment and transport.

Other medical emergencies include strokes (cerebrovascular accidents), diabetic coma or insulin shock, acute abdominal infections, and seizures. Prompt recognition and treatment by the paramedic are essential. Finally, treating the pediatric patient can be one of the most difficult emergencies, but saving a child's life or rescuing a child from permanent, disabling injury is very rewarding. The broad range of knowledge required of paramedics makes them a very special part of the health care team.

Diagnostic and Treatment Techniques

Three technologies that distinguish the paramedic from the basic EMT are intravenous therapy, advanced airway management, and defibrillation.

Intravenous (IV) therapy may be an important procedure during the resuscitation of a patient who is suffering from hypovolemia, burn injury, blood loss, heatstroke, shock, electrolyte imbalance, or many other medical and surgical conditions. IV therapy is also important in providing an avenue of medication delivery in many medical situations, such as cardiac arrest, seizures, and asthma attacks. IV therapy is an invasive procedure that requires extensive training in its use in order for the paramedic to maintain the necessary skill level. In addition, paramedics must be aware of the indication for the use of IV therapy, the maintenance of such therapy, and possible complications.

IV therapy works via the infusion of fluid other than blood or blood products into the vascular system. This technique is used to establish and maintain direct access to the circulation or to provide fluids in order to maintain an adequate circulating blood volume. Fluids used for IVs are often referred to as electrolyte solutions, because the chemical compounds they contain are electrolytes. The most common electrolyte solutions used are sodium chloride solutions; for example, NS is a normal saline solution containing 0.9 percent sodium chloride. Occasionally, paramedics use plasma expanders or colloids, including Dextran. A common intravenous fluid is D5W, which is a 5-percent dextrose solution. The procedure for starting an IV includes preparing the solution, selecting the proper catheter size, selecting and preparing the site, and performing the venipuncture (insertion of a needle into a vein). Local complications to IV therapy may include some pain from the needlestick, hematoma formation at failed IV sites, infection, accidental arterial puncture, nerve damage, and thrombophlebitis. Environmental complications include cold climates, which cause IV solutions to freeze, and the danger of a needlestick to medical personnel during disposal. Proper precautions and periodic retraining keep paramedics up to date in their skills.

Advanced airway management means placing a tube into the patient's airway to maintain an open passage, to prevent aspiration of foreign bodies and stomach contents, and to allow the delivery of oxygen-enriched air. Three types of devices are employed in advanced airway management to achieve these objectives: the endotracheal tube (ENT), the esophageal obturator airway (EOA), and the pharyngeotracheal airway. The use of any of these devices by paramedics requires the consent of a medical director and adherence to written protocols. These devices require skill and instruction for proper insertion and use.

The ENT is placed through a patient's mouth or nose and directly through the larynx between the vocal cords. The tube may be placed blindly through the vocal cords using sounds of labored respirations as a guide, or it may be placed by feel through the cords. After placement, a soft balloon cuff near the end of the tube is then inflated with approximately 10 cubic centimeters of air to seal the trachea and anchor the tube, so that air can be blown directly into the lungs. The ENT prevents aspiration and gastric distension. It facilitates airway suctioning and enables the delivery of high volumes of oxygen at higher-than-normal pressures. In addition, certain medications may be given down the tube. ENT placement and use are difficult skills to master, requiring considerable practice and expert initial instruction. Direct visualization of the vocal cords is an important skill to have in order to prevent tracheal damage. If intubation takes too long, the resulting delay in oxygenation may lead to brain damage. Constant monitoring of lung sounds is needed to ensure that the tube stays in place.

The EOA has been in use since 1973 to facilitate airway management in cardiopulmonary resuscitation. The EOA is a plastic, semirigid tube approximately 30 centimeters long and 13 millimeters in diameter. The lower end of the tube is smooth, rounded, and closed. The upper third of the EOA is designed to function as an airway. It has sixteen holes in its wall at the junction of the middle and upper sections; when properly inserted, these holes will lie at the level of the pharynx and provide free passage of oxygen-enriched air to the lungs. The lower two-thirds of the EOA should lie in the esophagus. The balloon surrounding the end of the tube is normally inflated to block the esophagus and prevent the regurgitation of stomach contents backward into the airway. The face mask that comes with the EOA is designed to fit snugly about the patient's nose and mouth and must provide a tight seal. The EOA is used only for short-term airway management. It should be removed when the unconscious patient awakens and is able to protect the airway or when ENT placement has been performed over the EOA. At the time that the balloon is deflated and the EOA is removed, there is a high risk of vomiting and/or regurgitation of gastric contents. The EOA is not to be used on patients who are awake, on small children, or on patients with known esophageal disease.

The pharyngeotracheal airway is designed to provide lung ventilation when placed in either the trachea or the esophagus. This device is designed to be inserted blindly into the oropharynx and esophagus by paramedics who have received training and are authorized to use it. A pharyngeotracheal airway is contraindicated in conscious or semiconscious patients with a gag reflex. It should not be used with children under the age of fourteen or with adults under five feet tall.

With the use of any of these airway devices, the patient may regain consciousness while intubated. Such patients will usually gag, choke, and grasp at the device in an attempt to remove it, often resulting in injury to the airway. The patient's hands must be immediately restrained while the airway device is removed.

Defibrillation is the delivery of an electric current through a person's chest wall and heart for the purpose of ending ventricular fibrillation. The device used for this procedure is called a defibrillator (also automated external defibrillator or AED); it is typically a portable, battery-powered instrument that is used to record cardiac rhythm and to generate and deliver an electrical charge. Defibrillation can be a lifesaving measure in the treatment of sudden cardiac arrest in which the heart is in an arrhythmia known as ventricular fibrillation or ventricular tachycardia (VT). These two conditions occur when cardiac muscle becomes oxygen deficient or is injured or dies,

causing the electrical system of the heart to be disturbed. Sometimes, the injured area of the heart begins to fire off uncoordinated electrical impulses. These irregular impulses can initiate abnormal beats called premature ventricular contractions (PVCs). If several of the PVCs occur close together, they produce the rhythm called ventricular tachycardia. If VT does not spontaneously convert back to a normal heart rhythm, it rapidly degenerates into ventricular fibrillation. The heart in VT beats faster and faster until its oxygen supply is depleted, at which point tissue injury begins and electrical impulses become completely uncoordinated and are fired at random.

If a defibrillator is applied to the patient and an electrical shock is given to the heart during the time of ventricular fibrillation, there is a good chance of restoring more normal electrical activity. This electrical countershock is thought to depolarize the cardiac muscle and conducting tissues instantaneously, thus resetting the electrical energies to the depolarized state. The patient's heart can then begin its normal conduction and contractions without having to contend with randomly generated electrical impulses. The electrical current delivered by defibrillators is measured in units called joules. In most protocols, the first shock is 200 joules, the second is between 200 and 300 joules, and the third and subsequent shocks are at the full 360-joule level. Paramedics using defibrillators need frequent continuing education in order to emphasize the practical skills of proper attachment of the electrodes, proper device operation, and recognition of cardiac arrhythmias.

Perspective and Prospects

Emergency medical services (EMS) in the United States had its beginnings in 1966. In that year, the Committees on Trauma and Shock of the National Academy of Sciences National Research Council jointly published *Accidental Death and Disability: The Neglected Disease of Modern Society*. This joint report brought public attention to the inadequate emergency medical care being provided to the injured and sick in many parts of the United States. Two federal agencies initiated reform measures: The Department of Transportation (DOT) initiated the Highway Safety Act in 1966, and the Department of Health, Education, and Welfare enacted the Emergency Medical Services Act in 1973. Both created funding sources to develop prehospital emergency care in an effort to eliminate the majority of prehospital deaths. Local EMS systems were established in the early 1970s. In the 1980s, practitioners took a hard look at what had been done in the past, and the focus changed from establishing EMS systems to developing educational programs to provide consistent levels of quality care to the sick and injured.

The EMS system is made up of various components that work together to provide the sick and injured with the best possible emergency care in the shortest possible time. The EMS system represents the combined efforts of the first responder, the EMT with basic life support skills, the EMT-paramedic with advanced life support skills, emergency department personnel, physicians, allied health personnel, hospital administrators, EMS system administrators, and the overseeing governmental agencies.

Emergency medical technology is an exciting field of study. Few areas offer more direct application of theory and skills. All the information received in an EMT class will be important when it comes to saving lives and lessening human suffering. Emergency medical technology combines theoretical information, practical skills, and common sense. Above all, the EMS person dealing with a patient must possess great compassion and understanding.

The certification of an EMT-paramedic is formal notice of certain privileges and abilities after the completion of specific training and testing. The possession of a certificate obligates the individual to conform to the standard of care of other certified emergency medical care personnel. Nearly every state exempts emergency medical care from the licensure requirements of the Medical Practices Act for nonmedical personnel. (Because many emergency medical care procedures may be construed by the public to be the performance of a medical act, the EMT must be protected legally in those situations.) The need for prehospital care providers is ongoing, and recruiting people to enter this field continues to be a challenge to the agencies that oversee this work.

—Jane A. Slezak, Ph.D.

See also Accidents; Arrhythmias; Burns and scalds; Cardiac arrest; Cardiopulmonary resuscitation (CPR); Choking; Critical care; Critical care, pediatric; Drowning; Electrocardiography (ECG or EKG); Emergency medicine; First aid; Fracture and dislocation; Heart attack; Heat exhaustion and heatstroke; Intravenous (IV) therapy; Respiration; Resuscitation; Shock; Strokes; Tracheostomy; Wounds.

For Further Information:

American Academy of Orthopaedic Surgeons. *Emergency Care and Transportation of the Sick and Injured.* Edited by Benjamin Gulli, Les Chatelain, and Chris Stratford. 10th ed. Sudbury, Mass.: Jones and Bartlett, 2011.

"EMTs and Paramedics." *Occupational Outlook Handbook.* Bureau of Labor Statistics, March 29, 2012.

Hamilton, Glenn C., et al. *Emergency Medicine: An Approach to Clinical Problem-Solving.* 2d ed. New York: W. B. Saunders, 2003.

Limmer, Daniel, et al. *Emergency Care.* 12th ed. Upper Saddle River, N.J.: Pearson/Prentice Hall Health, 2012.

Markovchick, Vincent J., and Peter T. Pons, eds. *Emergency Medicine Secrets.* 5th ed. Philadelphia: Mosby/Elsevier, 2011.

Rella, Francis J. *Manhattan Medics: The Gripping Story of the Men and Women of Emergency Medical Services Who Make the Streets of the City Their Career.* Hightstown, N.J.: Princeton Book Company, 2003.

Sanders, Mick J. *Mosby's Paramedic Textbook.* 4th ed. St. Louis, Mo.: Mosby/Elsevier, 2012.

Shapiro, Paul D., and Mary B. Shapiro. *Paramedic: The True Story of a New York Paramedic's Battles with Life and Death.* New York: Bantam Books, 1991.

Tangherlini, Timothy R. *Talking Trauma: Paramedics and Their Stories.* Jackson: University Press of Mississippi, 1998.

Paranoia

Disease/Disorder

Anatomy or system affected: Psychic-emotional system
Specialties and related fields: Psychiatry, psychology
Definition: Pervasive distrust and suspiciousness of others and a tendency to interpret others' motives as malevolent.

Causes and Symptoms

Paranoia is characterized by suspiciousness, heightened self-awareness, self-reference, projection of one's ideas onto others, expectations of persecution, and blaming of others for one's difficulties. Conversely, though paranoia can be problematic, it can also be adaptive. In threatening or dangerous situations, paranoia might instigate proactive protective behavior, allowing an individual to negotiate a situation without harm. Thus, paranoia must be assessed in context for it to be understood fully.

Paranoia can be experienced at varying levels of intensity in both normal and highly disordered individuals. As a medical problem, paranoia may take the face of a symptom, personality problem, or chronic mental disorder. As a symptom, it may be evidenced as a fleeting problem; an individual might have paranoid feelings that dissipate in a relatively brief period of time once an acute medical or situational problem is rectified.

As a personality problem, paranoia creates significant impairment and distress as a result of inflexible, maladaptive, and persistent use of paranoid coping strategies. Paranoid individuals often have preoccupations about loyalties, overinterpret situations, maintain expectations of exploitation or deceit, rarely confide in others, bear grudges, perceive attacks that are not apparent to others, and maintain unjustified suspicions about their relationship partner's potential for betrayal. They are prone to angry outbursts, aloof, and controlling, and they may demonstrate a tendency toward vengeful fantasies or actual revenge.

Finally, paranoia may be evidenced as a chronic mental disorder, most notably as the paranoid type of schizophrenia. In paranoid schizophrenia, there is a tendency toward delusions (faulty beliefs involving misinterpretations of events) and auditory hallucinations. Additionally, everyday behavior, speech, and emotional responsiveness are not as disturbed as in other variants of schizophrenia. Typically, individuals suffering from paranoia are seen by oth-

---

Information on Paranoia

Causes: May include psychological disorder (depression, schizophrenia), situational stress, drug intoxication or withdrawal, head injury, organic brain syndromes, pernicious anemia, B vitamin deficiencies, Klinefelter syndrome

Symptoms: Pervasive distrust and suspiciousness of others, tendency to interpret others' motives as malevolent, aloofness, heightened self-awareness, self-reference, blaming of others for one's difficulties, angry outbursts, controlling behavior

Duration: Acute to chronic

Treatments: Drug therapy, community-based therapy, cognitive and behavioral therapies

ers as anxious, angry, and aloof. Their delusions usually reflect fears of persecution or hopes for greatness, resulting in jealousies, odd religious beliefs (such as persecution by God, thinking they are Jesus Christ), or preoccupations with their own health (such as the fear of being poisoned or of having a medical disorder of mysterious origin).

Paranoia may best be understood as being determined by a combination of biological, psychological, and environmental factors. It is likely, for example, that certain basic psychological tendencies must be present for an individual to display paranoid feelings and behavior when under stress, as opposed to other feelings such as depression. Additionally, it is likely that certain physical predispositions must be present for stressors to provoke a psychophysiological response.

Biologically, there are myriad physical and mental health conditions that may trigger acute and more chronic paranoid reactions. High levels of situational stress, drug intoxication (such as with amphetamines or marijuana), drug withdrawal, depression, head injuries, organic brain syndromes, pernicious anemia, B vitamin deficiencies, and Klinefelter syndrome may be related to acute paranoia. Similarly, certain cancers, insidious organic brain syndromes, and hyperparathyroidism have been related to recurrent or chronic episodes of paranoia.

In terms of the etiology of chronic paranoid conditions, such as paranoid schizophrenia and paranoid personality disorder, no clear causes have been identified. Some evidence points to a genetic component; the results of studies on twins and the greater prevalence of these disorders in some families support this view. More psychological theories highlight the family environment and emotional expression, childhood abuse, and stress. In general, these theories point to conditions contributing toward making a person feel insecure, tense, hungry for recognition, and hypervigilant. Additionally, the impact of social, cultural, and economic conditions contributing to the expression of paranoia is important. Paranoia cannot be interpreted out of context. Biological, psychological, and environmental factors must be considered in the development and maintenance of paranoia.

Treatment and Therapy

Three major types of therapies are available to treat paranoia: pharmacotherapies, community-based therapies, and cognitive-behavioral therapies. For acute paranoia problems and the management of more chronic, schizophrenia-related paranoia, pharmacotherapy (the use of drugs) is the treatment of choice. Drugs that serve to tranquilize the individual and reduce disorganized thinking, such as antipsychotics, phenothiazines and other neuroleptics, are commonly used. With elderly people who cannot tolerate such drugs, electroconvulsive therapy (ECT) has been used for treatment.

Community-based treatment, such as day treatment or inpatient treatment, is also useful for treating chronic paranoid conditions. Developing corrective and instructional social experiences, decreasing situational stress, and helping individuals to feel safe in a treatment environment are

primary goals.

Finally, cognitive-behavioral therapies focused on identifying irrational beliefs contributing to paranoia-related problems have demonstrated some utility. Skillful therapists help to identify maladaptive thinking while unearthing concerns but not agreeing with the individual's delusional ideas.

Perspective and Prospects

Certain life phases and social and cultural contexts influence behaviors that could be labeled as paranoid. Membership in certain minority or ethnic groups, immigrant or political refugee status, and, more generally, language and other cultural barriers may account for behavior that appears to be guarded or paranoid. As such, one can make few assumptions about paranoia without a thorough assessment.

Clinically significant paranoia is notable across cultures, with prevalence rates at any point in time ranging from 0.5 to 2.5 percent of the population. It is a problem manifested by diverse etiological courses requiring equally diverse treatments. Increased knowledge about the relationship among paranoia, depression and other mood disorders, schizophrenia, and the increased prevalence of paranoid disorders in some families will be critical. As the general population ages, a better understanding of more acute paranoid disorders related to medical problems will also be necessary. Better understanding will facilitate the development of more effective pharmacological and nonpharmacological treatments that can be tolerated by the elderly and others suffering from compromising medical problems.

—*Nancy A. Piotrowski, Ph.D.*

See also Antianxiety drugs; Anxiety; Delusions; Hallucinations; Post-traumatic stress disorder; Psychiatric disorders; Psychiatry; Psychiatry, child and adolescent; Psychiatry, geriatric; Psychoanalysis; Schizophrenia; Shock therapy; Stress.

For Further Information:

Anderson F., and D. Freeman. "Socioeconomic Status and Paranoia: The Role of Life Hassles, Self-Mastery, and Striving to Avoid Inferiority." *The Journal of Nervous and Mental Disorders* 201, no. 8 (August, 2013): 698-702.

Barlow, David H., ed. *Clinical Handbook of Psychological Disorders*. 4th ed. New York: Guilford Press, 2008.

Bloom, Floyd E., M. Flint Beal, and David J. Kupfer, eds. *The Dana Guide to Brain Health*. New York: Dana Press, 2006.

Ellett, L. "Mindfulness for Paranoid Beliefs: Evidence From Two Case Studies." *Behavioural and Cognitive Psychotherapy* 41, no. 2 (2013): 238-242.

Graham, George. *The Disordered Mind: An Introduction to Philosophy of Mind and Mental Illness*. New York: Routledge, 2013.

Kring, Ann M., et al. *Abnormal Psychology*. 11th ed. Hoboken: John Wiley & Sons, 2010.

Munro, Alistair. *Delusional Disorder: Paranoia and Related Illnesses*. New York: Cambridge University Press, 1999.

Robbins, Michael. *Experiences of Schizophrenia: An Integration of the Personal, Scientific, and Therapeutic*. New York: Guilford Press, 1993.

Siegel, Ronald K. *Whispers: The Voices of Paranoia*. New York: Simon & Schuster, 1996.

Venter, Bruce. *Paranoid Schizophrenia My Label, My Life: How I Escaped the Strait Jacket of Serious Mental Illness.* Bloomington: AuthorHouse, 2012.

Paraplegia

Disease/Disorder
Anatomy or system affected: Legs, nervous system, spine
Specialties and related fields: Neurology
Definition: A motor or sensory loss in the lower extremities, with or without involvement of the abdominal and back muscles.

Information on Paraplegia

Causes: Spinal cord injuries, usually resulting from vehicle or sporting accidents, gunshot wounds, falls
Symptoms: Total or partial paralysis with loss of motion, sensation, and reflexes below lesion; urinary retention; absence of perspiration in paralyzed parts
Duration: Permanent or temporary
Treatments: Spinal alignment and stabilization, laminectomy, drug therapy (nitrofurantoin, vitamin C, analgesics and narcotics)

Causes and Symptoms

Paraplegia, the loss of motor and sensory function in the lower body, results in paralysis that may be complete or incomplete, spastic or flaccid, symmetric or asymmetric, and permanent or temporary. Almost half of the 10,000 to 12,000 spinal cord injuries reported each year result in paraplegia. This condition occurs twice as often in men as in women, and the incidence is highest between ages sixteen and thirty-five. Most spinal cord injuries result from trauma, especially automobile, motorcycle, and sporting accidents; gunshot wounds and falls also contribute. Less common causes are nontraumatic lesions, such as spina bifida, scoliosis, and chordoma.

In many patients, the onset of total or partial paralysis is immediate, resulting in loss of motion, sensation, and reflexes below the level of the lesion, with urinary retention and absence of perspiration in the paralyzed parts. In some patients, careful questioning and gentle examination are necessary to determine the extent of motor or sensory loss. Spinal cord injuries with motor and sensory loss may result in bowel, bladder, and sexual dysfunctions, depending on the level of the lesion and whether damage to the cord is complete or incomplete. In an incomplete spinal cord injury, perianal sensation, voluntary toe flexion, or sphincter control is still present. In a complete spinal cord injury, lack of sensation or voluntary muscle control is apparent and persists for twenty-four hours. Any return of functional muscle power distal to the injury is unlikely.

Diagnosis requires a clinical history, neurologic examination, and computed tomography (CT) scans. A lumbar puncture may rule out blocked cerebrospinal fluid circulation. Laboratory studies include a complete blood count (CBC), prothrombin time, electrolytes, twenty-four-hour urine for creatinine clearance, serum creatinine, and urinalysis. Weekly urine samples for culture and sensitivity are advisable during the entire rehabilitation period.

Treatment and Therapy

The four goals of treatment for any spinal cord injury are restoration of normal alignment for the spine, early assurance of complete stability of the injured spinal area, decompression of compressed neurologic structures, and early rehabilitation to an active and productive life.

Treatment begins at the scene of the accident by not moving the patient until the spine and head have been stabilized through strapping the patient to a board. Even after reaching the hospital, the patient is not removed from the board but placed on a stretcher while still strapped to it. Such stabilization helps prevent reversible damage from becoming permanent through additional injury to the neuraxis. Supportive treatment corrects systemic shock and controls local hemorrhage. Insertion of a Foley catheter ensures uninterrupted urine drainage.

Whenever possible, the care of spinal cord injuries emphasizes conservative treatment, such as closed reduction of fractures. However, unstable fractures and fracture dislocations require fusion following reduction, combined with recumbent immobilization until healing occurs. Bone fragments pressing on the spinal cord may require laminectomy (surgical removal of the vertebral arch). Drug therapy may include nitrofurantoin to prevent bladder infection; large doses of vitamin C to enhance utilization of protein and help minimize infection by acidifying the urine; diazepam, baclofen, or dantrolene sodium to relieve skeletal muscle spasms from upper motor neuron disorders; and, sparingly, analgesics and narcotics to relieve pain. The extent of paralysis cannot be accurately assessed until a year after the spinal cord injury.

—*Jane C. Norman, Ph.D., R.N., C.N.E.*

See also Accidents; Emergency medicine; Hemiplegia; Laminectomy and spinal fusion; Nervous system; Neuralgia, neuritis, and neuropathy; Neuroimaging; Neurology; Neurology, pediatric; Paralysis; Physical rehabilitation; Quadriplegia; Spinal cord disorders; Spine, vertebrae, and disks.

For Further Information:

Asbury, Arthur K., et al., eds. *Diseases of the Nervous System: Clinical Neuroscience and Therapeutic Principles.* 3d ed. New York: Cambridge University Press, 2002.
Bromley, Ida. *Tetraplegia and Paraplegia: A Guide for Physiotherapists.* 6th ed. New York: Churchill Livingstone/Elsevier, 2006.
Fehlings, Michael G. *Essentials of Spinal Cord Injury: Basic Research to Clinical Practice.* New York: Stuttgart, 2013.
Iansek, Robert, and Meg. E. Morris, eds. *Rehabilitation in Movement Disorders.* Cambridge: Cambridge University Press, 2013.
Kohnle, Diana. "Paraplegia." *Health Library,* November 28, 2012.
Victor, Maurice, and Allan H. Ropper. *Adams and Victor's Principles of Neurology.* 9th ed. New York: McGraw-Hill, 2009.

Parasitic diseases

Disease/Disorder
Anatomy or system affected: All
Specialties and related fields: Environmental health, epidemiology, family medicine, internal medicine, public

health, virology

Definition: Diseases borne by parasites, or organisms that live within "host" organisms; parasites travel to their hosts via vectors that may include fleas, mosquitoes, rats, and other animals.

Key terms:

commensalism: a relationship in which one symbiont, the commensal, benefits from a host symbiont, but the host neither benefits nor is harmed by the commensal

host: a living plant or animal harboring or affording subsistence to a parasite

hyperparasitism: a relationship in which parasites act as hosts to other parasites

mutualism: a relationship between symbionts in which both members benefit from the association

parasitism: a relationship in which one symbiont, a parasite, harms its host symbiont or in some way lives at the expense of the host

phoresis: when two symbionts "travel together" but neither is physiologically dependent on the other

symbiont: any organism involved in a symbiotic relationship with another organism

symbiosis: a relationship in which two symbionts live in close association with each other; commonly, one symbiont lives in or on the body of the other

Types of Parasites

Parasites are organisms that take up residence, temporarily or permanently, on or within other living organisms for the purpose of procuring food. They include plants such as bacteria and fungi; animals such as protozoa, helminths (worms), and arthropods; and forms such as spirochetes and microscopic viruses.

The study of parasitism is a study of symbiosis. Symbiosis occurs when two organisms, known as symbionts, live in close association with each other, usually with one organism living in or on the body of the other. Such a living arrangement is called a symbiotic relationship. In a symbiotic relationship, the symbionts are usually, but not always, of different species, and the relationship need not be beneficial or damaging to either organism.

Often, two symbionts will exist together merely as traveling companions. Such a symbiotic relationship is called phoresis. In such cases, neither partner is physiologically dependent on the other, but the smaller of the two organisms has simply attached itself for the ride. Examples of phoresis are bacteria carried on the legs of a cockroach and fungus spores on the feet of ants and beetles.

If a situation exists in which both symbionts benefit from an association, the partnership is referred to as a mutual relationship. In most cases, mutualism is obligatory because both symbionts have evolved to a point at which they are physiologically dependent on each other and the survival of both symbionts requires a continuous interrelationship. Such a relationship exists between termites and the protozoan fauna that live in their guts. Termites are unable to digest cellulose fibers, because their bodies cannot produce the proper enzyme, but protozoa that live in a termite's gut synthesize the ingested cellulose fibers and excrete a fer-

Information on Parasitic Diseases

Causes: Infection with parasites, often through vectors

Symptoms: Wide ranging; may include fever, malaise, vomiting, inflammation, joint pain, muscle aches, diarrhea

Duration: Acute to chronic

Treatments: Drug therapy, supportive care

mented product that nourishes the host termite. The protozoa benefit by living in a stable, secure environment, with a constant supply of food, and the termite is supplied with sustenance.

Another form of mutualism that is not obligatory is called cleaning symbiosis. In this instance, certain animals, called cleaners, remove other parasites, injured tissues, fungi, or invading organisms from a cooperating host. Examples of cleaning relationships include birds that groom the skins of rhinoceroses and the mouths of crocodiles, and tiny shrimp that remove parasites from the body surfaces of fish.

When one symbiont benefits from its relationship with its host but the host neither benefits nor is harmed, the condition is called commensalism. Examples of commensals are pilot fish and remoras, which attach themselves to turtles or other fish, using their hosts as transportation and scavenging food left over when the hosts eat; in no way, however, do they harm their hosts or rob them of food. Another example of commensalism exists between humans and the amoeba *Entamoeba gingivalis*. This amoeba lives in the human mouth, feeding on bacteria, food particles, and dead epithelial cells, but it never harms its human host. The amoeba is transmitted from person to person by direct contact and cannot exist outside the human mouth.

When one member of a symbiotic relationship actually harms its host or in some way lives at the expense of the host, it is then a parasite. The word *parasite* is derived from the Greek *parasitos*, which means "one who eats at another's table" or "one who lives at another's expense." A parasite may harm its host by causing a mechanical injury, such as boring a hole into it; by eating, digesting, or absorbing portions of the host's tissue; by poisoning the host with toxic metabolic products; or by robbing the host of nutrition. It has been found that most parasites inflict a combination of these conditions.

The majority of parasites are obligate parasites-that is, they must spend at least a portion of their lives as parasites to survive and complete their life cycles. Most of these obligate parasites have free-living stages outside their hosts in which they exist in protective cysts or eggs. Certain symbionts are referred to as facultative parasites, which means that the organism is not normally parasitic, but if the proper situation arises, it becomes a parasite. The most common facultative parasites are those that are accidentally eaten or enter a host through a wound or body orifice. One facultative parasite whose infection of humans is almost always fatal is the amoeba *Naegleria*, which is responsible for

Common Human Parasites

Virus	Bacterium	Amoeba
Fungus	Head louse	Bedbug
Cat flea	Tick	Mosquito
Roundworm	Hookworm	Tapeworm

Any organism that, temporarily or permanently, lives on or in another organism for the purpose of procuring food is considered a parasite; these parasites may cause infection in their human hosts.

amebic meningitis. Many obligate parasites are also hyperparasites. Hyperparasitism exists when parasites play host to other parasites; for example, the malaria-causing parasite *Plasmodia* is carried in mosquitoes, and juvenile tapeworms live in fleas.

Parasites that live their entire adult lives within or on their hosts are called permanent parasites. Other parasites, such as mosquitoes and ticks, are called temporary parasites because they feed on their hosts and then leave. Temporary parasites are actually micropredators that prey on different hosts, or on the same host at different times, as the need for nourishment arises. There are many parallels between parasitism and predation in that both parasites and predators live at the expense of their hosts or prey. Parasites, however, do not normally kill their hosts, because to do so results in their own death. It is the mark of a well-adapted parasite to produce as few pathological conditions in the host as possible.

Despite the knowledge that parasites are a major cause of disease, it is wrong to assume that an animal hosting a parasite must ultimately be in danger. The healthiest human or wild animal is probably harboring some type of parasite, and while the host and parasite may live for years without interfering in each other's existence, at any given time, the healthy host can fall victim to a disease brought on by the parasite, or some change in the host may destroy the parasite.

Whether the host reacts to its symbiotic partner with indifference, annoyance, or illness is the result of many factors. The most important is how many parasites are being hosted. A single hookworm takes approximately 0.5 milliliter of blood per day from its host. This is about the same amount of blood lost when one pricks oneself with a needle. This amount of blood loss is so low that the host will never miss it and, in most instances, will not even know that

the parasite is there. If a host harbors five hundred hookworms, however, the blood loss per day becomes 250 milliliters, approximately one half pint, and the result is physically devastating to the host.

Causes and Symptoms

Medical parasitology is the study of human diseases caused by parasitic infection. It is commonly limited to the study of parasitic worms (helminths) and protozoa. The science places nonprotozoan parasites in separate disciplines, such as virology, rickettsiology, and bacteriology. The branches of parasitology known as medical entomology and medical arthropodology deal with insects and noninsect arthropods that serve as hosts and transport agents for parasites, as well as with the noxious effects of these pests. The study of fungi (molds and yeasts), including those that cause human disease, is called mycology.

Throughout history, human welfare has suffered greatly because of parasites. Fleas and bacteria killed one-third of the human population of Europe during the seventeenth century, and malaria, schistosomiasis, and African sleeping sickness have killed additional countless millions. Despite successful medical campaigns against yellow fever, malaria, and hookworm infections worldwide, parasitic diseases in combination with nutritional deficiencies are the primary killers of humans. Medical research suggests that parasitic infections are so widespread that if all the known varieties were evenly distributed among the human population, each living person would have at least one.

Most serious parasitic infections occur in tropical, less modernized regions of the world, and because most of the planet's industrially developed and affluent populations live in temperate regions, many people are unaware of the magnitude of the problem. On an annual basis, 60 million deaths occur worldwide from all causes; of these deaths, half are children under five years of age. Fifty percent of these, 15 million child deaths per year, are directly attributable to a combination of malnutrition and intestinal parasitic infection. It must be noted that less than 15 percent of the world's present population is served by adequate clean water supplies and sewage disposal programs, and that almost all intestinal parasitic infections are the result of ingesting food or water contaminated with human feces.

The transmission of parasitic diseases involves three factors: the source of the infection, the mode of transmission, and the presence of a susceptible host. The combined effect of these factors determines the dispersibility and prevalence of a parasite at a given time and place, thus regulating the incidence of a parasitic disease in a population. Because of host specificity, other humans are the chief source of most human parasitic diseases. The various manifestations of any human parasitic disease are a result of the particular species of parasite involved, its mode of transport, the immunological status of the host, the presence or absence of hosts, and the pattern of exposure.

Humans transmit parasitic diseases to one another through the intestinal tract, nose and mouth, skin and tissue, genitourinary tract, and blood. It is fecal discharge, however, that offers the most convenient and common means for a parasite or its ova and larvae to leave its host, since the majority of parasites inhabit the gastrointestinal tract. For this reason, the proper disposal of fecal material is the most important method of preventing the spread of parasitic disease. Since most parasites inhabit the intestinal tract, food and water are also important means of transmitting parasitic infections. The infective organism may be present in contaminated drinking water, in animal and fish flesh used as food, in human feces used as fertilizer, or on the hands of food handlers.

Arthropods are one of the main sources of parasitic diseases in humans. Arthropods act as both mechanical carriers of and intermediate hosts to many diseases-bacterial, viral, rickettsial, and parasitic-which they transmit to humans. In most tropical countries, basic preventive medicine for many devastating parasitic diseases depends on the control or eradication of insects and arachnids.

There are four major groups of parasites that most often invade human hosts: nematodes, trematodes, cestodes, and protozoa. Most nematodes, or roundworms, are free-living, and nematodes are found in almost every terrestrial and aquatic environment. Most are harmless to humans, but some parasitic nematodes invade the human intestinal tract and cause widespread debilitating diseases. The most prevalent intestinal nematodes are *Ascaris lumbricoides*, which infect the small intestine and affects more than a billion people; the whipworm *Trichuris trichiura*, which infects the colon and is carried by an estimated 500 million individuals; the human hookworms *Necator americanus* and *Ancylostoma duodenale*, which suck blood from the human small intestine and cause major debilitation among undernourished people; and *Enterobius vermicularis*, the human pinworm, which infects the large intestine and is common among millions of urban dwellers because it is easily transmitted from perianal tissue to hand to mouth.

Nonintestinal, tissue-infecting nematodes are spread most often by hyperparasitic bloodsucking insects such as mosquitoes, biting flies, and midges. The most common tissue-infecting nematode is *Trichinella spiralis*, the pork or trichina worm, which is the agent of trichinosis. Other important parasitic nematodes include *Onchocerca volvulus*, which is transmitted by blackflies in tropical regions and causes blindness, and the mosquito-transmitted filarial worms that are responsible for elephantiasis.

Trematodes, or flatworms, are commonly called flukes. Flukes vary greatly in size, form, and host living location, but all of them initially develop in freshwater snails. The human intestinal fluke, the oriental liver fluke, and the human lung fluke are all transmitted to humans by the ingestion of raw or undercooked aquatic vegetables, fish, or crustaceans. An important group of trematodes consists of the blood flukes of the genus *Schistosoma*, which enter the body through skin/water contact and are responsible for schistosomiasis.

Cestodes, commonly called tapeworms, are parasitic flatworms that parasitize almost all vertebrates, and as many as eight species are found in humans. The two most common cestodes-*Taenia saginata*, the beef tapeworm, and *Taenia solium*, the pork tapeworm-are transmitted to humans by infected beef or pork products obtained from livestock that grazed in fields contaminated by human feces, or by contaminated water. The resulting disease, cysticercosis, which is potentially lethal, develops mostly in the brain, eye, and muscle tissue. Another animal-transmitted cestode is the dog tapeworm, *Echinococcus granulosus*, which dogs ingest by eating contaminated sheep viscera and then pass on to humans, who ingest the parasite's eggs after petting or handling an infected dog. The human infestation of *E. granulosus* results in hydatid disease. Probably the most dramatic of the cestode parasites is the gigantic tapeworm *Diphyllobothrium latum*, which may reach a length of 10 meters and a width of 2 centimeters. This tapeworm is transmitted to humans by the ingestion of raw or undercooked fish. This tapeworm, like most cestodes, can be effectively treated and killed by drugs, but if the worm merely breaks, leaving the head and anterior segments attached, it can regenerate its original body length in less than four months.

Protozoa that can infect human hosts are found in the intestinal tract, various tissues and organs, and the bloodstream. Of the many varieties of protozoa that can live in the human intestinal tract, only *Entamoeba histolytica* causes serious disease. This parasite, which is ingested in water contaminated by human feces, is responsible for the disease amebiasis, also known as amebic dysentery. A less serious, though common, waterborne intestinal protozoan is *Giardia lamblia*, which causes giardiasis, a common diarrheal infection among campers who ingest water fouled by animal waste.

Another group of protozoa parasites specializes in infecting the human skin, bloodstream, brain, and viscera. *Trypanosoma brucei*, carried by the African tsetse fly, causes the blood disease trypanosomiasis (African sleeping sickness). In Latin America, infection by the protozoa *Trypanosoma cruzi* results when the liquid feces of the reduviid bug is rubbed or scratched into the skin; it causes Chagas disease, which produces often fatal lesions of the heart and brain. Members of the protozoan genus *Leishmania* are transmitted by midges and sandflies, and their parasitic infestation manifests in long-lasting dermal lesions and ulcers; the destruction of nasal mucous, cartilage, and pharyngeal tissues; or in the disease kala-azar, resulting in the destruction of bone marrow, lymph nodes, and liver and spleen tissue.

Two other types of protozoa are parasitic to humans. The first is the ciliate protozoa, which are mostly free-living, and of which only a single species, *Balantidium coli*, is parasitic in humans. This species is responsible for balantidiasis, an ulcerative disease. The second is the sporozoans, all of which are parasitic. Many species of sporozoans are harmful to humans, the most important being *Plasmodium*, the agent of malaria. The sporozoan parasite *Toxoplasma gondii*, the agent of toxoplasmosis, is responsible for encephalomyelitis and chorioretinitis in infants and children and is thought to infect as much as 20 percent of the world's population. *Pneumocystis* pneumonia, a major cause of death among persons with acquired immunodeficiency syndrome (AIDS), was formerly considered a result of sporozoan infection but is now thought to be fungal.

Perspective and Prospects

Because of their size, the large parasitic worms were among the first parasites to be noted and studied as possible causes of disease. The Ebers papyrus, written about 1600 BCE, contains some of the earliest records of the presence of parasitic worms in humans. In early Egypt, trichinosis, cysticercosis, and salmonellosis were all likely to be acquired from pigs. This knowledge is reflected in the law of Moses, later reinforced in the Qur'an, which forbids the eating of "unclean swine" or the touching of their dead carcasses-a clear indication that people knew of the relationship between parasitic worms and human disease. Persian, Greek, and Roman physicians were also familiar with various parasitic worms, and many of their early medical writings describe the removal of worm-induced cysts. The Arabic physician and philosopher Avicenna (979-1037 CE) was the first to separate parasitic worms into classifications: long, small, flat, and round.

The modern study of parasites began in 1379 with the discovery of the liver fluke, *Fasciola hepatica*, in sheep. During the eighteenth century, many parasitic worms and arthropods were described, but progress was slow prior to the invention and widespread use of the microscope. The microscope made possible the study of small protozoan parasites and allowed for detailed anatomic and lifecycle studies of larger parasites.

In 1835, *Trichinella spiralis*, the parasite responsible for the disease trichinosis, was described, and quickly thereafter knowledge concerning the parasitic worms of humans

began to accumulate. Many new species were discovered, prominent among which were the hookworm and the blood fluke.

Between 1836 and 1901, the first protozoan parasites of humans were recognized and described; among the most important of these were the parasites responsible for giardiasis, gingivitis, vaginitis, trichomoniasis, kala-azar, and Gambian trypanosomiasis (sleeping sickness).

Although arthropods had been recognized as parasites since early times, their role in transporting other parasites and in spreading disease was not noted until 1869, when the larval stages of the dog tapeworm were found in the dog louse. Further investigations led to the identification in 1893 of ticks as the transmitting agents of Texas fever in cattle. By 1909, parasitologists had observed the development of the malarial parasite in mosquitoes, had proved the transmission of yellow fever by the mosquito *Aedes aegypti*, and had linked the tsetse fly to African sleeping sickness, the tick to African relapsing fever, the reduviid bug to Chagas disease, and the body louse to the transmission of typhoid fever.Human Experience: Philosophy, Neurosis, and Elements of Everyday Life

In 2013 the American Academy of Neurology (ANN) published new guidelines for the treatment of neurocysticerosis, a tapeworm infection of the brain that can trigger epileptic seizures. The AAN, concerned with what appears to be an increase in the incidence of the disease, based their recommendations on a review of ten studies published between 1980 and 2010. An estimated 40,000 to 160,000 cases of neurocysticerosis occur annually in the United States

—Randall L. Milstein, Ph.D.

See also Amebiasis; Babesiosis; Bacterial infections; Bacteriology; Biological and chemical weapons; Bites and stings; Chagas' disease; Coccidiodomycosis; Dengue fever; Ehrlichiosis; Diarrhea and dysentery; Elephantiasis; Encephalitis; Fungal infections; Giardiasis; Insect-borne diseases; Leishmaniasis; Lice, mites, and ticks; Lyme disease; Malaria; Microbiology; Pinworms; Protozoan diseases; Rocky Mountain spotted fever; Roundworms; Schistosomiasis; Shigellosis; Sleeping sickness; Tapeworms; Toxoplasmosis; Trichinosis; Tropical medicine; Typhoid fever; Viral infections; Worms; Yellow fever.

For Further Information:

Despommier, Dickson D., et al. *Parasitic Diseases.* 5th ed. New York: Apple Tree, 2006.

Frank, Steven A. *Immunology and Evolution of Infectious Disease.* Princeton, N.J.: Princeton University Press, 2002.

Gittleman, Ann Louise. *Guess What Came to Dinner? Parasites and Your Health.* Rev. ed. New York: Putnam, 2001.

HealthDay. "Tapeworm-Linked Seizures May Be Rising in US, Doctors Say." *MedlinePlus,* April 8, 2013.

Klein, Aaron E. *The Parasites We Humans Harbor.* New York: Nelson Books/Elsevier, 1981.

MedlinePlus. "Parasitic Diseases." *MedlinePlus,* May 21, 2013.

Roberts, Larry S., and John Janovy, Jr., eds. *Gerald D. Schmidt and Larry S. Roberts' Foundations of Parasitology.* 9th ed. New York: McGraw-Hill, 2013.

Wilson, Brenda A., Abigail A. Salyers, et al. *Bacterial Pathogenesis: A Molecular Approach.* 3d ed. Washington, D.C.: ASM Press, 2011.

Parathyroidectomy

Procedure

Anatomy or system affected: Endocrine system, glands, neck

Specialties and related fields: Endocrinology, general surgery

Definition: The removal of all or part of the parathyroid gland or parathyroid tumors.

Indications and Procedures

The parathyroid glands are four structures attached to the rear of the thyroid gland, which is found in the neck. Their main function is the secretion of parathyroid hormone (PTH), a protein that regulates the concentration of blood calcium. Abnormalities in proper calcium concentration can lead to bone demineralization, neuromuscular problems, or renal (kidney) damage.

Parathyroidectomy is occasionally warranted under conditions of hyperparathyroidism: the excess secretion of PTH. Hyperparathyroidism most commonly results in excess resorption of bone calcium, causing skeletal pain or loss of height. The demineralization may also lead to fractures of the spine or long bones, which may be accompanied by extreme muscle weakness and frequent urination. Since the patient may be asymptomatic, diagnosis is most commonly made on the determination of excess serum and urine calcium. X-rays may also indicate bone abnormalities resulting from the resorption of calcium. The condition itself may be caused by hyperplastic (overactive or enlarged) glands, or in less common circumstances (2 percent of cases), hyperparathy- roidism may result from a parathyroid adenoma (a benign tumor on a gland).

Asymptomatic patients, or patients with only mildly elevated blood calcium, may not need treatment. Should symptoms become more severe, surgical procedures may be necessary, generally involving the removal of excess parathyroid tissue. If the hyperplasia involves all four parathyroid glands, three of the glands are usually removed, with resection of the fourth. If the cause of the PTH elevation is an adenoma, it is necessary to remove the tumor surgically.

Uses and Complications

Since the primary symptom of hyperparathyroidism is excess blood calcium, the removal of excess tissue may suddenly reduce calcium levels to normal. The rapid fall of calcium may cause a transient tetany (involuntary muscle contractions), but otherwise recovery from such surgery parallels any other surgical procedure. PTH and calcium levels must continue to be monitored postoperatively. If parathyroidectomy results in excessively low PTH levels, it may be necessary to provide lifelong diet supplements of calcium and vitamin D. Surgical complications include injury to the thyroid gland and/or to the vocal cords.

—*Richard Adler, Ph.D.; updated by*
Sharon W. Stark, R.N., A.P.R.N., D.N.Sc.

See also Endocrine disorders; Endocrine glands; Endocrinology; Glands; Hashimoto's thyroiditis; Hormones; Hyperparathyroidism and hypoparathyroidism; Thyroid disorders; Thyroid gland; Thyroidectomy; Tumor removal; Tumors.

For Further Information:

Braverman, Lewis E., ed. *Diseases of the Thyroid*. 2d ed. Totowa, N.J.: Humana Press, 2003.
Gardner, David G., and Dolores Shoback, eds. *Greenspan's Basic and Clinical Endocrinology*. 9th ed. New York: McGraw-Hill, 2011.
Melmed, Schlomo, et al., eds. *Williams Textbook of Endocrinology*. 12th ed. Philadelphia: Saunders/Elsevier, 2011.
Montemayor-Quellenberg, Marjorie. "Parathyroidectomy-Conventional." *Health Library*, June 13, 2013.
Montemayor-Quellenberg, Marjorie. "Parathyroidectomy-Minimally Invasive." *Health Library*, June 13, 2013.
Neal, J. Matthew. *Basic Endocrinology: An Interactive Approach*. Malden, Mass.: Blackwell Science, 2000.
"Parathyroid Gland Removal." *MedlinePlus*, December 10, 2012.
Rosenthal, M. Sara. *The Thyroid Sourcebook*. 5th ed. New York: McGraw-Hill, 2009.
Ruggieri, Paul, and Scott Isaacs. *A Simple Guide to Thyroid Disorders: From Diagnosis to Treatment*. Omaha, Nebr.: Addicus Books, 2004.

Parkinson's disease

Disease/Disorder

Anatomy or system affected: Dopaminergic neurons, midbrain, substantia nigra, nervous system, musculoskeletal system

Specialties and related fields: Neurology, geriatrics and gerontology, internal medicine, physical therapy

Definition: A progressive disease that results in a movement disorder characterized by tremor, muscular rigidity, and slow movement.

Causes and Symptoms

British physician James Parkinson, in his landmark 1817 paper titled "An Essay on the Shaking Palsy," recounted the cases of six patients who suffered from a long-term disease characterized by "involuntary tremulous motion, with lessened muscular power in parts not in action even when supported, with a propensity to bend their trunks forward from a walking to a running pace."

This shaking palsy described by Parkinson is now known as Parkinson's disease (PD) or paralysis agitans. The slowly progressing neurodegenerative condition is characterized by a movement disorder consisting of tremor, stiffness, and slowness of movement. PD may also be accompanied by other complications, such as cognitive dysfunction, psychiatric manifestations, and gastrointestinal issues, among others. It is the second most common neurodegenerative disease in the world after Alzheimer's disease, and its occurrence worldwide is estimated at 3 per 1000 people over the age of forty. Geographic variations in prevalence have also been noted, and there seems to be a discrepancy between the genders, with males showing a higher prevalence (especially in the age 50-59 group) and a worse phenotype than females (potentially due to estrogen levels). In the US alone, over 1 million people live with PD, and the numbers grows every year by more than 50,000 patients.

The cause of Parkinson's disease is idiopathic, meaning that its origin is unknown, but recent research has shown

Information on Parkinson's Disease

Causes: Unclear; likely involves genetic and environmental factors

Symptoms: Tremors, impaired gait, muscle rigidity, masklike facial appearance, impaired swallowing, difficulty with repetitive movement and manual dexterity

Duration: Chronic and progressive

Treatments: Alleviation of symptoms through chemotherapy, surgery, physical therapy

that there may be some genetic and environmental factors linked to the disease progression. About 5-10% of cases have been shown to be inherited with mutations in specific genes (GBA, LRRK2, and SNCA, among others) linked to an increased risk of developing PD. Certain chemicals and pesticides have also been linked to an increased risk of PD, while smoking may actually have a protective effect against PD (due to nicotine's potential as a therapeutic chemical).

The symptoms of PD are caused by death of specific cells in the brain. Dopaminergic neuron death in the substantia nigra of the midbrain leads to a lack of inhibitory action, which in turn causes excess nerve impulses to fire to the motor nerves. This lack of inhibition leads to too much stimulation, producing both the resting tremor and rigidity seen in PD patients. Neuropathologically, there is a loss of pigmentation in the substantia nigra –from the lack of dopaminergic neurons and neuromelanin—and potential depositing of Lewy bodies, which are aggregates of cytotoxic protein (alpha-synuclein). These changes in the brain are believed to cause the physical symptoms PD patients experience.

PD manifests slowly, typically first on one side of the body and then on both sides, and targets movement before causing symptoms throughout the body. As previously mentioned, the hallmark symptoms are:

- *Resting tremors*: shaking without having an activity or intention induce tremors
- *Bradykinesia*: slow body movement with overall weakness
- *Rigidity*: inability to move with ease due to increased resistance

A late symptom in many PD cases is a poor sense of balance and posture; this is tested clinically by pulling backwards on a standing patient, which causes PD patients to take several steps to regain their balance or even fall. Parkinson's disease is not limited to the above three symptoms as it is a highly complex condition—additional symptoms include changes in cognition, hallucinations, and potential dementia; psychiatric manifestations such as emotional changes, mood disorders, and anxiety; insomnia and other sleep disturbances; olfactory dysfunction and rhinorrhea; and gastrointestinal problems such as constipation and dysphagia.

Clinically, physicians use the Movement Disorder Society-Sponsored Revision of the Unified Parkinson's Disease Rating Scale (MDS-UPDRS), a comprehensive scale that includes both motor and non-motor symptoms, to help diagnose Parkinson's disease and identify its severity.

Treatment and Therapy

While there is currently no cure for Parkinson's disease, there are pharmacological approaches a physician can take to ameliorate a PD patient's symptoms and to help achieve patients' goals. The most widely used drug for improving motor symptoms and quality of life in early PD is levodopa, a precursor to dopamine which helps replace and increase the lost levels of dopamine in PD patients. It is commonly administered with carbidopa to alleviate the nausea that may come with levodopa administration. Levodopa takes approximately 30 minutes to start working, and lasts about 4-5 hours in the bloodstream. Dopamine agonists (pramipexole, ropinirole), and monoamine oxidase B (MOAB) inhibitors such as selegiline can also help with motor symptoms, but have fewer motor complications. Depending on the patient, side effects of these medications can include increased impulses, excessive somnolence, and psychotic episodes. The doses for these treatments can be modified by a trained specialist in PD, and non-motor symptoms may be alleviated during the course of the therapy with the appropriate drugs.

In late stages of the disease when medications no longer control the symptoms, a doctor may recommend deep brain stimulation (DBS), which is an experimental surgical treat-

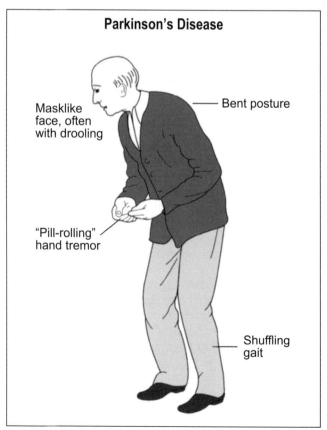

Parkinson's Disease

Masklike face, often with drooling

Bent posture

"Pill-rolling" hand tremor

Shuffling gait

Parkinson's disease, which often attacks older people, is characterized by debilitating symptoms that become more severe as the disease progresses.

In the News:
New Drug Treatments for Parkinson's Disease

Sinemet, a combination of levodopa and carbidopa, remains the drug of choice for treating Parkinson's. Carbidopa is a dopa decarboxylase inhibitor that keeps levodopa intact until it can enter the brain. Brain dopa decarboxylase converts the levodopa into dopamine, which substitutes for the dopamine missing as a result of Parkinson's disease. Neither carbidopa nor dopamine can enter the brain. A number of generic equivalents for Sinemet have been recently approved by the Food and Drug Administration (FDA). These generics make the most effective drug against Parkinson's disease more affordable.

Dopamine agonists are also used to treat Parkinson's disease. They stimulate cells much like dopamine does. In a preliminary study, a new dopamine agonist, 7-OH-DPAT, stimulated the production of new dopamine-producing nerve cells in the substantia nigra of rats. Pramipexole, a dopamine agonist already in use, has shown signs of the same effect. These drugs may eventually be used to stimulate production of new cells in the substantia nigra and thus to cure Parkinson's disease. Pramipexole may also be effective in treating depression in Parkinson's patients.

A new monoamine oxidase type-B inhibitor (MAOI), rasagiline, was approved by the FDA in 2006. MAOIs protect dopamine in the brain from the enzyme MAO. There are older MAOIs, such as selegiline, but this addition offers another tool for use against Parkinson's disease.

The catechol O-methyltransferase (COMT) inhibitor entacapone also protects dopamine in the brain from degradation. Entacapone is often prescribed with carbidopa/levodopa to protect dopamine in the brain, making lower doses of levodopa more effective. In 2003, the FDA approved a new drug, Stalevo, which combines carbidopa/levodopa and entacapone in a single pill, making the combination easier to take.

Two new drugs treat aspects of Parkinson's disease. Exelon was approved by the FDA in 2006 to treat the dementia that sometimes accompanies Parkinson's disease. Apokyn is the first drug approved to treat the periods of immobility suffered by some patients with advanced Parkinson's disease at the time that immobility strikes. Both drugs have serious side effects, however, and must be carefully managed. All drugs used to treat Parkinson's disease have undesirable side effects. Most are physiological, but some are psychological. For example, evidence is accumulating that pramipexole can stimulate compulsive gambling.

—*Carl W. Hoagstrom, Ph.D.*

probable, that remedial means might be employed with success." —*James Parkinson, 1817*

Two hundred years ago, Parkinson predicted that early PD could be successfully treated, though his proposed primitive treatment largely differs from the one we have today. Since its inception as the main PD treatment in 1975, carbidopa/levodopa therapy has improved the quality of life of many PD patients in their early stages, but researchers and physicians have not been able to find ways to stop disease progression since then. Different combinations of drugs that enhance the effects or extend the longevity of levodopa have been developed, but nothing has come close to eradicating this neurodegenerative disorder. In 2002, the FDA approved DBS as a measure to help PD patients, particularly after other treatment options have been exhausted. Since then, the FDA has approved other DBS-related devices as treatment options, but pharmacological advancements have remained relatively stagnant. However in a minor advance the FDA recently approved a new MAOB inhibitor, safinamide, as an additional drug to levodopa, when a patient is not responding to levodopa alone. Levodopa continues to be the gold standard.

Research into PD over the past decades has offered potential mechanism-related insights and genetic links, although this has not always translated into treatments. Animal models have been used for years to imitate Parkinson's; recently, with the advent of stem cell technologies, new human-based models attempt to predict disease mechanism and progression. Stem cells themselves have been touted as a potential treatment, though there is not enough data yet about the efficacy and currently poses dangerous risks. Gene-editing offers additional opportunities, though it has not yet been fully harnessed to slow disease progression or treat symptoms.

—*Brian Campos, BA*

For Further Information:

Gandhi, S., & Wood, N.W. (2010). Genome-wide association studies: the key to unlocking neurodegeneration? Nat Neurosci, 13(7), 789-794.

Gardner, J. (2013). A history of deep brain stimulation: Technological innovation and the role of clinical assessment tools. Social Studies of Science, 43(5), 707-728.

Goetz CG, Tilley BC, Shaftman SR, Stebbins GT, Fahn S, et al. (2008). Movement Disorder Society-sponsored revision of the Unified Parkinson's Disease Rating Scale (MDS-UPDRS): scale presentation and clinimetric testing results. Mov Disord., 23(15):2129-70.

Haaxma, C.A., Bloem, B.R., Borm, G.F., Oyen, W.J.G., Leenders, K.L., Eshuis, S.,... Horstink, M.W.I.M. (2007). Gender differences in Parkinson's disease. Journal of Neurology, Neurosurgery & Psychiatry, 78(8), 819-824.

Ma, C., Liu, Y., Neumann, S., & Gao, X. (2017). Nicotine from cigarette smoking and diet and Parkinson disease: a review. Translational Neurodegeneration, 6(1), 18.

Mayo Clinic Staff (2015, July 7). Parkinson's disease. Retrieved from: https://www.mayoclinic.org/diseases-conditions/parkinsons-disease/basics/definition/con-20028488

Parkinson, J. (2002). An Essay on the Shaking Palsy. The Journal of Neuropsychiatry and Clinical Neurosciences, 14(2), 223-236.

Parkinson's Disease Foundation (2017). Statistics on Parkinson's. Retrieved from: http://www.pdf.org/parkinson_statistics

ment that may lead to resting tremor suppression and improved quality of life. The surgery involves implanting an electrical device—a neurostimulator—that potentially blocks the uninhibited nerve signals, therefore improving tremors. The mechanism behind DBS' success is poorly understood, though theories have been posited about how it affects the brain.

Perspective and Prospects

"It seldom happens that the agitation extends beyond the arms within the first two years; which period, therefore, if we were disposed to divide the disease into stages, might be said to comprise the first stage. In this period, it is very

Power, J.H.T., Barnes, O.L., & Chegini, F. (2017). Lewy Bodies and the Mechanisms of Neuronal Cell Death in Parkinson's Disease and Dementia with Lewy Bodies. Brain Pathology, 27(1), 3-12. doi:10.1111/bpa.12344

Pringsheim, T., Jette, N., Frolkis, A., & Steeves, T.D.L. (2014). The prevalence of Parkinson's disease: A systematic review and meta-analysis. Movement Disorders, 29(13), 1583-1590.

Shah, V.V., Goyal, S., & Palanthandalam-Madapusi, H.J. (2017). A Possible Explanation of How High-frequency Deep Brain Stimulation Suppresses Low-frequency Tremors in Parkinson's Disease. IEEE Transactions on Neural Systems and Rehabilitation Engineering, PP(99), 1-1.

Tolosa, E., Marti, M.J., Valldeoriola, F., & Molinuevo, J.L. (1998). History of levodopa and dopamine agonists in Parkinson's disease treatment. Neurology, 50(6 Suppl 6), S2-10; discussion S44-18.

Patellofemoral pain syndrome
Disease/Disorder

Also known as: runner's knee, idiopathic anterior knee pain

Anatomy or system affected: Musculoskeletal system, kneecap

Specialties and related fields: Orthopedics, sports medicine, primary care, physical therapy

Definition: pain in the front of the knee, worsened with sitting, squatting or running for an extended period of time

Key terms:

patella: kneecap

femur: thigh bone

quadriceps: four muscles located in the front of the thigh, responsible for knee extension

Patellofemoral pain syndrome (PPS) is pain occurring in the front of the human knee, often due to wear and stress. The term *patella* is the kneecap, the bone cap of the knee joint, and *femoral* refers to the femur, or thigh bone. The patellofemoral joint is one of the two joints of the human knee, the other being the tibiofemoral. The syndrome can appear in one knee or in both knees. It is one of the most common injuries caused by running. Patellofemoral pain syndrome is also known as "runner's knee" or "jumper's knee," although it can occur in non-runners as well, and "anterior knee pain syndrome." It is not caused by a specific disease or condition. In addition to pain, another occasional symptom of PPS is popping or cracking sounds from the knee. In extreme cases, the knee may give way.

PPS is a clinical diagnosis, made usually by history and physical examination. X-Rays or MRIs are generally not considered necessary for a diagnosis of PPS, although in some cases they may be used to rule out other explanations for the pain, such as arthritis in patients over fifty years old or a dislocated patella or other injury. Patellofemoral pain syndrome is also distinguished from bursitis of the knee, which also causes pain in the area of the patella but has a completely different physical cause. Chrondomalacia patellae is sometimes treated as a synonym for PPS, but it can be distinguished as a syndrome specifically caused by the degeneration of cartilage of the knee joint. PPS must also be distinguished from patellofemoral osteoarthritis (PF OA), which generally occurs in older patients and also has characteristic radiographic findings including narrowed joint space and osteophytes, or bone spurs.

Causes and Symptoms

PPS is a multifactorial condition, but there are certain elements that can increase the risk of development of PPS. Repetitive exercise straining the knee can be one cause of PPS in addition to running and jumping, cycling, climbing stairs, and squatting. The onset of PPS is often associated with a change in exercise routine such as the addition of a new exercise that puts pressure on the knee joint. Patellofemoral pain syndrome is frequently encountered by specialists in sports medicine. However, exercise or other physical activity is not necessary for PPS, and it can also appear in sedentary people. Weakness or inflexibility of the quadriceps muscles in the thigh can cause PPS. Core strength deficiencies, which cause weakened pelvic stability, are also implicated in the development of PPS. Women are particularly vulnerable to PPS, as well as to other injuries of the knee, due to the slight incurve of a woman's hip bone, which increases the stress on the knee joint. Patellofemoral pain is often intermittent. It can appear during exercise or exertion, in extreme cases making exercise impossible, but it can also appear when going up or down stairs or after sitting for a long time in one position with the knee bent, as at a desk or at a movie or theater (known as the "theater sign"). Pain is often difficult for patients to localize.

One cause of PPS is poor tracking of the patella along the femur when the knee is bent, which in turn irritates the cartilage where the patella grinds against the femur rather than moving straight up and down. A slight misalignment of the patella aggravated by stress or repeated impact may lead to PPS. This may be caused by exercise or exertion with flat feet or poorly fitted shoes that increase the pronation, or rolling, of the foot, which again puts strain on the knee.

Treatment

To prevent PPS, some doctors recommend exercises to increase the flexibility and strength of the quadriceps. Runners should avoid very hard surfaces and only gradually add uphill running to their routines. Properly fitting shoes are also valuable in preventing PPS. Theater-goers can try

---

Information on
Patellofemoral Pain Syndrome (PPS)

Causes: repetitive knee strain, quadriceps weakness, diminished core strength, patellar tracking/ malalignment

Symptoms: anterior knee pain, "buckling," "creaking" or pain with standing after prolonged sitting

Duration: pain may be gradual or acute in onset and can continue unless treatment or preventive measures initiated

Treatments: rest, ice, activity limitation, NSAIDs, acetaminophen, physical therapy, stretches, quadriceps and core strengthening

to get aisle seats, so they have room to occasionally straighten their legs.

Once patellofemoral pain strikes, immediate treatments to reduce it include ice packs and rest. Non-steroidal anti-inflammatory drugs (NSAIDs) and acetaminophen are also used to soothe the pain, although they have little effect beyond a few hours. Long-term treatments for PPS are based on physical therapy and are successful in over half of all cases. They include strengthening of the quadriceps muscles to restore muscle balance, as well as restricting those activities that cause pain. Hip strengthening has also been shown to be of some effectiveness. Knee braces, which restrict the knee's range of motion, may be helpful, although the clinical evidence for this is weak. Evidence for the benefits of patellar taping, another commonly used treatment, is also weak. There are a very few extreme cases for which surgery is recommended. Exercises and stretches are a crucial way to reduce the likelihood of developing PPS again. There is also evidence to suggest that foot orthotics combined with physical therapy may be more effective in reducing PPS symptoms than physical therapy alone, but it is unclear as to which patient population benefits the most from this. The use of intra-articular corticosteroid injections for PPS pain relief has limited evidence.

If PPS is caused by exercise, some doctors recommend changing or minimizing exercise routines, particularly switching to activities that place less impact on the knee, such as swimming or cycling, as well as ensuring that the shoes used for exercise fit properly. Exercises involving squatting, such as burpees, are particularly aggravating and may need to be suspended. Practitioners of various alternative medicine techniques such as acupuncture, chiropractic, and Pilates claim the ability to treat PPS, but such claims are not backed by scientific evidence.

Perspective and Prospects

PPS is an active area of medical research. Research into PPS and other forms of anterior knee pain is funded by the Patellofemoral Foundation, a nonprofit organization founded in 2002 and headquartered in Farmington, Connecticut. The organization cosponsors an annual award for excellence in patellofemoral research along with the International Society of Arthroscopy, Knee Surgery and Orthopedic Sports Medicine and promotes knowledge of the patellofemoral joint among physicians and surgeons. There is also a biannual series of "Patellofemoral Pain Research Retreats and Clinical Symposia" held for physicians and other clinicians dealing with the problem.

—William E. Burns, PhD;
updated by Ananya Anand, MSc

For Further Information:
Berry, Tiffany, et al. "Effect of Pain On Hip and Knee Kinematics During a Prolonged Run in Female Runners with Patellofemoral Pain Syndrome." *ISBS-Conference Proceedings Archive.* 2014. Web. 8 Jan. 2016.
Hettrich, Carolyn, Daniel Liechti. "Patellofemoral Pain Syndrome." http://orthoinfo.aaos.org/topic.cfm?topic=A00680
LaBella, Cynthia. "Patellofemoral Pain Syndrome: Evaluation and Treatment." *Primary Care: Clinics in Office Practice* 31.4 (2004): 977-1003.
Papadopoulos, Konstantinos, et al. "A Systematic Review of Reviews in Patellofemoral Pain Syndrome. Exploring the Risk Factors, Diagnostic Tests, Outcome Measurements and Exercise Treatment." *Open Sports Medicine Journal* 9 (2015): 7-17.
Petersen, Wolf, et al. "Patellofemoral Pain Syndrome." *KneeSurgery, Sports Traumatology, Arthroscopy* 22.10 (2014): 2264-74.
Rogers, Thomas, et al. "Structured Rehabilitation Model for Patients with Patellofemoral Pain Syndrome." *Sports Injuries.* N.p.: Springer Berlin Heidelberg, 2014. 1-12.
Thomeé, Roland, Jesper Augustsson, and Jon Karlsson. "Patellofemoral Pain Syndrome." *Sports Medicine* 28.4 (1999): 245-62.
van der Heijden, Rianne A., et al. "Exercise for Treating Patellofemoral Pain Syndrome. An Abridged Version of Cochrane Systematic Review." *European Journal of Physical and Rehabilitation Medicine.* (2015): n. pag. Web. 8 Jan. 2016.
Waryasz, Gregory R, and Ann Y. McDermott. "Patellofemoral Pain Syndrome (PFPS): A Systematic Review of Anatomy and Potential Risk Factors." *Dynamic Medicine: DM* 7 (2008): 9. Web. 4 Jan. 2016.

Patent ductus arteriosus
Disease/Disorder
Anatomy or system affected: Cardiovascular system, heart, aorta, pulmonary system, lungs, circulatory system, pulmonary artery, ligamentum arteriosum
Specialties and related fields: Cardiology, pediatrics, neonatology, pulmonology
Definition: A condition in which there is failure of the ductus arteriosus to close after birth, resulting in a persistent connection between the aorta and pulmonary arteries. This allows blood to flow from the aorta to the pulmonary arteries.
Key terms:
auscultation: listening to the sounds of the heart, lungs, and other internal organs, typically with a stethoscope
congenital: disease or abnormality that is present at the time of birth
echocardiogram: ultrasound that is used to visualize the structures of the heart
neonatal respiratory distress: breathing disorder in newborns resulting from immature lungs that do not produce enough pulmonary surfactant
pulmonary hypertension: high blood pressure in the blood vessels of the lungs

Causes and Symptoms

Patent ductus arteriosus (PDA) is a common congenital (at birth) heart defect. Prior to birth, the fetus does not need blood to travel through the lungs for oxygenation. The developing fetus receives oxygen from the mother's circulation, and the ductus arteriosus (a blood vessel connecting the pulmonary artery to the descending aorta) remains patent, or open, to allow blood to bypass the fetus's non-functioning lungs. Once the baby is born and takes its first breath, blood vessels in the lungs open, allowing blood to flow to the lungs to pick up oxygen. After a few days, the ductus arteriosus typically narrows and closes, becoming the ligamentum arteriosum. PDA occurs when the opening of the ductus arteriosus does not close. The PDA allows blood to circulate from the aorta into the pulmonary arteries (a left-to-right shunt that sends oxygenated blood back to the lungs), and too much blood flows into the infant's lungs. This leads to pulmonary hypertension (high blood pressure in the lungs), which can lead to congestive heart failure.

Some infants are at a higher risk than others for developing PDA, but the exact etiology of the condition is unknown. PDA is more common in females than males, and it has been most commonly associated with premature birth, especially with neonatal respiratory distress syndrome. Neonatal respiratory distress syndrome is a breathing disorder common in premature infants caused by underdeveloped lungs. Maternal infection with Rubella (German measles) during pregnancy is also a significant risk factor for the development of PDA. Genetics and family history can be risk factors that predispose certain children to the condition. A family history of heart defects or genetic conditions, such as Down Syndrome (Trisomy 21) increase the risk of PDA. In addition, environmental factors may play a role. For example, infants born at altitudes higher than 10,000 feet (3,048 meters) are at a higher risk of developing PDA than those born at lower altitudes. PDA is also common in infants with other congenital heart defects such as transposition of the great vessels or pulmonary stenosis.

While there is no specific test that determines the onset of PDA, doctors can usually detect heart issues soon after birth by *auscultating* (listening to internal body sounds) the infant's heart with a stethoscope. A PDA will produce a characteristic heart murmur that is commonly described as a "continuous machine-like" murmur. Chest x-rays and echocardiograms (an ultrasound that tests the heart's function) will reveal an enlarged heart and evidence of increased blood flow to the lungs.

The most common symptoms of PDA include rapid or heavy breathing; shortness of breath; sweating; fatigue; poor feeding; and poor weight gain and growth. These symptoms vary according to the size of the PDA and whether the infant was born prematurely or full-term. However, some infants do not show any signs of PDA, especially if the PDA is small. Smaller PDAs may not cause major complications and may go undetected until the child reaches adulthood.

Larger PDAs cause a large amount of blood to flow from the aorta into the pulmonary arteries. Excess blood flow to the lungs leads to pulmonary hypertension. Pumping against this increased pressure causes the right ventricle of the heart to hypertrophy (become thicker), leading to heart failure very soon after birth. Thickening of the right ventricle can cause Eisenmenger syndrome. In this condition, a left-to-right shunt becomes a right-to-left shunt (when deoxygenated blood is sent to the body instead of the lungs), leading to *cyanosis* (bluish discoloration of the skin due to reduced oxygen in the blood).

Women who have PDA and become pregnant may face serious issues during pregnancy. They are at a higher risk for certain complications such as arrhythmia (abnormal heart rhythms), heart failure, and pulmonary hypertension.

Information on Patent Ductus Arteriosus

Causes: Premature birth, congenital rubella syndrome, genetic conditions, chromosomal abnormalities, high-altitude birth

Symptoms: Tachypnea (rapid breathing), dyspnea (shortness of breath), continuous machine-like heart murmur, poor feeding, poor weight gain, fatigue, cyanosis, heart failure

Duration: The abnormality can present in the first year of life and last into adulthood depending on the size of the defect

Treatments: NSAIDS, Indomethacin, trans-catheter coil, open-heart surgery

---

Treatment and Therapy

Infants typically need medication to help close the PDA. Some medications include nonsteroidal anti-inflammatory drugs (NSAIDs) such as indomethacin. Indomethacin blocks the hormone Prostaglandin E, which normally prevents the ductus arteriosus from closing, and should be administered a few days after birth. If medications do not work, catheterization or surgery may be required.

If the PDA does not close with medications, it may require trans-catheter coil closure. During the procedure, catheters (long thin tubes) are inserted into the femoral artery in the leg and guided to the PDA near the heart. A coil is then inserted through the catheter to plug up the PDA. Sometimes, open-heart surgery is needed to close the PDA. During surgery, known as a PDA ligation, the surgeon will open the chest to expose the PDA. The PDA is then either tied closed with sutures or clamped shut with metal clip.

After the PDA is closed, the patient usually does not have any other health complications or physical restrictions. The long-term prognosis for those with PDA is very good. No further medications or additional procedures generally are needed.

While a comprehensive prevention method does not exist, pregnant women can assume certain steps to ensure a healthy pregnancy that can help reduce the risks of PDA. Some of these include:

- Avoiding smoking, drinking alcohol, and taking drugs
- Alleviating stress
- Maintaining a healthy diet
- Exercising
- Receiving vaccinations
- Women with heart defects, genetic conditions, or a family history of such conditions should consult a physician or genetic counselor prior to becoming pregnant.

—*Steffan Kim, MD*

See also: Congenital rubella syndrome, Trisomy 21, murmurs, auscultation, NSAIDS, cardiac catheterization, Eisenmenger syndrome

For Further Information:

Kim, Luke K., and Jeffrey C. Milliken. "Patent Ductus Arteriosus (PDA)." *Medscape*. WebMD LLC. 16 Sept. 2015. Web. 14 Feb. 2016. http://emedicine.medscape.com/article/891096-overview

"Patent Ductus Arteriosus." *MedlinePlus*. U.S. National Library of Medicine. Web. 14 Feb. 2016. https://www.nlm.nih.gov/medline plus/ency/article/001560.htm

"Patent Ductus Arteriosus (PDA)." *American Heart Association*. American Heart Association, Inc. Web. 14 Feb. 2016. http://www.heart.org/HEARTORG/Conditions/CongenitalHeartDe fects/AboutCongenitalHeartDefects/Patent-Ductus-Arteriosus-PDA_UCM_307032_Article.jsp#. Vr3r3Pnyu70

"Patent Ductus Arteriosus (PDA)" *Lucile Packard Children's Hospital Stanford*. Stanford Children's Health. Web. 30 Aug. 2017. http://www.stanfordchildrens.org/en/topic/default?id=patent-ductus-arteriosus-pda-90-P01811. Accessed 4 Sep. 2017.

"Patent Ductus Arteriosus (PDA)." *Mayo Clinic*. Mayo Foundation for Medical Education and Research. 16 Dec. 2014. Web. 14 Feb. 2016. http://www.mayoclinic.org/diseases-conditions/patent-ductus-arteriosus/basics/definition/con-20028530

"What Is Respiratory Distress Syndrome?" *National Heart, Lung, and Blood Institute*. U.S. Department of Health and Human Services. Web. 14 Feb. 2016. https://www.nhlbi.nih.gov/health/health-topics/topics/rds

Pathology

Specialty

Anatomy or system affected: All

Specialties and related fields: Biochemistry, cytology, forensic medicine, histology, microbiology, oncology

Definition: The science that studies the changes to cells, tissues, and organs that result from the processes leading to diseases and disorders.

Key terms:

autopsy: the dissection and examination of a human body after death

congenital: referring to a condition present at birth; it may result from an inherited trait or damage before birth

disease: an abnormal condition of the body, with characteristic symptoms associated with it

etiology: the cause of a disease or disorder

homeostasis: the maintenance of a stable internal environment needed for the proper functioning of the body's cells

metabolism: the collective term for the chemical activities of the body's cells

Science and Profession

The science of pathology seeks to identify accurately the etiology of a disease and its development in the human body, which in turn leads to other studies focused on the diagnosis, treatment, and prevention of the disease.

A pathologist may be a medical doctor or hold a doctoral degree in a related field such as cell biology or microbiology. He or she may be employed in one of several different types of work, such as research, clinical, surgical, and forensic pathology. The human body is a complex structure and, as in all living organisms, its basic unit of function is the cell. Similar cells are organized into tissues, tissues form organs, and organs are grouped into systems. All systems in the body must work together to maintain homeostasis. If this internal stability is changed too drastically, a disease results. To understand a disease thoroughly-and ultimately to diagnose, prevent, or treat it-its pathogenesis must be understood. This term includes the cause of the disease, its method of damaging the body, and the changes resulting from its presence. A specific disease may have many causes, and its symptoms and severity may vary in different patients. Nevertheless, it is convenient to place a disease into one of seven groups based on its primary cause or manifestation in the body: genetic defects, infections, immune disorders, nutritional disorders, traumas, toxins, and cancers.

Genetic disorders are those caused by a defect in one or more genes. Genes, which are found on chromosomes, are duplicated and passed from one generation to another. Each gene is responsible for directing the manufacture of a protein. Every protein has a characteristic three-dimensional structure, on which its function depends. If a mutation occurs in a gene, the protein may function poorly or not at all. Although the pathogenesis of a genetic disease may involve devastating effects in the body, its origin may be traced to the function of a single protein. A person with hemophilia may bleed to death because of a lack of the gene for blood-clotting protein. In sickle cell disease, hemoglobin molecules are abnormal, which results in abnormal red blood cells and difficulty in transporting oxygen throughout the body. Changes in gene function occur throughout a person's life. Many degenerative changes associated with aging are believed to be caused by aging genes and the subsequent loss of cell, tissue, and organ function.

Infections are those diseases that are caused by other organisms, usually microorganisms such as viruses, bacteria, protozoa, or fungi. Such organisms, called pathogens, are parasitic on body tissues or fluids. The damage from pathogens may be direct, resulting from tissue destruction, or may be caused by the toxins that they produce. *Entamoeba histolytica*, for example, is a protozoan that is ingested in contaminated water or food. It begins feeding on the tissues of the intestine and may cause ulcerlike lesions in the intestinal wall. *Clostridium botulinum* is the bacterial species that causes botulism. Its deadly effects are attributable not to tissue destruction but to its production of a poison that attacks the nervous system.

Immune disorders include immune deficiencies, autoimmune diseases, and allergies. The body's immunity involves a complex system of checks and balances to protect against invasion by foreign cells or substances. It is the main defense against infectious diseases. When a person's immune system is not functioning properly, the body is unable to fight off infections. Some individuals are born with immune deficiencies. Others may acquire the deficiency later in life through the use of immunosuppressive drugs to prevent rejection of an organ transplant or because of an infectious disease such as acquired immunodeficiency syndrome (AIDS). Regardless of the primary cause of the immune deficiency, the patient may die as a result of an infection that would be considered harmless in the general population. Another group of immune disorders includes the autoimmune diseases. In these disorders, the immune system begins to make antibodies against the body's own tissues. For example, joint tissue is destroyed in rheumatoid arthritis, and nerve tissue is destroyed in multiple sclerosis. Allergies represent a third group of immune disorders. An allergic response is an overreaction to a substance that would ordinarily be considered harmless by the body. During this reaction, a chemical called histamine is released that causes such changes as rashes and upper respiratory symptoms. In more severe reactions, asthma or circulatory system collapse may occur.

Nutritional disorders include dietary deficiencies, excesses, and imbalances. Vitamins and minerals are needed to take part in certain chemical reactions in the body. In vitamin deficiencies, these reactions are blocked. For example, vitamin A is needed for the proper functioning of the nerve endings in the eye that are responsible for seeing black and white and in dim light; thus, a person with a vitamin A deficiency may develop night blindness. Proteins, carbohydrates, and fats must be ingested in sufficient amounts to supply energy and raw materials to build body tissue. Excessive consumption, however, is associated with such conditions as obesity, diabetes, and heart disease.

Trauma generally refers to injury done to the body by an external force, such as in an automobile accident. The damage to the body may be relatively minor but still have serious effects. Damage to a blood vessel may cause hemorrhaging and subsequent loss of blood. Injury to the brain or spinal cord may result in paralysis or loss of other body function. Physicians also use the word "trauma" to mean any occurrence that damages the body or organs. High fever, for example, may be said to cause trauma to the brain. Extreme emotions may also have effects on the body.

Toxins are poisons that may originate from the surroundings of an individual and be absorbed through the skin or inhaled. A person can be overcome by carbon monoxide from a defective furnace or automobile heater, for example. Toxins may also be ingested in water or food. Drug overdoses or accidental ingestion of household chemicals will also cause toxic reactions. Medical ecology is a field of medicine that concerns itself with the long-term toxic effects of chemicals released into the environment from plastics or other materials associated with modern life.

Cancers arise when the cell division process becomes abnormal. Ordinarily, cells in the body divide at a limited rate that is characteristic of a particular tissue. When cells divide rapidly in an uncontrolled manner and metastasize (spread) to other parts of the body, the condition is termed a malignancy or cancer. Cancers are grouped according to the type of tissue from which they develop. Carcinomas arise from epithelial tissue such as skin. Sarcomas arise from connective tissue such as bone or muscle. Leukemias result from abnormal and rapid reproduction of white blood cells in the bone marrow. Lymphomas are cancers of the lymphatic tissues, such as the lymph nodes or spleen. The severity of the cancer and the chances for recovery depend on the extent of the cancer when first diagnosed, the type of tissue or location involved, the speed at which the cells are dividing, and whether the cancer has spread to other areas of the body.

While it is convenient to place pathologies into separate groups, in reality their causes and effects overlap. An individual who is malnourished may have a weakened immune system and be vulnerable to infectious diseases. The immune system attacks not only foreign cells from outside the body but also abnormal cells arising within the body, such as cancer. Thus, patients with AIDS often develop cancer. Some individuals are at increased risk for cancer because of genetic factors called oncogenes. If these individuals smoke or eat unwisely, they may develop cancer, while others with the same inherited risk who adopt a prudent lifestyle do not. It is important for researchers and physicians to understand these complex pathological relationships so that they can diagnose and treat such conditions.

Diagnostic and Treatment Techniques

A pathologist must be familiar with the typical test values associated with body functions and with the microscopic appearance of healthy cells and tissues in order to be able to differentiate correctly a normal condition from a pathological one. This body of knowledge has involved the collection of tissues and the measurement of values gleaned from years of medical treatment and research. Although based on large populations, these values may be misleading. For example, the amounts of blood cholesterol were measured in Americans, and the average level of cholesterol was labeled "normal." In reality, this value has been shown to be unhealthy and linked to heart disease.

Research pathology concentrates on the basic study of diseases or disorders. This type of study usually focuses on the cellular and biochemical aspects of a disease. Information is exchanged with other researchers in an effort to gain a complete understanding of the etiology of a disease and the mechanisms by which it damages the body. Laboratory experiments may be performed to determine if the condition can be stopped or at least slowed.

Other pathologists are more closely associated with patient treatment. A clinical pathologist is involved in the diagnosis of disease through study of body fluids, secretions, and excretions. Such a person must be knowledgeable in hematology (the study of blood), microbiology, and chemistry. A surgical pathologist is responsible for testing samples of cells and tissues excised during surgery. In such a procedure, called a biopsy, a small section of tissue is taken from the affected area and sent to the laboratory. The pathologist then examines the sample using a microscope and determines whether the tissue is normal or whether it indicates the presence of cancer or some other disease state.

At one time, it was necessary to perform what was known as exploratory surgery if laboratory tests and x-rays did not lead to a diagnosis. Less invasive, and safer, techniques have been developed to eliminate that need. Fiberoptic methods involve the use of light shining through a flexible tube containing glass fibers. The flexible tube can be inserted through a body opening or through a small incision, allowing the physician to see internal cavities and determine if any visible abnormalities are present or to perform a biopsy. In some cases, the condition can be corrected without further surgery.

Many other tools and techniques are available to clinical and surgical pathologists. Some abnormalities can be observed directly, such as a rash or external tumor. Microscopes are used to detect changes that are too minute to be seen by the naked eye. Another tool used to diagnose disease or disorders is the medical x-ray, which can determine the presence of a broken bone, kidney stones, or dense tumors. Soft tissues are not so easily visualized using normal x-ray techniques. Ingestion of an opaque substance such as barium may help to delineate the outline of a structure such as the esophagus or intestine. Other medical imaging procedures, such as ultrasound, magnetic resonance imaging (MRI), and computed tomography (CT) scans, allow even more detailed visualization of body structures.

An autopsy pathologist examines the body after death. In a hospital setting, the purpose of an autopsy is usually to confirm or determine the natural cause of death. Even when the cause is known, an autopsy may be requested, since information obtained in this way may lead to better understanding of the pathological processes that resulted in death and suggest possible ways of preventing deaths in the future.

A forensic pathologist, also called a coroner or medical examiner, is an autopsy pathologist who works closely with the police and criminal justice officials. This relationship is especially important if there are suspicious circumstances surrounding the death or the discovery of the body, in order to determine whether the death has resulted from an intentional poisoning or a violent act. In some cases, a coroner must also attempt to identify the body. Such abnormalities in the body as scars, healed fractures, and dental cavities can aid in this effort. Samples of cells may be used for DNA fingerprinting, a comparison of genetic material from the deceased to that of someone believed to be a close relative, in an attempt to verify identification. If it is determined that a murder has occurred, the pathologist contributes to the investigation by determining such facts as the cause and time of death. Special care must be taken during any autopsy since the information may be used as legal evidence.

The correct diagnosis and identification of the etiology of a disease are essential to providing insight into possible treatments. Pathologists also play a key role in determining the mode of transmission. The following historical examples illustrate this application of pathology.

In the 1930s, it was discovered that the urine of some developmentally disabled children had a peculiar odor. Analysis of the urine showed the presence of an abnormal chemical that damaged the nervous system, resulting in mental deficiencies. The chemical was found to result from a failure of the body to make an enzyme necessary to break down the amino acid phenylalanine, which in turn was the result of a genetic defect, termed phenylketonuria (PKU). Simple blood and urine tests can determine the presence of this defect at birth. While this disease cannot be cured, those with PKU can be placed on a special diet low in phenylalanine, and so avoid the buildup of the amino acid and its resulting damage. In this genetic disease and others, once the precise mechanism of damage is found, efforts can be made to identify the presence of the gene and then to lessen its effects.

In July 1976, more than five thousand members of the American Legion attended a convention in Philadelphia, Pennsylvania. Within two weeks of returning home, nearly two hundred of them became ill, and twenty-nine of these died. Laboratory tests and autopsies identified the process that caused death as severe pneumonia accompanied by high fever but could not determine its origin. Although a pathogen was suspected, none could be found through microscopic examination of tissues or culture studies. Attention turned to the hotel and its air conditioning system in an attempt to determine if some toxin had spread through the air ducts, but no such substance was found. Several months later, a pathologist at the Centers for Disease Control in Atlanta, Georgia, was examining lung tissue sections taken from chick embryos and discovered the bacteria that had caused the illness, now known as Legionnaires' disease. Further tests showed them to be sensitive to the antibiotic erythromycin. When subsequent cases occurred, prompt diagnosis of the disease allowed the correct treatment to be given. The presence of these bacteria in water tanks associated with large air conditioning systems has led to preventive measures.

In 1981, the first cases of AIDS were identified. While the mode of transmission was discovered fairly quickly, it was not until 1986 that the human immunodeficiency virus (HIV) was identified. The pathogenesis of this disease begins with the infection of white blood cells, called helper T cells, that are an essential link between the identification of an invading pathogen and the production of antibodies by other cells called B cells. At first, the body begins to make antibodies against the virus as it would any other infectious disease. Then, over a period of several years, an increasing number of T cells are infected and destroyed. Eventually, the body loses the ability to make the antibodies necessary to fight all infectious diseases and to destroy cancer cells. After further study of the virus, researchers were able to discover a chemical, azidothymidine, or AZT (later called zidovudine), that could interfere with a key enzyme needed by the virus to reproduce. Although it could not cure the disease, the drug slowed its effects. AIDS research efforts are not aimed solely at attempts to kill the virus: by studying its pathogenesis, the means may be found to counteract the effects of the disease on the body's immune system.

Perspective and Prospects

In the early days of medicine, knowledge of pathology was limited to what could be observed directly through the human senses. Treatments were empirical, a matter of trying different drugs or procedures until one was found that worked. Most basic knowledge of human anatomy and physiology was lacking. Often, human autopsies were not permitted because of religious and cultural practices.

A culture's beliefs about disease influence medical practice. From the time of the ancient Greeks until the rise of modern medicine, various theories were accepted. Some believed that disease had supernatural origins. The term *influenza*, for example, came from the belief that the disease was caused by the influence of the stars. Others believed that the body's functions were dependent on fluids in the body, called humors. Bleeding was used to release the bad humors that were causing the disease.

By the seventeenth century, dissection of cadavers was practiced to identify completely the normal and abnormal gross anatomy of the human body. The microscope was developed and used to study human tissues. In the late nineteenth century, it was shown that microorganisms could cause disease, which in turn led to specific tactics aimed at prevention and treatment. With knowledge of the infectious process and the development of anesthesia, surgery became more widespread. This trend, in turn, increased the knowledge of disease processes in tissues and organs.

In the twentieth century, more sophisticated techniques were developed to focus on processes at the cellular level. The electron microscope allowed researchers to visualize structures within cells. Other research showed that series of chemical reactions, called metabolic pathways, are necessary for proper cell function. The comparison of these pathways in normal cells with those in abnormal cells enabled researchers to understand the pathogenic effect of toxins and many genetic diseases. The use of computers in medical analysis has increased the precision of laboratory tests and has permitted the detection of abnormal chemicals in smaller amounts than were possible before.

During the effort to map the human genome-that is, to identify and locate all the genes found on the forty-six human chromosomes-one of the techniques employed was to compare the chromosomes of individuals known to have genetic diseases with those who do not, and so identify the abnormal gene. Identification of oncogenes (cancer-causing genes) or genes linked to such diseases as diabetes mellitus and heart disease may alert individuals at high risk in time for them to get regular diagnostic tests or to change their lifestyles. Knowledge gained by taking the study of disease to the genetic level will ultimately lead to more effective treatments and prevention for these and other pathological conditions.

—Edith K. Wallace, Ph.D.

See also Autopsy; Bacteriology; Biopsy; Blood testing; Cancer; Cytology; Cytopathology; Dermatopathology; Diagnosis; Disease; Electroencephalography (EEG); Endoscopy; Epidemiology; Forensic pathology; Genetics and inheritance; Gram staining; Hematology; Hematology, pediatric; Histology; Homeopathy; Immunization and vaccination; Immunopathology; Inflammation; Invasive tests; Laboratory tests; Malignancy and metastasis; Microbiology; Microscopy; Mutation; Noninvasive tests; Oncology; Physical examination; Prion diseases; Prognosis; Serology; Signs and symptoms; Toxicology; Urinalysis; Veterinary medicine.

For Further Information:

Baden, Michael M. *Unnatural Death: Confessions of a Medical Examiner.* New York: Random House, 1989.
Corrigan, Gilbert. *Essential Forensic Pathology: Core Studies and Exercises.* Boca Raton: CRC Press, 2012.
Crowley, Leonard V. *Introduction to Human Disease: Pathology and Pathophysiology Correlations.* Boca Raton: CRC Press, 2012.
Gao, Zu-hua, ed. *Pathology Review.* Calgary: Brush Education, 2013.
Jensen, Marcus M., and Donald N. Wright. *Introduction to Microbiology for the Health Sciences.* 4th ed. Englewood Cliffs, N.J.: Prentice Hall, 1997..

King, Richard A., Jerome I. Rotter, and Arno G. Motulsky, eds. *The Genetic Basis of Common Diseases.* 2d ed. New York: Oxford University Press, 2002.
Kumar, Vinay, Abul K. Abbas, and Nelson Fausto, eds. *Robbins and Cotran Pathologic Basis of Disease.* 8th ed. Philadelphia: Saunders/Elsevier, 2010.
McCance, Kathryn L., and Sue M. Huether. *Pathophysiology: The Biologic Basis for Disease in Adults and Children.* 6th ed. St. Louis, Mo.: Mosby/Elsevier, 2010.
Parham, Peter. *The Immune System.* 3d ed. New York: Garland Science, 2009.
Shaw, Michael, ed. *Everything You Need to Know About Diseases.* Springhouse, Pa.: Springhouse Press, 1996.
Shtasel, Philip. *Medical Tests and Diagnostic Procedures: A Patient's Guide to Just What the Doctor Ordered.* New York: Harper & Row, 1991.

Patient-centered medical home

Health care system

Anatomy or system affected: Biopsychosocial

Specialties and related fields: Pediatrics, family and geriatric medicine, home health, evidence based practice

Definition: A team based health care delivery model led by a health care provider to provide comprehensive and continuous medical care to patients with a goal to obtain maximal health care outcomes.

The Patient-Centered Medical Home (PCMH) is a care model designed to enhance the care delivered to patients while still allowing attention to each individual's unique needs. The process of implementing a PCMH improves the quality, efficiency and effectiveness of care.

In a 2007 document entitled *Joint Principles of the Patient-centered Medical Home*, the American Academy of Family Physicians, the American College of Physicians, the American Academy of Pediatrics and the American Osteopathic Association defined the model to include patient access to a personal physician who leads the care team; a care team designed to provide comprehensive care at all stages of life from birth to end of life care; integrated and coordinated care that takes into consideration the patients ethnicity and culture; use of evidence based medicine to enhance patient outcomes; and, a commitment to access to care. The care team includes physicians, physician assistants, advanced practice nurses, social workers, nutritionists and others who interact with the patient to meet their total care needs. Smaller practices may link with others to deliver the comprehensive care needed.

As health care in the United States moves away from payment for numbers of patients treated to a payment system based on quality and outcomes of care, the need for change in the delivery system is evident. Patients and payers increasingly expect health outcomes are quality driven. Personalized care that is coordinated between specialists, especially with chronic diseases such as diabetes and heart disease, is critical. As payments are stretched, improved access to appropriate care rather than excessive care must become the norm. Physicians are experiencing stress from patients and payers for care that may or may not be reimbursed. Physicians want to deliver the best quality of care possible in a safe and effective manner, while remaining financially solvent.

The PCMH model enables a physician practice to be ready for changes in reimbursement structures such as merit based incentive payments (MIPs), alternative payment models (APMs), and accountable care organizations (ACO). The MIPS provides additional payment based on evidence-based and practice-specific quality measures reported to the payer. The APM provides incentive payments for specific conditions, care episodes or a population for high quality and cost efficient care. An ACO is a group of doctors, hospitals, and other health care providers, who work as a team to provide coordinated, high quality care to Medicare patients. As practices transition to PCMH models, cost savings and more efficient use of resources results. More primary and multi-specialty physician practices are developing a PCMH model in their practices as resources are stretched.

More recently, single specialty clinics, such as medical oncology practices, are developing PCMH models designed to coordinate the care cancer patients need from initial diagnosis to cure or end of life care. As the model becomes more accepted, other single disease specialties may attempt to adapt the model to their practice patterns.

Background

The PCMH is widely accepted as a model of excellence in primary care delivery. While the word home is used in the title, it is not a place but rather a way of organizing a care partnership between the physician and the patient. Working together with the care team, the patient develops a personalized care plan that addresses physical, mental, and supportive care needs. Care is considered to be 24/7; the patient has access to a provider round the clock. Medicine reconciliation, or reviewing all the medicines the patient is taking, is an important part of participation in a PCMH. Too often, patients see multiple doctors for a variety of conditions and may receive prescriptions that interact inappropriately causing more damage than good. Encouraging wellness by supporting appropriate health behaviors such as stop smoking and weight loss is also a part of this model of care.

The Patient-centered Medical Home is comprised of five components. The first is that it is comprehensive and meets most of a patient's physical and mental needs, including prevention, screening, acute and chronic treatment to end of life care. Patient-centered care focuses on the needs of the whole patient with emphasis on establishing a long term relationship with both patients and caregivers over time.

A significant complaint about the U.S. health system is that the care provided is often fragmented as multiple specialists provide care, often with little communication with other providers. Coordinated care is important to deliver optimal outcomes. Preventing multiple drug interactions, choosing non-invasive care over surgery, and managing side effects of multiple diseases are just a few reasons that coordinated care is needed.

Providing access to health care is a critical component of a healthy population. Access to care is often dependent on the type of private or government payments available. Patients without insurance are often severely limited in the care they receive or may even be denied care. Self-pay is not a realistic option as the cost of health care continues to rise dramatically. Insurance and government payers negotiate reduced rates for care, but self-pay patients are often expected to pay full price for care delivered.

Quality of care is important to the delivery of appropriate and safe outcomes. A PCMH is committed to the use of evidence based medicine and clinical practice guidelines. Clinical practice guidelines are often developed by consensus panels of subject experts based on extensively researched evidence and are considered to be the optimal care that needs to be delivered to a patient. Shared decision making with the patient, caregivers and other physicians involved in ongoing care enhances care delivery, safety and provides the most optimal outcome of treatment.

The U.S. Healthcare System is in dire need of overhaul to control costs and increase access to all citizens. Increasing access to appropriate care is critical. Care coordination is one method to better manage the patient population seeking care. The PCMH is one model that shows great promise going forward.

Implementation

The PCMH is generally considered to be based in the primary care practice and focuses on how care is organized and delivered. The five components necessary to develop the model are comprehensiveness, patient-centered, coordinated care between providers, providing patient access to care and quality and safety. A smaller practice may need to partner with others to develop a PCMH. Supportive functions necessary include a robust information technology system, a workforce with the attributes and attitude to put patients first, and financial stability as the system is implemented. Professional organizations and the Agency for Healthcare Research and Quality all have resources that can assist a physician practice to determine their readiness to develop a PCMH as do agencies that provide assessment and recognition programs.

Becoming recognized as a Patient-Centered Medical Home may enhance payment from providers by as much as a 10 percent payment increase. Recognition programs include a variety of agencies in different regions of the U.S. The Joint Commission Primary Care Medical Home Recognition Program, the Accreditation Association for Ambulatory Health Care Medical Home Program and the URAC Patient Centered Medical Home Recognition Program are just a few examples. The National Committee for Quality Assurance (NCQA) has a PCMH evaluation program that currently recognizes over 12,000 practices as meeting their standards. There are also more than 100 payers who support the NCQA recognition program with financial incentives. Reviewing the standards from these agencies will also assist in the steps needed to become a PCMH.

The Patient-centered Medical Home will continue to be an integral component of health care going forward. As both patients and payers demand more for their dollar, coordinating care that is appropriate, of high quality and safe will be important. The PCMH helps deliver this level of care.

—*Patricia Stanfill Edens, PhD, RN, LFACHE*

For Further Information:
Accountable Care Organizations. Centers for Medicaid and Medicare Services. Available from: https://www.cms.gov/Medicare/Medicare-Fee-for-Service-Payment/ACO/index.html.
Alternative Payment Model Overview (APM). Centers for Medicaid and Medicare Services. Available from: https://qpp.cms.gov/apms/overview.
American Academy of Family Physicians, American College of Physicians, American Academy of Pediatrics, American Osteopathic Association. Joint Principles of the Patient-Centered Medical Home. Available from: http://www.aafp.org/practice-management/transformation/pcmh.html.
Patient-centered Medical Home Recognition. National Committee for Quality Assurance. Available from: http://www.ncqa.org/programs/recognition/practices/patient-centered-medical-home-pcmh.
Patient-Centered Primary Care Collaborative. Defining the Medical Home, A patient-centered philosophy that drives primary care excellence. Available from: http://www.pcpcc.org/about/medical-home.
The Merit Based Incentive Payment System (MIPS). Centers for Medicaid and Medicare Services. Available from: https://www.cms.gov/Medicare/Quality-Initiatives-Patient-Assessment-Instruments/Value-Based-Programs/MACRA- MIPS-and-APMs/Quality-Payment-Program-MIPS-NPRM- Slides.pdf
U.S. Department of Health and Human Resources. Agency for Healthcare Research and Quality. Defining the PCMH. Available from: https://pcmh.ahrq.gov/page/defining-pcmh

Pediatrics

Specialty

Anatomy or system affected: All

Specialties and related fields: Family medicine, genetics, neonatology, nursing, perinatology, pulmonary medicine, urology

Definition: The field of medicine devoted to the care of children at birth and through childhood, puberty, and adolescence.

Key terms:

acute: referring to a short and sharp disease process

chronic: referring to a lingering disease process

congenital: inborn, inherited

full-term: referring to a gestation period of a full nine months

premature: referring to a birth that is less than full term

puberty: the time of hormonal change when a child begins the physical process of becoming an adult

Science and Profession

The practice of pediatrics begins with birth. Most babies are born healthy and require only routine medical attention. Many hospitals, however, have a neonatology unit for babies who are born prematurely, who have disease conditions or birth defects, or who weigh less than 5.5 pounds (even though they may be full-term babies). All these infants may require short-term or prolonged care by pediatricians in the neonatology unit.

The problems of premature babies usually center on the fact that they have not fully developed physically, although other factors may also be involved, such as the health and age of the mother, undernourishment during pregnancy, lack of prenatal care, anemia, abnormalities in the mother's genital organs, and infectious disease. A past record of infertility, stillbirths, abortions, and other premature births may indicate that a pregnancy will not go to full term.

Low birth weight in both premature and full-term babies is directly related to the incidence of disease and congenital defects and may be indicative of a low intelligence quotient (IQ). Between 50 and 75 percent of babies weighing under 3 pounds, 5 ounces are mentally disabled or have defects in vision or hearing. Recent studies also indicate an increase in neurological problems such as attention-deficit hyperactivity disorder and autism in these children.

Because the lungs are among the organs that develop late in pregnancy, many premature infants are unable to breathe on their own. Some premature babies are born before they have developed the sucking reflex, so they cannot feed on their own.

Hundreds of congenital diseases can be present in the neonate. Some are apparent at birth; some become evident in later years. Some may be life-threatening to the infant or become life-threatening in later years. Others may be harmless.

The child may be born with an infection passed on from the mother, such as rubella (German measles) or human immunodeficiency virus (HIV), the virus that causes acquired immunodeficiency syndrome (AIDS). Rubella may also infect the child in the womb, causing severe physical deformities, heart defects, mental disability, deafness, and other conditions. Genital herpes affects about 1,500 newborns in the United States each year and may cause serious complications. A herpes infection during the second or third trimester of a woman's pregnancy may increase the chance of preterm delivery or cesarean section. Group beta strep (GBS) infections are another serious problem for one of every 2,000 newborns in the United States. GBS may cause sepsis (blood infection), meningitis, and pneumonia.

Among the most prevalent congenital birth defects is cleft lip, which occurs when the upper lip does not fuse together, leaving a visible gap that can extend from the lip to the nose. Cleft palate occurs when the gap reaches into the roof of the mouth.

Various abnormalities may be present in the hands and feet of neonates. These can be caused by congenital defects or by medications given to the pregnant mother. Arms, legs, fingers, and toes may fail to develop fully or may be missing entirely. Some children are born with extra fingers or toes. In some children, fingers or toes may be webbed or fused together. Clubfoot is relatively common. In this condition, the foot is twisted, usually downward and inward.

Many congenital heart defects can afflict the child, including septal defects (openings in the septum, the wall that separates the right and left sides of the heart), the transposition of blood vessels, the constriction of blood vessels, and valve disorders.

Congenital disorders of the central nervous system include spina bifida, hydrocephalus, cerebral palsy, and Down syndrome. Spina bifida is a condition in which part of a vertebra (a bone in the spinal column) fails to fuse. As a result, nerves of the spinal cord may protrude through the spinal column. This condition varies considerably in severity; mild forms can cause no significant problems, while severe forms can be crippling or life-threatening. In hydrocephalus, sometimes called "water on the brain," fluid accumulates in the infant's cranium, causing the head to enlarge and putting great pressure on the brain. This disorder, too, can be life-threatening.

Cerebral palsy is caused by damage to brain cells that control motor function in the body. This damage can occur before, during, or after birth. It may or may not be accompanied by mental disability. Many children with cerebral palsy appear to be mentally disabled because they have difficulty speaking, but, in fact, their intelligence may be normal or above normal. Down syndrome is one of the most common congenital birth defects, affecting 1 in 200 infants born to mothers over age thirty-five. It is caused by an extra chromosome passed on to the child. The distinct physical characteristics of Down syndrome include a small body, a small and rounded head, oval ears, and an enlarged tongue. Mortality is high in the first year of life because of infection or other disease.

Cystic fibrosis is one of the most serious congenital diseases of Caucasian children. Because the lungs of children with this disease cannot expel mucus efficiently, it thickens and collects, clogging air passages. The mucus also becomes a breeding ground for bacteria and infection. Other parts of the body, such as the pancreas, the digestive system, and sweat glands, can also be impaired. A common congenital disorder among African American children is sickle cell disease. It causes deformities in red blood cells that clog blood vessels, impair circulation, and increase susceptibility to infection.

One of the major problems of infancy is sudden infant death syndrome (SIDS), in which a baby that is perfectly healthy, or only slightly ill, is discovered dead in its crib. In 2010 in the United States, over 2,000 infant deaths were reported as SIDS. The cause is not known. The child usually shows no symptoms of disease, and autopsies reveal no evidence of smothering, choking, or strangulation. Research indicates that rebreathing of carbon dioxide as well as exposure to secondhand cigarette smoke and other forms of indoor air pollution may greatly increase the risk of SIDS.

Infectious diseases are more prevalent in childhood than in later years. Among the major diseases of children (and often adults) throughout the centuries have been smallpox, malaria, diphtheria, typhus, typhoid fever, tuberculosis, measles, mumps, rubella, varicella (chickenpox), scarlet fever, pneumonia, meningitis, and pertussis (whooping cough). In more recent years, AIDS and hepatitis have become significant threats to the young.

Certain skin diseases are common in infants and young children, such as diaper rash, impetigo, neonatal acne, and seborrheic dermatitis, among a wide variety of disorders.

Fungal diseases of the skin occur often in the young, usually because of close contact with other youngsters. For example, tinea pedis (athlete's foot), tinea cruris (jock itch), and tinea corporis (a fungal infection that occurs on nonhairy areas of the body) are spread by contact with an infected playmate or by the touching of surfaces that harbor the organism. Similarly, parasitic diseases such as head lice, body lice, crabs, or scabies are easily spread among playmates. Some skin conditions are congenital. Between 20 and 40 percent of infants are born with, or soon develop, skin lesions called hemangiomas. They may be barely perceptible or quite unsightly; they generally resolve by the age of seven.

One form of diabetes mellitus arises in childhood, insulin-dependent diabetes mellitus (IDDM) or type 1. In the healthy individual, the pancreas produces insulin, a hormone that is responsible for the metabolism of blood sugar, or glucose. In some children, the pancreas loses the ability to produce insulin, causing blood sugar to rise. When this happens, a cascade of events causes harmful effects throughout the body. In the short term, these symptoms include rapid breathing, rapid heartbeat, extreme thirst, vomiting, fever, chemical imbalances in the blood, and coma. In the long term, diabetes mellitus contributes to heart disease, atherosclerosis, kidney damage, blindness, gangrene, and a host of other conditions.

Cancer can afflict children. One of the most serious forms is acute lymphocytic leukemia. Its peak incidence is between three and five years of age, although it can also occur later in life. Leukemic conditions are characterized by the overproduction of white blood cells (leukocytes). In acute lymphocytic leukemia, the production of lymphoblasts, immature cells that ordinarily would develop into infection-fighting lymphocytes, is greatly increased. This abnormal proliferation of immature cells interferes with the normal production of blood cells, increasing the child's susceptibility to infection. Before current treatment modalities, the prognosis for children with acute lymphocytic leukemia was death within four or five months after diagnosis.

In addition to the wide range of diseases that can beset the infant and growing child, there are many other problems of childhood that the parent and the pediatrician must face. These problems may involve physical and behavioral development, nutrition, and relationships with parents and other children.

Both parents and pediatricians must be alert to a child's rate of growth and mental development. Failure to gain weight in infancy may indicate a range of physical problems, such as gastrointestinal, endocrine, and other internal disorders. In three-quarters of these cases, however, the cause is not a physical disorder. The child may simply be underfed because of the mother's negligence. The vital process of bonding between mother and child may not have taken place; the child is not held close and cuddled, is not shown affection, and thus feels unwanted and unloved. This is seen often in babies who are reared in institutions where the nursing staff does not have time to caress and

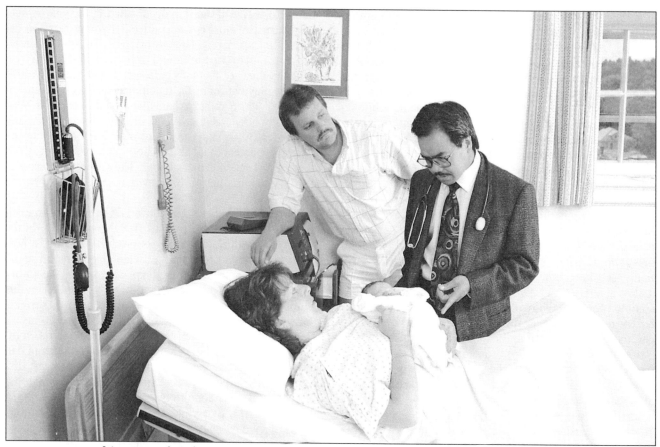

It is customary for pediatricians to visit newborns in the hospital in the days following delivery. (Digital Stock)

comfort infants individually.

Similarly, later in childhood, failure to grow at a normal rate can be caused by malnutrition or psychological factors. It could also be attributable to a deficiency in a hormone that is the body's natural regulator of growth. If this hormone is not released in adequate supply, the child's growth is stunted. An excess of this hormone may cause the child to grow too rapidly. Failure to grow normally may also indicate an underlying disease condition, such as heart dysfunction and malabsorption problems, in which the child does not get the necessary nutrition from food.

The parent and pediatrician must also ensure that the child is developing acceptably in other areas. Speech and language skills, teething, bone development, walking and other motor skills, toilet habits, sleep patterns, eye development, and hearing have to be evaluated regularly.

Profound mental disability is usually evident early in life, but mild to moderate disability may not be apparent until the child starts school. Slowness in learning may be indicative of mental disability, but this judgment should be carefully weighed, because the real reason may be impaired hearing or vision or an underlying disease condition. The diagnosis of neurological disorders, such as autism and attention-deficit hyperactivity disorder (ADHD), has greatly increased in recent years and poses a special challenge to both parents and pediatricians.

The battery of diseases and other disorders that may be-

set a child remains more or less constant throughout childhood. Puberty, however, begins hormonal changes that trigger new disease threats and vast psychological upheaval. As early as eight years of age in girls and after ten or eleven years of age in boys, the body begins a prolonged metamorphosis that changes the child into an adult. Hormones that were previously released in minimal amounts course throughout the body in great quantities.

In boys, the sex hormones are called androgens. Chief among them is testosterone, which is secreted primarily by the testicles. It causes the sexual organs to mature and promotes the growth of hair in the genital area and armpits and on the chest. Testosterone also enlarges the larynx (voicebox), causing the voice to deepen.

Girls also produce some testosterone, but estrogens and other female sex hormones are the major hormones involved in puberty. They cause the sexual organs to mature, the hips to enlarge and become rounded, hair to grow in the genital area and armpits, the breasts to enlarge, and menstruation to begin.

Many disease conditions can arise in association with the hormonal changes that occur during puberty, such as breast abnormalities and genital infections. Far and away the most common medical disorder at this time, however, is acne. Acne is a direct result of the rise in testosterone that occurs during puberty. About 85 percent of teenagers experience some degree of acne, and about 12 percent of these will develop severe, deep acne, a serious condition that can leave lifelong scars.

Important psychological changes also occur during puberty. The personality can be altered as the developing child begins to crave independence. Ties to the family weaken, and the teenager becomes closer to his or her peer group. Sexual feelings can be strong and difficult to repress. In modern Western society, this is usually the time when the teenager may begin to experiment with tobacco, alcohol, drugs, or other means of achieving a "high," although in some groups the use of these substances begins much earlier. Substance abuse is a major problem throughout society, but it is particularly devastating among young people.

Sexual activity among teenagers is widespread and, combined with inadequate education about health issues and limited access to care, has led to significant medical problems. The incidence of sexually transmitted infections (STIs) is higher among teenagers than any other group. Teenage pregnancy is one of the most challenging issues in modern society.

If the pregnant teenager who continues her pregnancy is from a disadvantaged family background, she is even more likely than other teen mothers to receive little or no prenatal care. Risks of delayed or absent prenatal care can include a fetus that is not properly nourished. Additional risks can arise from a mother who smokes, drinks alcohol, or takes drugs throughout the pregnancy. In these cases, the child often may be born prematurely, with all the physical problems that premature birth involves. Hospital care of these infants is extremely costly, as is the maintenance of the mother and child if the baby survives.

Another important issue of teenage sexuality is the rapid spread of HIV, both as a sexually transmitted infection and as an infection passed from mother to baby.

Diagnostic and Treatment Techniques

Pediatrics is one of the widest-ranging medical specialties, embracing virtually all major medical disciplines. Some pediatricians are generalists, and others specialize in certain disease areas, such as heart disease, kidney disease, liver disease, or skin problems.

Doctors and nurses specializing in neonatology, including advanced practice nurse practitioners with specialty certification in pediatrics or neonatology, have radically improved the survival rates of premature and low-weight babies. In neonatal care of the premature, the infant may have to be helped to breathe, fed through tubes, and otherwise maintained to allow it to develop.

Infectious diseases passed from the mother to the newborn child are a particular challenge. In some cases, such as with GBS and herpes infections, appropriate antibiotics and antiviral agents can be given. In others, such as with babies born with HIV, support measures and medications that help prevent the progress of the disease are the only procedures available.

Many birth defects and deformities can be repaired or at least ameliorated. Disorders such as cleft lip or palate, de-

formities of the skeletal system, heart defects, and other physical abnormalities often can be remedied by surgery. Certain structural malformations may require prosthetic devices and/or physical therapy.

The treatment of spina bifida depends on the seriousness of the condition; surgery may be required. With hydrocephalus, medication may be helpful, but most often a permanent shunt is implanted to drain fluids from the cranium. Before this technique was developed, the prognosis for babies with hydrocephalus was poor: More than half died, and a great many suffered from mental disability and physical impairment. Today, 70 percent or more live through infancy. Of these, about 40 percent have normal intelligence; the others are mentally disabled and may also have serious physical impairment.

There are no cures for cerebral palsy, but various procedures can improve the child's quality of life, exercise and counseling among them. Neither is there a cure for Down syndrome. If mental disability is profound, the child may have to be institutionalized. When a child with Down syndrome can be cared for at home in a loving family, his or her life can be improved.

SIDS continues to be a problem both in hospitals and in the home. The American Academy of Pediatrics' Back to Sleep campaign, in which parents are encouraged to place babies on their backs for sleeping, has been extremely successful, however, and has resulted in a decrease in the incidence of SIDS by 70 to 80 percent.

Managing the infectious diseases of childhood is one of the major concerns of pediatric providers, who are often called on to treat infections, for which they have a wide variety of antibiotics and other agents. Pediatric providers also seek to prevent infectious diseases through immunization. Medical authorities now recommend routine vaccination of all children in the United States against diphtheria, tetanus, pertussis, measles, mumps, rubella, poliomyelitis, pneumococcal pneumonia, *Hemophilus influenzae*, varicella, and hepatitis A and B. Vaccines are also available against rabies, influenza, cholera, typhoid fever, plague, and yellow fever; these vaccines can be given to the child if there is a danger of infection. Vaccines for diphtheria, tetanus, and pertussis are generally given together in a combination called DTaP. Measles, mumps, and rubella vaccines are also given together as MMR. Repeated doses of some vaccines are necessary to ensure and maintain immunity.

Skin disorders of childhood, including teenage acne, are usually treated successfully at home with over-the-counter remedies. As with any disease, however, a severe skin disorder requires the attention of a trained provider.

Patients with diabetes mellitus type 1 are dependent on insulin throughout life. It is necessary for the pediatrician or attending nurse to teach both the parent and the patient how to inject insulin regularly, often several times a day. Furthermore, patients must monitor their blood and urine constantly to determine blood sugar levels. They must also adhere to stringent dietary regulations. This regimen of diet, insulin, and constant monitoring is often difficult for the child to learn and accept, but strict adherence is vital if the patient is to fare well and avoid the wide range of complications associated with diabetes.

Other serious conditions are now considered to be treatable. Modern pharmacology has greatly improved the prognosis of children with leukemia. Similarly, many children with growth disorders can be helped by treatments of growth hormone.

Medications and other treatment modalities for the mental disorders of childhood have improved in recent years. Mentally disabled children can often be taught to care for themselves, and some even grow up to live independently. Children with behavioral problems may be helped by clinicians specializing in child psychology or psychiatry.

The problems of sexuality, sexually transmitted infections, and pregnancy among teenagers have provoked a nationwide response in the United States among medical and sociological professionals. Safer-sex programs have been launched, and clinics specializing in counseling for teenage girls are in operation to stem the rise in teenage pregnancies.

Perspective and Prospects

Pediatrics affects virtually every member of society. Diseases that once raged through populations of all ages are now being controlled through the mass immunization of children. Some diseases of childhood are not yet controllable by vaccines, but research in this area is ongoing.

Childhood health is directly related to economics. Middle-class and upper-class children have ready access to professional care for any problems that may arise. The medical and psychological needs of disadvantaged children, however, especially those who live in inner cities, are often neglected. Many of these children are not being immunized fully and remain susceptible to diseases that are no longer a problem among the middle and upper classes.

In an effort to improve the medical care of disadvantaged children, some vaccines are being made available at low or no cost to inner-city families. Programs educate parents and teachers about the need for a child to receive the full dosage of vaccine. Computerized records allow authorities to keep track of the immunization status of individual children and to alert their parents when a follow-up inoculation is due.

The psychological problems of inner-city children, as well as children who live in disadvantaged rural areas, are at least as serious as the bodily diseases that threaten them. They may live in a universe of violence, deprivation, and drug addiction, and they might lack a stable family environment and opportunities for advancement. Pediatric providers at all levels can advocate for these youth by becoming involved in medical, psychological, and sociological outreach programs to help disadvantaged children.

—*C. Richard Falcon;*
updated by Lenela Glass-Godwin, M.W.S.

See also Apgar score; Cardiology, pediatric; Childhood infectious diseases; Circumcision, male; Cognitive development; Congenital disorders; Critical care, pediatric; Dentistry, pediatric; Dermatology, pediatric; Developmental disorders; Developmental stages; Emergency medicine, pediatric; Endocrinology, pediatric; Family medicine; Gastroenterology, pediatric; Genetic diseases; Growth; Hema-tology, pediatric; Motor skill development; Neonatology; Nephrology, pediatric; Neurology, pediatric; Obesity, childhood; Optometry, pediatric; Orthopedics, pediatric; Perinatology; Psychiatry, child and adolescent; Puberty and adolescence; Pulmonary medicine, pediatric; Safety issues for children; Surgery, pediatric; Urology, pediatric; Well-baby examinations.

For Further Information:
American Academy of Pediatrics. http://www.aap.org.
Doyle, Barbara T., and E. D. Iland. *Autism Spectrum Disorders from A to Z*. Arlington, Tex.: Future Horizons, 2004.
Hay, William W., Jr., et al., eds. *Current Diagnosis and Treatment: Pediatrics*. 21st ed. New York: Lange Medical Books/McGraw-Hill, 2012.
Hoekelman, Robert, ed. *The New American Encyclopedia of Children's Health*. New York: New American Library/Dutton, 1991.
Kimball, Chad T. *Childhood Diseases and Disorders Sourcebook: Basic Consumer Health Information About Medical Problems Often Encountered in Pre-adolescent Children*. Detroit, Mich.: Omnigraphics, 2003.
Kliegman, Robert M., and Waldo E. Nelson, eds. *Nelson Textbook of Pediatrics*. 19th ed. Philadelphia: Saunders/Elsevier, 2011.
Litin, Scott C., ed. *Mayo Clinic Family Health Book*. 4th ed. New York: HarperResource, 2009.
Middlemiss, Prisca. *What's That Rash? How to Identify and Treat Childhood Rashes*. London: Hamlyn, 2002.
Nathanson, Laura Walther. *The Portable Pediatrician: A Practicing Pediatrician's Guide to Your Child's Growth, Development, Health, and Behavior from Birth to Age Five*. 2d ed. New York: HarperCollins, 2002.
Sanghavi, Darshak. *A Map of the Child: A Pediatrician's Tour of the Body*. New York: Henry Holt, 2003.
Taubman, Bruce. *Your Child's Symptoms: A Parent's Guide to Understanding Pediatric Medicine*. New York: Simon & Schuster, 1992.

Pellagra

Disease/Disorder

Anatomy or system affected: Nervous system, brain, digestive system, skin

Specialties and related fields: Nutrition, dietitian, global health, gastroenterology, cardiology, neurology, dermatology

Definition: A disease caused by a deficiency of niacin (Vitamin B3).

Key terms:

ataxia: loss of voluntary coordination of muscle movements producing gait abnormalities

dementia: chronic disorder of mental processes that results in memory loss, personality changes, and impaired reasoning

dermatitis: inflammation of the skin that can manifest in a variety of different ways depending on the etiology

Causes and Symptoms

Pellagra is a disease that results from a vitamin B3 (niacin) deficiency. Niacin is an organic compound that is required for the production of NAD (nicotinamide adenine dinucleotide) and NADP (nicotinamide adenine dinucleotide phosphate). NAD and NADP are important in many molecular processes, including cellular respiration, within the body, which is why pellagra produces broad symptoms and ultimately results in death if left untreated. Pellagra is commonly seen in South America, where the

Information on Pellagra

Causes: Vitamin B3 deficiency, tryptophan deficiency, alcoholism, chronic diarrhea, carcinoid syndrome, Hartnup's disease, medications

Symptoms: Diarrhea, dermatitis, dementia, death, confusion, sensitivity to sunlight, glossitis (inflammation of the tongue), aggression, ataxia (loss of coordination)

Duration: Pellagra can progress to death within 4-5 years if left untreated

Treatments: Nicotinamide, Vitamin B3 (niacin)

diet consists heavily of maize, a poor source of niacin and tryptophan. Pellagra is also seen in many developing countries where many patients are poor and malnourished.

There are two forms of pellagra. Primary pellagra occurs when the patient's diet lacks niacin. This can either be due to a direct dietary deficiency of niacin or a dietary deficiency of tryptophan, an amino acid that the body can convert to niacin. Secondary pellagra arises when there is adequate niacin and tryptophan in the patient's diet, but the patient is not able to absorb the niacin or convert the tryptophan to niacin. Secondary pellagra is usually seen in the setting of chronic diarrhea, Hartnup's disease (which prevents normal absorption of amino acids), carcinoid tumors (which will deplete tryptophan levels), or chronic alcoholism and liver damage leading to poor absorption. Isoniazid therapy, which is utilized to treat tuberculosis, can also cause pellagra. Isoniazid binds to and inactivates vitamin B6 so that it cannot be used in the synthesis of niacin.

The most important symptoms of pellagra are known as the 4 D's: diarrhea, dermatitis, dementia, and death. Dermatitis will present as alopecia (loss of hair), red skin lesions, and peeling, scaling, and thickening of skin that has been exposed to sunlight. Early mental changes include insomnia and fatigue, but eventually progress to dementia, hallucinations, and confusion. If left untreated, pellagra will typically kill within 4 to 5 years. Other symptoms include dilated cardiomyopathy (enlarged heart), glossitis (inflammation of the tongue), ataxia (loss of coordination), and aggressive behavior.

Treatment and Therapy

The diagnosis of pellagra can be made based on symptoms alone. Treatments for pellagra include nicotinamide and supplemental niacin. Nicotinamide is preferred to niacin due to the fact that niacin often produces unpleasant side effects such as itching, burning, and flushing of the skin. Nicotinamide can be given orally or by injection. The amount of nicotinamide administered and the frequency of administration is determined by the degree to which the pellagra has progressed. Improvements typically begin within days of starting nicotinamide therapy.

—*Steffan Kim*

See also: Hartnup's disease, carcinoid tumor, chronic alcoholism

For Further Information:
"Dr. Joseph Goldberger & the War on Pellagra." *Office of NIH History*, history.nih.gov/exhibits/Goldberger/index.html. Accessed 19 Oct. 2016.
Hegyi, Vladimir et al. "Dermatologic Manifestations of Pellagra." *Medscape*, 22 Feb. 2016, emedicine.medscape.com/article/1095845-overview. Accessed 19 Oct. 2016.
"History of Pellagra." *University of Alabama at Birmingham Reynolds-Finley Historical Library*, www.uab.edu/reynolds/pellagra/history. Accessed 19 Oct. 2016.
Ngan, Vanessa. "Pellagra." *DermNet New Zealand*, www.dermnetnz.org/topics/pellagra/. Accessed 19 Oct. 2016.
"The Origins of Maize: The Puzzle of Pellagra." *European Food Information Council*, Dec. 2001, www.eufic.org/article/en/artid/origins-maize-pellagra/. Accessed 19 Oct. 2016.
"Pellagra." *MedlinePlus*, medlineplus.gov/ency/article/000342.htm. Accessed 19 Oct. 2016.
"Pellagra." *PBS Learning Media*, wvia.pbslearningmedia.org/resource/odys08.sci.life.gen.pellagra/pellagra/. Accessed 19 Oct. 2016.

Pelvic inflammatory disease (PID)

Disease/Disorder

Anatomy or system affected: Genitals, reproductive system, uterus

Specialties and related fields: Gynecology, microbiology

Definition: A serious bacterial infection of the upper genital tract that is often sexually transmitted.

Key terms:

contact tracing: also known as partner referral; a process that involves identifying the sexual partners of infected patients, informing the partners of their exposure to disease, and offering resources for counseling and treatment

ectopic pregnancy: a pregnancy that occurs anywhere other than in the uterus; ectopic pregnancies can be life-threatening, since they can rupture and bleed profusely

laparoscopy: a minimally invasive surgical procedure performed through small incisions in the abdomen

polymicrobial infection: an infection caused by multiple microorganisms such as bacteria and viruses

sexually transmitted disease(STD): an infection caused by organisms transferred through sexual contact (genital-genital, oral-genital, oral-anal, or anal-genital); the transmission of infection occurs through exposure to lesions or secretions that contain the organisms

Causes and Symptoms

Pelvic inflammatory disease (PID) is a polymicrobial infection of the upper genital tract. The infectious microbes may be sexually transmitted organisms (such as *Neisseria gonorrhea, Chlamydiatrachomatis,* and *Mycoplasma genitalium*) and/or endogenous bacteria found in the vagina (e.g., staphylococci, streptococci, enteric bacteria, such as *Klebsiella* species, *Escherichia coli* or *Proteus* species, or anaerobic bacteria like *Bacteroides* species). These microorganisms can travel from the lower genital tract (vagina, cervix) into the upper genital tract (uterus, Fallopian tubes, ovaries, and pelvic cavity) and establish infection there. Occasionally, PID can occur via another mechanism, such as any infection and rupture of the appendix or lower gastrointestinal tract that causes spillage of bacteria into the pelvic cavity.

85 percent of PID cases are caused by sexually transmitter microorganisms or by bacteria that cause infections of the birth canal (vaginosis). The remaining PID cases are caused by normal microbial residents of the lower reproductive tract of females.

Approximately 106,000 outpatient visits and 60,000 hospitalizations each year are due to PID. Each female PID patient costs around $2,000 to treat, and this number can rise to $6,000 if she develops chronic pelvic pain.

Most cases of PID are asymptomatic. In cases where symptoms occur, the patient has lower abdominal or pelvic pain. The Centers for Disease Control and Prevention (CDC) stipulates the diagnostic criteria for PID, noting that the diagnosis is made on clinical findings rather than on laboratory evidence. During abdominal examination, the lower abdomen is tender to palpation. Upon pelvic examination, either the cervix is tender upon movement by the examiner or one or both ovaries or the Fallopian tubes are tender to palpation; both of these symptoms can be present as well. Other symptoms and signs of PID include fever and abnormal cervical discharge.

Laboratory tests can be helpful in establishing a diagnosis when clinical symptoms are ambiguous and in emphasizing the need for partner treatment. Tests include blood tests that suggest systemic inflammation (such as the erythrocyte sedimentation rate) and cultures or nucleic acid amplification tests for *N. gonorrhea* or *C. trachomatis*. With ultrasound or other imaging techniques, fluid collections associated with the Fallopian tubes, ovaries, or elsewhere in the pelvic cavity can be identified as consistent with PID. On rare occasions, PID can spread to the upper abdomen, leading to pain and tenderness in that area. In particular, the infection can affect the region surrounding the liver, leading to Fitz-Hugh Curtis syndrome.

Long-term consequences of PID can be significant and can occur in asymptomatic as well as symptomatic patients. PID can cause scarring of the reproductive tract leading to infertility. Damaged fallopian tubes can fill with fluid (hydrosalpinx) and cause pain and infertility. PID increases the risk for ectopic pregnancy, a potentially life-threatening condition. If the infection spreads beyond the reproductive tract, then organs such as the bowels may become involved in the infection as well. Any organs involved in the infection run the risk of becoming damaged and scarred and might abnormally adhere to other organs. In addition to the acute pain of PID, the disease can also lead to chronic pelvic pain, which can be difficult to treat. Women with a history of PID have an almost two-fold increase in the risk of ovarian cancer.

Treatment and Therapy

Pelvic inflammatory disease is usually treated in an outpatient setting, although severe cases require hospitalization and intravenous medications. Antibiotics are the first-line treatment for PID, which is most commonly treated empirically based on clinical suspicion. Because PID is polymicrobial, combinations of antibiotics, each targeted

---

Information on Pelvic Inflammatory Disease (PID)

Causes: Bacterial infection transmitted through sexual contact or from other areas of body

Symptoms: Usually asymptomatic; may involve lower abdominal or pelvic pain, fever, abnormal cervical or vaginal discharge; can lead to scarring, infertility, ectopic pregnancy

Duration: Chronic

Treatments: Antibiotics, abscess drainage if needed

---

at different bacteria, are given simultaneously. Drug regimens differ according to the severity of the disease. For severe PID, patients are usually treated in the hospital with cefotetan or cefoxitin combined with doxycycline, or clindamycin plus gentamicin. For mild to moderate PID, outpatient therapy is preferred and first-line treatments typically consist of ceftriaxone or cefoxitin/probenecid or cefotaxime plus doxycycline. Metronidazole is sometimes added to regimens as a third drug to cover anaerobic organisms and is always included if infection with the protozoan *Trichomonas vaginalis* is suspected. Unfortunately, the stomach discomfort caused by metronidazole can cause patients to stop taking it prematurely. Infections with *C. trachomitis* may warrant the inclusion of azithromycin, and for *N. gonorrhea* infections, ceftriaxone and doxycycline are particularly effective. Because of resistance, fluoroquinolone antibiotics (e.g., ciprofloxacin, moxifloxacin) are no longer used to treat gonorrhea infections. Patients are normally treated for 14 days.

Since PID is usually sexually transmitted, therapy involves counseling regarding the prevention of sexually transmitted infections (STIs) and safer sexual techniques. Condoms and other barrier techniques decrease the spread of STIs. Anal penetration followed by vaginal penetration during intercourse may increase the risk of infection of the female reproductive tract. Testing for other STIs, such as hepatitis B and C and syphilis; wet prep testing for bacterial vaginosis and trichomonas; and screening for human immunodeficiency virus (HIV) are all encouraged, since the risk factors for PID and other STIs are similar. Contact tracing is offered to notify sexual partners of their possible exposure to STIs and to encourage them to seek medical attention. Treatment of these partners can decrease reinfection of the patient from subsequent sexual encounters and prevent the partners from spreading infection to others. Having multiple sex partners is a risk factor for PID.

Perspective and Prospects

One of the first reports of PID was from ancient Greece and involved a case in which pus from the pelvis was drained through the vagina. However, it was not until the 1880s that the sequence of events starting with the ascension of lower genital tract infection to cause upper tract disease was recognized. With the widespread use of laparoscopy in the 1960s, a more accurate diagnosis of PID could be made, allowing clinicians to recognize that PID has many clinical presentations. Future prospects focus primarily on the prevention of PID, since treatment does not prevent many of the long-term effects. Prevention involves continued widespread screening of asymptomatic men and women at risk for STDs, as well as partner referral and safer-sex education. Studies have shown that the screening and treatment of asymptomatic women for STDs has reduced the prevalence of these infections in the general population in the United States, thus translating into a reduction in the incidence of PID. With these prevention techniques, there is hope that the morbidity and serious sequelae of PID will be reduced.

—Anne Lynn S. Chang, MD;
updated by Michael A. Buratovich, PhD

See also: Antibiotics; Bacterial infections; Chlamydia; Contraception; Ectopic pregnancy; Genital disorders, female; Gonorrhea; Gynecology; Infertility, female; Ovaries; Reproductive system; Sexually transmitted diseases (STDs); Uterus; Women's health.

For Further Information:

Holmes, King K., et al., eds. *Sexually Transmitted Diseases*. 4th ed. New York: McGraw-Hill Medical, 2008.

Kasper, Dennis L., et al., eds. *Harrison's Principles of Internal Medicine*. 16th ed. New York: McGraw-Hill, 2005.

"Pelvic Inflammatory Disease (PID) Treatment." *Centers for Disease Control and Prevention*, March 1, 2013.

Schuiling, Kerri Durnell, and Frances E. Likis. *Women's Gynecologic Health*, 2d ed. Sudbury, Mass.: Jones and Bartlett Learning, 2013.

Sutton, Amy L. *Sexually Transmitted Diseases Sourcebook*. Detroit, Mich.: 2013.

Sweet, Richard L., and Harold C. Wiesenfeld, eds. *Pelvic Inflammatory Disease*. New York: Taylor & Francis, 2006.

Vorvick, Linda J. "Pelvic Inflammatory Disease (PID)." *MedlinePlus*, September 12, 2011.

Workowski, Kimberly A. "Sexually Transmitted Diseases Treatment Guidelines 2010." *Centers for Disease Control and Prevention*, December 17, 2010.

Penile implant surgery

Procedure

Anatomy or system affected: Genitals, reproductive system
Specialties and related fields: General surgery, psychiatry, urology
Definition: The surgical placement of a prosthetic device inside the penis to make it rigid enough for penetration.

Key terms:

corpora cavernosa: two parallel erectile cylinders on the upper side of the penis that are filled with blood during a natural erection

corpus spongiosum: a third cylinder in the penis below the corpora cavernosa; the urethra passes through it and the glans penis forms the front end of the cylinder

erection: a complex phenomenon involving nerves, blood vessels, and the mind that leads to the entrapment of blood in the penis, making it rigid

glans penis: the head of the penis

impotence: the lack of sustained erection that is rigid enough for penetration in sexual intercourse

urethra: the channel through which urine and seminal fluid are passed; it starts at the bladder neck, goes through the shaft of the penis, and ends at the glans penis

Indications and Procedures

Penile implant surgery is performed when all other, nonsurgical means of treating impotence, or erectile dysfunction, have been exhausted or are not suitable for the patient. A thorough workup must be performed to diagnose the cause of the impotence, which can be psychogenic or organic. The term "psychogenic" is used when there are no anatomical, hormonal, or physiological problems with the patient's erectile mechanism; instead, the problem is in the patient's mind. Organic causes include poor blood flow to the penis, the inability of the erectile cylinders to trap blood in the penis (venous leak), or a problem with the nerves, which is seen in diabetic patients. Impotence may also result from a hormonal disturbance.

A penile implant, or penile prosthesis, is an artificial device, usually consisting of inflatable cylinders and a pump, that can simulate an erection in men who suffer from impotence that has a biological (rather than a psychological) cause. When the patient squeezes the pump in the scrotum, fluid from an implanted reservoir fills the cylinders.

Organic causes for impotence can be determined with certain tests, including an analysis of blood chemistry and hormone levels, as well as a test for the presence of erection during sleep. Finally, the physician may perform an invasive test in which a drug is injected into the penis so that the erectile response can be observed. Usually, less aggressive, nonsurgical treatments are tried first. If they fail, then penile implant surgery is considered.

There are two types of implants: One is semirigid and malleable, and the other is inflatable. Semirigid rods, the earliest type of penile prostheses, are inserted into the corpora cavernosa (erectile tissue) in the penis. The advantages of this type are a simple surgical technique, lack of mechanical failure, and low cost. The disadvantages include poor cosmetic results because of a permanently rigid penis, which is difficult to conceal, and extrusion of the penile implant. The malleable prosthesis is like a semirigid one except that it can be bent in the middle, so that concealment is not as difficult. Lifting the prosthesis upward makes it rigid. The design of these prostheses is based on a central wire with multiple springs that cause the penis to become erect when the prosthesis is pulled upward and the springs come into position so that they support one another.

The second group of penile prostheses are inflatable. These multicomponent prostheses contain two cylinders that fit in the corpora cavernosa. The fluid from a reservoir is pumped into the cylinders to achieve an erection. After the prosthesis has been used, the fluid is pumped back into the reservoir, and the penis becomes flaccid. There are two types of inflatable prosthesis: one in which the pump and the fluid reservoir are combined (two-component type) and one in which the pump is separate from the reservoir (three-component type). The advantage of this type of penile prosthesis is that it more closely mimics a natural erection, in hich the penis not only elongates but also expands in di- ameter. In addition, the penis is closer to a normal shape when in the flaccid state. The disadvantages are significantly higher cost, the chance of mechanical failure in the

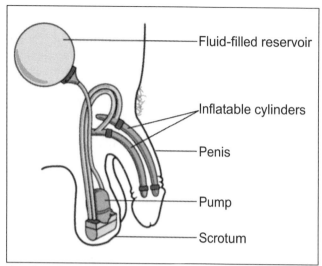

Fluid-filled reservoir

Inflatable cylinders

Penis

Pump

Scrotum

A penile implant is an artificial device, usually consisting of inflatable cylinders and a pump, that can simulate an erection in men who suffer from impotence that has a biological (rather than a psychological) cause. When the patient squeezes the pump in the scrotum, fluid from an implanted reservoir fills the cylinders.

connections and tubing, and the chance of leakage of fluid from the reservoir or the cylinders. The total time of the operation is slightly more for inflatable penile prostheses than semirigid and malleable prostheses.

The surgical approaches for the placement of a penile prosthesis are the same for semirigid, malleable, and inflatable types. In the infrapubic approach, the patient is placed on his back. An incision is made at the junction where the penis meets the body, just above the penis in the lower part of the abdominal wall. After the skin and fatty tissues are cut, the corpora cavernosa are exposed. While carefully protecting the nerve responsible for sensation in the penis, the surgeon opens and dilates the corpora cavernosa. The lengths of the corpora are measured, appropriate-length artificial cylinders are inserted, and the corpora are closed.

In the case of semirigid and malleable prostheses, the operation ends after the skin is closed. In the case of an inflatable penile prosthesis, however, two extra steps are taken. A place is created for the pump and reservoir. In a two-component inflatable penile prosthesis, a pocket is created for the combined pump and reservoir just underneath the skin of the scrotum, in an area that is easily accessible to the patient. In a three-component penile prosthesis, a pocket is created in thescrotum for the pump and a space is created for the reservoir in the lower part of the abdomen, above the pubic bone and in front of the bladder. The reservoir is connected to the pump, and in this fashion the placement of the prosthesis is completed. An appropriate amount of fluid is left in the reservoir based on the length of the cylinders. The penile prosthesis is evaluated for proper function and cosmetic appearance, and the incision is closed.

Uses and Complications

In the immediate postoperative phase, the cylinder of the inflatable penile prosthesis is left totally deflated so that a scar forms around the pump and reservoir that will allow

the normal function of the prosthesis in the future. After two weeks, the cylinders are cycled: The patient inflates his penile prosthesis for thirty to sixty minutes every day and then deflates it. In about six weeks, the pain should have subsided significantly so that the patient is ready to use his penile prosthesis for sexual intercourse. Close monitoring ensures that no infection develops, and the patient is asked to report to the doctor immediately if there is any redness or swelling in the area, which are signs of an impending infection. If an infection occurs, it is initially treated aggressively with antibiotics. If antibiotic therapy does not work, the penile prosthesis may have to be removed.

The complications associated with penile implants include infection, mechanical failure (resulting in the loss of pump or reservoir function), and inadvertent inflation of an inflatable penile prosthesis when the patient sits or stands up. In certain cases, the penile prosthesis can also migrate forward or backward. It can even perforate the corpora cavernosa and extrude through the penis, an emergency situation that needs to be corrected immediately. There is a remote possibility of gangrene of the penis if infection and extrusion take place simultaneously.

Perspective and Prospects

Penile implant surgery is an excellent procedure for patients who have problems with impotence that is not treatable with medication, in that the implant allows them to achieve an erection rigid enough for penetration. This surgery is more applicable in younger patients who have become impotent, either because of diabetes mellitus or after surgical treatment of prostate or rectal cancer, which can lead to damage of the nerves responsible for erection. An older age is not a contraindication for penile prosthesis, however, if the patient is in good physical condition and wants a penile prosthesis. In all cases, it is important that surgery be performed only after significant counseling with the patient, who should understand all the benefits and risks.

The technology involved in penile implant surgery has evolved since the 1970s, starting from a simple, rigid prosthesis and leading to an inflatable, multicomponent prosthesis. The incidence of mechanical failure in the multicomponent inflatable prosthesis is constantly decreasing, and some companies that manufacture this type now offer a lifetime warranty.

—Saeed Akhter, M.D.

See also Diabetes mellitus; Erectile dysfunction; Gender reassignment surgery; Genital disorders, male; Men's health; Prostate cancer; Psychiatry; Reproductive system; Sexual dysfunction; Testicular surgery; Urology.

For Further Information:

Buchanan, Jill. "Penile Prosthesis Insertion." *Health Library*, November 26, 2012.

Carson, Culley C., III. "Penile Prosthesis Implantation: Surgical Implants in the Era of Oral Medication." In *Erectile Dysfunction*, edited by Carson and Martin I. Resnick. Philadelphia: Saunders/Elsevier, 2005.

Carson, Culley C., III. *Urologic Prostheses: The Complete Practical Guide to Devices, Their Implantation, and Patient Followup*. Totowa, N.J.: Humana Press, 2002.

Ellsworth, Pamela, and Bob Stanley. *One Hundred Questions and Answers About Erectile Dysfunction*. 2d ed. Sudbury, Mass.: Jones and Bartlett, 2008.

Parker, James N., and Philip M. Parker, eds. *The Official Patient's Sourcebook on Impotence*. San Diego, Calif.: Icon Health, 2002.

"Penile Implants." *Mayo Clinic*, February 25, 2011.

Pryor, John P. *Urological Prostheses, Appliances, and Catheters*. New York: Springer, 1992.

Taguchi, Yosh, and Merrily Weisbord, eds. *Private Parts: An Owner's Guide to the Male Anatomy*. 3d ed. Toronto, Ont.: McClelland & Stewart, 2003.

Tanagho, Emil A., and Jack W. McAninch, eds. *Smith's General Urology*. 17th ed. New York: McGraw-Hill, 2008.

Wein, Alan J., et al., eds. *Campbell-Walsh Urology*. 10th ed. Philadelphia: Saunders/Elsevier, 2012.

Peptic ulcers. *See* Ulcers.

Perinatology

Specialty

Anatomy or system affected: All

Specialties and related fields: Embryology, neonatology, obstetrics, pediatrics

Definition: The branch of medicine dealing with the fetus and infant during the perinatal period (from the twenty-eighth week of gestation to the twenty-eighth day after birth).

Key terms:

amniotic fluid: fluid within the amniotic cavity produced by the amnion during the early embryonic period (two to eight weeks) and later by the lungs and kidneys

cesarean section: an incision made through the abdominal and uterine walls for the delivery of a fetus

fetus: the unborn offspring in the postembryonic period, from nine weeks after fertilization until birth

infant: a young child from birth to twelve months of age

ischemia: a local anemia or area of diminished or insufficient blood supply as a result of mechanical obstruction of the blood supply (commonly narrowing of an artery)

placenta: a fetomaternal organ that joins mother and offspring; it secretes endocrine hormones and selectively exchanges soluble, blood-borne substances through its interior structures

Rh: a human blood factor, originally identified in rhesus monkeys, that can be either positive (present) or negative (absent)

Science and Profession

Practitioners of perinatal medicine include physicians and advanced practice nurses with a specialty in perinatology (neonatal and pediatric nurse practitioners). They then complete additional training specifically related to the perinatal period (defined variously as beginning from twenty to twenty-eight weeks of gestation and ending one to four weeks after birth). The emphasis of perinatology is on a time period rather than on a specific organ system. The principal event of the perinatal period is birth. Prior to delivery, the perinatologist is concerned with the physiological status and well-being of both mother and fetus. Immediately after delivery, the perinatologist strives to maximize the newborn's chances for survival.

Diagnostic and Treatment Techniques

Prior to the birth, several diagnostic procedures are commonly employed by the perinatologist: ultrasonography, the measurement of fetal activity, and the evaluation of fetal lung maturity. Ultrasonography uses sound waves to create images. Sound waves are transmitted from a transducer that has been placed on the skin. Waves that are sent into the body reflect off internal tissues and structures, and the reflections are received by a microphone. Sound travels through tissues with different densities at different rates, which are characteristic for each tissue. Computers interpret the reflected sounds and convert them into an image that can be viewed. The images must be interpreted or read by someone with specialized training, usually a radiologist. Ultrasound does not involve radiation; thus it is not harmful to the fetus. Because sound waves are longer than radiation, the image generated is not as clear as that obtained with electromagnetic waves.

The measurement of fetal activity is important in evaluating fetal health. Fetal movement is normal; the earliest movement felt by the mother is called quickening. The diminution or cessation of fetal movement is indicative of fetal distress. Accordingly, movement is monitored by reports from the mother, palpation by the clinician, and ultrasound: Mothers report movements, individuals examining pregnant women can apply their hands to the abdomen and feel fetal movements, and ultrasonography can show breathing and other movements in real time using continuous video records of fetal movements.

Fetal lung maturity is assessed by measuring the relative amounts of lecithin and sphingomyelin in amniotic fluid. The concentration of lecithin increases late in fetal development, while sphingomyelin decreases. A lecithin-sphingomyelin ratio that is greater than two indicates sufficient fetal lung maturity to ensure survival after birth.

Labor and delivery are the primary events of the perinatal period. Factors that can lead to difficulties include abnormalities of the placenta and prematurity. The placenta can be abnormally located (placenta previa) or can separate prematurely (placenta abruptio). Normally, the placenta is located on the lateral wall of the uterus. Placenta previa is defined as a placenta located in the lower portion of the uterus. The placenta is compressed by the fetus during passage through the birth canal. This compression compromises the blood supply to the fetus, which causes ischemia and can lead to brain or other tissue damage or to death. This condition is usually managed by a cesarean section. Placenta abruptio refers to a normal placenta that separates prior to fetal delivery. This condition is potentially life-threatening to both mother and fetus; immediate hospitalization is indicated.

Prematurity is defined as delivery before the fetus is able to survive without unusual support. Premature infants are placed in incubators. A lack of body fat in the infant leads to difficulty in maintaining a normal body temperature; special heating is provided to offset the problem. Lung immaturity may require mechanical assistance from a respirator. An immature immune system makes premature infants especially susceptible to infections; strict isolation precautions and prophylactic antibiotic therapy address this problem.

Many factors contribute to increasing the risks normally associated with pregnancy and delivery: maternal size and age; drug, tobacco, or alcohol use; infection; medical conditions such as diabetes mellitus and hypertension; and multiple gestations. A woman with a small pelvic opening may be unable to deliver her child normally; the solution in this case is a cesarean section. The risk of genetic abnormalities increases with advancing maternal (and, to a lesser degree, paternal) age. Counseling prior to conception is indicated. Once an older woman becomes pregnant, amniotic fluid should be obtained to test for genetic abnormalities. The degree of surveillance is dependent on maternal age: The recommended frequency of medical checks increases for older women.

Alcohol intake during pregnancy can result in an infant who is both developmentally disabled and mentally retarded; smoking during pregnancy frequently leads to an infant with a low birth weight. Drug usage during pregnancy can lead to anatomic or mental impairment. Avoiding the use of all substances is the easiest way to eliminate problems completely; any drug should be used only under the guidance of a physician. Some viral infections such as German measles (rubella) early in pregnancy can cause birth defects. Immunization prior to conception will avoid these problems.

Diabetes mellitus can cause abnormally large intrauterine growth and babies (frequently more than 10 pounds and referred to as macrosomic) who are too large for normal delivery. Diabetes that commonly develops during pregnancy is called gestational diabetes. Medical monitoring to detect diabetes early is prudent. Appropriate medical management of preexisting diabetes minimizes problems associated with pregnancy. A macrosomic infant must be delivered with a cesarean section. Hypertension can also develop during pregnancy. Like diabetes, it can compromise both mother and fetus. Appropriate and aggressive medical management, sometimes including complete bed rest, is needed to control high blood pressure during pregnancy. Multiple gestations (such as twins or triplets) strain the supply of maternal nutrients to the developing fetuses. Because space is limited, multiple fetuses are usually smaller than normal at birth.

Rhesus disease, also known as Rh incompatibility, can complicate pregnancy. It can occur only in the child of a father whose blood type is Rh-positive and a mother whose blood type is Rh-negative, and it affects the blood supply of a fetus. The treatment includes the identification of both maternal and paternal blood types and the administration of Rho(D) immune globulin to the mother at twenty-six weeks of gestation and again immediately after birth. An affected infant may require blood transfusions; in a severe case, transfusions may be needed during pregnancy.

Perspective and Prospects

Management of a pregnancy requires specialized skills. As the number of risk factors related to either mother or fetus increases, the problems associated with pregnancy also increase. The care of a pregnant woman and her fetus requires input from many individuals with specialized training. Consequently, perinatology is very much a team effort. Together, the team members can ensure a safe journey through the perinatal period for a pregnant woman and a healthy transition to life outside the womb for a newborn infant.

—*L. Fleming Fallon, Jr., M.D., Ph.D., M.P.H.*

For Further Information:
Bradford, Nikki. *Your Premature Baby: The First Five Years*. Toronto, Ont.: Firefly Books, 2003.
Creasy, Robert K., and Robert Resnik, eds. *Maternal-Fetal Medicine: Principles and Practice*. 5th ed. Philadelphia: W. B. Saunders, 2004.
Cunningham, F. Gary, et al., eds. *Williams Obstetrics*. 23d ed. New York: McGraw-Hill, 2010.
Martin, Richard J., Avroy A. Fanaroff, and Michele C. Walsh, eds. *Fanaroff and Martin's Neonatal-Perinatal Medicine: Diseases of the Fetus and Infant*. 2 vols. 9th ed. Philadelphia: Mosby/Elsevier, 2011.
Moore, Keith L., and T. V. N. Persaud. *The Developing Human*. 9th ed. Philadelphia: Saunders/Elsevier, 2013.
"Pregnancy and Perinatology Branch (PPB)." *National Institute of Child Health and Human Development*, November 30, 2012.
Ruhlman, Michael. *Walk on Water: Inside an Elite Pediatric Surgery Unit*. New York: Viking-Penguin, 2003.
Sadler, T. W. *Langman's Medical Embryology*. 12th ed. Philadelphia: Lippincott Williams & Wilkins, 2012

Periodontal surgery

Procedure

Anatomy or system affected: Gums, mouth, teeth
Specialties and related fields: Dentistry, general surgery, orthodontics
Definition: Any surgical procedure involving tissues or bone associated with support of the teeth.

Indications and Procedures

Periodontal disease is the most common cause of tooth loss among persons middle-aged or older. Most periodontal problems originate as dental caries, or cavities, the decay and destruction of teeth by bacteria. While most common periodontal difficulties can be prevented or solved through regular visits to the dentist, if decay is untreated it may lead to serious dental problems. At their worst, periodontal problems may require surgery as part of the treatment.

If decay develops within the root area, a pus-filled abscess may develop. The first indication is an ache or throbbing in the area of the tooth. The gum may be tender and swollen. If the abscess begins to spread, local lymph nodes in the neck may become swollen, as well as that portion of the face. Without proper treatment, the abscess may damage the jawbone or even result in blood poisoning.

The abscess may be eliminated through a root canal procedure, in which the pus is drained and the canal cleaned and filled. If the infection has spread into underlying tissue, however, more general surgery may be required. In a procedure called an apicoectomy, both the root and the bone that covers the root may be drilled away by the oral surgeon. Antibiotics may also be administered to eliminate the infection completely.

Uses and Complications

Most periodontal problems begin with dental caries and gingivitis, an inflammation of the tissue of the gums by bacteria that are associated with the formation of caries. If these conditions are not treated by a dentist in their early stages, they may progress to more serious problems. In addition to the danger of abscess formation, pockets of infection may develop under the gums. Gingivectomy, a minor surgical procedure in which such sites of infection are removed, can usually treat cases that are not advanced.

In most instances, proper oral hygiene is sufficient to prevent problems. When necessary, surgical procedures can treat more advanced cases successfully. Complications are rare and are usually associated with bacteria that are able to survive in isolated crypts. Such sites offer threats of abscess formation. For this reason, the dentist or oral surgeon will monitor the results of the periodontal procedure for some months afterward.

—*Richard Adler, Ph.D.*

See also Abscess drainage; Abscesses; Cavities; Dental diseases; Dentistry; Endodontic disease; Gingivitis; Gum disease; Oral and maxillofacial surgery; Periodontitis; Plaque, dental; Root canal treatment; Teeth; Tooth extraction; Toothache.

For Further Information:
Chwistek, Marcin. "Root Canal." *Health Library*, Mar. 15, 2013.
Eley, Barry M., M. Soory, and Julius David Manson. *Periodontics.* 6th ed. Edinburgh, Scotland: Saunders/Elsevier, 2010.
Neff, Deanna M., and Laura Morris-Olson. "Periodontal Surgery-Open Flap." *Health Library*, June 4, 2012.
Neff, Deanna M., and Laura Morris-Olson. "Periodontal Surgery-Soft Tissue Graft." *Health Library*, June 4, 2012.
"Periodontal Plastic Surgery." *American Academy of Cosmetic Dentistry*, n.d.
Preus, Hans R., and Lars Laurell. *Periodontal Diseases: A Manual of Diagnosis, Treatment, and Maintenance.* Chicago: Quintessence, 2003.
Renner, Robert P. *An Introduction to Dental Anatomy and Esthetics.* Chicago: Quintessence, 1985.
Ring, Malvin E. *Dentistry: An Illustrated History.* New York: Abradale, 1992.
Rose, Louis F., et al., eds. *Periodontics: Medicine, Surgery, and Implants.* St. Louis, Mo.: Mosby, 2004.
Scully, Crispian, and Athanasios Kalantzis. *Oxford Handbook of Dental Patient Care.* 2d ed. New York: Oxford University Press, 2005.
Taintor, Jerry, and Mary Jane Taintor. *The Complete Guide to Better Dental Care.* New York: Checkmark Books, 1999.

Periodontitis

Disease/Disorder
Also known as: Pyorrhea, gum disease
Anatomy or system affected: Bones, gums, teeth
Specialties and related fields: Dentistry, orthodontics
Definition: A disorder of the teeth resulting from advanced gingivitis, inflammation and infection of the bones and the ligaments supporting the teeth.

Key terms:
calculus: mineralized dental plaque, which forms both above and below the gum line and harbors bacteria that produce toxins and cause the gums to become inflamed
dental plaque: a sticky substance, composed of millions of bacteria, that collects around and between teeth; a major cause of tooth decay and gum disease (gingivitis), it is hard to see because it is whitish colored like the teeth
gingivitis: a disorder involving inflammation of the gums (gingiva)
oral cancer: a disorder involving abnormal, malignant tissue growth in the mouth
periodontal ligament: the connective tissue structure that surrounds the root and connects it with the bone
periodontal pocket: a large pocket that forms between the teeth and gums; it collects plaque, calculus, and debris from food and other sources

Causes and Symptoms

Periodontitis is the advanced stage of gum disease (or periodontal disease) that occurs when the earlier stage of gum disease, gingivitis, is left untreated or if treatment is delayed. Gingivitis is caused by bacteria in plaque and tartar, which if left on the teeth for too long can inflame and infect the gums. In periodontitis, the infection and inflammation spread from the gums (gingiva) to the ligaments and bones that support the teeth. Dental plaque begins to spread down the roots of the teeth, and the gums become infected, which causes damage to the bone and fibers (periodontal ligament) that support the teeth. As the disease progresses, the gums pull away from the teeth, allowing more food and plaque to be trapped under them and inviting more damage to occur. In advanced stages of the disease, the teeth become increasingly loose, and shifting may occur because of widespread damage to the bone and ligaments holding the teeth in place. The bite may therefore shift, and there may be difficulty chewing. Loss of support causes the teeth to become increasingly loose and eventually fall out.

Periodontal disease can be caused by the use of smokeless tobacco. In the areas where the tobacco is held against the cheek, the tobacco and by-products cause irritation and infection of the gums. The gums begin to recede, and periodontal disease affects the teeth in the area. The area is also highly prone to oral cancer.

The early symptoms of periodontitis tend to resemble those of gingivitis, with mouth sores and swollen gums that are tender when touched but otherwise painless. Progressive symptoms include swollen gums that are bright red or reddish-purple. The gums may appear shiny and may bleed easily, and there may be odor to the breath.

Treatment and Therapy

Treatment methods for advanced (chronic) periodontal disease include aggressive oral hygiene instruction and reinforcement and evaluation of the patient's plaque control. Scaling and root planing to remove microbial plaque and calculus below the gum line, followed by surgery to reduce the depth of the periodontal pocket, is the most common office-based procedure to help manage the disease. Lesions

---

Information on Periodontitis

Causes: Untreated inflammation or infection of gums; may result from use of smokeless tobacco

Symptoms: Swollen gums that are tender, bright red or reddish-purple, shiny, and bleed easily; mouth sores; bad breath

Duration: Chronic, progressive if not treated

Treatments: Proper oral hygiene, plaque control (scaling, root planing, surgery), antibiotics

---

may be treated with adjunctive antimicrobial therapy and antibiotics. Long-term maintenance is necessary. Flossing, more frequent brushing, and mouthwashes are recommended to the patient between regular dental visits.

The long-term outcome of treatment may depend upon patient compliance and professional maintenance at appropriate intervals. If the primary teeth are affected, then the infection should be monitored closely in order to avoid possible attachment loss. The goals of periodontal therapy include altering or eliminating the causative microbes and contributing risk factors for periodontitis, thereby arresting advancement of the disease and preserving the teeth. Ultimately, it is desirable to prevent the recurrence of periodontitis. Because of the complexity of aggressive periodontal disease with regard to systemic factors, immune defects, and microbial flora, however, control may not be possible in all instances. In such cases, a reasonable treatment objective is to slow the progression of the disease.

Perspective and Prospects

Periodontitis is the primary cause of tooth loss in adults. This disorder is uncommon in childhood, but the incidence rate increases during adolescence. In addition to a lack of good oral hygiene, certain risk factors have been associated with periodontitis. It is more severe and occurs with a frequency two to five times greater among patients with diabetes mellitus. Smoking can increase the risk of developing severe periodontitis by a factor of three to six times, depending on smoking duration and number of cigarettes.

While periodontitis can be managed effectively with current surgical and nonsurgical therapies in some patients, other patients are less responsive to the treatment options available. Most people with periodontitis receive little or no treatment at all.

—*Jason A. Hubbart, M.S.*

See also Abscess drainage; Abscesses; Cavities; Dental diseases; Dentistry; Endodontic disease; Gingivitis; Gum disease; Halitosis; Oral and maxillofacial surgery; Periodontal surgery; Plaque, dental; Root canal treatment; Teeth; Tooth extraction; Toothache.

For Further Information:

Detienville, Roger. *Clinical Success in Management of Advanced Periodontitis*. Translated by Nicolai Johnson. Chicago: Quintessence International, 2005.

Edwardsson, S., et al. "The Microbiota of Periodontal Pockets with Different Depths in the Therapy-Resistant Periodontitis." *Journal of Clinical Periodontology* 26, no. 3 (1999): 143-152.

"Gum Disease." *MedlinePlus*, Apr. 25, 2013.

"Gum Disease Information." *American Academy of Periodontology*, 2013.

Healthnet: Connecticut Consumer Health Information Network. "Your Dental Health: A Guide for Patients and Families." *UConn Health Center*, Nov. 27, 2012.

Lamont, R. J., and H. F. Jenkinson. "Life Below the Gum Line: Pathogenic Mechanism of Porphyromonas Gingivalis." *Microbiology and Molecular Biology Reviews* 62, no. 4 (1998): 1244-1263.

Page, R. C. "The Role of Inflammatory Mediators in the Pathogenesis of Periodontal Disease." *Journal of Periodontal Research* 26 (1991): 230-242.

Page, R. C., and K. S. Kornman. "The Pathogenesis of Human Periodontitis: An Introduction." *Periodontology* 2000 14 (1997): 9-11.

"Periodontal (Gum) Disease: Causes, Symptoms, and Treatments." *National Institute of Dental and Craniofacial Research*, Aug. 2012.

Reynolds, J. J., and M. C. Meikle. "Mechanism of Connective Tissue Destruction in Periodontitis." *Periodontology* 2000 14 (1997): 144-157.

Rose, Louis F., et al., eds. *Periodontics: Medicine, Surgery, and Implants*. St. Louis, Mo.: Mosby, 2004.

Peristalsis

Biology

Anatomy or system affected: Abdomen, gastrointestinal system, intestines, stomach

Specialties and related fields: Gastroenterology, internal medicine

Definition: A series of muscular contractions that sweep along the gastrointestinal tract, causing a localized narrowing that pushes food and waste material from the mouth to the anus for excretion.

Key terms:

digestion: the mechanical and chemical process of breaking down food into small units called molecules, which are then absorbed into the bloodstream

distal: away from the point of origin; for example, the distal esophagus is the end toward the stomach

gastrointestinal motility: the spontaneous movement of the gastrointestinal tract; for example, it includes peristalsis but not chewing

gastrointestinal tract: the digestive tract; a tubelike series of organs that includes the mouth, pharynx, esophagus, stomach, small intestine, large intestine, and anus

involuntary muscle contractions: muscle contractions that occur unconsciously, such as those of the intestines

proximal: toward the origin; for example, the proximal esophagus is the end toward the throat

smooth muscle: muscle that when viewed under a microscope, does not have striations, which are stripes seen in skeletal muscle cells; smooth muscle contracts involuntarily

Structure and Functions

The gastrointestinal (GI) tract is a muscular tube about ten meters long. It includes the mouth, pharynx, esophagus, stomach, small and large intestines, and anus. The channel running through this tube is the lumen. Food travels through the GI tract to be broken down into molecules. These food molecules then pass through the lining of the GI tract into the bloodstream, a process called absorption.

Waste material that is not absorbed is eliminated as feces.

Since digestion, absorption, and elimination occur in different regions of the GI tract, the contents must be pushed aborally, meaning away from the mouth. This occurs by means of peristaltic contractions, which begin with a localized, circumferential narrowing of the lumen. From outside the organ, it would look as if someone had put a tight, invisible ring around the tract, causing a constriction. This constriction sweeps along the digestive tract, pushing the contents aborally. Peristaltic contractions require four major components: the muscular wall of the GI tract, nerve cells in the walls of the GI tract, nervous connections with the brain, and a relay system in the brain. These work together so that the contractions are coordinated on all sides of the lumen and move in the proper direction.

Most of the GI tract is lined with smooth muscle, which is controlled by a part of the nervous system that does not require any conscious effort in order to function. The wall of the digestive tract contains two layers of muscle. The inner layer consists of several layers of muscle cells arranged concentrically. In the outer layer, the cells are arranged longitudinally. When the inner layer of cells is stimulated by nerves, it contracts, producing a narrowing of the lumen that pushes material aborally. When the outer layer of cells contracts, it shortens the long axis of the GI tract, causing an increase in the diameter of the lumen. This enlargement is especially important in the esophagus, which must sometimes accommodate large pieces of food.

There are two networks of nerve cells in the wall of the GI tract. The important network that affects peristalsis is called the myenteric plexus and is located between the circular and longitudinal layers of muscle cells. It contains nerve cells that receive impulses from nerves coming from the brain and transmit those impulses to the muscle cells. One of the functions of this plexus is to help ensure that peristaltic contractions occur in the proper direction. It also enables peristalsis to begin after local distension of the esophagus. If a large piece of food is stuck in the esophagus, peristaltic contractions begin pushing the food down into the stomach.

Nervous connections between the esophagus and the brain influence peristalsis. Some neurons carry sensory information from the esophagus to the brain; this information is important for the brain to be able to sense discomfort in the esophagus. Other neurons carry information from the brain to the esophagus that can modulate the contraction strength and speed of peristalsis. A relay system in the brain stem is involved in the process of swallowing and may also play a role in controlling peristalsis. It is not yet clear to what degree peristalsis is governed by the brain as opposed to the smooth muscle cells or the myenteric plexus.

Peristaltic contractions are measured by means of an instrument called a manometer, which can be advanced into organs such as the esophagus. It monitors increases in intraluminal pressure (pressure inside the GI tract) caused by contractions. A tracing is obtained that plots pressure versus time. Different tracings are obtained for different regions of the esophagus. Thus, in a recording of peristalsis,

tracings of the proximal esophagus would show a transient increase in pressure, followed by an increase in pressure in the middle and then the lower esophagus.

Peristaltic contractions differ in the various regions of the GI tract and serve different purposes. In the esophagus, where peristalsis serves to propel food from the pharynx into the stomach, the main type of activity is called primary peristalsis. Initiated by swallowing, it propels material down toward the stomach. Primary peristaltic contractions can push a solid mass of food down the esophagus in about six seconds. With the aid of gravity, liquids do not need peristaltic contractions, as they can pour down the esophagus in one second. Between the lower end of the esophagus and the stomach is a narrowed region called the lower esophageal sphincter (LES). This is an area of muscular circular fibers that normally keep the junction between the esophagus and stomach closed. When food or liquids reach the lower esophagus, the LES relaxes, allowing them to pass into the stomach.

There are two main motility patterns in the stomach and small intestine: fasting and fed patterns. In the fasting pattern, there are long periods of relaxation that alternate with periods of intense, repeated peristaltic contractions. These contraction waves migrate along the stomach toward the small intestine. When viewed on a manometry tracing, they are called migrating motor complexes (MMCs). In the fed pattern, the motility response varies depending on the content of the meal. Solid meals cause different effects in different parts of the stomach. The proximal stomach is mainly for storing food after eating and for emptying stomach contents. After eating solids, the proximal stomach relaxes to accommodate the food. Later, it slowly contracts, emptying the material toward the small intestine.

The functions of the distal stomach are mixing food with stomach acid and enzymes and mechanically grinding solids into smaller pieces. Solids and liquids are also propelled by peristaltic contractions toward the pylorus, a narrow region separating the stomach from the small intestine. Only material that is finely ground will pass into the small intestine. The small intestine is about five meters long and moves the material coming from the stomach, called chyme, toward the large intestine. During the transit of chyme through the small intestine, water and nutrients are absorbed. Enzymes digest the food particles in chyme down into minute particles, or molecules. These molecules are absorbed through the lining of the small intestine into the bloodstream. Wastes that cannot be digested and absorbed pass to the large intestine, where more fluid is absorbed, leaving a semisolid material called feces.

The motility pattern of the small intestine is similar to that of the stomach during fasting: intermittent periods of peristalsis push material down toward the large intestine. The purpose of this fasting peristaltic activity is to sweep cellular debris and bacteria toward the large intestine. Otherwise, bacteria may overgrow in the small intestine and cause diarrhea. During the fed pattern, there are no prolonged quiescent periods between groups of peristaltic contractions as there are in the fasting state. The function of the fed state is to make sure that the chyme is mixed well with digestive enzymes and that it has an opportunity to come into contact with the absorptive surface of the intestinal wall. As with the rest of the GI tract, small intestinal motility is subject to the brain's control. If a person is placed in a dangerous situation, the brain will send signals to decrease intestinal motility, which will no longer be a priority.

In the large intestine, or colon, peristalsis slowly moves feces toward the rectum for elimination. The slow movement enables most of the water in the feces to be absorbed into the bloodstream. In the proximal large intestine, liquid feces are moved back and forth by contractions, eventually moving distally. In time, this material becomes more solid and moves intermittently toward the rectum. This intermittent peristalsis is called mass movement. It fluctuates during the day, increasing in frequency after meals. As the feces distend the rectum, a reflex occurs that stimulates passage of stool to the outside.

Disorders and Diseases

Peristalsis may not always progress normally; it may be absent, too vigorous, or uncoordinated. An example of a disorder involving lack of peristalsis is achalasia, which means "failure to relax." In this disease, the LES does not relax, thus impairing the passage of food into the stomach. Another characteristic of the disorder is aperistalsis, which is the absence of peristalsis of the esophagus. One common symptom of achalasia is dysphagia, which is a sensation of food sticking in the throat. Another symptom is regurgitation of undigested food during or just after eating, which often results in weight loss.

The cause of primary achalasia is unknown. Secondary achalasia may be due to infiltrating cancer, radiation damage, or other external factors; in Central and South America, the most common cause is Chagas disease, a parasitic infection. Achalasia is characterized by a reduction in ganglion cells, which are nerve cells that are normally present in the myenteric plexus of the esophagus. There may also

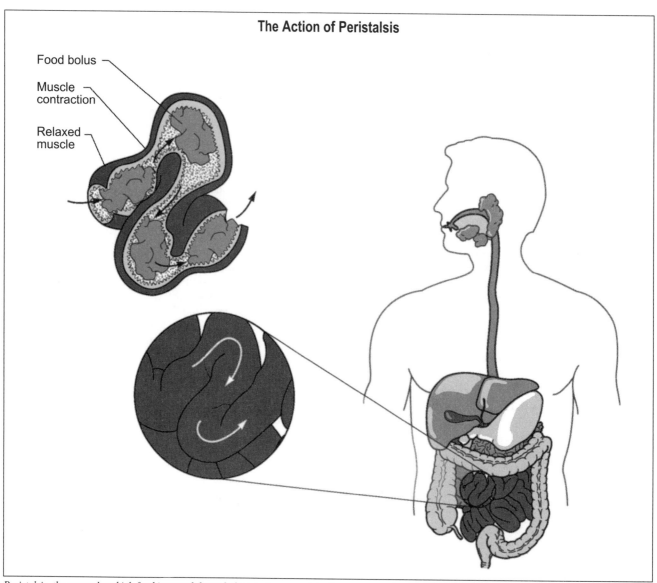

The Action of Peristalsis

Food bolus
Muscle contraction
Relaxed muscle

Peristalsis, the means by which food is moved through the intestines, consists of a constant series of contractions and relaxations of the intestinal walls.

be damage to the cell bodies of nerve cells in the brain that innervate the myenteric plexus. It may be that the damaged ganglion cells cause damage to the brain cells, or vice versa. A neural lesion in the LES can lead to a sphincter muscle that fails to relax appropriately, which in turn leads to obstruction of the passage of food. One result is that the esophageal body eventually becomes chronically dilated. Another factor leading to dilation of the esophagus is the loss of ganglion cells in the wall of its body, which results in the absence of peristalsis.

Achalasia usually begins during middle age. The predominant symptom is dysphagia in response to all solids and frequently liquids as well. Eating often causes chest discomfort to the point that people with achalasia lose weight because they avoid eating. Although regurgitation of undigested foods commonly occurs shortly after eating, it may occur hours later, especially when the patient lies down at night. Food contents may be regurgitated and inhaled, leading to nighttime coughing spells.

On manometry, the peristaltic waves normally seen after an act of swallowing are absent. Instead, there may be some low-pressure contractions appearing simultaneously in all parts of the esophagus. Their lack of orderly progression prevents the contractions from propelling food down the esophagus. The pressure in the lumen of the esophagus in the region of the LES may be elevated; often the LES is so tight that it is difficult to advance the manometry catheter through it. The LES also fails to relax normally after swallowing.

Treatment of achalasia rarely results in a return of peristalsis, but it may provide relief for the obstruction caused by a tight LES. Some drugs can relax the LES, but success with these is variable. Often, stretching of the LES with instruments called dilators is performed. The best dilator is a long instrument with an inflatable balloon at the tip. The dilator is advanced into the esophagus and through the LES. The balloon tip is positioned so that when the balloon is inflated, it stretches the LES. The LES needs to be stretched to the point of tearing the circular muscle in order to achieve a long-term reduction in LES pressure. This procedure is risky and may be complicated by the development of a large tear, creating a hole in the wall of the esophagus called a perforation.

Surgical cutting of the LES, called an esophagomyotomy, is more effective than dilation. The more reduction in LES tone that occurs, however, the more likely it is that the person will suffer from reflux of stomach acid. Although the stomach's lining is normally resistant to the irritating effects of acid, the esophagus may become irritated when exposed to chronic acid reflux. A common symptom of this reflux is heartburn, which is a sensation of hot material rising into the esophagus.

An example of too-vigorous peristalsis is esophageal spasm. There are a few different manometric patterns to esophageal spasm, the most consistent being one of intense contractions of the esophagus that do not sweep along its length but occur at the same time at different regions of the esophagus. During manometry, the esophagi of those patients with spasms are often very sensitive to stimulation with certain drugs, resulting in increased strength, or amplitude, of the contractions. Not only is there an exaggerated motor response in esophageal spasm but there may be an abnormal sensory component to the disorder as well. For example, loud noises or stressful mental tasks may cause an increase in the amplitude of contraction waves. Esophageal spasms tend to occur in middle age. The most common symptom is intermittent dysphagia that is variable in severity. It is not progressive and does not result in weight loss. Chest pain is a frequent complaint and may mimic that of a heart attack.

The diagnosis of esophageal spasm often requires manometry. Another useful diagnostic test is to attempt to re-create symptoms of spasm. For example, a drug known to cause smooth muscle contraction is administered. If symptoms similar to the presenting chest pain are re-created, then it is presumed that the pain was attributable to esophageal spasm. Various medications that relax smooth muscle have been used to treat these spasms, with moderate success. Once the medications are stopped, however, the symptoms recur.

Peristalsis requires both an intact myenteric plexus and well-coordinated connections with the central nervous system. Diabetics commonly suffer from neuropathy, a condition that damages various nerve cells in the body. This neuropathy is thought to be responsible for their various gastrointestinal motility disturbances. About 75 percent of diabetics can be shown to have esophageal peristaltic disturbances-up to one-third of diabetics suffer from dysphagia- although they are commonly not felt. Using manometry, an absence of coordinated peristaltic activity is usually found. Diabetics may have tertiary contractions, which are noncoordinated, nonpropulsive contractions of the wall of the esophagus.

Stomach, or gastric, motility is abnormal in about 25 percent of diabetics, resulting in disordered gastric emptying. Emptying of liquids may be normal, but emptying of solids is commonly delayed. There is commonly an absence of MMCs, which results in a decrease in the ability of the stomach to grind food. There may also be spasms of the distal stomach, causing obstructions of materials that would normally flow out of the stomach and into the small intestine. Another gastric disturbance is gastroparesis, a decreased ability of the stomach to propel food along, resulting in a sensation of fullness despite long periods of elapsed time between meals. Because of this, diabetics often have difficulty finishing an entire meal. They may also suffer from nausea, bloating, and vomiting after meals. Treatment of gastroparesis includes reduction of blood sugars if they are elevated. This may be accomplished by reducing food intake (if previously excessive) or increasing the dose of insulin. Medications called prokinetic drugs may increase gastric motor activity; examples of these drugs include metoclo- pramide, dromperidone, and cisapride.

The neuropathy suffered by diabetics may damage the nerves that normally stimulate intestinal reabsorption of fluid; this results in diarrhea, which affects 10 percent of diabetics. Other diabetics suffer from constipation, which may be caused by impaired peristaltic activity of the colon.

Perspective and Prospects

In 1674, the first case of what was probably achalasia was reported by Sir Thomas Willis, who called the disorder "cardiospasm." In 1937, F. C. Lendrum proposed that cardiospasm was attributable to incomplete relaxation of the LES, and he changed the condition's name to achalasia.

Throughout the twentieth century, study of peristalsis advanced in leaps and bounds. In 1927, E. Jacobson reported on an association between esophageal spasm and strong emotion; gastroenterologists continue to note a correlation between spastic disorders of the GI tract and anxiety. In 1938, E. M. Jones reported an experimental reproduction of esophageal spastic pain by the inflation of small balloons in the esophagus. The development of esophageal manometric techniques advanced significantly in the 1970s. These techniques have allowed a much more thorough understanding of gastrointestinal motility, which enables the development of better drugs to alter it. Therapeutic advances in treating disorders such as achalasia have been made, most notably starting in the 1940s, when A. M. Olsen performed pneumatic dilations of the esophagus.

One of the most practical advances for disorders involving decreased peristalsis has been the development of prokinetic drugs, which increase gastrointestinal motility. Metoclopramide was the first to be developed and is still in use. Cisapride may prove to be effective, especially because its effects do not wear off with chronic use, as do those of metoclopramide.

Perhaps the most important area of research into gastrointestinal motility is the study of the signals for smooth muscle contraction, such as which chemicals (neurotransmitters) are released by the nerve endings where they join up with nerve cells in the myenteric plexus or with the smooth muscle cells. More than fifteen hormones and neurotransmitters are known to affect gastrointestinal motility. Once their specific functions are better understood, researchers can try to develop drugs that mimic their effects, depending on whether an increase or a decrease in motility is desired.

In the United States, some motility disorders are very prevalent, such as irritable bowel syndrome (IBS). This disorder involves symptoms such as abdominal distension, abdominal pain relieved by bowel movements, bowel movements that become more frequent during pain episodes, constipation, and loose stools. IBS accounts for almost as many working days lost to illness as the common cold. It is the most common cause for referral to a gastroenterologist, making up 20 to 50 percent of their referrals. Surveys in the general population have shown that approximately 15 percent of Americans have symptoms to justify a diagnosis of IBS.

Most disorders of peristalsis are not deadly, but they can cause much discomfort. With better understanding of the neurology of the gut, as well as the acceptance of a model for understanding the disorders that includes attention to psychological and sociological effects on the GI tract, medicine will be able to better decrease the suffering that occurs with these disorders.

—*Marc H. Walters, M.D.*

See also Acid reflux disease; Chagas' disease; Colitis; Colon; Constipation; Crohn's disease; Diabetes mellitus; Diarrhea and dysentery; Digestion; Esophagus; Gastroenterology; Gastroenterology, pediatric; Gastrointestinal disorders; Gastrointestinal system; Intestinal disorders; Intestines; Irritable bowel syndrome (IBS); Obstruction; Rectum; Small intestine.

For Further Information:

Barrett, Kim E., Susan M. Barman, Scott Boitano, and Heddwen L. Brooks. *Ganong's Review of Medical Physiology*. 24th ed. New York: Lange Medical Books/McGraw-Hill Medical, 2012.

DiMarino, Michael C. "Esophageal Disorders." *Merck Manual Home Health Handbook*, October 2007.

"Esophagus Disorders." *MedlinePlus*, June 12, 2013.

Feldman, Mark, Lawrence S. Friedman, and Lawrence J. Brandt, eds. *Sleisenger and Fordtran's Gastrointestinal and Liver Disease: Pathophysiology/Diagnosis/Management*. 9th ed. 2 vols. Philadelphia: Saunders/Elsevier, 2010.

Kapadia, Cyrus R., Caroline R. Taylor, and James M. Crawford. *An Atlas of Gastroenterology: A Guide to Diagnosis and Differential Diagnosis*. Boca Raton, Fla.: Pantheon, 2003.

Peikin, Steven R. *Gastrointestinal Health: The Proven Nutritional Program to Prevent, Cure, or Alleviate Irritable Bowel Syndrome (IBS), Ulcers, Gas, Constipation, Heartburn, and Many Other Digestive Disorders*. 3d ed. New York: Perennial Currents, 2004.

Tortora, Gerard J., and Bryan Derrickson. *Principles of Anatomy and Physiology*. 13th ed. Hoboken, N.J.: John Wiley & Sons, 2012.

Peritonitis

Disease/Disorder

Anatomy or system affected: Abdomen, gastrointestinal system, intestines

Specialties and related fields: Bacteriology, critical care, emergency medicine, gastroenterology, general surgery, internal medicine, microbiology

Definition: An inflammation of the membrane lining the abdominal cavity (peritoneum), usually secondary to a bacterial infection.

Causes and Symptoms

Peritonitis is an acute condition that typically results from a bacterial infection of the membrane lining the abdominal organs or the abdominal cavity itself, known as the peritoneum. Primary bacterial peritonitis occurs because of a generalized infection, usually with *Streptococcus pneumoniae* with peritoneal seeding and is usually seen in adolescent girls. Secondary bacterial peritonitis, on the other hand, is caused by the rupture and perforation of a hollow organ of the gut, such as the appendix or a gastric ulcer. Other causes of peritonitis include postsurgical complications, catheter contamination in dialysis patients, and infection with enteric bacteria from the gut that cause pelvic inflammatory disease (PID) in women. A type called *spontaneous bacterial peritonitis* is a complication of ascites seen in chronic liver or kidney failure.

The clinical presentation of peritonitis may vary depending on the severity and source of infection and may range

---

Information on Peritonitis

Causes: Bacterial infection, rupture and perforation of organ (e.g., appendix) or gastric ulcer, postsurgical complications, catheter contamination, pelvic inflammatory disease (PID), complication of ascites in chronic liver or kidney failure

Symptoms: May include severe abdominal pain, fever and chills, diarrhea, inability to pass feces and urine, shock, worsening of renal failure, encephalopathy

Duration: Acute

Treatments: Supportive measures for respiration and circulation, surgery, antibiotics, intravenous fluids

---

from no symptoms to severe abdominal pain, fever and chills, diarrhea, inability to pass feces and urine, shock, worsening of renal failure, or encephalopathy. Typical bacterial peritonitis may be manifested by an extremely still patient who finds that even slight movement aggravates the pain. Physical examination may reveal tenderness over the abdomen with positive rebound tenderness, fluid in the abdominal cavity, and other signs of liver or kidney failure.

For diagnosis, needle aspiration (paracentesis) of the fluid from the abdominal cavity can be done for biochemical and microbiological analyses, including cell count, gram stain, and culture; ultrasound guidance may help in locating the abdominal fluid. Blood cultures may be helpful in some cases. If rupture of a hollow organ is the cause, an x-ray of the abdomen shows the presence of air under the diaphragm. Blood cultures are useful in diagnosing spontaneous bacterial peritonitis and primary peritonitis. Ultrasound examination is used to detect fluid in the abdomen.

Treatment and Therapy

The treatment of peritonitis depends on its presentation and cause. Supportive measures to secure adequate respiration and circulation are used for patients who are in critical condition. A ruptured internal organ is usually treated surgically after the patient is stabilized. Infection is managed with antibiotics. Inadequate or improper management of peritonitis may lead to abscess formation, intestinal obstruction, hepatorenal syndrome, encephalopathy, sepsis, and ultimately death.

Peritonitis is an emergency situation, and it is of utmost importance that the condition be diagnosed and treated at an early stage in order to avoid fatal complications. Any case of significant abdominal pain must be examined thoroughly and investigated to rule out peritonitis. The prognosis depends directly on the promptness of treatment.

—*Rashmi Ramasubbaiah, M.D.*

See also Abdomen; Abdominal disorders; Colon; Gastrointestinal disorders; Gastrointestinal system; Intestinal disorders; Intestines; Pelvic inflammatory disease (PID); Small intestine.

For Further Information:

Augustin, Rolf. *Peritonitis in CAPD*. New York: Karger, 1987.
Badash, Michelle. "Peritonitis." *Health Library*, October 31, 2012.
Conn, Harold O., Juan Rodés, and Miguel Navasa. *Spontaneous Bacterial Peritonitis: The Disease, Pathogenesis, and Treatment*. New York: Marcel Dekker, 2000.
Fry, Donald E., ed. *Peritonitis*. Mount Kisco, N.Y.: Futura, 1993.
Fry, Donald E. *Surgical Infections*. London: JP Medical Ltd., 2013.
Icon Health. *Peritonitis: A Medical Dictionary, Bibliography, and Annotated Research Guide to Internet References*. San Diego, Calif.: Author, 2004.
Kasper, Dennis L., et al., eds. *Harrison's Principles of Internal Medicine*. 16th ed. New York: McGraw-Hill, 2005.
"Peritonitis." *Mayo Clinic*, July 9, 2011.

Pertussis. *See* Whooping cough.

PET scanning. *See* Positron emission tomography (PET) scanning.

Pharmacology

Specialty

Anatomy or system affected: Blood, brain, cells, immune system, nervous system, psychic-emotional system

Specialties and related fields: Anesthesiology, biochemistry, cytology, endocrinology, family medicine, microbiology, oncology, preventive medicine, public health, toxicology

Definition: The science or knowledge of chemicals that affect biological processes.

Key terms:

pharmacist: a person with a license to dispense or sell drugs prescribed by a medical practitioner, such as a dentist, physician, or veterinarian

pharmacognosy: the preparation of medicinal agents from natural sources

pharmacologist: a scientist who studies pharmacology

therapeutics: the use of chemicals in the diagnosis, prevention, or treatment of disease

toxicology: the study of the effects of toxins (poisons) and their antidotes

Science and Profession

The science of pharmacology includes the history, source, physical and chemical properties, and biochemical and physiological effects of drugs (therapeutic chemicals, diagnostic chemicals, toxins, and related substances).

"Drug" is a noun in common usage, but it has complex meanings. "Drug" or "medicine" is often used today to indicate a therapeutic substance usually obtained from a pharmacy or drugstore. "Drug" also is used to indicate an illegal substance used for mood-altering effects. Historically, people made their own drugs from materials found naturally in plants, animals, and minerals; some people continue to do so. The term "drug" in this article will focus on the meaning as it is understood by scientists called pharmacologists. Any chemical can be thought of as a drug by a pharmacologist: A drug is simply a chemical that produces a change in a biological process.

Water and oxygen can be thought of as drugs, as can foods and poisons. "Drug," therefore, is a word to indicate an idea, concept, or perception about a chemical. When the chemical, such as oxygen, is causing a change in a biological process, then the chemical is acting as a drug. If the same chemical is causing a change in some other kind of system-for example, causing an iron rod to rust-then the chemical is not acting as a drug. Drugs may be found in nature or made by humans. Most of the chemicals used today as drugs are made by humans.

The biological process that is being changed by a drug may be one occurring in a sick person. Many drugs are used therapeutically-that is, to treat diseases-but pharmacologists do not limit drugs to therapeutic chemicals. They are interested in drug effects on any biological process, even healthy ones occurring in plants and microorganisms, as well as those in animals and humans.

All drugs, even therapeutic drugs, will have several effects on biological processes. Some of these effects are seen only at high concentrations. Unwanted effects, especially if they are injurious, are called adverse effects. A serious adverse effect, especially if it requires special medical treatment, may be considered a toxic reaction, or poisoning. Any chemical that produces an injurious effect, one that is detrimental to a biological process, is called a toxin. The severity of the toxic effect is based on the concentration of the toxic substance. Toxic substances in the environment are called pollutants.

The idea of drug concentration is very important. "Concentration" refers to the number of chemical molecules in a specified volume (such as a teaspoonful, an ounce, or a milliliter) of liquid or gas. Concentration is related to dosage and to the intensity of a drug's effect on a biological process. It is important to remember, however, that the effect of a drug on the body may vary considerably depending on the route of administration. For instance, if one were to eat a drug, then metabolism of the drug is usually very slow, whereas if one were to inject a drug into the bloodstream, then the effects of the drug are observed quite rapidly. Therefore, when pharmacologists discuss drugs and their effects, particularly on humans, they will also frequently discuss the route of administration to make the context of the effect clear.

Concentration and the related concept of dilution are easy to understand. Two spoonfuls of sugar in a glass of water form a more concentrated solution of sugar-water than one spoonful. The more concentrated sugar-water will taste sweeter. Since taste is a biological process caused by a chemical, the chemical (sugar) can be thought of as a drug. The concentration of the chemical affects the biological process. There is a limit, however, to the sweetness of a solution. At some point, more sugar added to the solution will not increase the sensation of sweetness. Adding more sugar may result in a "toxic" reaction of nausea and even vomiting.

There are also different kinds of sugars. When one says that some are sweeter than others, one means that sweeter sugars will be just as sweet at very dilute concentrations as less-sweet sugars at very high concentrations. Thus the first kind of sugar is said to be more potent than the second, even though the second can be just as sweet at high concentra-

tions. Some sugars, however, will not taste very sweet regardless of the concentration. This example illustrates principles that are shared by many drugs. It is important to understand that taking a double dose of a drug will not necessarily produce a double effect. It is also important to understand that a tiny dose of one drug can have the same, or even stronger, biological effect than a large dose of a similar drug.

Most therapeutic drugs act directly on special parts of cells within the body called receptors. A receptor is part of the cell structure, just as a hand is part of human anatomy. A receptor for a specific drug is always located at the same place within a cell, just as the hand is always located at the end of an arm. Yet there are different kinds of receptors, just as people have both hands and feet, found at various locations in cells. Many receptors are found on the cell surface; others are found inside cells. Some receptors are found only on certain types of cells.

Each type of receptor has a specific function, just as hands and feet have specific functions. When a drug "fits" a receptor, like a ball or a glove fits a hand, or how a key fits a lock, the receptor starts the biological process for which the drug is known. Different kinds of drugs can fit a single type of receptor, which explains why different drugs (for example, aspirin and acetaminophen) can have similar effects (relieve pain). Furthermore, one drug may be able to act on several different types of receptors. A receptor, however, can have only one biological response to all the drugs that act on it.

A drug acting on receptors in cells of one organ can affect distant organs. For example, a drug acting on brain cells may cause the nerves acting on blood vessels to increase blood pressure, which can change the heartbeat. The effect of a drug on receptors is usually temporary and should be reversible. In most cases in which a drug works through a receptor, the receptor releases the drug after the two have come together. If this release does not occur, the receptor is said to be blocked. The blockage of a receptor can be therapeutically beneficial, but it may sometimes lead to an adverse reaction.

In humans and animals, most drugs travel in the bloodstream to reach cell receptors. The drug enters the bloodstream after being applied to a body surface or after being swallowed, inhaled, or injected. The effect of the drug is eventually diminished because the body dilutes the drug, chemically alters it (so that it no longer has a pharmacological effect), and eliminates it. Chemical alteration of drugs usually occurs in the liver by a process called biotransformation. Elimination of most drugs, or their biotransformed relatives, usually occurs through the urine but may sometimes occur through secretions (sweat, tears, or breast milk), feces, or even exhaled gases.

Diagnostic and Treatment Techniques

Three examples of the use of therapeutic chemicals in the field of pharmacology are anesthesia, cardiac-enhancing drugs, and drugs that fight infections. These examples demonstrate the use of various classes of drugs and provide insight to the variety of drug action.

Anesthetics are chemical painkillers. They are very important drugs, because most diseases are accompanied by pain. Often, the first objective of a patient is to get relief from the pain, even though the anesthetic may do nothing to cure the disease. Pain is a sensation felt in the brain, not at the site of injury. Special nerves at the site of injury send a signal (nerve impulse) to the brain, where it is interpreted as pain occurring at a specific location in the body. Mild pain and severe pain are detected by different kinds of nociceptive (pain) nerves. As pain increases in severity, the brain not only perceives and interprets the pain but also sends out special autonomic signals.

Autonomic signals from the brain serve an extremely important function: They control body functions that do not require conscious thought, such as sweating, heart rate, blood pressure, digestion, and eye focus. Autonomic signals coordinate these functions and change them in response to conditions outside the body. When the body is threatened, such as when a person is frightened, autonomic signals prepare the body to fight or to flee the threatening situation. The pain of surgery causes the brain to send autonomic signals to put the body in a defensive state, resulting in sweating and increases in heart rate, breathing, and blood pressure. Additionally, all the muscles of the body will become tense. This defensive state is undesirable during surgery.

Drugs used to relieve pain without causing unconsciousness are called analgesics. Mild pain can usually be controlled with an analgesic such as aspirin. More severe pain may require an opioid analgesic such as morphine. Sometimes, the term "narcotic" is used as a synonym for opioid analgesics, but that term is often used in a legal context to indicate any chemical that can cause dependence (addiction). An analgesic changes the way in which the brain interprets a nociceptive stimulus. The most severe pain, such as that during surgery, is controlled by an anesthetic. An anesthetic may act at a specific site, such as on the nerves of a tooth; a local anesthetic such as novocaine blocks the transmission of the nociceptive stimulus to the brain. Other anesthetics, required for major surgery, cause a loss of consciousness; these are called general anesthetics. As with all therapeutic drugs, the action of an anesthetic is reversible.

A general anesthetic should perform several functions: It should alter the brain's interpretation of pain, cause a temporary amnesia that prevents remembrance of the nociceptive sensation, produce autonomic stability, and cause muscle relaxation. This is much to ask of a single drug. Therefore, general anesthesia is achieved by using several drugs, each capable of accomplishing one or more of the goals.

A general anesthetic agent usually works on nerve cells to provide pain relief and amnesia. These general functions are provided by both kinds of general anesthetics, those that are inhaled and those that are injected. Other drugs are used to control autonomic signals and to provide for muscle relaxation. When the surgery is completed, the patient returns to consciousness as the anesthetic agents are removed from the nerves. This is done by biotransformation and by excretion. Pain immediately after surgery will be controlled by an opioid analgesic. When the pain diminishes as healing progresses, it becomes milder and can be controlled with a nonopioid analgesic.

Drugs are also important in helping people recover from a myocardial infarction (heart attack). The heart is a pump that supplies blood to all cells of the body. Blood carries oxygen and nutrients to the cells and removes waste materials from them. The heart is a living muscle composed of cells, and blood vessels must supply each cell of the muscle. If a blood vessel in the heart becomes suddenly blocked, then the cells served by that blood vessel become starved and die. This is a heart attack. If only a small portion of the heart is injured, the person can survive the attack, especially if drugs are given that strengthen the heart.

An important class of drugs used to strengthen the heart is composed of the cardiac glycosides, such as digitalis. These drugs act to improve the ability of the heart cells to use calcium efficiently. Calcium is essential to maintaining a normal heartbeat. Because a heart attack is painful, it causes a defensive autonomic response from the brain. It is important to use analgesics to relieve the pain and other drugs to control the autonomic response. Another important therapy is to provide more oxygen to the heart. This is done directly, by administering oxygen, but it is also done by using drugs that can remove the blockage from the blood vessel. Since the blockage usually occurs when a blood clot forms in a damaged blood vessel, drugs that dissolve clots can sometimes open the blocked vessel and restore the flow of oxygen-rich blood to the starved cells. A person recovering from a heart attack will sometimes be given drugs to prevent another blockage. Some drugs prevent fatty deposits from forming in the vessels, while others act to slow down clot formation.

Drugs used to treat infection are designed to kill cells. Infection is caused by foreign microbes attacking the body. The microbes may be viruses, bacteria, fungi, or even parasitic worms. Antimicrobial drugs (antibiotics) are given to the infected person to destroy the foreign cells without damaging the patient's own cells. Therefore, the drug must be selectively toxic to the foreign cells. Few drugs are perfectly selective, however, and most have some toxic effects on the patient as well.

There are many ways to develop a selectively toxic drug, but selectivity usually depends on a unique feature of the invading foreign cells, such as the cell walls of bacteria. Human cells are surrounded by cell membranes. Bacteria have cell membranes as well, but they also have cell walls outside these membranes. If the bacterial cell wall is damaged, then the bacterium becomes weakened and can be killed by the body's defense mechanisms. Penicillin is an antimicrobial drug that damages the cell walls of many bacteria. Penicillin has very few adverse effects on the infected person, because human cells do not have cell walls. (Unfortunately, however, some people develop an allergic reaction to penicillin.)

Perspective and Prospects

In the prehistoric world, priests were called upon to intercede for persons suffering from disease and pain. As humans gained experience and developed a means of sharing that experience, especially through written records, it was noticed that certain components of the diet could reliably inflict or relieve pain; these were the first drugs. Similar effects could be obtained by inhaling natural materials or applying them to the skin through rubbing or injection. Such activities were thought to involve supernatural powers, however, and authority to use these drugs was still restricted to members of the priesthood, namely, medicine men or shamans.

Writings about the medicinal properties of natural materials can be found in Chinese, Egyptian, Greek, Indian, and Sumerian manuscripts, some of which are thought to be as much as six thousand years old. The Ebers Papyrus of Egypt (1550 BCE) contains more than eight hundred prescriptions using seven hundred drugs. It was known that some drugs were cathartics, some were diuretics, and others were purgatives, soporifics, or poisons. Yet factual knowledge about why these actions occurred was lacking, in large measure because knowledge of body function and chemistry was lacking. In this absence, people speculated that drug action was due to "essential properties" of the drug, such as warmth or wetness.

Only with the European Renaissance in the early sixteenth century was the domination of religion over intellectual inquiry challenged effectively. The scientific method was applied to questions about the natural world, both physical and living. In 1543, Andreas Vesalius published the first complete description of human anatomy. In the early seventeenth century, William Harvey discovered the circulation of blood, and Antoni van Leeuwenhoek discovered living cells with his microscope. In the eighteenth century, the chemistry of oxygen was established by Carl Scheele, Joseph Priestley, and Antoine Lavoisier, and by the end of the century, chemical methods were becoming available to separate pure drugs from crude natural concoctions. In 1806, Friedrich W. Serturner purified morphine from the opium poppy, and in 1856, Friedrich Wöhler isolated cocaine from coca. Also of great intellectual and economic significance was the 1828 synthesis by Wöhler of urea, the first of many chemicals which heretofore had been available only from living organisms. Hormones, general anesthetics, and the bacterial cause of infectious diseases were discovered.

Until the twentieth century, drugs were discovered empirically; they existed in nature and needed to be "found." The knowledge gained during the nineteenth century about how drugs worked enabled pharmacologists of the twentieth century to "design" drugs not found in nature. For example, Paul Ehrlich, a German scientist, announced in 1910 that he had successfully combined a dye that stains bacteria with the poison arsenic to create an antibacterial drug, arsphenamine (Salvarsan), that is highly effective in treating syphilis. In a similar way, the antibacterial sulfonamide chemicals were developed in the 1930s.

It was soon recognized that the powerful effect of pure drugs (in contrast to potions made from natural materials) had the potential to harm as well as to help, to kill or to cure. The safe use of these drugs required special knowledge, so government agencies were established in the twentieth century to regulate drug manufacture and distribution. The original Pure Food and Drug Act, passed by the United States Congress in 1906, imposed quality controls on drug manufacturers. In 1927, Congress created the Food, Drug, and Insecticide Administration (FDIA), to enforce the 1906 law. Until 1914, any drug could be obtained without a prescription; this was changed by the Harrison Narcotic Act. Further limitations on the sale of drugs to the general public came with the Food, Drug, and Cosmetic Act of 1938 and the Durham-Humphrey Amendment of 1951. The Controlled Substance Act of 1970 superseded the Harrison Narcotic Act.

With the passage of time, enforcement responsibilities were changed. The FDIA became the Food and Drug Administration (FDA) in 1931 and was transferred from the Department of Agriculture to what is now the Department of Health and Human Services. The Drug Enforcement Administration for controlled substances was established within the Justice Department.

At the beginning of the twenty-first century, drugs were available to alter personality, to cure some types of cancer, to influence the reproductive system, and to control the body's response to foreign materials such as transplanted organs. Many of these drugs were designed using powerful computers. Drugs were available to alter plant and animal ecosystems. The use of these drugs, such as the pesticide DDT and the wartime defoliant Agent Orange, had devastating effects on humans and the environment that required remedial action. Drugs were even being developed to alter cellular genetics.

—Armand M. Karow, Ph.D.;
updated by Nancy A. Piotrowski, Ph.D.

See also Acid-base chemistry; Aging: Extended care; Anesthesia; Anesthesiology; Antianxiety drugs; Antibiotics; Antidepressants; Antihistamines; Anti-inflammatory drugs; Aphrodisiacs; Bacteriology; Catheterization; Chemotherapy; Clinical trials; Critical care; Critical care, pediatric; Decongestants; Digestion; Drug resistance; Emergency medicine; Enzyme therapy; Enzymes; Fluids and electrolytes; Food and Drug Administration (FDA); Food biochemistry; Genetic engineering; Geriatrics and gerontology; Glycolysis; Herbal medicine; Homeopathy; Hormone therapy; Hormones; Laboratory tests; Melatonin; Metabolism; Microbiology; Narcotics; Oncology; Over-the-counter medications; Pain management; Pharmacy; Polypharmacy; Prescription drug abuse; Psychiatry; Psychiatry, child and adolescent; Psychiatry, geriatric; Rheumatology; Side effects; Sports medicine; Steroids; Substance abuse; Terminally ill: Extended care; Thrombolytic therapy and TPA; Toxicology; Tropical medicine; Veterinary medicine.

For Further Information:

American Pharmaceutical Association. *Handbook of Nonprescription Drugs.* 17th ed. Washington, D.C.: Author, 2012.

Brunton, Laurence L., et al., eds. *Goodman and Gilman's The Pharmacological Basis of Therapeutics.* 12th ed. New York: McGraw-Hill, 2011.

Griffith, H. Winter. *Complete Guide to Prescription and Nonprescription Drugs.* Revised and updated by Stephen Moore. New York: Penguin Group, 2013.

Liska, Ken. *Drugs and the Human Body, with Implications for Society*. 8th ed. Upper Saddle River, N.J.: Pearson/Prentice Hall, 2009.
Parrish, Richard. *Defining Drugs: How Government Became the Arbiter of Pharmaceutical Fact*. Somerset, N.J.: Transaction, 2003.
PDR for Nonprescription Drugs, Dietary Supplements, and Herbs. 33d ed. Montvale, N.J.: PDR Network, 2012.

Pharyngitis

Disease/Disorder
Also known as: Sore throat
Anatomy or system affected: Throat
Specialties and related fields: Otorhinolaryngology
Definition: Inflammation of the mucous membranes of the pharynx or throat, often caused by a viral infection or bacteria.

Information on Pharyngitis

Causes: Viral or bacterial infection, sinusitis, postnasal drip, mononucleosis, seasonal allergies, pollutants, smoking
Symptoms: Sore throat that is red, swollen, or puffy and may have white spots of pus; fever; coughing; swollen tonsils; throat scratchiness; pain when swallowing; and lymph node enlargement
Duration: Acute
Treatments: Pain medications, warm saltwater gargles, antibiotics, tonsillectomy if needed

Causes and Symptoms

Sore throat is the chief complaint of pharyngitis. The throat (pharynx) extends from the nasal passages above and behind the mouth to the esophagus in the neck. Viruses or bacteria infect the pharynx and cause it to swell. The throat often appears red, swollen, or puffy and may have white spots of pus. Fever and cough are also common, and examination may reveal swollen tonsils. Throat scratchiness, pain when swallowing, enlarged lymph nodes in the neck, cough, and irritation are also common in pharyngitis.

Bacteria and viruses that cause pharyngitis generally enter the body through the nose or mouth. The organisms are transmitted through direct contact with someone who has one of these infections and are passed in nasal secretions and saliva.

Viruses that cause the common cold (coronavirus and rhinovirus) or other respiratory diseases may also produce symptoms of pharyngitis. Additionally, sinusitis and postnasal drip may cause irritation of the pharynx. Pharyngitis associated with fever and the appearance of pus on the tonsils may indicate streptococcal pharyngitis, which can be diagnosed by a "quick antigen" test and confirmed by a culture. Persistent pharyngitis accompanied by malaise unresponsive to antibiotics may indicate mononucleosis or other nonbacterial causes such as seasonal allergies, the inhalation of pollutants such as household cleaners or automobile exhaust, and smoking or exposure to secondhand smoke.

Treatment and Therapy

Viral pharyngitis is treated with aspirin or over-the-counter pain remedies and warm saltwater gargles. Bacterial pharyngitis is treated with a course of antibiotics either orally or by injection. Proper nutrition is important. Zinc boosts the immune system and relieves soreness. Vitamin C strengthens the immune system and the mucous membranes, and beta carotene restores the integrity of mucous membranes and supports immune function. If the tonsils have been chronically infected, they may require surgical removal (tonsillectomy).

Perspective and Prospects

Approximately 40 to 60 percent of cases of pharyngitis are caused by a virus, and about 15 percent are associated with streptococcal bacteria. In the United States, children average five sore throats per year and strep infection every four years. The incidence of pharyngitis and strep is highest in children between the ages of five and eighteen. Pharyngitis is rare in children below three years of age. Adults experience an average of two sore throats per year and strep infection approximately every eight years. Worldwide, the incidence is higher.

Formerly, it was commonly regarded as therapeutic to remove tonsils surgically to prevent repeated cases of pharyngitis, especially in children. Modern medical opinion on the subject, however, indicates that removing tonsils has not resulted in fewer cases of pharyngitis; therefore, tonsillectomy surgery is performed less frequently than in the past.

—*Marcia J. Weiss, M.A., J.D.*

See also Allergies; Antibiotics; Bacterial infections; Coronaviruses; Mononucleosis; Mouth and throat cancer; Nasopharyngeal disorders; Otorhinolaryngology; Pharynx; Rhinoviruses; Sinusitis; Sore throat; Strep throat; Streptococcal infections; Tonsillectomy and adenoid removal; Tonsillitis; Tonsils.

For Further Information:
Carson-DeWitt, Rosalyn. "Viral Pharyngitis." *Health Library*, March 12, 2013.
Ferrari, Mario. *PDxMD Ear, Nose, and Throat Disorders*. Philadelphia: PDxMD, 2003.
Goldstein, Mark N. "Office Evaluation and Management of the Sore Throat." *Otolaryngologic Clinics of North America* 25 (August, 1992): 837-842.
Litin, Scott C., ed. *Mayo Clinic Family Health Book*. 4th ed. New York: HarperResource, 2009.
Morrison, Roger. *Desktop Guide to Keynotes and Confirmatory Symptoms*. Albany, Calif.: Hahnemann Clinic, 1993.
Parker, Philip M. and James N. Parker. *Pharyngitis: A Medical Dictionary, Bibliography, and Annotated Research Guide to Internet References*. San Diego, Calif.: ICON Health Publications, 2004.
Pechère, Jean Claude, and Edward L. Kaplan, eds. *Streptococcal Pharyngitis: Optimal Management*. New York: S. Karger, 2004.
Vorvick, Linda J. "Pharyngitis." *MedlinePlus*, January 8, 2012.

Pharynx

Anatomy
Also known as: Throat
Anatomy or system affected: Ear, gastrointestinal system, head, immune system, mouth, neck, nose, respiratory system, throat

Specialties and related fields: Internal medicine, otorhinolaryngology, pulmonary medicine, speech pathology

Definition: The cavity behind the nose and mouth through which air enters the lungs and food and water enter the esophagus.

Structure and Functions

The pharynx, or throat, is the tube-shaped passageway that begins at the back of the nasal cavity, extends downward behind the mouth, and terminates at the fork of the esophagus and trachea, or windpipe. It comprises three sections: the nasopharynx, just behind the nose; the oropharynx, behind the mouth; and the laryngopharynx or hypopharynx, the remaining area above the esophagus. The pharynx contains lymphatic tissue to fight infection: the adenoids in the nasopharynx and the tonsils in the oropharynx. The left and right Eustachian tubes connect the nasopharynx to the ears and balance air pressure between the middle and outer ear.

Food enters the pharynx from the mouth, while air enters from the nose and mouth. The act of swallowing begins as a voluntary contraction of muscles and continues involuntarily until food passes into the esophagus. In the laryngopharynx, the epiglottis, a flap of connective tissue, prevents food and water from entering the trachea, while the soft palate of the mouth rises to block the nasopharynx so that material stays out of the nose. During vocalization, the pharynx plays a role in shaping the sounds made by the vocal cords, located just below it in the larynx.

Disorders and Diseases

Most problems in the pharynx arise from infection and inflammation. Pharyngitis, or sore throat, is an acute infection, usually from a virus or streptococcus bacteria, that is most common in children. Similarly, tonsillitis is an infection of the tonsils, quinsy (peritonsillar cellulitis and abscess) affects tissue near the tonsils, and epiglottitis is a bacterial infection of the epiglottis. Abscesses, with or without inflammation, may also occur in the pharynx; cysts known as Tornwaldt cysts may occur in the midline of the nasopharynx; and contact ulcers may result from damage to the pharyngeal tissue caused by swallowing something chemically harsh or physically abrasive or jagged.

Although not common, throat cancers can occur in the nasopharynx and tonsils. They are usually squamous cell carcinomas and occur predominantly in males, usually due to smoking and alcohol consumption.

People with cleft palates may not have complete closure of the nasal passage during swallowing, a condition called velopharyngeal insufficiency. The condition can impair speech and give it a marked nasal sound.

—*Roger Smith, Ph.D.*

See also Common cold; Decongestants; Laryngectomy; Laryngitis; Mouth and throat cancer; Nasal polyp removal; Otorhinolaryngology; Pharyngitis; Plastic surgery; Respiration; Sinusitis; Smell; Sore throat; Strep throat; Tonsillectomy and adenoid removal; Tonsillitis; Tonsils; Voice and vocal cord disorders.

For Further Information:

Beers, Mark H., et al., eds. *The Merck Manual of Medical Information*. 2nd home ed. Whitehouse Station, N.J.: Merck Research Laboratories, 2003.

Parker, Steve. *The Human Body Book*. 2nd ed. New York: DK Adult, 2013.

PM Medical Health News. *21st Century Complete Medical Guide to Throat and Pharynx Disorders: Authoritative Government Documents, Clinical References, and Practical Information for Patients and Physicians*. Mount Laurel, N.J.: Progressive Management, 2004.

Sasaki, Clarence T. "Introduction: Throat Disorders." *Merck Manual Home Health Handbook*, July 2008.

Thibodeau, Gary A., and Kevin T. Patton. *Structure and Function of the Human Body*. 14th ed. St. Louis, Mo.: Mosby/Elsevier, 2012.

"Throat Disorders." *MedlinePlus*, June 16, 2013.

Phenylketonuria (PKU)

Disease/Disorder

Also known as: Phenylalaninemia, phenylpyruvic oligophrenia, Følling's disease

Anatomy or system affected: Blood, brain, liver, nervous system

Specialties and related fields: Biochemistry, embryology, epidemiology, genetics, neonatology, neurology, nutrition, pediatrics

Definition: A genetic disorder caused by a deficiency of the liver enzyme phenylalanine hydroxylase.

Key terms:

phenylalanine: an essential amino acid

phenylalanine hydroxylase: a liver enzyme that catalyzes the conversion of phenylalanine to tyrosine

tetrahydrobiopterin: a cofactor for the conversion of phenylalanine to tyrosine

Causes and Symptoms

Phenylketonuria (PKU) is a genetic disorder, occurring in about one in 10,000 births, that disrupts the metabolism of the amino acid phenylalanine. The disorder is caused by a deficiency of phenylalanine hydroxylase, a liver enzyme that catalyzes the conversion of phenylalanine to tyrosine. Since normal phenylalanine metabolism is blocked, the amino acid accumulates in blood and tissues, resulting in progressive, irreversible mental retardation and neurological abnormalities. Most forms of PKU are caused by a mutation-more than two hundred mutations are now characterized-in the gene for phenylalanine hydroxylase. A small percentage of infants with PKU have a variant form of the condition, known as malignant PKU. This disorder is caused by a defect in the synthesis or metabolism of tetrahydrobiopterin, a cofactor for the conversion of phenylalanine to tyrosine, or in other enzymes along the pathway. Without treatment, malignant PKU causes a progressive, lethal deterioration of the central nervous system.

Infants with classic and malignant PKU appear normal; however, if untreated, the condition severely impairs normal brain development and growth after a few months of age, causing mental retardation, seizures, eczema, and neurological and behavioral problems. Affected infants have plasma phenylalanine levels ten to sixty times above normal, along with normal or reduced tyrosine levels and high concentrations of the metabolite phenylpyruvic acid in their urine.

Newborns are screened routinely for PKU within the first three weeks of life, usually by using whole blood obtained from a heel prick. Elevated phenylpyruvic acid levels also can be detected in urine of infants with PKU after adding a few drops of 10 percent ferric chloride, resulting in a deep green color. Newborns often have transient PKU-elevated phenylalanine and phenylpyruvic acid levels in the first few weeks of life that normalizes-so classic PKU should be distinguished from transient conditions. Elevated phenylalanine levels that persist beyond a few weeks of life, accompanied by normal or low tyrosine levels, usually indicate an inborn error of metabolism. Malignant PKU is usually diagnosed by detecting biopterin metabolites in urine or showing that tetrahydrobiopterin supplementation restores normal phenylalanine and tyrosine levels.

Babies of mothers with PKU are at high risk of brain damage, impaired growth, and malformations of the heart and other organs. Managing maternal phenylalanine levels at near normal concentrations appears to be crucial to preventing these cognitive and neurological defects.

The clinical basis for the damaging effects of PKU on the brain is unclear. Elevated phenylalanine levels may interfere with brain myelination or neuronal migration during development. In addition, PKU decreases the levels of the neurotransmitters dopamine and serotonin, which may be the basis for its neurological effects.

Treatment and Therapy

The detrimental effects of PKU can largely be controlled by maintaining phenylalanine levels in the normal range through a strict low-phenylalanine diet. This complex diet, often supplemented with tyrosine, prevents the buildup of phenylalanine and its metabolites in body tissues. Children whose phenylalanine levels are regularly monitored and managed can achieve normal intelligence and development. In infants with malignant PKU, tetrahydrobiopterin or cofactor supplements are required to control phenylalanine levels successfully.

Treatment for PKU must begin at a very early age, before the first three months of life, and usually continue through adulthood, or else some degree of mental retardation or neurological abnormalities is expected. Screening newborns for PKU before three weeks of age is mandated in all fifty US states. Strict control of phenylalanine levels also is indicated for pregnant women with PKU because their babies are at high risk for severe brain damage.

The successful treatment of PKU depends on managing phenylalanine levels. However, the diet is complex and challenging to sustain over many years. Since phenylalanine is an essential amino acid, found in virtually all proteins, maintaining adequate nutrition is nearly impossible on a low-phenylalanine diet. The treatment requires rigorous protein restriction and the substitution of most natural proteins in meat, fish, eggs, and dairy products. Phenylalanine intake must not be too restricted, how-

---

Information on Phenylketonuria (PKU)

Causes: Genetic disorder
Symptoms: If untreated, irreversible mental retardation and neurological abnormalities, seizures, eczema, behavioral problems
Duration: Typically chronic, sometimes progressive
Treatments: Strict low-phenylalanine diet, drug therapy

---

ever, or else phenylalanine deficiency can occur.

In some cases, dietary treatment for PKU can be discontinued or made less restrictive as children age, without causing severe effects. In many cases, however, the ill effects of the disorder carry into adulthood unless dietary management is continued over the long term. Untreated adolescents and adults may exhibit behavioral or neurological problems, difficulty concentrating, poor visual-motor coordination, and a low intelligence quotient (IQ).

Perspective and Prospects

Phenylketonuria was the first inborn error of metabolism shown to affect the brain. This genetic disorder was discovered in the 1930s by Ivar Asbjørn Følling. Since its discovery, PKU has been controlled successfully by rigorous newborn screening programs and careful dietary management of phenylalanine levels in pregnant women and in children with the disease. Newer research has focused on improving medical formulations for low-phenylalanine diets and amino acid supplementation for children and adults.

In the 1980s, clinical trials examined the use of dialysis-like procedures that allowed the rapid breakdown of phenylalanine in the blood. The treatment applies to pregnant women with PKU or those with severely elevated phenylalanine levels resulting from stress or illness. In the late twentieth century, PKU became the focus of gene therapy research. Animal models of PKU have been successfully treated by introducing normal phenylalanine hydroxylase deoxyribonucleic acid (DNA) into the liver cells of mice. Since the underlying genetic defects are known in most cases of PKU, gene therapy appears a likely research focus for long-term treatment.

—*Linda Hart, M.S., M.A.*

See also Digestion; Enzymes; Genetic diseases; Intellectual disability; Metabolic disorders; Metabolism; Neonatology; Nervous system; Neurology, pediatric; Nutrition; Screening.

For Further Information:

Behrman, Richard E., Robert M. Kliegman, and Hal B. Jenson, eds. *Nelson Textbook of Pediatrics*. 19th ed. Philadelphia: Saunders/Elsevier, 2011.

Chopra, Sanjiv. *Dr. Sanjiv Chopra's Liver Book: A Comprehensive Guide to Diagnosis, Treatment, and Recovery*. New York: Simon & Schuster, 2002.

Kimball, Chad T. *Childhood Diseases and Disorders Sourcebook: Basic Consumer Health Information About Medical Problems Often Encountered in Pre-adolescent Children*. Detroit, Mich.: Omnigraphics, 2003.

Marlow, Amy. "Phenylketonuria." *Health Library*, November 26, 2012.

Martin, Richard J., Avroy A. Fanaroff, and Michele C. Walsh, eds. *Fanaroff and Martin's Neonatal-Perinatal Medicine: Diseases of the Fetus and Infant*. 9th ed. St. Louis, Mo.: Mosby/Elsevier, 2011.

MedlinePlus. "Phenylketonuria." *MedlinePlus*, May 13, 2013.

Moore, Keith L., and T. V. N. Persaud. *The Developing Human*. 9th ed. Philadelphia: Saunders/Elsevier, 2013.

National PKU News. *National PKU News*, March 2013.

Parker, James N., and Philip M. Parker, eds. *The Official Parent's Sourcebook on Phenylketonuria*. San Diego, Calif.: Icon Health, 2002.

Phlebitis

Disease/Disorder

Anatomy or system affected: Blood vessels, circulatory system

Specialties and related fields: General surgery, internal medicine, vascular medicine

Definition: The inflammation of a vein, often seen in conjunction with blood clots within the deep and superficial veins outside the heart.

Key terms:

embolus: a detached blood clot that may travel through the venous system to lodge in other major veins, such as a pulmonary embolus, which may cause blockage of the major blood vessels within the lungs

endothelial damage: disruption of the cellular lining of a blood vessel such as a vein; part of Virchow's triad

hypercoagulability: an increase in the ability of blood to clot or to change from a liquid state to a solid one; coagulation of blood is dependent upon activation of clotting agents within the body

stasis: stagnation of blood or the failure of blood to flow; venous stasis may be the result of obstructions to outflow from the veins

superficial thrombophlebitis: inflammation and clotting of the veins of the arms and/or legs that lie just beneath the surface of the skin and drain into the deep veins of the limbs

venous thrombosis: formation of a blood clot within the veins of the body

Causes and Symptoms

Phlebitis, meaning the inflammation of a vein, is a general term used to describe the presence of blood clots, or thrombi, in the veins of the body outside the heart. Blood clots because of the formation of clotting agents, such as fibrin. When blood clots within the body, there are three principal factors involved: damage to the venous endothelium, the cells that form the lining of the vein; venous stasis, or failure of the blood to flow; and hypercoagulability, or an increase in clotting factors in the blood. These three features associated with phlebitic episodes-endothelial damage, stasis, and hypercoagulability-are referred to as Virchow's triad (named for Rudolf Virchow, who in 1846 described the characteristics of thrombus formation in the deep veins of the lower extremities).

Patients with phlebitis will complain of swelling, tenderness, and inflammation of the affected limb. If the clot has formed in the veins just beneath the surface of the skin, they may feel a hard, cordlike structure in the segment of the vein that is filled with a thrombus. If the blood clot has not attached firmly to the wall of the vein, it may break loose and travel in the bloodstream to enter the vessels within the lung. These traveling clots are known as emboli and, depending on their size, they may either dissolve in the pulmonary vessels of the lung or block major vessels, preventing blood flow to that part of the lung. It has been shown that there is a greater risk of pulmonary embolism if the venous clots are formed in the leg veins above the knee than if phlebitis occurs in the calf veins.

To understand the factors that predispose the blood to clot within the body, it is necessary to understand the anatomy of the venous system and the mechanisms by which blood flows through the veins. Approximately 75 percent of the body's blood is found in the venous system, which is divided into three parts: the superficial veins, the deep veins, and the perforating, or communicating, veins. The superficial veins of the extremities are large, thick-walled, muscular structures that lie just beneath the skin. The deep veins are thin-walled and less muscular than the superficial veins. In the extremities, these deep veins are named after the arteries that they accompany. Blood is transported from the superficial to the deep veins by the communicating veins, or perforators. Thin, leaflike, bicuspid valves are found in most veins of the body, even in venules as small as 0.15 millimeter in diameter. These valves can open readily to allow blood to pass as it moves from the superficial to the deep veins on its return trip to the heart and can close rapidly to prevent blood flow from moving in the reverse direction. There are more valves in the veins of the calf than there are in the thigh veins, and no valves are found in the common iliac veins of the pelvis or in the inferior vena cava (the deep vein that transports blood through the abdomen).

The venous system must perform four important body functions. First, the veins must return blood that has been pumped through the arteries back to the heart. Additionally, the veins must be able to expand and contract so that they can regulate the increases and decreases in blood volume in the body. They must be responsive to the transport of blood during exercise and, along with the capillaries, play a major role in regulating body temperature.

Veins have the unique feature of being able to change their shape and size in order to respond to changes in pressure from within the vein (caused by increased fluid volume in the body) and to pressure from outside the vein (from tissue fluids and changes in pressure that occur as a result of gravity and the weight of the column of blood in the veins when one is standing or sitting up). As an example, when a hand is hanging at the side of the body, the veins on the back of the hand are full and visible because the veins are full of blood and the internal venous pressure is greater than the pressure from outside the vein. If the hand is raised over the head, the veins collapse because of the changes in internal venous pressure and gravitational and hydrostatic pressure, the pressures on the outside of the vein.

Blood is pumped under pressure by the heart to the arteries in order to supply nutrients and oxygen to the tissues. In

Information on Phlebitis

Causes: Damage to cells forming the lining of vein; failure of blood flow; increase in clotting factors in blood; use of oral contraceptives; long periods of inactivity; use of catheters; pregnancy

Symptoms: Swelling, tenderness, inflammation, presence of hard knot or lump

Duration: Acute to chronic

Treatments: Heparin infusion, anticoagulants, bed rest, leg elevation, moist heat

contrast, the heart has little influence on moving blood through the low-pressure veins of the body on its return trip. Blood is returned from the extremities to the heart and lungs by contraction of the calf muscles during exercise and by changes in the intra-abdominal and intrathoracic pressures that occur with respiration. For example, with a limb at rest, blood will flow toward the heart from the superficial system to the deep veins via the perforating veins as a result of the changes in abdominal and thoracic pressures that occur with breathing. With exercise, the calf muscles may exert more than 200 millimeters of mercury (mmHg) pressure on the large, saclike veins, the sinusoids in the sole, and the gastrocnemius veins of the calf, causing blood to move rapidly out of the foot and calf.

If the valves are incompetent such that the leaflets fail to meet when the valve closes, the column of forward-moving blood cannot be maintained in the segments of the veins between the valve sites. In this case, when one stops exercising, blood will flow backward toward the feet through the damaged valves, resulting in increased venous pressure at ankle level.

As one inhales, the diaphragm descends, compressing the inferior vena cava and stopping the flow of blood from the legs. With exhalation, the diaphragm rises and venous flow will continue toward the heart in a competent venous system. It is interesting that flow in the arms is under the control of intrathoracic, rather than intra-abdominal, pressure changes. Thus, with inhalation, the flow of blood from the arms increases as the pressure within the chest cavity is reduced. Upon exhalation, venous flow from the arms is impeded (which is in contrast to the respiratory effects that influence venous return from the legs).

As long as blood continues to circulate, the likelihood of clotting is reduced. There are, however, several risk factors that may cause changes in blood flow, damage to the vein wall, or hypercoagulability of the blood-the three features involved in venous thrombosis.

Venous thrombosis may occur as a result of obstructions to venous outflow from the limb. For example, taking a long trip by car, train, or airplane may require sitting for many hours without the freedom to walk around and exercise the calf muscles. Because the calf muscle pump is inactive, blood will pool in the veins of the legs. This failure of blood to flow, or venous stasis, places the individual at increased risk for clotting of blood in the calf veins. Similarly, patients who are prescribed bed rest because of acci-

dents, pregnancy, or critical illnesses and those patients who undergo long surgical operations are at risk for forming thrombi in the leg veins because of venous stasis and, as a result of the thrombosis, are also at risk for pulmonary embolism.

The incidence of phlebitis increases linearly with age. This fact is thought to reflect an increase in the diameter of the veins and the venous sinusoids within the calf muscles as a result of loss of elastic tissue in the vein walls. As the vein diameter increases, venous flow becomes sluggish. As an individual grows older, the muscle mass in the thigh and calf decreases and the calf muscle pump becomes less effective at moving venous blood toward the heart. This pooling of blood places elderly patients at risk for phlebitic episodes.

In the modern health care setting, the most common cause of phlebitis has been injury to the vein wall by intravenous catheters or by the infusion of drugs that cause inflammation of the venous endothelium. If a catheter is left in place for an extended period of time, infection may occur within the vein along its course, causing inflammation of the vein wall, venous stasis, and eventual thrombosis of the vein.

Inflammation of the vein may also occur as a result of venography, an invasive procedure used to determine if thrombi are present in the deep or superficial veins of patients. With this test, contrast dyes are injected into the veins to delineate the blood-flow patterns and venous anatomy and to define the segments of the vein where clots are present and are obstructing blood flow. Approximately 3 percent of patients have thrombi form in their veins following this diagnostic procedure. Approximately 8 percent of these patients will require hospitalization for treatment of postvenographic phlebitis.

Women who are taking oral contraceptives containing the hormone estrogen are thought to be at increased risk for phlebitis because of the decrease in the muscular tone of the vein wall and subsequent decrease in velocity of blood flow in the veins that results from the use of these drugs. Estrogen compounds may increase the surface adhesiveness of platelets, the blood cells that are responsible for clotting, causing them to stick together and form large clots that can block the veins. Additionally, estrogen compounds may influence chemicals within the blood that affect its ability to clot. Specifically, it is thought that these hormonal compounds affect clotting factors II, VII, VIII, and X and also cause a decrease in antithrombin III, a chemical that influences the production of thrombin, the principal factor controlling the formation of thrombi.

The influence of estrogen on the body's ability to control the production of appropriate levels of clotting factors is also noted during pregnancy and in the postpartum period. Phlebitis is diagnosed three to six times more frequently in women in the first four months following delivery than it is in women who have not become pregnant, as a result of estrogen-induced hypercoagulability of the blood. It is also interesting to note that women who deliver their babies by cesarean section are at increased risk for thrombophlebitis because of venous stasis occurring during the more prolonged recovery period that follows surgical delivery.

Treatment and Therapy

The symptoms of phlebitis-unilateral limb swelling, local inflammation, tenderness, and pain-may be associated with other medical conditions. Because there are no specific signs that are used to diagnose deep or superficial venous thrombosis, physicians misdiagnose phlebitis in approximately 50 percent of cases. As noted above, venography, once thought to be the standard for the identification of venous thrombosis, may actually predispose the patient to phlebitis. Noninvasive diagnostic techniques have been developed to demonstrate the presence, location, extent, and severity of the thrombotic process.

It has been shown that chemicals found naturally in the endothelial cells that line the veins can lyse, or dissolve, small clots. The veins of the calf have more lytic potential than the veins of the thigh and pelvis. In exercise, the compression of the calf muscles on the veins causes this material to be forced into the venous blood, thus helping to dissolve small thrombi.

Acute thrombosis of the deep veins above the knee usually requires hospitalization and infusion of heparin, a drug that prevents further clotting, allowing the body's mechanism to dissolve clots to act more quickly and effectively. If left untreated, clots in this location may continue to propagate toward the large pelvic veins or the inferior vena cava, or pieces of a thrombus, called emboli, may break off the clot and travel through the vena cava to enter the pulmonary circulation of the lungs. In many cases, pulmonary embolism is life-threatening.

Patients with clots in the deep veins of the legs are instructed to stay in bed with the leg elevated to prevent venous pooling, and moist heat is applied to the leg to promote local circulation of blood. Patients will continue to take anticoagulant drugs for several months following hospitalization to ensure that fresh clots do not form in the veins, and they are instructed to wear elastic compression stockings to promote venous circulation.

It has been shown that clots will resolve completely in approximately 70 percent of patients receiving anticoagulant therapy. The remainder of patients will continue to have obstructions of their veins because of a clot that did not lyse, and as a result of the phlebitic episode, the venous valves will become incompetent. These patients will continue to be at risk for phlebitis and frequently express complaints of having tired, aching, heavy legs. If damage to the valves is severe, venous pressure at ankle level is increased, and blood may be forced out of the veins into the surrounding tissues, causing ulcers to form.

Thrombosis of the superficial veins, frequently called thrombophlebitis, is most often treated with hot compresses and elevation of the leg to relieve the local venous inflammation. Care must be taken to ensure that the clot does not continue to extend toward the segment of superficial vein where it joins the deep venous system, because the patient would then be at risk for pulmonary embolism.

Attempts have been made to bypass segments of a thrombosed vein surgically and to transplant new valves in venous segments that have become incompetent as a result of postphlebitic valve damage. Such procedures, however, have been unrewarding. Anticoagulant and lytic therapies begun early in the thrombotic process appear to offer the best results with the least long-term sequelae for phlebitic patients.

Perspective and Prospects

It has been estimated that approximately two million people are affected by phlebitis each year in the United States and that there are approximately two hundred thousand deaths per year as a result of venous thrombosis. Autopsy data suggest that 1 to 2 percent of phlebitic patients will die from pulmonary embolism each year.

—*Marsha M. Neumyer*

See also Arteriosclerosis; Blood and blood disorders; Blood vessels; Bypass surgery; Circulation; Deep vein thrombobis; Embolism; Surgery, general; Thrombosis and thrombus; Varicose veins; Vascular medicine; Vascular system; Venous insufficiency.

For Further Information:

Bick, Roger L. *Disorders of Thrombosis and Hemostasis: Clinical and Laboratory Practice*. 3d ed. Philadelphia: Lippincott Williams & Wilkins, 2002.

Furtado, LuÃs Carlos do Rego. "Incidence and Predisposing Factors of Phlebitis in a Surgery Department." *British Journal of Nursing* (July 28, 2011): S16-25.

Icon Health. *Phlebitis: A Medical Dictionary, Bibliography, and Annotated Research Guide to Internet References*. San Diego, Calif.: Author, 2004.

Kohnle, Diana. "Phlebitis." *Health Library*, September 26, 2012.

Litin, Scott C., ed. *Mayo Clinic Family Health Book*. 4th ed. New York: HarperResource, 2009.

Loscalzo, Joseph, and Andrew I. Schafer, eds. *Thrombosis and Hemorrhage*. 3d ed. Philadelphia: Lippincott Williams & Wilkins, 2003.

Rutherford, Robert B., ed. *Vascular Surgery*. 6th ed. Philadelphia: Saunders/Elsevier, 2005.

"Thrombophlebitis." *MedlinePlus*, May 6, 2011.

Phlebotomy

Procedure

Also known as: Venipuncture

Anatomy or system affected: Arms, blood, blood vessels, cells, circulatory system

Specialties and related fields: Hematology

Definition: The collection of blood specimens for analysis.

Indications and Procedures

Phlebotomy is performed to acquire blood samples for microbiology, cytology, fluid analysis, or other testing. Blood collection tubes are drawn in a specific order to avoid cross-contamination of additives in tubes designed for specific tests. Collection tubes are color-coded according to the additives (if any) contained within them. An essential component of the procedure is the accurate labeling of tubes with information identifying the patient. Blood collection should be carried out only by a licensed phlebotomist.

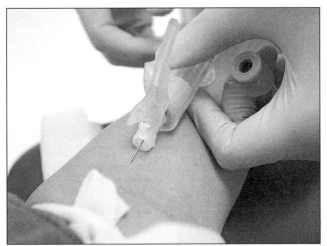

A phlebotomist draws blood from a patient. (© Francis Twitty/ iStockphoto.com)

A temporary tourniquet is applied to the arm three to four inches above the selected puncture site, the skin is cleaned with an alcohol or iodine wipe, and then a needle is inserted into a vein (venipuncture). Blood can also be collected from an artery or fingerstick, if appropriate. Often, the skin is palpated and the vein is traced with a finger, or the arm may be massaged until a superficial vein is readily apparent. After one or more tubes of blood (typically about ten milliliters in volume) are collected, a gauze sponge is applied until bleeding stops and then an adhesive bandage is applied. The tourniquet is immediately removed after the last tube to be drawn starts to fill. The entire procedure takes only a few minutes.

When smaller volumes of blood are required, collection can be accomplished by a simple fingerstick on the third or fourth finger of the nondominant hand, using a sterile lancet. The first drop of blood is wiped away, and then blood is collected into a capillary tube while the finger is gently massaged. After the fingerstick procedure, the patient normally is instructed to hold a small gauze pad over the puncture site for a few minutes to stop the bleeding. For blood collection on a newborn baby or infant, the heel is the recommended puncture site.

Uses and Complications

Phlebotomy is a routine procedure with minimal risks. Trained phlebotomists take precautions to protect themselves and the patient from exposure to blood-borne diseases and to prevent the occurrence of infection. These precautions include the use of rubber or latex gloves and only new, sterile disposable tubes and needles. Most frequently, blood is taken from the larger and fuller median cubital and cephalic veins of the arm; wrist and hand veins can also be acceptable. Certain areas are avoided in venipuncture: extensive scar tissue from burns or injury, the site of a previous mastectomy, regions of hematoma, sites of intravenous (IV) therapy and blood transfusion, cannula or fistula devices, and extremities suffering from edema. Some patients may experience light-headedness or even faint during blood collection; to prevent accidents, the patient remains seated during the brief procedure.

—Michael R. King, Ph.D.

See also Bleeding; Blood and blood disorders; Blood banks; Blood testing; Blood vessels; Circulation; Hematology; Hematology, pediatric; Laboratory tests; Transfusion.

For Further Information:
Garza, Diana, and Kathleen Becan-McBride. *Phlebotomy Handbook: Blood Collection Essentials.* 7th ed. Upper Saddle River, N.J.: Pearson/Prentice Hall, 2005.
Hoeltke, Lynn B. *The Complete Textbook of Phlebotomy.* 4th ed. Albany, N.Y.: Delmar, 2012.
McCall, Ruth E., and Cathee M. Tankersley. *Phlebotomy Essentials.* 5th ed. Baltimore: Wolters Kluwer/Lippincott Williams & Wilkins, 2012
"Venipuncture." *MedlinePlus*, August 31, 2011.

Phobias
Disease/Disorder
Anatomy or system affected: Psychic-emotional system
Specialties and related fields: Psychiatry, psychology
Definition: Excessive fears of certain objects, people, places, or situations.

Causes and Symptoms

Phobias can induce a state of anxiety or panic, often debilitating sufferers, restricting them from full freedom of action, career progress, or sociability. For example, a heterosexual person who fears talking with the opposite sex will have problems dating and progressing socially.

Fear serves an important and necessary function in life. It keeps one from putting a hand in a flame or walking into oncoming traffic. The fear of death and the unknown is commonplace; it causes many to dislike, even dread, passing by cemeteries, even though there is no logical reason. While many forms of fear are normal, if they occur out of context, in socially unacceptable manners, too severely, or uncontrollably, then the diagnosis is a phobia.

Many different phobias have been cited in the literature and have specific terms in dictionaries, constructed by prefixing the word "phobia" with Greek or Latin terms (such as acrophobia or claustrophobia). While their enumeration is an interesting pastime, phobias are serious conditions and should be treated by professional psychologists.

Phobias are caused by perceived dangerous experiences, both real and imagined. Sometimes, it is gradual: A worker may develop anxiety reactions to a boss over several weeks. Likewise, a single moment of terror can cause a lifetime of avoidance: A dog attack can generate cynophobia (fear of dogs) in a child. Children are especially susceptible to phobias, most of which are caused by fear of injury. The death of a close relative is difficult for children to understand and requires a delicate, sensitive, and honest explanation. Questions and expressions of feelings (often resentment) by the child should be encouraged and discussed. It is repression, unanswered questions, lack of supportive people, and guilt feelings that can lead to morbid attitudes and fantasies, by which phobias develop. Experiences in the past and associated fears remain dormant, to recur and be relived.

Information on Phobias

Causes: Psychological disorder
Symptoms: Feeling of anxiety or panic, impaired social interaction, impaired freedom of action
Duration: Often chronic
Treatments: Cognitive and behavioral therapy (e.g., controlled exposure to object of fear)

Anticipatory fears can also cause phobias. Driving trainees and beginning drivers often have phobic reactions, dreading possible accidents. Students, often the best or most conscientious ones, may spend sleepless nights worrying about the next day's examination. They fear experiences that may never occur, irrationally magnifying the consequences of their performance to one of absolute success or utter doom. Concentration produces positive results (that is, good grades), but obsession may cause paralyzing fear and pressure, even suicide. Several other theories exist regarding the cause of phobias.

Phobias can be classified into three primary groupings: simple phobias, social phobias, and agoraphobia. Simple phobias are directed toward specific things, animals, phenomena, or situations. Rodents, cats, dogs, and birds are common objects of fear. A swooping gull or pigeon may cause panic. Insects, spiders, and bugs can provoke revulsion. Many cultures have a fear of snakes. A phobia exists, for example, when a house is inspected several times each day for snakes; a phobic person may vacate a rural home for an urban dwelling in order to avoid them. Blood, diseased people, or hospital patients have caused fainting. Some vegetarians dread meat because of traumatic observations of slaughter. Fear of heights, water, enclosed spaces, and open spaces involves imagined dangers of falling, drowning, feeling trapped, and being lost in oblivion, respectively. These feelings are coupled with a fear of loss of control and harming oneself by entering a dangerous situation. Sometimes, a specific piece of music, building, or person triggers reactions; the initial trauma or conditioning events are not easily remembered or recognized as such.

Social phobias are fears of being watched or judged by others in social settings. For example, in a restaurant, phobics may eat in rigid, restrictive motions to avoid embarrassments. They may avoid soups, making noises with utensils, or food that requires gnawing for fear of being observed or drawing attention. Many students fear giving speeches because of the humiliation and ridicule resulting from mistakes. Stage fright, dating anxiety, and fear of unemployment, divorce, or other forms of failure are also phobic conditions produced by social goals and expectations. The desire to please others can exact a terrible toll in worry, fear, and sleepless nights.

Agoraphobia is a flight reaction caused by the fear of places and predicaments outside a sphere of safety. This sphere may be home, a familiar person (often a parent), a bed, or a bedroom. Patients retreat from life and remain at home, safe from the outside world and its anticipated perils. They may look out the window and fear the demands and expectations placed on them. They are prisoners of insecurity and doubt, avoiding the responsibilities, risks, and requirements of living. Many children are afraid of school, and some feign illness to remain safely in bed. Facing the responsibilities of maturation causes similar reactions.

Treatment and Therapy

Different schools of psychology espouse different approaches to the treatment of phobias, but central themes involve controlled exposure to the object of fear. Common core fears include fear of dying, fear of going crazy, fear of losing control, fear of failure, and fear of rejection.

The most effective approach to treating these disorders is a cognitive-behavioral strategy. With this approach, dysfunctional thinking is identified and changed through collaborative efforts between the patient and therapist. Additional dysfunctional behavior is identified and changed through processes involving conditioning and reinforcement.

Through an initial minimal exposure to the feared object or situation, discussion, and then progressively greater controlled contact, patients experience some stress at each stage but not at a level sufficient to cause a relapse. They will proceed to become desensitized to the object in phases. Therapists may serve as role models at first, demonstrating the steps that patients need to complete, or they may provide positive feedback and guidance. In either case, the role of the patient is active, and gradual exposure occurs. In the process, patients learn to adapt to stress and become more capable of dealing with life.

Other supervised therapies exist, some involving hypnosis, psychoanalysis, drugs, and reasoning out of one's fears. In dealing with phobics, it must be recognized that anyone can have a phobia. Patience, understanding, supportiveness, and professional help are needed. Telling someone simply to "snap out of it" increases stress and guilt.

—John Panos Najarian, Ph.D.;
updated by Nancy A. Piotrowski, Ph.D.

See also Antianxiety; Anxiety; Body dysmorphic disorder; Bonding; Death and dying; Depression; Emotions: Biomedical causes and effects; Neurosis; Nightmares; Post-traumatic stress disorder; Psychiatric disorders; Psychiatry; Psychiatry, child and adolescent; Psychiatry, geriatric; Psychoanalysis; Psychosomatic disorders; Separation anxiety; Stress; Stress reduction; Toilet training.

For Further Information:

Barlow, David H. *Anxiety and Its Disorders.* 2d ed. New York: Guilford Press, 2004. Examines the subject in the context of recent developments in emotion theory, cognitive science, and neuroscience. Reviews the implications for treatment and integrates them into newly developed treatment protocols for the various anxiety disorders.

Bourne, Edmond J. *The Anxiety and Phobia Workbook.* 4th ed. Oakland, Calif.: New Harbinger, 2005. This is an excellent self-help book for problems related to anxiety. It may also be helpful for family members seeking to understand anxiety better or to support those affected by anxiety.

Maj, Mario, et al., eds. *Phobias.* Hoboken, N.J.: John Wiley & Sons, 2004. Reviews the diagnosis, classification, pharmacotherapy, psychotherapy, and social and economic burdens of phobias.

Marks, Isaac M. *Fears, Phobias, and Rituals: Panic, Anxiety, and Their Disorders*. New York: Oxford University Press, 1987. This book draws on fields as diverse as biochemistry, physiology, pharmacology, psychology, psychiatry, and ethology to form a fascinating synthesis of information on the nature of fear and of panic and anxiety disorders.

Saul, Helen. *Phobias: Fighting the Fear*. New York: Arcade, 2001. Traces the historical and cultural roots of phobias, examining case studies and literature in the process.

Stewart, Gail B. *Phobias*. San Diego, Calif.: Thomson/Gale, 2005. Discusses phobias, especially as they relate to children. Includes bibliographical references and an index.

Phrenology

Specialty

Anatomy or system affected: Brain, skull

Specialties and related fields: Neurology, neuroscience, psychiatry, psychology

Definition: A discredited field that theorizes well-developed areas of the cerebral cortex of the brain, each with its own functional properties, corresponded to bumps on the skull. Likewise, a depression on the skull would indicate an underdeveloped faculty.

Key term:

theory of localization: a theory that stated the brain consisted of many specific areas that took on their own functional properties

Science and Profession

Phrenology was championed by Franz Joseph Gall (1758-1828), an Austrian physician and anatomist, who developed the theory that the size of cortical regions of the brain was correlated with specific talents such as inquisitiveness, destructiveness, secretiveness, and friendship. In addition, enhanced brain areas were reflected as enlarged bumps on the skull directly above it. In all, Gall believed he had located twenty-seven faculties that were unique to humans and nineteen that were found on some nonhuman animals. These special talents were referred to by Gall as "organs." The extra organs that humans possessed, according to Gall, were areas that corresponded to things such as wisdom, passion, and the sense of satire. Besides paying attention to the bumps on the cranium, the recesses were also important since they reflected the underdevelopment of specific talents.

Prior to the nineteenth century, there were was some discussion regarding how the brain was organized as a collection of many different neuroanatomical structures, each with their own functional properties. Gall is credited with developing this notion into the theory of localization. The theory of localization was proposed as an alternative to the theory of equipotentiality which held the belief that mental abilities depended on the whole brain rather than just a single isolated area. Phrenology benefited from the popularity of localization theory even though there was little empirical evidence to support its claims.

Another physician who popularized phrenology was Johann Spurzheim (1776-1832), a devoted follower and colleague of Frances Gall. They began to work together in 1804 in Vienna and shortly thereafter began to lecture extensively around the world. Spurzheim not only helped espouse Gall's ideas about phrenology, he also developed his own ideas and proposed several additional organs and distinguished between cognitive and emotional faculties. Eventually, after a series of lecture tours, which included a trip to the United States, Spurzheim became the leading proponent of phrenology. While in the United States, some of his lectures were directed towards physicians as a means to discuss possible clinical applications of phrenology. Yet, before these discussions could gain traction, Spurzheim died from typhoid fever in his mid-50s. His skull, at Spurzheim's request, was preserved and studied. It currently resides in the Warren Museum at Harvard Medical School.

In the United States, during the 1820s, phrenology gained acceptance from several professional groups as well as garnered interest from the general public. The Central Phrenological Society was formed in Philadelphia in 1822. Two years later the first American textbook on phrenology Elements of Phrenology was published. An American by the name of George Combe (1788-1858) wrote the Constitution of Man in 1827, which sold more than 100,000 copies. It has been reported that this book was one of the most popular books, in English, during this era. In addition, the psychograph was developed as a type of phrenology machine. It systematically measured thirty-two different points on the cranium and would list out which traits were more or less present on a five-point scale. The Psychograph Company operated from 1929-1937, and the psychograph machine could be found in department stores or theaters for the amusement of the general public.

Perspective and Prospects

While phrenology gained a meteoric rise in popularity, its collapse and eventual fall into disrepute came just as quickly. Perhaps the most ardent opponent against phrenology was Marie-Jean-Pierre Flourens (1794-1867), a French physiologist, who held a strong belief in experimental laboratory methods that were conducted mostly on animals (e.g., hens, ducks, frogs) to discredit not only phrenology, but the larger theory of localization in general. Flourens' book, Phrenology Examined, was his strongest attempt to show that bumps on the skull were in no way related to various skills. Today, phrenology is viewed as an amusing afterthought by the neuroscientific community.

—Bryan C. Auday, Ph.D.

See also Neurology: Neuroscience

For Further Information:

Finger, Stanley. *Origins of Neuroscience: A History of Exploration into Brain Function*. Oxford: Oxford University Press, 1994.

Kolb, Bryan, and Ian Q. Whishaw. *Fundamentals of Human Neuropsychology*. 6th ed. New York: Worth Publishers, 2009.

Horton Jr., Arthur MacNeill, and Danny Wedding. *The Neuropsychology Handbook*. 3rd ed. New York: Springer Publishing Company, 2008.

Lambert, Kelly G., and Craig H. Kinsley. *Clinical Neuroscience: Psychopathology and the Brain*. 2nd ed. New York: Oxford University Press, 2011.

Leek, Sybil. *Phrenology*. New York: Collier-Macmillan, 1970.

Zillmer, Eric A., Mary V. Spiers, and William C. Culbertson. *Principles of Neuropsychology*. 2nd ed. Belmont, CA: Thomson Wadsworth, 2008.

Physical examination

Procedure

Anatomy or system affected: All

Specialties and related fields: All

Definition: A step in the diagnostic process in which the physician makes general observations about the patient and examines structures of the patient's body through touching (palpation), tapping (percussion), and listening, usually with the aid of a stethoscope (auscultation).

Key terms:

auscultation: active listening, usually with the aid of a stethoscope, to sounds generated by the body

inflammation: irritation caused by such things as infection, injury, allergy, or toxins; symptoms include redness, swelling, warmth, pain, and drainage

organ system: structures of the body, in close proximity or distanced from one another, which together perform a function or functions

palpation: application of the hands, or touching, to determine the size, texture, consistency, and location of body structures

percussion: gentle tapping of the examiner's finger, which has been positioned on the patient; a hollow sound is heard over air-filled structures, while a dull thud is heard over solid areas or liquid-filled structures

sign: objective evidence of disease; a finding noted by the physician during the course of the physical examination

symptom: subjective evidence of disease, provided by the patient

Indications and Procedures

Physical diagnosis-the principles, practices, and traditions that form the foundation of the modern physical examination-has rightly been called an art. Usually taught during the first two years of medical training, the basic skills of observation, auscultation, palpation, and percussion are later augmented by hands-on experience with actual patients. For many students, this acquisition of physical diagnostic skills marks the point when they begin to feel like "real" doctors. Observation techniques may be overt or subtle, as a patient may have difficulty maintaining usual behavior if consciously aware of scrutiny. An examiner may even find it necessary to distract the patient in order to allow accurate assessment.

Auscultation, from the Latin *auscultare* (to listen), is generally performed with the aid of a stethoscope. Normal bodily functions generate sounds, the presence or absence of which may provide clues to health or illness. Palpation, from the Latin *palpare* (to touch softly), involves the application of the examiner's hands to the patient's body. This touching conveys information about the size, texture, consistency, temperature, and tenderness of physical structures. This person-to-person contact can also exert an important calming or reassuring effect on the patient. Percussion, from the Latin *percussio* (striking), entails a

gentle tapping of the examiner's finger, which has been placed on the patient. A resonant return is noted over hollow, air-filled structures. In contrast, solid or fluid-filled structures produce a dull fullness. A simple demonstration of this technique can be performed by partially filling a bucket with water. By tapping on the outside and noting the variations in sound, it is possible to estimate the fluid level without looking inside the bucket.

To some extent, the widespread use of sophisticated diagnostic imaging technologies has decreased the emphasis on physical examination skills in actual practice. This trend is unfortunate, because it lessens face-to-face contact between the patient and physician and may thus prove unsatisfying for both. It would be misleading, though, to view technological discoveries as competing only with the physical examination. Over the years, the usefulness of physical diagnosis has been enhanced by the availability of simple tools and elegant instruments that augment the examiner's biological senses. Common examples include the stethoscope, the oto-ophthalmoscope (a handheld halogen light source with interchangeable optics, used to view the inside of the eyes and ears), the reflex hammer, and the tuning fork. Indeed, the line separating physical diagnosis from other diagnostic procedures has been blurred as more portable devices find their way into the hands of the practicing physician.

During the physical examination, diagnostic techniques are applied in an interaction between the examiner and the patient at a unique moment in time. As such, the outcome depends on the skills of the individual examiner and on the patient's manifest physical characteristics. Changes in physical state over time are common; variation in physical examination findings over time is not unexpected. For example, heart murmurs, which are sounds generated by the heart, are graded on a scale from I/VI (one over six), designating a very faint murmur, to VI/VI (six over six), designating a murmur loud enough to be heard even without a stethoscope at a distance away from the patient. It is not uncommon for physicians, even cardiologists, who specialize in the heart, to disagree on the description of a murmur. In addition, a murmur itself can get louder or softer, or even disappear entirely with advancing age, exercise, pregnancy, or other factors. Physical diagnosis is an imprecise science. Medical educators have attempted to address this imprecision by modifying traditional instructional methods.

The physical examination should be considered within the larger context of medical information gathering. Customarily, it follows the collection of historical information about the patient's immediate and past health statuses. Like a road map, the history guides the scope and focus of the subsequent examination. This marriage of history taking and physical examination is colloquially referred to as the "H and P." Though not as often recommended as in the past, the annual complete (or head-to-foot) physical examination may come to mind when this topic is discussed. More commonly, a physical examination is directed and focused on particular regions or organ systems.

In the general screening examination of an apparently

healthy subject, a systematic survey is undertaken, following an assessment of structural and/or functional relationships. A structural division would involve examination of all the organ systems contained in or adjacent to a particular body part (for example, the foot), such as the bones, muscles, nerve supply, blood vessels, and skin. A functional examination of the cardiovascular organ system would include the heart, neck, lungs, abdomen, skin, and extremities, because manifestations of cardiovascular disease may be present in locations physically remote from the heart itself. A patient complaining of a specific problem undergoes a detailed examination of the organ systems or body structures most likely to be affected.

The sequential performance of a physical examination incorporates both structural and functional strategies. Though most examiners follow a similar framework, individual differences in physicians and patients result in a wide variety of acceptable patterns. Ideally, the process begins when the patient first arrives. Clues to a patient's overall level of independent function, such as mobility, dexterity, and speech patterns, may be noted. As the medical history is taken, the patient's level of alertness, as well as orientation to time, place, and self, often becomes apparent. The complete examination generally begins with the head, including the face and scalp. A survey of the skin surfaces may be accomplished with the patient completely naked, or it may be divided into discrete segments to be checked as the examination proceeds. Inspection of the eyes, ears, nose, and throat follow. Next, the neck, chest, and back are surveyed. A breast examination may be done at this time. After evaluation of the heart and lungs, the patient is asked to lie down for the abdominal examination. Genital organs may be checked at this time or may be deferred until a later part of the session. The neurologic inspection usually follows and entails the integration of findings from earlier parts of the examination with maneuvers specific to the neurological examination. In the mental status portion of the neurologic examination, formal evaluation of memory, orientation, speech patterns, and thought processes takes place. The musculoskeletal examination likewise integrates earlier findings with a detailed focus on bone and joint development and function. Finally, the extremities are checked. Upon completion of the history and physical, the diagnosis may be readily apparent or further evaluation may be needed.

Pertinent findings, whether normal or abnormal, are documented in the medical record and may be supplemented by diagrams or photographs if necessary. Depending on the purpose of the examination, these may be entered on a separate preprinted form with check-off spaces or simply noted in the chart. Computer technology allows the storage and retrieval of this information in a patient database file.

Uses and Complications

The application of physical examination techniques may be illustrated by considering three distinct cases: a child's

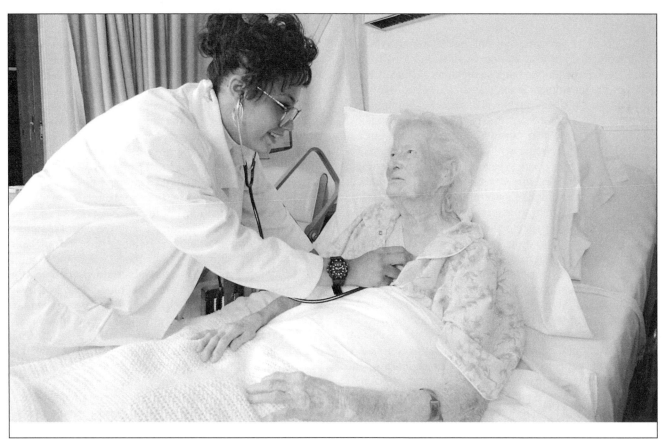

A physician uses a stethoscope to check a patient's airways. Such hands-on evaluation is important in diagnosis. (Digital Stock)

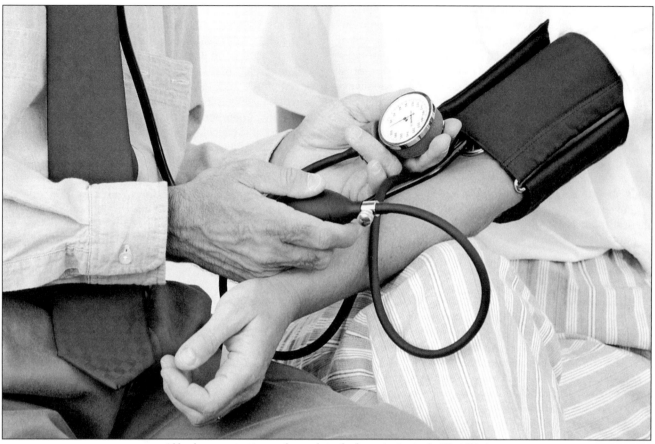

A blood pressure test is one of several standard examination tools. (PhotoDisc)

school physical, a routine gynecologic examination with a Papanicolaou (Pap) test, and the evaluation of a sprained ankle. Each has a unique purpose dictating the breadth and detail of the techniques employed. In the school physical, the purpose of the examination is to screen a symptom-free individual for signs of previously unrecognized medical conditions; thus, the survey is broad. The annual gynecologic examination with a Pap testing is more focused-screening for cervical cancer and other gynecologic illness, including sexually transmitted diseases-and will focus on the reproductive system. The evaluation of the sprained ankle is done to assess damage to an identified body part following a specific injury, and it will entail a detailed inspection of the affected area. How these underlying considerations influence the methods employed are apparent as each case is considered.

A child's school physical examination is preceded by a broad historical investigation of the individual's birth details, immunization status, social interactions, growth and development, and daily activity. Height and weight are measured and plotted on a growth chart to facilitate comparison with expected normal values for children of the same age and sex. In many cases, the actual numbers are of less importance than the trend relating repeated measurements. Vision and hearing screening are employed to identify defects that could interfere with school performance.

Vital signs-temperature, pulse, blood pressure, and breathing-are determined. Temperature is usually determined orally, though rectal or axillary (armpit) locations may be used. Although 37 degrees Celsius (98.6 degrees Fahrenheit) is often quoted as normal, a range of body temperatures can be found in healthy patients. Pulse rate is measured by palpation of the radial artery in the wrist. Circumstances may dictate performing this measurement in other locations, such as the carotid artery in the neck or the femoral artery in the groin. Most patients will have a pulse between sixty and one hundred beats per minute. Higher or lower numbers are common and may be related to athletic conditioning, medications, or illness.

Blood pressure is determined with the aid of a stethoscope and a sphygmomanometer (blood pressure cuff) and is expressed in millimeters of mercury. After pumping the cuff to a high pressure, the examiner slowly deflates the cuff while listening for the sounds of blood flow, usually in the brachial artery above the elbow. The onset and end of these sounds indicate the systolic and diastolic blood pressure measurements. A measurement of 120/80 (systolic over diastolic) is often considered normal, but acceptable blood pressures will vary among individuals. In this case, the normal blood pressure for a child is lower than for an adult. Breathing rate is checked by observation and varies, depending on age and medical conditions, from approximately twelve to forty breaths per minute. Infants and children have higher rates than adults.

Following the determination of vital signs, a general physical survey is performed. The head is inspected to confirm normal shape and absence of injury. Eye movements and response to light are noted, along with any inflammation. The ears, nose, and throat are checked for signs of inflammation or scarring. A puff of air may be used to test the mobility of the eardrum. Palpation of the neck may reveal enlargement of the thyroid gland or lymph nodes. The chest is observed for abnormalities, and auscultation of the lungs is performed to monitor air flow during breathing. The cardiac examination will focus on possible murmurs, sounds generated by turbulent blood flow. Since many murmurs are harmless, and many children will have a murmur noted at some point, careful auscultation is needed to define the nature of heart sounds. If a murmur is heard, the patient may be asked to perform certain maneuvers, such as standing up quickly or taking a deep breath and straining. These actions may cause the murmur to change in a way that allows recognition of its underlying cause.

Next, the abdomen is observed for symmetry and distension. By palpation, the examiner may discover enlargement of the liver or spleen. Percussion over the liver area may confirm enlargement of that organ. Auscultation of the sounds produced by the bowels may provide clues to increased or decreased intestinal function. An external genital examination is appropriate for boys and girls. Proper descent of the testicles into the scrotum should be ascertained for boys, while menstrual complaints may dictate an internal examination for girls. Scoliosis (curvature of the spine) or other abnormalities in neurological or musculoskeletal development may be found. Examination of the skin surface is especially important in children; in addition to birthmarks, signs of child abuse may be visible and require evaluation. The length of time needed for the entire screening process will vary. If the child is already known to the examiner and has been seen recently for other reasons, the examination itself may be brief. The presence of abnormal findings may require a lengthy, detailed evaluation.

An annual gynecologic examination and Pap testing is preceded by a directed gathering of the patient's medical and family history, focusing on the reproductive system. This completed, the patient is asked to lie on her back, with her feet apart in foot rests that extend from the table. Examination of the female genital tract begins with a survey of the external structures, the clitoris, labia, and vaginal opening. A discharge or surface lesions such as sores or warts may arouse suspicion of sexually transmitted disease. Since many women have some discharge normally, however, laboratory tests are often needed to establish the diagnosis of infection. To examine the internal structures of the vagina, the examiner uses a speculum, a metal or plastic instrument about five inches long and shaped like a duck's bill. A hinge in the back allows it to be opened after insertion into the vagina, permitting inspection of the cervix and the vaginal walls with the help of a bright light. At this time, the sample is taken from the cervix, usually with a small brush and wooden spatula. After removal of the speculum, the bimanual (literally, "two hands") examination is done.

Gloved, lubricated fingers are inserted into the vagina, while the other hand presses down from the outside of the abdomen. For many women, this is the most uncomfortable part of the examination, though sensitivity by the examiner can lessen the discomfort. The cervix, uterus, Fallopian tubes, ovaries, and bladder may be palpated. A rectovaginal examination is performed by placing one finger in the vagina and another finger of the same hand in the rectum. This allows palpation of the space between the vagina and the rectum, as well as of the rectum itself. A breast examination may be performed during the office visit. Although most women focus on lumps, other potential signs of breast cancer, such as bleeding from the nipple, a persistent rash around the nipple, skin dimpling, or retraction (turning in) of the nipple, are noted. Because breast cancer is most common in upper and outer quadrants of the breasts and may spread to lymph nodes in the armpit, palpation of these areas is prudent.

In the examination of an apparent ankle sprain, the presence of an abnormality is a given, and the evaluation is geared to the documentation of the extent of the injury to the ankle itself and to adjacent structures. Initial observation may reveal that the patient has obvious pain while walking into the examining area. Swelling and redness may be prominent. Palpation of the leg and ankle will likely elicit tenderness over the damaged ligaments, especially with movement. Intact circulation can be confirmed by placing the fingers over the arteries of the foot and noting strong pulses. Instability of the joint itself may be discovered by applying pressure in various directions. The possibility of nerve damage is assessed by testing sensation and the strength in the foot. Though this examination is directed toward a relatively limited area of the body, it may require considerable time because of the depth of detail involved.

Perspective and Prospects

The modern physical examination is the product of a gradual evolution rather than of a single discovery or invention. Though certain individuals are credited with the adoption of particular physical diagnostic techniques, the interpretation of bodily characteristics as indicators of health status has ancient roots that predate Hippocrates, who was born in 460 BCE on the island of Cos in Greece. From the Middle Ages until the eighteenth century, physical examination focused on the pulse, which was accorded much diagnostic significance, and the feces. The scientific foundations of current practices were uncovered in Europe during the late eighteenth century and early nineteenth century. René Laënnec (1781-1826), a French physician, is generally acknowledged as the originator of the stethoscope, which greatly enhanced the power of auscultation. Compared to modern instruments, it was crude, consisting of a straight rigid tube which was placed between the patient's body and the physician's ear. The use of percussion as a diagnostic technique is credited to Leopold Auenbrugger and Jean-Nicolas Corvisart des Marets, contemporaries of Laënnec. Since that time, many physicians have contributed to the body of knowledge that supports physical diagnosis, and texts on the subject are filled with descriptions of maneuvers and findings that bear their names: Sir William Osler, Moritz H. Romberg, Joseph F. Babinski, William Heberden, Antonio M. Valsalva, Franz Chvostek, and so on.

Though the patient's history and physical examination have excellent diagnostic power, the adoption of advanced imaging techniques may lead to less reliance on physical diagnostic techniques. Thus, traditional hands-on examination risks falling by the wayside. Reasons for adopting new medical technologies in its place are many and controversial. Like other skills, physical diagnosis requires ongoing use if the practitioner is to remain sharp. Physical examinations can be imprecise, with disagreement among competent examiners regarding the presence or absence of findings. In contrast, electromechanical systems may provide more consistent information, though the interpretation of this information is still subjective. It is easy to forget that laboratory or radiological findings by themselves have very limited usefulness. It is not unusual for test reports to note, "Clinical correlation is advised." In other words, test results must be interpreted in the light of the information that has been gathered about the patient through the history and the physical examination. The performance of a detailed evaluation can be time-consuming for the physician and the patient, especially when compared to requesting a test. Pressured by patient expectations or liability concerns, physicians may be reluctant to rely on the physical examination alone in lieu of a battery of confirmatory or exploratory scans or blood tests.

The consequences of this shift are likely to change the way in which the patient views the physician and the way in which the physician approaches the patient. Traditionally, the healing role has been intimately associated with the face-to-face meeting of doctor and patient, exemplified by the laying on of hands. From the patient's perspective, the concept of the personal physician, the familiar voice and touch of the healer who displays ongoing concern and compassion, should not be discounted. This therapeutic relationship will be compromised if physicians become mere brokers for imaging and testing services. With such an arrangement, there would be no reason for the doctor and patient even to see each other. Additionally, important diagnostic information may present itself in a manner that cannot be detected by a scan, such as a subtle clue in the patient's mannerisms or body language. Even a human examiner may have difficulty analyzing such vague information, but impressions can nevertheless contribute to the clinical evaluation. This suggests that the physical examination will continue to hold an important place in the physician's array of diagnostic tools.

—*Louis B. Jacques, M.D.*

See also Apgar score; Blood pressure; Diagnosis; Education, medical; Noninvasive tests; Nursing; Phlebotomy; Physician assistants; Pulse rate; Screening; Signs and symptoms; Well-baby examinations.

For Further Information:
Goldman, Lee, and Dennis Ausiello, eds. *Cecil Textbook of Medicine.* 23d ed. Philadelphia: Saunders/Elsevier, 2007.
Jarvis, Carolyn. *Physical Examination and Health Assessment.* 6th ed. St. Louis, Mo.: Saunders/Elsevier, 2012.
Pagana, Kathleen Deska, and Timothy J. Pagana. *Mosby's Diagnostic and Laboratory Test Reference.* 11th ed. St. Louis, Mo.: Mosby/Elsevier, 2013.
Shorter, Edward. *Bedside Manners.* New York: Simon & Schuster, 1985.
Siraisi, Nancy G. *Medieval and Early Renaissance Medicine.* 2d ed. Chicago: University of Chicago Press, 2009.
Swartz, Mark H. *Textbook of Physical Diagnosis: History and Examination.* 6th ed. Philadelphia: Saunders/Elsevier, 2010.
Tierney, Lawrence M., Stephen J. McPhee, and Maxine A. Papadakis, eds. *Current Medical Diagnosis and Treatment 2007.* New York: McGraw-Hill Medical, 2006.
Vorvick, Linda J. "Physical Examination." *MedlinePlus,* January 1, 2013.

Physical rehabilitation

Specialty

Anatomy or system affected: Bones, hips, joints, knees, legs, ligaments, muscles, musculoskeletal system, nerves, nervous system, spine, tendons

Specialties and related fields: Exercise physiology, orthopedics, osteopathic medicine, physical therapy, sports medicine

Definition: The discipline devoted to the restoration of normal bodily function, primarily of the muscles and skeleton.

Key terms:

atrophy: a wasting away; a diminution in the size of a cell, tissue, organ, or part

cutaneous: pertaining to the skin

edema: the accumulation of an excessive amount of fluid in cells or tissues

electromyography: an electrodiagnostic technique for recording the extracellular activity (action and evoked potentials) of skeletal muscles at rest, during voluntary contractions, and during electrical stimulation

gangrene: necrosis (tissue death) caused by the obstruction of the blood supply; may be localized in a small area or may involve an entire extremity

goniometry: the measurement of angles, particularly those for the range of motion of a joint

ischemia: a local anemia or area of diminished or insufficient blood supply caused by mechanical obstruction of the blood supply (commonly, narrowing of an artery)

musculoskeletal: pertaining to or comprising the skeleton and the muscles

physiatry: the branch of medicine dealing with the prevention, diagnosis, and treatment of disease or injury and the rehabilitation from resultant impairments and disabilities; uses physical agents such as light, heat, cold, water, electricity, therapeutic exercise, mechanical apparatus, and pharmaceutical agents

rehabilitation: the restoration of normal form and function after injury or illness; the restoration of the ill or injured patient to optimal functional level in the home and community in relation to physical, psychosocial, vocational, and recreational activity

vascular: relating to or containing blood vessels

Science and Profession

Physical rehabilitation has been defined as a scientific discipline that uses physical agents such as light, heat, water, electricity, and mechanical agents in the management and rehabilitation of pathophysiological conditions resulting from disease or injury. Rehabilitation involves the treatment and training of patients with the goal of maximizing their potential for normal living physically, psychologically, socially, and vocationally.

Historical records indicate that the Chinese used rubbing as a therapeutic measure as early as 3000 BCE Hippocrates also advocated rubbing in writings dated from 460 BCE; it was used by subsequent Roman civilizations. The Roman poet Homer wrote about hydrotherapy as a cure for Hector. Immersion in the Nile and Ganges rivers as an aid to healing has been practiced for centuries. Peter Henry Ling developed and published a scientific basis for therapeutic massage in 1812. Modern physical therapy was established in 1917 with the creation of the Division of Special Hospitals and Physical Reconstruction. This effort was directed at persons injured in World War I and included educational and vocational training programs.

Physical rehabilitation is known for its work in restoring function to traumatized limbs. Practitioners in the field work with persons of all ages: with children to overcome birth defects, with adults to restore muscular function lost from strokes, with the elderly to maintain as much of normal functioning as possible in the face of advancing age, and with postoperative patients to accelerate healing and a return to normal activities. In addition, emphasis is placed on preventing and treating athletic injuries-prevention through the teaching of exercises to strengthen specific body parts and treatment through the restoration of normal bodily movements.

Prevention is defined as the avoidance of sickness, disability, or injury. There are three types or levels of prevention: primary, secondary, and tertiary. Primary prevention refers to complete avoidance before any problem has developed. A good example of primary prevention is being immunized for a specific disease. Secondary prevention refers to attempts to limit the extent of a disease, disability, or pathological process. A convenient illustration of secondary prevention is an individual who quits smoking. Some damage may have been done to the lungs and other organs, but it is curtailed when an individual stops smoking. The extent of recovery for lost function depends on the degree of damage incurred before the cessation of the activity. Tertiary prevention refers to attempts to recover functions or abilities that have been lost or severely compromised. Physical rehabilitation is a form of tertiary prevention: Attempts are made to restore normality that has been lost as a result of an accident, disease process, or injury.

Physical rehabilitation employs individuals with a variety of training. Physiatrists are physicians who have specialized training in physical medicine and rehabilitation. They are usually the leaders of rehabilitation teams and direct many of the activities of other personnel. Physiatrists supervise the assessment of injured patients and actually conduct invasive tests such as electromyography. Physical therapists are specialists with some graduate-level training; in the United States, the scope of their activities is regulated by individual states and may vary from state to state. Typically, they operate alone but under the supervision or direction of a physiatrist, although in some states they are able to practice independently. Physical therapists carry out the treatment plan devised by a physiatrist and apply the therapeutic modalities. Speech and occupational therapists have specialized training in assisting patients in these particular areas. Speech therapists concentrate on overcoming language and speech difficulties, while occupational therapists specialize in providing injured persons with skills and training for new jobs. Therapy aides assist these specialists in completing some of the more routine aspects of rehabilitation. Their education ranges from one to four years of training after high school.

Diagnostic and Treatment Techniques

Individuals must be assessed prior to receiving physical rehabilitation. The assessment process begins with a complete history and physical examination. Subsequently, specific tests may be needed. Two common assessment tools are goniometry and electromyography. Goniometry refers to the measurement of joint motion. It is done by measuring angles of movement and is reported in degrees of arc. Electromyography is a technique that is used to evaluate the functioning of muscle units. Electrodes are placed in muscle groups. The nerve that controls the muscle is electrically stimulated, and the resultant muscle reaction is measured. Electromyography yields information concerning both the strength of muscle contractions and the speed of conduction along the nerve. These data help to pinpoint the basis of many muscular problems. As with all testing, patient-derived values are compared to standard norms to estimate pathology or lost function.

Other aspects of an injured patient are also assessed: speech and language, psychological makeup, and vocation. Speech and language are needed for communication. Strokes or other injuries can interfere with the ability to communicate. Depending on where they occur in the brain, strokes can have different effects; these must be identified. Language ability requires both neurological integrity and muscular control. Any deficit in either component can impair speech. A primary goal of rehabilitation is communication proficiency (both speech and language), which is a prerequisite for success in many jobs.

Psychological makeup is assessed to pinpoint personality problems that could impede normal interactions with the world or success in a job. Individuals requiring assistance in this area are referred to other professionals for specialized help. Vocational assessment is important because individuals sustaining strokes or serious injuries are frequently unable to return to their previous jobs. When a vocational recommendation has been made for a patient, a specific course of rehabilitation is created.

Four main therapeutic modalities are used in physical re-

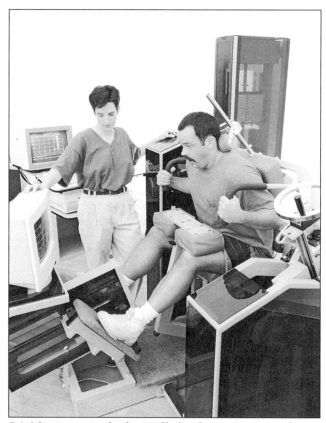

Rehabilitation may involve the use of high-tech equipment to control movements and to monitor results. (PhotoDisc)

habilitation: heat, diathermy, cold, and hydrotherapy. Heat increases the rate of cellular metabolism, thus increasing blood flow. Heat also has a sedative effect, relaxing the body part. Tissue repair occurs more rapidly with increased metabolism and circulation. Stress on the injured area is reduced, allowing tissue repair to proceed unimpeded. The net effect is to speed healing.

Heat is supplied by several methods. Compresses of cloth immersed in heated water have been used for centuries. Confining the heated water in a container provides heat in a dry form. Electric heating pads are more convenient because they can supply dry heat at a constant temperature for an unlimited length of time. Melted paraffin is occasionally used to concentrate heat in a specific location; this substance must be applied by a professional under controlled conditions. These modalities supply heat to the surface of skin; it penetrates passively, diminishing in intensity with increasing distance from the surface.

Infrared lamps provide heat that can penetrate to greater depths than heat sources applied to the surface of skin. Additional advantages include dryness and being able to position the body to be heated in any position. Because of its ability to penetrate, infrared light must be limited in exposure to avoid burns. It can also cause excessive drying of skin surfaces. Heat can also be supplied convectively, most often by immersion in warmed water. The stream of water can be directed at particular body parts, providing both heat and stimulation.

Diathermy is defined as deep heating. Deep tissues are heated because superficial heating produces only a few mild physiologic reactions. The problem is to avoid burning superficial tissues while heating deep structures. Three main methods are used to achieve this desired effect: shortwave, ultrasound, and microwave. In all three methods, energy is transferred and finally converted into heat when it reaches deep tissues. With shortwave, energy is transferred into deeper tissues by high-frequency current. Ultrasound uses high-frequency acoustic vibrations that penetrate into deep tissues. Microwave uses electromagnetic radiation to heat deeper tissues. Diathermy exploits all the advantages of heat: locally elevated temperatures, increased circulation, and decreased sensitivity of nerve fibers, which increases the threshold of pain. Diathermy is most useful in treating relatively deep muscular injuries. It cannot be used safely with sensory impairment because burning can occur, nor can it be used in joints that have been replaced with prostheses.

Cold creates physiological effects that are opposite to those of heat. Cooling decreases tissue metabolism. The application of cold slows blood circulation, which, in turn, tends to reduce tissue swelling caused by edema. Cold is more penetrating than heat. Too much cold, however, can become a problem. Cooling a large surface area of skin or lowering the core temperature of a body induces shivering, which causes the production of heat.

Cooling affects the nervous system. With cooling, the first cutaneous sense to be lost is light touch. Motor power is lost next. Pain and gross pressure are eventually lost with a sufficiently long application of cold. When ice is applied, an individual subjectively experiences an appreciation of the cooling, followed by a sense of burning or aching and, eventually, by cutaneous anesthesia. The total time needed to induce cutaneous anesthesia is between five and seven minutes. Cooled underlying muscle fibers lose some of their power; thus people are temporarily but noticeably weaker after cold is applied. The cooling of connective tissues around joints may diminish the ease and precision of movement.

Local cooling is used to reduce the unrestricted flow of fluid and blood into tissues after they have been traumatized. Cold reduces pain, both superficial and deep, and reduces reflex spasticity of muscles. Cold tends to preserve and extend the viability of tissues that have inadequate circulation, thus retarding the development of gangrene in an ischemic body part, which is most commonly seen in limbs.

There are reasons not to apply cold. Occasionally, individuals react to cold by abruptly increasing their arterial pressure. People who suffer from Raynaud's disease usually do not tolerate very well cold applied to their fingers or toes. The stiffness associated with rheumatoid arthritis is usually aggravated by cooling. Prolonged or excessive cooling can lead to frostbite. People who have experienced clinical hypothermia are must less tolerant of cold than those who have not had such an experience.

Several common methods exist for achieving therapeutic cooling: immersion, cold packs, cryokinetics, and a combination of local cooling and remote heating. Immersion is usually begun in cold water to which ice is steadily added. Total immersion is usually limited to ten or twenty minutes. The affected portion of the body is submerged in the chilled water. Cooling to a temperature above that of ice water may reduce muscular spasticity. Cold packs are often made by wrapping ice in a wet towel or plastic bag and applying it to the skin. Frozen cold packs should not be applied directly to the skin because they can cause locally severe tissue damage.

Cryokinetics is a procedure that combines cooling and exercise. Cooling is first accomplished by means of immersion or rubbing the skin over the affected part of the body with ice for five to seven minutes, so-called ice massage. The cooling produces a mild anesthesia that allows the individual to exercise the cooled body portion actively without pain. This method is considered to be particularly effective in recent acute muscle strains. The simultaneous application of heat and cold is sometimes effective. Heating an uninvolved portion of the body maintains the core temperature, which inhibits shivering, while cold applied to the injured portion of the body reduces pain. In theory, this arrangement allows cold to be applied for longer periods of time than would otherwise be possible. Because it is difficult to control heating and cooling simultaneously, however, this technique is not frequently used.

Hydrotherapy is the external application of water for therapeutic purposes. The water temperature can range from cold to hot. With immersion, water provides buoyancy, which relieves pressure on weight-bearing portions of the body. Water also provides resistance that is used in treating patients with motor weakness. Buoyancy alters the effect of exercises done in water by allowing a severely injured person to move; this provides psychological benefit and hope that the motion can eventually be done out of water. Brief application of cold has a tonic or stimulating effect, increasing blood pressure and the respiratory rate and stimulating shivering. Mild hot water provides sedation to irritated sensory and motor nerves, thus relieving pain caused by cramps and spasms in muscles. It also reduces stress, calming agitated or excited persons. The most common method of hydrotherapy is a whirlpool bath, which combines buoyancy, heat, and mechanical stimulation to the affected body part.

Massage and movement are key components of applied physical rehabilitation. Massage is the systematic and scientific manipulation of body tissues; massage is best performed by the hands. Massage has a sedative effect when constantly and steadily applied, and it leads to a decrease in muscular tension. Combined with heat or cold, the resulting relaxation facilitates the movement of injured body parts. Mechanically, massage stimulates the circulatory system, enhancing blood flow. The applied force of massage is effective in stretching muscle groups and breaking the adhesions between individual muscle fibers that limit motion. This same action mobilizes fluid and promotes its elimination. Massage does not develop muscle strength, however, and should not be used as a substitute for active exercise.

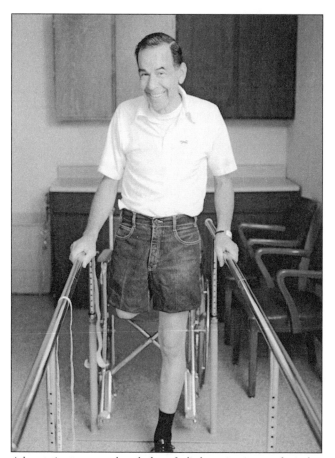

A devastating trauma such as the loss of a limb requires intense physical therapy to help the body adapt. (Digital Stock)

Therapeutic exercise is defined as the performance of movement to correct an impairment, improve musculoskeletal function, or maintain a state of well-being. Movement is the key: The energy to accomplish the movement can be supplied passively by a therapist or actively by an individual. Muscles are stretched with passive movement or contracted during the process of active flexion or contraction. Individuals with injuries that involve the nervous system may lose the function of any muscles supplied by the injured nerves. These muscles must be moved passively in order to avoid loss of muscle mass and function as a result of disuse atrophy. Muscles respond to stimulation. Thus, exercises are designed to strengthen injured muscles. Parts in adjacent body structures must be stabilized to maximize the benefit derived from exercise. Prolonged moderate stretching is more beneficial than momentary vigorous stretching. Movements and stretching should be within the pain tolerance of the patient in order to avoid injury to blood vessels.

Perspective and Prospects

Physical rehabilitation operates within a larger context of health care provision. The need for primary prevention is addressed by teaching correct methods for strengthening muscle groups to athletes and recreational fitness practitioners. Classes on first aid measures for treating common musculoskeletal injuries are taught by rehabilitation specialists such as physicians, therapists, and nurses. These classes are offered in schools and communities throughout the year. Physicians practicing occupational medicine also advocate primary prevention of musculoskeletal injuries associated with the work site. These professionals analyze working environments and recommend ways to restructure particular job tasks in order to reduce the chances of injury.

Secondary prevention is provided in office and hospital settings by professionals who treat injuries such as sprains, strains, and fractures. Care for acute injuries is usually accompanied by instruction in prevention in the hope that patients will avoid similar problems in the future. In the working environment, injured workers are provided with appropriate treatment and therapy and returned to work in an expeditious manner that is consistent with standards of proper care. This approach is usually best for all concerned, especially the injured worker. Such a case illustrates the many facets of rehabilitation. Normal physical functioning is returned with conventional therapy. Self-esteem is bolstered with return to meaningful work and previous income-earning capacity. Economically, the employer also benefits by having a trained and experienced worker on the job rather than having a skilled individual on disability and a less capable replacement worker on the job, both receiving payment.

Tertiary prevention involves the traditional rehabilitation activities that begin after treatment for a massive injury or chronic disease process. Frequently, such rehabilitation returns only a portion of lost functions. Nevertheless, this treatment has value, improving self-esteem and the quality of life for an injured person. It underscores, however, the greater importance of the avoidance and prevention of injuries.

Health can be viewed as being on a continuum. One end is defined by death, the final termination of health. All life constitutes the rest of the spectrum. Health is frequently defined as the absence of disease or infirmity. This definition is appealing in its simplicity but is difficult to use because it is based on the absence rather than the presence of something. The question of where good health ends and impaired health begins is probably highly individual and open for debate. The division point between good and bad or acceptable and unacceptable health status, however, does provide a useful beginning for the activities encompassed by physical rehabilitation. The recovery of lost or impaired function is the domain of this field. This goal is also consistent with the definition of tertiary prevention. Rehabilitation and prevention are complementary opposites. Together, they span the entire spectrum of health.

—*L. Fleming Fallon, Jr., M.D., Ph.D., M.P.H.*

See also Aging: Extended care; Allied health; Amputation; Back pain; Bionics and biotechnology; Birth defects; Braces, orthopedic; Cardiac rehabilitation; Chiropractic; Exercise physiology; Healing; Heart attack; Hydrotherapy; Muscles; Nursing; Occupational health; Orthopedic surgery; Orthopedics; Orthopedics, pediatric; Osteopathic medicine; Overtraining syndrome; Prostheses; Rotator cuff surgery; Speech disorders; Sports medicine; Strokes; Tendinitis; Tendon disorders.

For Further Information:
Braddom, Randall L., ed. *Physical Medicine and Rehabilitation.* 3d ed. Philadelphia: Saunders/Elsevier, 2007. Discusses physical therapy and medical rehabilitation. Includes a bibliography and an index.
DeLisa, Joel A., et al., eds. *Physical Medicine and Rehabilitation: Principles and Practice.* 4th ed. Philadelphia: Lippincott Williams & Wilkins, 2005. This standard textbook provides a comprehensive overview of rehabilitation. It is written for professionals but is accessible to laypeople. The subject entries are written by experts in their fields.
Fletcher, Gerald F., et al., eds. *Rehabilitation Medicine: Contemporary Clinical Perspectives.* Philadelphia: Lea & Febiger, 1992. An introduction to the subject of rehabilitation written for professional audiences. The writing is consistent and of high quality. The illustrations are unusually good.
Garrison, Susan J., ed. *Handbook of Physical Medicine and Rehabilitation: The Basics.* 2d ed. Philadelphia: Lippincott Williams & Wilkins, 2003. This text provides a good overview of the subject. Because it is written for students, it should be understandable to most readers. As an introduction to rehabilitation, it is well written.
Neumann, Donald A. *Kinesiology of the Musculoskeletal System: Foundations for Rehabilitation.* 2d ed. St. Louis, Mo.: Mosby/Elsevier, 2010. A text for physical rehabilitation students and clinicians that gives an introduction to terminology and basic concepts of kinesiology and reviews the structure and function of the musculoskeletal system and the biomechanical and quantitative aspects of kinesiology.
Sinaki, Mehrsheed, ed. *Basic Clinical Rehabilitation Medicine.* 2d ed. St. Louis, Mo.: Mosby, 1993. An introductory textbook for students in the field. Well written, has good illustrations, and should be readily understood by laypeople.

Physician assistants

Specialty

Anatomy or system affected: All

Specialties and related fields: Emergency care, family medicine, general surgery, geriatrics and gerontology, internal medicine, neonatology, nursing, public health

Definition: Health care providers who work under the supervision of licensed physicians and who are trained to perform physical examinations, diagnose illnesses, interpret laboratory tests, set fractures, and assist in surgeries.

Key terms:

American Academy of Physician Assistants (AAPA): a professional society founded in 1968 to promote the role of PAs in providing high-quality, cost-effective health care

Association of Physician Assistant Programs (APAP): a consortium of educational institutions that offer accredited PA programs, providing academic guidance and standards for member schools

fee-for-service (FFS): the traditional way of paying for medical care by billing patients when services are rendered (in contrast to the practices of health maintenance organizations)

geriatrics: the branch of medicine dealing with problems and diseases of aging

health maintenance organization (HMO): a group of general practitioners, specialists, and allied health professionals who provide medical services to subscribers paying a regular maintenance fee

pediatrics: the branch of medicine dealing with the development and diseases of children *primary care*: general medical services provided in family medicine, internal medicine, pediatrics, geriatrics, obstetrics, and emergency care (in contrast to specialists, such as urology or cardiac surgery)

Science and Profession

The training of physician assistants was initiated at the Duke University Medical Center in 1965. There was a persistent shortage of primary care physicians. At the same time, the thousands of medical corpsmen who were discharged annually from the military services were unable to convert their skills into civilian occupations. Four Navy veterans with medical experience, all men, were enrolled in a trial program to give them additional training. A new curriculum was developed on a week-by-week basis, using the educational resources of the medical school. The men were graduated after two years and found their professional niche as assistants to licensed physicians.

The program at Duke served as a model that spread quickly to other medical institutions. Start-up funds became available from government agencies such as the Veterans Administration, the Office of Economic Opportunity, and the Public Health Service. By 1972, there were twenty-six training programs in operation in the United States. Two years later, the number had grown to fifty-three. New professional organizations were formed to evaluate and accredit the educational programs and to develop certification examinations for the individual graduates. By the late twentieth century, fifty-seven accredited PA programs were available at medical schools and teaching hospitals and through the armed forces.

The American Academy of Physician Assistants (AAPA) has adopted the following official definition for "physician assistant":

> *Physician Assistants (PAs) practice medicine with supervision by licensed physicians. As members of the health care team, PAs provide a broad range of medical services that would otherwise be provided by physicians. It is the obligation of each team of Physician/PA to ensure that the PA's scope of practice is identified; that delegation of medical tasks is appropriate to the PA's level of competence; that the relationship of, and access to, the supervising physician is defined; and that a process of performance evaluation is established. Adequate and responsible supervision of the PA contributes to both high quality patient care and continued professional growth.*

The status of PAs as subordinates to MD's is clearly delineated in this job description.

By 2003 there were more than 45,000 PAs in the United States. Each year, PA training programs produce approximately 4,000 new graduates. PAs must pass a national certifying examination before they can begin to practice and be licensed by the state. The examination is open only to graduates of accredited programs. To maintain certification, PAs must complete one hundred hours of continuing medical education every two years and take a recertification exam every six years. These requirements are intended to ensure the continued competency of PAs as qualified medical professionals.

The typical PA student has a bachelor's degree and four years of health care experience prior to admission into the program. About half of the entering students previously were either nurses, emergency medical technicians (EMTs), medics in the military, or emergency room technicians. There is strong competition to enter PA programs, with five applicants turned down for every student accepted.

The training program for PAs normally lasts two years. It is like a shortened version of the medical school curriculum for MD's. The first year is composed of classroom and laboratory courses in anatomy, physiology, microbiology, and other basic sciences. Also, introductory instruction is given in pediatrics, obstetrics, general surgery, internal medicine, and emergency care. PAs often are in the same classes with medical students.

Second-year PA students are assigned to clinical rotations, seeing and treating patients under the supervision of a physician. The emphasis is on family medicine and other primary care. They receive a variety of practical experience by working in an individual physician's office, a nursing home, a hospital, a rural clinic, a large group practice, or an emergency room. Some PAs learn to assist in major surgery and to provide preoperative and postoperative care.

After graduation, PAs practice in almost all types of health care settings. The demand for their services is increasing rapidly. The United States Bureau of Labor Statistics (BLS) projected that the number of PA jobs would increase by 30 percent between 2010 and 2012, much faster than the average for all occupations.

Most PAs practice in primary care, where the shortage of qualified medical personnel is most severe. MD's who work in radiology, surgery, anesthesiology, gynecology, and other specialties have about double the median income of general practitioners. It becomes clear that a strong economic incentive exists for physicians to become specialists, leaving vacancies in primary care for PAs. Rural clinics, small towns, and inner-city hospitals have a particularly difficult time recruiting MD's for staff vacancies, so PAs are finding ready acceptance to fill the gap. PAs earn approximately 70 percent of the median net income of MD's in general family medicine. According to the Bureau of Labor Statistics, the median pay for PAs in 2010 was $86,410 per year.

The high cost of health care in the United States compared with other developed, industrial countries became a major political issue in the late twentieth century. In the United States, the ratio of MD specialists to general practitioners was 68 percent to 32 percent, whereas in Western Europe the ratio was roughly 50/50. Critics both within and outside the medical profession pointed to this imbalance in the United States as a major factor raising the cost of and limiting broad access to health care. During the 1980s, the number of new medical school graduates entering general practice declined from 36 percent to only 14 percent. The United States still produces an oversupply of specialists, while the shortage of primary care doctors continues to worsen. According to the Association of American Colleges, the US had 352,908 primary-care doctor in 2010, and the college association estimates that 45,000 more will be needed by 2020.

An outspoken editorial published in 1993 in the *Journal of the American Medical Association* addressed the issue of how to deal with an impending crisis in primary care. One recommendation was to increase the supply of PAs, nurse practitioners, chiropractors, and other nonphysician providers. These individuals would participate as team members alongside physicians in an integrated, cost-effective health care setting. Another suggestion to reduce total health care costs was to place more emphasis on preventive medicine. PAs have acquired a good reputation for advising patients about how to adopt healthier lifestyles.

Another proposal to deal with the primary care shortage would be to require a period of mandatory national health service for all medical school graduates. Such a policy could be justified by considering the substantial federal tax money that supports medical education. The US Congress would have to enact appropriate legislation. The experience of working on the staff of a community health facility would broaden the training of physicians, even if they go into specialty practice afterward.

Diagnostic and Treatment Techniques

After completing a two-year accredited training program and passing the certification examination, PAs are qualified to perform approximately 80 percent of the routine duties most commonly done by physicians. PAs can give general physical examinations; diagnose illnesses; determine treatments; give injections, immunizations, and catheterizations; interpret laboratory tests; suture wounds; set fractures; deal with medical emergencies; and assist in surgical operations. In most states, PAs can write prescriptions for medication.

PAs are not independent medical practitioners. By law or regulation, all PAs must have a licensed physician to supervise and be responsible for their work. It is not necessary, however, for the physician and the PA to be located in the same building or even in the same town. In rural communities, for example, state law generally allows such supervision to occur via telephone.

Suppose that a small town is being served by a clinic with three physicians, one of whom is about to retire. There are several smaller towns nearby with no medical service at all, and the nearest hospital is forty miles away. The Chamber of Commerce and other civic groups start a vigorous fundraising and advertising campaign to find a replacement for the retiring doctor, but with no success. Finally, one of the doctors contacts the state medical school to inquire about the possibility of hiring a PA.

From the point of view of the doctor, a PA can take care of routine school and employment physical examinations, minor acute illnesses, baby checkups, and so forth, so that the doctor can focus on more complex problems. The PA can also relieve the doctor by making rounds at the community nursing home. The PA would be expected to share in call duty on nights and weekends. The doctor could take time off for occasional vacations, medical meetings, or family obligations. To help the underserved nearby towns, a satellite clinic could be set up that would be staffed by the PA perhaps half a day each week.

From the point of view of the PA, medical practice in a small town brings some special rewards. The PA is accorded a position of prestige as a member of the small, professional community that includes teachers and lawyers. This situation is in strong contrast to urban health care, where the PA is a minor figure among hundreds of doctors and other hospital personnel. Furthermore, rural PAs are likely to see a wider variety of medical problems and, after establishing rapport with their supervising physician, are able to exercise more independent judgment about diagnosis and treatment.

In a small town, the doctor must emphasize the team concept of medical care, of which the PA is a valued member. The supervisory role of the MD needs to be clearly and formally established. The majority of PAs, for example, are insured by a rider on the physician's malpractice policy. To fit into the social environment, PAs have stated that it helps if they themselves grew up in a small town and if they are married. A large number of PAs have successfully found their medical role as primary care providers in rural communities.

A very different role is filled by PAs serving as surgical assistants in a hospital. With specialized training, they can act as assistants during surgery as well as provide preoperative and postoperative care.

When a surgery patient is admitted, surgical PAs can be assigned to write up the medical history and give an entrance physical examination. They can evaluate preoperative laboratory tests and inform the surgeon of any potential complications. They can spend time with the patient and family members to explain the intended procedure and to answer their questions.

During surgery, PAs can assist the surgeon with clamping and tying as needed. They should be familiar with various patient monitoring devices and should inform the surgeon if problems arise. After surgery, the PA can accompany the patient to the recovery room or intensive care unit (ICU).

During the patient's recuperation time in the hospital, PAs will make regular rounds. They can prescribe medications, change dressings, and generally free the surgeon from the more routine tasks of daily patient care. They can write the discharge orders, which then have to be reviewed and approved by the supervising surgeon.

Surgical PAs have become accepted as assistants in almost all kinds of surgery. For example, they can specialize in orthopedics, kidney transplantation, heart surgery, urology, and skin grafts for burn victims. They must receive appropriate on-the-job training with clinical instruction from their supervising physician to prepare for such surgical specialties.

Health maintenance organizations (HMOs) are another area of employment for a large number of PAs. HMOs are a popular, cost-effective alternative to the traditional fee-for-service (FFS) method of paying for health care. HMOs are prepaid health plans that provide medical, surgical, and hospital benefits to their members. Such a plan is usually offered as a fringe benefit of employment, with the company paying all or part of the monthly fee. When medical services are needed, the patient must come to doctors who are part of the HMO.

When PAs are hired by an HMO, they work under a supervising physician. PAs can examine patients, make a provisional diagnosis, initiate treatment, or refer a case to an appropriate specialist. In a primary care office, the majority of routine problems-a runny nose, infected wounds, or prenatal counseling-can be handled by the PA with little help. Access to staff doctors for consultation, however, is readily available.

From the viewpoint of the PA, working for an HMO brings increased job security. If the supervising physician happens to leave, the job of the PA continues. In a solo office, by contrast, when the physician leaves the PA has to look for a new position. Another advantage of HMO employment is the opportunity for professional growth through interactions with other health care staff members. Also, some PAs particularly like the diversity of experience at an HMO in providing primary care to all age groups, from infants to the elderly.

HMO administrators have reported that acceptance of PAs by patients generally has been good. Pamphlets are made available to explain the educational background of PAs, their subordinate status to physicians, and legal limitations on their level of responsibility. Malpractice suits against PAs have been relatively rare. Patients who insist on seeing an MD can be accommodated, but surveys have shown an equal degree of patient satisfaction with MD and PA services.

Depending on their individual interests and skills, PAs have established themselves in a wide variety of other health care settings. They can be found in geriatric practice, prison health programs, trauma centers, infant critical care units, and military hospitals or on American Indian reservations. Some PAs have gone into administration or public health management. New professional opportunities for PAs continue to evolve as their special contributions to health care are increasingly recognized.

Perspective and Prospects

The concept of the physician assistant was created in the 1960s in response to a shortage of primary care physicians and other health care workers. Medical corpsmen in the armed forces who entered civilian practice were men who wanted a new designation to distinguish them clearly from the nursing profession. With a relatively short training program, they were envisioned as physician's helpers, always working under MD supervision. The role of women in the workplace has changed greatly since the 1960s; consequently the PA profession is no longer dominated by men. According to the 2010 census report conducted by the American Academy of Physician Assistants, 62 percent of PAs were female and 38 percent were male.

By the 1990s, holding down medical costs had become a national priority. In the United States, about 13 percent of the gross national product was expended on health care in 2000, whereas comparable industrialized nations were able to provide broader coverage for their citizens at considerably lower expense. According to the Centers for Medicare and Medicaid Services, approximately 17.9 percent of the US gross domestic product (GDP) was spent on health care. The role of PAs in providing cost-effective medical services was widely recognized. Other issues besides cost, however, still need to be addressed.

A personnel crisis has arisen in the United States because of the relatively small fraction of physicians who choose to work in primary care and family medicine. By the 1990s, only about one-third of the country's nearly 500,000 MD's were general practitioners, with the rest becoming specialists. Such an imbalance results in a lack of access to medical services, especially in rural areas and among the urban poor. A shift in the medical workforce from specialization to primary care is needed to help these underserved groups.

Another issue in the cost and allocation of health care is the growing number of elderly people. Certain illnesses such as Alzheimer's disease, heart disease, and strokes are particular problems of aging. Cataract surgery of the eye is performed largely on older people and is the biggest single line-item expense in the Medicare program. The American Association of Retired Persons (AARP) has made the funding of long-term care facilities a major priority.

The training of doctors has been criticized for overemphasizing the treatment of illnesses while neglecting preventive measures. For example, few physicians take a course in nutrition. The harmful consequences of smoking, alcohol consumption, lack of exercise, and poor diet are clearly established. If the medical profession would provide counseling about better health habits to patients, eventually the cost of treatment could be decreased. Such counseling would not require the expensive time of an MD, who has gone through lengthy medical school and internship programs. It can be provided by a PA who has authoritative information and good communication skills.

Physician assistants, nurses, physical therapists, nurse practitioners, midwives, medical technologists, and other allied health professionals are all part of the total health care team, with different areas of responsibility. One commentator has stated that no one hires an electrical engineer to change a light bulb; similarly, it is not economical to use MD's for routine care that can be supplied by others. The role of PAs is an expanding one.

—*Hans G. Graetzer, Ph.D.*

See also Allied health; Anatomy; Education, medical; Emergency medicine; Family medicine; Health maintenance organizations (HMOs); Hospitals; Internal medicine; Laboratory tests; Managed care; Nutrition; Obstetrics; Pediatrics; Physical examination; Physiology; Preventive medicine; Surgery, general.

For Further Information:
Anderson, Susan M. *Selected Annotated Bibliography of the Physician Assistant Profession*. 4th ed. Arlington: Association of Physician Assistant Programs, 1993.

Arenofsky, Janice. "For a Healthy Prognosis: Examine a Career as a PA or CRNA." *Career World* 21 (1993): 26-30.

Ballweg, Ruth, Sherry Stolberg, and Edward M. Sullivan, eds. *Physician Assistant: A Guide to Clinical Practice.* 3d ed. Philadelphia: Saunders/Elsevier Science, 2003.

Dill, MJ, et al. "Survey Shows Consumers Open to a Greater Role for Physician Assistants and Nurse Practitioners." *Health Affairs* 32, no. 6 (2012): 1135-1142.

Greer, Kathleen. "PAs Envision Evolving Role at Annual AAPA Meeting." *Physician Assistant* 27, no. 7 (2003): 10-13.

Halter, Mary, et al. "The Contribution of Physician Assistants in Primary Care: A Systematic Review." *BMS Health Services Research* 13, no. 1 (2013): 223.

Hooker, Roderick S., and James F. Cawley. *Physician Assistants in American Medicine.* 2d ed. St. Louis: Churchill Livingstone/Elsevier, 2003.

Jones, J. Michael. *A Kernel in the Pod.* Philadelphia: Xlibris, 2002.

Lundberg, George D., and Richard D. Lamm. "Solving Our Primary Care Crisis by Retraining Specialists to Gain Specific Primary Care Competencies." *Journal of the American Medical Association* 270 (1993): 380-381.

Piemme, Thomas E, et al. *The Physician Assistant: An Illustrated History.* Gilbert: Acacia Corp, 2013.

Sacks, Terence J. *Opportunities in Physician Assistant Careers.* 2d ed. Chicago: UGM Career Books, 2002.

Workman, James. "Marcus Welby, PA." *Washington Monthly* 24 (1992): 26" 30.

Physiology

Biology
Anatomy or system affected: All
Specialties and related fields: All
Definition: The branch of biology dealing with the structures and functions of various systems in living organisms.
Key terms:

extracellular fluid: the internal environment of the human body that surrounds the cells; the fluid contains ions, gases, and the nutrients needed by cells for proper functioning and is constantly circulated throughout the body by the blood and into tissues by diffusion

homeostasis: the maintenance of a constant internal environment; the systems of the body work together to maintain a constant temperature, pH, oxygen availability, water content, ion concentrations, and so on

negative feedback: a homeostatic control system designed to respond to a stress by returning body conditions to normal physiologic levels

pH: a measure of the acidity or alkalinity of a solution; equal to the negative logarithm of the hydrogen ion concentration (as measured in moles per liter)

positive feedback: when a stimulus causes more of the same to occur; can be useful in some instances, such as with blood clotting and uterine contractions during childbirth

scientific method: a method of scientific investigation of a problem through observation, the formation of a hypothesis (a possible explanation to a problem), experimentation, and the reevaluation of data

The Fundamentals of Physiology

Physiology is a branch of science that applies to all living things. The goal of the physiologist is to understand the mechanisms leading to the proper functioning of organisms such as bacteria, plants, animals, and humans. Physiology is an important aspect of many of the medical sciences. In immunology, researchers seek to understand the functioning of the immune system. Cardiovascular scientists study the workings of the heart. Knowledge of the normal physiologic functioning of an organism is important in identifying the diseases that cause a deviation from the normal state.

Essential to the discovery of new data is the application of the scientific method of research. The first step in this method is observation. This involves examining a particular system or organism of interest, such as the transport of nutrients in a plant stem or the flow of air into the lungs of an animal, and initially observing a specific event or phenomenon. Asking why and how the event occurs leads to the next step-forming a hypothesis, or scientific question. A hypothesis is a possible explanation of the observation, which can be tested further to see if it is true. Testing, or experimentation, is the third step in the scientific method. The experiment involves setting up a controlled situation that directly tests the hypothesis in order to determine the cause-and-effect relationship between the hypothesis and the initial observation. As the experiment is conducted, the investigator makes further observations of the system's functioning and collects these findings as data. Following data collection and analysis comes the fourth step, making conclusions. The conclusion may or may not support the researcher's original hypothesis. To confirm the results further, more testing is often done. If, upon additional testing, similar conclusions are reached, the researcher may move on to the final step of the scientific method: publication. The experimental design, results, and conclusions are written down in a paper that is then submitted to a scientific journal. Publication permits other researchers to be informed of and evaluate the experiment and possibly to use the results to further their own research endeavors.

Applying this scientific method to the human model, it becomes apparent that the physiological conditions of the human body are in a state of dynamic equilibrium. While variables such as pH, ion and nutrient concentrations, and water content are constantly changing, they never differ significantly from their optimum level, unless the body is in a state of disease. Sensors, an integrating center, and effectors are important contributors to the regulation of these variables. Sensors are located throughout the body and are designed to monitor specific physiologic conditions. For example, baroreceptors monitor arterial blood pressure, chemorecep- tors monitor the concentrations of hydrogen ions and carbon dioxide in the extracellular fluid, and thermoreceptors monitor body temperature. The conditions of the body are then transmitted via nerve impulses to a particular integrating center located in the brain, spinal cord, or endocrine glands. The integrating center interprets the nerve impulses and determines if a response is required. To respond to a particular condition, the integrating center activates certain effectors. An effector is usually a muscle or a gland that, when activated, performs a specific function to return the body to normal physiologic conditions.

Extracellular fluid is also important in the maintenance of the above-mentioned variables. Two basic types of fluid compose about 60 percent of the human body. Two-thirds of the body's fluid is intracellular fluid (cytoplasm) and is found inside cells. The other one-third of the fluid is extracellular fluid and is located in the spaces between cells (interstitial fluid), in blood vessels (plasma), and in the lymphatic vessels (lymph). This fluid is constantly circulated throughout the human body in the blood and lymphatic vessels. The ions, gases, and nutrients in the fluid can easily diffuse out of the capillaries and into the adjacent cells, where they can be utilized in normal cell activities. Because the estimated one hundred trillion cells of the body are exposed to basically the same composition of extracellular fluid, it has been termed the body's internal environment.

The extracellular fluid is the medium of exchange of biologically important molecules and materials. Their concentration and availability is under the control of various organs and systems. For example, the kidneys play an important role in regulating the water content, ion and waste concentrations, and acid-base balance of the extracellular fluid. The gastrointestinal tract is responsible for digesting and making food available for absorption into the bloodstream. The liver maintains the normal glucose concentration in the blood through processes that store glucose, remove glucose from storage, or produce new glucose from other nutrients. The lungs aspirate to provide adequate oxygen and carbon dioxide exchange in the blood. An important job of the physiologist is to discover the mechanisms used by these and other organs to perform their respective functions.

Homeostasis and Feedback Systems

Each of the aforementioned variables has an optimum physiologic range over which the body can function normally. The systems of the body work together in an attempt to keep the body's internal environment within these normal ranges. This process is called homeostasis. Stress placed on the body-whether from the outside environment (heat, cold) or from within (disease, emotional reactions)-can lead to fluctuations in the internal environment. Significant deviations from the normal can lead to a state of disease in the body. To prevent these types of changes, the body has incorporated a number of control devices that are governed by the nervous and endocrine systems. The nervous system is constantly evaluating the state of the body and is able to detect when something is awry. When the body strays too far from its balanced condition, it responds in one of two ways. First, it may send nervous impulses to the proper organs that counteract the stress and return it toward its original state. Second, it may activate the endocrine system to release its chemical messengers or hormones that will bring the body back into balance.

The nervous and endocrine systems are also important components in the feedback systems that regulate the body's internal environment. The two basic types of feedback systems are called negative feedback and positive feedback. Negative feedback is a homeostatic control mechanism that responds to a stress-related change by returning a condition to its normal range. For example, an increase in the blood glucose level induces specific steps that reduce the glucose to its normal level. Positive feedback is designed to amplify the response given to a certain stress. For example, during childbirth, uterine contractions intensify as a result of a positive feedback system, thus enabling the birth of a baby. The majority of the feedback systems in the human body are negative, since in most instances (with a few, specific exceptions) a positive system is detrimental to the body.

Negative feedback. Often, several systems work together to monitor and regulate a particular physiologic condition. An excellent example of this can be seen in the negative feedback regulation of the mean arterial blood pressure. Baroreceptors are the monitoring devices for arterial pressure. They are composed of nerve endings located in the arterial wall of specific blood vessels, such as in the arch of the aorta and the neck area where the common carotid artery divides into the internal and external carotid arteries. Baroreceptors respond to the stretching of the arterial wall. These arteries undergo greater-than-normal stretching during times of high blood pressure and are more relaxed in times of low blood pressure.

Baroreceptors are constantly informing the brain of the status of the mean arterial pressure by sending out nervous impulses to the cardiovascular control center, located in the medulla of the brain. When the body is subject to stress that causes the blood pressure to rise, the elastic arterial walls experience an increase in the amount that they are stretched. The baroreceptors, being stretch receptors, respond to this change by increasing their output of nervous impulses to the brain. In contrast, a drop in blood pressure decreases arterial wall stretching, causing the baroreceptors to send out fewer impulses to the brain.

The nervous impulses from the baroreceptors travel to the cardiovascular control center in the brain via afferent neurons. The cardiovascular control center is a network of neurons that receive and integrate nervous impulses from a variety of other control centers. The cardiovascular control center is connected to the heart by both sympathetic and parasympathetic nerves and to the blood vessels primarily by sympathetic nerves. An increase in the rate of impulses from the baroreceptors (in response to an increase in arterial pressure) results in an increase in the amount of parasympathetic stimulation and a decrease in sympathetic stimulation. On the contrary, a decrease in the rate of impulses from the baroreceptors (in response to a decrease in arterial pressure) results in a decrease in the amount of parasympathetic stimulation and an increase in sympathetic stimulation.

To understand the significance of the stimulation of parasympathetic-versus-sympathetic nervous stimulation, a brief comment must be made as to the organization of the nervous system. The central nervous system (CNS) is made up of the brain, the brain stem, and the spinal cord. The peripheral nervous system (PNS) comprises the nerves that go into and leave the brain stem and spinal cord. The peripheral nervous system is further divided into a somatic portion and an autonomic portion. The somatic nervous system's sensory receptors transmit impulses to the CNS, which then sends impulses through motor neurons to the skeletal muscles. The autonomic nervous system monitors the condition of the internal organs via sensory nerves to the CNS and responds via motor nerves to glands and involuntary muscles. The parasympathetic and sympathetic nerves are the two types of motor nerves that make up the autonomic nervous system. In general, sympathetic nerves initiate the body's fight-or-flight response to stressful situations. Parasympathetic nerves are responsible for more vegetative functions, such as the ingestion and digestion of food.

The combinations of particular nerve activations and deactivations have particular effects on the state of the heart and peripheral blood vessels. As stated above, an increase in mean arterial pressure, as detected by the baroreceptors, invokes a response that increases parasympathetic stimulation of the heart and decreases sympathetic stimulation of the heart and blood vessels. This response serves to reduce the heart rate and the contractility of the heart, thus reducing cardiac output. In addition, blood vessels in the skin and muscles are allowed to dilate, reducing the total peripheral resistance of the blood. The direct relationship of the mean arterial pressure (MAP) to the cardiac output (CO) and total peripheral resistance (TPR) is represented by the formula "MAP = CO TPR." It can be observed that decreasing both CO and TPR results in a decrease in the MAP. This occurs to the point at which the MAP returns to its normal range. If the applied stress decreases the MAP as detected by the baroreceptors, parasympathetic stimulation decreases and sympathetic stimulation increases. This causes an increase in CO and an increase in TPR, resulting in an overall increase in mean arterial pressure.

Positive feedback. An example of positive feedback regulation can be seen in the process of childbirth. Weak, periodic uterine contractions begin during the third trimester of a human pregnancy. As the pregnancy progresses and the time comes for delivery of the baby, these contractions become stronger and increase in frequency. Such contractions are necessary for the expulsion of the baby and the placenta from the mother.

Contractions of the uterine muscles begin at the top, or apex, of the uterus and move down toward its base, at the location of the cervix. These contractions force the head of the baby onto the cervix and stretch it open in a process termed cervical dilation. Cervical stretching sends nerve impulses to the hypothalamus in the brain, which then stimulates the posterior pituitary gland to release the hormone oxytocin. Oxytocin makes the uterine contractions stronger and more rhythmic. Continued stretching of the cervix leads to an increase in the amount of oxytocin released by the pituitary. This positive feedback cycle continues until the baby is born, at which point the pressure on the cervix is removed and it can relax.

Perspective and Prospects

Physiology began more than two thousand years ago during the time of the ancient Greeks. The well-known philosopher Aristotle (384-322 BCE) was also a physiologist who made biological observations and described the blood vessels as part of a system with the heart at its center. He also believed that the heart was a furnace that heated the blood and that it was the body's seat of intellect. In the city of Alexandria, Herophilus (335-280 BCE) believed that the seat of intellect was the brain, not the heart. He studied arteries and veins and determined that arteries have thicker walls. Erasistratus (310-240 BCE) began his training under Herophilus. He believed that arteries served as air vessels and that the veins carried the blood, which was made in the liver from food. Several hundred years later, Galen (129-c. 199 CE) conducted an experiment that showed that blood, not air, flowed through arteries. Though some of his other ideas were later disproved, he left behind a considerable number of writings on physiology, medicine, and philosophy.

Galen's ideas were taught for many hundreds of years until the Renaissance. During this time, physiologists made important discoveries and observations that challenged the findings of Galen. Andreas Vesalius (1514-1564) was trained as a doctor and became a professor of surgery and anatomy at a medical school in what is now Italy. Vesalius's style of teaching was to dissect a cadaver as he lectured, and he included anatomical drawings in his written texts. He wrote what has become known as the first modern anatomy textbook, *De Humanis Corporis Fabrica* (the structure of the human body), published in 1543.

A few decades later, William Harvey (1578-1657) was born in England and later trained as a doctor. He also did some lecturing and wrote a study of circulation, *De Motu Cordis et Sanguinis in Animalibus* (on the motion of the heart and of blood in animals), published in 1628. Harvey viewed the heart as a pump that contracted to expel blood and discovered that the blood moved in a circular path in the body. He believed that the blood traveled from the right ventricle to the lungs and then to the left ventricle, not directly from the right to the left ventricle. He also theorized that air stayed in the lungs and did not move to the heart to meet the blood.

Joseph Priestley (1733-1804), an English chemist, investigated the processes of combustion and breathing. Priestley's experiments used a bell jar, a candle, a green plant, and a mouse. He observed that a candle placed under a bell jar went out, but could later be lit after a green plant was placed under the jar for several days. He also observed that a mouse placed under the jar died after some time. When placed under the jar with a green plant, however, the mouse lived for a longer period of time.

Using an early microscope, Robert Hooke (1635-1703) studied a piece of cork and coined the term "cells' for he compartments that he observed. Two hundred years later, German biologists Matthias Schleiden(1804-1881) and Theodor Schwann (1810-1882) proposed their cell theory. Their theory encompassed some of the essential ideas in biology and physiology, including that all organisms are made of cells which have similar metabolic processes and chemical components, that an organism's functions result from different cells working together, and that all cells have their origin in preexisting cells.

The invention of the thermometer allowed scientists to gain further insights into human physiology. With this investigation came the discovery that the human body maintains a relatively constant internal body temperature, despite changes in the temperature of its environment. The French physiologist Claude Bernard (1813-1878) used the words "milieu intérieur" to describe this constant internal environment of the human body. American physiologist Walter Cannon (1871-1945) later coined the term "homeostasis" to describe this condition.

Essential to investigations and discoveries that advance the field of physiology is the ever-changing nature of technology. Early research was conducted simply with observations of the unaided eye. Later discoveries developed glass lenses to form a light microscope which magnified images up to 1,000 times and opened up a world of tissues and cells that were previously indiscernible. Newer technology led to the formation of the electron microscope, which provided magnification of specimens greater than 100,000 times and revealed the intricacies of subcellular structures.

Technology has advanced to the growth of living cells and tissues in laboratory dishes. Cell culture allows the investigator to change or regulate the environment of the biological material and to determine the effect of such alterations on growth and reproduction. Techniques such as cytochemistry, autoradiography, and immunochemistry have been developed to stain or localize certain regulatory molecules or cellular structures, enabling the scientist to quantify their effects on cell physiology. Cell fractionation has been developed to separate cells into their various components or organelles, thus providing a way that a specific organelle can be studied in isolation. Genetic engineering is a powerful technology that allows the researcher to manipulate and alter the genes of cells that control their functions. All these techniques are frequently used in physiology research and are powerful forces that have expanded scientific understanding.

—*John L. Rittenhouse and Roman J. Miller, Ph.D.*

See also Anatomy; Cells; Cytology; Endocrinology; Exercise physiology; Fluids and electrolytes; Hormones; Kinesiology; Nervous system; Neurology; Sleep; Systems and organs.

For Further Information:
Costanzo, Linda. *Physiology Cases and Problems.* New York: Lippincott Williams & Wilkins, 2012.
Fox, Stuart Ira. *Human Physiology.* 11th ed. Boston: McGraw-Hill, 2010.
Ganong, William F. *Review of Medical Physiology.* 23d ed. New York: Lange Medical Books/McGraw-Hill Medical, 2009.
Guyton, Arthur C., and John E. Hall. *Guyton and Hall Textbook of Medical Physiology.* 12th ed. Philadelphia: Saunders/Elsevier, 2011.
Levitzky, Michael. *Pulmonary Physiology.* New York: McGraw-Hill Medical, 2013.
Preston, Robin R. *Physiology (Lippincott's Illustrated Review Series).* New York: Lippincott Williams & Wilkins, 2012.
Prosser, C. Ladd, ed. *Environmental and Metabolic Animal Physiology.* 4th ed. New York: Wiley-Liss, 1991.
Rhoades, Rodney, and Richard Pflanzer. *Human Physiology.* 4th ed. Pacific Grove, Calif.: Brooks/Cole, 2003.
Tortora, Gerard J., and Sandra Reynolds Grabowski. *Introduction to the Human Body: The Essentials of Anatomy and Physiology.* 6th ed. Hoboken, N.J.: John Wiley & Sons, 2007.

Phytochemicals

Biology
Anatomy or system affected: All
Specialties and related fields: Nutrition, preventive medicine
Definition: Nonnutritive chemicals that plants produce, providing health benefits to humans who eat foods derived from plants.

Protective Role and Abundance

People who eat a diet rich in fresh fruits, vegetables, and whole grains obtain some protection from various diseases because of the phytochemicals that the plants contain. Phytochemicals are not traditional nutrients, such as proteins, carbohydrates, or fats; nor are they vitamins or minerals. Instead, they are substances that plants produce to protect against environmental stresses, such as attack by fungi and other organisms, or to attract animal pollinators or seed dispersers. Many phytochemicals are plant pigments, giving fruits and vegetables their animal-luring colors. There are thousands of phytochemicals, and plant species vary widely in the kinds and amounts that they contain.

Many phytochemicals have antioxidant properties, meaning that they help protect cells from oxidative damage, which has been implicated in cancer, diabetes, heart disease, strokes, and other disorders. Some phytochemicals function in humans in ways similar to the female hormone estrogen.

Although diets rich in plant-based foods have been shown to result in lower incidences of a number of diseases, scientists have had difficulty pinpointing which of the many different phytochemicals are protective. It may be that the interaction of a variety of naturally occurring phytochemicals, rather than any particular ones, is the significant factor in promoting health.

Some Major Kinds

One important group of phytochemicals, the carotenoids, includes many antioxidants. Of the numerous health claims that have been made for these plant pigments, one of the few to be substantiated is that increased consumption of lutein, a carotenoid found in green leafy vegetables such as collards, kale, spinach, and broccoli, is associated with a lowered risk for macular degeneration, an eye disease associated with advanced age.

Flavonoids, pigments that belong to a major class of phytochemicals called polyphenols, are abundant in vegetables, fruits such as blueberries and raspberries, and beverages such as tea, red wine, and fruit juices. Some flavonoids, including the widely occurring group anthocyanins, have antioxidant properties. Flavonoids called isoflavones are plant estrogens plentiful in soy products.

Perspective and Prospects

The discovery that phytochemicals are important to human health was not made until late in the twentieth century, and research is still being done. Scientists do not advise taking dietary supplements of particular phytochemicals; rather, they recommend a diet high in a variety of fruits, vegetables, and whole grains. Taking concentrated forms of phytochemicals might be harmful over the long term.

—*F. Hill, Ph.D.*

See also Antioxidants; Food biochemistry; Nutrition; Preventive medicine; Supplements; Vitamins and minerals.

For Further Information:

American Institute for Cancer Research, ed. *Nutrition and Cancer Prevention: New Insights into the Role of Phytochemicals*. New York: Kluwer Academic/Plenum, 2001. Advances in Experimental Medicine and Biology 492.

Bao, Yongping, and Roger Fenwick, eds. *Phytochemicals in Health and Disease*. New York: Marcel Dekker, 2004.

Meskin, Mark S., Wayne R. Bidlack, Audra J. Davies, Douglas S. Lewis, and R. Keith Randolph, eds. *Phytochemicals: Mechanisms of Action*. Boca Raton, Fla.: CRC Press, 2004.

Meskin, Mark S., Wayne R. Bidlack, Audra J. Davies, and Stanley T. Omaye, eds. *Phytochemicals in Nutrition and Health*. Boca Raton, Fla.: CRC Press, 2002.

Meskin, Mark S., Wayne R. Bidlack, and R. Keith Randolph, eds. *Phytochemicals: Nutrient-Gene Interactions*. Boca Raton, Fla.: CRC Press/Taylor & Francis, 2006.

"Phytochemicals." *American Cancer Society*, January 17, 2013.

"Phytochemicals and Cardiovascular Disease." *American Heart Association*, May 1, 2013.

Webb, Denise. "Phytonutrients: The Hidden Keys to Disease Prevention, Good Health." *Environmental Nutrition* 26, no. 1 (January, 2003): 1-6.

Pick's disease

Disease/Disorder

Also known as: Frontotemporal dementia (FTD), lobar sclerosis, circumscribed brain atrophy, focal cerebral atrophy, semantic dementia, primary progressive aphasia

Anatomy or system affected: Brain, nervous system, psychic-emotional system

Specialties and related fields: Family medicine, geriatrics and gerontology, internal medicine, neurology, psychiatry, psychology

Definition: A brain disease causing shrinkage of tissue in discrete areas (focal lesions) in the frontal and temporal anterior brain lobes, thus reducing verbal reasoning and speech production.

Key terms:

anterior: referring to the front, in the direction of the face

autosomal gene: all nonsex, nongender determining chromosomes; a dominant autosome will carry the trait that is observed in the organism, such as hair color or height

frontotemporal lobes: the two frontal and two temporal lobes that are located toward the front and on both the left and right side of the brain; jointly, they have the primary responsibility for executive thinking, reasoning, social judgment, and auditory functions

Causes and Symptoms

Pick's disease, also called frontotemporal dementia (FTD), is similar to, but much rarer than, Alzheimer's disease. The current designation of the syndrome groups together Pick's disease, primary progressive aphasia, and semantic dementia. Some medical researchers believe that corticobasal degeneration and progressive supranuclear palsy should be added to FTD, which would then be called Pick complex. The differing terms reflect different theoretical models of the disease, and specialists are likely to continue to debate these models.

An autosomal dominant genetic trait is speculated as a specific cause in some cases of FTD. In these cases, there is a family history of someone showing symptoms of a frontal lobe dementia. Pick's disease is often inherited, though in many cases there is no evident family (genetic) history and the cause is unknown.

Onset is slow and insidious. Tissues shrink (atrophy) in the frontal and temporal brain lobes. FTD also causes some brain cells to develop abnormal fibers called Pick's bodies. The cells in these bodies have an abnormal amount of a protein called tau. Tau appears throughout the body's cells but exists in abnormally high amounts in Pick's bodies and in Pick cells that exist inside normal brain cells (neurons). These form elsewhere in the brain and are not limited to the frontotemporal regions. These fibers are generally straight and single, as compared to Alzheimer's neurofibrillary tangles, which tend to be paired and helical.

Though Pick's disease varies greatly in how it affects individuals, it has a common core or clusters of symptoms. Some or all may be present at different stages of the disease. Since the frontal lobes involve emotional and social functioning, the first notable cluster of symptoms usually causes behavioral and affective changes such as impulsivity, compulsive overeating or only eating one type of food, drinking alcohol to excess (when not a prior problem), rudeness, impatience, aggressiveness, social withdrawal, poor social interaction, inability to hold a job, inattention to personal hygiene, sexual exhibitionism, promiscuity, abrupt mood changes, emotional aloofness, environmental indifference, marked distractibility, decreased interest in daily activities, and being unaware of these changes (lack of insight). Deterioration in personality usually occurs before dementia itself is evident-that is, before there is evident memory loss. This is one way that specialists diagnose it as distinct from Alzheimer's disease, in which the early symptoms involve memory loss.

Changes in physical mobility and coordination (apraxia) can also appear as early symptoms. They can include increased muscle rigidity or stiffness, difficulty getting around, worsening coordination, generalized weakness, and urinary incontinence.

Another characteristic cluster of symptoms relates to worsening language, including reduced-quality speech, shrinking vocabulary, word-finding problems, difficulty understanding speech (receptive aphasia) or producing understandable speech (expressive aphasia), repeating words and phrases others use (echolalia), progressive loss of reading and writing, and possibly complete loss of speech (mutism).

Treatment and Therapy

At present, there are no medications that can effectively treat FTD, although several can help treat many of its symptoms. Medications used in Alzheimer's disease are not routinely prescribed because they often increase aggression in Pick's disease patients.

Maximizing quality of life is the key treatment, and many of the more disturbing behaviors respond well to medication, including aggression and agitation. In addition to adding medications for symptom control, discontinuation of medications that promote confusion or that are not essential to the care of the person may improve cognitive function. It is common for anticholinergics, analgesics, and central nervous system depressants to be discontinued. Because many of the functions that FTD affects are also affected by low levels of thiamine, thiamine supplementation is often recommended.

Behavior modification is often the treatment of choice in controlling unacceptable or dangerous behaviors. Rewarding and reinforcing appropriate, positive behaviors while ignoring inappropriate, negative behaviors (within the bounds of safety) can significantly influence how patients act and interact. Formal psychotherapy is seldom effective because it overloads patients" limited cognitive resources. Reality orientation, with repeated reinforcement of environmental and other cues, can reduce disorientation and agitation. Sensory functions, often overlooked, should be evaluated and augmented as needed, including hearing aids, eyeglasses, and cataract surgery.

In addition, good nursing and caregiving, guided occupation activities, and participation in support groups all can improve the management of this type of dementia. Family counseling and family psychoeducation often go a long way in fostering adaptive changes that are necessary to care for patients at home. It is also important for families of Pick's disease patients to obtain support to help them cope with a disease that is likely to have a prolonged, ever-demanding course. Visiting nurses or aides, volunteer services, adult protective services, and other community resources may be helpful in caring for the person. Legal advice may be appropriate early in the course of the disorder. Advance directives, power of attorney, health care proxy, and "do not resuscitate" orders can make dealing with the later stages of the disease easier.

Perspective and Prospects

Pick's disease affects about 1 out of 100,000 people, accounting for 0.4 percent to 2.0 percent of all cases of dementia. More common in women then men, it typically has an onset between ages forty and sixty, with a modal age of fifty-four, but it has been known to affect patients as young

> **Information on Pick's Disease**
>
> **Causes:** Shrinkage of brain tissue, abnormal fibers in brain cells (Pick's bodies)
> **Symptoms:** Behavioral and affective changes (impulsivity, compulsive eating, rudeness, impatience, aggressiveness, social withdrawal, poor personal hygiene, sexual exhibitionism, promiscuity, abrupt mood changes, aloofness, distractibility, lack of insight); physical disorders (muscle rigidity, poor coordination, weakness, incontinence); language disturbances (shrinking vocabulary, word-finding problems, difficulty understanding speech, echolalia, loss of reading and writing, mutism)
> **Duration:** Chronic and progressive
> **Treatments:** None; medications, behavioral therapy for symptoms

as twenty. A family history of FTD is considered a risk factor, although most Pick's patients have no family history of the disease.

The first description of the disease was published in 1892 by Arnold Pick. Until recently, it was thought that Pick's disease could not be distinguished from Alzheimer's disease during life. In accordance with major research criteria of German neuropsychiatry, Pick's atrophy was constructed as a full-blown disease entity in the 1920s. This concept gained acceptance in the German and Anglo-American scientific community and was the starting point for further investigations in the 1950s and 1960s.

Initial diagnosis is mostly based on history and symptoms, signs, and tests and by ruling out other causes of dementia, especially those with metabolic causes. The development of neuropsychological assessment procedures and the use of electroencephalograms (EEGs), computed tomography (CT) scans, and magnetic resonance imaging (MRI) scans are generally necessary in the prediagnostic workup of the disease. Functional brain imaging, such as single photon emission computed tomography (SPECT) or positron emission tomography (PET) scans, are often appropriate in some patients.

Patients with FTD or Pick's disease will show a progressive decline. Rapidly progressing forms may be fatal in two years; slower forms may take ten. The cause of death is often opportunistic infection or, less commonly, the general failure of total body systems.

Recent identification of pathogenic mutations in Alzheimer's disease and frontotemporal dementia has improved understanding of these dementias and is guiding the investigations that use animal and tissue culture models. Eventually, it is hoped that this research will result in developing medications that can treat, stop, and reverse these diseases.

—*Paul Moglia, Ph.D., and Anju Varanasi, M.D.*

See also Alzheimer's disease; Brain; Brain disorders; Dementias; Frontotemporal dementia (FTD); Memory loss; Neurology; Psychiatry; Psychiatry, geriatric.

For Further Information:
Carson-DeWitt, Rosalyn, and Rimas Lukas. "Dementia." *Health Library*, Sept. 27, 2012.
Frederick, Justin, "Pick Disease: A Brief Overview." *Archives of Pathology and Laboratory Medicine* 130 (July, 2006): 1063-1066.
"Frontotemporal Disorders: Information for Patients, Families, and Caregivers." *National Institute on Aging*, Mar. 13, 2013
Kertesz, Andrew, and David G. Munoz, "Frontotemporal Dementia." *Medical Clinics of North America* 86 (2002): 501-518.
Jasmin, Luc, and David Zieve. "Pick's Disease." *MedlinePlus*, Feb. 16, 2012.
"NINDS Frontotemporal Dementia Information Page." *National Institute of Neurological Disorders and Stroke*, Mar. 20, 2013.
"Non-Alzheimer's Forms of Dementia." In *The Mayo Clinic Guide to Alzheimer's Disease: The Essential Resource for Treatment, Coping, and Caregiving*. Rochester, Minn.: Mayo Clinic, 2005.

PID. *See* Pelvic inflammatory disease (PID).

Pigeon toes

Disease/Disorder

Also known as: In-toeing

Anatomy or system affected: Bones, feet, hips, joints, knees, legs, ligaments, muscles

Specialties and related fields: Orthopedics, pediatrics, physical therapy, sports medicine

Definition: Usually a temporary condition in which one or both feet point inward when the heels are placed in a normal standing position.

Causes and Symptoms

Pigeon toes sometimes occur in children as a normal phase of development. Patients walk forward on a straight path while a toe or toes turn toward the body's axis. In infants and toddlers, pigeon toes are usually caused by how their hips, legs, and feet were positioned in the womb. Heredity also influences how pigeon toes are caused.

Patients may have pigeon toes for several reasons. Some are pigeon-toed because their feet are curved. In-toeing can also be caused by stiff muscles that hinder leg flexibility. Many cases of pigeon toes are attributable to how hip, leg, knee, and ankle joints and bones are angled and rotated.

Rotated tibias cause in-toeing in what is termed internal tibial torsion. Internal femoral torsion refers to when femurs significantly rotate from the hip socket to knee, affecting foot placement. Sleeping and kneeling positions may exacerbate fetal rotation and angling. Infants' feet often attain correct alignment before they walk, but if they temporarily continue in-toeing, pigeon toes probably will not slow the development of movement skills.

Treatment and Therapy

Usually, pigeon toes improve as children age, particularly as they gain experience walking. Pigeon toes do not necessitate treatment unless they interfere with movement. Corrective shoes and braces designed for specific cases are sometimes prescribed for young children. Casts can straighten curved foot position. Exercises enhance movement by stretching and strengthening muscles and ligaments to support normal positions.

Information on Pigeon Toes

Causes: Normal development, curved feet, stiff leg muscles, angle and rotation of hip, leg, knee, and ankle joints and bones

Symptoms: Improper foot and leg alignment

Duration: Chronic during early childhood

Treatments: None unless condition interferes with movement; may include corrective shoes and braces, casts, exercises

---

Children who continue to display pigeon toes after walking for one year should be examined because pigeon toes and such hip abnormalities as dysplasia often occur simultaneously. Asymmetrical in-toeing should also be investigated. Medical professionals will measure body angles, observe patients' movement while standing and walking, and study wear patterns on their shoes to detect how the hips and legs might affect ankle and foot mobility. X-rays can detect related skeletal disorders. Examinations should look for possible neurological conditions and tumors that might cause in-toeing.

Children aged eight years or older may require additional medical intervention. If pigeon toes significantly hinder motion in older patients whose development did not resolve their pigeon toes, physicians may recommend surgical adjustments to enable patients to gain normal mobility. Such measures aid patients who desire involvement in athletic activities.

Perspective and Prospects

In the nineteenth and twentieth centuries, physicians routinely advised the use of corrective splints and shoes. Often these treatments reassured parents that toddlers' pigeon toes would not be a permanent condition. Beginning in the 1930s, many patients wore the Denis-Browne splint, in which shoes are rigidly affixed together by a metal bar at a set angle, while they slept.

By the early twenty-first century, such practices were not implemented as often because many physicians questioned the benefits of therapeutic devices expediting improvement. Most advised allowing pigeon toes to correct naturally during development.

—*Elizabeth D. Schafer, Ph.D.*

See also Bones and the skeleton; Braces, orthopedic; Feet; Flat feet; Foot disorders; Lower extremities; Orthopedic surgery; Orthopedics; Orthopedics, pediatric.

For Further Information:
Atanda, Alfred. "Common Childhood Orthopedic Conditions." *KidsHealth*, November 2011.
Atanda, Alfred. "In-toeing and Out-toeing in Toddlers." *KidsHealth*, November 2011.
Cailliet, Rene. *Foot and Ankle Pain*. 3d ed. Philadelphia: F. A. Davis, 1997.
Harkless, Lawrence B., and Steven M. Krych. *Handbook of Common Foot Problems*. New York: Churchill Livingstone, 1990.
Herring, John A., ed. *Tachdjian's Pediatric Orthopaedics*. 4th ed. 3 vols. Philadelphia: Saunders/Elsevier, 2008.

Klag, Michael J., et al., eds. *Johns Hopkins Family Health Book*. New York: HarperCollins, 1999.

Lippert, Frederick G., and Sigvard T. Hansen. *Foot and Ankle Disorders: Tricks of the Trade*. New York: Thieme, 2003.

Lorimer, Donald L., et al., eds. *Neale's Disorders of the Foot*. 7th ed. New York: Churchill Livingstone/Elsevier, 2006.

Skinner, Harry B, and Patrick J. McMahon. *Current Disorders and Treatment in Orthopedics*, 5th ed. New York: Lange Medical Books, 2013.

Pigmentation

Biology

Anatomy or system affected: Eyes, hair, skin

Specialties and related fields: Dermatology, environmental health

Definition: The coloration of human skin and eyes based on the presence and amount of five different pigments; the most important of these pigments, melanin, protects the body from ultraviolet radiation.

Key terms:

dermis: the layer of skin underneath the epidermis that contains hemoglobin and oxyhemoglobin

epidermis: the outer layer of the skin that contains melanocytes, which produce melanin

hypodermis: the layer of fat under the dermis that contains carotene

melanin: a protein that darkens the color of the skin and protects against ultraviolet radiation

melanoma: cancer of the melanocytes, the cells that produce melanin

ultraviolet radiation: radiation that is potentially damaging to the skin; it is not visible to humans

Structure and Functions

One of the most apparent human characteristics is the color of a person's skin. Five pigments play major roles: melanin, melanoid, carotene, hemoglobin, and oxyhemoglobin. Melanin occurs in the greatest variation and is the most important of the five; in large amounts, it can mask the effects of the other pigments.

Melanocytes are cells that convert tyrosine, an amino acid, into the black pigment called "melanin." The rate of production is controlled by a hormone called "melanocyte-stimulating hormone (MSH)," which is released by the anterior pituitary gland. About a thousand melanocytes occur on each square millimeter of the body (with the exception of the head and the forearms, which have twice as many). Interestingly, all human races vary greatly in color but tend to have the same number of melanocytes, which inherit different abilities to make melanin.

When humans are compared, an uninterrupted array of shades of skin color is found. Traits that show such continuous variation are thought to be controlled by several sets of genes (polygenetic inheritance). Thus, several sets of genes were believed to control the amount of pigmentation. In 2005, researchers at Pennsylvania State University found two variant expressions of a single gene that may be responsible for the observed distribution of human skin color.

Melanocytes convert tyrosine intomelanin by several chemical steps that involve the key enzyme tyrosinase. A functional tyrosinase molecule consists of different amino acids (the building blocks of proteins) and copper. Traces of copper are in the normal human diet and provide the amounts needed for the enzymes.

Tyrosine, the molecule that is converted to melanin, is one of twenty amino acids occurring in biological systems that chain together in various ways to make up different proteins. Eight of these amino acids are essential-that is, they must be present in the diet. The remaining twelve amino acids can be made by chemical modification of the others. Tyrosine is not an essential amino acid. Ample amounts of tyrosine occur in all meats and in most dairy products. If it is not taken into the body in sufficient amounts, however, it will be made from other amino acids. Either way, tyrosine is delivered to the melanocytes and changed into melanin. This product, with its high molecular weight, functions to protect the skin from excessive ultraviolet (UV) radiation.

UV radiation is an invisible part of the sun's radiation having wavelengths from one hundred to four hundred nanometers. Humans can see the colors of the spectrum from red through violet. Wavelengths of radiation that are slightly longer than red (infrared) cannot be seen but are detected by the body as heat. Wavelengths that are shorter than violet, such as UV, cannot be seen or felt. Nevertheless, UV radiation penetrates the body. In moderation, UV light is valuable for humans because the body uses its energy to synthesize vitamin D. Vitamin D allows the intestinal absorption of calcium to be used for skeletal growth and for nerve and muscle function.

UV radiation poses several risks. A sunburn involves UV radiation damage to epidermal skin cells, which release chemicals that dilate blood vessels, causing redness. Swelling and blistering may occur. When large numbers of cells are destroyed, the skin speeds up production of new cells, which forces the burned cells to peel off. UV radiation also can change the skin's collagen, a protein that holds tissues together in much the same way that concrete is reinforced by steel rods. The changes in the collagen, possibly by causing cross-linkage between fibers, can permanently wrinkle the skin. Finally, many researchers agree that UV light may also inhibit the immune response by damaging Langerhans cells in the epidermis. When damaged, these large cells lose their ability to alert the other cells of the immune system to infection. The most serious danger is that UV radiation may alter the genetic code within cells, causing cancer.

Melanin protects the cells of the body by blocking and absorbing UV light. People who have more melanin by heredity are not at as high a risk as those who are lighter. (This is not to say that dark-skinned people should not protect themselves from the sun.) In all cases, exposure to UV radiation immediately causes the skin to darken by causing oxygen to combine with the melanin that is already present. Exposure also increases the rate of melanin production and speeds its distribution to other cells, producing more darkening.

Melanocytes are found at the bottom of the outer layer of

the skin, which is called the "epidermis." They are also at the base of the shafts of hairs and in the eye, producing coloration of the iris and in the black membrane of the eye behind the retina. The pigment-producing melanocytes in the skin are found at the base of the epidermis among cube-shaped skin cells that cannot make pigment. About thirty-six of these epidermal cells occur for each melanocyte. Melanocytes have long extensions that reach out to protect the regular skin cells. Furthermore, melanin can also be transferred to epidermal cells. Skin color is also influenced by the distribution and size of the pigment granules in the melanocytes. Very dark skin tends to have single, large granules. Lighter skin tends to have clusters of two to four smaller granules.

On a larger scale, small uneven clusters of pigment are called "freckles." These spots of melanin show mostly in lighter-skinned people, are controlled by heredity, and appear with sun exposure to the skin. Because of this uneven distribution of melanin, other cells among the freckles are not protected and can easily be sunburned.

Moles (nevi) are larger, dark spots of melanin that tend to increase as a person ages. Two types occur: the pigment can be deposited into the dermis (intradermal nevi) or can be found between the dermis and the epidermis (junctional nevi). The first type of mole tends to be elevated and have hair growing from it. The second tends to be flat and very dark.

Large amounts of melanin in hair will cause it to be black. Lesser amounts make it brown, and still less causes it to be blond. White or gray hair has no melanin. Yet a separate gene for a reddish, iron-containing pigment can be inherited. If two of these recessive genes are present, then the hair will be red. Depending on the amount of melanin that is also present, such people range from almost purely red hair to a strawberry blond color to a reddish-brown (auburn). Larger amounts of melanin will cover the red pigment completely.

Lack of melanin in the iris of the eye will scatter light and cause the eye to reflect blue. Larger amounts cause the eye color to be darker. The pigment in the iris serves to block radiation that could sunburn the retina. In 1992, investigators at Boston College found that eye sensitivity increases when the amount of melanin is greater.

Melanin breaks down as it moves toward the outer layers of the epidermis, forming a chemical called "melanoid" in the process. Melanoid can be seen as a yellow color in the thick (calloused) skin of the palms of the hands and the soles of feet.

Carotene is a yellow-to-orange pigment that tends to accumulate in the layer of fat under the skin. This pigment is also responsible for the color of carrots, yellow vegetables, and the yellows in autumn leaves. When taken into the body, carotene is stored in the liver and converted into vitamin A, which is used in vision. Females usually store more carotene than males because of their higher percentages of fat. Asian peoples tend to have combinations of low melanin and higher carotene that produce a yellowish skin hue.

Hemoglobin and oxyhemoglobin are pigments that are found inside red blood cells. Hemoglobin is dark red but looks bluish through the skin. If hemoglobin combines with oxygen, it is called "oxyhemoglobin." Oxyhemoglobin is bright red. Skin color from this pigment varies with the amount of blood that is circulated at the surface of the dermis, the relative amounts of hemoglobin and oxyhemoglobin that are present, and the densities of other pigments. Hemoglobin and oxyhemoglobin affect the color of light-skinned people more than of darker people. The skin of lighter people generally looks reddish, with oxygen-poor veins appearing blue.

Rapid change of hair color, from dark pigmented to gray or white, is impossible because of the slow growth rate of hair. Melanin is deposited into the hair shaft at the root. The hairs grow outward at a rate of about thirteen millimeters a month. Hence, a loss of pigment production would take a long time to show. The myth of rapid change may be based on diseases that cause all the pigmented hair to fall out overnight, leaving only white hairs.

Disorders and Diseases

Pigmentation can be abnormal and associated with disease. Excess adrenocorticotropic hormone (ACTH) can increase melanin. ACTH contains several hormones, including MSH. Addison disease involves the overproduction of ACTH. Also, certain injuries such as burns, chemical irritations, or some infections may cause an increase in pigmentation, as can pregnancy. Injuries in which melanocytes are destroyed may result in scar tissue that lacks pigmentation. An excessive intake of carotene can cause light skin to turn orange, a condition called "carotenemia."

Skin cancer has increased over time. In the late twentieth century, the rate doubled every decade from the 1960s to the 1990s. The ozone layer, a thin layer of gas molecules consisting of three oxygen atoms, was being depleted by chemicals such as refrigerants that were released into the atmosphere. This layer protects life on the planet from the full shower of ultraviolet radiation that comes from the sun. In 2013, according to the World Health Organization, some two to three million skin cancers were being diagnosed annually. Any changes in the skin, such as a mole that changes in color or begins to grow, should be shown to a doctor. Although moles and other abnormalities in pigmentation are not usually dangerous, some may develop into melanomas.

Researchers have been trying to discover if it is possible to tan safely. Attempts have been made to develop better creams to block UV radiation. Skin cancer is less common among dark-skinned people; it has been reasoned that if melanin could be put into a skin cream, lighter-skinned people could have more of this natural protection. Unfortunately, many sources of melanin are expensive.

Presently, the best way to avoid skin cancer is to avoid the sunlight, especially when and where the light is most intense-at midday, near the equator, during the summer at other latitudes, at high altitudes, and in highly reflective environments such as sand or snow. Additional protection can be found by using a sunscreen lotion with a high sun-protection factor (SPF) of at least 15. SPF 15 permits fifteen times longer exposure before burning (compared to using no sunscreen), and SPF 30 is thought to protect even the fairest skins. The American Academy of Dermatology recommends using SPF 30 or higher.

Nevertheless, even with frequent applications of sunscreens, people may be putting themselves at risk of melanoma, the most serious skin cancer. Specifically, deoxyribonucleic acid (DNA) absorbs and can be directly damaged by the 280 and 315 nanometer range of UV radiation, and it was formerly assumed that this range, called UVB, was the only one about which people had to worry. Sunscreens were initially developed to block only UVB, the "burning rays." Data collected by Richard B. Setlow and his colleagues at Brookhaven National Laboratory in 1993, however, indicated that longer wavelengths, including some visible light and UVA (315-400 nanometers), can also damage DNA. Setlow suggested that melanin itself absorbs this energy, setting off chemical reactions that produce chemicals that then damage the melanocytes. This process may be the cause of melanoma. The current consensus is that people should protect themselves from all sunlight, using a broad-spectrum sunscreen lotion that protects against both UVA and UVB. The same risks apply to tanning salons.

Most melanomas are skin cancers. They can also be found inside the eye, as a black spot on the white of the eye, on the iris, or in the center of the field of vision. Treatment of such growths with radiation or surgical removal of the tumor are options. Removal of the entire eye may be necessary. Preventive measures include sunglasses that filter UV light. According to the American Academy of Ophthalmology, sunglasses should block 99 to 100 percent of UV radiation. Most manufacturers label their sunglasses.

In 1991, a controlled study was done in which injections of synthetic MSH were tested. The goal was to help prevent sunburn and skin cancer in high-risk individuals who tan poorly. Those receiving MSH showed significant tanning compared to those who received injections of a placebo. Some mild side effects occurred in the MSH group, including some brief flushing and vague stomach discomfort after the injection.

There are several irregularities of pigmentation. If the tyrosinase enzyme is missing, a person will produce no melanin. This condition is inherited among all races, and such a person is called an "albino" (Greek for "white"). Actually, the lack of melanin allows hemoglobin to determine the skin color. In some types of albinism, an affected individual produces reduced amounts of melanin, resulting in an appearance that is only slightly lighter than that found in the individual's family and ethnic community. All albinos have less protection from the sun and, in addition to the risks to the skin, have poor vision because of light reflections off the back of the eye that normally would be absorbed by pigment. With no pigment in the iris, they are also more likely to suffer damage to their retinal cells, resulting in blindness.

Especially in lighter-skinned people, a lack of hemoglobin (anemia) will cause paleness. If a person's body circulates more blood into the dermis, the skin will appear more reddish or flushed. This could signal that the body is attempting to cool itself or that a person is embarrassed. If the body is cold or emotionally shocked, it may reduce circulation of blood to the surface of the dermis and the individual will appear pale. Lack of normal sunlight can cause a person to slow the production of melanin. A person who is exercising by swimming in cold water may not circulate blood as quickly as it is needed, and the increase of hemoglobin may turn that person blue, a tone that is noticeable in people with both large and small amounts of melanin.

Perspective and Prospects

Scientists believe that the first humans probably had their origin in Africa and were darkly pigmented. As people migrated to the higher latitudes, where the radiation from the sun was less direct, having less pigment may have been adaptive. Less melanin would allow these people to synthesize needed vitamin D where there was less direct sunlight and less UV light. Before individuals began to migrate over long distances, populations were neatly distributed with darker skins near the equator and lighter skins in northern Europe. Inuits are an interesting exception: they have dark skin and live in a northern latitude. Their diet, however, has traditionally included fish livers with sufficient vitamin D.

The possibility of danger from the sun and other radiation is only a recent discovery. Ultraviolet radiation was discovered in 1801. By 1927, H. J. Muller showed in the laboratory that x-rays cause changes in the genetic code of fruit flies that can be inherited. Such changes, called "mutations," can be harmful. Further investigations showed that UV light, while not as dangerous as x-rays, can also cause mutations. The likelihood of mutation in an organism is proportional to the dose of radiation that is received; spacing out the exposure makes no difference.

Attempts to classify races by description of skin color have given little return. Paul Broca (1824-80) developed an elaborate table of twenty colors for cross-matching with the eyes and twenty-four colors for cross-matching with the skin. The color of the skin, however, is extremely difficult to judge: the color itself changes with environmental and physiological conditions, the ability of observers varies, and the lighting conditions under which comparisons are made can make a difference in the results.

To avoid some of these problems, studies have been performed with a device that measures the reflection of various wavelengths by the skin. In 1992, a study of members of the Jirel population in Nepal showed that the reflections from measurements of upper arm skin using three different wavelengths varied as if the reflective properties were controlled by only a single set of genes. Evidently, the use of various wavelengths gives little additional information about color differences.

—Paul R. Boehlke, Ph.D.

See also Albinos; Dermatology; Grafts and grafting; Plastic surgery; Skin; Skin cancer; Skin disorders; Skin lesion removal; Tattoo removal; Vitamins and minerals; Vitiligo.

For Further Information:

A.D.A.M. Medical Encyclopedia. "Skin - Abnormally Dark or Light." *MedlinePlus*, May 13, 2011.

"Albinism." *Mayo Foundation for Medical Education and Research*, April 2, 2011.

Balter, Michael. "Zebrafish Researchers Hook Gene for Human Skin Color." *Science* 310, no. 5755 (December 16, 2005): 1754-55.

Freinkel, Ruth K., and David T. Woodley, eds. *Biology of the Skin*. New York: Parthenon, 2001.

Greeley, Alexandra. "Dodging the Rays." *FDA Consumer* 27 (July/August, 1993): 30-33.

Greener, Mark. "Gene for Red Hair Could Shed Light on Skin Pigmentation." *Dermatology Times* 20, no. 12 (December, 1999): 19.

Guttman, Cheryl. "Pigmentation Disorders Common in Asians." *Dermatology Times* 20, no. 8 (August, 1999): 24.

"Health Effects of UV Radiation." *World Health Organization*, 2013.

Levine, Norman, ed. *Pigmentation and Pigmentary Disorders*. Boca Raton, Fla.: CRC Press, 1993.

Schalock, Peter C., ed. "Overview of Skin Pigment." *Merck Manual of Home Health Handbook*, January, 2013.

Turkington, Carol, and Jeffrey S. Dover. *The Encyclopedia of Skin and Skin Disorders*. 3d ed. New York: Facts On File, 2007.

"UV Radiation." *United States Environmental Protection Agency*, June, 2010.

Weedon, David. *Skin Pathology*. 3d ed. New York: Churchill Livingstone/Elsevier, 2010.

Pimples. *See* Acne.

Pinworms

Disease/Disorder

Also known as: *Enterobius vermicularis*, threadworms, seatworms

Anatomy or system affected: Gastrointestinal system, intestines, skin

Specialties and related fields: Dermatology, family medicine, pediatrics, public health

Definition: A common parasitic nematode that resembles a white thread approximately 0.5 inch in length.

Causes and Symptoms

Infestation with pinworm, a common name for the organism *Enterobius vermicularis*, is characterized by itching around the anus that becomes worse at night, causing sleeplessness, irritability, and general restlessness. There may also be vague gastrointestinal symptoms such as loose stools or nausea. Humans are the only host for the pathogen. Young children are most often affected, and the disease spreads easily to other members of the household.

Adult pinworms live in the large intestine. Females migrate to the anus and deposit eggs outside the body; this is the cause of the itching. Scratching often causes the eggs to be deposited on food and eaten or transferred directly to the mouth and swallowed. Newly hatched larvae migrate to the large intestine and lay eggs over a four-week period. Pinworm eggs are viable outside a host for up to two weeks.

Children typically complain of intense itching around the anal area at night. Scratching may cause bleeding in the region. Interrupted sleep may cause irritability during the day. Individual worms are not commonly seen. The most common diagnostic procedure is to apply a piece of pressure-sensitive cellulose tape to the anus and look for eggs

Information on Pinworms
Causes: Parasitic infestation
Symptoms: Itching around anus that becomes worse at night, sleeplessness, irritability, general restlessness, vague gastrointestinal symptoms such as loose stools or nausea
Duration: Acute
Treatments: Drug therapy, proper hygiene

under a microscope.

Pinworm infestation must be differentiated from fungal and yeast infections, allergies, and conditions caused by other species of worms. Fungal and yeast infections can be cultured. Allergies may include itching near the anus but usually involve other areas of the body as well. Analyzing their eggs or bodies can identify other species of worms.

Treatment and Therapy

Pinworm infestation is relatively easy to treat. Drugs requiring a physician's prescription are taken by mouth for three to five days and usually kill the pinworms. Antihistamines can be used to obtain relief from itching.

It is very important to wash one's hands thoroughly with soap and warm water after using the toilet and before meals. Fingernails should be closely trimmed to prevent injury when scratching and to minimize the chance of transferring eggs. All clothing of a patient should be washed after each use. Laundering bedding will kill pinworm eggs.

Although pinworm infestation is annoying, it is otherwise benign. A cure can be obtained readily using appropriate drug therapy. Repeated infestation is common, however, especially among children.

—*L. Fleming Fallon, Jr., M.D., Ph.D., M.P.H.*

See also Anus; Gastroenterology; Gastroenterology, pediatric; Gastrointestinal disorders; Gastrointestinal system; Insect-borne diseases; Itching; Parasitic diseases; Worms; Zoonoses.

For Further Information:

Badash, Michelle. "Pinworm." *Health Library*, September 10, 2012.

Despommier, Dickson D., et al. *Parasitic Diseases*. 5th ed. New York: Apple Tree, 2006.

Durani, Yamini. "Infections: Pinworm." *KidsHealth*, May 2011.

Gittleman, Ann Louise. *Guess What Came to Dinner? Parasites and Your Health*. Rev. ed. New York: Putnam, 2001.

Klein, Aaron E. *The Parasites We Humans Harbor*. New York: Nelson Books/Elsevier, 1981.

Litin, Scott C., ed. *Mayo Clinic Family Health Book*. 4th ed. New York: HarperResource, 2009.

Roberts, Larry S., and John Janovy, Jr., eds. *Gerald D. Schmidt and Larry S. Roberts' Foundations of Parasitology*. 7th ed. Boston: McGraw-Hill Higher Education, 2005.

Scheinberg, Dianne. "Pruritus Ani." *Health Library*, March 15, 2013.

Shannon, Joyce Brennfleck. *Contagious Diseases Sourcebook: Basic Consumer Health Information about Diseases Spread from Person to Person*. Detroit, Mich.: Onmigraphics, 2010.

Woolf, Alan D., et al., eds. *The Children's Hospital Guide to Your Child's Health and Development*. Cambridge, Mass.: Perseus, 2002.

Zieve, David, et al. "Pinworms." *MedlinePlus*, August 14, 2012.

Pituitary gland

Biology

Anatomy or system affected: Brain, endocrine system, glands

Specialties and related fields: Biochemistry, endocrinology, family medicine, nutrition, obstetrics, osteopathic medicine, pediatrics

Definition: An endocrine gland located at the base of the brain, just inferior to the hypothalamus.

Key terms:

adenohypophysis: another name for the anterior lobe of the pituitary gland

negative feedback: a common physiological process by which the product of a process feeds back to inhibit further stimulation (or reverse) the process

neurohypophysis: another name for the posterior lobe of the pituitary gland

positive feedback: a physiological process in which a product feeds back to stimulate the process, resulting in additional production or the continuation of that process

Structure and Functions

The pituitary gland is similar in size to a pea and has two lobes, the anterior (adenohypophysis) and the posterior (neurohypophysis). The anterior lobe accounts for a greater proportion of the total weight, approximately 80 percent. The pituitary gland is involved in the release of numerous hormones that have a multitude of effects throughout the body; as a result, it is often referred to as the "master" gland. The functions of the hormones released from the pituitary gland include reproductive functions (including childbirth and lactation), bone growth and development, and regulation of metabolic processes, body temperature, water balance, circulation, and blood pressure. Therefore, a normally functioning pituitary gland is essential to the health and maintenance of homeostasis in humans.

Hormones released from the anterior lobe of the pituitary gland include thyroid-stimulating hormone (TSH) or thyrotropin, growth hormone (GH), adrenocorticotropic hormone (ACTH), follicle-stimulating hormone (FSH), luteinizing hormone (LH), and prolactin (PRL). The hypothalamus, which is located just superior to the pituitary gland, regulates the release of hormones from the anterior pituitary gland by releasing hormones that travel through a blood network called the hypophyseal portal system to the anterior pituitary. For example, the hypothalamus releases growth-hormone-releasing hormone (GHRH), which travels to the anterior pituitary and stimulates the release of growth hormone. Alternatively, if the body wants to decrease the secretion of GH, the hypothalamus may do so by releasing growth-hormone-inhibiting hormone (GHIH), also known as growth-hormone-release-inhibiting hormone (GHRIH) or somatostatin. Another common inhibiting hormone released from the hypothalamus is prolactin-inhibiting hormone (PIH), which reduces the release of PRL from the anterior pituitary.

In contrast to the anterior lobe, the posterior lobe of the pituitary gland releases two hormones: oxytocin and antidiuretic hormone (ADH), which is commonly referred to as vasopressin. The release of these hormones is influenced by blood pressure, osmolarity of the blood, and other inputs, such as those from the nervous and reproductive systems.

Several hormones released by the pituitary gland stimulate other organs or tissues directly, resulting in changes in overall physiologic function. For example, GH increases protein synthesis and the related growth of muscles, bones, and tissues. GH also increases the release of glucose and fat breakdown to fuel these anabolic processes. PRL stimulates the mammary glands and causes lactation, and oxytocin also stimulates lactation and causes contraction of the uterine wall during labor. Finally, ADH causes the kidneys to reabsorb or retain water, aiding in the body's ability to regulate water balance and hydration levels.

Other hormones released by the pituitary gland stimulate the release of still other hormones from subsequent endocrine glands. These include TSH, which stimulates the thyroid gland to release thyroid hormones; ACTH, which stimulates the cortex of the adrenal glands to release cortisol; and the sex hormones FSH and LH, also called gonadotrophs, which stimulate the sex organs in males and females to release hormones involved in the production of sperm and the function of the menstrual cycle, respectively.

The release of most hormones from the pituitary gland is controlled by classic negative-feedback loops. In these systems, an increase in product feeds back to inhibit further stimulation of that system. Using the thyroid hormones as an example, the hypothalamus releases thyrotropin-releasing hormone (TRH), which stimulates the anterior pituitary to release TSH, which then causes the thyroid gland to release thyroid hormones. When circulating levels of thyroid hormones are higher than normal or necessary, they feed back to inhibit or slow the release of TRH from the hypothalamus and TSH from the anterior pituitary. Conversely, when circulating levels of thyroid hormones are low, they feed back to increase the release of TRH and TSH, which will ultimately increase the release of thyroid hormones from the thyroid gland. Therefore, there are several sites of control involved in the release of products from the pituitary gland.

A notable exception to this trend is the presence of a positive-feedback process involving the pituitary gland and the hormone oxytocin. In this system, the stretching of the cervix during labor causes the release of oxytocin, which increases contractions in the uterus to assist with the progression of labor and eventual childbirth. The oxytocin feeds back in a positive fashion by increasing the stretching of the cervix, which then leads to the release of even more oxytocin. This cycle continues until the child is born, at which time the stimulus of cervix stretch and the related oxytocin release both cease.

Disorders and Diseases

Pituitary dysfunction is typically characterized by an oversecretion or undersecretion of pituitary hormones. An overactive pituitary gland is an endocrine defect characterized by excessive growth in stature and mass, plus a variety of other symptoms, depending on which hormones are elevated. The increased hormone release from the pituitary gland is often attributed to a pituitary tumor. If this is the case, then the tumor may be treated with radiation therapy, surgical removal, or the use of an antagonist to decrease the release of pituitary hormones.

Individuals with underactive pituitary glands, or hypopituitarism, experience symptoms such as short stature, low body mass, infertility or reproductive difficulties (including the inability of women to lactate following childbirth), low energy levels, perpetual feeling of cold due to an inability to regulate body temperature, and fatigue. Hypopituitarism may also be caused by a pituitary tumor, as well as injury to or infection of the hypothalamus or pituitary gland. The treatment for hypopituitarism involves stimulating the release of hormones from the target organs or tissues, rather than stimulating the pituitary gland itself.

—*Kristin S. Ondrak, Ph.D.*

See also Brain; Endocrine disorders; Endocrine glands; Endocrinology; Endocrinology, pediatric; Glands; Hormones; Hypothalamus; Systems and organs.

For Further Information:

Baylis, P. H. "Posterior Pituitary Function in Health and Disease." *Clinical Endocrinology and Metabolism* 12, no. 3 (November 1983): 747-770.

Besser, G. M. "Pituitary and Hypothalamic Physiology." *Journal of Clinical Pathology Supplement (Association of Clinical Pathologists)* 7 (1976): 8-11.

Daniel, P. M. "Anatomy of the Hypothalamus and Pituitary Gland." *Journal of Clinical Pathology Supplement (Association of Clinical Pathologists)* 7 (1976): 1-7.

Freeman, Susan, L. "The Anterior Pituitary." In *Endocrine Pathophysiology*, edited by Catherine B. Niewoehner. 2d ed. Raleigh, N.C.: Hayes Barton Press, 2004.

Harris, G. W. "Neural Control of the Pituitary Gland: I. The Neurohypophysis." *British Medical Journal* 2, no. 4731 (September 8, 1951): 559-564.

Harris, G. W. "Neural Control of the Pituitary Gland: II. The Adenohypophysis, with Special Reference to the Secretion of ACTH." *British Medical Journal* 2, no. 4732 (September 15, 1951): 627-634.

Klibanski, Anne, and Nicholas Tritos, eds. "Pituitary Disorders." *Hormone Health Network*, May 2013.

"Pituitary Disorders." *MedlinePlus*, July 11, 2013.

Pityriasis alba
Disease/Disorder

Anatomy or system affected: Arms, back, neck, skin

Specialties and related fields: Dermatology, family medicine, histology, pediatrics

Definition: A common skin disorder that causes light-colored, scaly patches of skin on the face, neck, and arms.

Causes and Symptoms

Pityriasis alba is a nonspecific disorder of the skin regarded as a manifestation of atopic dermatitis. It may be triggered by drying agents, including the sun, wind, soap, and bathing. It typically manifests itself on the fragile skin of children between the ages of three and sixteen, usually appearing on the face but sometimes extending to the neck, arms, and trunk of the body. Several patches are typical,

---

Information on Pityriasis Alba

Causes: Unknown; related to atopic dermatitis triggered by drying agents (sun, wind, soap)

Symptoms: Light-colored spots on face, neck, arms, and trunk; sometimes itchy

Duration: A few months to three years, sometimes recurrent

Treatments: Self-resolving; alleviation of symptoms may include moisturizers, mild hydrocortisone cream, phototherapy

---

extending in diameter from 5 to 30 millimeters. The exact cause is unknown. Although annoying, the disease is not dangerous or contagious.

Pityriasis alba appears as slightly elevated round to oval spots that have little color. The spots are usually white but occasionally pale pink to light brown. The boundaries of the spots are generally uneven and not clearly visible. Being light-colored, the spots are most noticeable in the summertime, standing out from the tanned skin of a patient. As the disorder progresses over a few weeks, the affected areas often develop very fine powdery scales. Dry skin makes the rash worse.

Treatment and Therapy

Since the disorder eventually resolves on its own in almost all cases, treatment may not be necessary. It is important to keep the skin moisturized. A variety of lotions, creams, or ointments (such as Curel, Nivea, or Lubriderm) may be applied to the affected areas, particularly after bathing or exposure to the sun. If the rash is inflamed or itchy, then a mild hydrocortisone cream can be applied daily. For some patients, phototherapy improves the condition.

Pityriasis alba usually clears after a few months, but in some cases it can last up to three years. It typically takes at least several weeks in order for new healthy skin to develop and adjust its color back to normal. In some cases, the disorder will reappear from time to time. Some children experience the disease every summer, but over the years, their skin color eventually returns to normal.

Perspective and Prospects

Pityriasis is derived from the Greek *pityron*, which means "scales," while *alba* means "white." Therefore, pityriasis alba describes white, scaly patches. The rash is most often confined to the face, especially around the cheeks, mouth, and chin. About 20 percent of the time, it may also occur on the neck, arms, and chest. Occasionally, it may show up only on the arms and trunk of the body.

Care must be taken to distinguish pityriasis alba from other related skin disorders, particularly tinea versicolor and vitiligo. Tinea versicolor, a fungal infection, can be ruled out by examining flakes of skin from the affected areas with a potassium hydroxide test. In vitiligo, there is a well-defined border between normal skin and the diseased spots.

—*Alvin K. Benson, Ph.D.*

See also Dermatitis; Dermatology; Dermatology, pediatric; Rashes; Skin; Skin disorders.

For Further Information:
Berman, Kevin. "Pityriasis Alba." *MedlinePlus,* May 13, 2011.
Kimball, Chad T. *Childhood Diseases and Disorders Sourcebook: Basic Consumer Health Information About Medical Problems Often Encountered in Pre-adolescent Children.* Detroit, Mich.: Omnigraphics, 2003.
Leung, Donald Y. M., and Malcolm W. Greaves, eds. *Allergic Skin Disease: A Multidisciplinary Approach.* New York: Marcel Dekker, 2000.
Wolff, Klaus et al.. *Fitzpatrick's Color Atlas and Synopsis of Clinical Dermatology.* 7th ed. New York: McGraw-Hill Medical, 2013.

Pityriasis rosea

Disease/Disorder

Anatomy or system affected: Back, chest, skin

Specialties and related fields: Dermatology, family medicine, pathology

Definition: A skin disorder that manifests with a characteristic rash.

Causes and Symptoms

Pityriasis rosea is primarily a skin disease of children and young adults, with females being more commonly affected than males. The initial lesion is a characteristic eruption seen on the trunk called the herald or mother patch, as it signals the onset of lesions to come. This is a scaly pink plaque which is around one to two centimeters in diameter, slightly raised above the surface, with central salmon-colored wrinkles. This lesion should be differentiated from that of syphilis and ringworm.

The herald patch is followed in about two weeks by a crop of similar but smaller lesions all over the trunk. The pink scaly oval papules are distributed along the skin tension lines in the trunk and result in a so-called Christmas tree distribution. The lesions may be mild to moderately pruritic (itchy) and will resolve spontaneously in four to six weeks, without any specific treatment. Other symptoms may involve mild aches and fatigue.

The exact cause of this exanthem (eruptive disease) is not known, but it is believed to result from exposure to various viruses. Most patients appear to have a positive recent history of influenza or an upper respiratory tract infection. The eruption typically appears in spring and fall and appears to cluster among close contacts; however, it is not believed to be highly contagious.

Treatment and Therapy

There is no specific treatment for pityriasis rosea, and usually none is required, as the disease is self-limited and resolves without treatment in four to six weeks. Pruritus is usually mild and can be treated with antihistamines and calamine lotion. If itching is severe, then topical steroids and a short, tapered dose of systemic steroids may be administered. Ultraviolet B (UVB) radiation is another treatment option. Patients are also advised to avoid hot showers and strenuous activity, as sweat and water appear to exacerbate the rash.

Information on Pityriasis Rosea

Causes: Unknown; possibly exposures to viruses

Symptoms: Herald or mother patch, smaller scaly pink lesions on trunk; usually itchy

Duration: Four to six weeks

Treatments: Self-resolving; alleviation of symptoms may include antihistamines, calamine lotion, steroids, ultraviolet B radiation

---

Perspective and Prospects

The term *pityriasis* is derived from the Greek *pityron,* meaning "scales." The term, initially applied to include all those skin disorders that were characterized by fine scales, is presently used only with modifiers such as *rosea, alba,* or *versicolor. Rosea* means "pink," and therefore pityriasis rosea describes pink-colored, fine, scaly lesions.

It is important clinically to distinguish the herald patch from other skin conditions. Therefore, a blood test for syphilis should be included for differential diagnosis. Also, ringworm, which requires treatment with antifungal agents, should be ruled out.

About 3 percent of the patients with pityriasis rosea experience recurrences, and no systemic manifestations have been demonstrated.

—Rashmi Ramasubbaiah, M.D.

See also Dermatology; Dermatology, pediatric; Itching; Lesions; Rashes; Skin; Skin disorders; Viral infections.

For Further Information:
Chuh, Antonio A. T. "Pityriasis Rosea: Roles of the Dermatology Nurse." *Dermatology Nursing* 16, no. 2 (April 1, 2004): 130-136.
Parker, James N., and Philip M. Parker. *Pityriasis Rosea: A Medical Dictionary, Bibliography, and Annotated Research Guide to Internet References.* San Diego, Calif.: ICON Health Publications, 2004.
Kasper, Dennis L., et al., eds. *Harrison's Principles of Internal Medicine.* 18th ed. New York: McGraw-Hill, 2012.
Montemayor-Quellenberg, Marjorie. "Pityriasis Rosea." *Health Library,* September 26, 2012.
Rakel, Robert E., ed. *Textbook of Family Practice.* 8th ed. Philadelphia: W. B. Saunders, 2011.
Tapley, Donald F., et al., eds. *The Columbia University College of Physicians and Surgeons Complete Home Medical Guide.* Rev. 3d ed. New York: Crown, 1995.
Vorvick, Linda J. "Pityriasis Rosea." *MedlinePlus,* October 14, 2012.

PKU. *See* Phenylketonuria (PKU)

Placenta

Biology

Anatomy or system affected: Circulatory system, endocrine system, reproductive system, uterus

Specialties and related fields: Embryology, obstetrics

Definition: The organ that develops during pregnancy to connect the mother to the developing fetus through the umbilical cord.

Structure and Functions

The placenta is an important and unique organ that

develops in women only during pregnancy. The placenta connects a woman's body to the embryo and then the fetus through the umbilical cord. The cells that make up the placenta, called trophoblasts, function to control the degree of uterine invasion in the mother and the development of a nutrient, gas, and waste transport for the fetus. The fetus receives oxygen and nutrients from the mother and eliminates wastes through the placenta. The placenta is necessary for the development and survival of the fetus during pregnancy, but it must be delivered from the mother's body after the baby's birth. It is then termed the afterbirth.

In addition to its primary goal of transporting nutrients, oxygen, and waste between mother and fetus, the placenta also serves as a major endocrine organ. The placenta synthesizes and secretes sex steroid and protein hormones. One hormone in particular, human chorionic gonadotropin (hCG), is secreted by the placenta about one week after an egg has been fertilized (conception). This hormone stimulates the production of the steroid hormone progesterone, which is needed for survival of the baby. The detection of hCG in a mother's urine is the most common test for pregnancy.

Disorders and Diseases

In most pregnant women, the placenta forms and grows normally. In some cases, however, the placenta does not grow properly, is poorly positioned in the uterus, or does not function properly. It may be too large or small or connect abnormally. Placental problems are among the most common complications with pregnancy.

Placenta previa is a condition that occurs during pregnancy when the placenta implants in the lower part of the uterus and obstructs the cervical opening to the birth canal. The incidence of placenta previa is approximately one of two hundred births.

Placenta abruptio during pregnancy is a condition in which the placenta separates from the uterus before the fetus is born. This condition occurs in about one of every ninety deliveries. A woman is more likely to develop this condition if she has preeclampsia. The cause is not known, but preeclampsia usually occurs in the second half of pregnancy. Signs include high blood pressure, swelling, and protein in the urine. The risk of preeclampsia is higher in women carrying multiple fetuses, in teenage mothers, and in women older than age forty. Most women with preeclampsia still deliver healthy babies, but a rare few may develop a condition called eclampsia (seizures caused by toxemia), which is very serious for the mother and the baby. Approximately 8 percent of pregnant women will develop preeclampsia.

When the placenta fails to develop or function properly, the fetus cannot grow and develop normally; this is called placental insufficiency. The earlier in pregnancy that this occurs, the more severe the resulting problems. If placental insufficiency occurs for a long time during pregnancy, then it may lead to intrauterine growth retardation or restriction (IUGR), a condition in which the fetus does not grow as large as it should while in the uterus. These babies are very small for their gestational age. IUGR can be caused by decreased blood flow to the placenta, drug use, smoking, alcoholism, or placental abnormalities. A diagnosis can be made through ultrasound to measure fetal growth and a non-stress test that measures the heart rate and movement of the fetus. Between 3 and 5 percent of all pregnancies are complicated by IUGR caused by placental insufficiency. A baby with severe IUGR is more likely to have health problems in the newborn period, as well as throughout childhood.

Perspective and Prospects

The placenta is a unique organ essential for the birth of a child. The most common problems in pregnancy involve the placenta; fortunately, many are manageable. With preeclampsia, delivery of the baby is the best way to protect both the mother and the baby. This is not always possible, however, because it may be too early for the baby to live outside the womb. In this case, steps can be taken to manage the preeclampsia until the baby can be delivered, including decreasing blood pressure with bed rest or medicine. Fortunately, preeclampsia is usually detected early in women who obtain regular prenatal care, and most problems can be prevented. Most cases of IUGR cannot be prevented, especially if they are the result of genetic causes. Some cases can be prevented by taking the following precautions: abstinence from alcohol, tobacco, and illicit drugs; careful monitoring and early treatment for high blood pressure and diabetes; and a diet high in folate before and during pregnancy to protect against certain birth defects.

—*Thomas L. Brown, Ph.D.*

See also Childbirth; Childbirth complications; Embryology; Miscarriage; Preeclampsia and eclampsia; Pregnancy and gestation; Premature birth; Stillbirth; Ultrasonography; Umbilical cord; Uterus.

For Further Information:

Benirschke, Kurt, Graham Burton, and Rebecca Baergen. *Pathology of the Human Placenta*. 6th ed. New York: Springer, 2012.

Berven, Eirik, and Andras Freberg. *Human Placenta: Structure and Development, Circulation, and Functions*. New York: Nova Biomedical Books, 2010.

Harding, Richard, and Alan D. Bocking, eds. *Fetal Growth and Development*. New York: Cambridge University Press, 2001.

Kay, Helen H., D. Michael Nelson, and Yuping Wang. *The Placenta: From Development to Disease*. Chichester, England: Wiley-Blackwell, 2011.

Power, Michael L, and Jay Schulkin. *The Evolution of the Human Placenta*. Baltimore, Md.: Johns Hopkins University Press, 2012.

Tilly, Jonathan L., Jerome F. Strauss, and Martin Tenniswood, eds. *Cell Death in Reproductive Physiology*. New York: Springer-Verlag, 1997.

Wynn, Ralph M., and William P. Jollie, eds. *Biology of the Uterus*. 2d ed. New York: Plenum, 1989.

Plague

Disease/Disorder

Anatomy or system affected: Lungs, respiratory system

Specialties and related fields: Bacteriology, emergency medicine, environmental health, epidemiology, public health

Definition: An infection transmitted by fleas, which may prove fatal if left untreated.

Causes and Symptoms

Plague is caused by infection with a bacterium called *Yersinia pestis* (formerly *Pasteurella pestis*). *Yersinia pestis* is a gram-negative, bipolar-staining bacillus that predominantly infects rodents, with humans being accidental hosts. The disease is transmitted by the bite of a flea that has become infected after a blood meal from another animal with the bacterium in its bloodstream or by the ingestion of contaminated animal tissues.

There are three cycles that perpetuate plague in animals and humans. Sylvatic or wild plague is maintained in the wild rodent population, such as ground squirrels, rock squirrels, and prairie dogs. Urban rat plague occurs in developing countries, especially seaports, and is maintained by the infection of urban and domestic rats, which during epidemics may be as high as 10 percent of the rat population. Finally, there is pneumonic plague, a form of the disease limited to humans, which directly transmit the infection via infected aerosol droplets from a person with a lung infection.

The most common plague illness in humans is called bubonic plague. After an incubation period of two to eight days following the bite of an infected flea, there is a sudden onset of fever, chills, weakness, and headache. Within hours, extremely tender oval swellings one to ten centimeters in length appear in one anatomic area of lymph nodes, usually the groin, axilla (armpit), or neck. These buboes presumably result when the bacteria inoculated into the

Information on Plague
Causes: Bacterial infection transmitted through bite of infected flea
Symptoms: Sudden onset of fever, chills, weakness, headache; extremely tender oval swellings; pneumonia
Duration: Acute, often fatal if untreated
Treatments: Antibiotics, supportive care

skin by the infected flea migrate to the regional lymph nodes. Many of these patients will have bacteria intermittently present in the bloodstream during the acute stage of the illness.

Less common, but more severe, forms of the illness include septicemic and pneumonic plague. Septicemic plague occurs when the inoculated bacteria proliferate rapidly in the blood, overwhelming the patient before producing a bubo. Pneumonic plague may occur as a secondary pneumonia in bubonic plague, when the lung becomes infected by bacteria carried in the bloodstream, or as a primary pneumonia, through direct inhalation following exposure to a coughing plague patient. Septicemic and pneumonic plague are often fatal, especially if antibiotic therapy is delayed. Rarely, plague can be manifested as a pharyngitis resembling acute tonsillitis or meningitis.

Treatment and Therapy

A diagnosis of plague is suspected in febrile patients who have been exposed to rodents in areas of the world known to harbor the disease. The causative bacteria are usually

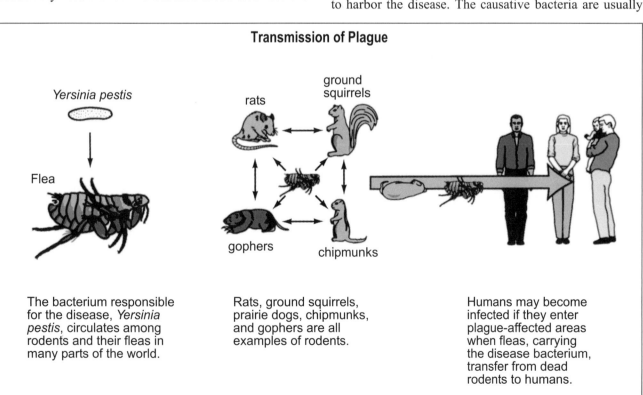

Transmission of Plague

Yersinia pestis

Flea

rats

ground squirrels

gophers

chipmunks

The bacterium responsible for the disease, *Yersinia pestis*, circulates among rodents and their fleas in many parts of the world.

Rats, ground squirrels, prairie dogs, chipmunks, and gophers are all examples of rodents.

Humans may become infected if they enter plague-affected areas when fleas, carrying the disease bacterium, transfer from dead rodents to humans.

A variety of small mammals, particularly rodents, carry the flea that transmits the plague bacterium Yersinia pestis.

identified by microscopic examination and culture of material obtained from aspiration of a bubo. Blood, sputum, throat swabs, or spinal fluid can be processed in a similar manner.

Quarantine, rat control, and insecticides to kill fleas have successfully controlled urban plague in many cities around the globe. Sylvatic plague has been more difficult to control because of the range and diversity of the world rodent reservoirs. A vaccine is available for selected high-risk individuals. Untreated plague has a mortality of more than 50 percent, but this high risk of death can be reduced by the early institution of antibiotic treatment with either streptomycin or tetracycline and the use of modern medical supportive care.

Perspective and Prospects

The first pandemic of plague began in Egypt or Ethiopia in 540 CE. and continued for sixty years, killing about one hundred million people. The second pandemic, called the Black Death, began in the fourteenth century in central Asia and then spread to Europe, where a quarter of the total population died. The world is currently in the third pandemic, which began in China during the 1890s when infected rats were inadvertently transported on ships to other countries in the Americas, Asia, and Africa.

Currently, between one thousand and two thousand cases are reported each year to the World Health Organization, with African countries leading the list in numbers of cases. The United States reports an average of one to seventeen cases per year, mostly from Arizona and New Mexico. American Indians seem especially susceptible to this disease.

—*H. Bradford Hawley, M.D.*

See also Bacterial infections; Biological and chemical weapons; Bites and stings; Epidemics and pandemics; Epidemiology; Insect-borne diseases; Pneumonia.

For Further Information:
Altman, Linda Jacobs. *Plague and Pestilence: A History of Infectious Disease*. Springfield, N.J.: Enslow, 1998.
Centers for Disease Control and Prevention. "Plague: Maps and Statistics." *Centers for Disease Control and Prevention*, April 23, 2013.
Chase, Marilyn. *The Barbary Plague: The Black Death in Victorian San Francisco*. New York: Random House, 2003.
Cook, Gordon C., and Alimuddin I. Zumla, eds. *Manson's Tropical Diseases*. 22d ed. Edinburgh: Saunders/Elsevier, 2009.
Desalle, Rob. *Epidemic! The World of Infectious Disease*. New York: New Press, 2000.
Farmer, Paul. *Infections and Inequalities: The Modern Plagues*. Updated ed. Berkeley: University of California Press, 2009.
Gottfried, Robert S. *The Black Death: Natural and Human Disaster in Medieval Europe*. New York: Free Press/Macmillan, 1983.
Mandell, Gerald L., John E. Bennett, and Raphael Dolin, eds. *Mandell, Douglas, and Bennett's Principles and Practice of Infectious Diseases*. 7th ed. Philadelphia: Churchill Livingstone/Elsevier, 2010.
MedlinePlus. "Plague." *MedlinePlus*, January 14, 2013.
Puzanov, Igor. "Plague." *Health Library*, November 2012.
Woods, Gail L., et al. *Diagnostic Pathology of Infectious Diseases*. Philadelphia: Lea & Febiger, 1993.

Plaque, arterial

Disease/Disorder
Also known as: Atheroma, atheromatous plaque
Anatomy or system affected: Blood vessels, circulatory system, heart
Specialties and related fields: Cardiology, internal medicine, vascular medicine
Definition: Fatty deposits within arterial walls.

Causes and Symptoms

Arterial plaques are caused by a buildup of cholesterol and cell debris within arterial walls. This process occurs over a period of decades, starting at local sites of arterial inflammation. Low-density lipoproteins carrying cholesterol (LDL-C) that infiltrate these sites are highly susceptible to oxidation, which activates another inflammatory response that summons macrophages (part of the immune system). The macrophages engulf the oxidized LDL-C and accumulate as bloated foam cells along with some other cells to become a fatty streak. A tug-of-war ensues in which cholesterol continues to accumulate while other processes remove it. When too much cholesterol accumulates, a scablike cap is formed, while other processes slowly calcify the plaque from the bottom up. This strategy works well as long as the cap does not crack; a cracked cap leaks debris into the artery, which triggers thrombosis (clotting). Blockage of a large coronary artery causes a heart attack; blockage of arteries feeding the brain causes a stroke. Clots that are not fully occlusive get degraded, but repeated rounds of plaque rupturing and recapping eventually cause stenosis (narrowing of the artery) and ischemia (oxygen starvation).

Treatment and Therapy

Treatment begins with lifestyle changes-exercising, managing stress, stopping smoking, lowering blood pressure, eating more fruits and vegetables. The next step is reducing high levels of LDL-C using statins, which also provide antioxidant, anti-inflammatory, and plaque-stabilizing benefits. Bile acid sequestrants and cholesterol absorption inhibitors are sometimes used as well. Fibrates and niacin are used to counteract LDL-C by boosting HDL-C, the high-density lipoprotein or "good" cholesterol. High blood

---

Information on Arterial Plaque

Causes: Hypercholesterolemia, hypertension, inflammation
Symptoms: None in early stages; in later stages, when blood flow impaired, then unusual fatigue, light-headedness, palpitations, feeling of pressure on chest (angina)
Duration: Chronic
Treatments: Lifestyle changes, statins, blood pressure medication

pressure is typically treated using diuretics, beta blockers, or angiotensin-converting enzyme (ACE) inhibitors. Thrombosis risk is reduced using low-dose aspirin or drugs such as warfarin, clopidogrel, and prasugrel. Stenosis can be treated using nitroglycerin, ranolazine, and calcium-channel inhibitors to help arteries dilate. A common surgical procedure is to physically open the artery using a catheter, often done in conjunction with implanting a stent to keep the artery propped open. Surgery can also be used to scrape out arteries or replace them.

Perspective and Prospects

Once plaques reach their later stages of development, they are extremely difficult, if not impossible, to remove. Prospects are best when lifestyle changes are initiated early in adulthood. Blood tests for assessing risk factors are invaluable; the most useful ones measure fasting levels of glucose, total cholesterol, LDL-C, HDL-C, triglycerides, homocysteine, and C-reactive protein (a marker of inflammation). Monitoring and controlling blood pressure is also vitally important.

—*Brad Rikke, Ph.D.*

See also Angina; Angiography; Angioplasty; Arteriosclerosis; Bypass surgery; Cardiac arrest; Cardiology; Cholesterol; Circulation; Claudication; Embolism; Endarterectomy; Echocardiography; Heart; Heart attack; Heart disease; Hypercholesterolemia; Hyperlipidemia; Hypertension; Ischemia; Phlebitis; Stents; Strokes; Thrombolytic therapy and TPA; Thrombosis and thrombus; Transient ischemic attacks (TIAs); Vascular medicine; Vascular system; Venous insufficiency.

For Further Information:

Crowley, Leonard V. *An Introduction to Human Disease, Pathology, and Pathophysiology Correlations.* 9th ed. Boston: Jones and Bartlett, 2013.
Mittal, Satish. *Coronary Heart Disease in Clinical Practice.* London: Springer, 2005.
Rosenblum, Laurie. "Atherosclerosis." *Health Library,* May 8, 2013.

Plaque, dental

Disease/Disorder
Also known as: Dental biofilm
Anatomy or system affected: Mouth, teeth
Specialties and related fields: Dentistry
Definition: Various kinds of bacteria that live in the mouth stick to each other and then to the tooth surface, both above and below the gums, causing tooth decay and gum disease.
Key terms:
gingivitis: inflammation of the gum tissue
periodontitis: inflammation of the tissues around the teeth
tartar: hardened, mineralized layers of dental plaque

Causes and Symptoms

Dental plaque begins to form when food that contains sugars and starches adheres to teeth. Bacteria that harmlessly live in the mouth feed on these carbohydrates and excrete acids. These acids dissolve the minerals in the enamel on the surfaces of teeth, leading to tooth decay. They also irritate the gums, causing gingivitis and periodontitis. When

> ## Information on Dental Plaque
> **Causes:** Bacterial buildup on teeth
> **Symptoms:** Slimy sensation to tongue
> **Duration:** Temporary until cleaned
> **Treatments:** Toothbrushing, professional cleaning, tooth scaling

dental plaque builds up, it can become mineralized; this form is called tartar. Plaque especially accumulates in the grooves of the molars, between adjacent teeth, and along the margin between the teeth and gums.

Susceptibility to tooth decay from dental plaque is dependent upon how clean the mouth is kept, whether fluoride is in the toothpaste and drinking water, the amount of moisture in the mouth, the composition of the diet, and heredity.

Plaque can be felt with the tongue as a slime on the surface of teeth. Because plaque is colorless and accumulates in areas that are difficult to see and reach, hasty toothbrushing may not effectively remove it. Disclosing tablets and solutions are available that contain a harmless dye to stain the bacteria, thereby indicating where plaque remains after brushing.

A study published by the *British Medical Journal* in 2012 linked poor oral hygiene and increased dental plaque to increased incidents of cancer deaths.

Treatment and Therapy

Removing dental plaque from teeth is important for good oral health. Teeth should be brushed thoroughly at least twice a day with a fluoride toothpaste. Dental floss should be used daily to remove bacteria and food from between teeth and under the gum line where a toothbrush may not reach. Mouthwash containing fluoride should be used to rinse away plaque and keep oral tissues moist. Sticky, sugary, and starchy foods and beverages should be limited; raw fruits and vegetables are good choices because they disrupt plaque buildup. Teeth should be professionally examined and cleaned every six months. In cases of stubborn tartar accumulation, tooth scaling by a dental professional may be required more frequently. In addition to antiseptics and antibiotics, som me dentists also use lasers to treat the growth of bacteria in pockets of gum near the teeth.

Perspective and Prospects

Tartar control toothpastes now contain pyrophosphates to inhibit mineralization along with antibacterial agents to control the bacteria population. Dentists are now offering sealants, a thin coating of plastic that is painted on the chewing surfaces of molars to prevent plaque from building up in the grooves.

—*Bethany Thivierge, M.P.H., E.L.S.*

See also Cavities; Dental diseases; Dentistry; Dentistry, pediatric; Endodontic disease; Fluoride treatments; Gingivitis; Gum disease; Periodontitis; Root canal treatment; Teeth; Teething; Toothache.

For Further Information:
Smiech-Slomkowska, Grazyna, et al. "The Effect of Oral Health Education on Dental Plaque Development and the Level of Caries-Related *Streptococcus mutans* and *Lactobacillus* spp." *European Journal of Orthodontics* 29 (April, 2007): 157-160.
Soderling, E. M. "Xylitol, Mutans Streptococci, and Dental Plaque." *Advances in Dental Research* 21 (August, 2009): 74-78.
Wahaidi, V. Y., et al. "Neutrophil Response to Dental Plaque by Gender and Race." *Journal of Dental Research* 88, no. 8 (August, 2009): 709-714.

Plasma

Anatomy

Anatomy or system affected: Blood, blood vessels, cells, circulatory system, endocrine system, heart, immune system, respiratory system, urinary system

Specialties and related fields: Biochemistry, cardiology, cytology, endocrinology, general surgery, hematology, internal medicine, microbiology, nutrition, serology, vascular medicine

Definition: The liquid component of the blood that transports the blood cells.

Structure and Functions

A clear, straw-colored liquid, plasma makes up about 55 percent of the total blood volume. Although its major component is water (90 percent by volume), plasma also contains glucose, proteins, clotting factors, hormones, carbon dioxide, and dissolved salts and minerals. The main proteins in plasma are albumin, globulins, and clotting proteins, particularly fibrinogen. Gamma globulin is an important component of the immune system. Mineral ions in plasma include sodium, potassium, chloride, bicarbonate, calcium, and magnesium. These electrolytes are essential in maintaining fluid balance, nerve conduction, muscle contraction, blood clotting, and pH balance in the body.

Suspended within the plasma are red blood cells (erythrocytes), five kinds of white blood cells (leukocytes), and platelets (thrombocytes). In addition to carrying these blood cells, plasma transports nutrients, waste products, antibodies, clotting agents, and chemical messengers to help maintain a healthy body. Plasma circulates dissolved nutrients throughout the body, where they are diffused by osmotic pressure into the tissues and cells that need them. It is also the main medium for transporting excretory products to the kidneys and lungs for elimination.

Disorders and Diseases

The most characteristic disease associated with plasma is hemophilia. It results from an inherited change in one of the clotting proteins (factor VIII), leaving it dysfunctional. This single change disrupts the chemical reactions necessary for clotting. As a result, patients with hemophilia experience bleeding, swelling, and bruising. Crippling defects may include recurrent hemorrhaging into joints and muscles and bleeding into body cavities.

Tests of the clotting function of plasma include analysis of indicators such as the prothrombin time and the partial thromboplastin time. These tests identify a deficiency of any of the clotting factors. Most cases involving abnormal bleeding can then be traced to specific defects. Hemophilia can be controlled by infusion of factor VIII that has been collected from donated blood or plasma.

Perspective and Prospects

The possibility of using blood plasma for transfusion purposes was reported in a medical journal by physician Gordon R. Ward in 1918. Due to the advantages that plasma has over whole blood with regard to shelf life and donor-recipient compatibility, the use of plasma for blood transfusions was advanced during the 1930s. During World War II, anatomist Charles Drew developed a modern, highly sterile system for processing, testing, and storing plasma in a blood bank. During the early twenty-first century, research suggests that exploring and measuring the plasma proteome (the proteins in plasma, of which there are known to be 289) can help track slow changes associated with disease, such as rheumatoid arthritis. The best therapeutic options and drugs available for treatment of the disease can then be implemented.

—*Alvin K. Benson, Ph.D.*

See also Bleeding; Blood and blood disorders; Blood testing; Circulation; Disseminated intravascular coagulation (DIC); Fluids and electrolytes; Hematology; Hematology, pediatric; Hemophilia; Pathology; Rh factor; Serology; Thrombocytopenia; Transfusion; Von Willebrand's disease; Wiskott-Aldrich syndrome.

For Further Information:
Berenson, James R. "Overview of Plasma Cell Disorders." *Merck Manual Home Health Handbook*, July 2008.
De la Rocha, Kelly, Igor Puzanov, and Brian Randall. "Plasmapheresis." *Health Library*, May 11, 2013.
"Hemophilia." *MedlinePlus*, June 26, 2013.
Schaller, Johann, et al. *Human Blood Plasma Proteins: Structure and Function.* New York: Wiley, 2008.
Trice, Linda. *Charles Drew: Pioneer of Blood Plasma.* New York: McGraw-Hill, 2000.
Valverde, José Luis, ed. *Blood, Plasma, and Plasma Proteins: A Unique Contribution to Modern Healthcare.* Amsterdam: IOS Press, 2006. Pharmaceuticals Policy and Law 7.

Plastic surgery

Procedures

Anatomy or system affected: All

Specialties and related fields: Dermatology, emergency medicine, general surgery, oncology, physical therapy, psychology

Definition: Plastic surgery uses such procedures as grafting and the implantation of prostheses in order to treat congenital defects and tissue or limb damage resulting from trauma; reconstructive surgery uses the techniques of plastic surgery to repair injured tissues or to reattach severed body parts, while cosmetic surgery employs these same methods to alter body shape or appearance for aesthetic purposes.

Key terms:

congenital: existing at birth; often used in reference to certain mental or physical malformations and diseases, which may be hereditary or caused by some influence during gestation

cosmetic surgery: the application of plastic surgical techniques to alter one's appearance for purely aesthetic reasons

debridement: the excision of contused and devitalized tissue from a wound surface

dermis: the second layer of skin, immediately below the epidermis; it contains blood and lymphatic vessels, nerves, glands, and (usually) hair follicles

epidermis: the outermost thin layer of skin that encompasses structures superficial to the dermis

granuloma: a nodular, inflammatory lesion that is usually small, firm, and persistent and usually contains proliferated macrophages

plastic surgery: the branch of operative surgery concerning the repair of defects, the replacement of lost tissue, and the treatment of extensive scarring; it accomplishes these ends by direct union of body parts, grafting, or the transfer of tissue from one part of the body to another

reconstructive surgery: the application of plastic surgical techniques to repair damaged tissues

turgor: fullness and firmness; the quality of normal skin in a healthy young person

Indications and Procedures

The intent of plastic, reconstructive, and cosmetic surgery is to restore a body part to normal appearance or to enhance or cosmetically alter a body part. The techniques and procedures of all three surgical applications are similar: extremely careful skin preparation, the use of delicate instrumentation and handling techniques, and precise suturing with extremely fine materials to minimize scarring.

Reconstructive surgery. Notable examples of reconstructive surgery involve the reattachment of limbs or extremities that have been traumatically severed. As soon as a part is separated from the body, it loses its blood supply; this leads to ischemia (lack of oxygen) to tissues, which in turn leads to cell death. When an individual cell dies, it cannot be resuscitated and will soon start to decompose. This process can be greatly slowed by lowering the temperature of the severed body part. Packing the part in ice for transport to a hospital is a prudent initial step.

An important consideration in any reconstructive procedure is site preparation. The edges, or margins, of the final wound must be clean and free of contamination. Torn skin is removed through a process called debridement. A sharp scalpel is used gently to cut away tissue that has been crushed or torn. All bacterial contamination must be removed from the site prior to closure to prevent postoperative contamination. Foreign material such as dirt, glass, gunpowder, metals, or chemicals must be completely removed. The margins of the wound must also be sharply defined. Superficially, this is done for aesthetic reasons. Internally, sharply defined margins will reduce the chances for adhesions to form. Adhesions are bands of scar tissue which bind adjacent structures together and restrict normal movement and function. Therefore, both the body site and the margins of the severed part must be debrided and defined. Reconstruction consists of the painstaking reattachment of nerves, tendons, muscles, and skin, which

are held in place primarily by sutures although staples, wires, and other materials are occasionally used. Precise alignment of the skin to be closed is accomplished by joining opposing margins. Postoperative procedures include careful handling of the wound site, adequate nutrition, and rest in order to maximize healing. Abnormalities in the healing process can lead to undesirable scarring from the sites of sutures. Such marks can be avoided with careful attention to correct techniques.

Bones are reconstructed in cases of severe fractures. The pieces are set in their proper positions, and the area is immobilized. Where immobilization is not possible, a surface is provided onto which new bone can grow. These temporary surfaces are made of polymeric materials that will dissolve over time.

Congenital anomalies such as a deformed external ear or missing digit can be corrected using reconstructive techniques. In the case of a missing thumb, a finger can be removed, rotated, and attached on the site where the thumb should have been. This allows an affected individual to write, hold objects such as eating utensils, and generally have a more nearly normal life. Similar procedures can be applied to replace a missing or amputated great or big toe. The presence of the great toe contributes significantly to balance and coordination when walking.

Prosthetic materials are implanted in a growing variety of applications. There are two basic types of materials used in prostheses, which are classified according to their surface characteristics. One is totally smooth and inert; an example is Teflon or silicone. The body usually encloses these materials in a membrane, which has the effect of creating a wall or barrier to the surface of the prosthesis. From the body's perspective, the prosthesis has thus been removed. With any prosthesis, the problem most likely to be encountered is infection, which is usually caused by contamination of the operative site or the prosthesis. Infection can also occur at a later, postoperative date because of the migration of bacteria into the cavity formed by the membrane. This is a potentially serious complication. A smooth prosthesis can also be used to create channels into which tissue can later be inserted. In such an application, the prosthesis may be surgically removed at some time in the future. A second type of prosthesis does not have a smooth surface; rather, it has microscopic fibers similar to those found on a towel. This type of surface prevents membranes from forming, contributing to a longer life for the prosthesis by reducing postoperative infections.

An important procedure in reconstructive surgery is skin grafting. A graft consists of skin that is completely removed from a donor site and transferred to another site on the body. The graft is usually taken from the patient's own body because skin taken from another individual will be rejected by the recipient's immune system. (Nevertheless, fetal pig skin is sometimes used successfully.) Skin grafting is useful for covering open wounds, and it is widely used in serious burn cases. When only a portion of the uppermost layer of the skin is removed, the process is called a split thickness graft. When all the upper layers of the skin are removed, the result is a full thickness graft. Whenever possible, the donor site is selected to match the color and texture characteristics of the recipient site.

A skin flap is sometimes created. This differs from a graft in that the skin of a flap is not completely severed from its original site but simply moved to an adjacent location. Some blood vessels remain to support the flap. This procedure is nearly always successful, but it is limited to immediately adjacent skin.

A wide variety of flaps has been developed. A flap may be stretched and sutured to cover both a wound and the donor site. Flaps may be created from skin that is distant to the site where it is needed and then sutured in place over the donor site. Only after the flap has become established at the new site is it cut free from the donor site. Thus, skin from the abdomen or upper chest may be used to cover the back of a burned hand, or skin from one finger may be used to cover a finger on the other hand. This two-stage flap process requires more time than a skin graft, but it also has a greater probability of success.

Plastic surgery. Plastic surgery consists of a variety of techniques and applications, often dealing with skin. Some common procedures that primarily involve skin are undertaken to remove unwanted wrinkles or folds. Folds in skin are caused by a loss of skin turgor and excessive stretching of the skin beyond which it cannot recover. Common contributors to loss of skin turgor in the abdomen are pregnancy or significant weight loss after years of obesity. Both women and men may undergo a procedure known as abdominoplasty (commonly called a "tummy tuck"). The skin that lies over the abdominal muscles is carefully separated from underlying tissue. Portions of the skin are removed; frequently, some underlying adipose (fat) tissue is also removed or relocated. The remaining skin is sutured to the underlying muscle as well as to adjacent, undisturbed skin. A major problem with this procedure, however, is scar formation because large portions of skin must be removed or relocated. The plastic surgeon must plan the placement of incisions carefully in order to avoid undesirable scars.

Plastic surgery is also used to reduce the prominence of ears, a procedure called otoplasty. In some children, the posterior (back) portion of the external ear develops more than the rest of the ear, pushing the ears outward and making them prominent. By reducing the bulk of cartilage in the posterior ear and suturing the remaining external portion to the base of the ear, the plastic surgeon can create a more normal ear contour. The optimal time to perform this procedure on children is just prior to the time that they enter school, or at about five years of age.

Cosmetic surgery. The most common site for cosmetic surgical procedures is the face. Correction may be desired because of a congenital anomaly that causes unwelcome disfigurement or because of a desire to alter an unwanted aspect of one's body. The cosmetic procedures that have been developed to correct abnormalities of the face include closure of a cleft lip or palate. The correction of a cleft lip is usually done early, ideally in the first three months of life. Closure of a cleft palate (the bone that forms the roof of the mouth) is delayed slightly, until the patient is 12 to 18 months old. These procedures allow affected individuals to acquire normal patterns of speech and language.

Among older individuals, common procedures include blepharoplasty and rhinoplasty. The former refers to the removal of excess skin around the eyelids, while the latter refers to a change, usually a reduction, in the shape of the nose. Both procedures may be included in the more general term of face lift. The effects of aging, excessive solar radiation, and gravity combine to produce fine lines in the face as individuals get older. These fine lines gradually develop into the wrinkles characteristic of older persons. For some, these wrinkles are objectionable. To reduce them-or more correctly to stretch them out-a plastic surgeon removes a section of skin containing the wrinkles or lines and stretches the edges of the remaining epidermis until they are touching. These incisions are placed to coincide with the curved lines that exist in normal skin. Thus, when the edges are sutured together, the resultant scar is minimized. Rhinoplasty often involves the removal of a portion of the bone or cartilage that forms the nose. The bulk of the remaining tissue is also reduced to maintain the desired proportions of the patient's nose. As with any plastic surgical procedure, small sutures are carefully placed to minimize scarring.

A third body area that is commonly subjected to cosmetic procedures is the breast. A woman who is unhappy with the appearance of her breasts may seek to either reduce or augment existing tissue. Breast reduction is accomplished by careful incision and the judicious removal of both skin and underlying breast tissue. Often the nipples must be repositioned to maintain their proper locations. A flap that includes the nipple is created from each breast. After the desired amount of underlying tissue is removed, the nipples are repositioned, and the skin is recontoured around the remaining breast masses.

Uses and Complications

Reconstructive, plastic, and cosmetic surgeries all have their complications, ranging from severe-such as the rejection of transplanted tissue-to minor but unpleasant-such as noticeable scars. In addition, there is an inherent risk in any procedure that requires the patient to undergo general anesthesia. With reconstruction, which involves the repair of damaged tissues and structures, the initial injuries sustained by the patient present further obstacles and dangers. The following examples from each type of surgery illustrate the risks involved.

For example, a surgeon who must perform a skin graft can choose between a split or a full thickness graft. A split thickness graft site will heal with relatively normal skin, thus providing opportunities for additional grafting at a later date. It also produces less pronounced scarring. A limitation of this technique, however, is an increased likelihood for the graft to fail. Full thickness grafts are stronger and more likely to be successful, but they lead to more extensive scarring, which is aesthetically undesirable and renders the site unsuitable for later grafts. The surgeon's decision is based on the needs of the patient and the severity of the injury.

The minimization of scarring is a major concern for many patients undergoing plastic surgery. The prevention of noticeable scars involves an understanding of the natural lines of the skin. All areas of the body have lines of significant skin tension and lines of relatively little skin tension. It is along the lines of minimal tension that wrinkles and folds develop over time. These lines are curved and follow body contours. As a rule of thumb, they are generally perpendicular to the fibers of underlying muscle. The plastic surgeon seeks to place incisions along the lines of minimal tension. When scars form after healing, they will blend into the line of minimal tension and become less noticeable. Furthermore, the scar tissue is not likely to become apparent when the underlying muscles or body part is moved. Undesirable scarring is a greater problem in large procedures, such as abdominoplasty, than in procedures confined to a small area, such as rhytidectomy (face lift), because of the difficulty in following lines of minimum tension when making incisions.

One of the most popular cosmetic procedures is breast enlargement. According to the American Society of Plastic Surgeons, 296,203 augmentation mammoplasties were performed in the United States in 2010, and the total number of women with implants in the United States is in the millions. Initially, the most commonly used prosthesis, or implant, was made of silicone. In some patients, silicone leaked out, causing the formation of granulomatous tissue. Such complications led to a voluntary suspension of the production of silicone prostheses by manufacturers and of their usage by surgeons. Different materials, such as polyethylene bags filled with saline solution or solid polyurethane implants, were soon substituted. Saline will not cause tissue damage if it leaks, and few adverse reactions to polyurethane have been reported. Silicone implants made a comeback in 2006, when the US Food and Drug Administration began approving them for use in women aged twenty-two years or older.

Perspective and Prospects

The origins of plastic, reconstructive, and cosmetic surgery are fundamental to the earliest surgical procedures, which were developed to correct superficial deformities. Without any viable methods of anesthesia, surgical interventions and corrections were limited to the skin. For example, present-day nose reconstructions (rhinoplasty) are essentially similar to procedures developed four thousand years ago. Hindu surgeons developed the technique of moving a piece

---

In the News: Wrinkle Treatment with Botox and Artefill

As a person ages, the collagen and elastin proteins in the skin that keep it supple and smooth begin to weaken. The skin begins to thin and lose fat, and gravity causes the skin to sag. Wrinkles and deep facial folds develop. While these changes once seemed inevitable and were reversible only through major plastic surgery, new products and treatments are rejuvenating aging faces. Two such products are Botox and Artefill (sold as Artecoll in countries outside the United States).

Botulinum toxin type A (Botox cosmetic) is a compound produced by the bacterium *Clostridium botulinum* and is the same toxin that causes the potentially lethal food poisoning known as botulism. When used to combat wrinkles, the toxin is highly purified and diluted thousands of times, then injected in very small, safe doses into facial muscles, particularly between the eyebrows and at the sides of the eyes. The toxin blocks the release of a chemical signal called acetylcholine from nerve cells, which normally leads to muscle contraction. Botox paralyzes the muscles to eliminate frowning and to relax the associated furrows and lines around the eyes and between the eyebrows. The effect lasts for three to four months or more, and then the procedure must be repeated to maintain the wrinkle-free appearance.

Botox was first approved for use in treating eye muscle disorders in 1989, and in April, 2002, the Food and Drug Administration (FDA) approved Botox for wrinkles, although it had been used legally to treat wrinkles prior to official approval. In 2001, more than 1.6 million Botox injections were given to an estimated 850,000 patients in the United States. The number of people using Botox is anticipated to increase over the next several years.

As an alternative to Botox treatment for wrinkles, Artefill has the advantage of being a long-term or potentially permanent treatment. Artefill is an injectable implant that contains tiny nonbiodegradable polymer microspheres of polymethylmethacrylate (PMMA) suspended in a solution containing 75 percent collagen. Artefill is injected into the wrinkle or facial fold, where the microspheres stimulate the body to produce its own collagen, which surrounds and encapsulates the microspheres. Within three to six months, the implant becomes permanently anchored in place by the body, where it plumps up the wrinkle.

Artefill has been used successfully to treat more than 200,000 patients outside the United States. Clinical trials of the implant in the United States were completed in September, 2001. In 2003, an FDA advisory panel recommended approval of Artefill for the treatment of wrinkles.

—*Karen E. Kalumuck, Ph.D.*

---

of skin from the adjacent cheek onto the nose to cover a wound. Similar procedures were developed by Italians using skin that was transferred from the arm or forehead to repair lips and ears as well as noses. Ironically, wars have provided opportunities to advance reconstructive techniques. As field hospitals and surgical facilities became more widely available and wounded soldiers could be stabilized during transport, techniques to repair serious wounds evolved.

Skin grafts have been used since Roman times. Celsus described the possibility of skin grafts in conjunction with eye surgery. References were made to skin grafts in the Middle Ages. The evolution of modern techniques can be traced to the early nineteenth century, when Cesare Baronio conducted systematic grafting experiments with animals. The modern guidelines for grafting were formulated in 1870. Instruments for creating split thickness grafts were developed in the 1930s, and applications of this procedure evolved during World War II.

Plastic, reconstructive, and cosmetic procedures have all become important in contemporary surgical practice. Reconstructive surgery allows the repair of serious injuries and contributes greatly to the rehabilitation of affected individuals. Cosmetic surgery can help individuals feel better about themselves and their bodies. Both use techniques developed in the broader field of plastic surgery.

There are both positive and negative aspects of plastic surgery. Positively, many individuals who sustain serious and potentially devastating injuries are able to return to relatively normal lives. Burn victims and those having accidents are more likely to return to normal activities and resume their occupations than at any time in the past. Miniaturization and new materials have extended the range of a plastic surgeon's skills. Negatively, there is growing criticism concerning the number of elective procedures undertaken for the repair of cosmetic defects.

The quest for perfection and physical beauty has prompted some critics to question the correctness of some unnecessary procedures. Although such procedures are not usually covered by insurance policies, their utilization has increased. The continuation of such activities invokes both ethical and personal considerations; there is no clearly defined, logical endpoint. Clearly, while plastic surgical techniques have benefited millions, there are opportunities for abuse. Society must decide if any limitations are to be placed on plastic surgical procedures and what they should be.

In the meantime, advances in materials, instruments, and techniques will benefit plastic, reconstructive, and cosmetic surgery. As but one example, the advent of magnification and miniaturization and the development of tiny instruments and new suture materials have allowed the reconstruction of many injury sites. Blood vessels and nerves are now routinely reattached and a mere nine individual sutures are required to join the severed portions of a blood vessel one millimeter in diameter.

—*L. Fleming Fallon, Jr., M.D., Ph.D., M.P.H.*

See also Age spots; Aging; Amputation; Birthmarks; Body dysmorphic disorder; Botox; Breast cancer; Breast disorders; Breast surgery; Breasts, female; Burns and scalds; Cancer; Carcinoma; Circumcision, female, and genital mutilation; Circumcision, male; Cleft lip and palate; Cleft lip and palate repair; Collagen; Cyst removal; Cysts; Dermatology; Dermatology, pediatric; Ear surgery; Face lift and blepharoplasty; Gender identity disorder; Gender reassignment surgery; Grafts and grafting; Hair loss and baldness; Hair transplantation; Healing; Jaw wiring; Laceration repair; Liposuction; Malignancy and metastasis; Mastectomy and lumpectomy; Melanoma; Moles; Obesity; Otoplasty; Otorhinolaryngology; Ptosis; Rhinoplasty and submucous resection; Skin; Skin lesion removal; Surgical procedures; Varicose vein removal; Varicose veins; Warts; Wrinkles.

For Further Information:
Grazer, Frederick M., and Jerome R. Klingbeil. *Body Image: A Surgical Perspective*. St. Louis, Mo.: Mosby Year Book, 1980.
Loftus, Jean M. *The Smart Woman's Guide to Plastic Surgery*. 2d ed. Dubuque, Iowa: McGraw-Hill, 2008.
MedlinePlus. "Plastic and Cosmetic Surgery." *MedlinePlus*, May 2, 2013.

Narins, Rhoda, and Paul Jarrod Frank. *Turn Back the Clock Without Losing Time: Everything You Need to Know About Simple Cosmetic Procedures*. New York: Three Rivers Press, 2002.
Rutkow, Ira M. *American Surgery: An Illustrated History*. Philadelphia: Lippincott-Raven, 1998.
Townsend, Courtney M., Jr., et al., eds. *Sabiston Textbook of Surgery*. 18th ed. Philadelphia: Saunders/Elsevier, 2012.
Weatherford, M. Lisa, ed. *Reconstructive and Cosmetic Surgery Sourcebook*. Detroit, Mich.: Omnigraphics, 2001.

Pleurisy

Disease/Disorder
Also known as: Pleuritis
Anatomy or system affected: Chest, lungs
Specialties and related fields: Emergency medicine, family medicine, internal medicine, pulmonary medicine
Definition: A syndrome of chest pain made worse by breathing.

Causes and Symptoms

The lungs sit within the chest wall just underneath the rib cage. The pleura is a very thin double lining covering the outer surface of the lungs and the undersurface of the ribs. During normal breathing, the lungs expand and relax, stretching their pleural membrane and moving it back and forth against the pleural membrane lining the rib cage. To minimize friction, a very small amount of fluid fills the space between them.

"Pleurisy" is a descriptive term that refers to chest pain with respiration. It occurs when the pleural membranes become irritated or inflamed. The pain is usually localized at the area of inflammation, but it can radiate toward the neck, shoulder, or abdomen. The pain may be mild discomfort or a severe stabbing or burning sensation. In addition to deep breathing, coughing or movements of the chest can exacerbate symptoms. Because of the pain, the patient may employ rapid, shallow breathing.

Patients with symptoms of a recent cold or respiratory infection likely have pleurisy caused by a virus; however, a

---

Information on Pleurisy

Causes: May include recent cold or respiratory infection; pneumonia; tuberculosis; trauma (muscle sprain, fractured rib); sickle cell disease; advanced kidney failure; recent heart attack; rheumatologic diseases (lupus, rhematoid arthritis); asbestos exposure; punctured lung; pulmonary embolism; lung cancer

Symptoms: Chest pain with respiration, ranging from discomfort or severe stabbing or burning sensation and worsened by coughing or chest movement; sometimes shortness of breath

Duration: One to two weeks

Treatments: Depends on cause; may include drainage of fluid, oxygen therapy, hospitalization

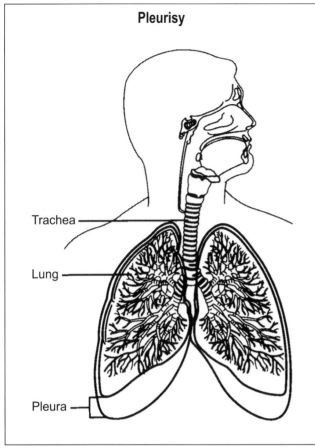

Pleurisy

Trachea

Lung

Pleura

The pleurae are the membranes that encase the lungs; pleurisy is the inflammation of one or both pleurae and may have a variety of causes.

more serious cause, such as pneumonia, may also be responsible. Tuberculosis is another infectious cause to be considered.

Patients with recent injuries to the chest or unusually strenuous activity may have pleurisy attributable to a muscle sprain or a fractured rib. Patients with sickle cell disease, advanced kidney failure, a recent heart attack, rheumatologic diseases such as lupus and rheumatoid arthritis, or asbestos exposure are also prone to pleurisy.

The most worrisome causes of pleurisy are pneumothorax (punctured lung), pulmonary embolism (blood clot in the lung), or lung cancer. These causes are more likely to be associated with shortness of breath, although this symptom is not reliably present.

Treatment and Therapy

Treatment of pleurisy depends on the underlying cause. In most cases, a chest x-ray is indicated. In some cases, a collection of fluid in the pleural space will be visible. However, patients with pleurisy may often have a normal chest x-ray. In concerning cases, particularly those associated with shortness of breath and abnormally low oxygen levels, further radiologic studies, such as a computed tomography (CT) scan or magnetic resonance imaging (MRI), may be necessary.

Pleurisy caused by viral infections, trauma, rheumatologic diseases, and sickle cell disease is generally

treated with pain medications, and the symptoms resolve within one to two weeks. Patients with kidney or heart disease may need drainage of the pleural fluid with a needle or tube placed into the pleural space through the back.

The more serious causes of pleurisy require specialized treatments based on the cause; typically, temporary oxygen supplementation is required, and sometimes hospitalization is necessary.

—*Gregory B. Seymann, M.D.*

See also Asbestos exposure; Chest; Embolism; Lung cancer; Lungs; Pneumonia; Pneumothorax; Pulmonary diseases; Pulmonary medicine; Pulmonary medicine, pediatric; Respiration; Sickle cell disease; Tuberculosis; Wheezing.

For Further Information:

Fishman, Alfred, ed. *Fishman's Pulmonary Diseases and Disorders.* 4th ed. New York: McGraw-Hill, 2008.

Marx, John A., et al., eds. *Rosen's Emergency Medicine: Concepts and Clinical Practice.* 7th ed. Philadelphia: Mosby/Elsevier, 2010.

"Pleurisy and Pleural Effusion." *InteliHealth*, April 19, 2011.

Porter, Robert S., et al., eds. *The Merck Manual Home Health Handbook.* Whitehouse Station, N.J.: Merck Research Laboratories, 2009.

Walsh, Beth. "Pleurisy." *Health Library*, September 1, 2011.

"What Are Pleurisy and Other Pleural Disorders?" *National Heart, Lung, and Blood Institute*, September 21, 2011.

Pneumocystis jirovecii

Disease/Disorder

Also known as: Pneumocystis carinii

Anatomy or system affected: Chest, lungs, respiratory system

Specialties and related fields: Microbiology, nuclear medicine, pulmonary medicine, radiology

Definition: A small fungus that normally lives in the respiratory tract of most people, but causes pneumonia in those with dysfunctional immune systems.

Key terms:

alveoli: terminal branchings of the respiratory tree that act as the primary sites of gas exchange in the lungs

immunosuppression: reducing the activity or efficiency of the immune system

Causes and Symptoms

Pneumocystis jirovecii, a single-celled fungus, commonly lives in the respiratory tracts of healthy people without causing any harm. However, in people whose immune systems do not work properly, *Pneumocystis jirovecii* can cause pneumonia. During World War II, premature and severely malnourished infants were diagnosed with *Pneumocystis jirovecii* pneumonia. Later, other cases were observed in immunosuppressed patients: cancer patients receiving chemotherapy, and transplant recipients being treated with immunosuppressants. Recently, *Pneumocystis jirovecii pneumonia* (PCP) has become the most common cause of death in patients with Acquired Immune Deficiency Syndrome (AIDS).

The life cycle of *Pneumocystis jirovecii* consists of three different stages: the trophozoite or trophic stage, the sporozoite or precystic form, and the cyst, which contains several

---

Information on *Pneumocystis Jirovecii*

Causes: Suppression of the immune system
Symptoms: Cough, fever, rapid breathing, shortness of breath
Duration: Variable
Treatments: Trimethoprim-sulfamethoxazole, clindamycin and primaquine, pentamidine, corticosteroids for lung inflammation

---

spores. Trophozoites live within the alveoli of the lung and are probably the infective form, and transmission occurs by means of airborne transmission.

The symptoms of PCP include shortness of breath upon exertion (dyspnea), fever, nonproductive cough, weight loss, chills, and, rarely, coughing up blood (hemoptysis). PCP patients also have an abnormally fast heart rate (tachycardia, over 100 beats per minute), rapid breathing (tachypnea, more than 20 breaths per minute), and mild crackles and course rattling (rhonchi) when they breathe.

Treatment and Therapy

The nonspecific nature of PCP symptoms necessitates other diagnostic tests to confirm the diagnosis. Observing the organism from respiratory tract fluid by means of various tissue stains provides the most definitive confirmation of PCP. Polymerase chain reaction (PCR) tests have been used successfully as well, but are not yet routinely available. Chest X-rays, computed tomography, or Gallium-67 scans can provide evidence that the patient has PCP, but are not conclusive.

Even though *Pneumocystis jirovecii* is a yeast-like fungus, it does not respond to antifungals, with the possible exception of echinocandin. The first choice for treatment consists of oral or intravenous trimethoprim-sulfamethoxazole (Septra, Bactrim, Sulfatrim). Patients with sulfa allergies or who have PCP infections that are resistant to trimethoprim- sulfamethoxazole should be given a combi-

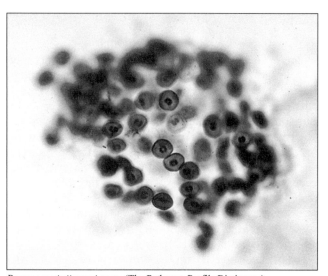

Pneumocystis jiroveci cysts. (The Pathogen Profile Dictionary)

nation of clindamycin and primaquine or intravenous pentamidine. Patients with severe inflammation and fluid in their lungs are treated with corticosteroids to clear their lungs so that they can breathe.

To prevent PCP (chemoprophylaxis), patients usually take trimethoprim-sulfamethoxazole, or dapsone, dapsone plus pyrimethamine, atovaquone, or aerosolized pentamidine. Smoking cessation can also decrease the rate of recurrent PCP infections.

AIDS patients who show the symptoms of PCP begin treatment immediately before completion of diagnostic tests. Babies born to mothers infected with Human Immunodeficiency Virus (HIV) begin preventative treatment 4-6 weeks after birth.

—*Michael A. Buratovich Ph.D.*

See also Immunology; Immunopathology; Lungs; Pulmonary medicine

For Further Information:

Gallant, Joel E. *Johns Hopkins HIV Guide.* Burlington, MA: Jones and Bartlett Learning, 2012.

Miller, Robert F., Laurence Huang, and Peter D. Walzer. "Pneumocystis Pneumonia Associated with Human Immunodeficiency Virus." *Clinics in Chest Medicine* 34, no. 2 (June 2013): 229-241.

Pneumonia

Disease/Disorder

Anatomy or system affected: Lungs, respiratory system
Specialties and related fields: Emergency medicine, epidemiology, family medicine, internal medicine, occupational health, public health, pulmonary medicine
Definition: An inflammation of one of several possible areas of the respiratory system, mainly in the lungs or bronchial passageways, resulting from bacterial or viral infection.

Key terms:

Gram's stain: a laboratory method for tracing the presence of certain bacteria in lung tissue; the procedure involves the observation of different levels of tissue discoloration as specific chemical reactions are induced

pleurisy: a secondary but very painful inflammation of the membranes that line the lungs and chest cavity; often accompanies pneumonia

Pneumocystis pneumonia: a form of pneumonia caused by the single-celled parasite *Pneumocystis carinii*; dangerous primarily to persons with impaired immunity mechanisms, particularly victims of acquired immunodeficiency syndrome (AIDS)

Streptococcus pneumoniae: commonly referred to as pneumococcus; the main bacteria responsible for pneumonia

Causes and Symptoms

Although modern medicine succeeded several generations ago in identifying the key viruses and bacteria responsible for pneumonia and in developing efficient medications for its treatment, a surprisingly high number of deaths from the complications of pneumonia continue to occur. In large part this is the case because pneumonia, which involves infection and inflammation in the respiratory system, occurs not only on its own but also as a complication brought about by other serious illnesses. In aged patients, especially, general deterioration of the body's resistance to bacterial or viral infection can lead in a final stage to death from pneumonia.

Just as the causes of pneumonia can vary, the disease itself may take different forms. Some sources postulate that pneumonia is not a single disease but a group of advanced lung inflammations. Because they are so similar in their symptoms and effects on the body, all members of this family of diseases are labeled as one form or another of pneumonia. Specific forms range from lobar pneumonia (caused by the bacterial invasion of *Streptococcus pneumoniae* into a single lobe of one lung) and bronchopneumonia (from *Haemophilus influenzae* bacteria colonizing in the bronchi) to viral pneumonia (which may be caused by complications originating from chickenpox or influenza virus). In all cases, symptoms include painful coughing, but other symptoms, such as high fever, reduced sputum production, or discolored (rust-tinged or greenish) sputum, may differ. It follows that the drugs that have been developed to treat pneumonia necessarily vary according to the variety of the disease involved.

Lobar pneumonia and bronchopneumonia are the two main classes of disease. The former occurs when an initial infection attacks only one lobe of one lung. Bronchopneumonia results from an initial inflammation in the bronchi and bronchioles (air passages to the lungs), which then spreads to the internal tissue of one or both lungs. Once the symptoms of pneumonia have become visible, any of the following may occur: fever, chills, shortness of breath, chest pains, or a painful cough that produces yellow-green or brownish sputum. These symptoms occur because of a condition called pleurisy, which is an inflammation of the membrane lining the lungs themselves and the general chest cavity area.

Some assumptions about the causes of pneumonia being limited to bacterial or viral sources have been altered. In particular, clinical observation of patients suffering from AIDS reveals that certain fungi, yeasts, or protozoa can cause pneumonia in these and other cases where immunodeficiency disorders are present.

Although it is apparent that pneumococci can thrive in various parts of the bodies of animals, particularly monkeys and humans, the process that leads to general infection and a concentrated and dangerous attack on the pulmonary system has been the subject of many medical investigations. It is nearly certain that the presence of the common cold virus in the upper respiratory tract can create the conditions needed for the movement of pneumococci from areas of the body where they may be generally present without causing harm (mainly in saliva) into the pulmonary system. Under conditions of normal health, many body mechanisms can stop a potential invasion of the pulmonary system. This process may involve nasal mucus, although it is not itself bactericidal (bacteria-killing), and other mucous membranes in the region of the larynx. Even beyond

---

Information on Pneumonia

Causes: Bacterial or viral infection
Symptoms: Lung inflammation, painful coughing, high fever, reduced sputum production, rust-tinged or greenish sputum
Duration: Acute
Treatments: Antibiotics (tetracycline, erythromycin), supportive care

---

the larynx and vocal cords, mechanical means associated with the upward sweep of hairlike protrusions called cilia on the inner linings of deeper respiratory membranes tend to protect the bronchial tree.

When normal protective processes are reduced, as when the cold virus is present, pneumococci may reach the lower respiratory zone and the parenchyma of the lung, where they settle and multiply. The metabolic products that accumulate as a result of this reproductive process begin to have injurious effects on the respiratory organs. Such injuries become actual lesions in the internal respiratory tissues. The process of infection that follows involves the deposition of fibrin in the adjacent blood and lymph vessels. This phenomenon actually tends to shield the invading organisms from the effects normally produced by antipneumococcal immune substances carried by the blood. If unchecked by medical treatment, reproduction of the invading pneumococci can lead to more extensive lesions. If tissue damage occurs, this can cause the formation of edema, a dangerous accumulation of fluids in spaces where fluids are not normally found. At a later stage of the disease, it appears that the pneumococci enter the interstitial and lymphatic tissues. The unchecked advance of pneumonia infection produces a general deterioration of vital breathing processes as excess fluids spread farther into the respiratory system. In weakened or immunocompromised individuals, this process can lead to death.

Treatment and Therapy

Medical treatment of the two main types of pneumonia is not the same. Lobar pneumonia requires treatment with penicillin. Bronchopneumonia, although also caused by pneumococcus bacteria, must be treated with different antibiotics. Most forms of pneumonia caused by viral infections, including psittacosis and mycoplasmal pneumonia, require one of two specific drugs: tetracycline or erythromycin. When viral pneumonia provides the basic disease to which bacterial infections in the lungs are added, however, antibiotics represent the main general means of treatment.

Since World War II, the progress of medical science in dealing with various types of pneumonia has been marked by the development of antimicrobial drugs that can be used in treating diagnosed cases of pneumonia. One of the earliest such drugs, which eventually turned out to be ineffective, was a derivative of quinine called Optochin. It was used for the first time on mice in 1912. Five years later, when the drug was applied to human patients, it was ob-

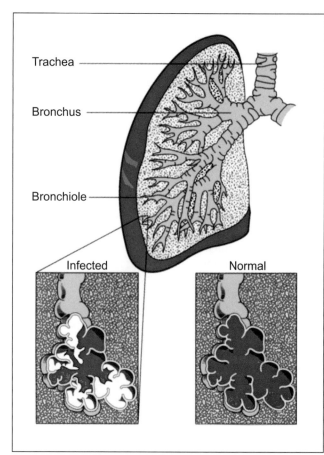

Trachea

Bronchus

Bronchiole

Infected   Normal

Pneumonia is actually a group of inflammatory diseases that affect the lungs; in lobar pneumonia, only one lobe of the lung is attacked, whereas in bronchopneumonia the bronchi and bronchioles, which lead to both lungs, are affected. The inset shows infection of the alveoli in lobar pneumonia.

served that the pneumococci were able to develop a surprising degree of resistance to these early antimicrobial substances. Thus, just as progress in the field of immunization had to wait for a later generation, so did effective drugs such as penicillin and other antibiotics that have become standard tools in the treatment of forms of pneumonia.

In most cases, advances in drug treatment to cure pneumonia have been strikingly successful. The phenomenon of the nonbacterial, nonviral version of *Pneumocystis* pneumonia arrived very soon after these successes. It posed a particular series of dilemmas for medical science in the 1980s and 1990s. This problem emerged when it became apparent that certain drugs that had been developed to treat pneumonia, in particular the drug combination of trimethoprim- sulfamethoxazole (TMP-SMZ), failed to achieve expected results in a rising number of cases of *Pneumocystis* pneumonia. This particular form of pneumonia turned out to be among the minority strains of the disease caused by single-celled microorganisms called protozoa.

The importance of *P. carinii* (also called *P. jirovecii*) in applied medical science soon extended beyond the restricted domain of pneumonia pathology. It had been discovered in 1909 in Brazil and was thought to affect only animals. This research involved local researchers led by the

Italian Antonio Carini, whose name was attached to the discovery. It was only much later, in the 1940s and 1950s, that the presence of *P. carinii* could be traced to pneumonia in human infants. This meant that a relatively unusual form of pneumonia belonged to limited number of cases caused not by bacteria or viruses but by fungi, yeasts, or microorganisms, specifically, single-celled protozoa. This form of pneumonia remained a relatively rare occurrence until the number of AIDS cases increased.

What appeared to be a near epidemic frequency of *P. carinii* was in fact a marker or indicator for discovering patients suffering from AIDS. This observation made it possible to immediately test for the presence of AIDS whenever cases of *P. carinii* appeared. Clinical experience during the 1980s revealed that at least 60 percent of all persons suffering from AIDS had contracted or would contract *P. carinii* pneumonia. The presence of *P. carinii* is now assumed to be associated with AIDS unless that diagnosis is excluded by a laboratory test.

It is important to note that relatively rapid advances made by medical researchers in preventing the spread of *P. carinii* and in treating the cases that did occur among infants led to a new appreciation for pneumonia. Applied research dating from 1958 and extending into the 1970s produced surprisingly effective agents to combat *P. carinii* pneumonia. This work led to the early application of drugs to people infected with human immunodeficiency virus (HIV). The concept of multiple drug therapy, patterned on TMP-SMZ, was also successfully applied in the field of cancer treatment.

Another drug, pentamidine, had been used to treat *P. carinii* pneumonia. When TMP-SMZ seemed to provide a superior treatment, pentamidine production was halted. When the potential utility of pentamidine in treating AIDS became apparent, the Centers for Disease Control and the Food and Drug Administration (FDA) had to take special action in 1984 to license an American supplier. This is how pentamidine quickly became widely available to treat individuals with AIDS. Pentamidine has also been successfully used as an effective treatment for a variety of viral diseases.

A side effect of these AIDS-related developments by the mid-1980s has been to reemphasize the importance of pneumonia. This renewed interest involves both treatments that are most appropriate for different types of pneumonia and research that is still needed to understand fully the role of this family of diseases in modern medicine and society.

Perspective and Prospects

Although modern medicine has not been able to reduce substantially or eliminate totally the number of cases of pneumonia, much has been learned about the disease and its causes. Scientific advances in the campaign to combat the effects of pneumonia in all areas of the world began with the first isolation of *Streptococcus pneumoniae* in France and the United States in 1880. The French discovery of pneumococci is associated with the laboratory of Louis Pasteur. Simultaneously, George Sternberg was completing work in the medical department of the US

Army. In the first decade after the isolation of pneumococci, many different researchers contributed to laboratory findings that linked these bacteria to inflammatory infections in the lungs of animals. They extended their research to include the effects on humans.

One of the most important early breakthroughs came in 1884 when the Danish researcher Hans Christian Joachim Gram developed a laboratory method for identifying specific bacteria in tissue specimens. This technique, called Gram's stain, revealed that different chemical reactions occur when samples of lung tissue and secretions from individuals ill with pneumonia and healthy persons are tested. The tissues stain very differently. The next step would lead to research into the phenomenon of phagocytosis, a process within pulmonary tissue that combats inapparent pneumococcus infection in healthy people. This specific discovery became linked with efforts to develop an immunization technology against pneumonia.

Until the 1980s, medical researchers used their knowledge of pneumonia mainly to develop methods of immunization against the disease. They also tried to diversify the drugs used in treating pneumonia. Efforts to produce a vaccine against pneumonia began with experiments by the German researchers George and Felix Klemperer, who tested antiserum in animals in 1891. The Klemperers were able to show that the offspring of adult rabbits which had been immunized were resistant to pneumococcal invasion and infection. Soon thereafter, they carried out the first injections of immune serum into human patients. This research ultimately led to the finding that there was no actual antitoxin or antibacterial property in the serum. Instead, it promoted phagocytosis, a process of encapsulation around pneumococci that aids in the immunological response of white blood cells in the body. The vaccine stimulates the body to create its own defenses.

In 1911 in South Africa, an experimental pneumonia vaccine program was undertaken. Although the specific program was not successful, the British physician and scientist Frederick Lister extended its theory. Unequivocal success with a pneumonia vaccine did not come until the last year of World War II. In 1945, C. M. MacLeod and several colleagues published research findings proving that pneumococcal infection in humans was preventable through the use of vaccines containing as many as fourteen specific antigens. These were termed capsular polysaccharides. The breakthrough that made those findings possible had been pioneered in 1930 when these antigens were injected into human beings for the first time. Previously, they had been used only in experiments with mice.

Pneumonia vaccines are critically important components of programs to prevent disease among older members of the population. In March 2013, the *American Journal of Medicine* published a study of 1,400 pneumonia patients over the age of fifty in which researchers found a correlation between pneumonia patients requiring hospitalization and an increased risk of decline their mental abilities. Experts recommend that the elderly receive a pneumonia vaccine each year. The death rate from pneumonia continues to rise, but not as quickly as the percentage of the population that is elderly. Pneumonia is one of the ten leading causes of death in the United States. In 1900, it was the second or third most common killer. Without vaccines, it might easily still be the second or third leading cause of death.

Children under the age of two are also at high risk for catching pneumonia. The World Health Organization reported in April 2013 that pneumonia was the leading cause of death in children worldwide, killing an estimated 1.2 million children younger than five each year. Only about 30 percent of the world's children with the disease receive antibiotics to treat it

—Byron D. Cannon, Ph.D.; updated by
L. Fleming Fallon, Jr., M.D., Ph.D., M.P.H.

See also Acquired immunodeficiency syndrome (AIDS); Avian influenza; Bacterial infections; Bacteriology; Bronchi; Bronchitis; Common cold; Coughing; Immunization and vaccination; Influenza; Lungs; Microbiology; Pleurisy; Pulmonary diseases; Pulmonary medicine; Pulmonary medicine, pediatric; Respiration; Severe acute respiratory syndrome (SARS); Streptococcal infections; Viral infections; Wheezing.

For Further Information:
Austrian, Robert. *Life with the Pneumococcus*. Philadelphia: University of Pennsylvania Press, 1985.
Badash, Michelle. "Pneumonia." *Health Library*, September 30, 2012.
Heron, Melonie. "Deaths: Leading Causes for 2009." *National Vital Statistics Reports* 61, no. 7 (October 26, 2012): 1-94.
Hughes, Walter T. Pneumocystis carinii *Pneumonitis*. 2 vols. Rev. ed. Boca Raton, Fla.: CRC Press, 1987.
Karetzky, Monroe, Burke A. Cunha, and Robert D. Brandstetter. *The Pneumonias*. New York: Springer, 1993.
MedlinePlus. "Pneumonia." *MedlinePlus*, May 20, 2013.
Niederman, Michael S., George A. Sarosi, and Jeffrey Glassroth. *Respiratory Infections*. 2d ed. Philadelphia: Lippincott Williams & Wilkins, 2001.
Papadakis, Maxine A., Stephen J. McPhee, and Michael W. Rabow, eds. *Current Medical Diagnosis and Treatment 2013*. New York: McGraw-Hill Medical, 2012.
Parker, James N., and Philip M. Parker, eds. *The Official Patient's Sourcebook on Streptococcus Pneumoniae Infections*. San Diego, Calif.: Icon Health, 2002.
Pennington, James E. *Respiratory Infections: Diagnosis and Management*. 3d ed. Hoboken, N.J.: Raven Press, 1994.
Preidt, Robert. "HealthDay: Pneumonia May Lead to Serious Aftereffects for Seniors." *MedlinePlus*, March 22, 2013.
West, John B. *Pulmonary Pathophysiology: The Essentials*. 8th ed. Philadelphia: Wolters Kluwer/Lippincott Williams & Wilkins Health, 2012.
World Health Organization. "Pneumonia (Fact Sheet No. 331)." *World Health Organization: Media Centre*, April, 2013.

Pneumothorax

Disease/Disorder

Anatomy or system affected: Chest, lungs, respiratory system

Specialties and related fields: Emergency medicine, pulmonary medicine

Definition: The collapse of a lung or portion of a lung as a result of the introduction of air or another gas or of fluid into the pleural space surrounding the lungs.

Key terms:

bronchoscopy: a medical procedure for viewing the inside of the lungs through a scope that is passed through the nose or mouth and into the lungs

bulla (bleb): a blister that develops on the surface of the lung

cyanosis: a bluish tinge to the skin, particularly on the fingers and toes, around the mouth, and the ear lobes as a result of inadequate oxygen to the tissues

subcutaneous emphysema: air that has leaked from the pneumothorax to under the skin

Causes and Symptoms

Pneumothorax is the result of anything that causes air or fluid, such as blood, to leak into the space between the two layers of pleura, which line the chest wall (parietal) and the lung tissue (visceral). For normal lung function there is negative pressure in this space. When air enters, the negative pressure is disrupted, and the atmospheric pressure presses on the lung tissue, deflating it. A pneumothorax can be mild and self-limiting, but a severe pneumothorax can collapse the whole lung and cause a shift in the location of the heart and great vessels. This is a life-threatening situation.

Pneumothorax is caused by trauma to the lung, medical procedures performed on the lungs, infant prematurity, existing lung disease, endometriosis in the chest, and bullae. Trauma includes anything that penetrates the chest wall, such as a stabbing, gunshot wound, or excessive blunt trauma to the chest. Medical procedures such as a bronchoscopy, cardiopulmonary resuscitation (CPR), liver or lung biopsy, chest surgery, and the insertion of chest tubes can cause a pneumothorax. Premature infants or infants who swallow meconium, newborn stool, can rupture their lungs attempting to breathe despite lung tissue that is sticking together. The presence of existing lung disease can increase the risk of developing a pneumothorax. These diseases include emphysema, asthma, chronic infections, tuberculosis, cystic fibrosis, cancer, and chronic obstructive pulmonary disease (COPD). An unusual cause of pneumothorax is the presence of endometriosis in the chest. This condition causes pneumothorax at the time of the menstrual cycle, when the endometrial tissue bleeds. Bullae develop due to local weakness in the lung tissue and can rupture with changes in atmospheric pressure, such as when scuba diving, flying, and mountain climbing. Most often bullae rupture for no apparent reason. Bullae are more common in cigarette smokers.

The symptoms of pneumothorax are shortness of breath, sharp pain in the chest, a feeling of tightness, cyanosis, dry cough, rapid heart rate, subcutaneous emphysema, and the sound of air moving through a penetrating chest wound. A primary pneumothorax is diagnosed by the symptoms; pulse oximetry, which measures oxygen saturation of the blood; auscultation, or listening to the lobes of the lungs through a stethoscope; and chest x-ray. A traumatic pneumothorax is related to a traumatic injury and a postmedical pneumothorax to a medical procedure.

Treatment and Therapy

A small pneumothorax will resolve on its own. It is treated with watchful waiting and repeated chest x-rays. If there is

---

Information on Pneumothorax

Causes: Trauma, medical procedures performed on lungs, infant prematurity, existing lung disease, endometriosis in chest, bullae

Symptoms: Shortness of breath, sharp pain in chest, feeling of tightness, cyanosis, dry cough, rapid heart rate, subcutaneous emphysema, sound of air moving through penetrating chest wound

Duration: One to four days, depending on severity and treatment

Treatments: Insertion of chest tube into intrapleural space, surgery

---

shortness of breath, then oxygen can be administered. If a pneumothorax does not resolve on its own, then a needle can be inserted through the chest wall into the pneumothorax (thoracentesis), and the air or fluid can be extracted. Another common treatment is the insertion of a chest tube with its tip in the intrapleural space. An airtight dressing is placed around the tube and the tube is drained into a system that includes a water seal in order to prevent the reintroduction of air. Gentle suction may be used to remove the air or any drainage present. Usually, the pneumothorax will resolve within two to three days, and then the tube can be removed. If the pneumothorax reoccurs after the suction is removed from the chest tube, then there is a more portable system called a Heimlich valve that can be used to continue chest drainage. This valve permits air or fluid to leave the interpleural space without permitting air to reenter.

If the pneumothorax does not improve, or if it reoccurs, then surgery may be required. Pleurodesis may be performed, particularly for ruptured bullae. In this procedure, a chemical irritant is used to create scar tissue to heal weakened spots in the lung. Surgery in the form of video-assisted thoracic surgery (VATS) can be performed to close the lung with staples. Open chest surgery is less commonly used to treat pneumothoraces.

In an emergency, a sucking or traumatic chest wound should be treated with an occlusive dressing to prevent the introduction of additional air into the chest. Ideally, this dressing should be sterile and have either petroleum jelly gauze or plastic to seal the wound.

Perspective and Prospects

Pneumothorax was first identified by Jean Marc Gaspard Itard, a student of Rene Laennec, in 1803. Laennec, himself, described the clinical picture of pneumothorax, in 1819. The first treatment of pneumothorax was thoracentesis. Both thoracentesis and chest tubes generally led to empyema, an infection in the pleural space because of the absence of aseptic technique. After the discovery of germ theory and aseptic technique by Ignaz Semmelweiss (1818-1865), Louis Pasteur (1822-1895), and Joseph Lister (1827-1912), pneumothorax could be treated with aseptic thoracentesis, or with surgery. Semmelweis discovered that hand washing between patients could limit the spread of infection after childbirth. Pasteur tested germ theory, and wrote about the microscopic germs that cause infection, both in the presence of air and in anaerobic tissue. Lister is referred to as the father of surgery because he introduced the use of chemicals to sterilize surgical instruments and to clean wounds. In 1875, G. E. Playfair developed water seal drainage for removing fluids from the chest, and in 1876, F. Cresswell Hewett used water seal drainage with chest tubes.

Tuberculosis was a scourge in the nineteenth century, and it frequently created a pneumothorax by eating through the lung. There were no antibiotics at this time, so treatment was limited, and most persons who developed tuberculosis died from it. In 1882, Italian physician Carlo Forlanini began to use pneumothorax for treatment of tuberculosis in an effort to rest the lung. This treatment was continued into the early twentieth century.

—*Christine M. Carroll, R.N., B.S.N., M.B.A.*

See also Asthma; Chest; Chronic obstructive pulmonary disease (COPD); Cystic fibrosis; Emphysema; Internal medicine; Lung cancer; Lung surgery; Lungs; Pleurisy; Pneumonia; Pulmonary diseases; Pulmonary medicine; Pulmonary medicine, pediatric; Respiration; Thoracic surgery; Tuberculosis.

For Further Information:

Alifano, Marco, et al. "Atmospheric Pressure Influences the Risk of Pneumothorax: Beware of the Storm!" *Chest* 131, no. 6 (July 26, 2007): 1877-1882.

Blavias, Allen J. "Pneumothorax-Series." *MedlinePlus*, March 22, 2013.

Chan, Stewart Siu Wa. "Tension Pneumothorax Managed Without Immediate Needle Decompression." *Journal of Emergency Medicine* 36, no. 3 (June 12, 2009): 242-245.

Chiu, Hsienchang Thomas, and Christine Kim Garcia. "Familial Spontaneous Pneumothorax." *Current Opinion in Pulmonary Medicine* 12, no. 4 (July 20, 2006): 268-272.

Dameron, Amanda L. "Pneumothorax." *Health Library*, March 15, 2013.

Mayo Clinic. "Pneumothorax." *Mayo Clinic*, April 5, 2011.

Podiatry

Specialty

Anatomy or system affected: Bones, feet, nails

Specialties and related fields: Dermatology, orthopedics, vascular medicine

Definition: The medical field that involves the diagnosis and treatment of diseases and abnormalities of the feet, ankles, and lower legs.

Key terms:

corticosteroid: a fatlike molecule (or steroid), produced by the adrenal gland or made synthetically, that can be used to treat inflammation

dysfunction: the disordered or impaired function of a body system, organ, or tissue

orthopedics: the surgical or manipulative treatment of any disorder of the skeletal system and the associated motor organs

orthotic device: a podiatric appliance or prosthesis that is used to correct a foot deformity

pharmacology: the aspect of biomedical science that studies therapeutic drugs, their administration, and their bioproperties

Science and Profession

The human foot, which is located at the end of the lower leg and connected to the leg by the ankle, is a very complex structure. Feet are designed to optimize both balance and mobility. Each foot is composed of twenty-six bones, ligaments that connect and articulate these bones, blood vessels that provide nutrients and oxygen, sensory nerves, and a very thick covering of tough, strong skin. Heredity and a lack of proper foot care frequently result in painful calluses, corns, bunions, enlarged joints, and ingrown toenails. In addition, a variety of diseases, such as diabetes mellitus and cardiovascular problems, can lead to many other serious foot dysfunctions.

Podiatrists-more correctly called doctors of podiatric medicine-examine, diagnose, and treat dysfunctions of the foot as well as related problems associated with the ankle and the lower leg. The first record of a process that was associated with podiatric medicine was the creation, in 100 BCE, of plasters that were used to treat corns at the Greek city of Smyrna. Although other records of podiatric treatments were found in antiquity and in the Middle Ages, the modern science of podiatry arose from the activities of the fourteenth century barber-surgeons of Europe.

In the United States, the first truly prominent modern podiatrist-then termed a chiropodist-was Isacher Zacharia. Zacharia, foot doctor to President Abraham Lincoln, published the first American podiatry text in 1862. Two other milestones in the history of American podiatry are the founding of the National Association of Chiropodists and the opening of the New York School of Chiropody. Both of these events occurred in 1912.

In 1958, the National Association of Chiropodists was renamed the American Podiatric Medical Association. From the New York School of Chiropody, whose first curriculum required only one year of chiropodic training, arose today's schools of podiatric medicine, which require a four-year study period and award to graduates the doctor of podiatric medicine (DPM) degree. This degree derives from a uniform curriculum that all schools follow.

There are more than sixteen thousand licensed podiatrists in the United States. These podiatric practitioners serve patients in American hospitals, in government health programs, and in the armed forces, though most of them are in private, individual practice. Furthermore, modern podiatric medicine is an accepted part of all major health insurance plans, of Medicare, and of Medicaid. To become a licensed DPM, it is first necessary to complete a four-year course of postgraduate study at a school of podiatric medicine.

Admission to all American podiatry schools requires the completion of at least three years of a solid bachelor's degree program, which must include a year each of biology, inorganic chemistry, and organic chemistry. Most podiatry school entrants have completed a bachelor's degree. In addition, a solid grade-point average and good scores on the Medical College Admissions Test (MCAT) are required for admission.

The first two years of podiatric professional education

use this background as a springboard that enables laboratory and lecture hall training in anatomy, biochemistry, physiology, pharmacology, diagnostic radiology, and numerous other biomedical sciences. The third and fourth years of training are dedicated to the acquisition of clinical expertise by practicing podiatric medicine in college or community clinics, in hospitals, and in the offices of experienced, well-established podiatrists.

Upon graduation, the new DPM usually completes a hospital residency encompassing three to four years. In the first year, clinical expertise is gained in podiatric orthopedics, biomechanics, and neurology. The first-year podiatry resident engages in supervised primary care, which involves observing, evaluating, and treating many dysfunctions of the feet, ankles, and lower legs. Minor podiatric surgery, such as the correction of a hammertoe, is also carried out during this training period. In the remaining residency years, the resident learns to carry out the more demanding aspects of podiatric surgery of the foot, ankle, and leg. During this time period, the podiatric resident becomes more independent and skilled.

Podiatric practitioners require licenses to practice. In the United States, these licenses are most often gained by passing state board examinations. Satisfactory scores on the separate tests given by the National Board of Podiatric Medical Examiners are also deemed satisfactory for podiatric licensing by many states. Renewal of podiatry licenses, however, requires that podiatrists undergo extensive continuing education aimed at keeping them at the cutting edge of the field.

Specialization is also possible for podiatrists. Podiatric specialists can be certified by the American Board of Podiatric Surgery, the American Board of Podiatric Medicine, or the American Board of Podiatric Public Health. Each of these podiatric specialty boards requires advanced clinical training, completion of written and oral examinations, and extensive experience in specific aspects of modern podiatric practice. Such board certification indicates that the individuals involved have met much higher standards than those required for licensing alone. Some podiatrists also belong to the American College of Foot and Ankle Surgery of the American Medical Association (AMA).

In modern practice, podiatric surgical procedures designed to prevent or correct podiatric deformities now supplant many of the more conventional methods that originally made up the expertise of most podiatric practitioners. In addition, numerous techniques that cause the improvement of the health and the function of the foot and the ankle, so as to preclude foot deformities, have become key aspects of the modern podiatric profession.

Diagnostic and Treatment Techniques

A thorough podiatric examination begins with the complete medical history of the patient, inspection of the patient's gait, and careful examination of both feet, the ankles, and the lower legs. When these procedures point to the diagnosis of a particular podiatric problem, x-ray examination, muscle testing, and neurological consultation may be carried out to search for more subtle problems that the initial examination suggested but did not prove.

Once a clear, complete diagnosis has been obtained, a treatment regimen-including physical therapy, various surgical treatments, medications, and the use of podiatric (orthotic) appliances-is prescribed. Often, all aspects of treatment are carried out in the podiatrist's office. Complex podiatric surgery, however, may require the use of a hospital surgical suite or its equivalent.

Among the podiatric problems most often seen are athlete's foot, bunions, calluses, corns, ingrown toenails, hammertoes, heel spurs, traumatic injuries to the ankles or feet, plantar warts, and complaints associated with arthritis, cardiovascular disease, or diabetes mellitus. In many cases-especially those engendered by athletics, diabetes, and cardiovascular problems-the podiatrist refers patients to other health practitioners, such as orthopedists, cardiologists, or endocrinologists. Increasingly, however, podiatrists and other specialists are beginning to work together as teams to solve such health problems.

Bunions are deformities of the big toes and their joints; they may or may not be painful, but they are almost always considered uncosmetic. When a bunion is not painful, it is usually treated by the use of an orthotic device that prevents further damage and pain. In cases where bunion pain is caused by inflammation, oral or injected anti-inflammatory drugs, such as corticosteroids, are often used for the shortest period of time needed to correct the problem. Such short-term treatment is made necessary by the potential health risks caused by this therapy, such as cardiovascular problems. In the most severe cases, surgery is used to remove the bunion. An incision is made near the bunion site, and a surgical burr is used to trim away the region of excess bone that is causing the problem. In cases where manipulative examination or x-rays show that the bunion problem is in the joint, much more complex surgery is required.

Corns and hammertoes may be considered together, as many corns are caused by hammertoes. Corns are not restricted to occurrence along with hammertoes, however, as they also arise spontaneously on any toe subject to inappropriate biomechanical stress. A corn (or heloma) is a skin protrusion-or thickening-atop or on the side of a toe. Corns can occur wherever a toe has been bent out of shape by a biomechanical problem or by a tight shoe. They can be quite painful. Hammertoe, a contracture of one of the toe joints, produces a toe malformation that makes wearing shoes painful and can lead to corns. Corns may be trimmed periodically or removed surgically. The treatment used by podiatrists depends on the severity of the problem seen. Similarly, hammertoes are corrected surgically. After treatment of these problems, it is important for the patient to wear shoes that fit appropriately, to use corrective orthotic devices that are prescribed, and to follow closely the instructions given by the podiatrist. Failure to do so can counteract the results of the podiatric treatment.

Calluses, like corns, are buildups of tough, thickened skin. Unlike corns, however, they occur most often on the bottoms of the feet. Calluses form to protect the foot from undue stress resulting from uneven weight bearing by the bottom of the foot. Therefore, they will form again after removal wherever the causative mechanical stress recurs. When a callus becomes painful, the appropriate treatment regimen varies greatly from case to case. Often, an orthotic device is used to produce evenness of weight bearing by the foot. In other cases, the callus is trimmed. In the most extreme cases, minor surgery is used to correct the anatomical defect in the metatarsal bone that is causing the problem. Again, success in callus treatment is optimized by carefully following the directions of the podiatrist. In the most severe instances, up to three months of diminished physical activity is required to enable complete healing of the trimmed metatarsal bones. Calluses may also occur at the back of the heel, as a result of tight shoes and dermatologic problems. These calluses are usually handled by trimming and subsequent purchase of more appropriate shoes.

Heel spurs, Achilles tendonitis, ankle problems, dermatologic problems of the foot, and diabetic/cardiovascular complications may also be treated by podiatrists. Furthermore, it should be recognized that podiatrists will often repair damaged bones, muscles, and tendons surgically. They can also prescribe medications and treat fractures or sprains by applying casts and braces.

Perspective and Prospects

Many advances in podiatric medicine have occurred in recent years. Most encouraging is the improved ability of podiatrists to handle severe foot problems. This improvement is largely attributable to advances in the field and to more thorough training both in professional school and in postgraduate experiences. The increasing positive interaction of podiatrists and other health care professionals in the treatment of dermatologic, cardiovascular, and diabetic problems is another great step forward.

It is believed that the job prospects for podiatrists will expand rapidly in the next fifty years, and there will be even greater success in the podiatric treatment of problems that are presently difficult to handle. It is also expected that additional podiatric medical schools will open to meet the need for more DPMs throughout the United States.

There are two main reasons for the excellent job prospects for podiatrists. First is the increase in the population of senior citizens. Because these individuals have had more wear and tear on their lower legs and feet than younger people, they have foot ailments that require treatment more frequently. Second is the increased interest in jogging and other sports in the general population, which will lead to more injuries that require podiatric intervention.

These factors are also expected to produce advances in the uses of orthotic appliances, generate sophisticated new diagnostic and surgical techniques, and lead to better cooperation between podiatrists and other health care professionals.

—*Sanford S. Singer, Ph.D.*

See also Athlete's foot; Bone disorders; Bones and the skeleton; Bunions; Corns and calluses; Feet; Flat feet; Foot disorders; Fungal in-

fections; Gout; Hammertoe correction; Hammertoes; Heel spur removal; Lower extremities; Nail removal; Nails; Orthopedic surgery; Orthopedics; Physical examination; Tendon disorders; Tendon repair; Warts.

For Further Information:

Alexander, Ivy L., ed. *Podiatry Sourcebook.* 2d rev. ed. Detroit, Mich.: Omnigraphics, 2007.
Copeland, Glenn, and Stan Solomon. *The Foot Doctor: Lifetime Relief for Your Aching Feet.* Rev. ed. Toronto, Ont.: Macmillan Canada, 1996.
Farr, J. Michael, ed. *Enhanced Occupational Outlook Handbook.* 7th ed. Indianapolis, Ind.: JIST Works, 2009.
Fink, Brett Ryan, and Mark S. Mizel. *The Whole Foot.* New York: Demos Medical, 2012.
Lippert, Frederick G., and Sigvard T. Hansen. *Foot and Ankle Disorders: Tricks of the Trade.* New York: Thieme, 2003.
Lorimer, Donald J., et al., eds. *Neale's Disorders of the Foot.* 7th ed. New York: Churchill Livingstone/Elsevier, 2006.
Rose, Jonathan D., and Vincent J. Martorana. *The Foot Book.* Baltimore: Johns Hopkins University Press, 2011.
Thordarson, David B., ed. *Foot and Ankle.* 2d ed. Philadelphia: Lippincott Williams & Wilkins, 2013.
Van De Graaff, Kent M., and Stuart I. Fox. *Concepts of Human Anatomy and Physiology.* 5th ed. Dubuque, Iowa: Wm. C. Brown, 2000.

Poisoning

Disease/Disorder

Anatomy or system affected: Gastrointestinal system, immune system, muscles, musculoskeletal system, nervous system, respiratory system, stomach

Specialties and related fields: Emergency medicine, environmental health, epidemiology, toxicology

Definition: Exposure to any substance in sufficient quantity to cause adverse health effects, from severe to fatal.

Key terms:

epidemiology: The study of the incidence of diseases or poisonings in affected populations

iatrogenic poisoning: poisoning resulting from medical treatment, which can include overdose, the administration of improper medication by the patient or prescribing physician, and adverse reactions

pharmacology: the science that deals with the chemistry, effects, and therapeutic use of drugs

syrup of ipecac: a plant extract that will induce vomiting when orally administered; the syrup can be used to induce vomiting after ingestion of a poisonous substance

toxicology: the science devoted to the study of poisons

toxidrome: a group of symptoms characteristic of a toxin or group of toxins that act on the same area of the nervous system

Causes and Symptoms

Probably the most accurate statement that can be made about the occurrence of poisoning in the United States is that the numbers vary widely depending on the information source and definition of poisoning. Incidents can be grouped into intentional poisonings, accidental poisonings, occupational and environmental poisonings, social poisonings, and iatrogenic poisonings. There is no single organization that collects and analyzes data from hospitals, physicians' offices, police and court records, and industrial accident and exposure records. One source has reported that as many as eight million people are accidentally or intentionally poisoned each year. It has been stated further that 10 percent of all ambulance calls and 10 to 20 percent of all admissions to medical facilities involve poisonings.

Many incidents of poisoning go unreported because a poison control center is not consulted or the effects are not severe enough to require extensive medical treatment. In other cases where exposure to the toxic agent involves constant contact to low but toxic levels of industrial chemicals, such as occupational or environmental exposures, symptoms may be subtle or confused with diseases that are associated with the normal aging process. The degree of illness and/or the number of premature deaths resulting from environmental exposure to naturally occurring or artificial toxic substances-radiation, chemical waste, and other toxins in the air, water, and food supply-is simply not known.

The most consistent and reliable sources of information on accidental poisoning in the United States are the annual statistics compiled by the American Association of Poison Control Centers. While poison control centers receive some calls related to intentional poisonings, 88 percent of the calls are considered accidental exposures. Combining all the poisoning types together, poison control centers are called concerning about 2.2 million human cases each year. It is important to note, however, that extrapolations from the number of reported poisonings to the number of actual poisonings occurring annually in the United States cannot be made from these data alone.

About 93 percent of exposures occur in the home, more than half involve children under six, and three-fourths involve ingestion. The great predominance of young children in the accidental poisoning category reflects the inquisitive behavior of that age group. For children under the age of one year, inappropriate administration of medications by the parents is the dominant cause of poisonings. For children over the age of five, exposure to toxic substances often represents the simple misreading of a medication label or the manifestation of family stress or even suicidal intent. These children have increased incidence of depressive symptoms and family problems compared to their nonpoisoned peer group.

Intentional poisoning of children also occurs-usually as a well-planned act of a psychologically disturbed parent. Although many of these incidents are clearly homicidal and abusive by design, some have received medical notoriety as cases of Münchausen syndrome by proxy. Münchausen syndrome itself is a psychiatric disorder in which the patient achieves psychological comfort from the attention and treatment received under the pretense of being afflicted with a serious or painful illness. In a variation of this condition, the psychiatric needs of an adult are fulfilled through an induced medical disorder in the child. For example, a parent might surreptitiously administer syrup of ipecac to his or her child, inducing unexplained vomiting and gastrointestinal disorders that requires extended hospital care. The phenomenon is rare but well documented in

---

Information on Poisoning

Causes: Exposure to biological, chemical, or environmental toxins; may be intentional, accidental, occupational, environmental, social, or iatrogenic

Symptoms: Varies; may include unconsciousness, disorientation, muscle spasms, seizures, swelling

Duration: Acute

Treatments: Emergency medical treatment (stabilization, life support mechanisms), antidotes and/or antiseizure medications, induction of vomiting

---

the medical literature and is classified as a form of child abuse.

Intentional poisonings are mostly suicide-related. The Centers for Disease Control and Prevention (CDC) reported that more than 38,000 Americans killed themselves in 2010. Of all suicides from 2005 to 2009, poisoning was the method chosen by almost 40 percent of women and about 12 percent of men. Although carbon monoxide (as in motor vehicle exhaust) is one of the most common agents used, intentional dosing with large quantities of drugs is also very frequently involved. Of the many thousands of drugs that could be used for overdose incidents, 90 percent of actual cases involve only about twenty products in nine drug groups. Most of these are addictive or abused drugs, including stimulants, antidepressants, tranquilizers, narcotics, sedatives or hypnotics, and antipsychotics. Alcohol alone is seldom lethal but is often consumed along with the more deadly drugs and may make the lethal effects possible.

Social poisoning is related to drug use or abuse, which can have significant societal consequences. There are hundreds of thousands of hospital and emergency room admissions each year for overdose treatment as well as for the indirect consequences of recreational drug use, such as violent crime, trauma, and vehicular accidents. Almost 400,000 drug-abuse-related emergency room visits were projected to have occurred in 1990 by the Drug Abuse Warning Network (DAWN), a federal government-sponsored data collection system. These figures do not include alcohol, however, unless it is mentioned as having been involved in a mixed drug exposure event.

The abuse of alcohol, the most widely available chemical intoxicant legally allowed for recreational use, is a major social problem in the United States. While a majority of the alcohol-consuming public demonstrates a lifelong pattern of little or moderate drinking without the development of addiction-related problems, it has been reported that a small percentage of the population (5 percent to 10 percent) drinks between one-third and one-half of all alcohol consumed. The causes of alcoholism involve a complex interaction of social, physiological, and genetic risk factors. In the United States, there are approximately 9 million people classified as chronic alcohol abusers, and according to the CDC, about 80,000 deaths per year are attributable to alcohol-related causes.

Tobacco use, although not as closely associated with

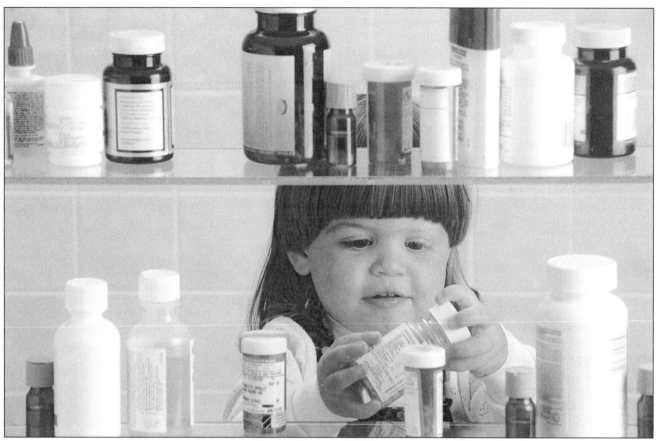

Childproof caps are essential in the prevention of accidental poisoning. (PhotoDisc)

criminal behavior and vehicular accidents as drugs and alcohol, has been connected with increased incidence of cancer, respiratory illnesses, and cardiovascular diseases. According to the World Health Organization, more than 5 million deaths worldwide per year are attributable to tobacco use. Both smoking and excessive alcohol consumption are becoming increasingly less socially accepted, but the continued wide acceptance of both alcohol and tobacco use obscures their potential to poison.

Treatment and Therapy

Emergency medical treatment of the poisoned patient is most often based on the relief of symptoms and the provision of life support. If the patient is awake and alert, a medical history is taken and a clinical examination is performed, both of which can help determine substance exposure. The medical staff must never assume that the patient is providing truthful information, especially if clinical impressions conflict with the patient account. If the patient is comatose, then stabilization and life support take immediate priority over determination of the specific toxic substance involved. The attending physician will want to prevent airway blockage and to maintain respiration and circulation, which may require mechanical aids for breathing assistance. Treatment of cardiac and blood pressure problems can be accomplished with drugs, fluid, or oxygen administration. If the patient is unconscious, the depth of central nervous system depression can be evaluated using a standard test of reactivity to light, sound, pain, and the presence or absence of normal body processes. If the patient is suffering from seizures, drugs that counteract these symptoms can be administered.

Although many hospitals offer in-house toxicology testing in a clinical laboratory, treatment usually must begin before results are available. For this and several other reasons, a comprehensive toxicology testing laboratory is not as useful an asset in the emergency treatment of poisoning as might be assumed. It would be impossible for any analytical laboratory to provide timely or cost-effective emergency identification of all potentially toxic substances. Instead, a more efficient strategy concentrates on analyzing those substances for which a specific antidote exists or for which specific medical procedures are required in a critical period of time. A very high percentage of drug overdose cases involve one of a group of six or eight drugs that will vary depending on locality. Pesticide poisoning, for example, is a more prevalent medical problem for rural than urban hospitals. Drug abuse is a problem in all localities, but the frequency and type of drugs abused vary. Regional preferences exist for PCP, cocaine, amphetamines, and opiates. Even prescription drug abuse depends on locality and the patient population.

Common pain relievers found in virtually every home medicine cabinet constitute a large number of both adult and pediatric poisoning incidents. Preparations containing aspirin, as well as nonaspirin analgesics containing acetaminophen (such as Tylenol), are possibly life-threatening when consumed in excess. Acetaminophen poisoning is particularly insidious since death from total and irreversible destruction of the liver will occur unless the antidote, a chemical called acetylcysteine, is administered within six hours of ingestion of a lethal dose. Since a specific antidote exists, most hospitals with emergency service will offer around-the-clock testing for acetaminophen levels in the blood. Aspirin, although not as lethal as acetaminophen, can be fatal if a sufficient amount is consumed. Its universal availability and common usage make aspirin a significant poisoning agent encountered in all localities. The symptoms of toxicity are related to aspirin's effects on temperature regulation, rate of breathing, and the body's ability to influence the acidity of the blood. Treatment involves monitoring the patient's vital signs and calculating the severity of the dose taken. Vomiting may be induced with syrup of ipecac, or charcoal (a very active adsorption agent) may be given orally to limit gastric absorption. Intravenous fluids may also be given to counteract the blood acidity changes.

Prescription drugs that are commonly overused or abused (antiepileptic medication, sedatives and tranquilizers, and antipsychotic or antidepressant drugs) are often routinely assayed in the hospital laboratory as part of the treatment process for patients receiving these medications. The levels in the blood can be monitored to determine the toxicity status of the patient. Usually, supportive care is sufficient for treatment until the drug clears the system. For certain tranquilizers and antidepressants, an antidote called flumazenil can be administered, but it must be used with caution.

Poisoning from an overdose of opiates or morphinelike drugs is a special treatment case. A specific antidote called naloxone can be administered if the patient is treated before irreversible respiratory depression occurs. Recovery is virtually instantaneous and dramatic, with a comatose patient becoming alert within seconds of naloxone administration. For this reason, the routine treatment of comatose patients includes the administration of opiate antidote even when the cause of the unconscious state is unknown.

Although heavy, long-term ethyl alcohol use invariably leads to liver dysfunction and a number of other organ disorders, alcohol is not usually life-threatening unless it is consumed in quantities sufficient to cause a coma. Death most commonly results from respiratory depression and related complications. Other types of alcohols, as well as antifreeze, can be involved in both accidental and intentional poisonings. Methanol or wood alcohol is a common industrial solvent found in materials around the home or work site; consumption can cause blindness and death. Isopropyl alcohol (or rubbing alcohol), although not as toxic as methanol, can also cause severe illness and death when consumed in sufficient quantities. Ethylene glycol, a common ingredient in antifreeze, is highly toxic and is especially attractive to small children and pets because of its sweet taste. It may also be consumed by alcoholics as an ethanol substitute. When not treated, its consumption can result in kidney failure. It is not the alcohols themselves that are the primary toxins but the degradation products called metabolites that form in the body in an attempt to eliminate the foreign substance. Ironically, the treatment for both methanol and ethylene glycol poisoning is administration of high doses of ethanol, which prevents the formation of toxic metabolites by the liver.

In the United States, lead poisoning is a major medical problem for children living in older, substandard housing; they can become exposed to large amounts of lead from the consumption of lead-based paint. (Even though such paints are no longer used in residential housing, many older buildings remain contaminated.) Another major source of exposure is inhalation of leaded gas fumes and exhaust. Other less common sources of lead poisoning include the consumption of food stored in leaded crystal or pottery or moonshine whiskey distilled in automobile radiators. Intentional gasoline sniffing by adolescents can also be a problem. Lead exposure is extremely hazardous because its effects are both severe and cumulative. Children are especially susceptible to lead poisoning because they absorb and retain more of this substance and have less capacity for excretion than adults.

The nervous system is a major site for lead toxicity, causing both psychological and neurologic impairment. The blood cell production can also be affected, with resulting anemia and decreased oxygen-carrying capacity. Because lead toxicity can result in behavioral and learning disorders that may already afflict children living in substandard conditions, sometimes poisoning cannot be detected by clinical symptoms alone and must be diagnosed through blood testing. Test data indicate that the level of lead associated with nervous system disorders is probably lower than previously believed. In the United States, a major screening effort has been financed by the federal government to detect high lead body deposits in children. The goal is to find affected children and to treat them before permanent damage occurs.

Perspective and Prospects

Poisoning has been a medical problem since the earliest times of human history. A tremendous variety of poisonous substances can be encountered in the natural world alone. It has been estimated that 200,000 plants and animals are known to be toxic to humans, some organisms producing as many as fifty or sixty toxins. The potential of almost any substance to be poisonous was recognized during the Renaissance by Paracelsus, a founder of modern toxicology, who stated, "All substances are poison; only the dose makes something not a poison." Many folk remedies and tribal medicine practices were derived from centuries of trial-and-error experiences with toxic plant and animal species in the environment. Historically, the development of the sciences of pharmacology and toxicology is closely related to the study of poisons.

As societies become more urban and technology-based, poisoning problems shift away from natural toxin exposures to those related to drugs and industrial chemicals. For many of these types of poisonings, sustaining the vital life processes until the toxin is cleared from the body is the only method of treatment. Specific antidotes are not available for many drugs or even for many natural poisons. Since a large number of toxins critically affect the nervous system, a diagnostic and treatment system has been developed based on the "toxidrome" concept. If a specific area of the nervous system can be shown to be affected, treatment can begin to counteract those effects even if the identity of the toxin is not known.

The symptoms of acute poisoning or overexposure to a toxic agent are likely to be treated as individual medical problems by physicians in an emergency medicine environment. Meanwhile, social poisons, which often do not create immediate medical emergencies, continue to exact enormous economic and medical costs to society over the long term; these poisoning problems have not been dealt with successfully by social, medical, or governmental agencies. In the case of environmental toxins, little if any well-established information on the long-term toxicity of these substances is available. The science of toxicology, particularly with regard to establishing the risk of exposure of a population to environmental toxins, often becomes a guessing game played by a governmental regulatory agency. Until societal and environmental poisonings can be better evaluated and controlled, they will continue to constitute serious economic and quality-of-life problems.
—*David J. Wells, Jr., Ph.D.*

See also Addiction; Alcoholism; Biological and chemical weapons; Bites and stings; Cyanosis; Domestic violence; Emergency rooms; Environmental diseases; Environmental health; First aid; Food poisoning; Iatrogenic disorders; Intoxication; Lead poisoning; Mercury poisoning; Münchausen syndrome by proxy; Nicotine; Over-the-counter medications; Poisonous plants; Prescription drug abuse; Smoking; Substance abuse; Suicide; Toxicology.

For Further Information:

Baselt, Randall C. *Disposition of Toxic Drugs and Chemicals in Man.* 9th ed. Foster City, Calif.: Biomedical, 2011.

Dart, Richard C., ed. *Medical Toxicology.* 3d ed. Philadelphia: Lippincott Williams & Wilkins, 2004.

Garriott, James C., ed. *Medicolegal Aspects of Alcohol Determination in Biological Specimens.* Littleton, Mass.: PSG, 1988.

Klaassen, Curtis D., ed. *Casarett and Doull's Toxicology: The Basic Science of Poisons.* 8th ed. New York: McGraw-Hill, 2013.

Morgan, Monroe T. *Environmental Health.* 3d ed. Belmont, Calif.: Thomson/Wadsworth, 2003.

"Poisoning." *MedlinePlus*, August 30, 2013.

Timbrell, John. *Introduction to Toxicology.* 3d ed. Washington, D.C.: Taylor & Francis, 2003.

Warren, Christian. *Brush with Death: A Social History of Lead Poisoning.* Baltimore: Johns Hopkins University Press, 2001.

Poliomyelitis

Disease/Disorder

Also known as: Polio

Anatomy or system affected: Brain, legs, muscles, musculoskeletal system, nerves, nervous system, spine

Specialties and related fields: Epidemiology, neurology, pediatrics, public health, virology

Definition: A contagious viral illness capable of causing meningitis and permanent paralysis; in response to a dra-matic increase in the frequency of cases in industrialized nations during the twentieth century, a vaccine was developed that has virtually eliminated this disease in Europe and the Western Hemisphere.

Key terms:

endemic disease: a disease that is usually present in a population and does not exhibit marked fluctuations in frequency from year to year

epidemic: a marked increase in the frequency of a disease, relative to the historical experience of the affected population

neurotropic virus: a virus that multiplies in neural tissues

serologic epidemiology: investigation of the history of disease exposure in a population by surveying the incidence of antibodies circulating in the bloodstream

subclinical infection: a disease process characterized by multiplication of the causative organism within the host and production of antibodies by the host without causing apparent illness

Causes and Symptoms

Poliomyelitis, or polio, is a contagious disease affecting humans and some nonhuman primates. It is caused by three closely related strains of a human enterovirus. In its most serious manifestation, it attacks nerve tissue in the spinal cord and brain stem, resulting in paralysis. Polio was one of the most feared diseases in developed countries in the twentieth century. A few medical researchers suspected the connection between the severe neurological symptoms of poliomyelitis and the more typical enteric form of the disease in the first decade of the twentieth century. A complete and accurate picture of the etiology of polio, however, was not demonstrated and accepted until the 1930s, when improved techniques for detecting viruses and antiviral antibodies enabled scientists to trace the disease in all of its phases.

The virus responsible for poliomyelitis is present in large numbers in the intestines of infected individuals. It is excreted in feces, from which it is spread to uninfected individuals through contaminated water, food, hands, and eating utensils and by flies and other filth-loving insects. Once it has been ingested, the poliovirus multiplies in the cells lining the intestine and invades the lymphatic system, producing swelling in the lymph nodes surrounding the intestine and in the neck. The symptoms of the disease at this stage may escape notice altogether, or the infected person may experience fever and a sore throat. These symptoms subside after two or three days as the body's immune system begins producing antibodies to overcome the virus. Most cases never proceed beyond this stage, termed the minor illness of polio.

In a minority of cases, after a period of several days in which a patient is asymptomatic, the minor illness is followed by the onset of neurological symptoms, signaling that the virus has invaded the spinal cord. Symptoms include pain and stiffness in the spine, lethargy, general muscular weakness, and flaccid (that is, not accompanied by spasms) paralysis of muscles, particularly of the legs. Paralysis of the legs occurs because the virus preferentially attacks neurons in the front or anterior horns of the spinal cord, including the motor nerves controlling the legs, and often affects one side more than the other. In the most severe cases, viral infection spreads from the spinal cord to the brain stem, attacking neurons serving the diaphragm and esophagus. Without aggressive medical intervention in the form of an artificial breathing apparatus, paralysis of the diaphragm is fatal.

In the absence of brain-stem involvement, a body's normal defenses usually overcome the viral infection. Since the body is unable to replace destroyed neurons, however, acute polio leaves the patient with permanent motor impairment ranging from mild muscular weakness to severe crippling disability. Aided by appropriate physical therapy during the recovery period, patients can usually regain some of the motor function lost during the active disease. As survivors of the polio epidemics of the 1940s and 1950s reached middle age in the late twentieth century, a late phase of the disease called postpolio syndrome was recognized. After decades of apparent normality, muscles affected by the initial paralytic attack experience gradual loss of function without evidence of renewed viral activity.

The proportion of cases resulting in permanent paralysis varies with the age structure of the population affected. Typically, no more than 10 percent of patients who experience a major illness including neurologic symptoms suffer such paralysis. Under premodern conditions, the latter probably accounted for less than 1 percent of the total cases, because subclinical infection, minor illness, and paralytic polio usually occurred in early childhood. Maternal antibodies provided protection for newborns, while a child's own immune system created antibodies following exposure. In this way, lifelong immunity to subsequent infection was acquired. With improving sanitation and an older susceptible population, however, this proportion gradually increased.

During an epidemic, polio is primarily spread by persons with mild and subclinical infections, who may be unaware that they are ill. Infectivity persists for two to three weeks after the onset of the intestinal disease. There is no evidence that lifetime carriers exist. It is virtually impossible to prevent the spread of an asymptomatic, fecally transmitted pathogen among young children in group settings by any behavioral means. Fortunately, vaccines have effectively eliminated polio as an epidemic disease in the developed world and in Latin America.

Treatment and Therapy

The history of efforts to prevent and treat poliomyelitis illustrates the changing attitudes of the medical community toward disease and the methods by which a once-important pathogen was virtually eliminated. Only time will tell whether the spectacular inroads made by medical science against poliomyelitis are permanent. Persons with compromised immune systems are reminders that vaccines cannot completely protect all individuals. They prevent health professionals from becoming complacent with respect to any infectious disease.

Information on Poliomyelitis

Causes: Viral infection

Symptoms: Swelling in lymph nodes surrounding intestines and in neck; in severe cases, pain and stiffness in spine, lethargy, general muscle weakness, paralysis (particularly of legs)

Duration: Acute to chronic

Treatments: Physical therapy, medical devices (splints, braces), prevention through vaccination

---

At the end of the nineteenth century, when epidemics of poliomyelitis first began to surface, medical science had made a number of important advances in the understanding and treatment of disease. First and foremost, the role of microorganisms in infectious disease was well established. Although viruses were still poorly defined, the principle that they were transmissible agents was understood. Second, although physicians had few specific remedies at their disposal, they had abandoned most of the drastic, plainly harmful remedies of earlier eras.

As polio became more and more prominent in morbidity statistics and the public imagination, the biomedical community responded on three different fronts. The first was an attempt to prevent transmission by quarantine measures and clinical studies. Scientists attempted to clarify the actual mode of transmission and the natural occurrence of the virus. Second, they attempted to treat paralytic cases in the acute and recovery phases. Lastly, scientists tried to develop a vaccine.

Quarantine measures were never very successful at controlling polio epidemics. Isolating critically ill patients in a sterile environment and restricting travel on the part of their family members, as was done in 1916 in New York, failed to quarantine people with mild infections, who were the main transmitters of the disease. Although the poliovirus can be found in untreated sewage, this was not a major source of infection in the United States. Flies can transmit the virus mechanically and thus may act as vectors, but fly eradication campaigns failed to have any effect on polio occurrence. In the period when it was incorrectly thought that the poliovirus entered through the nose, nasal sprays were touted as offering protection.

In the 1920s, the search for a cure emphasized the use of blood serum from individuals who had recovered from the disease. Theoretically, the idea was a sound one that had been used successfully for other diseases, but it proved ineffective in the case of polio, because the level of antibodies in the serum was not sufficiently high to have a therapeutic effect. More important, by the time patients developed paralytic symptoms, their bodies were already producing antibodies. Despite disappointing results, serum therapy was used extensively for fifteen years.

In 1920, Philip Drinker of the Harvard School of Public Health introduced the so-called iron lung, a respirator that mimicked the action of lungs by subjecting patients to fluctuations in air pressure. The iron lung gave some hope of survival to patients with paralysis of the diaphragm or lesions in the nervous centers of the brain that govern respiration. Its introduction was accompanied by misgivings that it would only serve to keep alive severely disabled patients who had no hope of survival outside a hospital. Such ethical concerns were justified, but artificial respirators also proved effective in temporarily treating acute cases of respiratory paralysis that subsided with time.

With respect to paralyzed limbs, advances in orthopedics in the early twentieth century allowed for surgical procedures that minimized twisting and deformity and for the design of braces that improved mobility. Observing that deformity could be lessened by bracing and immobilizing limbs at the onset of the paralytic form of the disease, doctors of the 1920s and 1930s had a tendency to encase polio victims, even those with little or no paralysis, in elaborate casts attached to pulley systems. Against this trend, Elizabeth Kenny, an Australian nurse, conducted what amounted to a crusade against immobilization and advocated active physical therapy in acute paralytic poliomyelitis.

In 1921, future president of the United States Franklin Delano Roosevelt was stricken with acute paralytic polio that left him with severe paralysis of both legs. Roosevelt later used his private fortune to establish a center for the rehabilitation of polio victims in Warm Springs, Georgia, where he had spent his convalescence. After he became president in 1933, Roosevelt became a leader in the fight against poliomyelitis. For several years, the principal charitable organization funding polio treatment and research in the United States was the president's Birthday Ball Commission, the immediate forerunner of the National Foundation for Infantile Paralysis (NFIP), better known under the name of its main fund-raising effort, the March of Dimes. Basil O'Conner, a personal friend of Roosevelt, headed both agencies.

Since an attack of polio in any of its forms confers lifelong immunity, researchers from the 1920s onward increasingly concentrated their efforts on developing a vaccine. Vaccines rely on dead or nonvirulent strains of a pathogenic agent to induce an immune response in a host. To produce a polio vaccine, one must have large quantities of poliovirus, and the only known source of poliovirus prior to 1938 was spinal cord tissue from infected monkeys or humans. In 1935, Maurice Brodie conducted human vaccine trials with a formalin-inactivated virus from monkey spinal cord. At the same time, John Kohler conducted trials with a virus that he claimed had been inactivated by repeated passage through many generations of monkeys. Brodie's vaccine was unsuccessful; Kohler's achieved notoriety as the suspected cause of several cases of paralytic polio.

After World War II, the NFIP concentrated its efforts on funding the development of an effective polio vaccine.

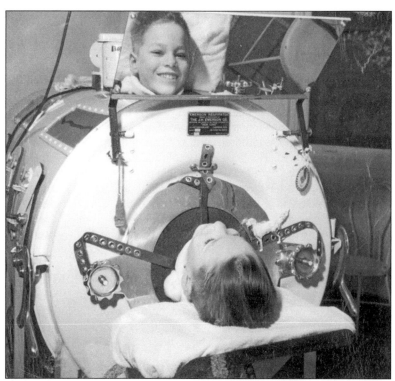

A boy with polio in an iron lung, circa 1955. (NMLM)

Thanks to the work of John Enders and others, a live poliovirus could be produced in tissue culture. Improved serological techniques enabled researchers to assess immunity in chimpanzees without sacrificing the animal. By 1950, a practical vaccination program was beginning to take shape under the direction of Jonas Salk, who headed the development of a formalin-inactivated injectable vaccine.

In 1954, with the collaboration of the National Institutes of Health and the US Census Bureau, the NFIP conducted a massive nationwide test of this inactivated Salk vaccine, involving 1.8 million children in the first, second, and third grades. In 1955, the number of new cases (or incidence) of polio among inoculated children was significantly lower than among controls, demonstrating that the vaccine was effective in clinical practice. Thereafter, the inoculation of children against polio became routine, and the incidence per 100,000 people declined dramatically-from 40 in 1952, the last major epidemic year, to 20 in 1955. The number of new cases per 100,000 people was 5 in 1959 and fewer than 1 in 1961 and subsequent years. There have been no domestically acquired cases of paralytic polio in the United States since 1987.

Salk's vaccine conferred only temporary immunity, requiring booster shots to be administered at yearly intervals. This made protection of the population cumbersome in industrialized countries and impractical in developing countries. The NFIP consequently turned its attention toward an effort, under the direction of Albert Sabin, to develop an orally administered attenuated viral preparation. The challenge was to develop a strain of virus that would multiply in the digestive system and stimulate antibody production but that could not attack the human nervous system. This effort was also supported by the World Health Organization (WHO). In 1957, an oral live virus vaccine was tested in Ruanda-Urundi (today Rwanda and Burundi). Between 1958 and 1959, field trials were conducted in fifteen countries, including the United States and the Soviet Union.

The Sabin oral vaccine confers longer-lasting immunity and is easier to administer, and therefore came to be used routinely to immunize children and adults against polio throughout the world. The WHO has exploited this advantage and undertaken a program of complete polio eradication. This program has been highly successful, and as of 2012, there were only three countries left in the world where polio was endemic (meaning not brought in from outside), down from more than 125 countries when the Global Polio Eradication Initiative was launched in 1988. The three remaining countries with endemic poliovirus are Nigeria, Pakistan, and Afghanistan. Six other countries in 2012 also reported isolated cases of polio, but they were either mild cases derived from the vaccine, or were brought into the country from outside. Altogether, 2012 saw fewer than 300 reported cases of polio worldwide.

Perspective and Prospects

There is evidence that poliomyelitis has afflicted human beings from the beginning of time. There is an Egyptian tomb painting of a priest with a withered leg, and descriptions of individuals with polio-like diseases occur in Greek medical literature. In general, however, polio seems to have been a rare disease; there are no records of epidemics of paralytic polio before the second half of the nineteenth century. The symptoms of paralytic polio are so distinctive and devastating that it is unlikely cases were overlooked.

In the early nineteenth century, a number of physicians published descriptions of cases in which a fever in infants or very young children was followed by paralysis of the lower limbs. At that time, polio was unknown among older children and adults. As a consequence, the disease came to be known as infantile paralysis. The occurrence was infrequent and sporadic, although Charles Bell, a distinguished English neurologist, recorded an account of an epidemic affecting all the three- to five-year-old children on the isolated island of St. Helena around 1830.

Between 1880 and 1905, several localized outbreaks of epidemic poliomyelitis occurred in rural Scandinavia. In 1894, the United States suffered its first major outbreak, in Rutland County, Vermont. In contrast to earlier experiences, significant numbers of older children and young adults were affected. It was also puzzling to epidemiologists that the outbreaks should have occurred in isolated rural areas rather than in urban centers. Ivar Wickman, a Swedish epidemiologist who tracked the course of the severe Scandinavian epidemic of 1905, obtained evidence for abortive and nonparalytic cases, and postulated that they were important to the epidemiology of the disease. His results were not taken seriously until thirty years later.

In 1916, the northeastern United States suffered one of the most devastating epidemics in the history of poliomyelitis, with more than nine thousand acute cases in New York City alone. Public health authorities, disregarding evidence that acute cases represented less than 10 percent of actual cases, instituted draconian quarantine measures that were largely ineffective. More than 95 percent of those affected in the 1916 epidemic were under nine years of age. By 1931, the date of the next major epidemic in the Northeast, the proportion of victims younger than nine had declined to 84 percent; by 1947, it had further declined to 52 percent. Poliomyelitis had somehow been transformed from an uncommon endemic disease affecting only very young children to a sporadic, rural epidemic disease that affected primarily but not exclusively children. Finally, it had become a widespread epidemic disease affecting all age groups in both rural and urban environments.

In 1905, when Swedish researchers attempted to show the existence of subclinical poliomyelitis infections, there was only one way to demonstrate polio in an unequivocal, scientifically rigorous manner. It involved filtering material from a diseased person to remove bacteria, inoculating the filtrate into the brain of a susceptible monkey, and waiting for paralysis to develop. Cost and logistics precluded large-scale tests. The trials that were conducted often failed because of inadequate sterility. In 1939, Charles Armstrong succeeded in propagating one of the three poliovirus strains in rodents, greatly facilitating research. In 1948, Enders and his colleagues succeeded in growing the poliovirus in tissue culture. In the meantime, reliable techniques for identifying antibodies to specific pathogens had been developed. This development enabled epidemiologists to determine which individuals had the live poliovirus in their bodies and which had developed immunity.

A series of studies conducted in the early 1950s among Alaskan Inuits, urban North Americans, and Egyptian villagers dramatically demonstrated the normal epidemiological pattern of polio occurrence and progress in three very different populations. Among Inuits living in Point Barrow, Alaska, only people over twenty showed antibodies to the virus, as a result of a known and devastating epidemic in 1930. In Miami, Florida, the proportion of persons with antibodies rose from 10 percent at age two to nearly 80 percent in adulthood. In Cairo, nearly 100 percent of the population over the age of three proved to have antibodies.

Therefore, the following epidemiological picture emerged. Before 1900, sanitary conditions in most of the world approximated those in Cairo, and most people contracted polio before the age of three. The vast majority of infections were subclinical, and paralytic cases occurred only sporadically in infants. As sanitation improved in the United States and Europe, the chances of contracting polio as an infant decreased. Thus, a pool of susceptible individuals of mixed ages arose, and epidemics occurred. Like mumps, measles, and other childhood illnesses, polio is more likely to cause severe illness in an adult than in a young child. For this reason, paralytic polio became a more serious health problem in Miami than in Cairo. Epidemics occurred first in rural areas in the United States and Scandinavia, where sanitation was relatively good and people were somewhat isolated from major population centers that served as sources of infection.

Defenders of the use of animals in biomedical research often cite the history of the conquest of poliomyelitis to support their point of view. From the earliest days of scientific poliomyelitis research until the discovery of tissue-culturing techniques for viruses in the 1940s, experimental work was dependent on monkeys. For many years, the only way of confirming that the virus was present was to inoculate a monkey with a suspected sample: If the monkey became paralyzed, the test was positive. Cultures were maintained through serial transfer from monkey to monkey, and the earliest vaccines were prepared from monkey spinal cord tissue.

The first successful tissue culture experiments involved fetal intestinal tissue. The experiments depended on having an available source of a characterized viral strain originally isolated from a human but maintained through several generations of transfer through animals. Even after the maintenance and characterization of viral strains and the production of virus for vaccines had moved from animal laboratories to test tubes of cultured cells, the first tests of the safety and efficacy of vaccines were performed with primates. Virtually every step in the conquest of polio involved experimental procedures.

Although the fight against poliomyelitis has been spectacularly successful, it would be unwise to be complacent about a disease that still exists in parts of the world and that is selectively virulent under modern urban conditions in developed nations. The percentage of schoolchildren, particularly those living in poorer neighborhoods, who receive routine vaccinations against childhood diseases is decreasing in the United States. Because of the availability of safe drinking water, children are no longer likely to naturally acquire immunity from subclinical infections.

In about 1 in 20 million cases, individuals will develop polio after receiving a vaccine. A naturally acquired case of polio is now exceedingly rare. The number of such cases is less than the number of cases of polio as a result of adverse reactions to the vaccine. For this reason, many parents are not having their children immunized against polio. These well-intentioned people are putting their children at an unnecessary risk of contracting the disease.

Other diseases that were once thought to be virtually extinct, such as measles and tuberculosis, are experiencing a resurgence because of declining commitment to public and community health and increasing numbers of people with compromised immune systems. Until the polio eradication campaign is complete, there is no guarantee that polio will be excluded from the list of resurgent diseases.

—*Martha Sherwood-Pike, Ph.D.; updated by*
L. Fleming Fallon, Jr., M.D., Ph.D., M.P.H.

See also Childhood infectious diseases; Enteroviruses; Epidemics and pandemics; Epidemiology; Immunization and vaccination; Meningitis; Paralysis; Viral infections.

For Further Information:
Blume, Stuart, and Ingrid Geesink. "A Brief History of Polio Vaccines." *Science* 288, no. 5471 (June 2, 2000): 1593-1594.
Carson-DeWitt, Rosalyn. "Poliomyelitis." *Health Library*, May 20, 2013.
Daniel, Thomas M., and Frederick C. Robbins, eds. *Polio*. Rochester, N.Y.: University of Rochester Press, 1997.
Garrett, Laurie. *The Coming Plague: Newly Emerging Diseases in a World out of Balance*. New York: Penguin, 1995.
Gould, Tony. *A Summer Plague: Polio and Its Survivors*. New Haven, Conn.: Yale University Press, 1997.
Hecht, Alan D., and Edward Alamo. *Polio*. New York: Chelsea House, 2003.
Munsat, Theodore L. "Poliomyelitis: New Problems with an Old Disease." *New England Journal of Medicine* 324 (April, 1991): 1206-1207.
Oshinsky, David M. *Polio: An American Story*. New York: Oxford University Press, 2005.
"Polio." *Centers for Disease Control and Prevention*, May 24, 2013.
"Poliomyelitis." *World Health Organization*, 2013.
Post-Polio Health International. http://www.post-polio.org.
Silver, Julie K. *Post-Polio Syndrome: A Guide for Polio Survivors and Their Families*. New Haven, Conn.: Yale University Press, 2002.

Polycystic kidney disease

Disease/Disorder

Anatomy or system affected: Blood vessels, brain, gastrointestinal system, kidneys, liver, pancreas
Specialties and related fields: Cardiology, gastroenterology, genetics, nephrology, urology
Definition: A genetic disorder characterized by multiple, bilateral, grapelike clusters of fluid-filled cysts that slowly replace much of the mass of the kidney, reducing kidney function and leading to renal failure.

Key terms:

acquired cystic kidney disease (ACKD): a condition that develops with long-term kidney problems, especially in patients who have been on dialysis for five years
autosomal dominant: referring to a disease for which an individual who carries the abnormal gene will have the disease; there is a 50 percent chance that a child will inherit the disease
autosomal recessive: referring to a disease for which an individual may carry the abnormal gene but not have the disease; a child will have the disease only if both parents passed on the gene
end-stage renal disease (ESRD): total chronic kidney failure

Causes and Symptoms

About 600,000 people in the United States have polycystic kidney disease (PKD), and 12.5 million suffer from it worldwide; it is the fourth leading cause of kidney failure. There are two major inherited forms of PKD, autosomal dominant and autosomal recessive, and a noninherited form called acquired cystic kidney disease (ACKD). The autosomal dominant type is the most common inherited form.

Autosomal dominant PKD has a slow onset, with symptoms usually developing between the ages of thirty and forty. Sometimes, symptoms do not appear until age seventy. Cysts grow out of the nephrons, the blood-processing units in the kidneys. High blood pressure occurs, and the

Information on Polycystic Kidney Disease

Causes: Genetic defect; long-term kidney damage associated with dialysis, end-stage renal disease

Symptoms: Cysts in kidneys, kidney enlargement, high blood pressure; may include pain in back and side, headaches, blood in urine, urinary tract infections, brain aneurysms, cysts in liver and pancreas, nail abnormalities, painful menstruation, varicose veins, hemorrhoids, joint pain, drowsiness, anemia

Duration: Progressive, usually fatal without treatment

Treatments: Alleviation of symptoms and prevention of complications; may include analgesics (aspirin, acetaminophen), antibiotics, iron supplements, blood transfusions, cyst drainage, dialysis, kidney transplantation

kidney enlarges as the cysts form. A normal kidney weighs 10 to 12 ounces and is the size of a human fist. A cyst-filled kidney can weigh as much as 22 pounds and can grow to the size of a football or larger. Healthy kidney tissue is destroyed as the cysts produce pressure on it, and renal failure eventually occurs. Once uremic symptoms appear, the disease is usually fatal within four years unless the patient receives dialysis or a kidney transplant. This destruction of kidney tissue may take as long as ten years.

Several other symptoms are associated with autosomal dominant PKD. Patients experience pain in the back and side, as well as headaches. Blood may appear in the urine, and urinary tract infections occur. Aneurysms in the blood vessels of the brain can also appear. Cysts may form in the liver and pancreas, and even the heart valves may be affected. Life-threatening bleeding into the abdominal cavity from cyst ruptures can occur. Other symptoms often associated with the disease are nail abnormalities, painful menstruation, joint pain, drowsiness, and anemia.

Autosomal dominant PKD is thought to occur equally in men and woman and in all races; however, some studies suggest that it occurs more often in white females than in African Americans. Diagnosis can be made by ultrasound, computed tomography (CT) scanning, and magnetic resonance imaging (MRI). Genetic tests are run to identify the presence of the autosomal dominant gene.

Autosomal recessive PKD usually affects children. Patients experience high blood pressure, urinary tract infections, and frequent urination. The liver, spleen, and pancreas are usually affected, resulting in low blood cell counts, varicose veins, and hemorrhoids. The child is usually smaller in size than average.

Autosomal recessive PKD can be diagnosed by ultrasound imaging of the fetus or newborn, which will reveal cysts in the kidneys. However, this procedure does not distinguish between the cysts of autosomal recessive and autosomal dominant PKD. Performing ultrasound examinations of relatives can be helpful in making a diagnosis.

The noninherited type of cystic disease is ACKD. It develops in kidneys as a result of long-term damage and bad scarring and is associated with dialysis and end-stage renal

disease (ESRD). About 90 percent of people who have been on dialysis for five years or more develop ACKD. People with ACKD may have underlying conditions such as glomerulonephritis or kidney disease associated with diabetes mellitus. The cysts of ACKD may bleed, and patients may develop renal cancer.

Treatment and Therapy

Polycystic kidney disease cannot be cured. The goals of treatment are the reduction of symptoms and the prevention of complications. Analgesics such as aspirin or acetaminophen (Tylenol) are used to treat the pain. If severe headaches occur, however, then an aneurysm may be involved. Therefore, the patient should see a physician before using over-the-counter medications.

Antibiotics are given to treat urinary tract infections, and high blood pressure is treated with proper diet, exercise, and medications as prescribed by a physician. Any symptoms of anemia are treated with iron supplements or blood transfusions.

Surgical drainage of cysts may be indicated because of pain, bleeding, infection, or obstruction. Because of the large number of cysts, surgery to remove them is not deemed proper. Eventually, the kidney may fail as a result of tissue destruction by the cysts, and dialysis and kidney transplantation become the only methods of treatment.

Perspective and Prospects

The first recorded case of polycystic kidney disease dates back to Stefan Bathory, the king of Poland who lived from 1533 to 1588. In the mid-1980s, the Polycystic Kidney Disease Foundation was formed.

Through extensive genetic research, a better understanding of PKD has been gained. In 1985, the first gene associated with autosomal dominant PKD was located on chromosome 16; in 1993, another was located on chromosome 4. Within three years, scientists isolated the proteins produced by these two genes, polycystin 1 and polycystin 2. Since then, scientists have identified the autosomal recessive PKD gene on chromosome 6.

Researchers are using mice bred with this genetic disease in an attempt to find a cure. In 2000, they reported that a cancer drug was successful in inhibiting cyst formation in mice with the PKD gene. The hope is that further testing will lead to safe and effective treatments for humans.

—*Mitzie L. Bryant, B.S.N., M.Ed.*

See also Cyst removal; Cysts; End-stage renal disease; Genetic diseases; Kidney cancer; Kidney disorders; Kidneys; Nephrectomy; Nephritis; Nephrology; Nephrology, pediatric; Pyelonephritis; Renal failure.

For Further Information:

Greenberg, Arthur, et al., eds. *Primer on Kidney Diseases*. 5th ed. Philadelphia: Saunders/Elsevier, 2009.

Kellicker, Patricia Griffin. "Polycystic Kidney Disease." *Health Library*, October 31, 2012.

MedlinePlus. "Kidney Cysts." *MedlinePlus*, May 20, 2013.

National Institute of Diabetes and Digestive and Kidney Diseases, National Institutes of Health. "Polycystic Kidney Disease." *National Kidney and Urologic Diseases Information Clearing House*, September 2, 2010.

National Kidney Foundation. *National Kidney Foundation*, 2013.

Parker, James N., and Philip M. Parker, eds. *The Official Patient's Sourcebook on Polycystic Kidney Disease*. San Diego, Calif.: Icon Health, 2002.

Schrier, Robert W., ed. *Diseases of the Kidney and Urinary Tract*. 8th ed. Philadelphia: Wolters Kluwer Health/Lippincott Williams & Wilkins, 2007.

Watson, Michael L., and Vicente E. Torres, eds. *Polycystic Kidney Disease*. New York: Oxford University Press, 1996.

Polycystic ovary syndrome

Disease/Disorder

Anatomy or system affected: Endocrine system, pancreas, reproductive system, skin

Specialties and related fields: Dermatology, endocrinology, family medicine, gynecology, nursing, nutrition, obstetrics, pathology, pediatrics, pharmacology, preventive medicine, psychology, public health

Definition: A complex disorder related to dysfunctional ovulation, endocrine abnormalities, and multiple cysts on the ovary that result in fertility difficulties. Polycystic ovary syndrome is related to obesity and diabetes and poses an increased risk for cardiovascular disease. In addition to these conditions, symptoms of hirsutism may be accompanied by depression or anxiety.

Key terms:

biguanide: a type of medication to lower blood glucose by increasing sensitivity to insulin and possibly lowering the liver's glucose production

gonadotropin: hormone secreted by the pituitary gland; the primary gonadotropic hormones are luteinizing hormone (LH) and follicle-stimulating hormone (FSH)

hirsutism: excess facial hair

hyperandrogenism: higher-than-normal levels of androgens in the blood

Causes and Symptoms

Polycystic ovary syndrome (PCOS) seems to be caused by a combination of genetics and environmental factors. Researchers are currently using candidate gene research to try to determine which genetic sequences may lead to susceptibility for PCOS. First-degree relatives of someone with PCOS are at higher risk of developing the condition themselves. Exposure to prenatal androgens may play a role, although this exposure may occur anywhere from the prenatal period through puberty. Additionally, in the prenatal period, the androgens appear to be from the fetus and not the mother.

Hyperinsulinemia and obesity both contribute to higher levels of androgens, called hyperandrogenism. Insulin may directly stimulate the production of androgens from the ovary, or it may indirectly affect androgen levels by inhibiting sex hormone-binding globulins. Obesity is associated with hyperinsulinemia.

The signs and symptoms can be ambiguous. The most common are related to the hyperandrogenism and include hirsutism (excess facial hair), infertility, and menstrual ir-

---

Information on Polycystic Ovary Syndrome

Causes: Environment and genetic risk factors not yet well defined

Symptoms: Hirsutism, hyperandrogenism, hyperinsulinemia, obesity, infertility, irregular menses

Duration: Chronic

Treatments: Diet for weight loss; medications, surgery

---

regularities. Acne and male-pattern baldness may also occur. The 1990 National Institutes of Health classification of PCOS requires disordered ovulation and clinical or biochemical evidence of hyperandrogenism. In 2003, the Rotterdam European Society of Human Reproduction and Embryology/American Society of Reproductive Medicine consensus workshop included having polycystic ovaries but suggested that two of these three symptoms were enough on which to base a diagnosis. Thus, a woman with PCOS may have disordered ovulation and polycystic ovaries with androgen excess, or androgen excess with polycystic ovaries but no disorder in ovulation. However, other scenarios are possible.

Hyperandrogenism can be evaluated through laboratory tests, including testosterone levels, sex hormone-binding globulins, and other androgen levels. However, these tests have not always reliably reflected PCOS symptoms. Ultrasound is used to detect the presence of polycystic ovaries and may include an assessment of follicle number and ovary size. Criteria for ultrasound evaluation include having twelve or more follicles that are two to nine millimeters in diameter or ovarian volume greater than ten cubic centimeters.

Treatment and Therapy

The main goal of treatment and therapy is to normalize menstrual cycles and ovulation and, if desired, achieve a successful pregnancy. The least-invasive approach to achieving this goal is weight loss in those who are overweight. Weight loss of 5 to 10 percent has been shown to have a positive impact on symptoms of PCOS-hirsutism, infertility, and menstrual irregularities as well as hyperinsulinemia. This goal can be achieved by a reduction in caloric intake and increased physical activity, although it is difficult to maintain.

Although weight loss is helpful, it may not alleviate all symptoms of PCOS in overweight females. In addition, only about half of those with PCOS are estimated to be overweight. Medications may be prescribed to achieve menstrual regularity or normalize blood glucose levels. Birth control medications will help to regulate menses if the woman is not trying to conceive. However, they may also result in weight gain and insulin resistance, which would be a negative effect for the PCOS treatment overall. Clomiphene citrate, a selective estrogen receptor modulator (SERM), may be prescribed to enhance the chances of conception, if this is desired. However, only 35 to 40 percent of women receiving this medication become pregnant. If clomiphene citrate fails to induce conception, then exogenous gonadotropins or laparoscopic ovarian surgery may be tried. However, gonadotropin therapy is associated with multifetus pregnancy, which is not found as often with surgery. However, regimens with low doses of gonadotropins have had some success over traditional doses in achieving single pregnancy. If these options fail to produce pregnancy, then in vitro fertilization is also an option.

For blood glucose normalization, oral hypoglycemic agents such as the biguanide metformin are usually prescribed. Some studies have suggested this medication may also enhance fertility, although other studies have found no such result. Current recommendations are to discontinue metformin when pregnancy is confirmed. Some suggest that metformin may be continued through pregnancy if type 2 diabetes is present. Nonsteroidal antiandrogen medications may help improve the symptoms of androgen excess, although they are not commonly used in adolescents. While several medications may improve hirsutism to some extent, nonpharmacological treatment can also be used, including waxing, electrolysis, bleaching, plucking, and heat or laser therapy.

Perspective and Prospects

First described by Irving F. Stein and Michael L. Leventhal in 1935, PCOS was for a time referred to as the Stein-Leventhal syndrome. At that time, surgical resection of the ovaries was fairly successful treatment, although complications with internal adhesions eventually made other treatments more desirable.

The prevalence of PCOS has been estimated from 2 to 30 percent of premenopausal women. While women of childbearing age were at one time believed to be the primary group afflicted with PCOS, adolescents are now also being diagnosed with the disorder. The diagnosis is somewhat more difficult because menses are often irregular until at least two years past menarche.

Polycystic ovaries by themselves have no long-term negative effects, although women with polycystic ovaries without the symptoms of the syndrome are at higher risk for hyperstimulation syndrome. Those with PCOS are at higher risk of complications associated with diabetes and cardiovascular disease. Depression and a reduced quality of life have been reported in women with PCOS, possibly as a result of difficulties with conception, dissatisfaction with appearance, and issues associated with chronic disease.

—*Karen Chapman-Novakofski, R.D., L.D.N., Ph.D.*

See also Cyst removal; Cysts; Diabetes mellitus; Genital disorders, female; Gynecology; Hormones; Hysterectomy; Infertility, female; Menopause; Menstruation; Obesity; Ovarian cysts; Ovaries; Pregnancy and gestation; Premenstrual syndrome (PMS); Puberty and adolescence; Reproductive system; Uterus.

For Further Information:

Dunaif, Andrea, et al., eds. *Polycystic Ovary Syndrome: Current Controversies, from the Ovary to the Pancreas.* Totowa, N.J.: Humana Press, 2008.

Franks, Stephen. "Polycystic Ovary Syndrome." *Medicine* 37, no. 9 (September, 2009): 441-444.

Hoeger, Kathleen M. "Role of Lifestyle Modification in the Management of Polycystic Ovary Syndrome." *Best Practice and Research: Clinical Endocrinology and Metabolism* 20, no. 2 (June, 2006): 293-310.

MedlinePlus. "Polycystic Ovary Syndrome." *MedlinePlus*, May 13, 2012.

Norman, Robert J., et al. "Polycystic Ovary Syndrome." *The Lancet* 370, no. 9588 (August 25, 2007): 685-697.

Radosh, Lee. "Drug Treatments for Polycystic Ovary Syndrome." *American Family Physician* 79, no. 671 (April 15, 2009): 671-676.

Polydactyly and syndactyly

Disease/Disorder

Also known as: Supernumerary digits, extra digits, polydactylia, polydactylism, hyperdactyly, syndactylia, syn- dactylism

Anatomy or system affected: Blood vessels, bones, feet, hands, skin

Specialties and related fields: General surgery, genetics, pediatrics, podiatry

Definition: Polydactyly is the presence of extra fingers or toes, while syndactyly describes two or more fingers or toes that are joined or fused together.

Key terms:

central or mesoaxial polydactyly: a complex form in which extra digits occur between the thumb and little finger or big toe and little toe

congenital: referring to a condition present at birth

digit: a finger or toe

postaxial polydactyly: an extra digit occurring near the little finger or little toe

preaxial polydactyly: an extra digit occurring near the thumb or big toe

Causes and Symptoms

Neither polydactyly nor syndactyly are serious congenital deformities, and they generally occur with no underlying or apparent cause. Both conditions may be genetic or inherited or may occur as a symptom of more than one hundred different inherited and developmental disorders. Sometimes there is not enough information to determine the cause, while other cases may be due to exposure during pregnancy to toxins such as cigarette smoking or the drug thalidomide or to poorly controlled diabetes during pregnancy. The hereditary aspects of the conditions are still being studied.

Polydactyly can vary from a poorly developed digit that is almost unnoticeable and without bone to a fully developed and functional digit. The condition occurs during fetal development when normal programmed cell death between digits fails to occur. In inherited cases, the genes responsible for the condition are dominant, which means that male and female children are equally likely to have the condition. Postaxial polydactyly is the most frequent form and accounts for about 75 to 80 percent of all cases. This type occurs in approximately one of every one thousand Caucasian births. African Americans are ten times more likely than any other ethnic group to have this type of polydactyly in the hand. One-half of polydactyly cases are bilateral, affecting both sides of the body, with the remainder of the cases affecting the left side almost twice as often as the right. Postaxial polydactyly is most often found in the hands and rarely found in both the hands and feet. People of Asian ancestry tend to have more occurrences of preaxial polydactyly, while central polydactyly is uncommon across all ethnic groups. All three types of polydactyly are believed to be inherited differently, although people in the same family may have different degrees of the condition.

In syndactyly, one or more digits fail to separate during fetal development. Syndactyly is one of the most common congenital malformations and occurs in about one of every 2,000 to 2,500 births. It is more common in males and Caucasians and usually affects the middle and ring fingers. In the toes, the condition most commonly affects the second and third toes. Incidents of syndactyly affect the left and right sides and the hands and feet equally and are usually bilateral. Syndactyly is described as either simple, in which the digits are fused by skin and soft tissue, or complex, in which the bones are also fused. The severity can range from incomplete webbing of the skin to sharing of the bones, nails, nerves, and blood vessels. Complicated syndactyly describes the addition of extra bones and unusual tendon or ligament development. Partial or incomplete syndactyly means that only part of the length of the digits are fused together. Complete syndactyly means that the entire length of the digits are fused together.

Treatment and Therapy

In most cases, polydactyly and syndactyly do not interfere with normal hand or foot function, and correction is done for cosmetic purposes. The conditions can be diagnosed at birth or by fetal ultrasound (sonogram). Once the condition is observed, physicians will normally require x-rays to determine its complexity.

In type A polydactyly, where the fully formed digit has bones, surgery is required when the baby is about a year old. In type B polydactyly, the digit is rudimentary, contains no bones, and is usually removed before the infant

---

Information on Polydactyly and Syndactyly

Causes: Genetic or inherited; may occur as symptom of more than one hundred different inherited and developmental disorders

Symptoms: In polydactyly, extra digit(s) varying from poorly developed without bone to fully developed and functional; in syndactyly, fusion of one or more digits

Duration: Lifelong unless corrected

Treatments: Surgery to remove extra digits or separate fused ones

---

leaves the hospital. Many people are unaware that they ever had polydactyly. Central polydactyly is more complex, may affect normal hand or foot function, and often requires multiple surgeries.

Multiple surgeries may be needed to separate the digits in complex or complicated cases of syndactyly, and the procedures are usually performed when the child is between six months and eighteen months old. Skin grafts are typically taken from the lower abdomen to cover the newly separated digits. If multiple digits are involved, then more than one surgery may be needed as only one digit is separated at a time. Some children also experience recurrent syndactyly, or "web creep," if there are complications in healing. In the feet, simple syndactyly is a cosmetic problem that is generally not treated unless surgery is desired.

Perspective and Prospects

Polydactyly and syndactyly have existed throughout history, and polydactyly is mentioned in the Bible in a description of a member of Goliath's family (2 Samuel 21:20). Italian painter Raphael (1483-1520) depicted polydactyly in at least six of his works, including *The Marriage of the Virgin* (1504) and *La Belle Jardiniere* (1507). The examination of polydactyly through several generations of a Berlin family by French mathematician, biologist, and astronomer Pierre-Louis Moreau de Maupertuis (1698-1759) is considered the first scientific analysis of a dominant inherited trait in humans.

Some famous polydactyls include King Charles VIII of France, Prime Minister Winston Churchill of England, Major League Baseball pitcher Antonio Alfonseca, Bollywood actor Hrithik Roshan, actress Gemma Arterton, jazz pianist Hampton Halls, blues guitarist Hound Dog Taylor, Roman era poet Volcatius Sedigitus, and possibly Anne Boleyn, one of Henry VIII's wives. A few famous syndactyls are Soviet leader Joseph Stalin; actors Ashton Kutcher, Dan Aykroyd, and Tricia Hefler; singer Rachel Stevens; and writers Rob Never and Mike Holderness. There is also some speculation that painter and inventor Leonardo da Vinci had syndactyly on his left hand.

—*Virginia L. Salmon*

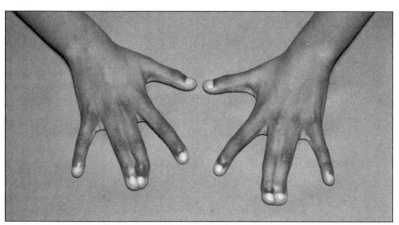

An example of syndactyly, a congenital fusion of the fingers. (St. Bartholomew's Hospital/Photo Researchers, Inc.)

See also Birth defects; Congenital disorders; Embryology; Genetic diseases; Lower extremities; Plastic surgery; Teratogens; Thalidomide; Upper extremities.

For Further Information:
Blereau, Robert P. "Polydactyly." *Consultant* 39, no. 12 (December, 1999): 3297.
Flatt, Adrian E. "Webbed Fingers." *Baylor University Medical Center Proceedings* 18 (January, 2005): 26.
Goldenring, John. "Webbing of the Fingers or Toes." *MedlinePlus*, December 1, 2011.
"True Polydactyly." *Consultant* 43, no. 10 (September 1, 2003): 1309.
Kaneshiro, Neil. "Polydactyly." *MedlinePlus*, November 7, 2011.
Vorvick, Linda J. "Repair of Webbed Fingers or Toes." *MedlinePlus*, August 11, 2012.
Wynbrandt, James, and Mark D. Ludman. "Polydactyly." In *The Encyclopedia of Genetic Disorders and Birth Defects*. 2d ed. New York: Facts On File, 2000.

Polyp removal. *See* Colorectal polyp removal; Nasal polyp removal.

Polymyalgia rheumatica
Disease/Disorder
Anatomy or system affected: Joints, immune system
Specialties and related fields: Rheumatology, internal medicine, gerontology
Definition: An inflammatory disorder of the joints and connective tissues of the shoulders, neck, and hips.
Key terms:
inflammation: the body's natural defense against an insult; characterized by heat, redness, swelling and pain to the area
steroids: an organic compound used as a treatment for treating inflammation
giant cell arteritis: a disease characterized by the inflammation of the arteries and veins that supply the head, neck and arms; it can cause headaches, jaw-pain and changes in vision
joints: a point where two or more bones join together

Causes and Symptoms

Polymyalgia rheumatica (PMR) is an inflammatory disorder of the joints and connective tissues of the shoulders, neck, and hips. The cause is unknown. The stiffness is typically worse in the morning, and PRM affects primarily older adults aged 50 and over. PMR can be associated with Giant Cell Arteritis (GCA); 15-30 percent of patients who have PMR will also have GCA. It is believed that they share some of the same disease processes, although the correlation is poorly understood. GCA is associated with cardiovascular events and should be treated promptly and seriously.

PMR is characterized by pain and stiffness in the shoulders, neck, and hip. The pain is worse in the mornings and with movement and is symmetric. Doing regular activities may be painful and/or challenging such as putting a shirt over one's head, or rolling over in bed in the morning. Pain is usually isolated to the joint and there may be joint swelling or point-tenderness. Muscle pain is usually not a common site of PMR. Overall constitutional symptoms may include fatigue, malaise, depression, and weight loss/gain. High fevers are uncommon, but point more to GCA than PMR.

Diagnosis is through evaluation of one's symptoms and some basic blood tests. The most common tests to check for PMR are called erythrocyte sedimentation rate (ESR) and C-reactive protein (CRP) tests. Both of these are markers for inflammation in the body. They are not specific to PMR, but can help paint the overall clinical picture.

Treatment and Therapy

Because PMR is an inflammatory disorder, the medications we use to treat PMR are an anti-inflammatory medicine called steroids. The optimal dose of steroids is tailored to each individual, but the goal is to give symptomatic relief on the lowest effective dose possible. Often, treatment for PMR must last several months. Patients often experience relief within the first few days of treatment.

Steroids are very effective, but also have several side effects that must be monitored closely. Of note, is the increased risk of osteoporosis with long-term use. For this reason, clinicians may advise patients to get routine screening for osteoporosis and take supplemental calcium and vitamin D to increase bone strength and decrease the risk of osteoporosis from steroid use. In addition, high blood pressure and diabetes are also associated with long-term steroid use and patients should be screened for these regularly.

Over-the-counter medications for pain such as ibuprofen and acetaminophen are not found to be effective in treating PMR.

Prognosis

PMR usually resolves spontaneously within months, but sometimes can last years. In these cases, side effects from the steroids need to be monitored closely. In addition, signs and symptoms of GCA such as headache, jaw pain, problems with vision, and fever should be evaluated regularly.

—*Maki Matsumura*

See also C-reactive protein, Erythrocyte sedimentation rate, Gerontology, Giant cell arteritis, Headache, Osteoarthritis, Pain, Rheumatoid arthritis, Rheumatology, Steroids

For Further Information:
Docken, W. *Polymyalgia Rheumatica.* Retrieved from http://www.rheumatology.org/Practice/Clinical/Patients/Diseases_And_Conditions/Polymyalgia_Rheumatica.
Hunder, G. "Clinical Manifestations and Diagnosis of Polymyalgia Rheumatica." *UpToDate,* edited by J.H. Stone and P.L. Romain. Retrieved from http://www.upto date.com/contents/clinical-manifestations-and-diagnosis-of-polymyalgia-rheumatica?detectedLanguage=en&source=search_result&search=polymyalgiarheumatica&selectedTitle=1~73& provider=noProvider.
Hunder, G. "Treatment of Polymyalgia Rheumatica." *UpToDate,* edited by UpToDate, edited by J.H. Stone and P.L. Romain. Retrieved from http://www.uptodate.com/contents/treatment-of-polymyalgia-rheumatica? detectedLanguage=en&source=search_result&search=polymyalgiarheumatica& selectedTitle=2~73&provider=noProvider.
Rovensky, Jozef, Burkhard F. Leeb, Howard Bird, Viera Stvrtinova, and Richard Imrich, eds. *Polymyalgia Rheumatica and Giant Cell Arteritis.* Germany: Springer-Verlag/Wein, 2010.

Polymyositis

Disease/Disorder
Anatomy or system affected: Muscular system
Specialties and related fields: Rheumatology
Definition: Polymyositis is an idiopathic disease of muscle inflammation. Myositis is the general category for inflammatory muscles diseases such as juvenile myositis, dermatomyositis, inclusion body myositis, and polymyositis. Referred to as inflammatory myopathies, the muscle inflammation can cause damage to the muscles. Referred to as inflammatory myopathy, the muscle inflammation can cause damage to the muscles. Polymyositis is considered to be an autoimmune disease. It can occur in persons of all ages, but is most common in middle childhood and in the twenties. Polymyositis is more common among women and girls. There are twice the number of cases in women than in men and boys. When the inflammatory condition of polymyositis is seen on the skin as well, this is termed dermatomyositis. The disease does not manifest immediately; rather, there is a gradual process of weakness over a three- to six-month period. Typically, there are remissions and exacerbations.

Key terms:

autoimmune: An autoimmune condition that is caused by the person's immune system. In this situation the immune system has failed to delete the T cells that are not recognizing "self" versus "non-self"

dysphagia: having difficulty swallowing due to muscle weakness

prognosis: the estimated good life or survival time as assessed by your physician

Causes and Symptoms

The main feature of polymyositis is the inflammation and the damage to the muscles that ensues. The person with polymyositis has white blood cells in the affected muscles. The inflamed muscles, caused by the disease, tend to release enzymes into the bloodstream. So, lab tests of the blood will demonstrate high levels of muscle enzymes. The muscles close to the trunk or torso are the main muscles affected. Usually there is symmetrical muscle weakness. Both the lungs and the heart can be affected by this condition. Problems in the lungs can cause dysphagia, shortness of breath, and infection. Heart problems are a little less common and can be a bad sign.

The primary symptom is the debilitating weakness, although it usually does not cause pain. There is a possibility that muscles of the body further away from the trunk can also become affected by the disease; if this occurs, it may only happen when there is a disease progression.

The disease may not be easily identified at first. Joint pain or weakness may be experienced as a general feeling of fatigue and exhaustion. Rising off a chair may be challenging as is the movement of raising one's arms to perform a simple action. Climbing stairs or lifting objects may feel extremely difficult or impossible. Likewise, when lying down, a person may find it difficult to get up. The weakness is felt in the torso or core area. Muscles of the hips, thighs, and shoulders are usually affected. Sometimes muscles may ache, and the body may be sensitive to touch. Dysphagia may occur, with the person finding it difficult to swallow. Further symptoms may include fever and weight loss. A skin irritation may be seen, such as a rash around the eyes (red or violet), on the knuckle area of the hand, on elbows, knees, neck, and chest. Some researchers think that polymyositis may be inherited. It appears that if a patient's family members have had neuromuscular problems, that the polymyositis may be inherited. It is also thought that it may be caused by a virus, such as cytomegalovirus.

Treatments and Therapy

The polymyositis diagnosis is verified by a series of tests. Following a full physical examination by a doctor, the patient will be sent for blood tests. Further testing may be conducted to ascertain the state of the nerves and muscles. The most critical tests are EMG (electromyography) and an MRI (magnetic resonance imaging) of the muscles affected, and a muscle biopsy. The blood test may demonstrate a high level of muscle enzymes, a CPK, and liver enzymes. Further testing may be conducted to ascertain the state of the nerves and muscles. There is also the theory that the person may have another autoimmune disease with similar symptoms.

Medications for polymyositis may comprise a number of prescriptions. The primary medication consists of immune system suppressants. Corticosteroids are typically prescribed, particularly as the first option to treat the illness. Their effectiveness relates to the ability to reduce muscle inflammation. When corticosteroids are not found to improve the condition, specialists may prescribe immunosuppressive medications. Medicines of this type include methotrexate, azathioprine, cyclosporine, tacrolimus, chlorambucil, mycophenolate, cyclophosphamide, and rituximab. If the symptoms are particularly debilitating the physician may put the patient on an infusion of immunoglobulins (IVIG).

Because of the muscular effects of the disease, doctors usually recommend a course of physical therapy to accompany medical treatment.

Perspective and Prospects

The cause of polymyositis remains elusive despite constant research. There is a possibility that hereditary factors may be responsible for polymyositis. As research continues and develops more insight into the immune system and related diseases. The hope is that understanding of the immune system and its functioning will facilitate deeper knowledge, and disease causes. There is a good prognosis for people who develop the disease in its early stages. Current research has revealed so far that immune system cells appear to invade muscle tissue at the onset of the disease, continuing to attack the muscles and causing damage. There is a good prognosis for people who develop the disease in its early stages. Possibilities of the disease becoming inactive happen often. In these instances, the process of rehabilitating the muscles can occur with beneficial results. Exercises to prevent the wasting away of unused muscles will be implemented with the aim of strengthening the affected and surrounding muscles.

Following are some organizations related to Polymyositis. In the United States, there are a number of organizations or associations providing information or support regarding muscle diseases such as polymyositis. These include: Muscular Dystrophy Association, National Institute of Arthritis and Musculoskeletal and Skin Diseases (NIAMS), Information Clearinghouse, National Institutes of Health, Myositis Association, and National Organization for Rare Disorders. Concerned patients or members of the public are always advised to consult with their doctors in addition to seeking medical information via public resources. Personal medical history is taken into account by a person's private doctor, physician, or specialist.

—Leah Jacob, MA;
updated by Christine M. Carroll, RN, BSN, MBA

For Further Information:

"Polymyositis and Dermatomyositis." *ArthritisResearch UK*, Arthritis Research UK, 2016. Web. 1 May 2016.

"Polymyositis." *Cleveland Clinic*, The Cleveland Clinic Foundation, 2015. Web. 1 May 2016.

"Polymyositis." *The Johns Hopkins Myositis Center*, Johns Hopkins Medicine, 2016. Web. 1 May 2016.

"Polymyositis (PM)." *MDA For Strength, Independence& Life*, Muscular Dystrophy Association, Inc., 2016. Web. 1 May 2016.

"NINDS Polymyositis Information Page." *National Institute of NeurologicalDisorders and Stroke*, National Institute of Neurological Disorders and Stroke, 2015. Web. 1 May 2016.

"Polymyositis-Adult." *The New York Times Health Guide*, 22 March 2013. Web. 1 May 2016.

"Polymyositis-Adult." *MedlinePlus*, U.S. National Library of Medicine, 26 April 2016. Web. 1 May 2016.

"Polymyositis." *Victoria State Government. Better Health Channel*, State Government of Victoria, Australia, 2016. Web. 1 May 2016.

MedicineNet. (2017) Polymyositis and Dermatomyositis Symptoms and Diagnosis. Retrieved on September 10, 2017 from http://medicinenet.com/polymyositis/article.htm

Pappu, Ramesh,MD, DPH. MBBS: Chief Editor. (22 November 2016) Polymyositis Clinical Presentation. Retrieved on September 10, 2017 from http://emedicine.medscape.com/article/335925-clinical

Polyps
Disease/Disorder

Anatomy or system affected: Abdomen, anus, bladder, gallbladder, gastrointestinal system, intestines, kidneys, nose, reproductive system, stomach, throat, urinary system, uterus

Specialties and related fields: Family medicine, gastroenterology, general surgery, genetics, gynecology, internal medicine, nephrology, otorhinolaryngology, proctology, pulmonary medicine, urology

Definition: Abnormal growths arising from mucous membranes anywhere in the body. A polyp is considered pedunculated if it is attached to the mucous membrane by a narrow, long stalk of tissue; if no stalk is present, then the polyp is said to be sessile.

Key terms:

colonoscopy: an endoscopic procedure used for visualization of the intestine

endoscopy: procedure with a flexible tube that allows direct viewing inside the body

inherited disorder: a disorder caused by an alteration of a gene and passed through families

Causes and Symptoms

The cause of polyps varies with the location of the polyp growth in the body. Symptoms are also site dependent.

Nasal polyps consist of inflamed tissue in the mucous membrane lining of the nose or sinuses. Causes of nasal polyps may be allergies, chronic infection, cystic fibrosis, and asthma. They usually develop around the ethnoid sinuses (inside the top of the nose) and may block the airway, resulting in difficulty breathing or shortness of breath because of obstruction. Breathing through the mouth, loss of the sense of smell, and a runny nose are common symptoms.

Vocal cord polyps are caused by mechanical injury such as shouting and usually occur on one vocal cord. Vocal cord nodules are not to be confused with polyps and are generally caused by chronic abuse such as singing. Symptoms include hoarseness and a breathy or raspy voice.

Stomach polyps are rare and are usually discovered by accident-for example, during an upper gastrointestinal endoscopy (a viewing of the interior of the stomach). Causes include *Helicobacter pylori* (*H. pylori*) bacteria or chronic gastritis (inflammation of the stomach) caused by an autoimmune response. Stomach polyps usually do not cause symptoms, but if symptoms occur they may include nausea, vomiting, abdominal pain, bleeding, or a feeling of fullness when eating even small amounts.

Colorectal polyps grow on the lining (mucous membrane) of the colon (also known as the large intestine) or rectum and may be caused by abnormal cell growth, heredity (family history or inherited disorder), or inflammatory diseases such as ulcerative colitis or Crohn's disease. Small polyps do not usually cause symptoms. If symptoms do occur, then they may include blood in a bowel movement, rectal bleeding, fatigue due to anemia from loss of blood, and pain.

Uterine polyps develop in the lining of the uterus and are caused by an overgrowth of endometrial cells. Occasionally, uterine polyps may slip through the cervix into the vagina, resulting in cervical polyps. The exact cause of uterine and cervical polyps is unknown, but may be related to the estrogen hormone level, chronic inflammation or clogged blood vessels in the cervix. Symptoms may include bleeding, heavy or irregular menstrual periods, a white or yellow discharge of mucus (leukorrhea), or there may be no symptoms.

Treatment and Therapy

The treatment for polyps varies by site. Medications, removal during colonoscopy (intestines), colposcopy (vagina and cervix) or other endoscopic procedures (throat, stomach, small bowel), and surgical removal are used. Biopsy of the polyp may also be done to determine if it is malignant (cancerous) or benign (not cancerous).

Information on Polyps

Causes: Varies with location; chronic allergies, hereditary factors, hormone levels, mechanical (overuse of vocal cords), uncontrolled cell growth from unknown causes

Symptoms: Varies with location; may include difficulty breathing, hoarseness, bleeding, pain, swelling

Duration: Until removed or minimized

Treatments: Medications, surgery

It is possible to prevent some polyps. Controlling allergies and managing chronic sinusitis may prevent nasal polyps. Vocal cord polyps are directly related to injury from yelling such as at a sporting event, so less abuse may lessen the potential for development. Stomach polyps caused by *H. pylori* may be controlled by treating the underlying bacteria and controlling gastritis may diminish the occurrence.

The goal of treatment for nasal polyps is to reduce the size of the polyp or to remove it. Because nasal polyps may occur in response to allergies or chronic sinusitis, medications such as corticosteroids (a drug that reduces inflammation), antihistamines, and antibiotics (a drug to fight infection) may be effective in shrinking the size of the polyp. If the polyp is in the sinus cavity, then endoscopic surgery using a small camera and tube inserted into the sinus allows the physician to remove the polyp.

Vocal cord polyps usually require surgical removal to restore the normal speaking voice. Voice therapy with a speech pathologist may be needed to prevent future occurrences. Stomach polyps require biopsy and, if there is concern, surgical removal. Medications to treat gastritis, including antibiotics, may be used. Routine colonoscopy and flexible sigmoidoscopy are recommended for routine cancer screening, and if a colorectal polyp is seen during the procedure, it is removed. If colorectal polyps are causing symptoms, then surgical removal either through colonoscopy or removal of a portion of the intestine may be needed. Uterine polyps may be watched, medications may be used to shrink them, or surgery may be used to remove them; if the polyps are cancerous, then a hysterectomy (removal of the uterus) is usually necessary.

Perspective and Prospects

Polyps are usually benign (not cancerous), but they can become malignant (cancerous) over time or in certain areas. Risk factors include age, obesity, family history, poor overall health (including allergies and chronic infections), stomach ulcer, infection, and inherited disorders such as cystic fibrosis or familial adenomatous polyposis. Prevention and screening, routine visits to the physician for health maintenance, and good health behaviors are important to prevent, recognize, or manage polyps. Prompt treatment is indicated if polyps cause symptoms or if a biopsy demonstrates malignant cells. Research is continuing on the causes of polyps and the influences that turn polyps from benign to malignant.

—*Patricia Stanfill Edens, Ph.D., R.N., FACHE*

See also Allergies; Colon; Colonoscopy and sigmoidoscopy; Colorectal cancer; Colorectal polyp removal; Colorectal surgery; Electrocauterization; Endoscopy; Gastroenterology; Gastrointestinal system; Intestinal disorders; Intestines; Nasal polyp removal; Nasopharyngeal disorders; Oncology; Otorhinolaryngology; Proctology; Rectum; Screening; Sense organs; Sinusitis; Smell; Uterus; Voice and vocal cord disorders.

For Further Information:

Bremmer, Hermann, et al. "Colorectal Cancers Occurring after Colonoscopy with Polyp Detection: Sites of Polyps and Sites of Cancers." *International Journal of Cancer* 133, no. 7 (October, 2013): 1672-1679.

Church, James M. "Laparoscopic versus Colonoscopic Removal of a Large Polyp." *American Journal of Gastroenterology* 104, no. 10 (October, 2009): 2633-2634.

Hellings, Peter W., and Hens Greet. "Rhinosinusitis and the Lower Airways." *Immunology and Allergy Clinics of North America* 29, no. 4 (November, 2009): 733-740.

Huber, Aaron R., and James F. Shikle. "Benign Fibroblastic Polyps of the Colon." *Archives of Pathology and Laboratory Medicine* 133, no. 11 (November, 2009): 1872-1876.

Lev, Robert, et al. *Adenomatous Polyps of the Colon: Pathobiological and Clinical Features*. New York: Springer-Verlag, 2012.

Maydeo, Amit, and Vinay Dhir. "The Gallbladder Polyp Conundrum: A Riddler on the Wall." *Gastrointestinal Endoscopy* 78, no. 3 (September, 2013): 494-495.

Thakkar, K., and D. S. Sihman, and M. A. Gilger. "Colorectal Polyps in Childhood." *Current Opinion in Pediatrics* 24, no. 5 (October, 2012): 632-637.

Porphyria

Disease/Disorder

Anatomy or system affected: Nervous system, skin

Specialties and related fields: Genetics, neurology, pediatrics

Definition: One of several rare genetic disorders caused by the accumulation of substances called porphyrins.

Causes and Symptoms

Porphyria refers to a group of diseases that share a common feature: a defect in the chain of chemical reactions that produce hemoglobin, the protein responsible for the transport of oxygen by the blood. These metabolic errors cause a buildup of porphyrins, resulting in two main types of illness: nervous system attacks and skin lesions.

There are two major groups of porphyrias: erythropoietic and hepatic. In erythropoietic porphyria, the porphyrins are synthesized in the bone marrow; in hepatic porphyrias, they are produced in the liver. Each of these porphyrias has several subtypes. For example, acute intermittent porphyria (AIP) is a hepatic porphyria most common in young adults and adults in early middle age. Its attacks are triggered by alcohol, certain drugs, and hormonal changes (such as those accompanying pregnancy). Some patients experience two to three episodes per year, while others may have as few as three in a lifetime.

Since all forms of porphyria are rare, a physician may not suspect the disease at first. The symptoms of porphyria include abdominal disturbances, nausea, vomiting, reddish urine, and prickling sensations in the hands and feet. The hallmarks that distinguish porphyrias, however, are the

---

Information on Porphyria

Causes: Genetic disorder; triggered by alcohol, drugs, sunlight

Symptoms: Nervous system attacks (mild mental confusion to delirium and hysteria), nausea, vomiting, reddish urine, prickling sensations in hands and feet, extreme photosensitivity of skin, skin lesions

Duration: Chronic with acute episodes

Treatments: Avoidance of triggering factors, protective clothing, drug therapy

---

skin and nervous system effects. Except for AIP, all the porphyrias cause extreme photosensitivity of the skin because the porphyrins that are deposited in the skin are excited by the ultraviolet aspect of sunlight. This reaction results in skin lesions, which may lead to disfigurement. The neurological disturbances of porphyria range from mild mental confusion to delirium and hysteria. If a porphyria is suspected, urine, stool, and blood tests are done to detect the presence of porphyrins.

Treatment and Therapy

Avoiding triggering factors is primary in the control of porphyria attacks. Alcohol and drugs, which may cause an attack, should be stopped. Protective clothing should be worn to prevent the irritating effects of sunlight. For certain porphyrias, drugs are available to suppress the formation of porphyrins. In the case of AIP, a simple increase in the consumption of carbohydrates is enough to inhibit the production of porphyrin-forming substances. The treatment of porphyrias is largely aimed at relieving its symptoms.

—*Robert T. Klose, Ph.D.*

See also Blood and blood disorders; Genetic diseases; Lesions; Metabolic disorders; Metabolism; Skin disorders.

For Further Information:

American Porphyria Foundation. http://www.porphyriafoundation.com.

Goldman, Lee, and Dennis Ausiello, eds. *Cecil Textbook of Medicine.* 23d ed. Philadelphia: Saunders/Elsevier, 2007.

Greer, John, et al., eds. *Wintrobe's Clinical Hematology.* 12th ed. Philadelphia: Wolters Kluwer/Lippincott Williams & Wilkins Health, 2009.

"Learning about Porphyria." *National Human Genome Research Institute,* April 18, 2013.

Parish, Kathy. "What's Wrong with This Patient?" *RN* 53, no. 7 (July, 1990): 43-45.

Parker, James N., and Philip M. Parker, eds. *The Official Patient's Sourcebook on Porphyria.* San Diego, Calif.: Icon Health, 2002.

"Porphyria." *Mayo Clinic,* May 7, 2011.

Rakel, Robert E., and Edward T. Bope, eds. *Conn's Current Therapy.* Philadelphia: Saunders/Elsevier, 2007.

Wood, Debra. "Porphyria." *Health Library,* November 26, 2012.

Positron emission tomography (PET) scanning

Procedure

Anatomy or system affected: All

Specialties and related fields: Biotechnology, nuclear medicine, radiology

Definition: A noninvasive imaging procedure in which a positron-emitting radiopharmaceutical is administered and a three-dimensional image of an organ, which accumulates the radiopharmaceutical, is obtained by detecting the radiation resulting from positron annihilation.

Key terms:

annihilation: the process whereby an electron and positron combine and their energy is converted into two photons traveling in opposite directions

positrons: a type of radiation, similar to electrons but with a positive charge, emitted by radioactive atoms

tomography: a procedure that yields images of body sections

Indications and Procedures

Positron emission tomography (PET) scanning permits the noninvasive determination of biological function, metabolism, and pathology following the administration of short-lived positron-emitting radiopharmaceuticals (radioactive pharmaceuticals). Positron-emitting radiopharmaceuticals are drugs that contain a radioactive atom that is transformed into a more stable atom by emitting a positron. A positron is a subatomic particle that has the same mass and charge as an electron, but the charge is positive rather than negative. When an energetic positron is emitted by a radioactive atom, it quickly loses its energy in the surrounding medium and comes to rest. The positron then combines with a free electron in the medium, the two particles are annihilated, and their energy is converted into two 511,000-volt-potential (511 keV) photons that travel in exactly opposite directions. The detection of these two photons in coincidence (simultaneously) by placing a ring of small radiation detectors around the patient is the basic principle used in PET scanning. The radiation detectors convert these light photons into electrical signals that are fed to a computer, which reconstructs the distribution of radioactivity in the desired organ and presents the information as an image on a video screen.

Uses and Complications

PET techniques are generally used to measure metabolic rates quantitatively in normal and abnormal tissues. The positron-emitting radionuclides oxygen-15, nitrogen-13, and carbon-11 are well suited for studying tissue metabolism because of their short physical half-lives and their ubiquitous presence in biomolecules. Oxygen-15 gas is useful for studying oxygen metabolism, whereas oxygen-15 water and oxygen-15 carbon monoxide are used to study blood flow and blood volume, respectively, in any organ. Fluorode- oxyglucose (FDG) labeled with fluorine-18 is another positron-emitting radiopharmaceutical that is useful in PET for the quantitative measurement of glucose metabolism. Glucose metabolism is high in brain tumors when compared to normal tissue. Hence, PET with fluorodeoxyglucose-18 is widely used in the detection of brain tumors and assessment of the degree of malignancy, since low-grade tumors are less metabolically active than high-grade tumors. Fluorodeoxyglucose-18 PET is also used to identify persistent tumors after surgery.

PET Scanning Techniques

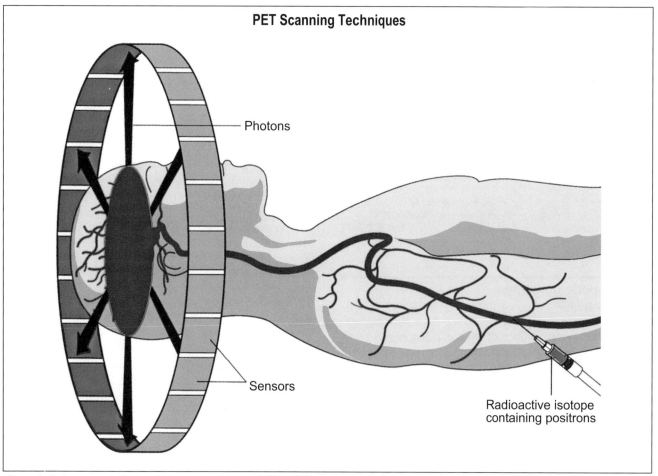

Photons

Sensors

Radioactive isotope
containing positrons

This method of scanning the brain, which can reveal the metabolic and chemical activity of tissue, is used to detect tumors, to evaluate damage resulting from strokes, and to diagnose and assess such conditions as Parkinson's disease, epilepsy, and certain mental illnesses.

The radiopharmaceuticals carbon-11 aminoisobutyric acid, rubidium-82 chloride, and gallium-68 citrate are useful for studying the blood-brain barrier permeability. This modality is also being used increasingly in patients with seizure disorders, dementia, and movement disorders. The application of PET in these cases may provide previously unavailable information about these diseases to help the practicing neurologist. PET imaging is also being used to understand the mechanisms behind normal brain processes. Among the mechanisms studied are language processing, speech, vision, and brain development. Recent improvements in whole-body PET scanning technology are useful in clinical oncology. This technique is being employed widely in the qualitative imaging of primary or recurrent tumors, lymph nodes, and distant metastases.

PET is also being used with increasing frequency to measure myocardial perfusion (heart function). A number of different perfusion agents labeled with rubidium-82, gallium-62, oxygen-15, and nitrogen-13 are being investigated. Some of these agents are being used to measure not only relative perfusion but also the absolute blood flow in selected regions of the myocardium. Carbon-11 palmitate is employed to determine cardiac fatty acid metabolism. These radiopharmaceuticals are generally safe because they involve low doses of radiation with minimal risks.

Perspective and Prospects

The most desirable radionuclides used in PET procedures-carbon-11, nitrogen-13, oxygen-15, and fluorine-18-can be produced only with a cyclotron. Because of their very short physical half-lives, a dedicated cyclotron and fully automated equipment for radionuclide separation are usually necessary. Radionuclides that emit positrons but do not require a nearby cyclotron for their production-such as copper-62, gallium-68, and rubidium-82-are receiving attention because of their reduced cost. Although PET scanning provides valuable diagnostic information that in many cases cannot be obtained using other modalities, the expensive nature of the highly technical equipment necessary may limit the availability of these procedures to specialized medical centers. The changing health care environment and the public demand for cost containment may hinder further advances in this area of diagnostic radiology. Technological advances in PET scanning instrumentation, however, may result in a markedly reduced cost for the procedure in the future.

—*Dandamudi V. Rao, Ph.D.*

See also Brain; Brain disorders; Imaging and radiology; Neuroimaging; Noninvasive tests; Nuclear medicine; Radiopharmaceuticals; Single photon emission computed tomography (SPECT).

For Further Information:

Christian, Paul E., Kristen M. Waterstram-Rich, eds. *Nuclear Medicine and PET: Technology and Techniques.* 7th ed. St. Louis, Mo.: Elsevier/Mosby, 2012.

Iturralde, Mario P. *Dictionary and Handbook of Nuclear Medicine and Clinical Imaging.* 2d ed. Boca Raton, Fla.: CRC Press, 2002.

Pagana, Kathleen Deska, and Timothy J. Pagana. *Mosby's Diagnostic and Laboratory Test Reference.* 11th ed. St. Louis, Mo.: Mosby/Elsevier, 2013.

"Positron Emission Tomography." *Health Library*, September 30, 2012.

"Positron Emission Tomography-Computed Tomography (PET/CT)." *RadiologyInfo.org*, March 28, 2013.

Preboth, Monica. "Use of PET in the Diagnosis of Cancer." *American Family Physician* 61, no. 8 (April 15, 2000): 2548.

Rao, Dandamudi V., et al., eds. *Physics of Nuclear Medicine: Recent Advances.* New York: American Institute of Physics, 1984.

Wolbarst, Anthony Brinton. *Looking Within: How X-Ray, CT, MRI, Ultrasound, and Other Medical Images Are Created.* Berkeley: University of California Press, 1999.

Postherpetic neuralgia

Disease/Disorder

Also known as: Neuropathy

Anatomy or system affected: Nerve cells, nerve roots, dermatome body, neurologic system, integument system

Specialties and related fields: Neurology, dermatology, infectious disease, and internal medicine

Definition: A condition that can potentially produce severe pain in a specific nerve root/dermatome that was once previously exposed to the herpes zoster virus (chicken pox-shingles). Neuralgia is the pain that is produced from a nerve that is inflamed or enduring destruction from a disease process. In the case of postherpetic neuralgia, the nerve damage is produced by the reactivation of the herpes zoster virus.

Causes and Symptoms

The persistent nerve pain that accompanies postherpetic neuralgia/neuropathy can be precisely linked to a previous exposure to the herpes zoster-varicella virus. The virus has the unique potential to reside dormant within the body of a previously infected nerve. Under normal conditions, our immune system protects us from the dormant virus ever becoming active. However, when an individual is under stress and/or the immune system is unable to function effectively, the virus can be reactivated. Reasons for the immune system's inability to function effectively are vast. More common reasons for this to occur include, but are not limited to, the effect of medications (steroids, antirejection drugs in organ transplants, chemotherapy agents), a diagnosis of cancer or simply the exposure to the zoster virus again without sufficient immunity to ward off the disease process.

Precisely, once the nerve cell fiber (neuron) has been exposed to the varicella virus (chicken pox) and some of the virus particles can settle into clusters in the nerve cells, these are called sensory ganglia. Here they remain for many years in an inactive (latent) form. The sensory ganglia can be located adjacent to the spinal cord and brain. These specialized cells relay information to the brain about what the body is presently sensing, specifically the sensations of heat, cold, touch, and pain.

The main task of the nerve cell fibers is to send a message to the brain when the nerve is stimulated. When the nerve stimulation has been altered by a previous infection with the varicella virus (zoster), then there can be an alteration in the way the brain perceives or receives this nerve's message. In other words, the nerve may produce the sensation of pain in the brain because of the damage it has sustained from the virus. In addition, when the virus is reactivated it can go on to destroy even more nerve tissue and the pain can become worse or even linger in this nerve indefinitely. The pain may be described as "burning" or "stabbing" in nature, even perceived as traveling within the nerve cell fiber's pathway. In the beginning, the pain may be described as mild and progress very rapidly to severe or intolerable pain. Once the individual perceives the sensation of pain, the skin around this affected area may produce a rash or erupt in blisters or vesicles. This is because the viruses multiply within the nerve fiber pathway that communicates with the skin surface. This syndrome is often referred to as shingles.

Our knowledge of the human system has increased tremendously. We understand better now how an alteration in one system can inherently affect another system. This is an excellent example of this process. It is for this reason that elderly and sick individuals are affected more by this disease. The duration is short term to chronic.

Treatment and Therapy

The treatment for postherpetic-neuropathy/neuralgia may involve multiple modalities. These may include indefinite pharmacologic therapy with antiviral medications, such as Acyclovir (Zovirax®), Valcyclovir (Valtrex®), Famciclovir (Famvir®). Tricyclic antidepressants (Nortriptyline®) are also widely employed early in the disease's progression. Another medication sometimes prescribed is the anticonvulsant/ antiseizure medication gabapentin (Neurontin®). Topical local anesthetics sometimes provide mild relief from the painful stimuli (Lidocaine®). These latter medications are available as creams or subcutaneous patches. The pain may be controlled with various analgesic medications including opioids and other controlled substances. Unfortunately, the sequale may be complex, and any patients may require continued follow-up with pain management services indefinitely.

A shingles vaccine has been encouraged since May 2006 to all individuals exposed to the varicella virus in the past if they are over the ages of 50. The U.S. Food and Drug Administration (FDA) approved a VZV vaccine (Zostavax®) that is widely employed in the United States. This is a preventive measure for the disease, not a treatment once the disease has progressed.

Future Expectations

Much research is being devoted to this area at present. The National Institute of Health (NIH) and various pharmaceutical companies are devoting research efforts in this area.

The employment of the shingles vaccine has been effective in slowing the prevalence of the disease and newer modalities in the area of pain control also provide positive gains in this area.

—*Mary Frances McGibbon*

For Further Information:

American Chronic Pain Assn (ACPA): http://www.theacpa.org

BRAIN: http://www.ninds.nih.gov

National Institute of Neurological Disorders and Stroke. "Shingles: Hope Through Research." http://www.ninds.nih.gov/disorders/shingles/detail_shingles.htm

National Shingles Foundation (For Research on Varicella Zoster): http://www.vzvfoundation.org

---

Postpartum depression

Disease/Disorder

Anatomy or system affected: Endocrine system, psychic-emotional system

Specialties and related fields: Gynecology, obstetrics, psychiatry, psychology

Definition: A physical and emotional condition that may be life-threatening, involving the symptoms of depression occurring from a month to a year following childbirth and thought to be caused in part to dramatic hormonal shifts occurring in conjunction with childbirth.

Causes and Symptoms

For most women, the symptoms of depression are fairly common in the first week after childbirth. According to *Healthy Children* magazine, approximately 70 to 80 percent of women who have given birth experience what are often called the "baby blues" or the "fourth-day blues." These symptoms often disappear or lessen without medical intervention within one or two weeks following birth. In contrast, postpartum depression (PPD) is more severe and longer lasting. It occurs in about one in every ten women who have given birth. Additionally, an important distinction between baby blues and PPD is that the blues typically do not interfere with the mother's ability to care for a baby, whereas PPD can affect the ability of the mother to care for her child and herself.

PPD symptoms often include sadness, restlessness, guilt, unexplained weight changes, insomnia, frequent crying, irrational fears, irritability, decreased energy and motivation, and even lessened feelings of self-worth. Doctors also look for the presence of a depressed mood or a significantly diminished interest or pleasure in nearly all activities. Postpartum depression also commonly interferes with a mother's ability to care for the baby.

A personal or family history of depression, bipolar disorders, or other mental illnesses puts one at higher risk for PPD. Other factors that seem to play a role are an unwanted pregnancy, a complicated or difficult labor, a fetal anomaly, a lack of social support, and a temporary upheaval, such as a recent move, death of a loved one, or job change. Women who have previously suffered from depression following the birth of a child have an increased risk of becoming depressed following a subsequent delivery. In women with a history of PPD, the risk of recurrence is about one in three

---

Information on Postpartum Depression

Causes: Hormonal imbalance, psychological factors, sleep deprivation, physical or sexual difficulties

Symptoms: Fatigue, depression, insomnia, frequent crying, irrational fears, irritability, guilt, inability to care for infant

Duration: Typically about one to several months

Treatments: Antidepressants, counseling

---

to one in four.

PPD is best understood as resulting from several causes. One factor is that the sudden change in body hormones caused by childbirth can affect the mother's mood. There is also a psychological sense of anticlimax after an event that has been anticipated for many months. Many new mothers are very tired, and some are a little apprehensive and lacking confidence about the challenges of motherhood. Another factor is the sudden change that may occur in lifestyle and an associated feeling of shrunken horizons, especially if the mother had been working before the birth. Additionally, environmental, social, and sexual difficulties can predispose some women to develop PPD.

PPD may be accompanied by a rare but very severe symptom known as postpartum psychosis. Symptoms may include dramatic mood swings, delusional thoughts about the baby, hallucinations, and severe sleep disturbances. Often a danger with this condition is that the mother contemplates or fears that she will kill her child. When such symptoms develop, immediate care is vital, as it will protect both the mother and the child. Additionally, immediate care will help to reduce the distress of the mother, which will in turn help her to regain her health more quickly and return to healthy mothering after treatment.

Treatment and Therapy

It is important for all new mothers to be aware of the baby blues and the more serious problem of PPD. Awareness of the possibility of PPD may encourage expectant mothers to better care for themselves psychologically and to prepare in advance for what may be a psychologically and physically challenging first few weeks of motherhood. In terms of prevention, it is important for new mothers to avoid becoming too tired and to obtain assistance in baby and household care as much as possible. The loving support of a husband or significant other, relatives, and close friends is extremely helpful. The baby's father can take turns caring for the baby when the baby is unsettled or distressed. During the day, friends or family can help with shopping or looking after the baby while the mother rests.

If the depression develops and persists, a physician should be consulted for an evaluation of PPD. Antidepressant medication, such as sertraline hydrochloride (Zoloft), is usually effective if administered in the early stages of depression. Counseling is also beneficial to PPD sufferers. In severe cases, in which postpartum psychosis develops or the level of depression becomes life-threatening, admission to a psychiatric hospital for treatment may be necessary. Finally, it is important to note that anyone receiving medications, especially antidepressants, should be in regular contact with their physicians. Side effects, such as increased thoughts of suicide, may be an associated risk.

—*Alvin K. Benson, Ph.D.;*
updated by Nancy A. Piotrowski, Ph.D.

See also Antidepressants; Anxiety; Depression; Hallucinations; Hormones; Pregnancy and gestation; Psychiatric disorders; Psychiatry; Psychosis; Women's health.

For Further Information:

Bennett, Shoshana S., and Pec Indman. *Beyond the Blues: A Guide to Understanding and Treating Prenatal and Postpartum Depression*. Rev. ed. San Jose, Calif.: Moodswings Press, 2006.

Kleiman, Karen R., and Valerie D. Raskin. *This Isn't What I Expected: Overcoming Postpartum Depression*. Boston, Mass.: Da Capo, 2013.

Lundberg-Love, Paula K., Kevin L. Nadal, and Michele Antoinette Paludi. *Women and Mental Disorders*. Santa Barbara, Calif.: Praeger, 2012.

Nason, Juliana K., Patricia Spach, and Anna Gruen. *Beyond the Birth: A Family's Guide to Postpartum Mood Disorders*. Seattle: Postpartum Support International of Washington, 2012.

Nicholson, Paula. *Postnatal Depression: Facing the Paradox of Loss, Happiness, and Motherhood*. New York: Wiley, 2001.

O'Hara, Michael W. *Postpartum Depression: Causes and Consequences*. New York: Springer, 1995.

Postpartum Support International. http://www.post partum.net.

Sebastian, Linda. *Overcoming Postpartum Depression and Anxiety*. Omaha, Nebr.: Addicus Books, 2006.

Post-traumatic stress disorder

Disease/Disorder

Also known as: Shell shock, combat neurosis, battle fatigue
Anatomy or system affected: Psychic-emotional system
Specialties and related fields: Psychiatry, psychology
Definition: A maladaptive condition resulting from exposure to events beyond the realm of normal human experience and characterized by persistent difficulties involving emotional numbing, intense fear, helplessness, horror, reexperiencing of trauma, avoidance, and arousal.

Causes and Symptoms

Post-traumatic stress disorder (PTSD) is said to occur when a person experiences symptoms such as intense fear, helplessness, or horror following exposure to a traumatic event (an event outside the range of normal human experiences). The traumatic event may involve threatened death, serious injury, or other threat to physical integrity; witnessing the death of or threat to another person; or learning about the death of or threat to a family member or close friend. Events such as natural disasters (earthquakes, mudslides, fires, floods, tsunamis, tornados), war, domestic violence, crime, accidents, and medical procedures may trigger the development of PTSD. PTSD is the only disorder in the *Diagnostic and Statistical Manual of Mental Disorders* (DSM) with a cited etiology.

PTSD involves reexperiencing the trauma, avoidance of things that remind the person of the trauma, and an uncomfortable state of arousal usually connected to readiness to avoid rexexperiencing a trauma. Reexperiencing includes recurrent and intrusive thoughts, recurrent distressing dreams, feeling as if the event is happening again, intense psychological distress at exposure to any reminders (internal or external) of the event, or intense physical reactivity to any reminders of the event. Persistent avoidance includes anything associated with the event, as well as a numbing of general responsiveness. Such numbing may be indicated by several of the following: avoiding thoughts, feelings, or conversations associated with the event; avoiding activities, places, or people that remind one of the event; forgetting an important aspect of the event; experiencing markedly diminished interest or participation in significant activities; feeling detached or estranged from others; having a restricted range of feelings, such as not being able to love; or feeling that the future is foreshortened. Increased arousal includes at least two of the following: difficulty with sleep; irritability or outbursts of anger; difficulty concentrating; hypervigilance; or exaggerated startle response. The reexperiencing, avoidance, and arousal start after the traumatic event, last more than one month, and cause clinically significant distress or impairment in social, occupational, or other important areas of functioning.

The course of the disorder varies, with some individuals not experiencing symptoms until years later, but most individuals experience symptoms within three months of the initial trauma. If the trauma occurs early in life, it may have profound effects on stress response throughout the individual's lifetime.

Persons with PTSD may describe painful guilt feelings about surviving when others did not, or about what they had to do to survive. Their phobic avoidance of situations or activities that resemble or symbolize the original trauma may interfere with interpersonal relationships and lead to marital conflict, divorce, or job loss.

The likelihood of developing PTSD increases as intensity and physical proximity to the event increase. Recent immigrants from countries where there is considerable social unrest and civil conflict may have elevated rates of PTSD. The disorder may occur at any age. Women are more likely to develop PTSD than men; this gender difference is thought to exist in part because some traumatic events that women experience occur directly to their persons.

Not everyone who experiences a significant trauma will develop PTSD. Individual differences in terms of immediate post-trauma assistance and support, long-term social support, stress response, physical health, and other biological factors may explain a lack of occurrence in some individuals.

Treatment and Therapy

Treatments for PTSD include individual therapy, group therapy, antianxiety and antidepressant drugs, and eye movement desensitization and reprocessing (EMDR). Combinations of therapies can also be effective. In general, the sooner the victim of PTSD receives treatment, the greater are the chances of complete recovery. It is important

Information on Post-traumatic Stress Disorder

Causes: Exposure to traumatic event

Symptoms: May include recurrent and intrusive thoughts; reliving of traumatic event; intense psychological distress with exposure to reminders of event; recurrent disturbing dreams; difficulty sleeping; irritability or outbursts of anger; detachment; difficulty concentrating; hypervigilance; exaggerated startle response

Duration: Often chronic with acute episodes

Treatments: Individual therapy, group therapy, antianxiety medications, antidepressants

to note, however, that complex techniques such as trauma debriefing and critical incident debriefing should be attempted only by well-trained persons. Discussing traumatic events in a way that is not sensitive to the experience of the victim may retraumatize them, so caution is advised. For untrained persons, the best way to help someone affected by a trauma is to help them get to a qualified treatment professional as quickly as possible. This is especially important because research has suggested that treatment delivered soon after the trauma may reduce the overall negative impacts of the trauma.

Psychotherapy can help the person come to grips with the traumatic event. Different approaches are used, including exposure (or imaginal) therapy, anxiety management/ relaxation training, cognitive therapy, and supportive psychotherapy. Also, hypnosis, journaling (such as thought diaries and grief letters), creative arts, and a critical-incident stress debriefing may be used in treating PTSD, either alone or in conjunction with psychotherapy.

Group therapy, in which victims of PTSD can share their experiences and gain support from others, is especially helpful. Groups are typically small (six to eight persons) and are often composed of individuals who have undergone similar experiences. Also, marital and family therapy or parent training may be used in treating PTSD.

In general, the goals of psychotherapy include facilitating victims' emotional engagement with the trauma memory, helping them organize a personal trauma narrative, assisting them in correcting dysfunctional cognitions that often follow trauma, helping them develop increased trust in others, and decreasing their emotional and social isolation. The therapist typically provides empathy, validation, safety, consistency, and sensitivity to cultural and ethnic identity issues.

Antianxiety and antidepressant drugs can relieve the physiological symptoms of PTSD. The major pharmacological agents include benzodiazepines, serotonin receptor partial agonists, tricyclic antidepressants, MAO inhibitors, and selective serotonin reuptake inhibitors. Because of the many biological abnormalities presumed to be associated with PTSD, and because of the overlap between symptoms of PTSD and other comorbid disorders, almost every class of psychotropic agent has been administered to PTSD patients. Whether it includes individual or group therapy, drugs, or some combination of these three, the treatment approach must be tailored to the individual PTSD sufferer and his or her unique situation.

EMDR is a newer therapy for PTSD. It combines many aspects of the other therapies described and works to facilitate reprocessing of traumatic information and experience. Guided discussion and therapeutic work may involve specific eye movements while remembering different aspects of the traumatic event. It is suggested that this type of activity creates an orienting response that facilitates trauma processing. The technique requires a high level of skill and sophistication and should be used only by appropriately trained professionals. EMDR is very highly recommended for trauma and remains a topic of great research interest.

It is important to remember that PTSD, like many other mental health disorders, may not occur in isolation. Comorbidity, or the presence of more than one disorder, is the rule rather than the exception with PTSD. Depressive disorders, substance use disorders, and other anxiety disorders are the disorders most likely to occur with PTSD. Treatment must address the comorbid conditions when they are present. PTSD can be reliably assessed through semi-structured interview and self-report measures. Treatment typically occurs on an outpatient basis, but it also may occur on an inpatient basis if the symptoms are severe.

Perspective and Prospects

PTSD was observed in World War I, when some soldiers had intense anxiety reactions to the horrors they were experiencing. At that time, it was called combat neurosis, shell shock, or battle fatigue. It was formally diagnosed as an anxiety-based personality disorder in the 1960s among Vietnam War veterans, but it is no longer considered a personality disorder and is instead seen as an anxiety disorder. It is also now known that traumatic events may include not only war but also violent personal assault, kidnapping, terrorist attacks, torture, natural or human-made disasters, severe automobile accidents, or different aspects of life-threatening illness. For children, sexually traumatic events may include sexual experiences that were developmentally inappropriate, even if no threatened or actual violence occurred. PTSD may be especially severe when the trauma is of human origin (for example, torture) and directly related to damage to one's person.

Promising research identifying change to the stress response system in younger persons following trauma, as well as gender differences in trauma response, are expected to fuel greater understanding of the mechanisms of trauma response. Such knowledge will in turn be useful for developing new drug, biological, and interpersonal therapies for children and adults and for both women and men.

—Lillian M. Range, Ph.D.;
updated by Nancy A. Piotrowski, Ph.D.

See also Accidents; Antianxiety drugs; Anxiety; Domestic violence; Psychiatric disorders; Psychiatry; Stress; Stress reduction.

For Further Information:

American Psychiatric Association. *Diagnostic and Statistical Manual of Mental Disorders: DSM-5*. 5th ed. Arlington, Va.: Author, 2013.

Bremner, Douglas J. *Does Stress Damage the Brain? Understanding Trauma-Related Disorders from a Neurological Perspective*. New York: W. W. Norton, 2002.

EMDR Institute, 2011.

Foa, Edna B., Terence M. Keane, and Matthew J. Friedman, eds. *Effective Treatments for PTSD: Practice Guidelines from the Society for Traumatic Stress Studies*. 2d ed. New York: Guilford, 2009.

Horowitz, Mardi J., ed. *Essential Papers on Post-traumatic Stress Disorder*. New York: New York University Press, 1999.

McNally, Richard J. *Remembering Trauma*. Rev. ed. Cambridge, Mass.: Harvard University Press, 2005.

National Center for Posttraumatic Stress Disorder. US Department of Veterans Affairs, May 21, 2013.

"Post-Traumatic Stress Disorder." *MedlinePlus*, May 14, 2013.

"Post-Traumatic Stress Disorder." *National Institute of Mental Health*, Dec. 3, 2012.

Riley, Julie Smith, and Brian Randall. "Post-Traumatic Stress Disorder." *Health Library*, Mar. 15, 2013.

Schiraldi, Glenn R. *Post-traumatic Stress Disorder Sourcebook*. 2d ed. New York: McGraw-Hill, 2009.

Sidran Institute-Traumatic Stress Education and Advocacy, 2013.

Postural orthostatic tachycardia syndrome (POTS)

Disease/Disorder

Also known as: Chronic orthostatic intolerance

Anatomy or system affected: Cardiovascular system, heart, blood vessels, circulatory system

Specialties and related fields: Cardiology, Neurology

Definition: Condition characterized by decreased volume of blood returning to the heart when standing up, resulting in symptoms such as an excessively increased heart rate.

Key terms:

autonomic nervous system: regulates involuntary actions for bodily functions (such as breathing, heart rate, and digestion)

tachycardia: fast heart rate

Causes and Symptoms

In postural orthostatic tachycardia syndrome (POTS), the body is unable to regulate blood flow through vessels due to dysautonomia (dysfunction in the autonomic nervous system). This results in symptoms such as dizziness or a fast heart rate upon standing. POTS is characterized by orthostatic intolerance, the inability to stand or sit vertically without developing symptoms that are alleviated when lying down. Signs include the heart rate increases by 30 beats per minute or is more than 120 beats per minute within 10 minutes of standing up. Orthostatic hypotension is another sign, which is a sustained decrease in systolic blood pressure 20 mmHg or diastolic blood pressure 10 mmHg within 3 minutes of standing or tilting the head upwards to>60 degrees.

Normally, the autonomic nervous system allows the body to function without conscious effort. Standing, for example, is facilitated by a large amount of blood automatically falling to the lower parts of the body. Changes in heart rate, vessels, and muscle, for example, ensure that blood is distributed to the upper parts of the body. In POTS, a defect exists in these automatic set of processes, so not enough blood is able to go to organs such as the brain and heart. This causes symptoms of fatigue, headache, and even fainting when standing up.

Tests and clinical signs can lead to a diagnosis of POTS. In the tilt table test, for example, patients strapped on a table are tilted to mimic standing up, and heart rate and blood pressure changes are monitored.

The exact causes and mechanisms of POTS are unknown. Some individuals acquire the condition after exposure to a virus, such as the Epstein-Barr virus in mononucleosis. Other individuals can acquire POTS after brain trauma or severe injuries. POTS can have multiple, complex causes. Primary causes of POTS include nitric oxide exposure, neuropathy, and certain viruses. Physical deconditioning, a decline in bodily function that can occur from a significant injury or from a chronic disease, is also considered a primary agent. Secondary causes of POTS include anemia, adrenal disorders, Ehlers-Danlos syndrome, Lyme disease, tumors, and more.

Treatment and Therapy

Since the specific causes of POTS is still unknown, treatment focuses on managing symptoms. Diet, exercise, and medication are three avenues for addressing primary POTS. Diets with a high sodium intake and low gluten intake have been shown to be effective in some patients; alcoholic beverages should be avoided as it may worsen symptoms of low blood pressure and dizziness, but fluid intake such as water should increase to help alleviate symptoms.

Exercise therapy may help improve overall well-being and is based on the theory that it may play a part in resetting the autonomic nervous system. Medications can also be used for managing or reducing the symptoms of POTS, but there is currently no silver bullet for curing the disease. An approach that does not involve medications includes raising the head of the bed onto a firm foundation (such as blocks) to help decrease the risk of dizziness when rising from the bed in the morning. Avoiding triggers, such as extreme temperatures, can be beneficial.

Perspective and Prospects

POTS affects nearly half a million people in the United States, with a majority of them females. The prognosis for POTS is generally favorable. Many individuals experience mild symptoms and can continue with their daily activities. However, others may be significantly impaired. Some people's symptoms improve with lifestyle changes such as exercise, diet, and medication; still, others' symptoms unfortunately persist and do not improve with treatment.

POTS is sometimes referred to as an "invisible illness" because it is not one, defined condition, but rather a constellation of conditions with a similar physiological state. There exists a spectrum of symptoms and clinical manifestations of POTS, so treatment varies from one person to the next. Because patients report fatigue to be the most significant symptom, they may experience reduced quality of life, a more sedentary lifestyle, and less energy to engage in daily activities. POTS may be misdiagnosed as anxiety, depression, or another psychological condition. Diagnosis is often delayed, with one survey reporting taking more than two years for half of patients with POTS to be diagnosed.

Continuing Research

Early twenty-first century research is investigating more effective medications for POTS. Clinical trials have found that pyridostigmine, a drug that typically is given to patients with myasthenia gravis to treat muscle weakness, can ameliorate tachycardia and maintain blood pressure among patients with POTS.

Another study, led by researchers at the University of California, San Diego, are investigating the drug Ivabradine. It is currently used to treat chronic heart failure, but also has been shown to treat tachycardia, so the researchers hypothesize that Ivabradine will reduce tachycardia among patients with POTS.

Researchers at Vanderbilt are investigating whether stimulating the vagus nerve can decrease POTS symptoms. The vagus nerve is responsible for involuntary functions of the human body, such as heart rate. These researchers are studying the impact of stimulating the vagus nerve on heart rate as a potential mode of treatment for individuals with POTS.

—*Anna Delamerced*

For Further Information:
Effect of Ivabradine on Patients With Postural Orthostatic Tachycardia Syndrome (POTS). (2017). Retrieved from http://clinicaltrials.gov/ct2. (Identification No. NCT03182725)

Jiawei, L., et al. (2015). The Value of Acetylcholine Receptor Antibody in Children with Postural Tachycardia Syndrome. *Pediatric Cardiology, 36*(1), 165-170. doi.org/10.1007/s00246-014-0981-8

Kanjwal, K., et al. (2011). Pyridostigmine in the treatment of postural orthostatic tachycardia: a single-center experience. *Pacing Clin Electrophysiol, 34*(6), 750-5. doi: 10.1111/j.1540-8159.2011.03047

Kaufmann H & Freeman R. Postural tachycardia syndrome. *UpToDate.* March 2015, http://www. uptodate.com/contents/postural-tachycardia- syndrome.

Low, P., et al. (2009). Postural tachycardia syndrome (POTS). *J Cardiovasc Electrophysiol, 20*(3), 352-8. doi: 10.1111/j.1540-8167.2008.01407

Transdermal Vagal Stimulation for POTS. (2014). Retrieved from http://clinicaltrials.gov/ct2. (Identification No. NCT02281097)

Prader-Willi syndrome

Disease/Disorder

Anatomy or system affected: Bones, brain, endocrine system, genitals, glands, heart, musculoskeletal system, psychic-emotional system, teeth

Specialties and related fields: Cardiology, dentistry, family medicine, genetics, neurology, pediatrics, pharmacology, psychiatry, pulmonary medicine

Definition: A disorder caused by a deletion in chromosome 15, characterized by developmental and cognitive delays, overeating resulting in obesity, and behavioral difficulties.

Causes and Symptoms

Prader-Willi syndrome is caused by a spontaneous deletion involving chromosome 15. Although this disease is genetic in nature, most parents of children with Prader-Willi syndrome have normal chromosomes. Some research indicates an association between the disease and fathers employed at the time of conception in fields associated with hydrocarbons, such as lumbermen, chemists, or mechanics. That connection might implicate an environmental trigger in some cases.

Prader-Willi syndrome occurs in one in 12,000-15,000 births and affects both genders and all races. Newborns with the disease appear floppy, with low muscle tone. They often had a low birth weight, and males may have undescended testicles. Small genitalia are common, as are small hands and feet. These babies feed poorly and display poor motor development. Mental retardation is common, ranging from mild to severe.

Between the ages of two and four, children with Prader-Willi syndrome develop an insatiable need to eat. They will do anything to get food and will eat without control. Obesity and other related health problems are major concerns for these patients. Many patients also suffer from behavioral disorders related to excessive eating, compulsive or repetitive behaviors, tantrums, and psychiatric disorders including depression and, in extreme cases, psychoses.

Treatment and Therapy

Primary treatment for Prader-Willi syndrome centers on the many health concerns related to obesity, in addition to meeting the educational, social, and emotional needs of patients as they grow and mature. Studies indicate an abnormally high level of the hormone ghrelin in these patients. It is the only appetite-stimulating hormone produced in the stomach and was touted in the early twenty-first century as a possible breakthrough in treatment.

Dietary restrictions, including types of food and portion control, are critical with these patients. Since they are unable to control their cravings for food, cooperation among family, school personnel, and community members is es-

---

Information on Prader-Willi Syndrome

Causes: Spontaneous genetic deletion, possibly with environmental trigger

Symptoms: Low birth weight, decreased muscle tone, small genitalia, undescended testicles, small hands and feet, short stature, poor motor development, mental retardation (ranging from mild to severe), insatiable need to eat, behavioral disorders, psychiatric disorders

Duration: Lifelong

Treatments: Alleviation of symptoms; may include dietary restrictions and regular exercise to avoid obesity, growth hormone, special education (speech, behavioral, and psychiatric therapy)

sential. Regular exercise is also recommended. Because patients with Prader-Willi syndrome are often small in stature, growth hormones are often used to facilitate growth and decrease the percentage of body fat, thus helping improve both strength and agility in patients. Special education services, including speech, behavioral assistance, and psychological or psychiatric services, are also important components of treatment.

Perspective and Prospects

Prader-Willi syndrome was first defined as a syndrome by Andrea Prader, Alexis Labhart, and Heinrich Willi in 1956. Prader and Willi refined the syndrome in 1963. Since the mid-twentieth century, researchers have focused on the influences of hormones and genetics in the development and treatment of this disease. Treatments evolved based on increased knowledge of how genes and hormones influence human biology and behavior.

—*Kathleen Schongar, M.S., M.A.*

See also Birth defects; Dwarfism; Environmental diseases; Genetic diseases; Growth; Intellectual disability; Obesity; Obesity, childhood; Psychiatric disorders; Psychiatry; Psychiatry, child and adolescent; Psychosis.

For Further Information

American Psychiatric Association. *Diagnostic and Statistical Manual of Mental Disorders: DSM-5.* 5th ed. Washington, D.C.: American Psychiatric Association, 2013.

Cassidy, Susanne B. "Prader-Willi Syndrome." *Journal of Medical Genetics* 34 (1997): 917-923.

Jones, Kenneth Lyons. "Prader-Willi Syndrome." In *Smith's Recognizable Patterns of Human Malformation.* 6th ed. Philadelphia: Saunders/Elsevier, 2006.

MedlinePlus "Prader-Willi Syndrome." *MedlinePlus,* May 13, 2013.

Prader-Willi Syndrome Association USA.*Prader-Willi Syndrome Association USA,* n.d.

Sadock, Benjamin J., and Virginia A. Sadock. *Kaplan and Sadock's Concise Textbook of Clinical Psychiatry.* 3d ed. Philadelphia: Wolters Kluwer/Lippincott Williams & Wilkins, 2009.

Precocious puberty

Disease/Disorder

Also known as: Sexual precocity, gonadotropin puberty, pubertas praecox

Anatomy or system affected: Musculoskeletal system, nervous system, psychic-emotional system, reproductive system

Specialties and related fields: Endocrinology, family medicine, genetics, neurology, pediatrics

Definition: The early onset of puberty caused by the premature secretion of sex hormones, resulting in the commencement of sexual maturation prior to age eight in girls and age ten in boys.

Key terms:

gonads: ovaries in girls and testes in boys

hormones: chemicals produced by glands such as the thyroid, pituitary, or adrenals that stimulate bodily changes or growth and that regulate body functions

hypothalamic hamartomas: tumors in the hypothalamic region of the brain, which are usually benign

hypothalamus: the region of the brain that stimulates glands to secrete hormones

idiopathic: having an unidentified cause

puberty: secondary sexual development that involves the maturation of the reproductive system and is typified by significant physical growth

Causes and Symptoms

Secondary sexual development is commonly known as puberty. It is typically characterized by growth of pubic and underarm hair, acne, and rapid physical development until about age eighteen. During puberty, a boy also grows facial hair, his penis and testes enlarge, and he begins to produce sperm. A girl develops breasts and begins to menstruate and ovulate.

Puberty is the result of hormonal changes triggered by the hypothalamus region of the brain. The brain releases luteinizing hormone-releasing hormone (LHRH) in periodic bursts, which causes the pituitary gland to secrete gonadotropin-releasing hormone (GnRH). Gonadotropins stimulate the ovaries in girls and the testes in boys to secrete sex hormones. These hormones-estrogen and progesterone in girls and testosterone in boys-start the sexual maturation process and stimulate rapid physical growth.

Puberty usually begins at about age twelve in boys and age eleven in girls. Approximately one in every ten thousand children begins puberty abnormally early, between infancy and approximately age nine. This condition, known as precocious puberty, affects both sexes but is two to five times more common among girls than boys. Early onset of puberty is also more likely to occur in overweight children.

In addition to prematurely developing secondary sexual characteristics, children with precocious puberty are initially tall for their ages. Left untreated, however, they rarely reach their full adult height potential because the same sex hormones that trigger early growth also end it prematurely. Males often grow no taller than 5 feet 2 inches, and many females remain under 5 feet. Precocious puberty frequently results in adolescent behaviors such as moodiness, irritability, and aggressiveness, as well as the early development of a sex drive. Children with precocious puberty reach sexual maturity at varying rates, and some characteristics may even begin to regress to their normal state.

When an underlying cause for precocious puberty cannot be determined, the condition is known as idiopathic precocious puberty. About 80 percent of cases in females and 40 percent of male cases are idiopathic. Common causes for precocious puberty that can be identified include genetic disorders or tumors in the hypothalamic region of the brain. Such tumors, known as hypothalamic hamartomas, are usually benign. Between 5 and 10 percent of boys with precocious puberty genetically inherit the condition from their fathers or indirectly from their maternal grandfathers. This genetic transmittal of precocious puberty only occurs in about 1 percent of girls with the condition. Less common causes of precocious puberty include other kinds of brain tumors, ovarian tumors or cysts, and adrenal gland disorders such as adrenogenital hyperplasia or congenital adrenal hyperplasia. Precocious puberty can

Information on Precocious Puberty

Causes: Hormonal imbalance; possibly linked to genetic disorders, tumors in hypothalamus, adrenal gland disorders, hydrocephalus, radiation therapy, nervous system disorders, McCune-Albright syndrome

Symptoms: Premature development of secondary sexual characteristics; above-average height until adulthood but failure to reach full growth potential, moodiness, irritability, aggressiveness, early development of sex drive

Duration: Chronic

Treatments: Hormonal therapy

also be caused by pituitary lesions, hydrocephalus, radiation therapy, nervous system disorders such as neurofibromatosis, thyroid disorders (specifically severe hypothyroidism), and a rare condition called McCune-Albright syndrome.

Children with precocious puberty are often self-conscious about their early physical and sexual development, since they appear older than their ages. Mental development is not affected by the condition, however, so children with precocious puberty are usually not as emotionally mature as they appear.

Treatment and Therapy

Underlying causes of precocious puberty, if known, are often difficult or impossible to treat. Surgical removal of noncancerous hypothalamic hamartomas and other brain tumors, for example, may not be feasible and rarely halts sexual development. Other causes such as neurofibromatosis are incurable, and treatments for conditions such as adrenal disorders may not stop the effects of precocious puberty.

Therefore, many forms of precocious puberty are treated by changing patients' hormonal balance. Synthetic hormones called LHRH analogs and gonadotropin-releasing hormone agonists (GnRHa) block the body's production of sex hormones and thus slow down or stop pubertal symptoms. The synthetic hormone histrelin acetate, also known by its brand name Supprelin, has been shown to be effective in reducing early sexual changes in both sexes and to slow bone growth. Leuprolide acetate, sold under the brand name Lupron-Depot PED, is another successful treatment for this condition. Daily injections of these drugs are stopped when the patient reaches the appropriate age for onset of puberty.

Synthetic versions of GnRH or LHRH interrupt the chain of hormonal events that result in sexual maturation. Some research, however, suggests a link between these therapies and bone mineral density loss. Treatments are administered in daily or monthly injections.

Girls with precocious puberty caused by congenital adrenal hyperplasia can be treated by suppressing the hormone known as ACTH with a glucocorticoid. Precocious puberty associated with McCune-Albright syndrome can be treated with testolactone, which blocks the production of estrogens. Some forms of precocious puberty involving the gonadotropins can be treated with the hormone suppressant nafarelin acetate.

Genetic counseling is recommended for families of patients with inherited precocious puberty. Psychological counseling may also benefit patients, since they may not fit in with peers because of the physical ramifications of the condition.

Perspective and Prospects

Previous treatments for precocious puberty included the use of synthetic progesterone, an artificial version of a sex hormone secreted by the ovaries. Synthetic progesterone frequently stops menstruation and reduces breast size in girls, but it has little or no effect on boys. Unfortunately, it fails to stop rapid growth in either sex. Synthetic progesterone can also result in several serious side effects.

Experimental treatments for idiopathic precocious puberty include a combination of spironolactone and testolactone for male patients, as well as another drug called deslorelin or Somagard for either sex.

—Cheryl Pawlowski, Ph.D.;
updated by Lenela Glass-Godwin, M.W.S.

See also Endocrine system; Endocrinology; Endocrinology, pediatric; Growth; Hormones; Menstruation; Puberty and adolescence; Sexuality.

For Further Information:
Carel, J. C., et al. "Treatment of Central Precocious Puberty by Subcutaneous Injections of Leuprorelin 3-Month Depot (11.25 mg)." *Journal of Clinical Endocrinology and Metabolism* 87, no. 9 (September, 2002): 4111-4116.
Creatsas, George, George Mastorakos, and George P. Chrousos, eds. *Adolescent Gynecology and Endocrinology: Basic and Clinical Aspects.* New York: New York Academy of Sciences, 2006.
Dowshen, Steven. "Precocious Puberty." *KidsHealth from Nemours,* October, 2012.
Grave, Gilman D., and Gordon B. Cutler, Jr., eds. *Sexual Precocity: Etiology, Diagnosis, and Management.* New York: Raven Press, 1993.
Henry, Helen L., and Anthony W. Norman, eds. *Encyclopedia of Hormones.* 3 vols. San Diego, Calif.: Academic Press, 2003.
Huffman, Grace Brooke. "Reassessing the Age Limit of Precocious Puberty in Girls." *American Family Physician* 61, no. 6 (March 15, 2000): 1850.
Kronenberg, Henry M., et al., eds. *Williams Textbook of Endocrinology.* 12th ed. Philadelphia: Saunders/Elsevier, 2011.
McCoy, Krisha. "Precocious Puberty." *Health Library,* September 30, 2012.
National Institutes of Health. "Puberty and Precocious Puberty: Overview." *NIH: Eunice Kennedy Shriver National Institute of Child Health and Human Development,* April 3, 2013.
Walvoord, Emily C., and Ora Hirsch Pescovitz. "Combined Use of Growth Hormone and Gonadotropin-Releasing Hormone Analogues in Precocious Puberty: Theoretic and Practical Considerations." *Pediatrics* 104, no. 4 (October, 1999): 1010-1014.

Preeclampsia and eclampsia

Disease/Disorder

Anatomy or system affected: Circulatory system, endocrine system, kidneys, nervous system, reproductive system

Specialties and related fields: Gynecology, nephrology,

neurology, obstetrics, vascular medicine

Definition: Preeclampsia is a serious complication of pregnancy, occurring any time from the middle stages of pregnancy to just after birth, characterized by hypertension and proteinuria. Eclampsia is a potentially fatal condition, likewise occurring any time from the middle stages of pregnancy to just after birth, characterized by seizures or coma that has no other apparent cause.

Key terms:

hemolytic anemia: a type of anemia caused by the destruction of blood cells

perinatal: referring to the period beginning in the twenty-eighth week of pregnancy and ending twenty-eight days after birth

proteinuria: the presence of protein (typically albumin) in the urine

---

Information on Preeclampsia and Eclampsia

Causes: Unknown; risk factors include first pregnancy, personal or family history of disorder, age younger than eighteen or older than forty, more than one fetus, obesity, and certain diseases (polycystic ovarian syndrome, diabetes, kidney disease, hypertension, autoimmune disorders)

Symptoms: For preeclampsia, high blood pressure, proteinuria, headaches, abdominal pain, vision problems; for eclampsia, convulsive seizures, organ damage, sometimes coma or death

Duration: Chronic during pregnancy

Treatments: Strict bed rest, balanced salt solution, sedatives, blood pressure medications, magnesium sulfate, diazepam, diuretics, delivery of baby as soon as possible

---

Causes and Symptoms

Preeclampsia, also known as toxemia of pregnancy or pregnancy-induced hypertension, is a serious condition that affects 6 to 8 percent of pregnant women, and is a leading cause of premature delivery, maternal death, and perinatal child death. The condition can arise any time from the twentieth week of pregnancy to the first week after birth. A woman is diagnosed with preeclampsia if she has elevated blood pressure in addition to proteinuria. The blood pressure of preeclampsia patients generally exceeds 140/90; however, an increase in systolic pressure by 30 or an increase in diastolic pressure by 15-even if the 140/90 cutoff is not reached-when accompanied by other characteristic symptoms is sufficient for a diagnosis of preeclampsia. Headaches, abdominal pain, and visual disturbances may accompany the disorder. Patients who have normal blood pressure prior to pregnancy but suffer from increased blood pressures as described above are said to suffer from pregnancy-induced hypertension (PIH).

Preeclampsia may lead to HELLP syndrome, characterized by *h*emolytic anemia, *e*levated *l*iver enzymes, and a *low p*latelet count. HELLP syndrome typically occurs in the last trimester, with women complaining of nausea, vomiting, and abdominal pain. In severe cases, the syndrome leads to intravascular blood clotting, kidney failure, liver failure, respiratory failure, systemic failure, and death.

Eclampsia, the most dangerous complication of preeclampsia, is characterized by convulsive seizures that may lead to coma or death. Organ damage, particularly in the kidneys, liver, brain, and placenta, may occur.

The risk of preeclampsia is higher in women experiencing their first pregnancy, or their first pregnancy with a different partner; women with a personal or family history of the disorder; women younger than eighteen or older than forty; those carrying two or more fetuses; women with a body mass index (BMI) greater than 30; women with polycystic ovarian syndrome; or women with other conditions such as diabetes, kidney disease, hypertension, or autoimmune disorders. Recent evidence indicates that the existence of high blood pressure, obesity, or diabetes prior to pregnancy is likely to predispose a pregnant woman to preeclampsia.

The cause of preeclampsia and eclampsia is not usually known. Kidney disease or other conditions that raise blood pressure may trigger the condition. Genetics may be important. An abnormal maternal immune response to fetal tissue may also play a role in triggering preeclampsia and eclampsia. The functioning of the placenta (which develops from the membrane known as the chorion) seems to play an important part in the development of preeclampsia. If it becomes hypoxic (oxygen-deprived), the placenta is believed to release as-yet-unidentified toxic substances into the maternal circulation, leading to the development of preeclampsia.

Treatment and Therapy

If caught early, mild cases of preeclampsia can be treated with strict bed rest, either at home or in the hospital if the condition does not improve. In more severe cases, bed rest should be accompanied by intravenous (IV) administration of balanced salt solution, such as Ringer's solution; sedatives; medication to control blood pressure; and, if necessary, medication to control seizures, such as magnesium sulfate. Diuretics may also be required. Once the woman's condition is stabilized, delivery should be accomplished, either vaginally or by cesarean section. Eclampsia and HELLP syndrome should be treated in the same way. If magnesium sulfate fails to control seizures, then drugs such as diazepam should be administered. While delivery of the fetus is often essential for the survival of both the mother and the baby, it frequently results in extremely premature infants who then face a large cadre of challenges associated with their prematurity.

Women treated for preeclampsia and related disorders should be monitored for other symptoms, including headaches, blurred vision, abdominal pain, vaginal bleeding, and loss of fetal heart sounds. Symptoms should resolve themselves within six hours after delivery.

Perspective and Prospects

Although preeclampsia was first described as early as the

nineteenth century, little progress has been made since in determining its cause. Recent research has focused on a number of potential factors. Among them are genetics, because of the relationship between a family history of the disorder and the risk of developing it. Some researchers have suggested nutrient deficiencies as a cause, but evidence for a nutritional relationship has been equivocal. Hormonal imbalances have been suggested as a cause, as have interruptions of the blood supply to the placenta, immune system responses to fetal tissue or attempts to repair perceived damage to vascular tissue, calcium deficiencies, and a host of other factors, including preexisting conditions such as lupus, diabetes, sickle cell disease, and kidney diseases.

Researchers seeking the cause of preeclampsia have recently focused on the placenta. Deprivation of vascular growth factors, such as vascular endothelial growth factor (VEGF), inhibits vascular development in the placenta, which adversely affects the developing fetus. Abnormal concentrations of VEGF have also been shown to cause nephron damage in the kidney.

With growth factors, hormones, nutrients, or myriad other compounds and conditions possibly playing a role in triggering preeclampsia and eclampsia, it is clear that much more work needs to be done.

—*David M. Lawrence;*
updated by Robin Kamienny Montvilo, R.N., Ph.D.

See also Blood pressure; Cesarean section; Childbirth; Childbirth complications; Embryology; Hypertension; Obstetrics; Placenta; Pregnancy and gestation; Premature birth; Proteinuria; Seizures; Toxemia; Vascular medicine; Vascular system; Women's health.

For Further Information:
Barden, Anne. "Pre-eclampsia: Contribution of Maternal Constitutional Factors and the Consequences for Cardiovascular Health." *Clinical and Experimental Pharmacology and Physiology* 33, no. 9 (September, 2006): 826-830.

Basso, Olga, et al. "Trends in Fetal and Infant Survival Following Preeclampsia." *Journal of the American Medical Association* 296, no. 11 (September 20, 2006): 1357-1362.

Gabbe, Steven G., Jennifer R. Niebyl, and Joe Leigh Simpson, eds. *Obstetrics: Normal and Problem Pregnancies.* 6th ed. Philadelphia: Elsevier/Saunders, 2012.

Lindheimer, Marshall D., James M. Robert, and F. Gary Cunningham, eds. *Chesley's Hypertensive Disorders in Pregnancy.* 3d ed. Amsterdam; Boston: Academic Press/Elsevier, 2009.

National High Blood Pressure Education Program. *Working Group Report on High Blood Pressure in Pregnancy.* Bethesda, Md.: National Institutes of Health, National Heart, Lung, and Blood Institute, 2000.

NIH. "Preeclampsia and Eclampsia: Condition Information." *NIH: Eunice Kennedy Shriver National Institute of Child Health and Human Development,* November 30, 2012.

Redman, Chris, and Isabel Walker. *Pre-eclampsia-The Facts: The Hidden Threat to Pregnancy.* New York: Oxford University Press, 1997.

Savitsky, Diane. "Pre-eclampsia." *Health Library,* March 14, 2013.

Pregnancy and gestation
Biology
Anatomy or system affected: Abdomen, reproductive system, uterus

Specialties and related fields: Embryology, gynecology, obstetrics

Definition: The development of unborn young within a woman's uterus and the accompanying physical, biochemical, and developmental changes that occur to both mother and child from conception until birth as genetic material from each parent is joined to create a unique individual.

Key terms:
amniotic sac: the sac that surrounds the fetus in the uterus and is filled with amniotic fluid

blastocyst: the fertilized egg after it has divided several times to form a hollow ball of cells in one of the earliest stages of development

cervix: the constricted lower end of the uterus

chorion: the membrane in the embryo that further differentiates into the placenta and umbilical cord

chromosomes: rodlike structures inside cells that carry the genetic material

embryo: the unborn child from the second through the eighth week of development

endometrium: the lining of the uterus

Fallopian tube: the structure that leads from the internal cavity of the uterus to the ovary

fetus: the unborn child from the eighth week after fertilization until birth

placenta: the organ that connects the mother to the embryo or fetus through the umbilical cord and is necessary for the child's nourishment

trimester: a division of pregnancy into three equal time periods of about thirteen weeks

Process and Effects
Pregnancy begins conception or fertilization with the fusion of an egg and sperm within a woman's body and continues until childbirth, typically thirty-eight weeks later. This gestational time is divided into three approximately equal periods called trimesters, each associated with specific physical and biochemical hallmarks.

Prior to conception, a mature egg, or ovum, ruptures from a fluid-filled follicle within the ovary and is swept into the Fallopian tube by large fringes on the tube that caress the ovary's surface. The empty follicle is transformed into a structure called the corpus luteum which secretes hormones that help to prepare the woman's body for pregnancy. If the ovum is fertilized within twenty-four hours, pregnancy will occur. If it is not fertilized, the uterine lining will be shed during menstruation.

Sperm ejaculated into a woman's vagina travel through the cervix and uterus and into the Fallopian tubes. Only about 200 of the original 500 million sperm delivered to the woman may reach the vicinity of the ovum. Enzymes in the sperm heads dissolve protective outer layers of the egg. When one sperm finally breaks through the plasma membrane, the innermost covering of the ovum, chemical changes on the surface of the ovum prevent additional sperm from entering. The genetic material contained in the sperm and ovum fuse. If the fertilizing sperm is a gynosperm, which carries an X chromosome, then the baby will be female; if it is an androsperm, which carries a Y chromosome, then the baby will be male.

About twelve hours after fusion of the genetic material, the first cell division occurs. Divisions continue at intervals of twelve to fifteen hours, doubling the number of cells each time, and the fertilized ovum is now called a blastocyst. The blastocyst is gently guided through the Fallopian tube to the uterus by the beating of the millions of tiny hairs, called cilia, that line the inner surfaces of the Fallopian tubes. This journey to the uterus takes about three days.

Upon arriving in the uterus, the blastocyst "explores" the endometrium, the uterine lining, for an appropriate site to settle. Prior to this implantation in the endometrium, the blastocyst ruptures from the clear protective sheath that helps to prevent it from settling in the Fallopian tube. By ten to fourteen days after fertilization, the blastocyst implants securely within the endometrium and the embryonic stage begins. At this point, it consists of several hundred cells and is about the size of the head of a pin.

After implantation, chemical signals produced by the blastocyst prevent the mother's immune system from recognizing the blastocyst as a foreign invader and destroying it. Other chemical signals cause the endometrium to thicken and extend blood vessels to the blastocyst for nourishment from the mother. The uterine wall softens and thickens, and the cervical opening is sealed with a mucus plug.

At this point, the cells of the blastocyst divide into two distinct clusters: One part will form the embryo itself, and the other part will join with the woman's tissue to form the placenta, the structure that will provide nourishment from the mother to the growing embryo. These early placental cells produce the hormone human chorionic gonadotropin (hCG). This hormone signals the ovary to cease ovulation and stimulates it to produce the hormone progesterone, which prevents menstruation and causes the endometrium to grow even thicker.

During the second week after fertilization, a cavity surrounding the embryo begins to form. This is destined to become the amniotic sac, which will contain the shock-absorbing amniotic fluid in which the fetus floats during development. At this time, the hCG being produced by the blastocyst and ovaries can be detected by pregnancy tests.

Three weeks after conception, the size of the embryo is about 2 millimeters (0.08 inch). The embryonic cells have divided into germ layers, distinct groupings of cells that are destined to produce specific body parts. The rudimentary brain appears at the end of a long tube. The heart is forming and will be beating within a week. At this point, the mother has missed her menstrual period and may be experiencing symptoms of pregnancy, such as nausea, heartburn, and tender breasts.

During the fifth through seventh weeks of embryonic development, massive physical changes occur. The crown-to-rump length of the embryo increases to around 1.25 centimeters (0.5 inch). The embryo's face, trunk, and limbs grow, and by the end of this period distinct fingers and toes are formed. The backbone is in place, and ribs begin to de-velop, as do skin, eyes, and all of the organ systems and the circulatory system. At this point, the placenta is connected to the embryo by the umbilical cord, and placental cells penetrate the blood vessels of the endometrium to provide transit of nutrients from the mother's bloodstream to the embryo. The placenta also filters out some potentially dangerous substances from the mother's bloodstream and aids in disposing of embryonic waste products.

By the eighth week of development, the embryo is about 4 centimeters (1.5 inches) long, weighs about 14 grams (0.5 ounce), and is composed of millions of cells. All organs are formed, and the embryo is officially called a fetus. The woman's uterus has increased in size, and her waistline may begin to enlarge. At this point, hormonal shifts stabilize, which frequently relieves morning sickness and other discomforts of early pregnancy.

Growth and organ system interconnection continue during the third month of fetal life, and the cells of the immune system are formed. During the fourth month, facial features develop, and the fetus may begin to respond to sound. Hair on the head and the eyebrows coarsens and develops pigment. The distinction between male and female fetuses becomes apparent with a visible vagina or penis. Sixteen to eighteen weeks after fertilization, the mother may feel the first fetal movements. She has gained several pounds, and changes in her body shape are readily visible. Frequently, this second trimester is associated with feelings of joy and minimal discomfort.

The third trimester is largely a period of growth for the fetus. Its weight increases rapidly. The fetus becomes very active within the amniotic fluid and responds to sound from both within and outside the mother. The weight gain may put incredible stress on the mother's body, and pressure on internal organs may cause frequent urination, heartburn, and difficulty breathing and sleeping.

Normal pregnancies vary from thirty-eight to forty-two weeks long. The lungs are the final organs to mature, and by the end of the eighth month all organ systems are established and functional. The fetus continues to gain weight until the end of pregnancy. At this time, the fetus will weigh around 3 kilograms (7 pounds) and have a crown to rump length of approximately 37 centimeters (14.4 inches). The end of pregnancy is heralded by the beginning of uterine contractions, and frequently by the rupture of the amniotic sac and expulsion of its fluid. Labor leads to the birth of a unique individual created from the developmental programs contained in the genetic material inherited from each parent.

Complications and Disorders

Since the developing embryo or fetus is dependent on the placental connection to the mother for nourishment, its health is directly tied to the diet and lifestyle of the mother. Any environmental substance that may cause a developmental defect is known as a teratogen. Women must take care to avoid teratogens such as drugs or nicotine during pregnancy. Pregnant women must ingest adequate levels of protein, vitamins, and iron to remain healthy and have a healthy baby. Smoking during pregnancy has been linked to to heart defects, and it decreases the amount of oxygen available to the fetus, which causes poor growth. Consumption of alcohol is associated with a host of defects collectively called fetal alcohol syndrome. Whether any level of alcohol consumption is safe during pregnancy is not yet known. The use of drugs such as marijuana and cocaine during pregnancy increases the likelihood of stillbirths and unhealthy babies.

The loss of a fetus before the twentieth week of pregnancy is called a miscarriage. The most common cause of miscarriage during the first trimester is a major genetic defect in which the embryo has missing or extra chromosomes and therefore cannot develop normally. Other common causes are physical abnormalities in the embryo, a malformed uterus in the mother, an "incompetent" cervix that opens as the fetus enlarges, scarring of the uterus, and hormonal deficiencies. Increasing age of the mother, smoking, and alcohol and drug consumption are also correlated with miscarriage. To prevent future miscarriages of a nongenetic cause, hormone therapy, medications, and surgery are options.

Ectopic pregnancies occur when the fertilized egg implants in the wall of the Fallopian tube instead of in the uterus. The growing embryo may rupture the tube, endangering the mother's life and necessitating emergency surgery and possible loss of that Fallopian tube. Unruptured ectopics can be treated with medication or laparoscopic surgery. Scarring of the Fallopian tube from an infection can narrow this passage and cause ectopic pregnancy, as can early "hatching" of the blastocyst from its protective covering.

Neural tube defects result from a problem in the ectodermal layer of the embryo resulting in improper closure of the brain and spinal cord in early embryonic development. The outcomes of this defect are anencephaly (absence of a complete brain and part of the skull), a lethal condition, or spina bifida (portions of the spinal cord protruding from the spine), which can vary from mild to severe. These disorders seem to occur in families with a history of neural tube defects in pregnancy. Folic acid, an important component of prenatal vitamins, can reduce the risk of neural tube defects.

Neural tube defects can be detected prenatally by ultrasound, in which high-frequency sound waves are bounced off the contents of the uterus. The echoes are converted to an image, or sonogram, on a screen. Another test for neural tube defects is the alpha fetoprotein test, which measures levels of a fetal protein in the mother's blood; high levels indicate a neural tube defect.

Down syndrome, which results from the presence of one extra chromosome number 21, is the leading cause of mental retardation in the United States and occurs in about 1 in every 800 live births. Many other genetic disorders are caused by missing or extra chromosomes. Some inherited diseases are attributable to errors in small pieces of chromosomes. Examples of these sorts of disorders include cystic fibrosis, hemophilia, Tay-Sachs disease, and sickle cell disease. Many of these genetic diseases can be detected by

prenatal tests.

Amniocentesis is performed between the fifteenth and seventeenth weeks of pregnancy. A needle is inserted through the mother's abdomen, and a sample of the amniotic fluid is removed. Fetal cells present in the fluid are cultured for two to three weeks. The fetal cells are then analyzed for chromosome complement or tested for small genetic changes that can result in specific genetic diseases. Occasionally amniocentesis is done in the third trimester to determine fetal lung maturity when delivery of a premature infant is expected. Chorionic villus sampling provides a similar means to examine the genetic material of the fetus. This test is performed as early as the eighth week of pregnancy when a small piece of the chorionic villus, a tissue of embryonic origin that surrounds the early placenta, is removed and genetic analysis is immediately performed. Prenatal diagnosis of a chromosome abnormality or genetic disease allows the parents to terminate the pregnancy or to prepare for the birth of an affected child.

Infections acquired by a pregnant woman may be only inconveniences for her, but they may have severe consequences for an unborn child. Rubella, or German measles, can cause fetal death or severe impairment during the first trimester and permanent hearing loss during the second trimester. Vaccination prevents contraction of rubella, but cannot be given during pregnancy. Cytomegalovirus (CMV) can cause physical and mental retardation, blindness, and deafness to the fetus if the mother first contracts CMV during pregnancy. Toxoplasmosis is an infection that can cause serious fetal consequences including miscarriage, stillbirth, and neonatal death if contracted in pregnancy. Avoidance of gardening where cats defecate and avoiding any contact with cat litter are measures counseled to pregnant women to reduce risk. Transmission of the sexually transmitted diseases syphilis and gonorrhea to the fetus can be prevented with antibiotic therapy. Human immunodeficiency virus (HIV), the virus that causes acquired immunodeficiency syndrome (AIDS), can be transmitted from mother to fetus through the placenta. Newborns with AIDS have a host of disorders and usually die within one or two years.

Rh factor is a substance on the surface of red blood cells. Individuals with and without this substance are Rh positive and Rh negative, respectively. If a woman is Rh negative and has an Rh-positive fetus, during delivery some of the baby's blood cells will enter the woman, and her body will manufacture antibodies to destroy the foreign cells. If with a subsequent pregnancy the fetus is Rh positive, these antibodies could attack and destroy the fetus. This problem is avoided by bloodtyping of mother and fetus during the first pregnancy and by administering Rh0(D) immune globulin (human), which destroys the fetal red blood cells entering the mother before her body can produce antibodies. Hence, future pregnancies are not at risk for Rh incompatibility.

A host of medical problems in the mother can develop during pregnancy that could jeopardize both her health and the health of her fetus. Blood pressure problems develop in about 7 percent of pregnant women as a result of the enormous changes in blood volume and pressure. The largest danger is that the fetus will not receive enough oxygen, which may lead to growth problems or sudden death during the final months of pregnancy. Preeclampsia is a cluster of symptoms related to high blood pressure, including edema (swelling caused by water retention) and kidney malfunction. Eclampsia (convulsions and coma) is life-threatening and needs emergency treatment. Bed rest, diet modifica-

tion, close monitoring by a physician, or hospitalization may be prescribed for mild to severe cases of high blood pressure during pregnancy.

The effect of the hormones induced by pregnancy on the production of insulin, which regulates sugar levels in the body, is not well understood. In some pregnancies, insulin levels are not regulated properly, which results in gestational diabetes. Untreated, this can result in loss of the fetus

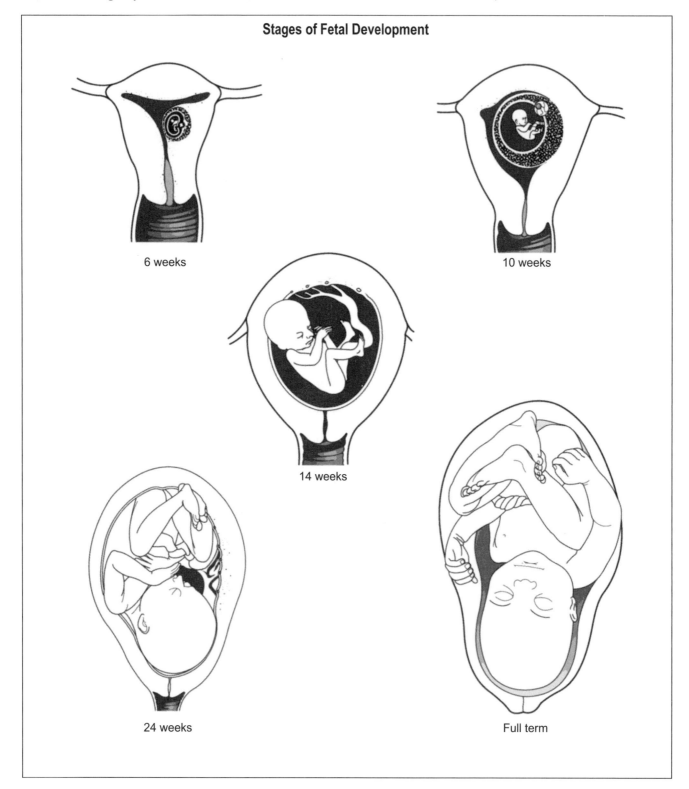

Stages of Fetal Development

6 weeks

10 weeks

14 weeks

24 weeks

Full term

late in pregnancy, the birth of a baby with high body fat content and an immature pancreas, or maternal convulsions and coma. Proper medical intervention and monitoring can correct or ease the effects of gestational diabetes on both mother and fetus.

Up to half of pregnant women develop anemia, a deficiency in red blood cells, because of a lack of iron or folic acid. The demand for the production of red blood cells in both mother and fetus leads to this disorder, which can cause poor growth in the fetus and increased susceptibility to infection, fatigue, and severe bleeding during childbirth for the mother. Proper diet and dietary supplements can alleviate anemia.

Perspective and Prospects

Until the mid-twentieth century, what was known about fetal development was derived mainly from the study of miscarriages. The development and use of ultrasound techniques in the 1960s allowed a more accurate picture of developmental progression of normal, active fetuses, and such techniques subsequently became indispensable for the detection of some developmental abnormalities.

While physicians had been able to sample the amniotic fluid surrounding a fetus since the late nineteenth century, it was not until 1970 that they discovered that the fluid contained fetal cells which could be analyzed for chromosomal composition. At this time, amniocentesis became a tool for prenatal genetic analysis and sex determination and a routine test for pregnant women over the age of thirty-five, who are at a higher risk of carrying a fetus with a genetic abnormality. The liberalization of abortion laws in the United States in the 1960s gave parents of abnormal fetuses the option of pregnancy termination. In the early 1980s, chorionic villus sampling allowed much earlier detection of genetic defects and facilitated decision making for the expectant parents.

In the 1980s, some physicians began performing surgery on fetuses within the mother's uterus to correct problems threatening the life of the fetus, such as kidney disorders. Advanced monitoring and intervention techniques have virtually eliminated maternal deaths during pregnancy and childbirth. Increased knowledge about infectious and toxic agents and about the ill effects of certain lifestyle habits upon a developing fetus has led to better education and prenatal care for both mother and fetus. Because of career and personal considerations, older women frequently wish to begin families. Medical advances have made it not uncommon for women past the age of forty to conceive for the first time and give birth to healthy infants.

Much research has been focused on the initial stages of pregnancy and infertility. Techniques have been developed to circumvent damaged Fallopian tubes. In the procedure called in vitro fertilization, a woman is given hormones to induce ovulation. Several mature eggs are removed from her ovaries and fertilized in a glass dish. The resulting blastocysts are then implanted into the woman's uterus. In some cases in which a woman is unable to carry the fetus herself, a surrogate mother has been used as an "incubator"

for the embryo. Unused embryos fertilized in vitro are stored in a deep freeze and may be thawed for future use. Early embryos have been separated into individual cells, which then develop into genetically identical blastocysts, each with the potential to become an infant. These technological advances have raised a host of ethical questions concerning disposal of the embryos and their genetic manipulation.

Human reproductive research is focused on the reversal or circumvention of infertility, the alleviation of maternal and fetal distress, and the prenatal detection and treatment of genetic disease. The knowledge gained about reproduction serves to enhance a sense of awe and wonder at the beauty and complexity of the gestational process.

—Karen E. Kalumuck, Ph.D.;
updated by Robin Kamienny Montvilo, R.N., Ph.D.

See also Abortion; Amniocentesis; Assisted reproductive technologies; Birth defects; Blurred vision; Breast-feeding; Cesarean section; Childbirth; Childbirth complications; Chorionic villus sampling; Conception; Contraception; Ectopic pregnancy; Embryology; Endometriosis; Fetal surgery; Gamete intrafallopian transfer (GIFT); Genetic counseling; Genetic diseases; Genital disorders, female; Gestational diabetes; Gynecology; In vitro fertilization; Infertility, female; Infertility, male; Mastitis; Menstruation; Miscarriage; Multiple births; Ovaries; Pap test; Placenta; Postpartum depression; Preeclampsia and eclampsia; Premature birth; Reproductive system; Sexual differentiation; Sperm banks; Stem cells; Sterilization; Stillbirth; Teratogens; Toxemia; Tubal ligation; Ultrasonography; Umbilical cord; Uterus; Women's health.

For Further Information:

Cunningham, F. Gary, et al., eds. *Williams Obstetrics*. 23d ed. New York: McGraw-Hill, 2010.

Curtis, Glade B., and Judith Schuler. *Your Pregnancy Week-by-Week*. 6th ed. Cambridge, Mass.: Da Capo Press, 2008.

Eisenberg, Arlene, Heidi E. Murkoff, and Sandee E. Hathaway. *What to Expect When You're Expecting*. 4th ed. New York: Workman, 2009.

Hales, Dianne, and Timothy R. B. Johnson. *Intensive Caring: New Hope for High-Risk Pregnancy*. New York: Crown, 1990.

Harris, A. Christine. *The Pregnancy Journal: A Day-to-Day Guide to a Healthy and Happy Pregnancy*. San Francisco: Chronicle Books, 2009.

Hotchner, Tracie. *Pregnancy and Childbirth*. Rev. ed. New York: Quill/HarperCollins, 2003.

Lees, Christoph, Karina Reynolds, and Grainne McCarten. *Pregnancy and Birth: Your Questions Answered*. Rev. ed. New York: DK, 2007.

Moore, Keith L., and T. V. N. Persaud. *The Developing Human*. 8th ed. Philadelphia: Saunders/Elsevier, 2008.

Morales, Karla, and Charles B. Inlander. *Take This Book to the Obstetrician with You: A Consumer's Guide to Pregnancy and Childbirth*. Rev. ed. New York: St. Martin's Press, 1998.

Murkoff, Heidi. Sharon Mazel. What to Expect When You're Expecting. New York: Workman Publishing Company, 2008.

Nilsson, Lennart. *A Child Is Born*. Text by Lars Hamberger. Translated by Clare James. 5th ed. London: Jonathan Cape, 2009.

Simkin, Penny. April Bolding. Ann Keppler. Janelle Durham. *Pregnancy, Childbirth, and the Newborn: The Complete Guide*. Hopkins, Minnesota: Meadowbrook Press, 2010.

Tsiaras, Alexander, and Barry Werth. *From Conception to Birth: A Life Unfolds*. New York: Doubleday, 2002.

Van Katwijk, C., and L. L. H. Peeters. "Clinical Aspects of Pregnancy After the Age of 35 Years: A Review of the Literature." *Human Reproduction Update* 4, no. 2 (March/April, 1998): 185-194.

Pregnancy test
Procedure
Anatomy or system affected: Ovaries, Uterus, Reproductive system
Specialties and related fields: Endocrinology, Obstetrics, Gynecology, Family Medicine
Definition: A urine or blood test used to evaluate whether or not a woman is pregnant.

Indications and Procedures

Pregnancy tests are a rapid, inexpensive, and accurate way to assess whether or not a woman is pregnant. Pregnancy occurs when a sperm fertilizes an egg after sexual intercourse. The newly fertilized egg implants in the wall of the uterus about 6-12 days after fertilization. This implantation causes a hormone called human chorionic gonadotropin (hCG) to be released. After implantation, hCG continues to be released by the placenta triggering other physiological changes that occur throughout pregnancy. It can be detected in the blood and urine of a pregnant woman. It is not present in males or non-pregnant females, which makes the test very reliable. HCG is the basis for pregnancy tests available over the counter in most drugstores and in medical settings. Pregnancy tests can reliably detect the presence of hCG 1-2 weeks after the first missed period. It is possible to detect the presence of hCG sooner, but the test results may be less accurate with higher false negative rates. For women without regular menstrual cycles, pregnancy tests may detect hCG about 3 weeks after sexual intercourse.

Pregnancy tests usually come in the form of a stick, strip, or cassette. There are also electronic forms available. The test is usually performed by urinating on the stick/strip or dropping urine into a reservoir on the cassette. Each of these methods contains antibodies designed specifically to target hCG. In the presence of hCG, these antibodies bind the hormone and undergo a chemical reaction to turn blue. If hCG is detected, this means the test is positive for pregnancy.

While the majority of pregnancy tests detect hCG in urine, hCG can also be detected in blood. HCG can be detected in blood about 1 week after ovulation, which is sooner than in urine. The blood test is also less convenient as it requires getting blood drawn in a medical center, and it usually takes longer to obtain these results. Usually, the urine hCG test is preferred in medical settings unless there are other indications for a blood test to verify the results.

Uses and Complications

There are several ways to perform a pregnancy test depending on the brand of the test. Some of the common ways to perform pregnancy tests are: urinating directly onto a stick or strip, dipping the strip into a cup of urine, or using a dropper to drop urine onto a cassette. Usually after applying the urine, it takes a few minutes for the reaction to complete and display the results. In most tests, if hCG is present the antibodies will bind and turn blue, which can be visualized in the form of a line or a cross. Electronic pregnancy tests may also display words like "pregnant" or "not pregnant." The readings may vary depending on the brand of the test so be sure to read and follow the directions provided.

HCG pregnancy tests are most accurate starting 1 week after a missed period. They may detect pregnancy earlier, but the results may be less accurate. There will be a higher false negative rate because it takes time for hCG levels to build up to a detectable range after its initial release. There is evidence to suggest that digital pregnancy tests may be both easier to use and more accurate for early home pregnancy tests than strips or cassettes.

While pregnancy tests are generally reported to be 99% accurate, it is possible to obtain false positive or false negative results. False positive results may be due to loss of a pregnancy soon after implantation in the uterine lining, medications that contain hCG (e.g. fertility drugs), or medical problems with the ovaries. False negatives as mentioned above may be due to taking the test too soon after fertilization. HCG levels increase over time so if an initial pregnancy test is negative, rechecking in 1-2 weeks may improve the accuracy of results. Checking the strip too early before the antibody reaction can fully develop or using dilute urine may also cause false negative results. Urine is most concentrated in the morning, so tests taken first thing in the morning may be slightly more accurate. If you have mixed positive and negative results, you may need to follow up with a health care provider to obtain a blood test or an ultrasound to verify pregnancy.

—*Kathleen Chung, BA*

For Further Information:
ELISA for Home Pregnancy Test. (n.d.). Retrieved October 27, 2017, from http://www.elisa-antibody.com/ELISA-applications/home-pregnancy-test
Parenthood, P. (n.d.). When to Take a Pregnancy Test | Options, Cost and Accuracy. Retrieved October 27, 2017, from https://www.plannedparenthood.org/learn/pregnancy/pregnancy-test
Tomlinson, C., Marshall, J., & Ellis, J. E. (2008). Comparison of accuracy and certainty of results of six home pregnancy tests available over-the-counter. Current Medical Research and Opinion, 24(6), 1645-1649. doi:10.1185/03007990802120572
Knowing if you are pregnant. (2017, February 01). Retrieved October 27, 2017, from https://www.womenshealth.gov/pregnancy/you-get-pregnant/knowing-if-you-are-pregnant

Premature birth
Disease/Disorder
Anatomy or system affected: Reproductive system, uterus
Specialties and related fields: Embryology, neonatology, obstetrics, pediatrics, perinatology
Definition: Premature birth is childbirth occurring before the thirty-seventh week of pregnancy; premature infants are those babies born before this time.

Babies born later than the thirty-seventh week of pregnancy and before the forty-second week are known as term or full-term infants, and birth anywhere during this period is within the window of normal gestation. By definition, babies born at or before the thirty-seventh week are called preterm or premature infants. (Babies born beyond the forty-second week are post-term infants.)

Every pregnancy and birth carry risk to both infant and mother. Preterm and premature infants, however, are at high risk. They have both a lower survival rate and more medical complications with potential lifelong effects than term babies. By 2013 in the United States, nearly one-half million babies were born prematurely each year, which constitutes a 36 percent increase since 1980, according to Centers for Disease Control. These infants make up the majority of the low-weight births that occur annually.

Developmental prematurity and survivability. Prior to twenty-four weeks of gestation, fetuses are not considered to have developed sufficiently to live outside the womb. Somewhere between twenty-four and twenty-eight weeks of gestation, however, the fetus does become viable, although any baby born between twenty-four and thirty weeks is called very premature. Very premature babies constitute about 1 percent of all live births in the United States. The lengths of these infants range from eleven to eighteen inches, and weights can range from one pound, five ounces to almost four pounds. At this stage of development, a few ounces more or less make a big difference in the baby's ability to survive. Neonates at two pounds have little better than a one in two chance of survival; infants at 3.5 pounds have better than a nine in ten chance.

Babies born between thirty-one and thirty-six weeks of gestation are moderately premature and make up between 4 and 6 percent of live births in the United States each year. These babies do well, with a 90 to 98 percent survival rate, and weigh from a little more than three to almost four and one-half pounds. Typical lengths range from sixteen to nineteen inches.

Parents who expect their very premature baby who reaches five to nine weeks of age to resemble a moderately premature baby born at thirty-five weeks will be disappointed. The very premature still appear much less like babies, are significantly lighter, and remain behind developmentally. They are often unready to be bottle-fed or breast-fed or to sleep in an open crib, and they are always less alert and have less behavioral control than the moderately premature. Simply reaching the same number of chronological weeks as moderately premature babies does not negate the substantial differences in their developmental beginnings.

Borderline premature infants are born during weeks thirty-seven or thirty-eight and constitute 16 to 20 percent of all live births in the United States. These babies are much like full-term newborns: They have almost the identical survival rate (98 percent) and approach average weights. Nevertheless, they are still at greater risk for respiratory distress syndromes, jaundice, unstable body temperatures, and a variety of problems associated with feeding.

The causes of prematurity and preterm births. Although many conditions result in premature birth, not all causes are known. Some well-known causes include toxemia in the mother (a multistage disease that begins with high blood pressure and rapid fluid retention and may progress to brain hemorrhage, seizure, and coma), placenta previa (when the placenta implants in the lower uterus), placenta abruptio

---

Information on Premature Birth

Causes: Wide ranging; may include toxemia, placenta previa, placenta abruptio, rupture of amniotic sac, incompetent cervix, multiple births

Symptoms: Low birth weight, developmental delays, reduced alertness, reduced behavioral control, greater risk for respiratory distress syndrome, jaundice, feeding problems

Duration: Acute

Treatments: Placement in neonatal intensive care unit, use of incubators, drug therapy to hasten physical development of organs

---

(when a normally positioned placenta detaches from the uterus), premature membrane rupture (when the tissue containing the amniotic fluid tears or leaks before labor begins), incompetent cervix (when the cervix opens mid-pregnancy), and multiple births (twins, triplets, and so on). Some of the recent increases in premature births can be attributed to more older women giving birth and to the alarming rise of obesity in the United States, both risk factors according to researchers.

Some mothers blame themselves for the premature births of their infants. While it is natural to look for a cause and a target to vent the often-powerful feelings associated with prematurity, it is the rare mother who deliberately causes her baby to be born earlier than necessary. While some factors in the mother-such as high blood pressure, diabetes mellitus, sickle cell disease, and kidney diseases-can contribute to prematurity, these are not volitional conditions and the mother is not at moral fault in any way. She did not will these conditions, and she did not intend for her baby to be born prematurely. In fact, some causes do not involve the mothers at all, but the babies themselves, including congenital defects, intrauterine illnesses, and defective placentas.

The vast majority of women will never deliver prematurely. Those who do, however, run about a 30 percent chance of having a second premature birth (according to the March of Dimes). In the rush to understand and find answers to prematurity, it is important not to overinvest in probability statistics and comparative risk factor data, which include race (for example, African Americans have a higher prematurity rate than whites), paternity (for example, a few individual men seem to father premature babies even with different mothers without risk factors themselves), and even a woman's own mother's exposure to biochemicals (such as diethylstilbestrol, or DES). It is extremely important to realize that many women who are formally classified as high-risk mothers have normal deliveries of full-term babies, and that others, who are healthy and without known risk factors, deliver premature, preterm babies.

In 2003, scientists announced an exciting discovery in the search for preventing premature birth. More than three hundred high-risk pregnant women-those who had given birth prematurely before-were given weekly injections of

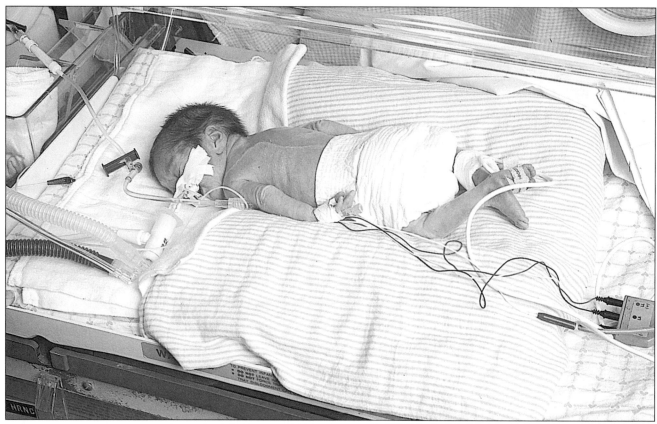

A premature infant in a neonatal intensive care unit. (SIU School of Medicine)

the hormone progesterone. This therapy reduced the chance of preterm birth by 34 percent, a number that elated the study's researchers. The use of progesterone therapy has been especially effective in the cases of women with short cervixes. Another study in 2002 suggested that measures used to detect early labor-including a medical device worn on the abdomen to record contractions, ultrasound examinations of the cervix, and a test for a chemical called fetal fibronectin-seem not to work very well in preventing preterm birth, leading researchers to continue to seek ways to predict and prevent premature delivery. Early detection of labor is important because it can allow doctors to prescribe antibiotics, medication to slow the contractions or help the fetus develop more quickly, or bed rest.

The psychological impact. There may be no event with a greater impact on a person's life than becoming a parent, and few events in a parent's life equal the impact of seeing one's tiny, struggling, helpless, and high-risk baby. It is common for parents to have been forewarned of the baby's chances, especially if the infant is very premature. They may, in fact, have begun to prepare themselves psychologically for the death of their baby even as the baby clings to life outside the womb. They may try to protect themselves from bonding to one whose death may be imminent. Parents who expected a bundle of joy can fear that even if their baby lives, he or she will be handicapped, sickly, malformed, and never able to live a life as an independent, functioning, and happy adult.

Parents sometimes confess to not knowing whether they

want their baby to live or die, and they feel guilt for not knowing. Their distress, confusion, and contradictory feelings can overwhelm them. Their babies may not look much like the babies they had pictured or prepared for, and they may not feel much like parents. Premature birth can be a crisis rarely equaled in a parent's life.

Some couples react and adapt successfully, while others do not. Nearly all parents of premature infants experience various forms of shock, denial, anger, guilt, and depression. Researchers who study and compare parents who cope better and worse have learned that those parents who accept and express their whole range of emotions (versus only the emotions that they believe they are supposed to have), who seek further information, who accept help in their caring for the babies, and who begin to develop an early relationship with their babies adapt to the crisis well and successfully.

Premature infants were thought, at one time, to be inactive, unaware, and inert. Research and anecdotal observation strongly support the view that these infants are acutely sensitive to their environment, though they usually respond in ways too subtle to be perceived casually. When parents are present, even on the outside of the incubator wall, their babies behave differently, tolerate feedings better, and heal more quickly and completely.

—*Paul Moglia, Ph.D.*

See also Birth defects; Childbirth; Childbirth complications; Intensive care unit (ICU); Multiple births; Placenta; Postpartum depression; Pregnancy and gestation; Stillbirth; Teratogens; Toxemia; Uterus.

For Further Information:

Bradford, Nikki. *Your Premature Baby: The First Five Years.* Toronto, Ont.: Firefly Books, 2003.

Curtis, Glade B., and Judith Schuler. *Your Pregnancy Week-by-Week.* 7th ed. Cambridge, Mass.: Da Capo Press, 2011.

Gabbe, Steven G., Jennifer R. Niebyl, and Joe Leigh Simpson, eds. *Obstetrics: Normal and Problem Pregnancies.* 6th ed. Philadelphia: Churchill Livingstone/Elsevier, 2012.

Gaines, Tami C. *Preemie Parents: Twenty-Six Ways to Grow with Your Premature Baby.* South Portland, Maine: Sellers, 2011.

Goepfert, Alice. *Management of Preterm Birth: Best Practices in Prediction, Prevention, and Treatment.* Philadelphia: Saunders, 2012.

Hotchner, Tracie. *Pregnancy and Childbirth.* Rev. ed. New York: Quill/HarperCollins, 2003.

Hynan, Michael T. *The Pain of Premature Parents: A Psychological Guide for Coping.* Lanham, Md.: University Press of America, 1987.

Martin, Richard J., Avroy A. Fanaroff, and Michele C. Walsh, eds. *Fanaroff and Martin's Neonatal-Perinatal Medicine: Diseases of the Fetus and Infant.* 2 vols. 9th ed. Philadelphia: Mosby/Elsevier, 2011.

Oh, William. *Evidenced-Based Handbook of Neonatology.* Hackensack, N.J.: World Scientific, 2011.

Ramsay, Sharon M., and Regina M. Santella. "The Definition of Life: A Survey of Obstetricians and Neonatologists in New York City Hospitals Regarding Extremely Premature Births." *Maternal and Child Health Journal* 15 no. 4 (May, 2011): 446-52.

Simkin, Penny, Janet Whalley, and Ann Keppler. *Pregnancy, Childbirth, and the Newborn: The Complete Guide.* 4th ed. Minnetonka, Minn.: Meadowbrook Press, 2010.

Premenstrual syndrome (PMS)

Disease/Disorder

Also known as: Menstrually related mood disorder (MRMD), premenstrual tension, late luteal phase disorder (LLPD), premenstrual dysphoric disorder (PMDD)

Anatomy or system affected: Breasts, psychic-emotional system, reproductive system

Specialties and related fields: Family medicine, gynecology, psychiatry, psychology

Definition: A disorder characterized by the cyclic recurrence of physical and behavioral symptoms during the days between ovulation and the first few days of menstruation.

Key terms:

endorphins: hormones, found mainly in the brain, that bind to opiate receptors, reducing the sensation of pain and affecting emotions

luteal phase: the second half of the menstrual cycle after ovulation; during this phase, the corpus luteum secretes progesterone

menses: the monthly flow of blood and cellular debris from the uterus that begins at puberty in women

premenstrual dysphoric disorder (PMDD): a severe form of premenstrual syndrome characterized by affective symptoms causing significant disturbances in relationships or social adaptation

progesterone: a hormone produced in the ovary that prepares and maintains the uterus for pregnancy

serotonin: a neurotransmitter involved in sleep, depression, and memory

Causes and Symptoms

Several causes of premenstrual syndrome (PMS) have been proposed. Changes in hormone levels during the luteal phase of the menstrual cycle, when the ovaries are making progesterone, may deplete neurotransmitters such as enkephalins and endorphins, which are responsible for a sense of well-being; gamma-aminobutyric acid (GABA), which aids in relaxation; and serotonin, which stimulates the central nervous system. The disorder may be more likely to occur in women who have enhanced sensitivity to progesterone, a disposition related to serotonin deficiency. PMS may be related to excess prostaglandin, a hormone-like substance that may affect blood pressure and metabolism and smooth muscle activity. Some evidence suggests that women with PMS have lower blood levels of allopregnanolone, a by-product of progesterone that plays a role in mood.

Up to 85 percent of women experience mild to moderate forms of PMS. Another 5 percent of women have symptoms so severe that they interfere with daily activity and may be diagnosed with premenstrual dysphoric disorder (PMDD). In some women, symptoms of PMS increase with age, perhaps because serotonin levels are altered with changes in estrogen levels.

PMS symptoms can be subdivided into physical, behavioral, and psychological. Physical symptoms include fatigue; headache; breast tenderness and swelling; back and abdominal pain; acne; heart palpitations; bloating; weight gain; nausea; muscle and joint pain; water retention; swelling of ankles, feet, and hands; and decreased tolerance to noise or light. Behavioral symptoms include fatigue, insomnia, dizziness, changes in sex drive, cravings for salty or sweet food, and increased appetite. Psychological symptoms include irritability, anger, depressed mood, crying, anxiety, tension, mood swings, and lack of concentration, confusion, forgetfulness, restlessness, loneliness, decreased self-esteem, and tension. The symptoms of depression, anxiety disorders, perimenopause, and thyroid dysfunction are similar to PMS. A distinguishing feature of PMS is its cyclic occurrence.

Researchers at the University of California, San Diego suggests the following criteria for diagnosing premenstrual syndrome: At least one psychological (affective) and physical (somatic) symptom occurs during the five to seven days before menses in each of the previous three cycles, and symptoms are relieved during days four through thirteen of the menstrual cycle. The National Institute of Mental Health and the American Psychiatric Association give similar diagnostic criteria. Blood tests are not necessary for the diagnosis of PMS. Laboratory studies such as a blood count or thyroid function tests may be recommended to screen for other medical conditions that cause fatigue, such as anemia and thyroid disease.

Treatment and Therapy

Treatment for premenstrual syndrome can be divided into three categories: nonpharmacologic therapy, dietary supplementation, and pharmacologic therapy.

Information on Premenstrual Syndrome (PMS)

Causes: Unknown; possibly depletion of neurotransmitters resulting from hormonal changes and sensitivities

Symptoms: Physical (fatigue, headache, breast tenderness and swelling, back and abdominal pain, muscle and joint pain, weight gain, water retention, acne, nausea, palpitations); behavioral (insomnia, dizziness, changes in sex drive, cravings for salty or sweet food, increased appetite); psychological (irritability, anger, depression, anxiety, mood swings, lack of concentration, confusion, forgetfulness, restlessness, decreased self-esteem)

Duration: Often chronic with acute episodes

Treatments: Patient education; exercise; adequate sleep; stress avoidance; dietary changes (increased complex carbohydrates, decreased sodium and caffeine); vitamin E supplements; calcium carbonate supplements; diuretics (spironolactone); antianxiety medications (benzodiazepines); selective serotonin reuptake inhibitors; hormonal therapy (Gonadotropin-releasing hormone agonists, oral contraceptives); Non-steroidal anti-inflammatory drugs (NSAIDs)

Nonpharmacologic therapies include patient education, supportive therapy, and behavioral interventions. Women who receive educational materials about PMS may gain an increased sense of control and relief of symptoms. Supportive therapies include relaxation and cognitive-behavioral therapy. A therapist may also be able to teach coping methods. Behavioral interventions include keeping a daily symptom diary. Each day for three months, a woman records in a diary and ranks any health complaints on a scale of "none at all" to "extreme." The PMS pattern is an increase in symptoms during the fourteen days before menstruation and then a decrease in symptoms within one hour to a few days after bleeding begins. In addition to keeping the diary, exercising thirty minutes a day (to stimulate the release of enkephalins and endorphins and to reduce swelling through sweat), sleeping six to eight hours every night, avoiding stress, and making dietary changes may help symptoms. Increasing the intake of complex carbohydrates (fruits, vegetables, and whole grains) may relieve mood-related symptoms by boosting the level of tryptophan, a precursor of serotonin. Lowering sodium intake can reduce bloating, fluid retention, and swelling. Restricting caffeine consumption may reduce irritability and insomnia.

Vitamin E supplements may reduce breast pain. Vitamin E as a dietary supplement is also a potentially beneficial antioxidant and poses minimal risk. Calcium carbonate supplementation may also improve PMS symptoms.

Nonprescription drugs, such as diuretics for bloating and analgesics for pain, may diminish the symptoms of PMS. Prescription treatments for PMS include antianxiety medication such as the benzodiazepines, which mimic the effects of GABA to relieve irritability; selective serotonin reuptake inhibitors (SSRIs), which increase serotonin levels; hormone treatments such as gonadotropin-releasing hormone (GnRH) agonists and birth control pills that stop the production of estrogen and progesterone; spironolactone, a diuretic that relieves breast tenderness and fluid retention; and nonsteroidal anti-inflammatory drugs (NSAIDs), or prostaglandin inhibitors, for pain such as headache.

Some treatments that have no proven benefit in relieving the symptoms of PMS include: Progesterone, antidepressant drugs such as Tricyclic Antidepressants (TCA), Monoamine Oxidase Inhibitors (MAOI), lithium, and popular dietary supplements such as evening primrose oil, essential free fatty acids, and ginkgo biloba.

Perspective and Prospects

Hysteria (literally, "wandering womb") was described in Egypt in about 1900 BCE as an abnormality of the uterus caused by its "migration" to different parts of the body, resulting in various symptoms, such as headache and swollen feet. The term "premenstrual tension" was first used by mental health professionals in the 1930s.

Research on PMS gained momentum in the 1980s. Whereas only one article on PMS appeared in 1964, 425 articles were published on the topic between 1988 and 1989. What had once been considered a pseudocondition, with PMS as a catchall phrase for up to 150 symptoms occurring before menstruation, was recognized as a medical disorder. Research has focused on biomedical and psychosocial causes and treatments.

—Elizabeth Marie McGhee Nelson, Ph.D.;
updated by Uzma Shahzad, M.D.,
and Christi N. Gandham, D.O.

See also Gynecology; Hormones; Menstruation; Stress; Stress reduction; Women's health

For Further Information:

Dalton, Katharina, and Wendy Holton. *Once a Month: Understanding and Treating PMS.* 6th ed. Alameda, CA.: Hunter House, 2000.

Dickerson, Lori M., J. Mazyck, and Melissa H. Hunter. "Premenstrual Syndrome." *American Family Physician* 67, no. 8 (April, 2003): 1743-1752.

Hahn, Linaya. PMS: *Solving the Puzzle-Sixteen Causes of PMS and What to Do About It.* Evanston, IL: Chicago Spectrum Press, 1995.

Taylor, Diana, and Stacey Colino. *Taking Back the Month: A Personalized Solution for Managing PMS and Enhancing Your Health.* New York: Perigee, 2002.

Vliet, Elizabeth Lee. *Screaming to Be Heard: Hormonal Connections Women Suspect and Doctors Still Ignore.* New York: M. Evans, 2001.

Yonkers, Kimberly A., and Robert F. Casper. "Clinical Manifestations and Diagnosis of Premenstrual Syndrome and Premenstrual Dysphoric Disorder." *UpToDate,* edited by Robert L. Barbieri, William F. Crowley, Jr., and Kathryn A. Martin.

Presbyopia

Disease/Disorder

Anatomy or system affected: Eyes, visual system

Specialties and related fields: Ophthalmology, optometry

Definition: Presbyopia is an age-related eye condition that causes progressive difficulty seeing objects at near distances.

Presbyopia (prez-bee-OH-pee-ah) refers to an eye condition that makes it difficult to see close objects. The word presbyopia comes from Greek words meaning, "to see like an old person." It is a natural part of the aging process that usually becomes noticeable between the ages of forty and fifty. The condition is normal, common, and unpreventable. It results from age-related changes to the lens of the eye that cause difficulty focusing on objects at close distances. People with presbyopia often hold books at arm's length to read them and find it challenging to see fine print in dim lighting. Glasses, contacts, and surgery can compensate for presbyopia, but there is no known way to prevent it.

Causes and Symptoms

Normal vision occurs when light rays enter the eye through the clear outer layer called the cornea. Light rays travel through the pupil, the black area at the center of the eye, and through the lens behind it. The lens is a transparent structure that changes shape to bend or refract light rays so they can be focused on the retina at the back of the eye. In order for clear images to be formed, light must be directly focused on the retina so that light-sensing nerve cells can transmit electrical impulses to the brain to be interpreted. Light that is focused behind or in front of the retina will be perceived as blurry.

As part of normal aging, the crystalline material of the lens hardens and becomes less flexible. The lens also continues to grow with age, making it more difficult for muscles surrounding the lens to change its shape. As a result, the lens becomes less effective at focusing light rays. The lens focuses light behind the retina instead of directly on it, producing a fuzzy image.

The changes that cause presbyopia develop gradually over time. People as young as thirty-five may find it harder to read fine print on labels or menus in a darkened restaurant. People with presbyopia often hold books at arm's length to read them or experience eyestrain when reading for long periods of time. People also notice blurred vision when switching from distance to near viewing. These problems are worse in dim light and can lead to headaches.

The most common risk factor for presbyopia is age; nearly everyone over the age of forty will develop the condition on some level. Some diseases can increase the risk of developing presbyopia before the age of forty-known as premature presbyopia-including diabetes, cardiovascular disease, and multiple sclerosis. Drugs such as antihistamines, diuretics, and antidepressants also can cause premature presbyopia. There is no known way to prevent presbyopia from developing.

Although presbyopia is a normal process of aging, people generally seek help when vision impairment affects their ability to work or enjoy everyday activities. An eye doctor can diagnose the condition during a general eye exam. During the exam, the physician will determine whether the symptoms are caused by presbyopia or another refractive eye condition such as hyperopia, myopia, or astigmatism, or abnormalities in other structures of the eye such as the cornea or retina. Components of the exam may include a visual acuity test, refraction test to measure glasses or contacts prescription, slit lamp examination, or dilated retinal exam. Presbyopia can occur in conjunction with other eye conditions, but a complete eye exam ensures that the correct treatment will be prescribed.

Treatment and Therapy

Many people who experience presbyopia correct it easily with reading glasses. These "readers" provide additional focusing strength to compensate for the loss of lens refraction during close work such as reading or sewing. Readers are readily available at many retail and convenience stores in a variety of price ranges and strengths. When selecting readers, people are recommended to choose the weakest strength that allows them to read without strain. Charts are often on display near readers to assist with this choice. Reading glasses may also be purchased from an eye doctor, who will ensure that they are the correct strength.

Whether purchased by prescription or over the counter, reading glasses may be worn over contact lenses to correct presbyopia and any other refractive error. In addition, bifocal and trifocal glasses are available to correct two or more problems with one pair of glasses. These types of lenses have one part powered for distance vision and another part for close vision.

Contact lenses also can be prescribed to allow multifocal vision. These lenses are weighted so that the prescription for distance viewing is in place when gazing out and the prescription for close vision is in place when looking down. Another option for contact lens wearers is to wear one contact with a prescription that corrects for distance vision while the other corrects for close work. In time, the brain adapts to choose the correct eye for the task at hand. This technique is known as monovision. Regardless of the method of correction chosen, corrective lenses need to be adjusted over time to compensate for additional changes to the eye from the aging process.

Presbyopia may also be corrected by surgical procedures collectively known as refractive surgery. LASIK surgery, which uses a laser to reshape the clear surface of eye, can be used to induce monovision, with one eye correcting for distance and the other correcting for close work. Future enhancements to the procedure may result in laser surgery that will create multifocal corrections, much like built-in bifocals. Conductive keratoplasty (CK) uses radio waves to adjust the curve of the cornea and can improve close vision, but its effects are temporary. Artificial lenses implanted into the cornea called corneal inlays are being studied as a way of providing additional refraction. Finally, surgically replacing the natural lens with an artificial one using techniques from cataract surgery can provide multiple focal lengths to minimize the focusing error caused by presbyopia. Further research is still being done to refine these techniques and develop new ways of correcting presbyopia.

—Claudine Yee, ScB

For Further Information:

"How the Eye Works as a Camera." *American Macular Degeneration Foundation*. Web. https://www.macular.org/eye-camera

"Eye Exams 101." *American Academy of Ophthalmology*, 25 May 2012. Web. https://www.aao.org/eye-health/tips-prevention/eye-exams-101

Boyd, Kierstan. "What Is Presbyopia?" *American Academy of Ophthalmology*, 1 Sep 2016. Web. http://www.aao.org/eye- health/tips -prevention/what-is-presbyopia

"Facts about Presbyopia." *National Eye Institute*, Oct 2010. Web. https://nei.nih.gov/health/errors/presbyopia

"Presbyopia." *Mayo* Clinic, 17 Oct 2014. Web. http://www.mayo clinic.org/diseases-conditions/presbyopia/basics/ definition/con-20032261

Boyd, Kierstan. "Presbyopia Treatment." *American Academy of Ophthalmology*, 1 Sep 2016. Web. http://www.aao.org/eye-health /diseases/presbyopia-treatment

Papadopoulos, Pandelis A and Papadopoulos, Alexandros P. "Current Management of Presbyopia." *Middle East African Journal of Ophthalmology*. 2014 Jan-Mar; 21(1): 10-17. https://www.ncbi.nlm.nih.gov/pmc/articles/PMC395903

Preventive medicine

Specialty

Anatomy or system affected: All

Specialties and related fields: All

Definition: The medical field that seeks to protect, promote, and maintain the health and well-being of individuals and defined populations and to prevent disease, disability, and premature death.

Key terms:

aerospace medicine: the medical specialty concerned with the health of the operating crews and passengers of air and space vehicles, together with support personnel

environmental medicine: the branch of medical science that addresses the impact of chemical and physical stressors and biological hazards on the individual or group in a community

epidemiology: the study of the incidence endence, distribution and determinants of disease in populations; includes attributes, such as gender, age, race, occupation, and social factors; and characteristics of disease, including but not limited to risk factors, incubation, infectivity, and chronicity

incidence: the number of new illnesses or newly diagnosed cases of disease, or events occurring within a specified period of time in a specific population

occupationalmedicine: a medical specialty focused on providing all levels of preventive medical services to working men and women in order to preserve, maintain, or restore health and well-being

prevalence: the actual number of individuals or live cases at a particular time with a disease or a given characteristic of a disease

public health: the well-being of humankind, both as a community and as individuals, accomplished by using scientific skills and beliefs that assist in health maintenance and health improvement

risk factors: the situations, circumstances, or conditions that increase the probability of the occurrence of disease or accident

Science and Profession

Modern preventive medicine is considered to exist at three levels within the health-care community. The initial level also known as primary prevention, has as its purpose to maintain health by removing the causes of or by protecting the community or individual from agents of disease and injury. These activities are no longer limited to the prevention of infection; yet they now include improvement in the environment and behavioral changes to reduce risk factors that contribute to chronic disease and injury. Examples of primary prevention are immunization programs. Other examples include risk reduction. For example, to reduce the risk of heart attack, one should refrain from smoking, be active, and reduce dietary fat intake-all wise primary prevention actions. Environmental risk reduction includes halting the loss of atmospheric ozone, reducing air and water pollution, and developing environmentally friendly technologies.

Secondary prevention seeks to detect and correct subclinical, adverse health conditions before they become manifest as disease, by reversing, halting, or retarding the disease process. A frequently used secondary prevention technique is health screening. Examples of secondary prevention aimed at detecting disease and early pathological changes include blood pressure measurement for hypertension (high blood pressure), fasting blood sugar screening for diabetes, mammography for breast cancer, PSA levels that detect prostate cancer, and glaucoma screening. In industry, a hearing test is used as a tool to prevent noise-induced hearing loss among the workforce. Once a potential health problem is identified, clinical preventive medicine techniques can be instituted to reverse the condition or prevent further progression.

Tertiary prevention attempts to minimize the adverse effects of conferred disease and disability. Coronary bypass surgery, vocational rehabilitation following a cerebrovascular accident (CVA), and treatment of an incapacitating mental illness are examples.

Specialists in the field of preventive medicine typically focus their efforts within the paradigms of primary and secondary prevention. In epidemiological terms, primary prevention results in a reduction of the incidence of a disease (the new cases occurring over time). Secondary prevention, on the other hand, results in a reduction of the prevalence of a disease (the number of actual people suffering from a particular illness at a given point in time).

Most health providers practice some degree of preventive medicine services. Pediatricians and pediatric nurse practitioners are practicing preventive medicine when they conduct "well-baby evaluations" and ensure that immunizations are current. Family medicine and primary care providers are promoting such services when they perform Pap testing or order mammograms. When smoking cessation is discussed as part of a clinical management plan and health care providers prescribe nicotine-patch regimens, that too is preventive medicine.

In the United States, approximately one thousand physicians specialize in general preventive medicine. Some use epidemiological methods to design and develop prevention programs that may feature a single intervention or may constitute a strategy that includes a multitude or matrix of screening technologies and interventions. Other preventive-medicine specialists including physician assistants and advanced practice nurses, provide services in a clinical setting by ordering a history and physical examination, which may include age- and gender-specific screening tests. The clinical preventive medicine specialist then can counsel the patient on lifestyle alterations recommended to preserve or improve health.

Within the United States, another field in preventive medicine is occupational medicine. Practicing in industry or private clinic settings, specialists in this field are concerned about preventing injury and illness as a result of the physical, biological, and chemical hazards that are present in the workplace. Should workers be injured or made ill as a result of their employment, the occupational health providers manage their treatment, rehabilitation, and return to work. Aerospace medicine providers limit their practice to those involved in the aeronautical and space transportation fields, including flight crews, support personnel, and passengers. The major task of these providers is to protect this population group from the adverse environmental conditions of flight, including pressure changes, reduced availability of oxygen, thermal stressors, accelerative forces, and psychosocial factors that might compromise performance.

Diagnostic and Treatment Techniques

An example of the application of preventive medicine is a comparison of the leading causes of death in the United States in 1900 with those in 2000. There was a major shift from deaths attributable to infectious disease at the beginning of the twentieth century to deaths attributable to chronic diseases that are often a reflection of individual lifestyle. Preventive medicine has proven itself effective in altering both the cause of death and the age at which death occurs. Accompanying this increased shift to chronic diseases such as cancer and heart disease, moreover, is a significant increase in the life expectancy of the population during the same century. Preventive medicine's focus is now on reducing morbidity and mortality from chronic diseases and accidents, particularly those in which an individual's lifestyle increases the risk for illness and death.

Disease prevention and health promotion are the two pillars supporting the discipline of preventive medicine. Beginning in 1987, a consortium was convened to begin to address a preventive medicine strategy to improve the health of Americans. The Institute of Medicine of the National Academy of Sciences worked with the US Public Health Service and numerous organizations to formulate health objective goals to be attained by the beginning of the twenty-first century. Once goals and objectives were established, the next task was to devise methods, technologies, and strategies to achieve the objectives by the year 2000. The resulting report was titled *Healthy People 2000: National Health Promotionand Disease Prevention Objectives* (1991).

The implementation of what was then known about disease prevention and health promotion was the central challenge. Good health is the result of reducing needless disease, injury, and suffering, resulting in an improved quality of life. A strategy of *Healthy People 2000* was to combine scientific knowledge, professional skills, community support, individual commitment, and the public will to achieve good health. This plan required reducing premature death, preventing disability, preserving the physical environment, and enabling Americans to develop healthy lifestyles.

Leading Causes of Death in the United States

1900	2000
1. Pneumonia and influenza	1. Heart diseases
2. Tuberculosis	2. Cancer and other malignant tumors
3. Diarrhea, enteritis, and ulceration of the intestine	3. Strokes
4. Heart diseases	4. Chronic lower respiratory diseases
5. Senility (ill-defined or unknown)	5. Accidents
6. Strokes	6. Diabetes mellitus
7. Nephritis	7. Pneumonia and influenza
8. Accidents	8. Suicide
9. Cancer and other malignant tumors	9. Chronic liver disease and cirrhosis
10. Diphtheria	10. Homicide

Three broad goals were detailed in *Healthy People 2000*: first, increase the healthy life span for Americans; second, reduce health disparity among Americans; and third, achieve access to preventive services for all Americans. A number of examples of the types of programs required to attain these goals were provided.

Tobacco use is the most important single preventable cause of death in the United States, accounting for more than four hundred thousand deaths annually. This loss of life is the equivalent of crashing two commercial jumbo jet airliners filled with passengers every day throughout the year. Smoking is a major risk factor for heart and lung disease; cancer of many organs, including the lungs, pancreas, and bladder; and stomach ulcers. Passive or environmental tobacco smoke is a recognized cause of cancer for exposed nonsmokers, and children in smoke-filled homes experience more ear infections. Tobacco use during pregnancy increases the risk of prematurity and low birth weight.

More than 3 million injuries occur annually in the US private sector, according to the Bureau of Labor Statistics; preliminary reports for 2013 indicate that more than four thousand deaths were attributable to work-related injuries. The occupations with the highest injury rates include mining, construction, agriculture, and transportation. The prevention of occupational disease and injury requires engineering controls, improved work practices, use of physical protective equipment, and monitoring of the work environment to identify emerging chemical and physical hazards.

In 2011 in the United States, nearly 575,000 people died from cancer. Nearly one in three Americans will experience a form of this disease. Research has helped to identify many risk factors related to cancer causation, such as tobacco use, low fiber intake, excess fat intake, sunburn, alcohol use, and exposure to chemical carcinogens. Information, education, and early detection have important roles in reducing both the incidence and the prevalence of cancer. Pap sampling, prostate examinations, mammography, and oral examinations are secondary prevention procedures that allow for early diagnosis and treatment. Such screening procedures, coupled with education and lifestyle changes, have the potential to reduce cancer rates significantly.

Healthy People 2010 (2000), like its predecessors, was developed through a broad consultation process, built on scientific knowledge and designed to measure programs over time. Its two primary goals included helping individuals of all ages increase life expectancy and improve their quality of life and eliminating health disparities among different segments of the population. The healthy life expectancy at birth increased slightly from 2000-1 to 2006-7 from about seventy-seven years of age to about seventy-eight among the overall population. There were no significant changes in health disparity across race and ethnicity in 70 percent of the objective areas. *Healthy People 2020* includes similar objectives to previous *Healthy People* reports, but also includes several new areas of focus, including adolescent health; lesbian, gay, bisexual, and transgender health; and sleep health. Improvement in health disparities tracked in Quality & Disparities Report 2014 has demonstrated im-

provement from 2010 to 2015 among uninsured adults from 18-64 years across all racial and ethnic groups and poverty levels (Cohen & Martinez, 2015; Access and Disparities in Access to Health Care, 2016).

Achieving the many objectives of *Healthy People* requires the dedicated commitment of preventive medicine specialists and the broader medical community. Enhanced effectiveness and efficiency of clinical preventive services, screening procedures, immunizations, consultation, and counseling can be achieved only through close relationships between the physician and both the community and the individual. To assess whether the goals and objectives for the prevention of disease and health promotion for the year 2010 were realistic, it would be helpful to review a success in the application of preventive medicine. Many of the objectives for 2010 were not met, but pesticide exposure, for example, was one area that showed marked improvement, from more than twenty-three thousand doctor's office visits in 1998 to less than fifteen thousand in 2008, though the total fell short of the 2010 target of less than twelve thousand visits. Another area in which preventative medicine seemed to be effective was the reduction of adolescent pregnancies, specifically among the black population. In 1996, the rate of pregnancy per one thousand girls between the ages of fifteen and seventeen was about 130; by 2005, the rate was less than eighty.

Coronary artery disease and its resultant heart attacks are preventable. A large national clinical trial of preventive medicine procedures known as MRFIT (multiple risk factor intervention trial) not only demonstrated the value of risk factor reduction in preventing disease but also demonstrated that the impact of established disease could be reversed. A subgroup of the MRFIT population made up of those who had established coronary artery disease at the start of the study had 55 percent fewer fatalities than did the control group when both were followed over seven years.

Preventive medicine interventions are not only cost-effective but relatively inexpensive as well. For example, coronary artery bypass surgery or a heart transplant costs many times more than preventive medicine rehabilitation and lifestyle modification programs. The same advantages also accrue for the prevention of strokes. Reducing salt intake, controlling high blood pressure, correcting obesity, performing regular exercise, and quitting smoking reduce the risk of stroke. The evidence clearly shows that preventive medicine reduces the death rate for heart attack and stroke and enhances quality of life.

Clinical preventive services have been designed based on the best available scientific evidence to promote the health of the individual while remaining practical and cost-effective. The 1989 publication of the *Guide to Clinical Preventive Services* (a document that has been updated several times) by the US Preventive Services Task Force was a major milestone on the road toward reducing premature death and disability. It has been well established that the majority of deaths among Americans under the age of sixty-five are preventable. The guide is the culmination of more than four years of literature review, debate, and synthesis and provides a listing of the clinical preventive services that clinicians should provide their patients. More than one hundred interventions are proposed to prevent sixty different illnesses and medical conditions. The guide is intended to be used by preventive medical specialists and other primary care clinicians. The recommendations are based on a standardized review of current scientific evidence and include a summary of published clinical research regarding the clinical effectiveness of each preventive service.

Although there have been sound clinical reasons for emphasizing prevention in medicine, studies have repeatedly demonstrated that physicians often fail to provide these services. Busy clinicians frequently have inadequate time with the patient to recommend or deliver a range of preventive services. Furthermore, until the publication of this guide, considerable controversy had existed within the medical community as to which services should be offered and how often. In the past, there was skepticism regarding the value of certain preventive interventions and their ability to reduce morbidity or mortality significantly. One result of this review process has been the clear evidence that reducing the incidence and severity of the leading causes of disease and disability is dependent on the personal health practices of individuals. The periodic health examination was once frequently referred to as an annual examination.

The *Guide to Clinical Preventive Services* tailors this examination to the individual needs of the patient and considers factors such as age, gender, and risk. Consequently, a uniform health examination is not recommended. The examination for those between forty and sixty-four years of age is scheduled on a one- to three-year basis, with the more frequent examinations scheduled for those in high-risk groups. Although the examination is not comprehensive, it is focused on identifying the leading causes of illness and disability among people in this age group. During the physical examination, particular attention would be paid to the skin of those individuals at high risk for excessive exposure to sunlight or with a family or personal history of skin cancer. A complete oral cavity examination would be appropriate for individuals using tobacco or consuming excessive amounts of alcohol. Counseling would be provided on such items as diet and exercise, substance abuse, sexual practices, and injury prevention.

According to the National Diabetes Clearinghouse, approximately 28 million persons in the United States suffer from diabetes; however, 7 million of them are unaware of their condition. Diabetes is the seventh leading cause of death in the United States, accounting for nearly seventy thousand deaths per year. In addition, it is the leading cause of kidney failure, blindness, and amputations. The detection of diabetes in asymptomatic persons provides an opportunity to prevent or delay the progress of the disease and its complications. The *Guide to Clinical Preventive Services* recommends an oral glucose tolerance test for all pregnant women between the twenty-fourth and twenty-eighth weeks of their pregnancy. Routine screening for diabetes in asymptomatic nonpregnant adults, using blood or urine tests, is not recommended. Periodic fasting blood sugar measurements may be appropriate in persons at high risk for diabetes mellitus, such as the markedly obese, persons with a family history of diabetes, or women with a history of diabetes during pregnancy.

Perspective and Prospects

In the mid-nineteenth century, John Snow provided one of the best examples of preventive medicine by applying what could be called observational epidemiology. During a rather severe cholera epidemic in London, Snow observed an unusual pattern of disease that appeared to be dependent on the particular water supply company providing water to the neighborhood. Recognizing that there was a high incidence of cholera in the Broad Street area, he was able to determine that most of the disease was associated with those families depending on the Broad Street pump for their drinking water. It has been said that he simply removed the handle on the pump and was able to control the epidemic in that area. His discovery occurred before there was a clear understanding of the relationship of bacteria or germs to infectious disease.

Another historic example of the application of preventive medicine was the control of smallpox. In the late eighteenth century, Edward Jenner observed that the milkmaids in the English countryside were not scarred by the scourge of smallpox. On further examination, he determined that these young women had years earlier been infected with cowpox and thus had been spared the more serious smallpox infection. He then advocated intentional infection with the cowpox vaccine. Years later, using this preventive medicine application, the World Health Organization was able to institute a worldwide eradication of smallpox. The last case of smallpox reported in the world was in October, 1977, marking the first time that a major human disease had been eradicated. Neither the control of cholera in London by Snow nor the eradication of smallpox resulted from medical or surgical treatment of a disease. These results were obtained because of the application of the principles of preventive medicine and public health.

—*Roy L. DeHart, MD, MPH;*
updated by Carolynn Bruno

See also: Acupressure; Acupuncture; Aging: Extended care; Allied health; Alternative medicine; Aromatherapy; Biofeedback; Braces, orthopedic; Cardiac rehabilitation; Cardiology; Centers for Disease Control and Prevention (CDC); Chiropractic; Cholesterol; Chronobiology; Colon therapy; Disease; Echocardiography; Electrocardiography (ECG or EKG); Environmental health; Exercise physiology; Family medicine; Genetic counseling; Genetics and inheritance; Geriatrics and gerontology; Holistic medicine; Homeopathy; Host-defense mechanisms; Hypercholesterolemia; Immune system; Immunization and vaccination; Immunology; Mammography; Meditation; Melatonin; National Institutes of Health (NIH); Neuroimaging; Noninvasive tests; Nursing; Nutrition; Occupational health; Osteopathic medicine; Pharmacology; Pharmacy; Physical examination; Physician assistants; Phytochemicals; Preventive medicine; Psychiatry; Psychiatry, child and adolescent; Psychiatry, geriatric; Screening; Self-medication; Serology; Spine, vertebrae, and disks; Sports medicine; Stress reduction; Telemedicine; Tropical medicine; Yoga.

For Further Information:

Access and Disparities in Access to Health Care. Content last reviewed May 2016. Agency for Healthcare Research and Quality, Rockville, MD. http://www.ahrq.gov/research/findings/nhqrdr/nhqdr15/access.html

Cohen RA, Martinez ME. Health insurance coverage: early release of quarterly estimates from the National Health Interview Survey, January-June 2015. Hyattsville, MD: National Center for Health Statistics; November 2015. http://www.cdc.gov/nchs/data/nhis/earlyrelease/Quarterly_estimates_2010_2015_Q12.pdf

Davies, Kevin. "Powering Preventative Medicine." *Bio-ITWorld* 10, no. 5 (September/October, 2011): 27-30.

Granello, Paul F. *Wellness Counseling*. Boston: Pearson, 2012.

Greenberg, Raymond S., et al., eds. *Medical Epidemiology*. 4th ed. New York: Lange Medical Books/McGraw-Hill, 2005.

Hales, Dianne. *An Invitation to Health Brief*. Updated ed. Belmont, Calif.: Wadsworth/Cengage Learning, 2010.

Halperin, William, and Edward L. Baker, eds. *Public Health Surveillance*. New York: Van Nostrand Reinhold, 1992.

Hood, Leroy, James R. Heath, Michael E. Phelps, and Biaoyang Lin. "Systems Biology and New Technologies Enable Predictive and Preventative Medicine." *Science* 306, no. 5696 (October, 2004) 640-43.

Jeste, Dilip V., and Carl C. Bell. *Preventative Psychiatry*. Philadelphia: Saunders, 2011.

Lee, Philip R., and Carroll L. Estes, eds. *The Nation's Health*. 7th ed. Sudbury, Mass.: Jones and Bartlett, 2003.

Litin, Scott C., ed. *Mayo ClinicFamily Health Book*. 4th ed. New York: HarperResource, 2009.

Payne, Wayne A., Dale B. Hahn, and Ellen Mauer. *Understanding Your Health*. 12th ed. New York: McGraw-Hill, 2013.

US Department of Health and Human Services. *Healthy People 2020: Health Understanding and Improving*. Washington, DC: Government Printing Office, 2010.

Wallace, Robert B., ed.*Wallace's Maxcy-Rosenau-Last Public Health and Preventive Medicine*. 15th ed. New York: McGraw-Hill, 2008.

Primary care
Health care system

Primary care is a patient's entry point into the health care system. A primary care practitioner can be one of several different types of medical professionals and usually provides for the patient's basic medical care and coordinates care with other providers for more complex health situations. The primary care practitioner is the one the patient sees for routine exams and common conditions such as ear or throat infections. It is usually the primary care practitioner who diagnoses more serious and/or chronic conditions such as heart disease or diabetes and refers the patient to a specialist for specific care for these conditions.

Background

A primary care practitioner is usually the person individuals refer to as their "doctor". This medical practitioner may be a physician, an internist, a nurse practitioner, or a physician's assistant. Some patients choose a primary care provider often referred to as a PCP—who has the educational background to deal with specialized populations. These may include pediatricians for children, family health providers, adult health providers and individuals specializing in gerontology for older adults.The PCP provides for all of the patient's primary health care needs. These include well-checks or check-ups, routine immunizations, screening, and care for common illnesses such as viruses, muscle and joint pains, skin eruptions and other infections. The primary care provider will also be the first point of contact for many sudden illnesses or injuries that do not require emergency room care.

It is often the primary care provider who diagnoses more serious illnesses or determines that a person's health concern requires a specialist's care. For instance, a patient who complains of foot pain may be referred to a podiatrist for more in-depth care. The routine tests ordered by a primary care provider either as part of an annual medical exam or in response to a health issue can also identify more serious illnesses that require follow-up with a specialist.

A primary care practitioner may also treat a patient for certain chronic conditions, such as high blood pressure, diabetes controlled or uncontrolled gastric problems, musculoskeletal issues, and others. It is important to keep your PCP involved in your care especially if you are referred to a specialist. This involvement provides coordination of care that can help prevent errors and improve health outcomes.

Overview

The focus of primary care is on the overall health of the individual rather than on one particular system or part of the body. The PCP coordinates care for the patient, directing the patient to specialists when needed while serving as a central point of contact that can avoid duplication of care and help prevent errors. For example, a patient who has pain in both a foot and a shoulder may see a podiatrist for the foot problem and an orthopedic specialist for the shoulder. If the two specialists are coordinating with the PCP, they might discover that both are prescribing similar pain medications for the patient, which could lead to medical complications.

The PCP is also an advocate for the patient when that patient is enmeshed in the larger health care system. A hospitalized patient who has concerns that are not being addressed by a surgeon and a patient who is having difficulty getting a health insurance claim paid can both benefit from the knowledge and intervention of the primary care provider.

Another important function of a primary care provider is a focus on prevention. Their emphasis on the overall health of the patient means that the PCP makes a point of being aware of what routine tests or immunizations the patient may need. They can also take note of other potential health risks, such as smoking, alcohol consumption, and weight issues, and provide guidance and care to help the patient avoid future health issues.

Medical fields include more primary care physicians than specialists. This means that PCPs help provide greater accessibility to health care for a wider portion of the public. They can also provide some level of specialized care for those who would otherwise go without, such as patients without insurance or low-income patients who lack the funds for copayments for specialists. This helps to increase access to care and improve the overall quality of health care available in an area.

The intervention of the PCP can also help to minimize the number of specialist visits that are required, either by identifying and initiating treatment for conditions before they become serious or by performing some of the follow-up that might otherwise be handled by a specialist. This care helps to improve the patient's overall health and reduce health care costs. The level of trust that can be built between a practitioner and a patient he or she sees regularly can also benefit health care outcomes by encouraging patient cooperation with treatment.

While primary care can be an important facet of improved health care availability and outcomes, reduced costs, and greater patient satisfaction, some potential issues exist. One is the lack of available PCPs. The need for more primary providers is outstripping the supply of new practitioners in the United States,. It can also be difficult to attract primary care providers to rural areas where income levels and the scarcity of specialists and medical facilities makes the need greatest.

—*Janine Ungvarsky;*
updated by Geraldine Marrocco

For Further Information:

"Choosing a Primary Care Provider." *MedlinePlus, US National Library of Health,* 14 Aug. 2015, http://medlineplus.gov/ency/article/001939.htm. Accessed 20 Dec. 2016.

Gordon, Mara. "Why I'm Becoming a Primary Care Doctor." *The Atlantic,* 18 Sept. 2014, http://www.theatlantic.com/health/archive/2014/09/why-im-becoming-a-primary-care-doctor/ 379231/. Accessed 20 Dec. 2016.

"Primary Care." *American Association of Family Physicians,* http://www.aafp.org/about/policies/all/primary-care.html. Accessed 20 Dec. 2016.

"The Primary Care Medicine Clerkship." *Vanderbilt University Medical Center,* https://medicine.mc.vanderbilt.edu/primary-care-definition. Accessed 20 Dec. 2016.

"Primary Care vs. Non-Primary Care Specialties." *American Association of Colleges of Osteopathic Medicine,* http://www.aacom.org/become-a-doctor/med-students/career-planning/career-options/pc-vs-non-pc. Accessed 20 Dec. 2016.

"What Is Primary Care?" *Johns Hopkins Bloomberg School of Public Health,* http://www.jhsph.edu/research/centers-and-institutes/johns-hopkins-primary-care-policy-center/definitions.html. Accessed 20 Dec. 2016.

"What is Primary Health Care?" *University of Bristol,* http://www.bristol.ac.uk/primaryhealthcare/whatisphc.html. Accessed 20 Dec. 2016.

"What's a Primary Care Physician?" *KidsHealth by Nemours,* http://kidshealth.org/en/parents/primary-care-physician.html. Accessed 20 Dec. 2016.

Prion diseases

Disease/Disorder

Anatomy or system affected: Brain, nervous system

Specialties and related fields: Epidemiology, neurology, pathology, public health

Definition: A variety of fatal neurological illnesses, inherited or transmissible, that are associated with abnormalities in proteins, called prions.

Key terms:

ataxia: the inability to control muscle movements

bovine spongiform encephalopathy (BSE): a prion disease of cattle; also called mad cow disease

Creutzfeldt-Jakob disease (CJD): a human prion disease found worldwide

dementia: a condition of deteriorated intellectual ability

encephalopathy: any abnormality in the structure or function of the brain

knockout mouse: mouse in which a specific gene has been inactivated or "knocked out"

kuru: a human prion disease formerly found in Papua New Guinea

prion: a protein that can assume an abnormal conformation, aggregate, and disrupt brain function

spongiform: shaped like or resembling a sponge

Causes and Symptoms

Prion diseases, also called transmissible spongiform encephalopathies, are progressive neurodegenerative disorders in humans and animals that lead to progressive memory loss, personality changes, and impaired motor control (ataxia). The diseases are almost always fatal. Human prion diseases include Creutzfeldt-Jakob disease (CJD), new variant Creutzfeldt-Jacob disease (vCJD), kuru, Gerstmann-Straussler-Scheinker syndrome, and fatal familial insomnia. Animal prion diseases include scrapie, chronic wasting disease (CWD), transmissible mink encephalopathy, feline spongiform encephalopathy, ungulate spongiform encephalopathy, and bovine spongiform encephalopathy (BSE), popularly known as mad cow disease.

While symptoms of scrapie have been noted in sheep and goats for hundreds of years, it was not shown to be transmissible until the 1930s. CJD was first noted in the 1920s, kuru in the 1950s, and BSE in the mid-1980s. Daniel Carleton Gajdusek began studying kuru in 1955 and won the Nobel Prize in Physiology or Medicine in 1976 for his work. Stanley B. Prusiner coined the term "prion" in 1982; he was awarded the Nobel Prize in 1997. Most scientists believe prions are the sole cause for transmissible spongiform encephalopathies.

The diseases are caused by misshapen versions of proteins called prions. Prions clump together and can proliferate by inducing shape changes in normal proteins. As prions aggregate, they cause spongelike lesions in the brain and disrupt brain function. The resultant illnesses are referred to as spongiform encephalopathies, which can be either inherited or transmissible. Prions are found in all species, from yeast to humans, but their normal role is not known. Their evolutionary persistence in so many species implies that they must serve an important purpose, although knockout mice lacking prions do not appear to be adversely affected.

Inherited spongiform encephalopathies are primarily attributed to mutations in the prion gene, leading to abnormally shaped proteins that aggregate over time to cause the brain damage and neurological symptoms characteristic of the diseases. Transmissible diseases occur when a susceptible animal is inoculated with a fragment or an extract of diseased tissue. Inoculation may occur by intravenous

---

Information on Prion Diseases

Causes: Genetic inheritance (mutation of prion gene); transmission through consumption of infected animal tissue, tissue transplants, contamination of surgical instruments, pharmaceuticals derived from human cadavers

Symptoms: Dementia and ataxia, leading to death

Duration: Several weeks or months

Treatments: None

---

transmission, such as via a blood transfusion, or orally by consumption of infected tissue or bodily fluids, such as saliva.

Prions are unusual in that the protein is the infectious agent; typical infectious agents, such as bacteria or viruses, contain nucleic acids, either ribonucleic acid (RNA) or deoxyribonucleic acid (DNA). While the infectious agent's mode of action is not fully understood-and what is understood is not universally accepted-researchers announced in 2003 that they had discovered a new way of identifying an antibody specific to prions. This discovery has important implications for understanding how prions propagate and, in turn, for manipulating the prions for the creation of a vaccine.

These diseases have been described in humans, cattle, sheep, deer, elk, mink, domestic cats, and wild felines, and they have been experimentally induced in monkeys, hamsters, and mice. Prion diseases are usually species-specific. However, the diseases in mink, domestic cats, and wild felines are attributed to consumption of feed derived from diseased animals (usually hooved animals), and a variant in humans is associated with the consumption of meat from cattle with BSE.

The most common animal prion disease is scrapie, found in sheep and goats. It is named for the intense itching that causes sheep to rub against hard objects, scraping off the wool. It also causes staggering, tremors, and blindness. It has been known for more than 250 years in Britain and other countries of western Europe. It has been reported in most sheep-raising countries with a few notable exceptions, such as Australia and New Zealand. It first appears at two to five years of age, can last longer than six months, and is eventually fatal. It is generally accepted that it is an infectious disease in which genetics also plays an important role. It has not been shown to be transmissible to humans and poses no risk to human health.

The most famous prion disease in animals is bovine spongiform encephalopathy (BSE). First noted in British cattle in 1986, it causes nervousness, aggression, and symptoms similar to scrapie. It appears in adult cattle between two and eight years of age and is fatal. The BSE epidemic, which peaked in 1992 and affected more than 200,000 animals, was apparently caused by feed containing protein from animals with prion disease. A ban on incorporating ruminant-derived protein into cattle feed appeared to be bringing the epidemic to an end in Great Britain by the early twenty-first century, although there was a troubling increase in cases in continental Europe.

The best-known prion disease in humans is Creutzfeldt-Jakob disease (CJD), which occurs worldwide at a rate of about one per million persons. Its symptoms include dementia and ataxia, leading to death. The disease may be classified as sporadic, familial (inherited), iatrogenic (acquired through a medical procedure), or variant. The sporadic form, which accounts for the majority of cases, appears in the elderly and has an unknown etiology. The inherited form (5 to 10 percent of cases) is primarily attributed to mutations in the gene for prions, making them more susceptible to aggregation in the brains of affected individuals. The iatrogenic form can be caused by tissue transplants, contaminated surgical instruments, and pharmaceuticals derived from human cadavers.

The new variant form of CJD (vCJD) was first described in 1996; it differed from the sporadic form by affecting younger individuals and having slightly different symptoms and duration; it has been associated with eating beef from cattle infected with BSE. As of 2011, a total of 176 cases of vCJD had been identified in Great Britain since 1986, all of them fatal; far smaller numbers of cases have been reported in other countries. Because of a long time course and an incompletely known cause, it is uncertain how many will be affected by this new variant form.

Treatment and Therapy

No effective treatment for prion diseases existed as of the early twenty-first century. Researchers have speculated that human prion diseases might be treated by preventing normal proteins from adopting the abnormal shape, by interfering with the interaction between abnormal and normal proteins, or by destabilizing the shapes of abnormal proteins. Research has identified hundreds of molecules that seem to deter the formation of prions, prolonging the survival times of laboratory animals, but much more testing remains to be done before human drug therapies become available. Thus far, the only treatments are aimed at symptoms, such as opiates for pain and anticonvulsants to lessen neuromuscular problems.

Perspective and Prospects

Concerns over prion diseases have increased in North America since the discovery of BSE in cattle from Canada and the United States. A screening program is in place to help detect infected cattle, but critics of the programs in both countries argue that it is not rigorous enough to provide adequate protection of the nations' food supplies. Despite the concerns over human health effects, considerable work remains to be done simply to achieve a better understanding of the origins, transmission, and pathogenesis of prion diseases.

—James L. Robinson, Ph.D.;
updated by David M. Lawrence

See also Brain; Brain disorders; Chronic wasting disease (CWD); Creutzfeldt-Jakob disease (CJD); Food poisoning; Mutation.

For Further Information:

Badash, Michelle. "Creutzfeldt-Jakob Disease." *Health Library*, March 15, 2013.

Booss, John, Margaret Esiri, and Margaret M. Esin, eds. *Viral Encephalitis in Humans*. Washington, D.C.: ASM Press, 2003.

Brown, David R., ed. *Neurodegeneration and Prion Disease*. New York: Springer, 2005.

Council for Agricultural Science and Technology. *Transmissible Spongiform Encephalopathies in the United States*. Ames, Iowa: Author, 2000.

Ferry, Georgina. "Mad Brains and the Prion Heresy." *New Scientist* 142, no. 1927 (May 28, 1994): 32-36.

"Prion Diseases." *Centers for Disease Control and Prevention*, December 10, 2012.

"Prion Diseases." *National Institute of Allergy and Infectious Diseases*, 2013.

Prusiner, Stanley B. "The Prion Diseases." *Scientific American* 272, no. 1 (January, 1995): 48-57.

Prusiner, Stanley B., ed. *Prion Biology and Diseases*. 2d ed. Woodbury, N.Y.: Cold Spring Harbor Laboratory Press, 2004.

Schwartz, Maxime. *How the Cows Turned Mad*. Translated by Edward Schneider. Berkeley: University of California Press, 2003.

Spencer, Charlotte A. *Mad Cows and Cannibals: A Guide to the Transmissible Spongiform Encephalopathies*. Upper Saddle River, N.J.: Prentice Hall, 2004.

Proctology

Specialty

Anatomy or system affected: Gastrointestinal system, intestines

Specialties and related fields: Gastroenterology, internal medicine, oncology

Definition: The branch of medicine that treats diseases of the colon, rectum, and anus.

Key terms:

anal incontinence: the inability to control defecation

colitis: inflammation of the mucous membranes of the colon

diverticulum: a pouchlike, weakened region of the colon wall that can cause pain and bleeding

endoscope: a lighted, flexible, hollow instrument used for examination and the placement of surgical instruments

fascia: connective tissues such as tendons and ligaments

hemorrhoids: dilated blood vessels in the anus or rectum that are itchy and painful

occult blood: fecal blood, as detected by microscopic or chemical testing

polyp: a tumorlike growth, such as of the colorectal mucous lining

rectal prolapse: the protrusion of the rectum through the anus

Science and Profession

The term "proctology" arises from the Greek *proktos*, meaning "anus." In 1961, this field was renamed colon and rectal surgery. The original term, which is still in wide use, will be employed for simplicity. Specialists in proctology are surgeons who are expert in surgery of the colon, rectum, anal canal, and perianal area near the anus. They also carry out surgery of other tissues and organs close to and involved in serious colorectal disease. Moreover, proctologists have special skill in endoscopy of the rectum and colon for the diagnosis and medical treatment of these regions. Proctology involves emergency situations less frequently than many other specialties. Consequently, the hours of these specialists are relatively regular, although no shorter than those of other physicians.

Many conditions encountered by proctologists are clear-cut in diagnosis and treatment. Hence, they often have the satisfaction of providing patients with quick, effective relief of serious pain and discomfort.

Training a proctologist is time-consuming, involving a five-year residency in general surgery, followed by a one-to two-year fellowship in colon and rectal surgery. The specialty is not easily entered because its practitioners are not numerous and there are usually several applicants for each open training position.

The main organ treated in proctology is the large intestine, or colon. This portion of the digestive tract starts at the cecum, a pouch joined to the small intestine. At the far end of the cecum, the colon is subdivided into ascending, transverse, and descending regions. Together, these regions absorb water and minerals from food that has not been digested and absorbed by the stomach or small intestine. The result is feces, which are stored in the colon for elimination from the body. The ascending colon extends upward on the right side of the abdominal cavity and is called the right colon. The transverse colon crosses from right to left in the cavity, and the descending colon (left colon) passes downward along the cavity's left side, ending in the rectum. The short, S-shaped portion of the left colon above the rectum is the sigmoid colon.

The entire colon is made of pouches whose complex series of contractions and expansions moves its contents through quite slowly, enabling optimum water and mineral recovery. The sluggish colon movement enables bacteria to thrive, sometimes causing uncomfortable gas. Normal synchronization of the digestive system leads to absorption of most of this gas, however, as well as the transfer of feces into the rectum for storage and a defecation reflex that releases feces at varied but appropriate intervals. Also synchronized with these digestive processes is the production of both mucus and bicarbonate, which help to propel colon contents through the large intestine and neutralize acid made by bacteria in the colon. These events usually prevent damage to the colorectal system or diseases of its components.

The digestive system does not exhibit frequent dysfunction in early life. Therefore, proctologists for the most part see middle-aged or elderly patients. Furthermore, 60 percent of the problems that they encounter are anorectal, and 40 percent are associated with a diseased colon. Conditions that are often treated by proctologists include, but are not restricted to, anal fissures, cancers, colitis, diverticular disease, hemorrhoids, pilonoidal disease, and polyps.

Diagnostic and Treatment Techniques

Thorough colorectal examination starts with a medical history to ensure the clarification of potential problems. Then the proctologist checks the perianal region for abnormalities such as dermatitis, abscesses, hemorrhoids, or lesions that may prove to be tumors. This is followed by digital examination with a lubricated glove, after a warning to patients that this procedure will result in the urge to defecate and cause some discomfort. Tissue irregularity, nodules, or tender areas are sought, and the prostate gland in men and the cervix in women are examined. To ensure complete exploration, a fecal sample is obtained and tested for the presence of occult blood. Other clinical tests of colon, rectum, and related tissues, including biopsy, are also carried out as needed.

Anal fissures may be discovered during this portion of the examination. An anal fissure is a linear tear of the lining of the anal canal, usually originating in the anorectal region. These fissures are common causes of acute anal pain, cutting or burning sensations beginning at defecation and continuing more mildly for several hours. They are thought to arise from trauma to the anal canal caused by large, dry, hard feces. Other causes of anal fissures include persistent diarrhea, inflammatory bowel disease (IBD), syphilis, leukemia, and anorectal cancer. The treatment of choice is the use of fecal softeners, increased fluid intake, and application of steroids. Surgery is usually carried out only for cases in which treated fissures do not heal.

Pilonoidal disease may also be detected; this is the formation of pits that contain pubic hair that has become trapped under the skin. If an abscess results, the problem is handled by its drainage under local anesthesia. Cleaning out of the pit and the removal of causative hair are also useful. Surgery is required only if the problem becomes chronic.

Anorectal cancers are relatively uncommon. They are treated in an individualized fashion with a varying combination of surgery, chemotherapy, and radiation therapy. Often, they are squamous cell carcinomas. In a smaller number of cases, melanomas, for which the survival rate is less than 5 percent, will occur. Other types of serious anorectal cancers include Paget's disease and basal cell carcinomas. These cancers have better survival rates.

Rectal prolapse, passage of the rectum through the anus, is another common anorectal problem. It is seen either in children under the age of two years or in the very elderly. In childhood, the problem is frequently attributable to anatomic underdevelopment, which cures itself. In adults, rectal prolapse may be partial or complete. Complete rectal prolapse results in the externalization of the entire rectum, bleeding, and excessive mucus discharge.

Rectal prolapse eventually causes anal incontinence, which may become irreversible. For cases in which a patient is feeble, the rectum is first manipulated to return it to a more normal placement. Then, a tightening steel or plastic loop is inserted under the skin at the anal opening to prevent future prolapse. When patients are robust enough for surgery, the rectum is often secured internally by a mesh sling anchored to internal fascia.

The treatment of internal or external hemorrhoids is another major aspect of proctological practice. Internal hemorrhoids are rarely painful because they are covered by insensitive colon mucosa tissue. The external variety, however, are rich in nervous tissue and may be very painful. Internal hemorrhoids are classified into four stages ranging from the relatively innocuous first-degree hemorrhoids, which do not prolapse, to fourth-degree hemorrhoids, which always prolapse.

Treatment for internal hemorrhoids, which depends on the severity of the bleeding and discomfort, ranges from education about proper diet and bowel habits to surgical removal (hemorrhoidectomy). Surgical removal is most often accomplished with a banding technique in which a tight rubber band is placed around the base of the hemorrhoid. Banding normally results in the sloughing off of dead tissue and the creation of a scar that prevents future problems. In cases of severe external hemorrhoids, banding is not used because it is too painful. Instead, more complex surgical excision is required.

Such symptoms as occult blood and lower abdominal pain may signal the need for a colon examination. Barium enemas and colonoscopy are the visualization techniques that are utilized. With a barium enema, a solution of radiopaque barium salt is placed into the colon after fasting and preliminary washing enemas have cleansed the organ. Then the colon containing the radiopaque solution is examined by X-ray techniques. This procedure can reveal diverticula, many colon cancers, large polyps, and other severe colorectal problems.

Colonoscopy, in its various forms, has become a mainstay in the diagnosis of colorectal disease. It is particularly valuable in finding smaller polyps, less developed cancers, and colitis. In addition, because patients who have had colon polyps removed have a one-in-four chance of new polyps forming within the next five years, colonoscopy provides minimally invasive and valuable follow-up. It can also prove useful in the follow-up of cancers and of inflammatory bowel disease.

Furthermore, an endoscope may be used to remove a smaller polyp directly or to determine that a large polyp or extensive carcinoma must be removed by laparoscopy or laparotomy. Colonoscopy is generally safe, and the entire large bowel from rectum to cecum may be examined with little risk to a patient. Moreover, endoscopic surgery greatly reduces hospital stays, recovery time, and the frequency of postsurgical mortality. The most common problems associated with colonoscopy are infrequent colon perforation as a result of diverticula, limited endoscopic access to the colon because of scarring from previous surgery, and flare-ups of ulcerative colitis.

Diverticular disease is quite common after the age of fifty. It is caused by small saclike pouches in the colon, often arising after colon spasms. In mild cases, diverticula can be observed by barium enema in patients exhibiting nonspecific abdominal pain and gas. In many instances, bleeding will occur. In some cases, diverticulitis (widespread diverticular infection and inflammation) can lead to serious colon blockage requiring colostomy, and in those cases where perforation occurs, peritonitis will result. Diverticulitis is most common in the lower left colon, originating in the sigmoid region. It may be painful enough to justify the nickname left-sided appendicitis.

Polyps, masses arising from the bowel wall, are asymptomatic in many cases but may cause bleeding and pain when they are large. The larger that a polyp becomes, the greater is the risk that it will become cancerous. Polyps are often identified after rectal bleeding and/or cramps and abdominal pain lead to barium enema and colonoscopy. They are then removed completely via colonoscopy or laparoscopy, depending on their size. Thereafter, it is suggested that the entire colon be examined via colonoscope at intervals dependent on symptoms over a five-year period. Polyps tend to recur and may be associated with cancer.

More than 50 percent of colorectal cancers occur in the sigmoid colon and rectum. These very common visceral cancers are seen most in people over the age of sixty. Treatment is usually surgical removal of the diseased area, and barring spread to noncolon sites, the five-year survival rate is near 90 percent. Considerable variation exists in the size, location, and treatment of this very serious disease. Disease that has spread beyond the colon wall requires chemotherapy or radiation, or both, and the prognosis is not as good.

Major aspects of colitis are Crohn's disease in the colon (most often ileocolitis), ulcerative colitis, and spastic colon. Crohn's disease often appears in early life and is associated with fever, pain, and diarrhea. There is no permanent cure for this baffling disease, which recurs repeatedly. Treatments used include diet manipulation, immunosuppressive drugs, steroids, antibiotics (when colitis is accompanied by bacterial infection), and surgery (when intractable pain and bowel obstruction require it).

Ulcerative colitis is another disease that may appear in early life. It is recurrent, varies in severity from mild to fatal, and in less severe cases manifests as intermittent attacks of bloody diarrhea. Treatment varies as with Crohn's disease. Particularly dangerous is toxic colitis; very severe cases require immediate surgery.

Spastic colon, or irritable bowel syndrome (IBS), is a much milder form of colitis. It has no known anatomic cause, but emotional factors or other causes of hormone imbalance have been proposed. Periodic abdominal pain, constipation, and/or diarrhea are its usual symptoms. Happily, more than half of colitis complaints are attributable to this relatively mild problem, which is treated by diet modification, observation, and painkillers once the possibility of more serious types of colon disease has been eliminated by physical examination and other methodologies.

Perspective and Prospects

Many advances in proctology have occurred since the 1970s, including the wide use of screening for occult blood in stools, which is easily done and often provides early detection of colorectal cancer. In addition, sophisticated endoscopic and laparoscopic techniques have been developed. The use of various types of endoscopes has enabled the precise examination of the colon and rectum, allowing the detection of colorectal problems that once would have gone unnoticed even after barium enema and related radiologic techniques were used. Furthermore, endoscopic surgery via colonoscopy and laparoscopy has reduced the severity of surgical intervention and the size of incisions, decreased hospital stays and recovery time, and resulted in higher surgical survival rates and facile follow-up after surgery.

The development of fiber-optic systems to be used with video camera techniques has improved colorectal examinations. Proctologists can review data rather than relying on single-shot views through a colonoscope. Such video records and their ongoing improvement may constitute the most significant innovations in colorectal diagnosis and surgery.

The development of additional clinical tests and drug therapy, including the wide use of steroids and immunosuppressive drugs, has also made some colorectal diseases much more manageable; examples are improved treatment of Crohn's disease and ulcerative colitis. Further advances in drug therapy, laparoscopy, and clinical testing may be major foci of future advances in this field.

—*Sanford S. Singer, Ph.D.*

See also Anus; Colitis; Colon; Colonoscopy and sigmoidoscopy; Colorectal cancer; Colorectal polyp removal; Colorectal surgery; Crohn's disease; Diverticulitis and diverticulosis; Endoscopy; Fistula repair; Gastroenterology; Gastrointestinal disorders; Gastrointestinal system; Hemorrhoid banding and removal; Hemorrhoids; Internal medicine; Intestines; Physical examination; Rectum; Urology.

For Further Information:

Beers, Mark H., et al., eds. *The Merck Manual of Diagnosis and Therapy*. 18th ed. Whitehouse Station, N.J.: Merck Research Laboratories, 2006.

Brown, Steven R. *Contemporary Coloproctology*. London: Springer, 2012.

Classen, Meinhard, G. N. J. Tytgat, and C. J. Lightdale, eds. *Gastroenterological Endoscopy*. 2d ed. New York: Thieme Medical, 2010.

Corman, Marvin L. *Colon and Rectal Surgery*. 5th ed. Philadelphia: Lippincott Williams & Wilkins, 2005.

Doherty, Gerard M., and Lawrence W. Way, eds. *Current Surgical Diagnosis and Treatment*. 13th ed. New York: Lange Medical Books/McGraw-Hill, 2010.

Givel, Jean-Claude, and Neil James Mortensen. *Anorectal and Colonic Diseases: A Practical Guide to Their Management*. London: Springer, 2010.

Kapadia, Cyrus R., James M. Crawford, and Caroline Taylor. *An Atlas of Gastroenterology: A Guide to Diagnosis and Differential Diagnosis*. Boca Raton, Fla.: Pantheon, 2003.

Peikin, Steven R. *Gastrointestinal Health*. Rev. ed. New York: Quill, 2001.

Taylor, Anita D. *How to Choose a Medical Specialty*. 5th ed. New York: Elsevier, 2012.

Progeria

Disease/Disorder

Also known as: Hutchinson-Gilford syndrome, Werner's syndrome

Anatomy or system affected: All

Specialties and related fields: Cardiology, pediatrics, vascular medicine

Definition: Rare disorders characterized by many aspects of premature aging.

Causes and Symptoms

There are two major, unrelated types of progeria: Hutchinson-Gilford syndrome, which begins in infancy, and Werner's syndrome, which develops in late adolescence to young adulthood. Recessive inheritance has been demonstrated for Werner's syndrome, whereas a dominant gene is a suspected source in Hutchinson-Gilford syndrome. Underlying causes have been difficult to determine, although an impaired ability to cope with free radicals appears to play a role in the degenerative course found in each disease.

Hutchinson-Gilford syndrome is characterized by superficial aspects of aging such as deteriorated skin, baldness, repeated nonhealing fractures, and vascular diseases, in addition to short stature and minimal subcutaneous fat. Arteriosclerosis and heart disease lead to a median age of death of thirteen. Werner's syndrome occurs more frequently, with the following symptoms: short stature, thin extremities, a squeaky voice, cataracts, an increased risk of diabetes mellitus, heart disease, tumors, hearing loss, and the loss of bone and teeth. Death usually occurs by the middle forties. Neither disorder is simply accelerated aging. For example, the central nervous system is relatively unaffected in both diseases.

Treatment and Therapy

No known cure exists for either progeria disease. Suggested treatments include antioxidant supplements (for example, vitamin E), growth hormone therapy, and gene therapy. Therapies have focused on providing a supportive environment and treating the symptoms to make the disorders less painful. Among these treatments are surgery, skin grafting (if skin ulceration occurs), and analgesic drugs.

Perspective and Prospects

Hutchinson-Gilford syndrome was first described by Jonathan Hutchinson in 1886. Hastings Gilford named the disorder progeria in a 1904 article. The first cases of Werner's syndrome were reported in the 1950s.

There are hopes for an eventual genetic solution to progeria diseases. The only definitive prospect for sufferers, however, is premature death.

—*Paul J. Chara, Jr., Ph.D.*

See also Aging; Death and dying; Genetic diseases.

For Further Information:

Judd, Sandra J., ed. *Genetic Disorders Sourcebook: Basic Consumer Information About Heritable Disorders*. 4th ed. Detroit, Mich.: Omnigraphics, 2010.

Gormley, Myra Vanderpool. *Family Diseases: Are You at Risk?* Baltimore: Genealogical Publishing, 2002.

Parker, James N., and Philip M. Parker, eds. *Progeria: A Medical Dictionary, Bibliography, and Annotated Research Guide to Internet References*. San Diego, Calif.: Icon Health, 2004.

Lewin, Benjamin. *Genes*. 9th rev. ed. Sudbury, Mass.: Jones and Bartlett, 2008.

Lewis, Ricki. *Human Genetics: Concepts and Applications*. 10th ed. Dubuque, Iowa: McGraw-Hill, 2012.

Milunsky, Aubrey. *Heredity and Your Family's Health*. Baltimore: Johns Hopkins University Press, 1992.

"Progeria." *MedlinePlus*, August 4, 2011.

Progeria Research Foundation. http://progeriaresearch.org/.

Prognosis

Procedure

Also known as: Future outlook

Anatomy or system affected: All

Specialties and related fields: All

Definition: A medically educated guess that helps to determine the probability of a patient's final outcome concerning a disease, illness, injury, or affliction. A prognosis may refer to a patient's quality of life, quantity of life, or both.

Key terms:

favorable: indicating that a better outcome is more likely to occur; the opposite is not favorable or unfavorable

future: any period of time from twenty-four hours later to ten or twenty years later

mortality: relating to death

Screening and Diagnosis

Every diagnosis has a prognosis. The diagnosis of any disease (tuberculosis, acquired immunodeficiency syndrome, chickenpox), any chronic condition (asthma, vitiligo, alopecia, cardiomegaly, multiple sclerosis), any cancer (melanoma, osteosarcoma, breast cancer, testicular cancer, lymphoma), any reaction to a bite or sting (rabies, spider or wasp venom, scabies), any medical emergency (gunshot wound, stabbing, motor vehicle accident), or any symptom or medical circumstance (hypothermia, dizziness, pregnancy) will create the need for a prognosis.

A prognosis may be described in words, numbers, charts, percentages, or graphs. If the chances of surviving or eliminating a given medical circumstance are good, then the prognosis is termed favorable. If not, then it may be said that the prognosis is poor or that the prognosis has become not favorable. Other possible words include excellent, good, fair, unfavorable, not good, failing, bleak, dim, or taking a turn for the worse. A prognosis may also be stated by how the patient is now compared to the expected outcome: For example, the situation may be critical now, but if the patient continues improving, he or she will have a favorable outcome.

A numerical prognosis is often given in the form of a

number scale of 1 to 10, or 1 to 100. The health care provider will state if the number 1 is the best case or the worst case in each scenario. A numerical prognosis may also be explained by using percentages. For example, the patient has a 25 percent chance that the disease will return or, conversely, a 75 percent chance that the disease will disappear. An example of long-term prognosis is that the patient's five-year outlook has a 90 percent chance of a full recovery.

Future Outlook

Many factors are taken into consideration when determining a prognosis. A certain factor may help improve a prognosis favorably, while others may affect a prognosis unfavorably. The following factors all influence a patient's prognosis: type of disease or illness, type of injury or affliction, nutritional habits, weight factor or obesity, current medications, exercise, alcohol consumption, smoking, work environment, care of or neglect of general overall health, previous health history, family history, race, gender, sexual orientation, age, financial status, education, religion, and culture. For example, by avoiding alcohol consumption and avoiding smoking, the patient can help to create a more favorable prognosis.

Early detection of any condition, disease, or illness will help to improve the odds of producing a more favorable prognosis. For example, according to the American Cancer Society, early breast cancer detection saves thousands of lives each year. This information can encourage women earlier in life to perform monthly self-breast examinations and to seek routine annual breast exams by their health care provider. Routine physicals are also helpful in finding afflictions such as high blood pressure early, so that patients may be given medications to help improve the long-term prognosis for a healthier life.

Early intervention also includes the point at which care is first administered, which can be a determining factor in the favorability of a prognosis. For example, if a patient has a heart attack and cardiopulmonary resuscitation (CPR) is administered within the first three minutes, then the patient will have a more favorable outlook for a good recovery (a better prognosis). If the patient does not receive any CPR until ten minutes after the heart attack, however, then the prognosis is not very good in terms of the patient surviving. In addition, the more severe an injury that may include extensive blood loss, the lower the chances of survival.

Understanding the Disease or Condition

Patient education is beneficial in helping produce a more favorable, long-term prognosis for any patient. This education may come in the form of pamphlets or books dispensed by the health care provider. Patients may also educate themselves through medical online sources or books pertaining to a particular situation.

In general, certain diseased or traumatized organs tend to have a less favorable prognosis, such as the liver, lungs, kidneys, ovaries, testicles, and pancreas. Certain diseases have their own stages of prognosis. For example, cancers that are detected while the patient is in stage 1 are considered more easily treatable and often the prognosis is more favorable if the disease is treated early, versus cancers that are found in stage 4. Stage 4 cancers have spread to other organs and may be difficult to control or stop. Stage 4 cancers often have a prognosis of not favorable (more likely resulting in death); if treated at this later stage, these cancers also have a greater tendency toward reoccurring.

Treatment Plans

Every treatment plan, therapy, or medication has the potential to alter a prognosis. Some alternative therapies that may be incorporated into treatment to help improve a prognosis include acupressure, acupuncture, herbal remedies, meditation, guided imagery, massage therapy, laughter, biofeedback, chiropractic, energy healing, yoga, Tai Chi Chuan, breathing and relaxation techniques, and a positive mental outlook.

The Morbidity and Mortality Weekly Report (MMWR) analyzes data and calculates statistics from every death that occurs. These lists can help the health care provider determine a treatment plan and a prognosis. By knowing a prognosis and understanding its recovery rate, a patient can make an informed decision regarding a treatment plan.

—*Suzette Buhr, R.T.R., C.D.A.*

See also Allied health; Alternative medicine; Biopsy; Blood testing; Cancer; Cardiac rehabilitation; Death and dying; Diagnosis; Disease; Epidemiology; Hospice; Imaging and radiology; Invasive tests; Laboratory tests; Noninvasive tests; Physical examination; Physical rehabiliation; Screening; Signs and symptoms.

For Further Information:
American Heart Association. "Cardiac Arrest." *American Heart Association*, February 2, 2013.
Centers for Disease Control and Prevention. "*MMWR*: Summary of Notifiable Diseases." *Morbidity and Mortality Weekly Report*, May 31, 2012.
Centers for Disease Control and Prevention. "*MMWR Weekly*: Current Volume (2013)." *Morbidity and Mortality Weekly Report*, June 21, 2013.
Morra, Marion, and Eve Potts. *Choices: The Most Complete Source Book for Cancer Information.* 4th ed. New York: HarperCollins, 2003.
Seaman, Andrew M. "Patient Communication Has Room to Grow." Reuters Health Information. *MedlinePlus*, May 27, 2013.

Prostate cancer

Disease/Disorder

Anatomy or system affected: abdomen, lymphatic system, reproductive system

Specialties and related fields: immunology, oncology, radiology, urology

Definition: Malignancy occurring in the prostate gland that is the deadliest cancer for men in the United States.

Key terms:

benignprostatic hyperplasia (BPH): enlargement of the prostate gland that often accompanies aging

orchiectomy: removal of the testes

prostate-specific antigen (PSA): a protein released from the prostate gland and is associated with prostate hyperplasia and/or prostate cancer

prostatectomy: the surgical removal of the prostate gland

single nucleotide polymorphisms: DNA sequences differing by a single nucleotide base pair

Causes and Symptoms

The normal human prostate gland is a walnut-sized male organ composed of glandular tissue and a thick coat of muscle tissue called the prostatic capsule. Located near the rectum just below the bladder, it secretes various components of semen: an alkaline fluid that makes sperm more viable after intercourse; substances that cause semen to "clot" temporarily helping to keep sperm in the female reproductive tract; and fibrolysin, a substance that later breaks down the semen clot and enables the sperm to move on and ensure fertilization. The urethra empties the urinary bladder and passes through the prostate gland. The prostate frequently enlarges in later life. When this occurs, it presses on and constricts the urethra, a disease which is called benign prostatic hyperplasia (BPH). While in most men BPH is at most uncomfortable, the hyperplasia sometimes results in difficult and painful urination, leading to the necessity for surgical intervention or even removal of the prostate gland.

Much more problematic is prostate cancer. Most often, prostate cancer is detected in asymptomatic men who are found to have lumps within the prostate during a routine rectal examination by a urologist. Regrettably, cancers detected in this way are often in a fairly advanced and dangerous stage of growth. Hence, some medical professionals recommend yearly urologic examinations after the age of forty (others say after fifty), along with clinical testing, so that early detection can prevent the most serious consequences of the disease.

An important adjunct of such testing is the blood test for prostate-specific antigen (PSA). PSA is a glycoprotein produced only by the cells of the prostate, and its levels in the blood sometimes correlate with the presence of malignancy. Normal values are under 4 nanograms per milliliter. Approximately 25 percent of men whose blood PSA levels are 4 to 10 nanograms per milliliter are diagnosed with prostate cancer. If diagnosed early, the cancer is treatable because the tumors are small and localized. When PSA levels exceed 10 nanograms per milliliter, about 70 percent of test patients are found to have the disease, their cancers are larger, and the prognosis is less favorable. Recent studies, however, have shown that the precise PSA level is frequently not an indication of cancer since men with relatively high PSA levels frequently have BPH but not cancer. A low PSA value is not necessarily indicative of being cancer-free. Research indicates that PSA may aid in detection, it does not reduce mortality. Some physicians recommend against the PSA test since it may lead to over diagnosis and excess treatment. Another blood test for prostate cancer is the measurement of acid phosphatase. This method is a less sensitive and a less reliable indicator of the disease when used alone. Done in conjunction with PSA testing, however, its increased levels are a good indicator of the extent of the metastasis.

Physical examination, ultrasound and magnetic reso-

Information on Prostate Cancer

Causes: Unclear; possibly genetic factors, environmental toxins, hormonal influences

Symptoms: Initially asymptomatic; in later stages, may include hard nodules in prostate gland, decreased urine flow, painful urination

Duration: Acute, possibly recurrent

Treatments: Surgery, radiation therapy, hormonal therapy, cryotherapy

nance imaging can aid in the diagnosis of prostate cancer, but biopsy is the best way to detect the cancer. A biopsy is performed if there are other possible signs such as a lump found during digital examination and/or a high PSA.

Risk factors associated with prostate cancer are obesity, advancing age, race (African Americans have a higher incidence than do Caucasian Americans.), family history, and a diet high in red meat and milk. Genome-wide association studies have identified single nucleotide polymorphisms that increase risk. A number of genes have been implicated as being associated with the cancer, but no single gene has yet been shown to be causative. Five to ten percent of prostate cancers are thought to be hereditary. Several studies have implicated papilloma virus as a possible cause, but these studies are controversial and are inconclusive. By pinpointing a cause, it may become possible to diagnose those men at particular risk, as well as to identify a target for treatment.

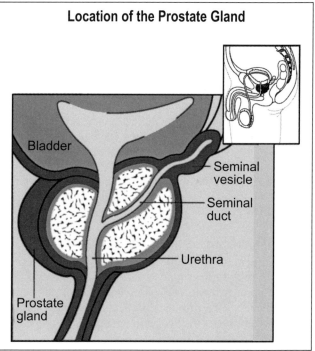

Location of the Prostate Gland

Bladder

Seminal vesicle

Seminal duct

Urethra

Prostate gland

The prostate is one of the major sites where cancer develops in older men; the inset shows the location of the prostate gland in the male reproductive system.

In the News: Possible Viral Cause of Prostate Cancer, Genetic Marker Reveals Higher Risk

Researchers have identified the presence of a virus in some prostate cancer patients. Previously, such a virus associated with this cancer had been known to occur only in mice. If prostate cancer is considered an infectious disease, then this discovery that could lead to new strategies of treatment and diagnosis for this most common major cancer afflicting adult men. Eric Klein and colleagues presented their finding at the 2006 American Society of Clinical Oncology prostate symposium. The discovery was made possible through the development by Joe DeRisi and associates of a novel "gene chip" that contains twenty thousand fragments of viral deoxyribonucleic acid (DNA). While this initial study involved samples from only eighty-six cancerous prostates, current research is aimed at studying hundreds more cancer samples to identify a virus that could be screened in patient blood samples.

In other work, Kari Stefansson and coauthors published a finding in the June, 2006, issue of *Nature Genetics* that demonstrated a common genetic variant associated with prostate cancer. They found that a specific marker located on chromosome 8 is significantly more frequently observed in men with prostate cancer, based on population samples collected from Iceland, Sweden, and the United States. This genetic variant was found in approximately 8 percent of prostate cancer cases studied and is significantly more associated with malignant prostate cancer cases. It had previously been reported that African Americans have a particularly high rate of incidence of prostate cancer and are more likely to die from the disease than are American men of European descent. The genetic variant discovered by Stefansson and coworkers is consistent with this previous finding, since the genetic marker appeared four times more frequently in prostate cancer patients of African descent.

—*Michael R. King, Ph.D.*

Treatment and Therapy

The treatment of localized prostate cancer is controversial and ranges from surveillance to various types of radiation treatment to hormone therapy to removal of the entire prostate (radical prostatectomy). In radical prostatectomy, the entire prostate, the nearby seminal vesicles, and the vas deferens are removed. This removes both the prostate, the focus of the cancer, and the nearby male sexual tissues that are most likely to be sites of cancer metastasis. When this procedure is carried out with prostate-confined tumors, cancer recurrence is less than 2 percent. In many cases, radiation therapy, which is viewed as less radical, is carried out on these cancers, and ten-year survival rates approach 70 percent.

For more severe or metastasized tumors, surgery and radiation treatment are followed by a number of hormone regimens. The latter include androgen deprivation, rationalized by the fact that most prostate tumors are androgen-dependent. The most common hormones used are pituitary antagonists that prevent testicular androgen secretion. Removal of the testes (orchiectomy, or castration) is another, more radical treatment. The result of castration can be un-pleasant physically and psychologically, but is the most effective treatment for immediately removing the source of the antigens the cancer needs to grow. The five- to ten-year survival rate for men found to have non-metastasized prostate cancer is viewed as good by many physicians, and the survival rates of those with more severe cancers are improving because of the discovery of better therapeutic drugs. If the cancer has metastasized to the bones, pain relief medication and bisphosphonates are often used.

Perspective and Prospects

Prostate cancer first became common in the 1960s. In North America, it is the most common cancer detected in men. In 2009, just over 200,000 men in the United States were found to have the disease, and nearly 30,000 died from it. More than 40 percent of American men fifty years of age or older who were autopsied after death from other causes were found to have prostate cancer as well. The incidence of prostate cancer varies among the races, being highest among African Americans. Overall, 3 to 4 percent of American men are expected to die from prostate cancer.

Current research is focused on identifying genes associated with the disease and the development of targeted therapy.

—*Sanford S. Singer, PhD;*
updated by Richard Adler, PhD
and Charles L. Vigue, PhD

See also: Aging; Cancer; Carcinogens; Chemotherapy; Genital disorders, male; Malignancy and metastasis; Men's health; National Cancer Institute (NCI); Prostate enlargement; Prostate gland; Prostate gland removal; Radiation therapy; Reproductive system; Tumor removal; Tumors; Urinary disorders; Urinary system; Urology.

For Further Information:
Bayoumi, Ahmed M., Adalsteinn D. Brown, and Alan M. Garber. "Cost-Effectiveness of Androgen Suppression Therapies in Advanced Prostate Cancer." *Journal of the National Cancer Institute* 92, no. 21 (November 1, 2000): 1731-1739.
Bostwick, David G., Gregory T. MacLennan, and Thayne R. Larson. *Prostate Cancer: What Every Man—and His Family—Needs to Know.* Rev. ed. New York: Villard, 1999.
Dollinger, Malin, et al. *Everyone's Guide to Cancer Therapy.* 5th ed. Kansas City, Mo.: Andrews McMeel, 2008.
Ellsworth, Pamela. *One Hundred Questions and Answers About Prostate Cancer.* 3d ed. Sudbury, Mass.: Jones and Bartlett, 2013.
Marks, Sheldon. *Prostate and Cancer: A Family Guide to Diagnosis, Treatment, and Survival.* 4th ed. Cambridge, Mass.: Da Capo Lifelong, 2009.
Marx, Jean. "Fused Genes May Help Explain the Origins of Prostate Cancer." *Science* 310 (October 28, 2005): 603.
McCoy, Krisha, and Rebecca J. Stahl. "Prostate Cancer." *Health Library*, September 19, 2012.
Nordqvist, Christian. Prostate cancer: Symptoms, risk factors, and treatment. Medical News Today, July 18, 2017. http://www.medicalnewstoday.com/articles/150086.php
"Prostate Cancer." *American Cancer Society*, September 4, 2012.
"Prostate Cancer." *Centers for Disease Control and Prevention*, May 8, 2013.

Prostate enlargement

Disease/Disorder

Also known as: Benign prostatic hyperplasia or hypertrophy (BPH)

Anatomy or system affected: Reproductive system, urinary system

Specialties and related fields: Endocrinology, urology

Definition: A common condition in which the prostate gland enlarges as a man matures.

Key terms:

benign: not recurrent or malignant; associated with favorable outcomes

cytokines: proteins that influence communication and interactions between cells; examples include interleukins, lymphokines, and cell-signaling molecules such as tumor necrosis factor, transforming growth factor, and interferons

endocrine: a term applied to organs or cells that produce hormones

enzyme: a protein that enhances the rate of chemical changes in living cells

gene: the basic unit of a chromosome carrying the information for a specific protein that is inherited

hormone: a chemical substance produced by an endocrine organ or cells that causes specific effects on the structure and function of the target organs or cells

inflammation: the body's defensive response to injury or infection; includes many factors in the process, including white blood cells and cytokines

laser: an instrument that generates a small intense beam of light that is used in surgery and other medical procedures

malignant: having the features of uncontrolled growth, invasion, and spreading; associated with unfavorable outcomes

phytomedicine: the use of plant substances as alternative treatment for medical diseases and conditions

tissue: a group of similar cells with a specific function

transurethral: across or through the urethra

Causes and Symptoms

Prostate enlargement is also known as benign prostatic hyperplasia or hypertrophy (BPH). Benign refers to the non-malignant nature of the condition. The prostate gland is a walnut-sized organ located below the bladder, the organ in which urine is stored. The prostate surrounds part of the urethra, which is a long tube that transports urine from the bladder to the outside of the body. The gland has a role in both the male reproductive system and the urinary system. The prostate adds secretions to semen, an alkaline fluid that neutralizes the acidic environment of the female reproductive system and provides nutritional elements for the sperm. BPH symptoms occur in more than half of men in their sixties and more than 90 percent of men in their eighties.

Prostate enlargement begins to develop in men at around age fifty. No single factor fully explains the condition, but many factors are known to be involved in BPH, including hormones, cell growth, and genetics. The hormones involved are the female hormone estrogen and the male hormones (androgens) testosterone and dihydrotestosterone (DHT). Men produce testosterone and a small amount of estrogen throughout their lives. The testosterone level decreases as men age and the relative amount of estrogen increases. Scientists have shown that the addition of estrogen to androgen increases BPH development in animals and that there is an increased ratio of female to male hormone (estrogen/androgen ratio) in prostatic tissue with BPH. DHT is another androgen that is related to BPH. It has been shown that men who do not have the enzyme (protein) that converts testosterone to DHT have small-sized prostate glands throughout their lives. Older men continue to produce DHT in the prostate, and this hormone may affect cell growth in the prostate. Moreover, studies have shown that BPH occurs in many men with a positive family history for prostate enlargement.

The prostate gland is surrounded by a tissue lining called the capsule. As the prostate enlarges against its surrounding capsule, the whole structure presses against that part of the urethra that the prostate surrounds; this constricts (obstructs) the urethra and affects the bladder. The bladder wall thickens and becomes more irritable. The symptoms of BPH result from the urethral obstruction and resulting bladder irritation and functional decline. Urethral obstruction causes voiding hesitancy, intermittency, weak stream, dribbling, and straining. Bladder irritation causes more sensitivity to smaller amounts of urine, resulting in more frequent urination, especially at night. Eventually, the bladder may weaken and its function may be affected adversely. The bladder can lose its ability to completely empty the stored urine during voiding; this can lead to acute urinary retention in the bladder.

Treatment and Therapy

The patient may notice the symptoms of BPH first and schedule an appointment with his doctor for evaluation. BPH diagnostic assessment includes a number of steps. A detailed medical history, focusing on the symptoms of the urinary system, will be obtained. A questionnaire such as the American Urological Association Symptom Index will help the doctor decide the severity of the symptoms. A physical examination will be performed, including a digital rectal examination, in which a gloved finger is inserted into the rectum to evaluate the size and condition of the prostate. A urine test to check for blood or signs of urine infection and a blood test to evaluate whether the kidneys are affected will be done as well.

Other tests may be recommended to determine if the symptoms are associated with the bladder or kidney or if cancer is present. One such test, postvoid residual urine volume, measures how much urine is left in the bladder after urination. The two tests that can determine the degree of blockage in urine flow are uroflowmetry, which measures the rate and amount of urine passed, and pressure-flow studies, which assess bladder pressure during voiding. In some cases, imaging of the kidney, bladder, and prostate may be necessary with x-rays, ultrasound, or cystoscopy, in which an instrument is passed through the urethra and used to view the interior of the bladder. A test for prostate-specific antigen (PSA) may also be recommended. PSA is a protein that is produced by prostate cells; it is often elevated in patients with prostate cancer but may also be increased in BPH.

Treatment of BPH includes conservative measures

Information on Prostate Enlargement

Causes: Unknown; factors include hormones (estrogen, androgens), cell growth, genetics

Symptoms: Constriction of urethra and bladder irritation resulting in urination problems (voiding hesitancy, intermittency, weak stream, dribbling, straining, frequency, infections)

Duration: Chronic

Treatments: None (watchful waiting), medications (alpha-blockers, enzyme inhibitors of 5-alpha-reductase, herbal remedies), surgery to remove tissue or gland

(watchful waiting), medical options (both conventional and alternative), surgical procedures, and minimally invasive therapies. The patient's decision is usually based on the effects of the BPH symptoms on his quality of life and on weighing the risks and benefits of available interventions. If the symptoms are severe and the urinary or reproductive tract is affected, however, then BPH needs to be treated.

BPH symptoms that do not bother the patient can be managed with watchful waiting. There is no active treatment involved, and the patient will see his doctor at least once a year to determine whether the symptoms are staying the same, improving, or worsening.

Medical options include taking conventional drugs such as an alpha-blocker or enzyme inhibitors of 5-alpha-reductase. Alpha-blockers relax the smooth muscles of the bladder neck and prostate. Examples of alpha-blockers include terazosin (Hytrin), doxazosin (Cardura), tamsulosin (Flomax), and alfuzosin (Uroxatral). The side effects of these drugs include dizziness, fainting, headache, tiredness, and low blood pressure. Enzyme inhibitors of 5-alpha-reductase prevent the conversion of testosterone to DHT, which in turn can decrease prostate growth. There are two drugs approved by the Food and Drug Administration (FDA) in this category, finasteride (Proscar) and dutasteride (Avodart). Their side effects include decreased libido, ejaculatory problems, and erectile dysfunction.

Alternative medications consist of herbal remedies. Studies on saw palmetto, a fruit extract from the American dwarf palm tree, have yielded equivocal results on its efficacy as a BPH treatment. Systematic reviews of beta-sitosterol plant extract, cernilton from rye grass pollen, and Pygeum bark extract from African plum tree showed that there is some BPH symptomatic improvement with these supplements. Better-designed studies for these remedies, however, may not confirm this favorable result, as was seen in the case of saw palmetto.

Surgical management of BPH includes transurethral resection of the prostate (TURP), transurethral incision of the prostate (TUIP), open surgery (prostatectomy), and laser surgery. TURP is the most common surgical option; the surgeon uses an instrument called a resectoscope to remove enlarged prostate tissue through the urethra. TUIP usually involves placing two deep incisions in the prostate where it meets the bladder neck; this decreases the resistance to urine flow from the bladder. Prostate tissue is not removed in this procedure. Prostatectomy, or prostate gland removal, is done in some cases; this involves removing the enlarged prostate in an open surgery. Laser surgery vaporizes the prostate tissue causing obstruction.

Minimally invasive procedures for treatment of BPH symptoms include application of heat from various sources to eliminate excessive prostatic tissue, such as transurethral needle ablation of the prostate (TUNA), transurethral microwave thermotherapy (TUMT), transurethral vaporization of the prostate (TUVP), water-induced thermotherapy, high-intensity ultrasound energy therapy, and interstitial laser coagulation. Removal of obstructing prostate tissue by these methods can allow better urinary flow. Mechanical approaches such as balloon dilation and urethral stent placement dilate the obstructed area of the urethra. Balloon dilation involves placing a catheter with a balloon at its tip through the urethra; the balloon is inflated in the area of obstruction. Urethral stents are placed in the obstructed urethral area to dilate the narrowed section for better urinary flow.

As with medical treatments, surgical management and minimally invasive procedures have risks and benefits. The risks include bleeding, infection, and impotence. The best therapy for BPH is not the same for all patients. The treatment options will depend on the severity of symptoms, the risks and benefits of the therapy, and the general health condition of the patient. A satisfactory management plan to treat BPH symptoms can be accomplished in a partnership between the patient and his physician.

Perspective and Prospects

The development of prostate enlargement is multifactorial, and the specific steps involved in its progression are still unresolved. Research studies are ongoing to evaluate the processes involved in the development of this condition. For example, chronic inflammation has been implicated in BPH. Studies have shown that tissue specimens from enlarged prostates have pro-inflammatory cells and cytokines. One cytokine implicated in BPH development is transforming growth factor beta. TGF-beta is involved in the cell signaling that causes an increase in expression of some genes in BPH, such as the gene called GAGEC1. This gene is a member of the GAGE family. The proteins expressed by these genes are associated with male and female reproductive organs such as the prostate, testis, Fallopian tubes, uterus, and placenta, as well as in cancers of the prostate, testis, and uterus. Unraveling these molecular processes in BPH may lead to the design of new therapeutic modalities for an enlarged prostate.

Recently, studies evaluating combination therapy, such as using both an alpha-blocker and a 5-alpha-reductase inhibitor for treatment of BPH and its related symptoms, have been carried out. One such study is the Medical Therapy of Prostate Symptoms Study (MTOPS), which showed that the clinical progression of BPH is delayed and symptoms are reduced by combination therapy. Clinical guidelines from authoritative sources such as the American Urological Association, the Agency for Healthcare Research and Quality, and the International Consultation on BPH still recommend that a patient discuss the risks and benefits of combination therapy with his physician. For example, the risks of side effects from two medications and the economic burden of purchasing two medications should be balanced with the benefits derived from the combination therapy.

The search for novel drugs to treat an enlarged prostate continues, including the development of more selective alpha-blockers and 5-alpha-reductase inhibitors (both steroidal and nonsteroidal). The factors that are involved in the development of BPH, such as cytokines, growth factors, estrogen, and androgen hormone receptors, are being evaluated as targets for potential therapeutic options. Some studies have also shown that botulinum neurotoxin (Botox) injection can shrink the prostate and reduce levels of PSA. However, such use of Botox is off-label and currently not approved for BPH by the FDA. Significant basic research regarding the mechanisms by which Botox affects the prostate and evidence-based data for use of Botox in BPH are needed.

Current studies in managing an enlarged prostate also include evaluation of specific aspects of herbal preparations such as saw palmetto and other alternative phytomedicine products. Moreover, treatment of BPH by surgical and minimally invasive procedures are still being compared with regard to clinical efficacy, related complications, and optimal energy sources for heat. The future will certainly bring more answers about the biological basis of enlarged prostate as well as even better treatment options.

—*Miriam E. Schwartz, M.D., M.A., Ph.D., and Shawkat Dhanani, M.D., M.P.H.*

See also Aging; Endocrinology; Genital disorders, male; Glands; Hormones; Hyperplasia; Men's health; Prostate gland; Prostate gland removal; Reproductive system; Urinary disorders; Urinary system; Urology.

For Further Information:

Alan, Rick. "Benign Prostatic Hyperplasia." *Health Library*, September 27, 2012.

Chuang, Yao-Chi, and Michael B. Chancellor. "The Application of Botulinum Toxin in the Prostate." *Journal of Urology* 176, no. 6 (December, 2006): 2375-2382.

DiPaola, Robert S., and Ronald A. Morton. "Proven and Unproven Therapy for Benign Prostatic Hyperplasia." *New England Journal of Medicine* 354, no. 6 (February 9, 2006): 632-634.

"Enlarged Prostate." *MedlinePlus*, September 19, 2011.

Komaroff, Anthony, ed. "Prostate Gland." In *Harvard Medical School Family Health Guide*. New York: Free Press, 2005.

McVary, Kevin T., ed. *Management of Benign Prostatic Hypertrophy*. Totowa, N.J.: Humana Press, 2004.

"Prostate Disorders." In *The Merck Manual Home Health Handbook*, edited by Robert S. Porter, et al. Whitehouse Station, N.J.: Merck Research Laboratories, 2009.

"Prostate Enlargement: Benign Prostatic Hyperplasia." *National Kidney and Urologic Diseases Information Clearinghouse*, March 23, 2012.

Rous, Stephen N. *The Prostate Book: Sound Advice on Symptoms and Treatment*. 3d ed. New York: W. W. Norton, 2002.

Prostate gland

Anatomy

Anatomy or system affected: Endocrine system, glands, reproductive system

Specialties and related fields: Endocrinology, oncology, urology

Definition: One of several accessory reproductive glands; its main function is to secrete into semen vital additive components that increase the fertilizing potential of sperm.

Key terms:

andrology: study of the physiological functions relating to male reproductive capacity

bulbourethal gland: the bulbous portion of the male urethra adjacent to the posterior prostate zone

gonad: the male or female organ (testis or ovary, respectively) in which the essential gametes are formed for reproduction

hyperplasia: a state of hormonal stimulation causing an increase in the number of cells in a tissue, resulting in an oversized organ

prostate-specific antigen (PSA): protein associated with the prostate gland

prostatoglandular carcinoma: the general pathological nomenclature for cancers located in the prostate gland

vas deferens: the duct that carries the male seminal fluid

Structure and Functions

The prostate is the largest of several glands that are referred to as the accessory glands of the male reproductive tract, the others being the seminal vesicles and the bulbourethral glands. Unlike the latter two, which evolved morphologically in smaller pairs, the prostate evolved as a single gland, approximately four centimeters in diameter in adults. It surrounds the urethra, the tubular tract that carries both semen and urine. During the early embryonic stage of life, both urinary organs and accessory sex glands are formed, through the cell-division process, out of the same original source of specialized cells in the intermediate mesoderm (called the nephrotome) and the cloaca.

In fact, up to a certain point in the growth of the human embryo, it is not possible to distinguish the pattern that will lead to formation of the male and female gonads. Following what is called the ambisexual stage, the undifferentiated gonad, or reproductive terminus, begins to evolve into a male or female reproductive organ, becoming either a testis or an ovary. Then, in the male, the three accessory sex glands begin to form. Their eventual key functions in the reproductive process will not begin, however, until the onset of puberty in the individual's growth cycle. Male puberty, or sexual maturity, is initiated when secretions from the testis and pituitary gland activate secretions from other organs, including the prostate gland. It is at this stage that elevated levels of androgenic steroids in the body cause the prostate to attain its full size and begin to secrete the fluids that are essential in the male reproductive function.

The function of all necessary reproductive glands, and of the prostate gland in particular, is to secrete fluids that affect the fertilization potential of the spermatozoa in the seminal fluid as it passes from its source in the testicles through the vas deferens duct. The vas deferens joins the urethra at a point just before the latter is encased by the prostate gland. Thereafter, the urethra serves as a channel for passage of seminal fluid through the penis.

When the adult prostate gland is functioning efficiently, the prostatic secretions that pass into the vas deferens should make up about 30 percent of the volume of the male seminal fluid. Although the process of prostate secretion after puberty is continuous, the composite elements of these secretions may vary. One notable variation in content occurs during moments of sexual excitement. A comparison of "resting" prostatic fluids with fluids obtained from ejaculation resulting from sexual stimulation suggests that the latter contains a higher level of certain enzymes, particularly acid phosphatase, than the former.

All "resting" prostatic fluid is only slightly basic, with an approximate pH of 7.2. The pH level may increase to 7.7 in men suffering from prostatitis. The main components of the fluid include diastase, an enzyme of the amylase group; proteolytic enzymes, especially fibrinolysin; citric acid; acid phosphatase, also an enzyme; cephalin, a chemical group containing amino acids that is found mainly in nervous-system tissues; cholesterol; magnesium; zinc; and calcium. In humans, but not necessarily in all mammals, calcium is more highly concentrated in prostatic fluid than in the blood plasma.

There are other differences between humans and other mammals with respect to the glandular origins of separate component elements of seminal fluid. Whereas citric acid originates in the human prostate gland, in other species it may come from the seminal vesicles, as is the case for boars, or it may flow in generally equal amounts from each of the accessory sex glands, such as in rabbits and guinea pigs. In all cases, citric acid is synthesized by chemical reactions within the originating glands.

There is general agreement that the fertilizing potential of spermatozoa is enhanced when combinations of these various prostatic fluid constituents join the flow of semen. No evidence has been found of an identifiable target effect by any one specific element, although tests of relative concentrations of citric acid in semen suggest an influence on the activity level of testicular hormones, especially androgen. Additionally, with regard to the fertilization potential of male spermatozoa carried in the seminal fluid, citric acid reacts chemically with other component elements in ways that may delay the coagulation of seminal plasma or contribute to its capacity to be absorbed at the appropriate time in the fertilization process.

Research has also tentatively established that the fertilization potential of spermatozoa may depend on levels of zinc contained in secretions from the prostate gland. One chemical effect of zinc is to slow the breakdown of genetically vital chromosomes in individual sperm cells. This function of zinc has not been tied directly to potential fertility levels, however, since surgical removal of the section of the prostate where zinc is in the highest concentration (the dorsolateral portion of the gland) has not changed repro-

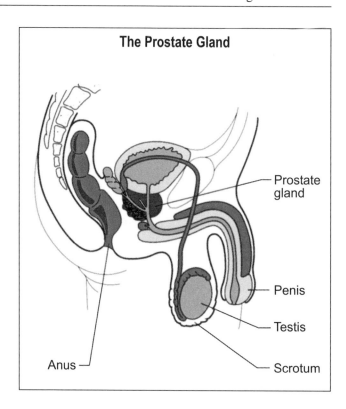

The Prostate Gland

Prostate gland

Penis

Testis

Scrotum

Anus

ductive capacities in laboratory rats. Because prostate surgery involving human patients is almost exclusively connected with attempts to arrest prostate cancer, no research data have been recorded that can be compared with experiments performed on animals.

One area of research that has established irrefutable evidence in connection with fertility levels deals with the effects of certain drugs on the functioning of the accessory sex glands, including the prostate. Tests on morphine and methadone users, for example, have shown a definite reduction in the volume of human seminal ejaculate. Methadone, and in some cases morphine, can actually cause a reduction of the weight and volume of the testes, seminal vesicles, and prostate glands of laboratory mice. Specific constituent elements of prostate secretions that appear to be reduced when drugs such as morphine sulfate are administered include prostatic fructose and different forms of glucose that contribute to metabolic activity in the prostate gland itself.

In addition to medical or self-administered drugs, chemicals that enter the body through the food chain, such as the pesticide DDT, can also affect the functioning of the prostate. In mice, the testosterone metabolic process, which is very much dependent on the prostate, has been shown to be significantly retarded when DDT is administered under close controls. Dieldrin is another pesticide that affects the ability of prostate tissue in mice to absorb testosterone.

Disorders and Diseases

In general terms, diseases of the prostate gland tend to fall into two main categories: nonproliferative and proliferative. The latter category is characterized by two forms of dangerous physical change in the tissues of the gland itself: lesions and neoplasms (or tumors).

Diseases of the nonproliferative type, although painful and potentially quite dangerous to the patient's health, may be treated by modern medical means. One subgroup in this category is congenital anomalies. Some of these have slowly developing symptoms and may be discovered only when some other difficulty, such as urinary irregularities or infertility, is the initial cause for the doctor's examination. The most common form of anomaly is the congenital cyst, which occurs as a result of obstructions in the normal flow of secretions through the prostate gland. Secretion blockage is sometimes caused by irregular development of the parenchyma, the functioning tissues of the gland itself. Subsequent development of a cyst in the prostate itself further impedes the normal flow of secretions within and from the gland.

Congenital cysts usually occur in the prostatic utricle, an oblong protrusion measuring about three millimeters that is palpable when a medical doctor performs a rectal examination. The abnormality is generally discovered in patients in their early twenties. In newborn infants, the fact of recent estrogenic stimulation in utero can have the temporary effect of making the utricle three times its eventual normal length. If the prostatic utricle does not shorten during childhood and early adulthood, examining doctors will be alerted to the existence of a cyst and the possible need for surgical intervention.

A second form of nonproliferative disease in the prostate involves the formation of tiny calculi, or stones, inside the gland. True prostatic calculi are generally rare, but they may occur when prostatic secretions are altered by one of several possible factors, including infection or some form of metabolic dysfunction. Altered secretions can lead to abnormal chemical deposits inside the organ. These deposits in turn attract mineral concentrations, particularly of calcium salts, the main component of calculi.

Although pathology texts list up to five forms of proliferative tumors that can attack the accessory reproductive glands, the prostate gland itself is mainly vulnerable to two out of the five: prostatic carcinoma and primary prostatic sarcoma. More common and less dangerous proliferative lesions (inflammations, not tumors) affecting the prostate involve many different forms of hyperplasia. Although the causes of such lesions can vary, their effect may be summarized as inflammation leading to either the obstruction of normal secretions originating in the prostate or the potentially harmful addition to prostate secretions of foreign by-products of the inflammatory process.

The most common proliferative lesion of the prostate, nodular prostatic hyperplasia (NPH), leads directly to urological disease, usually in middle-aged and elderly males. Its high incidence is reflected in the widespread need for some form of prostate surgery among men over fifty. The disease derives its name from the fact that it displays multinodular areas of inflammation, which makes it difficult for specialized surgeons to localize areas demanding attention. Doctors are still uncertain of the exact origins of NPH and the complexities of hormonal phenomena associated with the disease. It appears, however, that NPH is a combination of the more simply diagnosed prostatic hyperplasia (prostate enlargement) and a hypertrophy (tissue constriction) of the inner zones of the prostate gland itself.

Although these various forms of lesions affect a high percentage of the adult male population, the greatest pathological menace associated with the prostate gland involves malignant tumors. Prostatic cancers represent the second most common form of cancer occurring among American males, with more than two hundred thousand cases diagnosed each year in the United States. Early diagnosis can usually result in treatment and cure. Because of the difficulties associated with diagnosis and the complexities of possible treatments, however, a large percentage of those suffering from prostate cancers die from the disease.

There is a problem of extended delay in the appearance of symptoms; approximately 70 percent of the total recorded cases remain locally latent for years. Yet even the prostatoglandular tumors that have clinical manifestations are often discovered too late for effective medical intervention.

Doctors looking for symptoms of prostate cancer, beyond those that might appear in physical examination via the rectum, pay particular attention to several likely warning signs. These include possible malignant repercussions stemming from prostatic lesions, especially NPH; sacral, lower back, or upper pubic pain; excessive urinary retention; and uneven or interrupted urinary flow. In recent years, screening for prostate cancer has involved measuring the prostate-specific antigen (PSA) level in a blood sample. PSA levels in males with a normal prostate generally measure around two nanograms or less. Elevated levels may indicate the presence of a tumor. The test remains inexact, however, since even a benign prostatic hypertrophy (BPH), or prostate enlargement, may result in an increase in PSA values.

If a physician suspects the presence of cancer in the prostate region, three forms of biopsy may be used. The most accurate method involves actual surgical opening and removal of sections for laboratory biopsy. This method is the most expensive, however, and is recommended mainly when physicians are convinced that a radical prostatectomy should probably follow initial surgical intervention, for reasons that may not be limited to concerns about cancer. Of the other two methods of diagnosis, core needle biopsy and needle aspiration biopsy, the former has a slightly higher level of accuracy, while the latter is safer and generally has fewer complications.

A complicating factor that makes prostate cancers among the most difficult to treat is similar to what has been observed with NPH. In NPH, which is a proliferative lesion, multinodular development complicates localization of the diseased area for treatment. In the case of prostatoglandular carcinoma, approximately 30 percent of diagnosed patients have diffused, as opposed to focal, growth development patterns. In such cases, radical prostatectomy, despite the fact that it usually leaves the patient impotent, is generally believed to be the best course of action.

A second, less common category of prostate cancer is referred to as primary prostatic sarcoma. Although this disease represents only 2 percent of all prostate cancers, it differs from the more common prostatic carcinoma in that it may occur in male patients of any age and has been diagnosed in infants as young as four months. Another serious factor is that if this form of cancer appears in the prostate, it frequently extends directly to other adjacent organs or structures, primarily the bladder, seminal vesicles, or rectum.

Perspective and Prospects

Although statistics show that as of 2009, prostate cancer was the most common cause of cancer among men and the second most common cause of cancer death among men, the medical world remained divided over questions of prognosis. Doctors called upon by the National Cancer Institute hesitated to reach a consensus about the central question of relative success rates of radiation treatment versus surgical intervention. Part of the problem, the institute learned, was that because patients are most often diagnosed at an advanced age-according to the American Cancer Society, as of 2012, the average age at diagnosis was sixty-seven-data gathered on their physical condition do not provide sufficiently random samplings for comparison with the population as a whole. A main reason for apparent dissatisfaction with too-focused data is that, because of the typically late discovery of prostate cancer, one central consideration in choosing between surgery or radiation treatment is rendered less vital; past a certain stage in advanced adulthood, diminished sexual reproductive capacity also diminishes patient sensitivity to the possibility that surgical removal of cancerous growth in the prostate will almost certainly bring about impotence.

Significant research has addressed the possible causes of prostate cancer. In a significant number of cases, researchers have observed a specific form of deoxyribonucleic acid (DNA) translocation in cells making up the tumor, lending support to the belief many forms of such cancers result from certain mutations. In the future, observation of such specific mutations from biopsy material may allow for improved methods of screening.

—*Byron D. Cannon, Ph.D.;*
updated by Richard Adler, Ph.D.

See also Aging; Cancer; Colorectal surgery; Endocrine glands; Endocrinology; Genital disorders, male; Glands; Hormones; Malignancy and metastasis; Men's health; Oncology; Prostate cancer; Prostate enlargement; Prostate gland removal; Puberty and adolescence; Reproductive system; Semen; Urinary disorders; Urinary system; Urology; Vas defrens.

For Further Information:

American Cancer Society. http://www.cancer.org

Blute, Michael. *Mayo Clinic on Prostate Health: What to Do about Prostate Enlargement, Inflammation and Cancer.* 2d ed. Rochester, Minn.: Mayo Clinic, 2003.

Fox, Arnold, and Barry Fox. *The Healthy Prostate: A Doctor's Comprehensive Program for Preventing and Treating Common Problems.* New York: John Wiley & Sons, 1996.

McClure, Mark W. *Smart Medicine for a Healthy Prostate: Natural and Conventional Therapies for Common Prostate Disorders.* New York: Avery, 2001.

Marieb, Elaine N. *Essentials of Human Anatomy and Physiology.* 10th ed. San Francisco: Pearson/Benjamin Cummings, 2011.

Marx, Jean. "Fused Genes May Help Explain the Origins of Prostate Cancer." *Science* 310 (October 28, 2005): 603.

"Prostate Diseases." *MedlinePlus*, May 20, 2013.

Westheimer, Ruth, and Pierre Lehu. *Sex for Dummies.* 3d ed. Hoboken, N.J.: John Wiley & Sons, 2006.

Yeo, Lehana, et al. "The Development of the Modern Prostate Biopsy." *InTechOpen*, December 2, 2011.

Zangwill, Monica, and Igor Puzanov. "Conditions InDepth: Prostate Cancer." *Health Library*, October 11, 2012.

Prostate gland removal

Procedure

Also known as: Prostatectomy
Anatomy or system affected: Endocrine system, glands
Specialties and related fields: General surgery, oncology, proctology, urology
Definition: A surgical procedure to remove all or part of an abnormal prostate gland.

Key terms:

cauterization: a means of sealing blood vessels with heat; used to prevent bleeding

impotence: the inability to achieve an erection

incision: a cut made with a scalpel during a surgical procedure

incontinence: the inability to retain urine

prostate: a gland in males that surrounds the urethra and secretes a fluid into the ejaculate

urethra: the tube that connects the urinary bladder externally

Indications and Procedures

The removal of the prostate gland, or prostatectomy, may be performed when enlargement of the gland blocks or reduces the outflow of urine. Removal may also be indicated in prostate cancer or inflammation of the prostate (prostatitis).

Enlargement of the prostate gland, also known as benign prostatic hyperplasia (BPH), may affect men over the age of fifty. Because the prostate gland is situated so that it surrounds the urethra, when it enlarges, it can compress the urethra and reduce the flow of urine. Symptoms usually include gradual reduction in the ability to urinate effectively. Since the flow of urine out the urethra is obstructed by the enlarged gland, the patient experiences difficulty starting urination and a weak stream.

In early stages, the urinarybladder muscle becomes heavier and stronger in order to compensate for the increased resistance in the urethra. Eventually, however, the bladder is unable to expel all the urine and becomes distended. This urinary retention can cause abdominal swelling and a perceived urgency to urinate. In fact, the bladder may contract frequently and cause a need for frequent urination. This is one sign of bladder muscle failure and the need for medical attention. In some patients, there may be incontinence as a result of the leakage of small volumes of urine.

Prostate cancer is a malignant growth of the prostate gland. Most patients with prostate cancer are in their seventies; this condition also occurs in middle-aged men. The symptoms that develop are similar to those of BPH. Diagnosis is usually made by a digital rectal examination, ultrasonography, prostate biopsy, and a blood test for prostatic-specific antigens.

The treatment for both BPH and prostatic cancer involves medical management and surgical removal of all or part of the gland. In BPH, finasteride (Proscar) can be used to reduce the size of the gland and diminish symptoms. Prostate cancer can sometimes be managed using drugs that block or reduce the production of testosterone. Such agents include flutamide (Eulexin) and leuprolide. If medical management is not effective, surgical removal of the gland is usually indicated.

The most common surgical procedure for the removal of part of the prostate gland is transurethral resection of the prostate (TURP), which is performed using an instrument called a resectoscope. The patient is first anesthetized using spinal or general anesthesia. Then the resectoscope is inserted into the urethra at the tip of the penis and directed up toward the prostate gland. The resectoscope allows the surgeon to view the urinary bladder and prostate and insert a cutting instrument or heated wire into the area of the prostate to be removed. As the gland is cut away, it is removed from the urethra by suction. Any bleeding that may occur is stopped by a cauterizing electrode, which seals the vessels. After the prostate gland has been removed, the surgeon withdraws the resectoscope and inserts a catheter into the bladder to drain urine and any remaining blood or tissue.

If a more radical procedure than transurethral resection is needed, as in cases of prostate cancer, then retropubic prostatectomy is performed. This operation requires that the patient be anesthetized. The surgeon makes a horizontal incision just above the pubic hairline into the abdominal cavity and exposes the urinary bladder and prostate gland. A cut into the capsule that encases the gland is made, and the surgeon begins to remove the prostate gland. To drain excess fluid from the pelvic cavity, the surgeon places a temporary flexible tube near to where the prostate was excised. Bleeding vessels are cauterized, and the abdominal wall is sutured. A urethral catheter is inserted and left in place to aid in draining the bladder of blood and urine. An alternative to retropubic prostatectomy is perineal prostatectomy, in which the prostate is accessed through an incision in the perineum, the area between the scrotum and anus; this procedure is less common, because it carries a higher risk of nerve damage. Another option is laparoscopic prostatectomy, in which four or five very small incisions are made in the abdomen, through which computer-guided instruments and a camera are inserted to perform the procedure.

Uses and Complications

After removal of the urethral catheter, the patient is encouraged to drink large amounts of fluids and to pass urine. Occasionally, the patient may experience frequent and painful urination but should still consume adequate amounts of liquids to help clear the urinary tract of blood and other postoperative debris. A few patients will continue to have incontinence for several weeks.

More severe complications include intra-abdominal bleeding from surgery, infections, and blood clots that obstruct urine outflow from the bladder. Bleeding within the pelvic and abdominal cavities is usually detected and corrected during surgery. If it occurs after prostatectomy, a second operation may be required to find and stop the bleeding. Most infections of the urinary tract can be adequately treated with appropriate antibiotic therapy. Urinary obstruction resulting from a blood clot can be washed out with a catheter in the urethra.

Approximately 10 to 20 percent of men undergoing retropubic prostatectomy experience impotence. This complication is more common in older patients, and can often be treated with drugs such as Viagra.

For most men, the hospital stay is about two days for transurethral resection of the prostate, two to three days for open surgery, and overnight for a laparoscopic procedure. Several weeks after the surgery the patient can resume all activities, including intercourse. Most men are sterile, however, immediately after either procedure because most of the sperm and seminal fluid are expelled backward into the urinary bladder (retrograde ejaculation). The ejaculate is then excreted with the urine during the next urination.

—*Matthew Berria, Ph.D.,*
and Douglas Reinhart, M.D.

See also Aging; Biopsy; Cancer; Colorectal surgery; Endocrine glands; Genital disorders, male; Glands; Incontinence; Malignancy and metastasis; Men's health; Oncology; Prostate cancer; Prostate enlargement; Prostate gland; Radiation therapy; Reproductive system; Urinary disorders; Urinary system; Urology.

For Further Information:
American Medical Association. *American Medical Association Family Medical Guide.* 4th rev. ed. Hoboken, N.J.: John Wiley & Sons, 2004.
Bangma, Ch. H., and D. W. W. Newling, eds. *Prostate and Renal Cancer, Benign Prostatic Hyperplasia, Erectile Dysfunction, and Basic Research: An Update.* Boca Raton, Fla.: Parthenon, 2003.
Griffith, H. Winter. *Complete Guide to Symptoms, Illness, and Surgery.* Rev. 6th ed. New York: Perigee, 2012.
McPhee, Stephen J., and Maxine A. Papadakis, eds. *Current Medical Diagnosis and Treatment.* 50th ed. Los Altos, Calif.: Lange Medical, 2011.
Neff, Deanna M. "Prostatectomy." *Health Library,* September 26, 2012.
"Simple Prostatectomy." *MedlinePlus,* March 28, 2011.
"Transurethral Resection of the Prostate." *Health Library,* September 26, 2012.
Wein, Alan J., et al., eds. *Campbell-Walsh Urology.* 10th ed. Philadelphia: Saunders/Elsevier, 2012.
Zollinger, Robert M., Jr., and Robert M. Zollinger, Sr. *Zollinger's Atlas of Surgical Operations.* 9th ed. New York: McGraw-Hill, 2011.

Prostheses

Treatment
Anatomy or system affected: All
Specialties and related fields: Biotechnology, cardiology,

dentistry, dermatology, general surgery, occupational health, oncology, ophthalmology, orthopedics, physical therapy, plastic surgery

Definition: Artificial replacements for missing, malformed, diseased, or damaged human parts.

Key terms:

amputation level: the site and type of amputation

anaplastology: the art and science of artificially restoring parts of the body or face with lifelike and aesthetic prostheses

biosynthetics: materials that are both biological (found in nature) and synthetic (artificial)

osseointegration: a process in which bone grows around embedded titanium fixtures; the stabilized fixtures eventually support dental or facial prostheses

prosthetist: someone who designs, fabricates, and fits prostheses

residual limb: the limb remaining after amputation

teratogen: an agent that interferes with normal embryonic or fetal development

thermoplastic: a plastic that can be shaped when heated and that becomes rigid when cooled; it can be modified repeatedly for prosthesis fittings

thermoset: a plastic offering structural stability; it cannot be reshaped once cooled

Indications and Procedures

Traditionally, prostheses are defined as artificial replacements for missing, malformed, diseased, or damaged human parts. However, partly as a result of biomedical engineering feats, scientists and practitioners disagree as to what defines a prosthesis. Some think that only external devices that are mechanical, such as artificial limbs, are prostheses. Others think that internal devices, such as hip or knee replacements, or internal parts that are biological, such as transplanted organs and parts of organs, are prostheses. Finally, some think biosynthetic materials, such as artificial skin substitutes, qualify. Hence, the broadest definition could include artificial limbs, eyes, and noses; biosynthetic materials; organ transplants; heart valves; penile implants; bladder pumps; wigs; and dental appliances.

Body parts may be ruined or their function impaired as a result of disease, aging, congenital malformation, or trauma. Common diseases that may result in loss of limbs or destruction of tissue are diabetes, cancer, and vascular disease. Osteoarthritis erodes cartilage in the spine and joints and is common among older people. Congenital anomalies arising from exposure to teratogens during embryonic or fetal development may impair function. Trauma from accidents and war is a major cause of damage. Every week, land mines maim approximately twelve hundred people worldwide, many of them children. Generally, a prosthesis is prescribed if normal function or appearance can be partially or completely restored.

The most common prostheses are replacements for amputated limbs or parts of limbs. More than 70 percent of amputations in the United States are caused by peripheral vascular disease in which blood flow is partially or completely obstructed in blood vessels beyond the chest. Peripheral vascular disease includes arteriosclerosis (hardening of the arteries), thromboembolism (blockage of a blood vessel), and complications from diabetes, a chronic metabolic disease.

Amputations involve the disarticulation of joints (such as through the hips) and the transection of long bones. About two-thirds of lower leg amputations in the United States are at a level below the knee and include transtibial (across the lower leg bone), ankle, foot, and toe amputations. About a third of leg amputations are transfemoral (across the thigh bone). Most amputees are over sixty-five years of age and have peripheral vascular disease; a large proportion of these amputees have diabetes.

A lower extremity prosthesis comprises several components. A socket fits around the residual limb and transmits force for standing and walking. A sheath, sock, and liner serve as an interface between limb and prosthesis, offering protection and comfort, especially for people with peripheral vascular disease or sensitive skin. A suspension system secures the socket to the residual limb for safe ambulation. There may be a knee joint with a single axis and hinge, or a polycentric axis with changing centers of rotation. A pylon or tube connects the socket to the terminal device and may absorb, store, and release energy. The terminal device, such as a foot or ski, can respond to changing terrain if dynamic. For each component, a prosthetist selects the appropriate type after evaluating several factors, including the patient's upper body strength, trunk control, balance, posture, motivation, vocation, and hobbies and sports, as well as cost and aesthetics. Sometimes, at the patient's behest, a more lifelike prosthesis is designed instead of one that functions optimally and is easy to maintain.

About 90 percent of upper extremity amputations are the result of traumatic injury sustained by men between the ages of twenty and forty. Commonly, injury results from accidents with machines (especially farm machines), frostbite, and electrical burns. Prostheses for upper extremities range from being entirely cosmetic to optimally functional. There are two types of functional prostheses: body-powered (involving cable systems) and myoelectric. The latter use surface electrodes to translate energy from muscle contractions to prosthetic elbows, wrists, and hands.

In general, the level of amputation is linked to the degree of function that may be restored by a well-designed prosthesis and appropriate rehabilitation. For example, as the level rises from toes to hips, it becomes increasingly difficult to fully restore mobility and locomotion. Also, it is easier to restore the function of lower limbs than of upper limbs-primarily because of complex hand movements for grasping and manipulating.

Prostheses can replace parts of the face when plastic surgery is not a viable option. Sometimes, neither function nor appearance can be restored by more surgery. The patient may not be able to afford or refuses to endure more plastic surgery and elects instead to wear a prosthesis. Facial prostheses include ears, noses, midfacials, orbitals (eyes and lids), and artificial eyes. An anaplastologist, a member of a

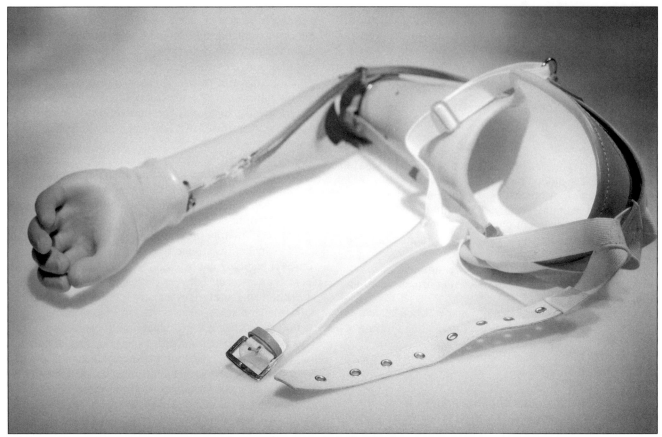

An arm prosthesis. (Stockbyte)

craniofacial rehabilitation team, custom designs a prosthesis for the tissue site after considering the symmetry of the face, its proportions, and anatomical landmarks. After sculpting and molding, a prosthesis is made of silicone rubber tinted to resemble the patient's skin color.

Medical adhesives can keep a facial prosthesis in place. However, a more secure method involves osseointegrated implants of titanium posts. After bone grows around the posts, abutments or extensions are added surgically to support a bar; the prosthesis is clipped to the bar to hold it in place. Sometimes magnets are used. Osseointegrated implants are an important improvement over adhesives in that a person who wears a facial or dental prosthesis is less likely to be embarrassed by losing it in public. Regardless of the method of securing the prosthesis, it must be taken off at night. Both the skin and the prosthesis need to be cleaned daily.

Uses and Complications

People who use prosthetic devices for ambulation expend more energy than do able-bodied people. For example, the energy expended in using a unilateral prosthesis (for one limb or segment) varies directly with the level of amputation. Lower energy costs (related to effort) are associated with longer residual limbs, unilateral rather than bilateral amputation of both limbs or segments, intact knee(s), and loss of limb(s) to trauma rather than vascular disease. Someone with a unilateral transtibial amputation will expend about 9 to 20 percent more energy walking than does an able-bodied person, whereas someone with a bilateral transfemoral amputation may expend almost 300 percent more energy. It is interesting to note that the effort to walk with crutches may be greater than with a prosthesis. Thus, the prognosis for successful ambulation may be better for a nonambulatory patient when fitted with a prosthesis rather than crutches.

Some of the common problems associated with prosthetic devices include initial pain, sensitivity, and edema (swelling) of the residual limb after surgery; discomfort when learning to use a prosthesis; problems with balance and gait (pattern of walking); the breakdown of skin where it comes into contact with an ill-fitting prosthesis; and the effort necessary for donning and doffing (putting on and taking off) a prosthesis. Some types of components are too challenging for the debilitated or the elderly. For example, donning the traditional suction suspension system for holding a transfemoral prosthesis in place requires strength, good balance, and cardiovascular fitness. Some of the dynamically responsive components are bioengineering marvels, but they are heavier and require relatively more strength to use than do traditional counterparts. In general, components suitable for athletes and laborers are not suitable for the weak and sedentary.

People who wear a facial prosthesis depend on its realism and attractiveness for psychological comfort in social settings. The quality of the prosthesis depends a great deal on the artistry of the anaplastologist. When successfully crafted, the prosthesis allows the wearer to feel confident in public whenever ordinary social distances are involved, such as when passing people on the street or making a purchase in a store. However, the prosthesis is detectable close up and may be a source of anxiety for the wearer in more intimate settings.

Although a facial prosthesis may allow a person to "pass" as normal looking, it may not restore the ability to communicate emotion nonverbally or the ability to speak clearly. Even if communication is possible, people may look away, thus disregarding any facial cues. Other difficulties arise when the face has been so damaged that normal eating behavior is impossible or embarrassing. This represents a serious challenge because a great deal of human social interaction involves food; the inability or unwillingness to share food can disrupt families and ruin friendships. The disfigured person may insist on eating alone. The worst consequence of facial disfigurement is social isolation, which leads to depression. However, mutual help groups and nonprofit networks, such as Let's Face It USA, can offer social support and information.

Typically, a facial prosthesis will last about two years, more with careful care. Over time, the silicone yellows when exposed to ultraviolet light, pollutants, and oil. The condition of both the prosthesis and the wearer's skin needs to be monitored regularly by a health care specialist.

Perspective and Prospects

Early versions of today's facial prostheses were crafted by two inspired artists during World War I. Captain Derwent Wood, an English sculptor working out of Britain's Third London General Hospital, was dismayed by the number of suicides committed by men disfigured in trench warfare. After multiple reconstructive surgeries, the men had healed physically but were ashamed of their faces. In response to their plight, Captain Wood made full or partial masks based on photographs taken before their injuries. He made very thin masks of galvanized copper lined with silver, which he painted with oils to approximate the coloration of their skin. Eyeglasses often held the masks in place.

Anna Coleman Ladd, a Boston sculptor in France with the American Red Cross, created masks using similar methods. The soldiers were particularly appreciative of the eyelashes, mustaches, and whiskers made of fine copper threads. If the mouth had been damaged, Ladd parted the lips of the mask just enough to allow a cigarette holder.

Today, facial prostheses are more lifelike and more securely attached to the face. Although there have been tremendous advances in reconstructive surgery and biosynthetic skin substitutes, facial prostheses are still necessary for some patients disfigured, for example, by cancer treatments or burns.

The earliest prosthetists for limbs were blacksmiths, armor makers, artisans, and amputees themselves. War was often the occasion for ingenuity. For example, during the Civil War thousands of amputees needed limb replacements. Wounded men made their own peg legs or crutches.

Replacement limbs and feet from mail-order catalogs were less crude and were made of carved or milled wood covered in rawhide that was glued in place.

Major scientific and technical advances were made in prosthetic design after World War II and the Vietnam War. The National Academy of Sciences organized a conference in 1945 to call attention to the needs of the wounded and to the lack of scientific innovation in the field of prosthetics. An intense research program was sponsored by the Office of Scientific Research and Development, and later by the Veterans Administration. The result was several design breakthroughs, such as the patellar tendon-bearing prosthesis for transtibial amputation and the quadrilateral socket and hydraulic swing-phase knee for transfemoral amputation. After the Vietnam War, myoelectric control systems for upper extremity prostheses and modular endoskeletal lower extremity prostheses were developed. (Endoskeletal refers to a prosthesis in which the pylon is covered with an anatomically shaped, soft foam covering.)

In the early twentieth century, prostheses were made primarily of wood and leather. By the end of the century, major advances in materials science for the aerospace and marine industries yielded stronger and more lightweight materials, many of which were adopted by prosthetists.

Some of the major innovations in prosthetic design depended on the development of thermosetting plastics, which were important for suction socket suspension systems, and transparent plastics, which improved diagnostic fittings. For example, transparent test sockets are used to evaluate potential weight-bearing areas on residual limbs, and transparent face masks are used to evaluate thermal injuries. Other advances in materials engineering, such as the development of carbon composites, contributed to the design of high-performance prosthetic feet for athletes.

Today, leather is still used for suspension straps, belts, and limb cuffs, but there exists an armamentarium of interesting materials useful for prostheses, such as steel, aluminum, titanium, and magnesium alloys; thermoplastics; thermosetting materials; foamed plastics; and viscoelastic polymers.

In the 1960s, computer-aided design and manufacture (CAD/CAM) systems revolutionized the fabrication of prostheses. Using CAD/CAM, surface contours of residual limbs are digitized by reading casts with a probe or scanner. The subsequent numerical models are used for computer-guided fabrication. By the early twenty-first century, medical imaging methods, such as computed tomography (CT) scanning and magnetic resonance imaging (MRI), were used in CAD/CAM systems. This was a major advance because CT and MRI allow the prosthetist to see underlying skeletal and soft tissue structures. Before the incorporation of medical imaging, the prosthetist relied on surface contour maps and palpation (feel) of the residual limb to evaluate anatomical structure. It is likely that advances in medical imaging will contribute further to innovative prosthetic design and fabrication in the future.

—*Tanja Bekhuis, Ph.D.*

See also Accidents; Amputation; Bones and the skeleton; Circulation; Critical care; Critical care, pediatric; Diabetes mellitus; Emergency medicine; Grafts and grafting; Lower extremities; Oncology; Orthopedic surgery; Orthopedics; Orthopedics, pediatric; Physical rehabilitation; Plastic surgery; Transplantation; Upper extremities; Vascular medicine; Vascular system.

For Further Information:

Hughes, Michael J. *The Social Consequences of Facial Disfigurement.* Brookfield, Vt.: Ashgate, 1998.

Lusardi, Michelle M., and Caroline C. Nielsen. *Orthotics and Prosthetics in Rehabilitation.* 3d ed. Philadelphia; London.: Saunders, 2012.

MedlinePlus. "Artificial Limbs." *MedlinePlus*, May 2, 2013.

Newell, Robert. *Body Image and Disfigurement Care.* New York: Routledge, 2000.

Ott, Katherine, David Serlin, and Stephen Mihm, eds. *Artificial Parts, Practical Lives: Modern Histories of Prosthetics.* New York: New York University Press, 2002.

Schaffer, Erik. "Overview of Limb Prosthetics." *The Merck Manual Home Health Handbook*, May 2007.

Seymour, Ron. *Prosthetics and Orthotics: Lower Limb and Spinal.* Philadelphia: Lippincott Williams & Wilkins, 2002.

Vorvick, Linda J. "Prosthesis." *MedlinePlus*, January 21, 2013.

Protein

Biology
Anatomy or system affected: All
Specialties and related fields: Biochemistry, nutrition
Definition: An important dietary nutrient with many essential functions in the body.

Structure and Functions

Proteins are composed of twenty-two different amino acids in various combinations joined together in a chain. The human body can synthesize fourteen amino acids, known as inessential amino acids, whereas the other eight, known as essential amino acids, must be provided by the diet. Proteins from dietary sources are considered complete or incomplete based on their amino acid content. Complete proteins provide all eight essential amino acids, whereas incomplete proteins have low amounts of, or are missing, at least one essential amino acid. Only fish, meat, poultry, eggs, cheese, and other foods from animal sources contain complete proteins. Peanuts, soy, nuts, seeds, green peas, legumes, and some grains provide the richest plant proteins. Omnivores typically eat a sufficient variety of foods to consume adequate essential amino acids. Vegetarians ensure sufficient amino acid intake by consuming a variety of plant proteins.

Every cell in the body contains protein. Proteins are essential for cell structure and function and comprise major components of skin, tissues, muscles, and internal organs. Dietary protein, one of three types of nutrients used for energy, is required for the building, maintenance, and repair of body tissue. Growth and development during childhood, adolescence, and pregnancy depend on proteins. Proteins participate in all cellular functions, such as acting as enzyme catalysts and transport and storage molecules. They also provide mechanical support and immune protection, generate movement, transmit nerve impulses, and control growth and differentiation. Important classes of proteins include enzymes, hormones, and antibodies.

Disorders and Diseases

Protein deficiency is relatively rare in developed countries, although poverty can prevent adequate protein consumption. Protein deficiency can result from stringent weight loss diets or in older adults. Severe protein deficiency is fatal. In developing countries, protein deficiency causes the disease known as kwashiorkor, which includes symptoms such as apathy, diarrhea, inactivity, failure to grow, fatty liver, and edema. Since the body cannot store protein, too much protein can also be harmful, with a high-protein diet potentially leading to high cholesterol or other diseases and possible effects on kidney function. Excess protein may also result in immune system hyperactivity, liver dysfunction, bone loss, and obesity. Proteins contribute to food allergies, with many people allergic to proteins in milk (casein), wheat (gluten), or proteins found in peanut, shellfish, or other seafoods.

Perspective and Prospects

A nutritionally balanced diet provides adequate protein. The average diet in the United States includes nearly twice the amount of protein required to maintain a healthy body. Although it was once believed that vegetarians needed to combine proteins by consuming all amino acids in the same meal, it is now realized that benefits of protein combining can be achieved over a longer period of time. In May 2013, the New York University Fertility Center published a study showing that women undergoing fertility treatment increased their chances of conception by increasing the amount of protein in their diets.

—*C. J. Walsh, Ph.D.*

See also Antioxidants; Carbohydrates; Cholesterol; Digestion; Food biochemistry; Gastroenterology; Gastroenterology, pediatric; Gastrointestinal system; Kwashiorkor; Macronutrients; Malabsorption; Malnutrition; Metabolism; Nutrition; Obesity; Obesity, childhood; Phytochemicals; Proteinuria; Supplements; Vitamins and minerals; Weight loss and gain; Weight loss medications.

For Further Information

"Can High-Protein, Low-Card Diet Boost Fertility Treatment?" *MedlinePlus*. May 6, 2013.

"Dietary Proteins." *MedlinePlus*. July 18, 2013.

Duyff, Roberta Larson. *American Dietetic Association Complete Food and Nutrition Guide.* Hoboken, N.J.: John Wiley & Sons, 2006.

Marshall, Keri. *User's Guide to Protein and Amino Acids.* Laguna Beach, Calif.: Basic Health Publications, 2005.

"Protein in diet." *MedlinePlus*. May 5, 2011.

Shils, Maurice E., Moshe Shike, A. Catharine Ross, and Benjamin Caballero. *Modern Nutrition in Health and Disease.* 10th ed. Philadelphia: Lippincott Williams & Wilkins, 2005.

Proteinuria

Disease/Disorder
Also known as: Albuminuria
Anatomy or system affected: Kidneys, urinary system
Specialties and related fields: Nephrology, urology
Definition: Disorder involving the elimination of abnormally high amounts of protein in the urine. It is typically defined as the excretion of more than 150 milligrams of protein in the urine per day.

Causes and Symptoms

Proteinuria is a disorder that does not have a unique cause. The excretion of abnormally high amounts of protein in the urine can have a number of benign causes, in which case the disorder is likely transient. These causes include dehydration, acute illness, and overexertion. In other instances, proteinuria is the result of a problem within the kidneys. This type of proteinuria is more severe, as well as chronic. Proteins play an important function in the body and are routinely carried in the bloodstream. Since proteins are large molecules, they are not routinely filtered out by the kidneys into the urine. When the glomeruli (the filtering mechanisms within the kidneys) are damaged for any reason, these large protein molecules do pass through the filters and into the urine to be eliminated.

Proteinuria has no symptoms early in its course. One of the earliest signs of proteinuria is the foamy appearance of urine in the toilet. This foamy appearance is caused by the abnormally high amount of protein. As the disorder progresses, the symptoms progress to the development of edema (an accumulation of fluid causing swelling). As a result of the loss of protein from the bloodstream, less fluid is carried in the bloodstream, with more remaining in the tissues. As a result, edema appears in the hands and/or the feet and in the abdominal area.

Treatment and Therapy

The diagnosis of proteinuria is made based on the collection of urine samples. In the past, it required the collection of a twenty-four-hour urine specimen, with the diagnosis of proteinuria being made if more than 150 milligrams of protein were excreted per day. More recently, the diagnosis of proteinuria has been made based on one urine sample by determining a urine albumin (protein) to creatinine (waste product) ratio. More than 30 milligrams of albumin per milligram of creatinine is indicative of proteinuria. Whenever proteinuria is present, additional tests of kidney function are indicated. Chronic proteinuria is often indicative of chronic kidney disease.

Treatment of proteinuria is dependent on treating the underlying problem. Dietary modifications may be made to control glucose, sodium, and protein intake. Medications may be used to treat diabetes and hypertension. The most commonly used medications are angiotensin-converting enzyme (ACE) inhibitors. Diuretics may be used as well in order to help the kidneys eliminate excess fluid.

Perspective and Prospects

Proteinuria was first alluded to, although unnamed, by Hippocrates around 400 BCE when he described bubbly urine as a symptom of kidney disease. Over the next two thousand years, there were multiple allusions to foaming urine in the scientific and medical literature, indirectly linking it to kidney disease and to dropsy (tissue swelling because of retention of excessive amounts of fluid). In 1814, an English physician, John Blackall, published a book on dropsy in which he directly established a link between that condition and proteinuria (using the actual term). Shortly

---

Information on Proteinuria

Causes: Dehydration, fever, inflammatory process, medications, pregnancy-induced hypertension, hypertension, diabetes, glomerular disease

Symptoms: Foamy urine earlier in disease; edema in hands, feet, abdomen later in disease

Duration: Acute or chronic

Treatments: Medication (antihypertensives), treatment of underlying disorders

---

thereafter, fellow English physician Richard Bright published *Reports of Medical Cases* (1827), in which he identified edema and proteinuria as the major symptoms of nephritis (inflammation of the kidney, also known as Bright's disease). Since that time, proteinuria has been considered to be an early and major symptom of kidney disease.

—*Robin Kamienny Montvilo, R.N., Ph.D.*

See also Diuretics; End-stage renal disease; Hypertension; Kidney disorders; Kidney transplantation; Kidneys; Nephrectomy; Nephritis; Nephrology; Nephrology, pediatric; Polycystic kidney disease; Protein; Pyelonephritis; Renal failure; Urinalysis; Urinary disorders; Urinary system; Urology; Urology, pediatric.

For Further Information:

Brenner, Barry M., ed. *Brenner and Rector's The Kidney*. 9th ed. Philadelphia: Saunders/Elsevier, 2012.
Glassock, R. J. "Focus on Proteinuria." *American Journal of Nephrology* 10, suppl. 1 (1990): 88-93.
"Proteinuria." *National Kidney and Urologic Diseases Information Clearinghouse*, September 2, 2010.
Strasinger, Susan J., and Marjorie Schaub Di Lorenzo. *Urinalysis and Body Fluids*. 5th ed. Philadelphia: F. A. Davis, 2008.

Proteomics

Specialty

Anatomy or system affected: All

Specialties and related fields: All

Definition: The study of the proteome, the collective body of proteins expressed from genes at any given point in time in any given cell, tissue, or organism. Proteomes differ for each kind of organism and are quite dynamic, changing their protein composition in response to such factors as aging, diet, exercise, medication, and disease.

Key terms:

mass spectrometry: a very sensitive technique that accurately measures protein or peptide mass; proteins are then identified by matching this information to the predicted mass for proteins and peptides from all genes thought to encode protein and held within genomic databases

microarrays: miniature plastic or glass chips upon which tiny amounts of biological material are permanently spotted in a gridlike array; in proteomics, protein microarrays, holding thousands of individual protein samples, are used to test for drug binding, antibody binding for diagnostic test development, or interactions with other proteins to determine function

subproteomes: proteomes within proteomes, such as the mitochondrial proteome as a subproteome of a cell, which, in turn, is a subproteome of a tissue; subproteomes can be functionally defined and transient in nature, resulting from medications, exercise, and changes in diet

two-dimensional gel electrophoresis: a technique that can separate thousands of proteins in complex mixtures through a polyacrylamide gel matrix in two dimensions, first by isoelectric point and second by molecular weight

Methodologies

Proteomics focuses on developing a proteome profile for any given cell, tissue, or disease through three main perspectives. Functional (quantitative) proteomics aims to identify, quantify, and localize proteins within proteomes. Structural proteomics aims to develop a precise three-dimensional structure of each protein in normal and abnormal states, which is vital to clinical diagnostics and drug discovery. Mapping protein-protein interactions aims to understand how proteins interact with one another in complexes, forming networks and pathways of biological activity to understand how diseases originate and progress.

Proteome size, complexity, and dynamics are the current biggest challenges to proteomics. For this reason, this field is closely tied to technological advances. The use of robotic techniques has led to processing hundreds of thousands of extremely small samples every day, which is called high-throughput. To profile proteomes, they must first be isolated, their proteins separated and then purified through large-scale two-dimensional polyacrylamide gel electrophoresis and/or mass spectrometry. Protein structural information is then determined using protein sequencing, mass spectrometry, and/or x-ray crystallography. Assigning protein function within a proteome involves protein and/or antibody microarray analyses to determine biochemical pathway involvement and any protein-protein interactions. Typically, laboratories will specialize in one of these approaches. All laboratories, however, must be able to integrate the information that they find with the discoveries of others. The creation of databases that hold, organize, and link the massive amounts of proteomic information generated to genomic information has been made possible only through advances in bioinformatic computer technology.

Medicine and Proteomics

Most diseases create alterations in cellular function. Complex diseases such as cancer, heart disease, and diabetes cannot be treated effectively if the underlying cause and proteins responsible remain unknown. However, the current practice of biomedical research is unable to identify these changes or determine how they relate to disease processes quickly enough to develop the needed diagnostics and treatment. Identifying proteomic components that are specific for a disease (biomarkers) is a major effort of proteomic research. The aim is to develop diagnostic kits that detect the very early phase of a disease. Within populations, the diagnosis, prognosis, treatment, origins, and progression of a disease are public health issues overseen by

epidemiologists. Genetic epidemiology is a new discipline that is closely following proteomic progress to develop better public health policies and planning. Proteomics is also expected to identify targets for new drugs.

In the early stages of development, proteome profiling has already shown that the human cardiac proteome is reproducibly and uniquely altered for different heart diseases and disorders. Biomarkers specific to prostate and breast cancer have been identified. These first studies encouraged proteomic researchers to turn to disease proteomic profiling. Because most diseases create protein alterations in blood plasma long before symptoms appear, proteomic serum and plasma profiling is a major research effort. Researchers have identified a blood plasma proteomic profile for ovarian cancer that appears to predict the disease accurately. Other researchers have turned to the proteomic profiling of pathogens, such as antibiotic-resistant bacteria or those organisms causing malaria or stomach ulcers. The goal is to identify biomarkers for use as drug targets and for the development of diagnostic kits.

One promising application of proteomic technology is in the area of early detection of disease. Historically, the identification and examination of disease markers has been based on individual proteins, which is not always reliable. For example, the assay for prostate-specific antigen (PSA) is used to screen for prostate cancer, but levels of this antigen may also be raised in benign conditions of the prostate, and other unrelated conditions can lead to false-positive results for this screen. Thousands of small proteins can be analyzed simultaneously using proteomic microarrays, and these results may suggest patterns of disease that may be useful for early detection. The potential therefore exists to use a panel of diagnostic markers, rather than a single protein, to identify a given disease state more accurately.

Perspective and Prospects

The origins of proteomics can be traced to the technique of separating complex mixtures of proteins by two-dimensional polyacrylamide gel electrophoresis in the mid-1970s. Refinement of the technique and the addition of protein sequencing methods enabled identification of the separated proteins. In the 1990s, advances in mass spectrometry provided a highly accurate, sensitive analysis of proteins capable of handling thousands of samples.

The final impetus for proteomic research was a direct outcome of the technological advancements of the Human Genome Project, including microarray analyses, the concept of high-throughput, and a paradigm shift in biological science research. Paramount was the recognition that the protein products of a gene, not the gene itself, are responsible for cellular processes. It became clear that the function of proteins in cellular pathways and processes could not be deduced from the deoxyribonucleic acid (DNA) sequence alone. Efforts quickly turned to studying all proteins and their functions in the context of genetics and diseases. As an emerging discipline, proteomics represents a new research form that is more global and integrative than traditional protein research in the past, which concentrated on the study of single proteins.

Currently, the concern among researchers is the sequestering of data generated in proteomic research for private company use or through aggressive patenting of results. Because of the complexity of the research, it is considered necessary for all to share their data in a public forum. The Human Proteome Organization (HUPO) was created to orchestrate cooperative sharing of both private and academic research efforts. First and foremost is the recognition that research must focus on what constitutes a normal proteome before assessing disease states, including defining the range of variability in normal proteomes as a result of age, ethnicity, and physiology. HUPO considers the human serum, liver, and brain to be the most important organs for proteomic profiling in the hope that these studies will lead to new drugs, diagnostics, and a basic understanding of cellular function. In whatever form proteomics takes, it is expected to change the practice of medicine drastically.

—*Diane C. Rein, Ph.D., M.L.S.;*
updated by Jeffrey A. Knight, Ph.D.

See also Aging; Biochemistry; Bioinformatics; Biostatistics; Cells; Disease; DNA and RNA; Epidemiology; Genetic diseases; Genetics and inheritance; Genomics; Laboratory tests; Mutation; Preventive medicine; Protein.

For Further Information:

Berman, Helen M., David S. Goodsell, and Philip E. Bourne. "Protein Structures: From Famine to Feast." *American Scientist* 90, no. 4 (July/August, 2002): 350-51.

Campbell, A. Malcolm, and Laurie J. Heyer. *Discovering Genomics, Proteomics, and Bioinformatics.* 2d ed. San Francisco: Pearson/Benjamin Cummings, 2007.

Divan, Aysha, and Janice Royds. *Tools and Techniques in Biomolecular Science.* New York: Oxford University Press, 2013.

Dreger, Mathias. "Proteome Analysis at the Level of Subcellular Structures." *European Journal of Biochemistry* 270, no. 4 (February, 2003): 589-99.

Ezzell, Carol. "Proteins Rule." *Scientific American* 286, no. 4 (April, 2002): 40-47.

Fulton, Kelly M., and Susan M. Twine. *Immunoproteomics: Methods and Protocols.* New York: Humana Press, 2013.

Hanash, Sam. "Disease Proteomics." *Nature* 422, no. 6928 (March 13, 2003): 226-32.

Merrill, Stephen A., and Anne-Marie Mazza, eds. *Reaping the Benefits of Genomic and Proteomic Research: Intellectual Property Rights, Innovation, and Public Health.* Washington, D.C.: National Academies Press, 2006.

Neha, Sharma, and S. L. Harikumar. "Use of Genomics and Proteomics in Pharmaceutical Drug Discovery and Development." *International Journal of Pharmacy and Pharmaceutical Sciences* 5, no. 3 (July, 2013): 24-28.

Patterson, Scott D., and Ruedi H. Aebersold. "Proteomics: The First Decade and Beyond." *Nature Genetics,* supp. 33 (March, 2003): 311-23.

Pierce, Benjamin A. *Genetics Essentials: Concepts and Connections.* New York: W. H. Freeman, 2013.

Sali, Andrej, et al. "From Words to Literature in Structural Proteomics." *Nature* 422, no. 6928 (March 13, 2003): 216-25.

Sellers, Thomas A., and John R. Yates. "Review of Proteomics with Applications to Genetic Epidemiology." *Genetic Epidemiology* 24, no. 2 (February, 2003): 83-98.

Wulkuhle, Julia D., Lance A. Liotta, and Emanuel F. Petricoin. "Proteomic Applications for the Early Detection of Cancer." *Nature Reviews Cancer* 3, no. 4 (April, 2003): 267-75.

Protozoan diseases

Disease/Disorder

Anatomy or system affected: Gastrointestinal system
Specialties and related fields: Microbiology, public health
Definition: Disease caused by protozoa, a diverse group of free-living, unicellular animals that function as parasites.

Key terms:

excyst: The escape of the organism from a protective, thick-walled resting structure called a cyst that has been swallowed by parasite's host.

flagellate parasites: parasitic protozoa that move by means of a whip-like structure called a flagellum.

parasite: any organism that lives on or in another organism of another species, which is known as the host, and derives nutrition from the host.

protozoa: single-celled, eukaryotic organisms that are highly diverse and move by means of pseudopods, flagella, or cilia.

Causes and Symptoms

Protozoa exist in almost every ecological niche. As parasites, they infect all species of vertebrates and many invertebrates, adapting to nearly all available sites within their hosts' bodies. There are nearly sixty-six thousand known species of protozoa; half of these are represented in the fossil record, and about ten thousand of the living species are known to be parasitic. Unlike many other parasites, protozoa replicate within their hosts to produce hundreds of thousands of their kind within several days of infection. Because of their variety, adaptability, and reproductive rates, parasitic protozoa exert a major influence on human existence.

The phylum Protozoa is subdivided into four subphyla, but only the subphylum Sarcomastigophora is of real concern to humans. Within this subphylum are the twelve genera of parasitic protozoa that cause diseases in humans and their domestic animals, the most important of which are *Trypanosoma, Leishmania, Trichomonas, Entamoeba, Eimeria, Toxoplasma, Babesia, Theileria, Giardia,* and *Plasmodium.*

The most startling characteristic of parasitic protozoan diseases in humans is the sheer number of cases that exist. For example, a conservative estimate suggests at least two hundred million persons harbor the protozoan *Entamoeba,* which causes amebic dysentery. Of this number, approximately 50 million people, globally, suffer from amebic colitis or more invasive infections that have spread to other organs. One to two billion humans are estimated to be infected with *Toxoplasma,* the protozoan that cause toxoplasmosis. *Trypanosoma,* the agents of sleeping sickness and Chagas disease, infect fifteen to twenty million people worldwide; *Giardia,* two hundred million; and *Leishmania,* which are responsible for the disease kala-azar, one to two million. The most important of all protozoan diseases, said to be the greatest killer in history, is malaria, which is caused by the parasite *Plasmodium* and results in the death of two to three million people annually.

Protozoa that infect humans are commonly found in the

intestinal tract, various tissues and organs, and the bloodstream. Of the many protozoa that reside in the human gut, only invasive *Entamoeba histolytica* causes serious disease. *E. histolytica* parasites are transmitted by the ingestion of water contaminated with human feces that contain *E. histolytica* cysts that pass through the stomach and excyst in the small intestine to form trophozoites. The trophozoites invade the innermost layer of the colon and cause the disease amebiasis or, its severe form, amebic dysentery. If the disease spreads by way of intestinal veins to the liver, the result can be hepatic amebiasis, or the infection can spread to the lungs, heart or brain. Although the majority of *E. histolytica* infections produce no symptoms, it can produce highly invasive infections. Another waterborne intestinal protozoan familiar to campers and vacationers is the flagellate *Giardia lamblia*, which causes giardiasis. Giardiasis results in a mild-to-serious, long-lasting diarrhea. It is usually acquired from the ingestion of water fouled by animal waste. It can also be transmitted by human sources and, if the outbreak occurs in a closed population, frequently results in a rapidly spreading infection.

A few flagellate parasites infect the human skin, bloodstream, and viscera. The flagellate *Trypanosoma cruzi* is the agent of Chagas disease, a major cause of debilitation and chronic heart disease among poorly housed populations of Central and South America. *T. cruzi* is transmitted when the liquid feces of an insect (genus *Triatoma*) are scratched into the skin or rubbed in the eye. In Africa, the tsetse fly carries the parasitic agents of the disease trypanosomiasis, also known as African sleeping sickness. The disease is generated by the flagellate parasites *Trypanosoma brucei gambiense* and *T. brucei rhodesiense*, which infect the bloodstream and can be fatal if they cross the blood-brain barrier.

Parasitic flagellates of the genus *Leishmania* are transmitted by bloodsucking midges and sandflies and result in macrophage infection. Cutaneous leishmaniasis is characterized by infected macrophages in the skin, resulting in long-lasting skin lesions. A similar condition, mucocutaneous leishmaniasis, common to the Amazon Basin, begins as skin ulcers and often progresses to the destruction of nasal mucosa, cartilage, and soft facial and pharyngeal tissues. Visceral leishmaniasis, or kala-azar, infects the spleen, liver, bone marrow, and lymph nodes.

Only one species of ciliate protozoa is parasitic in humans: *Balantidium coli*, a free-living, large protozoan covered with rows of cilia. It is found in the large intestine, where it can cause the ulcerative disease balantidiasis. The group of protozoa known as sporozoans are all parasitic and include many deadly parasites of humans: *Isopora*, *Sarcocystis*, *Cryptosporidium*, and *Toxoplasma*. *Toxoplasmagondii*, the agent of toxoplasmosis, is of great medical concern. It is estimated to infect between 20 and 50 percent of the world's population, and it can penetrate the placenta and subsequently infect the fetus of pregnant women who lack the proper antibodies. The most important sporozoans, however, are the agents of malaria.

Information on Protozoan Diseases

Causes: Parasitic infection
Symptoms: Wide ranging; may include chills, fever, sweating, anemia, spleen enlargement, gastrointestinal disorders, skin lesions
Duration: Acute to chronic
Treatments: Drug therapy, supportive therapy

Malaria is a disease caused by a group of sporozoans in the genus *Plasmodium* that infect the human liver and red blood cells. Malaria is characterized by periodic chills, fever, and sweats, leading to anemia, enlargement of the spleen, and complications that result in death, especially among infants. The parasites are transmitted to humans by the bite of any of sixty species of infected *Anopheles* mosquitoes. The disease is found in all tropical and temperate regions, but control efforts have eliminated it from North America, Europe, and the northern Asian continent. Despite control efforts and effective medical treatments, malaria is historically the greatest killer all human infectious diseases, and it remains the single most dangerous threat to humankind from an infectious agent. More than one million children die of malaria in Africa yearly.

Treatment and Therapy

Treatment is generally by antiprotozoal agents, antibiotics, or both, with the specific agent or agents depending on the type of protozoa. Amebiasis treatments usually combine metronidazole or alternative agents (e.g., tinidazole, ornidazole, and nitazoxanide) with so-called "luminal agents," such as paromomycin, diiodohydroxyquin or diloxanide furonate to kill any cysts. *Giardia* infections are also treated with metronidazole, or tinidazole, nitazoxanide, albendazole, mebendazole, paromomycin, or quinacrine. *Trichomonas* infections are treated with metronidazole or tinidazole. Balantidiasis is treated with metronidazole, paromomycin, tinidazole or tetracycline. Toxoplasmosis is treated with pyrimethamine combined with either sulfadiazine, clindamycin, atovaquone, or azithromycin. Leucovorin is also prescribed to protect the bone marrow from the toxic effects of pyrimethamine. The drugs of choice to treat cryptosporidiosis are nitazoxanide or paromomycin.

Leishmaniasis treatments vary, depending on the region of world from which the infection was contracted. The available agents include pentavalent antimonials (sodium stibogluconate and meglumine antimoniate), which contain the metalloid antimony, paromomycin, amphotericin B, and a newer drug, miltefosine. An even newer drug, benznidazole, was approved by the FDA in August, 2017, for the treatment of Chagas disease.

Various treatments for malaria exist and vary according to the type of malaria and where it was contracted. Chloroquine is an effective treatment for *Plasmodium falciparum* infections in Haiti, the Dominican Republic, Central America west of the Panama Canal, and most of the Middle East. Outside of these regions, *P. falciparum* are resistant to chloroquine, and artemisinin-based combination therapies (ACTs) are used. For *P. vivax* or *P. ovale* infections (Mexico and Central America), primaquine is the drug of choice. Malaria infections acquired outside endemic areas (e.g., Southeast Asia) are treated with ACTs, quinine-based regimens, mefloquine, or atovaquone-proguanil. Prophylactic treatments, which are used to prevent travelers from being infected with malaria, include doxycycline, atovaquone-proguanil, mefloquine, chloroquine (for use only when traveling to regions with chloroquine-sensitive malaria), and primaquine for areas where *P. vivax* and *P. ovale* are endemic.

—*Randall L. Milstein, PhD;*
updated by Michael A. Buratovich, PhD

See also: Bites and stings; Chagas' disease; Diarrhea and dysentery; Epidemiology; Giardiasis; Insect-borne diseases; Leishmaniasis; Lice, mites, and ticks; Malaria; Microbiology; Parasitic diseases; Sleeping sickness; Toxoplasmosis; Trichomoniasis; Tropical medicine; Zoonoses.

For Further Information:

Behnke, Jerzy M., ed. *Parasites: Immunity and Pathology; The Consequences of Parasitic Infection in Mammals*. New York: Taylor & Francis, 1990.

Dhawan, Vinod K. "Amebiasis." *Medscape*, May 22, 2017.

Despommier, Dickson D., et al. *Parasitic Diseases*. 5th ed. New York: Apple Tree, 2006.

Engleberg, N. Cary, Victor DiRita, and Terence S. Dermody, eds. *Schaechter's Mechanisms of Microbial Disease*. 5th ed. Philadelphia: Lippincott Williams & Wilkins, 2013.

Frank, Steven A. *Immunology and Evolution of Infectious Disease*. Princeton, N.J.: Princeton University Press, 2002.

Gutteridge, W. E., and G. H. Coombs. *Biochemistry of Parasitic Protozoa*. Baltimore: University Park Press, 1977.

Herchline, Thomas E. "Malaria." *Medscape*, October 26, 2016.

Nazer, Hisham. "Giardiasis." *Medscape*, February 15, 2016.

Roberts, Larry S., John Janovy Jr., and Steve Nadler. *Gerald D. Schmidt and Larry S. Roberts' Foundations of Parasitology*. 9th ed. New York: McGraw-Hill, 2013.

Stark, Craig G. "Leishmaniosis." *Medscape*, May 15, 2017.

Psoriasis

Disease/Disorder

Anatomy or system affected: Skin

Specialties and related fields: Dermatology, internal medicine

Definition: A chronic skin disease in which red, scaly patches develop, overlaid with thick, silvery-gray scales, causing physical discomfort as well as damage to self-esteem.

Key terms:

dermatologist: a physician who treats the skin and its structures, functions, and diseases

dermis: the layer of skin directly beneath the epidermis, consisting of dense connective tissue and numerous blood vessels

epidermis: the outermost part of the skin, composed of four or five different layers called strata

methotrexate: a powerful drug, originally developed to treat cancer, that is used to treat patients with severe cases of psoriasis

psoralens: chemicals found in plants that make the skin more sensitive to light

PUVA: a treatment for psoriasis in which the patient is exposed to ultraviolet A (UVA) light after receiving one of the psoralens

stratum corneum: the outermost layer of the epidermis; its cells are normally dead, hard, and removed by normal bathing

ultraviolet light: invisible light composed of waves that are shorter than the ordinary light waves able to be seen by humans

Causes and Symptoms

Psoriasis is a common skin problem that afflicts approximately two of every hundred people, affecting males and females with relatively equal frequency. Although it affects all races, it is most prevalent among northern Europeans. This stubborn, chronic, and as yet incurable disease most commonly appears in one's teens or twenties, although it can appear in early childhood. While 70 percent of those who develop psoriasis do so by the age of twenty, there is another common danger period in the fifties and sixties, with a large number of patients developing their first symptoms at that time.

There are several different types of psoriasis, making diagnosis difficult. By far the most widespread is the plaque type; because it accounts for 95 percent of all cases, this type is also called common psoriasis. Plaque-type psoriasis gets its name from the appearance of the patches of affected skin. Each patch resembles a plaque or small disk stuck to the body's surface. These dull, wine-colored patches of abnormal skin are often rounded or oval; they may be very irregular in shape when several nearby patches join together. The surface of each thickened patch is rough and scaly, with the scales ranging in color from red to white to the most typical silvery gray. These psoriatic plaques can be small (the size of coins) or become palm-sized and larger. Whatever their final size, they generally begin as purple or reddened areas the size of a pinhead. The original areas expand in size, usually for a few weeks, until they reach a stable phase and stop expanding. The average size of a plaque in the stable phase is between two and three inches. A patch of stable psoriasis may eventually grow pale, become less scaly, and disappear completely, or it may begin to enlarge for no apparent reason. Even those plaques that have disappeared may be reactivated and reappear in the same place at some later time.

Certain parts of the body seem most prone to psoriatic lesions, namely the elbows, the knees, the scalp, and the lower back. The patches may appear elsewhere, including the genitals and the buttocks, but the face, hands, and feet are rarely affected. Severe cases may cover the entire chest or back. In a few cases, psoriasis is symmetrical, appearing in the same area on the left and right sides of the body simultaneously. The patches are, however, more likely to develop in a random, scattered manner. Almost 50 percent of patients with psoriasis have lesions on their scalps. When these plaques are very large and widespread, they are difficult to treat and very difficult to hide. Although very uncomfortable, scalp psoriasis does not affect the growth of hair or cause baldness. It can cause a temporary thinning of the hair, but the hair grows normally again once the disease is controlled by medication. About one-third of psoriasis patients have affected fingernails and toenails. The diseased nails show pits or pinpoint indentations, loosening, thickening, and a yellowish discoloration. Surprisingly, in some people the condition remains on the nails alone, never developing elsewhere.

In addition to psoriasis of the nails, there are several rare and unusual types of psoriasis that are quite different from the common or plaque type. These include flexural or inverse, guttate, pustular, and erythrodermic psoriasis. Flexural psoriasis appears in folds and creases on the body and is often found on people who are particularly overweight and who are in their mid-forties or older. The patches tend to be very moist rather than scaly and are particularly sore and uncomfortable. Guttable psoriasis consists of an enormous number of highly scattered but minute plaques. It is extremely rare and occurs between the ages of eight and sixteen. Although the spots usually clear up in a few weeks, they sometimes recur or change into the large lesions of common psoriasis. Pustular psoriasis is the only form of the disease that occurs on the palms of the hands or the soles of the feet. It was named for the yellow or white pus-filled spots that form on the skin and eventually drop off. These spots form when enormous numbers of white blood cells invade the skin even though there is no infection present and, therefore, no need for these infection-killing cells. Erythrodermic psoriasis literally means "red skin." This very rare condition is so named because the entire body is covered by flaming red patches that do not turn scaly. Since the extensive nature of this condition makes internal temperature control very difficult and dehydration inevitable, it can be very dangerous and may require hospitalization.

Common psoriasis, by comparison, is not dangerous or life-threatening. It is usually not painful and does not even cause itching in most patients. It is, however, very annoying because of its unsightly appearance and its tendency to flare up repeatedly. Once the disease has appeared, it stays with the person for life, improving or worsening periodically. After periods of relative quiet, during which the skin may appear quite normal, patients with psoriasis experience new eruptions and scaling for no apparent reason. Plaques continue to form for an unpredictable amount of time, until the condition spontaneously quiets down again.

The source of the plaques is a failure in the mechanism by which normal skin renews itself. Ordinarily, the cells at the base of the epidermis reproduce themselves at a slow and steady rate. They then move upward in about twenty-eight days, changing chemically, dying, and detaching from the surface, the stratum corneum. In psoriatic skin, however, there is a huge increase in the number of basal cells in the epidermis, which reproduce so rapidly that they push upward to the surface in only four days, forming thick disks of sticky, abnormal cells. Below the epidermis, the dermis of a patient with psoriasis is also abnormal. Its normally fine blood vessels are wide and extremely twisted, which results in the red appearance of the plaques and causes bleeding to occur easily when the skin is bumped or scratched. An unusually high number of the white blood cells called neutrophils and T lymphocytes are also present. They move up into the epidermis, creating inflammation and swelling within the plaques.

Long before modern dermatology discovered these disturbing facts about the structure and the functioning of psoriatic skin, it was noted that the disease does seem to run in families. If one parent has the problem, there is a one-in-three chance that a child will eventually be afflicted; if both parents have the disease, the risk for their offspring is one in two. With nonidentical twins, there is a 70 percent chance that if one has psoriasis, they both will; with identical twins, the figure can be as high as 90 percent, according to some studies. Investigators suspect that psoriasis is not handed down by a simple pattern, such as with eye color inheritance. It seems more likely that the condition results from a combination of several genetic factors from each parent, much like the manner in which height and intelligence are inherited.

Treatment and Therapy

More than 90 percent of psoriasis patients can be cleared significantly of their lesions or even made lesion-free by the medicines and methods developed by modern technology. For minor outbreaks, limited to a small area of the body, the first choice for treatment is a corticosteroid cream or ointment applied directly to the plaques. Corticosteroids are hormones, produced by the adrenal glands, that are able to reduce inflammation. Corticosteroids are produced in the laboratory and combined with other chemicals to reduce inflammation even more effectively by decreasing blood flow to the psoriatic lesions. Dermatologists have a large variety of such preparations ranging from mild to extremely potent. They must find one that is strong enough to suppress the inflammation but not so strong that it causes unwanted side effects.

There are two major undesirable side effects of corticosteroid therapy. Psoriatic skin absorbs all substances more easily than normal skin; the excess hormones enter the bloodstream and can change the output of hormones by the pituitary and adrenal glands, dangerously altering the body's chemical balance. The other danger is to the skin itself, which becomes abnormally thin, easily damaged, and prone to infections. Another drawback to the use of corticosteroids is the tendency for the psoriatic plaques to reappear soon after the creams or ointments are discontinued.

Many patients find relief from a completely different class of medications, those which contain tar. This thick, black, oily liquid is produced from coal. It contains thousands of chemical substances, and biochemists do not know which of those substances actually help to heal the skin. Tar-containing ointments, creams, gels, shampoos, and bath additives are useful for removing the scales without worrisome side effects. A major drawback, however, is their tendency to stain clothing, bedding, bathroom tiles, and bathtubs. Some staining can be avoided by covering the treated skin area with bandages, cotton underwear, or a shower cap. In addition to the staining, many patients find the tar odor quite unpleasant; pharmaceutical companies are constantly trying to improve this aspect of these quite effective products.

A third type of preparation is particularly effective for removing very thick scales. These medications contain a compound called salicylic acid. Like the corticosteroids, salicylic acid ointments and gels are most effective when they are in contact with the plaques for a long period of time. After treatment, it is often recommended that patients cover their lesions with plastic gloves, plastic bags (for the feet), or taped-down plastic wrap for four to eight hours.

Patients with psoriasis have noted for years that exposure to the sun is very helpful in clearing their lesions. Daily sunlight exposure is effective for as many as 80 percent of patients. This treatment is relatively accessible for at least part of the year and inexpensive compared to the various medications available. Given the increased risk of skin cancer, it is strongly recommended that patients have repeated but brief sun exposures and avoid sunburn by using creams and lotions. Although sun exposure is helpful to most patients with common psoriasis, it rarely helps and can even worsen the pustulate and erythrodermic types. Since too much exposure to sunlight will damage rather than help any skin, even plaque-type patients are advised to stop their sun exposure once the psoriasis has improved.

For patients in many climates, sunbathing is possible for only a few months of the year. The development of sunlamps for use at home or in a dermatologist's office, hospital, psoriasis care center, or tanning parlor has made this therapy possible all year round. Because of the danger of severe sunburns, sunlamp treatments remain controversial. To reduce their danger, a dermatologist must carefully determine the amount of time of each treatment, the precise distance from the lamp, and the appropriate frequency of treatments for each individual patient to achieve maximal and safe results.

The curative effect of sunlight depends on the presence of the very short wavelength part of the light, called ultraviolet. It is ultraviolet B (UVB) waves that help heal psoriasis, possibly by slowing down the high growth rate of cells in the epidermis. Both natural sunlight and sunlamps contain UVB and, therefore, have the potential to help psoriasis. They also have the potential, however, to burn the skin.

Patients with severe psoriasis may require the use of ultraviolet A (UVA) waves from a special kind of sunlamp. The patient is given a dose of a psoralen, a substance that makes the skin more light-sensitive, and is then exposed to UVA inside a full-body light cabinet. Thirty treatments may be required to completely clear the skin. The psoralen is often given in tablet form, although some patients suffer fewer side effects if it is painted onto the skin or if they bathe in it. The early side effects of PUVA (psoralen plus UVA) treatment include nausea, itching, colored blotches on the skin, and occasional worsening of the psoriasis. More worrisome are the possible later side effects: skin cancer and the development of cataracts in the eyes. The danger of developing cataracts also exists from natural sunlight and UVB sunlamps; patients using any light therapy must use excellent sunglasses that block out all rays harmful to the eyes.

For the patient with widespread psoriasis who is not responsive to corticosteroids, tar preparations, or the various light therapies, the drug methotrexate is effective in more than 80 percent of patients. This powerful drug was originally developed to treat various kinds of cancer because it slows down the process of cell multiplication. Thus the psoriatic epidermal cells are prevented from reproducing and forming the scaly plaques. Often methotrexate must be taken for six months or a year, in pill form or by injection, to have a significant impact on an extensive case. Such a dosage poses a risk of numerous and serious side effects, including persistent feelings of sickness, indigestion, and diarrhea. Frequent tests are necessary to monitor the condition of the blood, since methotrexate can interfere with the bone marrow's production of normal blood cells. Most important, periodic liver biopsies, the removal of sample liver cells by means of a special needle, are necessary because methotrexate can cause irreversible damage to this crucial organ. It is very important that a pregnant woman never take methotrexate or that a woman never become pregnant while taking it. The drug's ability to interfere with cell growth can cause many abnormalities in a developing embryo or fetus. Similar fetal abnormalities can be caused by the drugs called retinoids.

For patients with pustular and erythrodermic psoriasis, the retinoids etretinate and acitretin can be very useful, if side effects are carefully monitored. Some dermatologists have been especially successful combining PUVA and etretinate therapies; the improvement in the psoriasis is greater than with either alone, while the lower dosage of each minimizes risk and side effects.

Another medication effective in treating severe psoriasis is cyclosporine. It has brought dramatic improvement to patients with lifelong disabling symptoms. Many people, however, can tolerate the drug only for short periods. Because of its potential to cause high blood pressure and kidney damage, as well as an increased risk of cancer, this medicine is prescribed only with extreme caution.

All the many therapies described can bring partial or total clearing of lesions and even result in the remission of the disease for a period of time. Until the cause of psoriasis is completely understood, however, it is likely that no permanent cure will be developed.

Perspective and Prospects

Descriptions of psoriasis are found in the records of the earliest known civilizations. The term "psora" comes from the ancient Greek language. Psoriasis was considered a form of leprosy in biblical times. Despite this ancient history and extensive modern research, however, the exact cause of psoriasis is still unknown. Unlike many human diseases, psoriasis does not afflict any animals; therefore, it cannot be studied through controlled laboratory testing.

Early work on psoriasis by dermatologists centered on differential diagnosis. This is the ability to distinguish psoriasis from various rashes caused by fungi, such as ringworm, and from the many forms of eczema or dermatitis caused by allergies. Skin biopsies developed by oncologists can now determine that the condition is not a cancer; the portion of skin removed, when placed under a microscope, will clearly show the dermal and epidermal appearance characteristic of psoriatic skin.

While skin scientists have proven that psoriasis is not contagious, it has been known since the 1930s that many cases develop soon after strep throat and other upper respiratory infections. The bacteria involved are not the cause of the psoriasis, however, but rather a trigger for the development of a condition for which the patient is genetically predisposed. Another trigger, excessive scratching or rubbing of the skin, can precipitate outbreaks in susceptible people; this is named the Koebner phenomenon, for its discoverer. With the help of neurologists and psychologists, it has been proven that the disease is not caused by "nerves," yet stress of all kinds is definitely able to make its symptoms worse, and patients must be helped to lower their stress levels if they are to keep the disease under control.

Nutritionists have searched for ways to use diet to help psoriatics, but to no avail. Although no particular foods either help or hinder the course of the disease, most dermatologists now recognize that drinking alcohol can both precipitate and aggravate the disfiguring plaques.

Immunologists have been very involved in the study of psoriasis even though it is not an allergic reaction to any substance in one's environment. In the late twentieth century, they pursued many possible connections between the streptococci bacteria that cause strep throat, the white blood cells called T lymphocytes that seek to destroy them, and the development of psoriasis. They believe that, in predisposed people, chemicals from the bacteria cause the T lymphocytes to give off substances that trigger the skin's uncontrolled and excessive production of epidermal cells.

Geneticists have been searching diligently for the source of the predisposition to psoriasis. Among the genes children receive from their parents are those that build particular proteins on their white blood cells called human leukocyte antigens (HLAs). Out of the hundreds of different HLAs that one can possibly inherit, those who develop psoriasis always seem to possess similar combinations. The identification of the genes responsible for HLAs and the role of those genes in precipitating psoriasis may bring about major improvements in the treatment and possibly a cure for this disease afflicting millions of people throughout the world.

—*Grace D. Matzen*

See also Dermatitis; Dermatology; Eczema; Lesions; Light therapy; Rashes; Scabies; Skin; Skin disorders; Skin lesion removal.

For Further Information:

"An Overview of Psoriasis and Psoriatic Arthritis." *National Psoriasis Foundation*, Feb. 2011.

"About Psoriasis." *National Psoriasis Foundation*, 2013.

Camisa, Charles. *Handbook of Psoriasis.* 2d ed. Hoboken, N.J.: John Wiley & Sons, 2004.

Cram, David L. *Coping with Psoriasis: A Patient's Guide to Treatment.* Omaha, Nebr.: Addicus Books, 2000.

Freinkel, Ruth K., and David T. Woodley. *Biology of the Skin.* New York: Parthenon, 2001.

Mackie, Rona M. *Clinical Dermatology.* 5th ed. New York: Oxford University Press, 2003.

Marks, Ronald. *Psoriasis.* 2d rev. ed. London: Sheldon Press, 1994.

Parker, James N., and Philip M. Parker, eds. *The Official Patient's Sourcebook on Psoriasis.* San Diego, Calif.: Icon Health, 2004.

"Psoriasis." *MedlinePlus*, May 6, 2013.

Shuman, Jill, and Purvee S. Shah. "Psoriasis." *Health Library*, Feb. 25, 2013.

Turkington, Carol, and Jeffrey S. Dover. *The Encyclopedia of Skin and Skin Disorders.* 3d ed. New York: Facts On File, 2007.

Weedon, David. *Skin Pathology.* 3d ed. New York: Churchill Livingstone/Elsevier, 2010.

"What Is Psoriasis?" *National Institute of Arthritis and Musculoskeletal and Skin Diseases*, Sept. 2009.

Psychiatric disorders

Disease/Disorder

Anatomy or system affected: Brain, psychic-emotional system

Specialties and related fields: Psychiatry

Definition: Clusters of psychological or behavioral symptoms that cause a person to experience serious emotional distress or significant mental impairment; these symptoms must be unusual or unexpected, or the patient must show evidence of more than one behavior that deviates from normal social expectations.

Key terms:

biomedical model: a way of viewing and understanding psychiatric disorders which emphasizes customary medical practice in identifying and treating a particular disorder from which a person suffers

diagnostic codes: the method used in the *Diagnostic and Statistical Manual of Mental Disorders* (DSM) to record psychiatric diagnoses for statistical and administrative purposes

multiaxial classification: the classification system used in the DSM to account for several factors when making psychiatric diagnoses, including present condition, developmental/personality disorders, physical disorders, life stresses, and overall functioning

neuroscience: the scientific specialization that seeks to understand mental processes, occurrences, and disturbances in terms of underlying mechanisms in the brain and the nervous system

psychodynamic model: a way of viewing and understanding psychiatric disorders which emphasizes the recognition and treatment of underlying psychological and developmental traumas

psychopharmacology: the use of drugs to study effects on brain chemistry; drugs are used to treat mental disorders, study brain chemistry, and promote new disease classifications

psychosocial treatment: a significant specialization in treating people with psychiatric disorders through employing principles of psychology, human behavior, family and group dynamics, and social and occupational learning

somatic treatment: the treatment of people with psychiatric disorders using specialized drugs and electroconvulsive therapy; some major drug groups used are antidepressants, antipsychotics, antimanics, anxiolytics, and psychostimulants

Causes and Symptoms

Many centuries ago, physicians began to understand that psychiatric disorders such as depression arose from abnormalities in brain structure or chemistry. As the field of psychiatry developed, medicine has had a profound influence in establishing the biomedical model to define and treat mental disorders. Sigmund Freud and other influential psychiatrists working in the late nineteenth century broadened the understanding of how emotional pain and trauma experienced during a person's childhood can contribute profoundly to the occurrence and course of mental disorders. The medical influence on the field of psychiatry was deepened and broadened by the contribution of neuroscience. Scientists who began studying the brain more intensively, beginning in the early twentieth century, proved the relationship of brain function to speech, learning, comprehension, memory, emotional regulation, and other important human abilities. Technologies developed in the late twentieth century, such as functional magnetic resonance imaging (fMRI) and genetic testing, have furthered psychiatrists' understanding of the biological, genetic, and neurological basis of a number of mental disorders.

Despite long and exacting efforts to understand mental illness, much remains to be explored. While psychiatrists would prefer to base their diagnoses on knowing the causes and the biological or neurological mechanisms of mental disorders, this knowledge has proved to be elusive. Therefore, most psychiatric diagnoses are based on the psychiatrist recognizing a pattern of symptoms and a typical course of disease. During World War II, psychiatrists realized that their colleagues differed widely in how they recognized and described various mental illnesses. Bureaucratic and professional forces coalesced in a drive to make the diagnosis of psychiatric disorders more systematic. In 1952, the American Psychiatric Association issued a manual that sought to clarify the diagnostic process. Unfortunately, the early manuals proved to be impractical and were largely ignored by psychiatrists. This changed when a more rigorous effort culminated in the publication of the third edition of the *Diagnostic and Statistical Manual of Mental Disorders* (DSM-III) in 1980. This text became widely accepted as the standard reference for psychiatrists to use when diagnosing psychiatric disorders. The manual has been strengthened and revised several times; a fifth edition,

known as DSM-5, was published in 2013. Scientists and clinicians continue their work on the manual to correct flaws, incorporate research findings, and explore new areas. However, shortly before the publication of the DSM-5 in May 2013, the US National Institute of Mental Health issued a statement condemning the DMS-5's "lack of validity," noting that "DSM diagnoses are based on a consensus about clusters of clinical symptoms, not any objective laboratory measure." While psychiatrists agree that standard definitions of psychiatric disorders are needed to clarify their thinking, permit easier communication, improve treatment planning, and stimulate further research, a growing number of psychologists recognize the need for more accurate diagnostic criteria that are based on genetic, neurophysiological, and biological measures. While psychiatrists agree that a more accurate diagnostic system based on biomarkers is needed, the technology and research to establish such diagnostic criteria are not yet available. Therefore, the symptom-based diagnostic criteria put forth in the DSM-5 remain the most widely used in the field of psychiatry.

When using the DSM-5, psychiatrists must find that the person exhibits specific signs and symptoms and has maintained this clinical picture for a sufficient length of time to warrant being diagnosed with a psychiatric disorder. The DSM-5 assigns a specific code for each psychiatric diagnosis, which facilitates administrative and statistical work. The diagnostic codes in the DSM-5 are compatible with the coding system used in the ninth edition of the International Classification of Diseases (ICD-9-CM), published by the World Health Organization. This coding system uses five-digit numerical codes. Contributing environmental factors are represented in the DSM-5 through an expanded set of ICD-9-CM codes, which provide clinicians with a way to indicate other issues that are affecting the presentation or course of treatment of the primary mental disorder. The tenth edition of the International Classification of Diseases (ICD-10-CM) is scheduled to be released in 2014. The ICD-10-CM coding system uses a combination of letters and numbers in its codes, and the DSM-5 contains both the ICD-9-CM and the ICD-10-CM coding systems to facilitate the transition to the ICD-10-CM coding system.

Furthermore, the DSM-5 combined the first three axes of the multiaxial diagnostic system used in the fourth edition of the DSM (DSM-IV-TR) into one list that includes all disorders. The DSM-IV-TR had listed clinical disorders on five separate axes, with Axis I referring to the principal disorder, Axis II indicating any additional personality disorder that might affect the Axis I disorder, Axis III indicating any medical problems that might affect the presentation or treatment of the principal disorder; Axis IV noting any psychosocial or contextual factors, and Axis V noting any disability. The DSM-5 introduced a nonaxial diagnostic system, combining Axes I, II, and III into one list, with an expanded set of ICD-9-CM codes to note any psychosocial or environmental factors and disability (formerly Axes IV and V).

Several major diagnostic categories of psychiatric disor-

Information on Psychiatric Disorders

Causes: Genetic and environmental factors, medications, substance abuse

Symptoms: Wide ranging; may include emotional distress, mental impairment, abrupt changes in mood or personality, anxiety, depression, manic behavior, substance abuse, difficulty sleeping

Duration: Acute to chronic

Treatments: Depends on type and severity; may include drug, psychosocial, somatic, and adjunctive therapies

ders are shown in the DSM-5. These include neurodevelopmental disorders; schizophrenia spectrum and other psychotic disorders; bipolar and related disorders; depressive disorders; anxiety disorders; obsessive-compulsive and related disorders; trauma- and stressor-related disorders; dissociative disorders; somatic symptom and related disorders; feeding and eating disorders; sleep-wake disorders; sexual dysfunctions; gender dysphoria; disruptive, impulse-control, and conduct disorders; substance-related and addictive disorders; neurocognitive disorders; and paraphilic disorders. This listing demonstrates the breadth of problems that are seen and treated by psychiatrists and other mental health practitioners.

Research shows that, on average, 26.2 percent of adults in the United States will experience one or more psychiatric disorders in a given year. Globally, approximately 10 percent of the adult population will have a psychiatric disorder, although psychologists believe the actual rates of mental illness are underreported in many developing countries. The most common disorders are anxiety disorders and mood disorders, such as depression.

Researchers learned that people who experience their first symptoms later in life generally have a better chance of recovering, but almost all people who suffer from a psychiatric disorder will experience distressing symptoms for several years. More men than women, the data show, have suffered a psychiatric disorder at some point in life, although women are more likely than men to experience anxiety or mood disorders. According to researchers, the differences in prevalence among the races may be more reflective of survey methods than of ethnic origins. Higher rates of mental illness are found among people who are poor and who fail to complete high school. People who suffer from one psychiatric disorder were found by researchers to be at a high risk (60 percent) for having another mental health disorder at some time during their lives.

Treatment and Therapy

Making an accurate diagnosis of psychiatric disorders is essential to treating problems properly, since many can be improved through the application of psychosocial, somatic, drug, and adjunctive therapies. For example, it is said that most people who suffer from major depression can be treated successfully with brief psychotherapy, a course of medication, or a combination of both. The somatic technique of exposing a person each day to a bank of bright lights (light therapy) has been used successfully to treat seasonal affective disorder (depression associated with a specific season, especially winter). Many depressed people and their families have been helped by the adjunctive therapy of participating in a support group.

The use of laboratory tests to clarify psychiatric diagnosis is growing in importance. Only a few disorders can be revealed by laboratory tests, but research is being conducted to validate such testing and to increase its scope and usefulness. Some tests are done routinely to rule out medical problems that may be causing the psychiatric problems the person is experiencing or to ensure that the patient can take needed medication.

Drugs have been used in the United States to treat psychiatric disorders since the early 1950s, and new medications are introduced frequently. The distressing thought disturbances experienced by people suffering from schizophrenia have been treated with antipsychotic drugs. Antipsychotics also are used to treat psychotic symptoms such as the hallucinations and delusions experienced by some people who are suffering from depression or other mood disorders. Several classes of antipsychotics have been developed. Lithium carbonate is the drug most commonly used to treat people suffering from bipolar disorders, in which patients experience swings in mood from the highs of mania to the lows of depression. Various classes of antidepressants such as tricyclics and monoamine oxidase inhibitors (MAOIs) are used to treat people suffering from depression. Many people experiencing symptoms associated with anxiety disorders have been helped through the use of benzodiazepines and other anxiolytics. Central nervous system stimulants (psychostimulants) are used to treat narcolepsy, a disorder in which people have trouble staying awake. Psychostimulants also are used to treat attention-deficit disorder (ADD), because the stimulants have the paradoxical effect of reducing the behaviors that disrupt classroom work and life at home. The drugs decrease excessive physical activity and have been shown to improve an individual's attention to adult guidance, increase attention span and memory, and lessen the individual's tendency to be distracted from tasks and to act impulsively. The person with ADD also is helped with behavior management techniques and careful control of the environment to reduce sources of external stimulation.

Unfortunately, the use of drugs in treating psychiatric disorders is not problem-free. Almost all psychopharmaceuti- cals have side effects that can be serious enough to prevent their use in treatment. A growing number of psychiatrists have expressed their concern over what they believe to be widespread overdiagnosis and overtreatment for psychiatric disorders in the United States; many patients respond well to simple lifestyle changes, such as increased physical activity or brief therapeutic interventions, so psychiatrists should prescribe psychopharmaceutical medications judiciously. Some people must take other prescription drugs that preclude the use of the drug needed to treat the psychiatric disorder. The possibility of overdose by people who have thoughts of taking their lives can limit the use of possibly toxic drugs. Some people are not helped by drug therapy, are reluctant to take drugs, or fail to take drugs properly. For such people, it is fortunate that other forms of treatment can be used.

Many people who suffer from psychiatric illness have been helped by trained psychotherapists, such as psychiatrists, psychologists, social workers, counselors, and members of the clergy. Many forms of psychotherapy are practiced. The aims of psychotherapy can be to help the person deal well with life's stresses and crises, confront and resolve psychological conflict, avoid interpersonal problems, and find more satisfaction and fulfillment in life. Psychotherapy is delivered to individuals, couples, families, and other groups. More emphasis is being placed on conducting psychotherapy only for a limited time, because this approach is preferred by most patients and their insurance companies and because research results support its effectiveness.

Behavioral therapy can be used to help the person to change specific behaviors that cause problems. Behavioral therapy has been used to treat several psychiatric disorders, including alcohol and drug dependence, anxiety, phobias, autism spectrum disorders, and eating disorders. Systematic desensitization has been used to help people who have irrational fears, or phobias. The patient is gradually introduced to the situation that elicits the fearful response and is taught to use relaxation techniques to reduce anxiety and to bring fears under personal control. In behavior modification programs, unwanted behavior is defined, targeted, reduced, and eliminated. At the same time, the person is rewarded for behaving properly.

Electroconvulsive therapy (ECT), formerly called shock therapy, is used generally to treat people with severe depression who have not responded to less intrusive treatment methods. In ECT, the patient is exposed to an electric current that is passed through electrodes taped to the scalp. The current causes the person to experience a brief seizure, usually for less than a minute. This treatment method has been used for many years, and several improvements have been made to make the procedure safer and less damaging to the person's memory.

Treatment of psychiatric disorders is usually delivered in the community where the affected person lives. In the United States, legislation in the 1960s caused federal funds to be used to build and staff community mental health centers. Many health insurance providers will pay part of the fees charged by private therapists, which allows some people to afford their services. Alcohol and drug treatment programs generally offer people either short-term residential or outpatient services. Many people are served in institutional settings, such as mental hospitals and nursing homes. Some use services provided by governmental funding.

Many people who have suffered psychiatric disorders recover completely; investigators find a 38 percent remission rate. The researchers were surprised to learn that people are most likely to recover from alcohol and drug abuse, gener-

alized anxiety, and antisocial personality. Complete freedom from distressing symptoms and episodes is less likely for those who suffer from mania, obsessive-compulsive disorder (in which the person performs repetitive rituals to allay anxiety caused by disturbing thoughts or fears), and schizophrenia (a disorder typified by thought disturbances such as hallucinations and delusions, mood changes, communication problems, and unusual behaviors). However, with a combination of pharmacological and psychosocial treatments and interventions, 70 to 90 percent of patients with psychiatric disorders experience a reduction of symptoms and improved quality of life, even without achieving full remission.

A large number of people who suffer mental illness have never been treated. Researchers estimate the economic cost of untreated psychiatric disorders in the United States to be more than $100 billion each year.

Perspective and Prospects

Early medical documents show that mental illness has always been an area of significant concern. Symptoms of mental illness were described in the Bible, and they were studied and treated in classical times. Interest in understanding mental disorders waned during the medieval period, when it was thought that sufferers were possessed by demons or were being punished by God. Mentally ill people were often maltreated and incarcerated. Finally, the foundation was laid in the late sixteenth century for a more complete understanding of psychiatric disorders: In 1586, Timothy Bright, a physician, published the first English-language text on mental illness, entitled *Treatise of Melancholie*.

In late eighteenth-century France, Philippe Pinel took over the management of a hospital for insane men and not only advocated more humane treatment of mentally ill people but also took steps to free them from the chains and other punishing devices that they were forced to endure. Pinel instituted the scientific study of mental illness. He tracked the prevalence of mental disorders, conducted studies to learn the natural course of mental illness, and established a treatment model followed by the more progressive psychiatric facilities.

The brain was studied even more intensely in the nineteenth century. During this era, scientists made important contributions to the understanding of how certain parts of the brain are responsible for specialized functions. They learned that particular brain regions are related to speech and language, movement, sensations, learning, understanding, and emotions. Emil Kraepelin correlated information about the age of onset, natural course, and length of time of particular mental disorders. He used the information that he organized to develop the first classification system of psychiatric disorders. Among the maladies he named were dementia praecox (now called schizophrenia), dementia in the elderly (now called Alzheimer's disease), and manic-depressive illness (bipolar disorder).

While neuroscientists were making significant contributions to the understanding of the brain, psychiatrist

Sigmund Freud was advancing his study of hysteria and its connection with childhood trauma. He used hypnosis and free association to release and resolve underlying misconceptions and fears and to give the patient relief from debilitating trauma and its associated symptoms. He also produced theories on psychological function and structure and on psychotherapy.

During the twentieth century, psychiatrists drew on a broad array of disciplines to improve the diagnosis and treatment of psychiatric disorders, including the study of brain chemistry, biology, structure, and functioning. Advances in neuroimaging techniques allowed scientists to study and sometimes diagnose brain dysfunction. Specialized drugs were developed to be used in the treatment of specific mental disorders. Since 1952, the American Psychiatric Association has published a series of diagnostic and statistical manuals designed to bring order to the study, diagnosis, and treatment of psychiatric disorders. Psychiatrists continue to work toward developing more accurate diagnostic criteria and more effective treatments for psychiatric disorders.

—Russell Williams, M.S.W.;
updated by Nancy A. Piotrowski, Ph.D.

See also Addiction; Alcoholism; Alzheimer's disease; Amnesia; Antianxiety drugs; Antidepressants; Anxiety; Asperger's syndrome; Autism; Bipolar disorders; Body dysmorphic disorder; Brain; Brain damage; Delusions; Dementias; Depression; Domestic violence; Eating disorders; Emotions: Biomedical causes and effects; Factitious disorders; Frontotemporal dementia (FTD); Gender identity disorder; Geriatrics and gerontology; Grief and guilt; Hallucinations; Hypochondriasis; Intoxication; Light therapy; Memory loss; Midlife crisis; Morgellons disease; Neurology; Neurology, pediatric; Neurosis; Neurosurgery; Obsessive-compulsive disorder; Panic attacks; Paranoia; Pharmacology; Phobias; Pick's disease; Postpartum depression; Post-traumatic stress disorder; Prader-Willi syndrome; Prescription drug abuse; Psychiatry; Psychiatry, child and adolescent; Psychiatry, geriatric; Psychoanalysis; Psychosis; Psychosomatic disorders; Schizophrenia; Seasonal affective disorder; Sexual dysfunction; Sexuality; Shock therapy; Sibling rivalry; Stress; Stuttering; Substance abuse; Suicide.

For Further Information:
American Psychiatric Association. *Diagnostic and Statistical Manual of Mental Disorders.* 5th ed. Arlington, Va.: American Psychiatric Association, 2013.
Black, Donald W., and Nancy C. Andreasen. *Introductory Textbook of Psychiatry.* 5th ed. Washington, D.C.: American Psychiatric Press, 2010.
North, Carol S., and Sean H. Yutzy. *Goodwin and Guze's Psychiatric Diagnosis.* 6th ed. New York: Oxford University Press, 2010.
Insel, Thomas. "Transforming Diagnosis." *National Institute of Mental Health*, April 29, 2013.
Kring, Ann M., et al. *Abnormal Psychology.* 11th ed. Hoboken, N.J.: John Wiley & Sons, 2010.
Oltmanns, Thomas F., et al. *Case Studies in Abnormal Psychology.* 9th ed. Hoboken, N.J.: John Wiley & Sons, 2012.
Sadock, Benjamin J., Virginia A. Sadock, and Pedro Ruiz, eds. *Kaplan and Sadock's Comprehensive Textbook of Psychiatry.* 9th ed. Philadelphia: Lippincott Williams & Wilkins, 2009.

Psychiatry
Specialty
Anatomy or system affected: All
Specialties and related fields: Critical care, family medicine, geriatrics and gerontology, neurology, pharmacology, preventive medicine, public health
Definition: A medical field concerned with the diagnosis, epidemiology, prevention, and treatment of mental and emotional problems.
Key terms:
anxiety disorders: conditions in which physical and emotional uneasiness, apprehension, or fear is the dominant symptom
bipolar disorders: problems marked by mania or mania with depression; historically known as manic-depressive disorders
dementias: disorders characterized by a general deterioration of intellectual and emotional functioning, involving problems with memory, judgment, emotional responses, and personality changes
depressive disorders: problems involving persistent feelings of despair, weight change, sleep problems, thoughts of death, thinking difficulties, diminished interest or pleasure in activities, and agitation or listlessness
personality disorders: pervasive, inflexible patterns of perceiving, thinking, and behaving that cause long-term distress or impairment, beginning in adolescence and persisting into adulthood
psychiatric diagnosis: a clinical labeling process involving the focused study of symptom patterns; physical, emotional, and personality factors; significant relationships; and recent events
psychotic: referring to a disabling mental state characterized by poor reality testing (inaccurate perceptions, confusion, disorientation) and disorganized speech, behavior, and emotional experience
psychotropic drugs: substances primarily affecting behavior, perception, and other psychological functions
schizophrenic disorders: mental disturbances characterized by psychotic features during the active phase and deteriorated functioning in occupational, social, or self-care abilities

Science and Profession
Psychiatrists receive training in biochemistry, community mental health, genetics, neurology, neuropathology, psychopathology, psychopharmacology, and social science. They complete medical school, a four-year residency in psychiatry, and two or more years of specialty residency. Specialty residencies focus on particular treatment methods (such as psychoanalysis) or methods of diagnosis and treatment for particular groups of clients (such as children, adolescents, or elders).

As diagnosticians and treatment providers, psychiatrists must be excellent observers of behavior and be knowledgeable about how nutritional, physical, and situational conditions can be related to mental or emotional problems. An ability to consult with other professionals is also important. Psychiatrists often receive patients from other professionals (general practitioners, psychologists, emergency room staff) and often request diagnostic, legal, case management, and resource advice from other professionals (psychologists, attorneys, social workers). In situations involving abuse, neglect, incompetency, and suicide, such consultation relationships are critical for appropriate referral and treatment.

Given this preparation, psychiatrists are able to diagnose and treat a wide variety of disorders. Some of the most common disorders treated in adult populations include disorders of anxiety (such as phobias, panic attacks, obsessive-compulsive behavior, acute and post-traumatic stress) and mood (such as depressive and bipolar problems). Personality, schizophrenic, substance abuse, and dementia-related disorders also are treated frequently by psychiatrists. Such conditions are described in detail in the American Psychiatric Association's (APA's) *Diagnostic and Statistical Manual of Mental Disorders: DSM-5* (2013).

Diagnostic and Treatment Techniques

A well-formulated psychiatric diagnosis facilitates treatment planning for mental and emotional disorders. Psychiatric diagnoses, however, are very complex. Previously, the APA used a axial system to diagnose psychiatric disorders. Axis I pertained to clinical conditions diagnosed in infancy, childhood, or adolescence; Axis II summarized problems related to personality and intellectual disability; and Axis III described any general medical conditions that are related to a person's mental problems and that may also warrant special attention. However, in *DSM-5* these axes are grouped by chapter. In *DSM-IV* Axis IV summarized psychological, social, and environmental problems that may affect the diagnosis, prognosis, or treatment of a person's mental problems. Axis V was used to give a standardized, overall rating of how well the person was functioning with his or her disorder; this axis has been dropped entirely.

Once a diagnosis is formulated, a treatment plan is composed. Usually, it involves some combination of medicinal and psychotropic drugs, bibliotherapy, dietary and behavior change recommendations, and psychotherapy for the affected individual and possibly members of his or her family. Treatment compliance is critical, particularly when psychotropic drugs are involved. As such, psychiatric treatment often involves frequent contacts and an aftercare plan of continued visits with the psychiatrist or a support group able to encourage follow-through on the treatment recommendations.

Perspective and Prospects

The concepts of mental health and illness have been in human cultures since ancient times. As early as 2980 BCE, priest-physicians were noted for their treatment of spirit possession involving madness, violence, mutism, and melancholy. In those times, such problems were thought to originate from external, supernatural forces. Later, during the rise of Greco-Roman philosophies in medicine, such states of mind began to be explored more as disturbances of the brain and less as the result of supernatural causes. As such, treatments began to develop greater reliance on methods such as vapors, baths, diets, and emetic and cathartic drugs.

Over time, the field of psychiatry has matured and taken on a major role in medicine. Research into the mind-body relationship has clarified how the mind can influence the healing of medical conditions, as well as how certain medical conditions are rooted in psychological, social, and environmental problems, rather than in a person's biology alone. Additionally, advances in the development of psychotropic drugs have played a major role in the treatment of disabling conditions long thought to be untreatable, such as schizophrenic and bipolar disorders.

In the future, psychiatry is expected to continue developing a broad variety of specialty areas. New techniques for working with children, adolescents, elders, and individuals with particular medical problems or of a particular gender or cultural background are developing rapidly. Finally, understanding the relationship between psychiatric disorders across the life span is likely to increase, as is the need to develop treatments for complex scenarios involving multiple diagnoses.

—*Nancy A. Piotrowski, Ph.D.*

See also Addiction; Aging; Aging: Extended care; Alcoholism; Alzheimer's disease; Amnesia; Anorexia nervosa; Antianxiety drugs; Antidepressants; Anxiety; Asperger's syndrome; Attention-deficit disorder (ADD); Autism; Bipolar disorders; Body dysmorphic disorder; Brain; Brain damage; Brain disorders; Bulimia; Chronic fatigue syndrome; Circumcision, female, and genital mutilation; Delusions; Dementias; Depression; Domestic violence; Eating disorders; Electroencephalography (EEG); Emergency medicine; Emotions: Biomedical causes and effects; Euthanasia; Factitious disorders; Family medicine; Fatigue; Frontotemporal dementia (FTD); Gender identity disorder; Gender reassignment surgery; Geriatrics and gerontology; Grief and guilt; Hallucinations; Hypnosis; Hypochondriasis; Incontinence; Intellectual disability; Intoxication; Light therapy; Memory loss; Midlife crisis; Neurology; Neurology, pediatric; Neurosis; Neurosurgery; Obesity; Obsessive-compulsive disorder; Panic attacks; Paranoia; Pharmacology; Phobias; Pick's disease; Postpartum depression; Post-traumatic stress disorder; Prader-Willi syndrome; Prescription drug abuse; Psychiatric disorders; Psychiatry, child and adolescent; Psychiatry, geriatric; Psychoanalysis; Psychosis; Psychosomatic disorders; Schizophrenia; Seasonal affective disorder; Sexual dysfunction; Sexuality; Shock therapy; Sleep disorders; Speech disorders; Stress; Stress reduction; Substance abuse; Sudden infant death syndrome (SIDS); Suicide; Terminally ill: Extended care.

For Further Information:

American Psychiatric Association. *Diagnostic and Statistical Manual of Mental Disorders: DSM-5*. Arlington, Va.: Author, 2013.

Andreasen, Nancy C., and Donald W. Black. *Introductory Textbook of Psychiatry*. 5th ed. Washington, D.C.: American Psychiatric Press, 2011.

Kring, Ann M., et al. *Abnormal Psychology*. 12th ed. Hoboken, N.J.: John Wiley & Sons, 2012.

Mazure, Carolyn M., ed. *Does Stress Cause Psychiatric Illness?* Washington, D.C.: American Psychiatric Press, 1995.

Muskin, Philip R., Patricia L. Gerbarg, and Richard P. Brown. *Complementary and Integrative Therapies for Psychiatric Disorders*. Philadelphia: Saunders, 2013.

Preston, John, and James Johnson. *Clinical Psychopharmacology Made Ridiculously Simple*. 7th ed. Miami: MedMaster, 2012.

Sadock, Benjamin J., and Virginia A. Sadock, eds. *Kaplan and Sadock's Comprehensive Textbook of Psychiatry*. 9th ed. Philadelphia: Lippincott Williams & Wilkins, 2009.

Semple, David, and Roger Smyth. *Oxford Handbook of Psychiatry*. New York: Oxford University Press, 2013.

Tomb, David. *Psychiatry*. 7th ed. Philadelphia: Wolters Kluwer/Lippincott Williams & Wilkins, 2008.

Psychiatry, child and adolescent

Specialty

Anatomy or system affected: Brain

Specialties and related fields: Psychiatry, child and adolescent psychology, neuroscience (brain research)

Definition: Subspecialty of psychiatry focusing on the diagnosis and treatment of disorders affecting thinking, emotions and behavior of children and adolescents

Key terms:

pathophysiology: biological processes that lead to the development of a disease

cognitive behavioral therapy: psychotherapy which aims to change distorted ways of thinking in order to improve behavior and mood; usually relatively short-term and focused

dialectical behavior therapy: psychotherapy which encourages older adolescents to take responsibility for their own problems and learn how to manage intense emotions

family therapy: psychotherapy which identifies and manages issues in the family and their interactions with the patient

interpersonal therapy: psychotherapy which focuses on improving interpersonal relationships

play therapy: psychotherapy which uses tools such as drawing, toys and dolls to help children understand and control their feelings and thoughts

psychodynamic psychotherapy: psychotherapy which focuses on understanding the motivating factors behind a child's behavior and feelings

Science and Profession

In the United States, child and adolescent psychiatrists must undergo three years of residency training after medical school in general psychiatry and neurology, followed by a further two years of specialty training in child and adolescent psychiatry.

The general psychiatry training includes in-depth study of the structure and function of the brain as well as neurological processes; epidemiology, genetics, and pathophysiology of psychiatric disorders; and treatments (including cognitive behavioral therapy and psychiatric drugs). The child and adolescent specialty training encompasses normal child and family development, mechanisms of psychiatric disorders affecting children and adolescents, and treatment. Psychiatric disorders affecting this group of individuals are ADHD, autism, mental retardation, mood disorders, learning disabilities, eating disorders, drug dependency, and conduct disorder (delinquency).

Doctors who complete the general psychiatry training can take the certification examination and, upon passing, will become certified in general psychiatry by the American Board of Psychiatry and Neurology (ABPN), which is accredited by the Accreditation Council for Graduate Medical Education. The ABPN also offers subspecialty certification in child and adolescent psychiatry.

Besides or beyond subspecialty training and certification, some child and adolescent psychiatrists choose to become involved in community psychiatry or to start a research career. Both of these paths entail further training, for example, in a community hospital or as a postdoctoral fellow in a university or research institute.

Diagnostic and Treatment Techniques

Diagnosis of psychiatric disorders is complicated because of the multitude of factors at play in psychiatric disorders, which include physical/biological, emotional, social and environmental factors. Diagnosis of such disorders in children and adolescents is further complicated by the effects of developmental processes. The Diagnostic and Statistical Manual of Mental Disorders (DSM), published by the American Psychiatric Association, is a reference book used by many psychiatrists. Now in its fifth edition, the DSM-5 contains revised diagnostic criteria to more accurately reflect the manifestation of psychiatric disorders in children and adolescents.

Psychotherapy is a commonly used technique to alleviate symptoms and improve functioning in children with psychiatric disorders. It encompasses several different types of therapy, including: 1) cognitive behavioral therapy; 2) dialectical behavior therapy; 3) family therapy; 4) group therapy; 5) interpersonal therapy; 6) play therapy; and 7) psychodynamic psychotherapy. All types of psychotherapy utilize communication to effect change in the individual's behavior and emotions.

For some children and adolescents, clinicians may decide to prescribe medications in combination with psychotherapy. Many medications have different effects in children than in adults, which should be taken into consideration when prescribing and monitoring treatment. Medications used to treat children and adolescents include antidepressants for depression, anxiety, and pain; benzodiazepines for anxiety disorders; stimulants for ADHD; as well as antipsychotics for bipolar disorder, schizophrenia, post-traumatic stress disorder, and obsessive compulsive disorder.

Similar to the situation in adults, the effects of medications vary from one individual to another. In addition, medications such as the class of antidepressants known as selective serotonin reuptake inhibitors (SSRIs) have been linked to an increased risk of suicidal thoughts and behavior in adolescents. However, a large 2007 study of clinical trials involving children with major depression or anxiety who were treated with antidepressants showed that the benefits probably outweighed the risks. This study was partially sponsored by the National Institute of Mental Health.

Perspective and Prospects

Starting in the 19th century, when influential thinkers of the day began to write about mental disorders in children, child and adolescent psychiatry has progressed from a burgeoning field to a fully-fledged subspecialty of psychiatry. In the 1950s, cognitive behavioral therapy, tricyclic antidepressants, and the first antipsychotics were developed. The first professor of child psychiatry was Lanfranco Ciampi, who assumed his position in 1923 in Argentina. In 1930, the first child psychiatry department was established in the

United States at Johns Hopkins Hospital. In 1937, the International Association for Child and Adolescent Psychiatry and Allied Professions (IACAPAP) was formed as the International Committee for Child Psychiatry. Since then, the field has continued to evolve and grow in numbers and recognition. One challenge that modern-day child and adolescent psychiatrists face is in defining their role with respect to other related healthcare professionals-whether they should be primarily therapists, prescribers of medication, or coordinators of a team of professionals who are each responsible for different aspects of treatment.

—Ing Wei Khor

For Further Information:

American Academy of Child & Adolescent Psychiatry. https://www.aacap.org/AACAP/Medical_Students_and_Residents/Medical_Students/What_is_Child_and_Adolescent_Psychiatry.aspx. Accessed September 10, 2017.

Massachusetts General Hospital Psychiatry Academy. http://mghcme.org/topics. Updated 2017. Accessed September 10, 2017.

American Board of Psychiatry and Neurology, Inc. Become Certified. https://www.abpn.com/become-certified. Accessed September 10, 2017.

National Institute of Mental Health. https://www.nimh.nih.gov/health/topics/mental-health-medications/index.shtml. Updated October 2016. Accessed September 10, 2017.

Psychiatry, geriatric

Specialty

Anatomy or system affected: All

Specialties and related fields: Critical care, family medicine, geriatrics and gerontology, neurology, pharmacology, preventive medicine, public health

Definition: A subspecialty of psychiatry which deals with the diagnosis and treatment of psychiatric syndromes experienced by older people.

Key terms:

acute confusion syndrome: a transient condition caused by the action of various biological stressors on vulnerable older persons, who may experience inattention, disorganized thinking, other cognitive impairments, and emotional problems

anxiety: a condition characterized by nervousness or agitation; in older people, it is often caused by the existence of a psychiatric disorder such as depression, a general medical condition such as hypothyroidism, or a side effect of medication

depression: a condition characterized by a persistent mood of sadness, weight loss, greatly decreased interest in life, and sometimes psychotic episodes; biological factors, family history of depression, underlying medical problems, and medication side effects all can contribute to these symptoms

hypochondriasis: a condition in which the patients believe strongly that they are suffering from one or more serious illnesses, even when this belief is unsupported by medical evidence

insomnia: disturbed sleep, which occurs in older people more often than in any other age group; insomnia in older people can be caused by many factors, such as dysfunctional sleep cycles, breathing problems, leg jerking,

underlying medical and psychiatric disorders, and the side effects of medication

memory loss syndrome: a condition in which a person gradually but progressively loses capacity in many cognitive areas, but especially in the ability to remember; Alzheimer's disease is considered the most common factor causing serious memory loss in older people

suspiciousness: a range of symptoms from increasing distrust of others to paranoid delusions of conspiracies; changes related to aging are thought to be major factors causing increased suspiciousness in older people

Science and Profession

Growing numbers of old and very old people and the increased complexity of diagnosis and treatment of this age group have driven the growth of geriatric psychiatry. Psychiatrists who specialize in working with the geriatric population note that the psychiatric problems experienced by older people often fit poorly in the diagnostic categories set down in the *Diagnostic and Statistical Manual of Mental Disorders: DSM-IV-TR* (4th ed., 2000). The interplay among declining physical health, decreasing mental functioning, social withdrawal and isolation, and vulnerability to stress makes proper diagnosis and appropriate treatment more difficult. In response to this complexity, practitioners of geriatric psychiatry tend to take a broader approach to diagnosis and to use an interdisciplinary model in developing a treatment plan. The profession of geriatric psychiatry has developed most in Great Britain and Canada but is attracting growing numbers of practitioners in the United States and other Western countries.

Diagnostic and Treatment Techniques

Geriatric psychiatrists tend to follow the lead of specialists in geriatric medicine, who have found that taking a syndromal approach to diagnosis appears to work better with older patients. Among the psychiatric syndromes used by geriatric psychiatrists are acute confusion, anxiety, depression, hypochondriasis, insomnia, memory loss, and suspiciousness. Special attention must be given by geriatric psychiatrists to the older person's overall ability to function, general health status, social support system, family history, and preexisting conditions. Geriatric psychiatrists are forced to acknowledge the role played by changes in the brain as it ages and to separate changes that are relatively benign from those that pose real threats to the patient. Hospitalization and significant medical intervention tend to occur more often in the later stages of a person's life, and geriatric psychiatrists are aware that these events can have a great impact on the patient's mental well-being.

When they can, geriatric psychiatrists draw readily upon the help of other health-care providers in treating elderly persons, including the use of specially qualified clinical psychologists, social workers, nurses, occupational therapists, speech pathologists, dietitians, and physical therapists. Improving the understanding of family members and providing them with supportive advice and services can be an important part of the overall treatment plan.

Perspective and Prospects

In the United States, federal funding has expanded for qualified providers, such as clinical psychologists and social workers, to render mental health services to older people, especially those who live in long-term care facilities. Funds have increased for the proper training of those who provide mental health services to older people. Examinations have been established to show evidence of "added qualifications" in geriatric medicine and psychiatry. More textbooks and specialty journals devoted to geriatric mental health are now in circulation. The federal government has sponsored important national conferences on various aspects of geriatric mental health. With the costs of hospital and long-term care continuing to rise, more emphasis has been given to preventive services and day-care services.

Furthermore, some hospitals have established specialized geropsychiatric units to improve diagnosis and treatment and to decrease the time that older people spend in the hospital. Services are expected to increase for adult children who care for older parents with mental illnesses. Research efforts have increased concerning the causes and appropriate treatment of psychiatric problems in older people. Older people are becoming healthier as they learn more about how mental health and physical health are affected by the way in which one lives. They are advised to stop smoking, eat a better diet, exercise more, and continue to take an active part in family and community life. All these trends are expected to continue in the future.

—*Russell Williams, M.S.W.*

See also Addiction; Aging; Aging: Extended care; Alcoholism; Alzheimer's disease; Amnesia; Antianxiety drugs; Antidepressants; Anxiety; Bipolar disorders; Brain; Brain damage; Brain disorders; Chronic fatigue syndrome; Delusions; Dementias; Depression; Domestic violence; Electroencephalography (EEG); Emergency medicine; Emotions: Biomedical causes and effects; Euthanasia; Factitious disorders; Family medicine; Fatigue; Frontotemporal dementia (FTD); Geriatrics and gerontology; Grief and guilt; Hallucinations; Hypnosis; Hypochondriasis; Incontinence; Intellectual disability; Intoxication; Light therapy; Memory loss; Neurology; Neurosis; Neurosurgery; Obesity; Obsessive-compulsive disorder; Panic attacks; Paranoia; Pharmacology; Phobias; Pick's disease; Polypharmacy; Prescription drug abuse; Psychiatric disorders; Psychiatry; Psychoanalysis; Psychosis; Psychosomatic disorders; Schizophrenia; Sexual dysfunction; Sexuality; Shock therapy; Sleep disorders; Speech disorders; Stress; Stress reduction; Substance abuse; Suicide; Terminally ill: Extended care.

For Further Information:

Andreasen, Nancy C., and Donald W. Black. *Introductory Textbook of Psychiatry.* 5th ed. Washington, D.C.: American Psychiatric Press, 2011.

Bee, Helen L., and Barbara L. Bjorklund. *The Journey of Adulthood.* 7th ed. Upper Saddle River, N.J.: Prentice Hall, 2011.

Birren, James E., and K. Warner Schaie, eds. *Handbook of the Psychology of Aging.* 7th ed. Boston: Academic Press/Elsevier, 2011.

Birren, James E., R. Bruce Sloane, and Gene D. Cohen, eds. *Handbook of Mental Health and Aging.* 2d ed. San Diego, Calif.: Academic Press, 1992.

Blazer, Dan G., and David C., eds. Steffens. *Essentials of Geriatric Psychiatry.* Washington, D.C.: American Psychiatric Publishing, 2012.

Blazer, Dan G., David C. Steffens, and Ewald W. Busse, eds. *The American Psychiatric Publishing Textbook of Geriatric Psychiatry.* 4th ed. Washington, D.C.: American Psychiatric Publishing, 2009.

Lavretsky, Helen, Martha Sajatovic, and Charles F. Reynolds, eds. *Late-Life Mood Disorders.* New York: Oxford University Press, 2013.

Miller, Mark D., and LalithKumar K Solai, eds. *Geriatric Psychiatry.* New York: Oxford University Press, 2013.

Sadock, Benjamin J., and Virginia A. Sadock, eds. *Kaplan and Sadock's Comprehensive Textbook of Psychiatry.* 9th ed. Philadelphia: Lippincott Williams & Wilkins, 2009.

Whitbourne, Susan Krauss, ed. *Psychopathology in Later Adulthood.* New York: Wiley, 2001.

Psychoanalysis

Treatment

Anatomy or system affected: Psychic-emotional system

Specialties and related fields: Psychiatry

Definition: A psychotherapeutic technique, developed by Sigmund Freud, in which the analyst helps the patient to uncover and resolve unconscious conflicts in order to treat personality disorders and/or deviance.

Key terms:

classical psychoanalysis: the method developed by Freud to help patients achieve insight into why they develop maladaptive ways of relating to others and experience disabling psychological symptoms

dreams: warnings sent from the superego to protect the ego from id impulses

instinctual drives: libido (the seeking of gratification of sexual impulses) and aggression (the seeking of gratification of destructive impulses)

neurosis: a psychic disturbance and defect from childhood that develops into a particular pattern of emotional illness and dysfunctional behavior

Oedipus complex: the experience of having sexual feelings toward the parent of the opposite sex, which is found in young children

psyche: the human mind, which according to Freud is divided into id, ego, and superego; the id contains instincts and repressed feelings, the ego directs everyday behavior, and the superego guides the ego

psychoanalyst: a person, usually a psychiatrist, who has received several years of postgraduate training and supervised practice in using psychoanalysis to diagnose and treat clients

psychosis: a condition occurring when a person's id impulses chronically defeat the control of the ego; schizophrenia and bipolar disorders are two examples of psychoses

transference: the tendency of a person who developed unsatisfying parental relationships to repeat this pattern unconsciously with others; psychoanalytic treatment depends on the development of transference between client and analyst

The Theoretical Basis of Psychoanalysis

Psychoanalysis is a method that is used to understand the workings of the human mind. Adherents to psychoanalysis believe that many forces operate to influence and shape the mind, including some that exist beneath the level of conscious awareness and control. Psychoanalysis permits scientists to observe and collect information about the mind, to develop and test scientific hypotheses about mental processes, and to use the scientific wisdom gained to diagnose and treat mental illnesses. Psychoanalytic theory helps psychiatrists and other mental health practitioners understand more about human emotions and psychological development. Though many psychoanalytic concepts were first developed only in the late nineteenth century, psychoanalysis has made significant and lasting contributions to modern psychiatry and continues to enhance its development.

The precepts of psychoanalysis have been subjected to much scientific scrutiny and criticism. As befits any scientific discipline, psychoanalytic theory has been revised periodically to account for new information, observations, and insights. Psychoanalytic theory also is seen as contributing to other scientific disciplines, such as neurology, the social sciences, and psychology. Psychoanalysis has also broadened understanding in the humanities, the arts, philosophy, ethics, and religion. Psychoanalysis clearly has had a profound and lasting impact upon a broad span of human interests and activities.

Psychoanalytic theory is largely a product of the efforts of Sigmund Freud (1856-1939) to link the physical processes of the human brain with the psychological manifestations of the human mind. While Freud was frustrated in his ultimate goal of demonstrating clearly the relationship between the two, his work informs the same search today. Therefore, an understanding of early and evolving psychoanalytic theory remains important to psychiatry and psychotherapy.

To begin developing an understanding of the complexities of psychoanalysis, one needs to be familiar with basic information about psychoanalytic theory. The discussion that follows will touch on instinctual drives, the architecture of the mind, psychological development, mental defense mechanisms, and the psychoanalytic classification of mental illness.

Human behavior is driven from early infancy on by the operation of basic instincts. Freud believed that the primitive and evolving physical needs of humans stimulate instinctual drives. He said instincts possess four essential characteristics: source, impetus, aim, and object. Instincts arise from a particular bodily area, generate varying amounts of energy, aim for gratification, and are directed at particular objects, such as other people. Libido, one of these instincts, drives humans to seek pleasure and provides gratification during all the several stages of human development, beginning with the infant sucking at the mother's breast. Later in his work, Freud expressed his belief that humans possess an aggressive instinct, which appears to be aimed at the destruction of the self and others. His formulation of dual and dueling instincts, as with much of his work, continues to evoke controversy in psychoanalytic circles.

Freud believed that the libido instinct is expressed early in life and continues to be expressed during several stages

as a prelude to mature psychosexual development. Infants first experience the oral stage, which centers on feeding. Libido is gratified during the act of nursing, and success experienced at this stage helps the infant develop a sense of trust and self-reliance. Older infants proceed to the anal stage, centering on the retention and expulsion of feces and urine. Successful experience during the anal stage equips children with what they need to develop personal autonomy, independence, guiltless initiative, self-assurance, and willingness to cooperate. Children then move to the phallic stage, finding a new interest in genitalia. Freud's theories about this stage are controversial, and many have been repudiated. He said that the penis holds the interest of both sexes, but girls form an early sense of inadequacy when they see that they do not have one (penis envy). Early sexual feelings are directed, according to Freud, toward the parent of the opposite sex (Oedipus complex). Parents regard these feelings as unacceptable and send signals to the children, who must repress their sexual urges. Boys act out of fear of castration, while girls act out of fear of loss of parental love and of envy of the boy's penis. Children who successfully negotiate this stage are said to have developed a firm basis for sexual identity, uninhibited curiosity, a sense of mastery, and the formation of conscience. Next comes the latency period, from ages five to thirteen, during which previous attainments are integrated and consolidated. Key elements of adaptive behavior develop during this stage. The teenage years are said to be spent in the genital stage, during which the child separates gradually from dependence on parents and begins to attach to new love objects and more mature interests. This stage culminates successfully in a sense of personal identity and acceptance.

Through Freud's study of and work with hysteria, a condition in which emotional conflicts are transformed into bodily maladies, he became convinced that the human mind contains dynamic forces that often oppose one another. For example, a person who experiences significant trauma in early childhood, and the painful emotions that attend it, can mentally oppose or repress memories of the trauma and the traumatic emotions. The repressed memories and emotions remain embedded in the unconscious regions of the mind until they are revived and re-experienced when stimulated by a later event. Thus, the force of emotional material that was repressed but never forgotten can exceed the force used by the conscious mind to hold the memories at bay. The concepts of repression and the needful recognition of repressed material continue to be important principles guiding psychoanalysis.

Freud conceived of the human mind, or psyche, as having three parts: id, ego, and superego. The basic instincts and repressed Oedipal urges of human beings reside in the id. Freud saw the id as a totally undifferentiated mass of energy, constantly seeking gratification without the constraints of reality or morality. In contrast, he saw the ego as being well organized, governed by an accurate perception of the external environment, and honoring certain principles of socially acceptable behavior. The ego seeks to form gratifying relationships with other people. At the same time, the ego must defend itself against the primitive urges of the id. The superego is the last division of the mind to form, which it does through successful resolution of the Oedipus conflict. It forms what is called the conscience and imposes control through guilt. The superego often operates during dreams, Freud said, sending warnings when the ego fails to defend properly against id impulses. Most work of the id and the superego is carried out unconsciously, while much of the ego's work operates at the conscious level.

After Freud had seen his theories confirmed in his clinical and personal experience, he felt comfortable in setting out his thoughts on psychopathology. Among the disorders that he identified were various types of neuroses, phobias, perversions, character disorders, personality disorders, psychoses, hypochondriasis, depressive states, and schizophrenia. He believed that mental illness is caused mainly by intrapsychic conflicts that are poorly managed by the mind or by abnormal mental processes and structures.

Indications and Procedures

In relation to medical science and, more specifically, to psychiatry, psychoanalysis is used to diagnose and treat emotional illness.

In diagnosis, psychoanalysts have purposes that differ considerably from those of general psychiatry. The analyst uses diagnosis to determine the patient's potential for analysis, the usefulness of analysis in treating the particular emotional problem experienced by the patient, the patient's level of incapacity, the likelihood that the patient will improve, and the likelihood that the analyst will be able to understand and help the patient. Other mental health specialists typically compare the signs and symptoms demonstrated or described by the patient to those cataloged in the American Psychiatric Association's *Diagnostic and Statistical Manual of Mental Disorders: DSM-5* (5th ed., 2013) and assign a diagnosis that best fits the patient. The psychoanalytic approach to diagnosis, conversely, is based on what the analyst can learn about the patient's inner experiences, especially unconscious conflicts and fantasies.

Psychoanalysis is considered to be the treatment of choice for younger adults suffering from chronic emotional illness not helped by less intensive therapies. People who suffer from hysteria, obsessive-compulsive neuroses, sexual perversions, and certain personality disorders are seen as the best candidates for psychoanalysis. To be considered for psychoanalysis, patients must demonstrate an ability to develop a reasonably good relationship with an analyst and must be willing and able to withstand a long, intensive course of treatment. Psychoanalysis is also expensive, and patients must be able to pay for treatment. Some, but not all, third-party payers will bear part of the cost of psychoanalysis; unfortunately, third-party review of the case compromises analyst-patient confidentiality. Patients who are psychotic or who are alcoholics or drug addicts are considered poor candidates for psychoanalysis. Older adults may have personalities too rigid to tolerate analysis, and others have an illness too minor to justify such treatment. Patients who

are chronically and deeply depressed may be unsuitable candidates for analysis, as are those who have failed to establish appropriate relationships with both parents. Patients must be deemed able not only to enter analysis but also to tolerate termination of therapy. Patients who need urgent intervention to preserve health and life are not good candidates for analysis; neither are those who have little opportunity to make changes in their lives. Because many factors enter into consideration, analysts give some patients a trial period of analysis before accepting them for treatment.

When a patient enters into psychoanalysis, the patient and analyst must resolve certain practical issues, such as setting up appointment times, payment schedules, and other policy matters. The patient must be willing to spend an hour a day, four or five days a week, for as long as five years to complete analysis.

The analyst and patient must be able to form a therapeutic relationship secure enough to withstand the test of time and the stress of treatment. Early on, the patient and analyst must endure as the patient anxiously defends the ego and resists plunging into deeper emotional material. Eventually, so-called transferenceneurosis emerges. Patients reexperience and often project onto the analyst infantile desires and conflicts. The process of returning to more primitive emotional states is called regression, and analysts must be skillful in helping the patient to avoid its inherent dangers.

Free association is used to deepen the regression. The analyst instructs the patient to talk freely about issues of current concern and to continue talking about whatever associations come into the patient's awareness, making no effort to censor or restrain the monologue. Despite a patient's apparent willingness to follow the analyst's direction, the patient's resistance to uncovering certain material begins to be demonstrated with silences, pauses, stammers, corrections, slips of the tongue, and so on. The analyst remains alert to these signals of resistance, as the shape of the resistance shows the nature of the neurosis. The analyst gives interpretations of the resistance and related unconscious material; for progress to be made, the interpretation must be accurate, and the patient must accept and make use of it. The patient must work through painful emotional conflicts and find ways to resolve them more satisfactorily. "Working through" consumes much of the time spent in analysis.

The analyst often employs several psychological maneuvers to help patients during analysis. The analyst might offer suggestions, in an effort to induce a mental state that opposes the patient's experiences, expectations, or concept of reality. For example, the analyst may assure the patient that working through repressed emotions will enable the patient to enjoy a more productive life. The analyst may manipulate the patient to facilitate recovery of or to neutralize early unconscious material. The analyst can help the patient by clarifying material that the patient may know only in a semiconscious, disorganized way. The term "countertransference" describes the variety of responses felt by the analyst toward the patient; the analyst must resolve such feelings satisfactorily in order to continue the analytic process.

Dreams are said to be the "royal road to the unconscious," and the analyst will often encourage the patient to recall dreams experienced the preceding night. Dreams not only process waking experiences but often offer clues as to unconscious reactions, wishes, and conflicts as well. The analyst offers interpretations of the dreams in order to bring unconscious material and patterns to the conscious awareness of the patient.

The couch on which the patient reclines during sessions is a trademark of psychoanalysis; it is used rarely in any other form of psychotherapy. The analyst typically is positioned outside the visual range of the patient. This arrangement is considered to be essential in encouraging regression and projection.

As the patient and analyst struggle together to help the patient bring repressed material into awareness, the patient may achieve greater self-understanding and increased ability to find more satisfactory resolutions to emotional conflicts.

The analyst begins to prepare the patient for termination as the active phase of the analysis comes to a close. Patients must be weaned well from dependence on the analyst and the analytic situation. While the patient may have relived and worked through many primitive wishes and conflicts, the continuing work of resolving conflicts as they arise rests primarily with the patient's ability to work through them independently.

The outcome of psychoanalysis can be difficult to evaluate, but success has been defined as having helped a patient improve adjustment to life, realize a certain amount of contentment, give happiness to others, deal more confidently with inevitable stresses, and maintain mutually satisfying relationships with others. In addition, the patient should experience a reduction in neurotic suffering and inhibitions, have fewer dependency needs, have increased potential for success in all significant areas of life, and function at a more mature level.

Perspective and Prospects

Psychoanalysis was born in the wake of evidence that hysteria can be caused by repressed memories or unconscious wishes. People who suffer from hysteria, now known as conversion disorder (functional neurological symptom disorder), develop physical symptoms such as paralysis or blindness in an otherwise healthy body. Sigmund Freud was influenced by the work of French neurologist Jean-Martin Charcot (1825-1893) and fellow Viennese physician Josef Breuer (1842-1925), both of whom were trying to find effective treatments for hysteria. Charcot relied on the use of hypnosis, while Breuer allowed patients to empty their minds, in an early version of free association. In 1895, Breuer and Freud published accounts of their theories and successful cures of patients suffering from hysteria. Freud also was influenced by the work of others on the hierarchy of the nervous system, philosophical concepts of the unconscious mind, posthypnotic suggestion, and the organization of the brain. He was a prolific author and teacher who fostered the careers of several followers.

Many of those who learned from and were influenced by Freud later developed their own variations or new areas of emphasis within Freudian psychoanalysis. Closer study of the role of the ego in emotional disorders led to the development of ego psychology, which enhanced the understanding of the defense, coping, and adaptive mechanisms of the ego. Others chose to emphasize the role of parents and other significant early childhood caregivers in the subsequent development of emotional health and illness. Still others developed what is known as self-psychology, a variant which emphasizes the importance of a person's cohesive sense of self and emotional well-being; the sense of self is either fostered or hindered by interpersonal relationships formed throughout life. Other variants that draw on the psychoanalytical principle include psychodynamic, insight-oriented, relationship, and supportive psychotherapies. Marital, group, and family therapy also depend heavily on an understanding and application of psychoanalytical theory. Generally speaking, most psychotherapeutic interventions used today are grounded in the psychoanalytic precepts developed by Freud and refined by students of his work.

Classical psychoanalysis is still practiced in the United States, but its use is limited by the relatively few properly trained analysts, the time and expense involved in the treatment process, the lack of widely accepted proof of its superiority as a treatment method, and the demand for brief intervention by patients of psychotherapy and those who pay for it. Modern practitioners of psychoanalysis are concerned by several trends: the ascendence of biological approaches to understanding and treating mental illness, the unwillingness of insurers to pay for psychoanalysis, the growing number of nonphysician analysts, the growing skepticism about its effectiveness, and the establishment of a universal system of psychiatric diagnosis that largely ignores the psychoanalytic perspective.

—*Russell Williams, M.S.W.*

See also Brain; Depression; Emotions, biomedical causes and effects; Hypochondriasis; Neurosis; Obsessive-compulsive disorder; Phobias; Psychiatric disorders; Psychiatry; Psychiatry, child and adolescent; Psychiatry, geriatric; Psychosis; Schizophrenia; Sibling rivalry.

For Further Information:

American Psychiatric Association. *Diagnostic and Statistical Manual of Mental Disorders: DSM-5.* 5th ed. Arlington, Va.: Author, 2013.

American Psychiatric Association Commission on Psychiatric Therapies. *The Psychiatric Therapies.* Washington, D.C.: Author, 1984.

American Psychoanalytic Association. "About Psychoanalysis." *American Psychoanalytic Association,* 2009-2013.

Clark, Ronald. *Freud: the Man and the Cause.* London: Paladin Grafton Books, 1987.

Gay, Peter. *Freud: A Life for Our Time.* London: Little, 2006.

Milton, Jane., Caroline Polmear, and Julia Fabricius. *A Short Introduction to Psychoanalysis.* Los Angeles: SAGE, 2011.

Mishne, Judith Marks. *The Evolution and Application of Clinical Theory: Perspective from Four Psychologies.* New York: Free Press, 1993.

Sadock, Benjamin J., and Virginia A. Sadock, eds. *Kaplan and Sadock's Comprehensive Textbook of Psychiatry.* 9th ed. Philadelphia: Wolters Kluwer Health/Lippincott Williams & Wilkins, 2009.

Stern, Daniel N. *Interpersonal World of the Infant: A View from Psychoanalysis and Development Psychology.* London; New York: American Psychoanalytic Association, 2008.

Psychosis

Disease/Disorder
Anatomy or system affected: Psychic-emotional system
Specialties and related fields: Psychiatry
Definition: The most severe mental disorder, in which the individual loses contact with reality and suffers from such symptoms as delusions and hallucinations.

Causes and Symptoms

The individual with a psychosis displays disordered thinking, emotion, and behavior. The individual fails to make sense of his or her surroundings, reacts inaccurately to them, and develops false thoughts or ideas about them. The resulting behavior can be described as peculiar, abnormal, or bizarre. Psychosis runs in families and most often first appears in late adolescence or early adulthood. There are some psychoses with medical and physical causes and some for which the cause is unknown. The treatment of psychoses involves removing or correcting the causes of the psychoses when possible. Psychosis describes a group of symptoms that can be part of several formal psychiatric diagnoses that include schizophrenia. Psychotic symptoms are characterized by delusions, hallucinations, disturbances of movement, and/or speech disturbances.

Delusions are false beliefs that are held despite strong evidence to the contrary. An example of an extreme delusion might be a man's belief that someone has planted a radio transmitter in his brain that sends signals to creatures on Mars. Hallucinations are false sense perceptions that, like delusions, are held despite strong evidence to the contrary. Hallucinations can involve any of the five senses. Examples of extreme hallucinations include feeling as if one is covered by ants, seeing green cows walking through the wall, hearing voices that do not exist, and smelling a constant odor when none exists.

Disturbances of movement can occur with psychoses. For example, a woman may become very exaggerated in her movements or, conversely, may become motionless for periods of time. These disturbances of movement are clearly bizarre and unnatural. Finally, speech disturbances are very common in psychoses. A man might speak in a way that is not understandable to others. He may carry on a conversation in which he believes that he is communicating normally but without making sense to others. Alternatively, speech might be clear but the individual shifts from one unrelated idea to another without being aware of doing so. Another psychotic symptom is severe emotional turmoil described as intense shifting moods with accompanying feelings of being confused.

Information on Psychosis

Causes: May include brain disturbances resulting from thyroid disorders, negative drug reactions, infections, epilepsy, tumors, and circulatory disorders (e.g., strokes); certain prescription and illegal drugs
Symptoms: Delusions, hallucinations, disconnection from reality, speech and movement disturbances
Duration: Acute to chronic
Treatments: Medication; individual, group, and family psychotherapy; hospitalization

---

Approximately 2 percent of all people will develop a psychosis sometime during their life. Although psychoses typically first appear in late adolescence or early adulthood, they may begin in middle to late life as well. The symptoms are apparently equally common in males and females. Because there is a strong family pattern to psychoses, some have suggested a genetic predisposition, and such evidence has been found. Environmental factors, however, such as home environment, parenting, and traumatic life events, may also play a role in some psychoses.

Treatment and Therapy

Psychoses are often categorized as organic or functional, which provides a way to communicate the cause of a psychosis and thereby the appropriate treatment. Organic psychoses are attributable to disturbances in the brain. These psychoses can be attributed directly to a problem in the structure, functioning, or chemistry of the brain. Various physical conditions and abnormalities can lead to psychosis, including thyroid disorders, drug reactions, infections, epilepsy, tumors, and circulatory disorders (for example, strokes). The treatment of organic psychoses involves removing or correcting the causes of the psychoses. In the case of a psychosis caused by a disorder of the thyroid gland, the individual might be prescribed medications to correct the thyroid problem or have the gland surgically removed. Certain prescription and illegal drugs can cause a psychosis; these include cocaine, alcohol, heart medications, and pain medications. In these situations, the psychotic symptoms are often eliminated when the medication or drug is discontinued. Organic psychoses may be the result of deteriorating physical conditions, such as Alzheimer's disease. Such a psychosis is typically nonreversible and is treated with tranquilizing medications to decrease the individual's discomfort and disruptive behaviors.

Functional psychoses are those psychoses for which no organic causes can be found. Often the psychotic symptoms are part of a more traditional psychiatric condition such as schizophrenia or depression. The mainstay of the treatment of functional psychoses is medication therapy. As with the organic psychoses in deteriorating physical conditions, tranquilizers are the most appropriate first-line treatment for psychotic symptoms. The goal of therapy is to decrease the frequency and disruption of psychotic thoughts and behaviors.

Individual, group, and family psychotherapy are also a

major part of treating individuals with functional psychosis or organic psychosis in deteriorating physical conditions. These therapies help to ensure compliance with the medication therapy, decrease the tendency for relapse, and can even lead to the reduction in the amount of medication required to relieve the individual's symptoms. The goal of psychotherapy is to help the individual maintain functioning.

Occasionally, the patient with a psychosis may require inpatient hospitalization. The experience of hallucinations or delusions can be particularly distressing and can lead to a severe depression. Furthermore, these hallucinations and delusions might be of a homicidal or suicidal nature. While hospitalization is not required in treating individuals with psychosis, when individuals become a danger to themselves or to others, a brief inpatient hospitalization may be required to stabilize the patients and return them to a higher state of functioning. During hospitalization, patients are treated with medication therapy along with individual, group, or family therapy until they can be safely returned to their environments. Occasionally, patients with psychoses have multiple episodes during their lives, requiring numerous inpatient hospitalizations. In May 2013, Georgia Health Sciences University in Augusta, Georgia, published a study linking urinary tract infections (UTIs) in patients with psychosis. According to the study, which was presented at the American Psychiatric Association's 2013 Annual Meeting, prevalence of UTIs was higher in patients with a history of psychosis.

—*Oliver Oyama, Ph.D.*

See also Addiction; Alcoholism; Delusions; Dementias; Depression; Domestic violence; Hallucinations; Intoxication; Neurosis; Paranoia; Prader-Willi syndrome; Prescription drug abuse; Psychiatric disorders; Psychiatry; Psychiatry, child and adolescent; Psychiatry, geriatric; Schizophrenia; Side effects; Substance abuse; Suicide.

For Further Information:

American Psychiatric Association. *Diagnostic and Statistical Manual of Mental Disorders: DSM-IV-TR*. 4th ed. Arlington, Va.: Author, 2000.

Barlow, David H., ed. *Clinical Handbook of Psychological Disorders*. 4th ed. New York: Guilford Press, 2008.

Bloom, Floyd E., M. Flint Beal, and David J. Kupfer, eds. *The Dana Guide to Brain Health*. New York: Dana Press, 2006.

Kring, Ann M., et al. *Abnormal Psychology*. 11th ed. Hoboken, N.J.: John Wiley & Sons, 2010.

Moskowitz, Andrew.Â *Psychosis, Trauma and Dissociation: Emerging Perspectives on Severe Psychopathology*. New York: Wiley, 2008. Print.

Torrey, E. Fuller. *Surviving Schizophrenia: A Manual for Families, Patients, and Providers*. 5th ed. New York: Collins, 2006.

Torrey, E. Fuller.Â *Surviving Schizophrenia: A Manual for Families, Patients, and Providers*. 5th ed. New York: Harper Perennial, 2006. Print.

Psychosomatic disorders

Disease/Disorder
Anatomy or system affected: All
Specialties and related fields: Psychiatry, psychology
Definition: Physical disorder influenced by psychological stressors, or disorders characterized by symptoms that result from unconscious psychological factors instead of an underlying medical condition.

Causes and Symptoms

In the 1950s, the diagnosis of "psychosomatic disorders" was coined to refer to medical conditions for which there were no clear medical causes, but there was a subtle distinction between psychological processes and physical illness in its definition. The current understanding of medical illness has progressed, however, and health professionals now understand that psychological or sociological factors contribute to most medical illnesses. Thus, the diagnosis of psychosomatic disorders has undergone refinement and more specific diagnostic classification. The two related psychiatric diagnostic classifications are "psychological factors affecting medical condition" and "somatoform disorders."

Psychophysical disorders. The diagnosis of psychological factors affecting a medical condition (also occasionally referred to as psychophysiological disorders) describes any physical condition or disorder that is influenced by psychological factors. These psychological factors can range from true psychiatric disorders such as depression to emotional stressors in the person's environment such as the death of a loved one, anger toward a coworker, or the inability to cope with normal life changes. The more common environmental stressors can lead to the initiation or the exacerbation of physical conditions, including headache, ulcer, asthma, arthritis, acne, irritable bowel syndrome, diabetes mellitus, muscular disorders, and essential hypertension. In certain cases, such as headache, the stressor causes the onset of symptoms. In others, such as diabetes, the stressors might cause a worsening of already existing symptoms because of their influence on the person's attitude about the illness and the resultant quality of life, the willingness or the ability of the person to comply with treatment, or the person's capacity to understand the illness and its treatment. For example, in a situation in which a person is faced with the death of a loved one, it would not be unusual to see a corresponding increase in headache frequency or uncontrolled blood sugar levels in the diabetic.

Somatoform disorders. Somatoform disorders are the second diagnostic classification subsumed under the old psychosomatic disorders category. In somatoform disorder, a person displays symptoms that suggest a physical disorder, but no medical evidence exists for such a disorder. In these cases, it is believed that the person possesses psychological stresses, conflicts, or needs that manifest themselves in physical symptoms. The distinction between somatoform and psychophysiological disorders is that in psychophysiological disorders the person has an identified physical illness or disorder that is influenced by psychological stress. In somatoform disorders, there are only physical symptoms and no physical findings or known mechanisms to diagnose any physical illness or disorder.

People with somatoform disorders are presumably unable to tolerate certain forms or intensity of emotional stresses, leading to an expression of their emotional dis-

Information on Psychosomatic Disorders

Causes: Psychological stressors, genetic or environmental factors

Symptoms: Wide ranging; may include headaches, paralysis, seizures, coordination problems, visual disorders

Duration: Acute to chronic

Treatments: Psychiatric medications, physical and emotional relaxation skills, psychotherapy

tress through physical symptoms. These disorders typically afflict people in their adolescence or young adult years and cause considerable disruption in life. The symptoms or focus on physical attributes are not intentionally produced or controlled. They are, at the time, outside the person's capacity to control them. There is no known cause for these disorders, and because they occasionally run in families, some have speculated that environment or genetics may play a role.

An example of a somatoform disorder is conversion disorder. People with conversion disorder display an alteration or loss of physical functioning characterized most often as paralyses, seizures, coordination problems, or visual problems. No physical causes are found for these symptoms. Instead, psychiatric evaluation suggests that the symptoms serve a role in helping the person cope with some type of stress, conflict, or need. A person might become temporarily blind or paralyzed in the right arm as an unconscious way of dealing with an upcoming stressful situation, such as a marriage.

Another somatoform disorder is somatization disorder. People with this disorder complain of unexplained symptoms for which no physical evidence exists. Such people believe that they have acquired a serious physical disorder and often seek out many health care providers to locate a cause for their symptoms. The disorders are often very disruptive to the person's life and quite costly in terms of medical expenses.

Treatment and Therapy

Treatment for psychophysiological disorders can include using psychiatric medications to manage intense depression or anxiety; educating the patient about the relationship between stressors and physical illness; challenging maladaptive health care beliefs or any unrealistic assumptions or expectations that the person might possess; teaching physical and emotional relaxation skills; developing and utilizing social support from others in the person's life; and instructing the patient in personal skills to manage better the event or situation causing the stress. These treatments can be very effective with psychophysiological disorders.

Treatment for somatoform disorders involves the use of individual, group, or family therapy to address the stresses, conflicts, or needs that are believed to be at the root of the problem. When patients identify the underlying problems, change their thoughts about these problems, and learn skills to deal more adaptively with them, their physical symptoms typically subside.

Perspective and Prospects

The relationship between the mind and the body has intrigued humankind for centuries. Beliefs about the contribution of the mind in the functioning of the human body have had a mixed history. Scientists and clinicians currently appreciate the influence of psychological and social factors in physical illness and dysfunction, but this has not always been the case. Theories of personality and its influence on health and illness can be found in ancient writings as early as 400 BCE. In the late sixteenth and early seventeenth centuries, the view that psychological factors could influence physical illness lost favor as the medical profession began an era of strict scientific study of the body and bodily processes. During this era, an illness or treatment would be considered legitimate only if a scientific explanation could be found for the process. Because of the limits of scientific methodology at the time, many of the traditional beliefs of this mind-body link were abandoned. The mind and body were theoretically separated until the early twentieth century, which saw the introduction of the field of psychobiology and the scientific study of the influence of the mind on the body.

—Oliver Oyama, Ph.D.

See also Antianxiety drugs; Anxiety; Depression; Factitious disorders; Hypochondriasis; Midlife crisis; Münchausen syndrome by proxy; Neurosis; Panic attacks; Phobias; Psychiatric disorders; Psychiatry; Psychiatry, child and adolescent; Psychiatry, geriatric; Psychoanalysis; Stress; Stress reduction.

For Further Information:

American Psychiatric Association. *Diagnostic and Statistical Manual of Mental Disorders: DSM-5.* 5th ed. Arlington, Va.: Author, 2013.

Asaad, Ghazi. *Psychosomatic Disorders: Theoretical and Clinical Aspects.* New York: Brunner/Mazel, 1996.

Asmundson, Gordon J. G., et al., eds. *Health Anxiety: Clinical and Research Perspectives on Hypochondriasis and Related Conditions.* New York: Wiley, 2001.

Gatchel, Robert J., and Edward B. Blanchard, eds. *Psychophysiological Disorders: Research and Clinical Applications.* Washington, DC: American Psychological Association, 1998.

Mate, Gabor, and T. Miller. *When the Body Says No: Understanding the Stress-Disease Connection.* New York: Wiley, 2003.

Phillips, Katherine A., ed. *Somatoform and Factitious Disorders.* Washington, DC: American Psychiatric Association, 2001.

Safer, Diane A., and Lukas Rimas. "Somatization Disorder." *Health Library,* Mar. 27, 2013.

Smith, G. Richard, Jr. *Somatization Disorder in the Medical Setting.* Rockville, Md.: Department of Health and Human Services, Public Health Service, Alcohol, Drug Abuse, and Mental Health Administration, National Institute of Mental Health, 1990.

"Somatoform Disorders." *FamilyDoctor.org,* Feb. 2010.

"Stress." *MedlinePlus,* May 22, 2013.

Pterygium/Pinguecula

Disease/Disorder

Also known as: Surfer's eye

Anatomy or system affected: Eyes

Specialties and related fields: Ophthalmology, optometry

Definition: A thickening of conjunctiva of the eye that grows onto the cornea (pterygium) or degeneration of a portion of the conjunctiva (pinguecula).

Key terms:

conjunctiva: the clear, moist membrane that coats the inner surfaces of the eyelids and the outer surface of the eye

cornea: the clear front window of the eye that transmits light into the eye

sclera: the tough white outer covering over the eyeball that extends over most of its surface

---

Information on Pterygium/Pinguecula

Causes: Ultraviolet radiation exposure causes the conjunctiva to degenerate (pinguelcula) or thicken and overgrow (pterygium)

Symptoms: Redness, tearing, dry and itchy eyes, blurring of vision

Duration: Usually arises around 20-40 years of age and remains for the rest of patient's life

Treatments: Artificial tears and ointments, optical steroids, surgery

---

Causes and Symptoms

When ultraviolet radiation from sunlight irradiates the conjunctiva, it can damage and kill conjunctival cells. Repeated sunlight exposure can sometimes produce small accumulations of dead and damaged conjunctival cells combined with degraded matrices that appear as yellowish-white deposits that sometimes calcify. Such a deposit is called a pinguecula (plural, pingueculae). Alternatively, in response to continued conjunctival cell death, the cells divide to replace the dead cells. Repeated damage to the conjunctiva can hyperactivate this healing response and a nontumorous growth of conjunctival cells, called a pterygium, thickens the conjunctiva and eventually grows over the cornea. In some cases pingueculae precede pterygia.

Pterygium and pinguecula occur with increasing frequency in climates that approach the equator. Those who live in dry, dusty environments, fishermen, surfers, and farmers experience increased rates of pterygium and pinguecula. Some studies have found that smoking increases the rates of pterygium and alcohol consumption increases the rates of pinguecula. Although pterygium and pinguecula can arise in anyone, they are rarely seen in those younger than 20 years old. People over 40 show the highest prevalence of pterygium and pinguecula and those between the ages of 20-40 have the highest incidence.

Treatment and Therapy

In most cases, pterygium and pinguecula do not cause any symptoms and require no treatment. Pingueculae tend to grow slowly and may, in some cases, appear unsightly, in

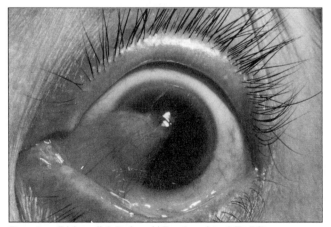

Pterygium. (Liebergall & Paskowski Eye Associates MD, PC)

which cases they can be surgically removed. Pinguelculae can also cause some eye discomfort and in such cases over-the-counter artificial tear products (e.g., Refresh Tears, GenTeal) or lubricating ointments (e.g., Refresh P.M., Hypo Tears) can provide relief. Infrequently, pingueculae can become inflamed (pingueculitis), which are effectively treated with prednisone eye drops (Pred Fotre).

Pterygium often requires no treatment unless it overgrows the cornea and deforms or scars it. In such cases, the pterygium significantly affects patient's sight and surgical extirpation can potentially restore normal sight to the eye. Unfortunately, simple excision has a high rate regrowth of the pterygium (24-89 percent). To prevent regrowth, radiation therapy and chemical agents such as mitomycin C, 5-fluorouracil, and thiotepa have been applied to the eye prior to surgery. Secondly, the sclera is covered with either amniotic membrane or a small piece of conjunctiva cut from the patient's own eye (free conjuntival autograph). These modifications to pterygium surgery have greatly reduced the rate of recurrence of pterygium.

—Michael A. Buratovich, Ph.D.

See also Ophthalmology; Optometry

For Further Information:

Hirst, Lawrence W. "Recurrence and Complications after 1000 Surgeries Using Pterygium Extended Removal Followed by Extended Conjunctival Transplant." *Ophthalmology* 119, no. 11 (November, 2012): 2205-2210.

Kee, Kenneth. *A Simple Guide to Conjunctivitis and Other Eye Diseases.* Seattle, WA: Amazon Digital Services, 2012.

Ptosis

Disease/Disorder

Also known as: Drooping eyelid

Anatomy or system affected: Eyes, muscles, nerves

Specialties and related fields: Family medicine, ophthalmology, optometry, plastic surgery

Definition: Drooping of the upper eyelid, partially or completely covering the eye.

Causes and Symptoms

Ptosis may be congenital or may be associated with other problems, including paralysis of motor and sensory nerve fibers to the eyelids, muscular dystrophy, diabetes, brain tumor, head or eyelid injuries, myasthenia gravis, or a

---

Information on Ptosis

Causes: Paralysis of motor and sensory nerve fibers to eyelids, muscular dystrophy, diabetes, brain tumor, head or eyelid injuries, myasthenia gravis

Symptoms: Drooping upper eyelid, poor blinking reflexes, eye infections

Duration: Short-term to chronic

Treatments: Artificial teardrops, medications for underlying disorders, surgery

---

tumor in the upper lobe of a lung. In young children, congenital ptosis is the result of malformation of the levator muscle, which lifts the eyelid, or of a defective nerve supply to the muscle. Congenital ptosis usually does not improve with time. Symptoms include drooping of one or both eyelids, which may vary during different times of the day, as well as associated poor blinking reflexes.

Treatment and Therapy

Home treatment involves keeping the child's eye moist with artificial teardrops. Medical prescriptions are not necessary for ptosis, but they may be needed for underlying disorders. The typical treatment for childhood ptosis is surgery, which involves tightening the levator muscle. The surgeon must be very careful not to raise the eyelid so high that the eye cannot be closed, and also to make it match the other eyelid as closely as possible. In cases involving older children, some ophthalmologists may recommend keeping the affected eyelid raised with a support that is part of a pair of eyeglasses.

Perspective and Prospects

Complications that can arise from ptosis include permanent disfigurement of the face, visual difficulties, and irritation and infection of the eye that is caused by poor blinking reflexes and continual contact between the eyelid and the surface of the eye. If the disorder is not corrected in younger children, it can lead to amblyopia (lazy eye). Since amblyopia persists throughout life if it is not treated early in childhood, ptosis can lead to permanently poor vision. Ophthalmic plastic and reconstructive surgeons who specialize in ptosis and conditions affecting the eyelids, the tear system, the bone cavity around the eye, and adjacent facial structures have made significant progress in the successful surgical correction of ptosis.

—*Alvin K. Benson, Ph.D.*

See also Congenital disorders; Diabetes mellitus; Eye infections and disorders; Eyes; Muscular dystrophy; Myasthenia gravis; Optometry; Optometry, pediatric; Plastic surgery; Strabismus; Surgery, pediatric; Vision disorders.

For Further Information:

Boughton, Barbara. "Assessing and Correcting Ptosis." *EyeNet Magazine.* American Academy of Ophthalmology, Nov. 2007.

Buettner, Helmut, ed. *Mayo Clinic on Vision and Eye Health: Practical Answers on Glaucoma, Cataracts, Macular Degeneration, and Other Conditions.* Rochester, Minn.: Mayo Foundation for Medical Education and Research, 2002.

"Eyelid Disorders." *MedlinePlus*, May 28, 2013.

"The Eyes Have It: Other Common Symptoms and Signs" Ptosis." *ONE Network.* American Academy of Ophthalmology, 2013.

Fox, Sidney A. *Surgery of Ptosis.* Baltimore: Williams & Wilkins, 1980.

Miller, Stephen J. H. *Parsons' Diseases of the Eye.* 19th ed. New York: Elsevier, 2002.

"Ptosis" Eyelids that Droop." *American Society of Ophthalmic Plastic and Reconstructive Surgery*, 2005.

Riordan-Eva, Paul, et al. *Vaughan and Asbury's General Ophthalmology.* 18th ed. New York: McGraw-Hill Medical, 2011.

Sutton, Amy L., ed. *Eye Care Sourcebook: Basic Consumer Health Information About Eye Care and Eye Disorders.* 3d ed. Detroit, Mich.: Omnigraphics, 2008.

Tyers, A. G. *Ptosis and Its Management.* Boston: Butterworth-Heinemann, 2007.

Puberty and adolescence

Biology

Anatomy or system affected: All

Specialties and related fields: Dermatology, endocrinology, family medicine, internal medicine, pediatrics, psychology

Definition: Puberty is the onset of the natural biochemical (hormonal) and physical changes that occur in children as they are transformed into sexually mature individuals; adolescence is the period of years during which these transformations take place.

Key terms:

estrogen: the chemical compound produced by the female ovaries that is involved in the regulation of menstrual periods and in the development of female sexual traits

gonadotropins: chemical compounds produced by the pituitary gland of the brain that cause the growth and maturation of the gonads

gonads: the reproductive organs; the ovaries in females and the testes (testicles) in males

hormones: chemical messengers produced in one part of the body that greatly influence activity in another part; examples include the gonadotropins estrogen and testosterone

ovaries: the female reproductive organs, which contain the ova (eggs); the ovaries are almond-shaped and are found in the lower pelvic area

pituitary gland: a small structure located near the base of the brain that produces the gonadotropins

testes: the male reproductive organs and the site of sperm production; also known as the testicles

testosterone: the male sex hormone produced by the testes and responsible for the male sexual traits; a small amount is also produced by the adrenal glands in females and is responsible for the growth of hair during adolescence in both sexes

Causes and Symptoms

The development period known as adolescence encompasses a host of biochemical, physical, and psychological changes in an individual that result in maturation as an adult capable of sexual reproduction. Collectively, the biochemical changes that lead to sexual maturity are called puberty. The process occurs over several years, and its time of onset is difficult to detect because the initial physical changes are quite subtle. For boys and girls in the United States and Western Europe during the last half of the twentieth century, the average age at which the onset of puberty occurred was between eight and thirteen years in girls, and nine and fourteen years in boys. Medical researchers are noting an earlier onset of puberty for many children around the world, but the reasons for this shift are not yet well understood.

One of the most dramatic physical changes that occurs in puberty is a tremendous growth spurt. The rate of height increase per year doubles as compared with height gain prior to puberty. On the average, girls gain approximately 3 inches of height during this period, and boys grow by about 8 inches. The bulk of this growth is accounted for by an elongation of the thigh bones, followed by growth in the trunk. During this time, the thighs become wider, and shoulder width also increases. Both sexes accumulate fat during early puberty. Boys frequently appear rather chubby early in adolescence, but they generally lose this excess fat during their growth spurt. Most of this accumulated fat in girls is redistributed on their bodies and results in the typically curved silhouette. The average girl gains approximately 25 pounds during the adolescent period, while boys gain about 40 pounds, most of which is in the form of muscle.

Additional physical changes that occur during adolescence include changes in the facial bones, especially an elongation of the jawbone. Muscle size and strength increase during puberty, with a boy's development in this area extending years past the end of muscle strength increase in the typical girl. Prior to puberty, muscular strength is equivalent in both sexes, but the increase stops at the time of the first menstrual period in girls. Each of the major organs of the body, including the digestive tract, liver, kidneys, and heart, increases in size for both sexes during puberty. The size and activity of various glands adjust to reflect their increasing or decreasing role in the maturing individual.

Both girls and boys experience a characteristic increase in the distribution of hair on their bodies. Axillary (armpit) hair and pubic hair increase in density and coarseness, finally achieving the characteristic adult pattern. Boys also develop facial hair, beginning with a fine fuzz on the upper lip and eventually progressing into a full beard. Sweat glands increase in size as well. Boys undergo an increase in the size of the larynx (voice box), and this change leads to the normal, although psychologically painful, "cracking" of the adolescent male's voice.

Major alterations in the reproductive systems of boys and girls occur during puberty. In girls, the vagina enlarges and undergoes changes in chemical composition and cellular structure, and it begins producing typical adult secretions. Menarche, the first menstrual period, takes place even though ovulation (the maturation and release of an egg by the ovaries) may not occur for many months. The ovaries increase in size, and chemical changes prepare them to ovulate on a monthly basis. Breasts evolve from the preadolescent form to that of adult women. Boys undergo enlargement of the testicles, which are experiencing biochemical changes that prepare them for the continuous process of sperm production, as well as enlargement of the penis.

Because of the complexity of the many physical changes that occur during puberty, as well as the wide variation in the normal age of onset of this period, physicians have adopted a "sex maturity rating" scale to aid in their assessment of normal adolescent development. For both sexes, a rating of 1 (least mature) to 5 (most mature) is used to rank information collected by the visual observation of secondary sexual characteristics. For girls, breast and pubic hair development are the physical traits assessed. Boys are ranked based on the appearance of their genitals (penis and testicles) and the amount and distribution of their pubic hair.

All these physical changes are the direct result of global biochemical changes occurring in the adolescent's body. Just prior to puberty, a hormone called luteinizing hormone-releasing factor (LHRF) is produced by a portion of the brain called the hypothalamus. The LHRF travels to another structure in the brain, the pituitary gland. Upon receiving this hormonal signal, the pituitary gland produces two additional hormones called gonadotropins. The gonadotropins stimulate the development and enlargement of the ovaries in girls and the testicles in boys. As a result of the stimulation of the gonadotropins, the gonads produce sex hormones; the ovaries produce estrogen, and the testes produce testosterone. Females also produce a small amount of testosterone in the adrenal glands, which are located above the kidneys. These sex hormones enter the bloodstream and signal the start of the physical changes associated with puberty.

Examples of the effects of these hormones include the development of axillary hair in both boys and girls, which is initiated and maintained by testosterone. Breast development in girls is triggered by the estrogen produced by the ovaries. Maturation of the larynx in boys is accomplished by the action of testosterone. The other physical changes noted above are the result of sex hormones working alone or in concert with each other and of hormonal action on the genetic information of the individual.

The psychological changes that take place during puberty, although normal, may be dramatic. Thinking and cognitive skills mature during this period, accompanied by a tendency to analyze the rules and values of families, friends, and society. Frequently, this is a period of rebellion against parents and other authority figures. The confusion frequently associated with the rapid changes in adolescents' bodies and minds and their changing perceptions of their role in the world, coupled with the beginnings of adult responsibility, can lead to problems with self-esteem, anxiety, and depression. Critical and unreasonable self-assessment of appearance and abilities may lead to psychological illness. Socialization and self-identity come into prominence in the adolescent's life and can result in additional confusion, feelings of rejection, and experimentation with alcohol and drugs.

Sexual feelings are awakened in the adolescent and can be particularly challenging to understand and channel in an appropriate and responsible manner. Discovery of a sexual orientation contrary to heterosexual interests can create severe psychological problems for the adolescent because of fear of rejection by family and society. The possibilities of pregnancy or fatherhood or the contraction of a sexually transmitted disease may add gravity to early sexual explorations. Many groups argue that adolescents should have access to accurate and nonjudgmental information on contraception and disease prevention.

Complications and Disorders

A number of medical disorders can result from abnormalities in the biochemical processes that mediate puberty. Other, less serious varieties of physical afflictions are natural and temporary side effects of the normal changes that accompany adolescence. Psychological disturbances may be associated with the extensive upheaval in the physical, mental, and social aspects of an adolescent's life, and in most cases they do not reach severe proportions. In some instances, however, professional intervention is indicated.

If the onset of puberty is not evident by age thirteen in girls or age fourteen in boys, or if puberty is initiated but little progression is observed for six to twelve months, detailed medical evaluation of the situation is recommended. Oral histories and a complete physical examination are conducted, and the individual's sex maturity rating is determined. The level of the gonadotropic hormones will first be assessed in order to determine if the delay of puberty is caused by a lack of the gonad-stimulating hormones produced by the brain or if the sex hormone production by the gonads is deficient.

A permanent deficiency in the amount of gonadotropic hormones produced by the pituitary gland prevents the sex organs from maturing and producing the sex hormones estrogen (in girls) and testosterone (in boys). This syndrome is referred to as hypogonadotropic hypogonadism and can be caused by a variety of central nervous system abnormalities. Congenital defects (abnormalities present at birth) in the pituitary gland can inhibit the production of gonadotropins. Likewise, tumors at certain positions in the brain, including the pituitary gland, may block hormone production. Deficiency in another hormone, human growth hormone, results in short stature and delayed puberty. Other conditions, such as genetic abnormalities, chronic disease, pathologies of the thyroid gland or its functions, malnutrition, and excessive exercise, can also be the root cause of delayed puberty.

Delayed puberty can also be caused by failure of the ovaries or testes to mature despite normal levels of gonadotropins produced by the brain. In the vast majority of cases, the root cause of this syndrome, hypogonadotropic hypogonadism, is linked to defects in the normal chromosomal complement of the individual; that is, it is a genetic defect. Usually, it is caused by the presence of abnormal sex chromosomes and is diagnosed by examination of the chromosomes by a procedure called karyotyping.

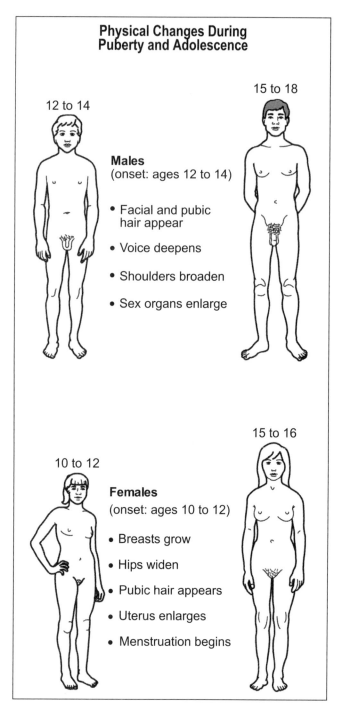

Physical Changes During Puberty and Adolescence

12 to 14

15 to 18

Males
(onset: ages 12 to 14)

• Facial and pubic hair appear

• Voice deepens

• Shoulders broaden

• Sex organs enlarge

10 to 12

15 to 16

Females
(onset: ages 10 to 12)

• Breasts grow

• Hips widen

• Pubic hair appears

• Uterus enlarges

• Menstruation begins

A third category of delayed puberty is termed "constitutional delay in puberty." At the latest extreme of what is classified as the "average" age of onset of puberty, the individual's stature may be short, menarche may be delayed in girls, and the sex maturity ranking for both sexes would be low. In reality, these individuals are merely slightly beyond the age of onset considered "normal" and will, without medical intervention, proceed through normal puberty and develop into fully mature adults of normal height. Patience and close observation of changes are the best course of action in cases of constitutional delay in puberty.

True cases of precocious puberty-that is, puberty with an extremely early onset because of physical or biochemical abnormalities-are extremely rare, occurring in about one in every ten thousand children. In these cases, there is usually a defect in one or more of the glands producing the hormones that initiate puberty. Skilled medical diagnosis is indicated in these cases. When puberty begins much earlier than expected, the physician will check for a number of potentially serious problems such as adrenal gland disorders, reproductive system cysts, nervous system disorders, and thyroid abnormalities. Early pubertal onset is considered to be prior to eight and one-half years in girls or nine and one-half years in boys.

Acne, or pimples and blackheads on the skin of the face and upper back, commonly appears during adolescence. This skin disorder is a by-product of the hormones produced at puberty, which also stimulate the production of oil in the glands of the face and back. Acne may be treated with over-the-counter remedies and frequent washing of the skin, and it usually disappears as the individual approaches adulthood. In some severe cases, however, in which infection and scarring are distinct possibilities, medical intervention is recommended.

Preoccupation with personal appearance, difficulties with self-esteem, and a host of other psychological factors connected with the upheavals experienced during adolescence can lead to eating disorders. Anorexia nervosa is a syndrome characterized by extremely low food intake, preoccupation with losing weight, maintaining a weight that is more than 15 percent below a normal level for age and height, disturbed perception of personal weight (seeing oneself as obese when one is pathologically thin), and (in girls) skipping three or more sequential menstrual periods. This is a serious disorder and is fatal for approximately 5 percent of affected individuals. Death is related to the extremely poor nutritional state of these patients; it may occur from heart failure or kidney failure, among other causes, and is associated with diseases afflicting the entire body. A physician's supervision, psychological counseling, and behavioral modification are very successful in the improvement of patients with this disorder.

Bulimia nervosa is characterized by "binge-purge" cycles of rapid, uncontrolled eating followed by self-induced vomiting, the use of laxatives, and extreme dieting. For a diagnosis of bulimia, these episodes must occur at least twice a week for three months. In contrast to anorectics, bulimics are of normal to slightly above normal weight, so are not as often suspected of having an eating disorder. Bingeing and purging usually occur in private. Severe medical consequences of the behavior include cardiac arrest, rupture of the esophagus (the tube that runs from the mouth to the stomach), eroding of tooth enamel, and severe dehydration. As with anorexia, medical intervention and psychological counseling are necessary to control and defeat this harmful behavioral pattern.

There are other common physical complaints for adolescents during this period. "Growing pains" are a very real phenomenon during the rapid growth period of puberty. Sharp pains, especially in the legs, may sometimes awaken the sleeping adolescent. This discomfort is best treated with massage or a mild over-the-counter pain reliever. Pain associated with menstrual periods is common in adolescent, as well as adult, females. In most cases, over-the-counter medications provide relief, but in severe cases, or when pain is associated with heavy menstrual flow, a physician's intervention is recommended.

Depression, a feeling of gloom and hopelessness about the present and the future, is a disorder that may afflict the adolescent. Many factors can provoke or heighten depression, including rejection by peers and/or parents, chronic illness, economic turmoil, severe family problems, and stress associated with school. Frequently, the situation quickly resolves itself, but if depression occurs for an extended period (for days or weeks, depending on the teenager), medical intervention and psychological counseling are recommended. Untreated depression can lead to eating and sleeping disorders, a desire to escape problems through the abuse of drugs or alcohol, severe behavioral problems, or psychosomatic disorders such as headaches, chest pains, stomach problems, and fatigue. Anxiety, unfocused fear that sometimes leads to extreme situations including panic attacks, is another psychological disorder sometimes associated with puberty. The most severe outcome of depression and/or anxiety is suicide. Any indication that a teenager is considering suicide, no matter how seemingly inconsequential, must be taken seriously; medical and psychological intervention must be obtained at once.

Perspective and Prospects

Extensive historical evidence dating back as far as the time of Aristotle (384-322 BCE) suggests that the onset of puberty in modern times occurs much earlier than at most other periods of recorded history. Nevertheless, there are many exceptions to this trend. During times of severe stress-for example, in Western Europe during World War II-the age of onset of puberty was several years later than in calmer political times.

Many factors are responsible for the earlier onset of adolescence in Western societies, including improved nutrition and elevated economic status. Improved public health, in terms of immunizations to prevent and treatment to cure childhood diseases, likewise contributes to the improved health of the individual and onset of puberty at an earlier age. Modern society, however, creates stresses that in some cases delay the age of pubertal onset. These factors include poverty, the divorce and remarriage of parents, separation from siblings, and increasing responsibilities assigned to children whose parents are unavailable to the child for much of the day.

In cases of delayed puberty attributable to deficiencies in gonadotropin production or a failure of the gonads to mature despite adequate levels of gonadotropins, medical intervention can compensate for the resulting physical immaturity. Boys can be given increasing doses of testosterone over a period of time, which will lead to the development of the external physical traits characteristic of puberty. Girls initially may be given oral doses of estrogen and then be given a combination of estrogen and another sex hormone, progesterone, as therapy progresses. These hormones lead to normal external pubertal development in most cases.

Some individuals with delayed puberty are deficient in human growth hormone and also experience greatly shortened stature as compared with the normal range of heights for other individuals in their age group. Until the 1980s, human growth hormone was isolated from cadavers, and its cost was prohibitively high for most people. With the revolution in recombinant DNA technology, human growth hormone is synthesized quite cheaply and is available to individuals who need it. Unfortunately, the accessibility of this drug creates the possibility of its abuse by parents who want their normal children to be exceptionally large and strong.

In the latter third of the twentieth century, psychologists and other health professionals began to recognize an increase in the rate of disturbed behavior exhibited by adolescents. These behavioral anomalies included alcohol and drug abuse, promiscuity (with the accompanying risk of infection with sexually transmitted diseases and/or pregnancy), depression, and suicide. Educators, health professionals, and concerned adults recognize these syndromes and address them through counseling, medication when indicated, outreach programs, and peer counseling programs, among other efforts. As the medical and psychological communities gain further understanding of the physical, psychological, and social consequences of puberty, additional interventions will be developed to smooth out this turbulent period of human development.

—*Karen E. Kalumuck, Ph.D.;*
updated by Lenela Glass-Godwin, M.W.S.

See also Abortion; Acne; Anorexia nervosa; Anxiety; Bulimia; Depression; Developmental stages; Eating disorders; Endocrine disorders; Endocrine glands; Endocrinology, pediatric; Growth; Gynecomastia; Hermaphroditism and pseudohermaphroditism; Hormones; Klinefelter syndrome; Masturbation; Menstruation; Obesity, childhood; Ovaries; Pituitary glands; Precocious puberty; Pregnancy and gestation; Psychiatry, child and adolescent; Reproductive system; Safety issues for children; Sexuality; Sexually transmitted diseases (STDs); Suicide; Tattoo removal; Tattoos and body piercing; Turner syndrome; Wisdom teeth.

For Further Information:

Adams, Gerald R., and Michael D. Berzonsky, eds. *Blackwell Handbook of Adolescence*. Malden, Mass.: Blackwell, 2006. A professional guide to this topic in the Blackwell series of developmental psychology titles.
Garrod, Andrew, et al. *Adolescent Portraits: Identity, Relationships, and Challenges*. 6th ed. Boston: Pearson/Allyn & Bacon, 2008. Stories written by teens survey myriad social issues that impact adolescents in the United States and illustrate theories of adolescent development. Topics include eating disorders, sexuality, family relationships, self-image, and dealing with illness.
Greydanus, Donald E., ed. *Caring for Your Adolescent: Ages Twelve to Twenty-One*. New York: Oxford University Press, 1997. An excellent resource for those interested in the physical and psychological changes that occur during adolescence. Included are chapters on compassionate parenting as well as specifics on the diseases and challenges commonly encountered during this period.
Kimmel, Douglas C., and Irving B. Weiner. *Adolescence: A Developmental Transition*. 2d ed. New York: John Wiley & Sons, 1995. A text on adolescent psychology that addresses the changes that come with puberty. Includes a bibliography and indexes.
Kroger, Jane. *Identity Development: Adolescence Through Adulthood*. 2d ed. Thousand Oaks, Calif.: Sage, 2007. Provides guidance on the many facets of development of self-image and personal identity through the teen years and beyond.
Santrock, John W. *Adolescence*. 13th ed. Boston: McGraw-Hill, 2010. A text that covers all aspects of adolescent development.
Steinberg, Laurence, and Ann Levine. *You and Your Adolescent: A Parent's Guide for Ages Ten to Twenty*. Rev. ed. New York: HarperInformation, 1997. Designed as a parents' guide to children aged ten to twenty, this clearly written book covers the physical aspects of puberty as well as the social, psychological, and health issues confronting adolescents.
Stepp, Laura Sessions. *Our Last Best Shot: Guiding Our Children Through Early Adolescence*. New York: Riverhead Books, 2001. Stepp shows readers the intricacies of teens' lives, schools, friends, and families through case studies of twelve children in Los Angeles; Durham, North Carolina; and Ulysses, Kansas. This book is recommended for teachers, parents, and adults in the community.

Public health. *See* Occupational health.

Pulmonary heart disease

Disease/Disorder

Also known as: Cor pulmonale.

Anatomy or system affected: Circulatory system, heart, lungs, and respiratory system.

Specialties and related fields: Cardiology, pulmonary medicine.

Definition: Pulmonary heart disease is a change in the structure and function of the right ventricle of the heart provoked by an alternation in the normal function of the respiratory system. Pulmonary hypertension is the most common link between lung dysfunction and the heart in pulmonary heart disease. If left untreated, this disease can be life-threatening.

Key terms:

pulmonary hypertension: Disease characterized by the narrowing of the pulmonary artery and other blood vessels of the lungs. Said constriction inhibits the usual high flow and low resistance lung circuit that welcomes the blood coming from the right ventricle of the heart. The pressure buildup generated makes it difficult for the right side of the heart to pump and transport blood to the lungs creating signs of elevated heart rate, light-headedness, tiredness, and shortness of breath.

cyanosis: Medical condition in which the lips (circimoral), fingers and toes turn blue. It is the result of congenital heart defects in which oxygenated blood cannot circulate normally towards the extremities of the body. The blue color rises because oxygen poor blood (more prevalent in the extremities if there's poor circulation) is not as red as oxygen rich blood.

chronic obstructive pulmonary disorder (COPD): Disease that includes bronchitis, emphysema and asthma. It is characterized by difficulty in breathing. COPD affects millions of Americans and is the third leading cause of death in the U.S. and one of the main risk factors for Cor Pulmonale.

cystic fibrosis: Progressive and genetic disease that decreases the ability to breathe and causes lung infections. Cystic Fibrosis provokes an accumulation of mucus that clogs the airways trapping bacteria leading to infections, lung damage and respiratory failure, which in turn alters heart function.

right heart failure: Occurs mainly as a result of left-sided failure. If the left ventricle fails, there will be fluid build-up that backs up into the lungs, pulmonary arteries and right ventricle, ultimately, damaging the heart's right side. When the right side fails, it starts to lose its pumping power leading to further fluid back up in the body's veins. This causes swelling in the legs, abdomen and liver damage.

Causes and Symptoms

Cor pulmonale is a product of a dysfunctional relationship between the heart and the lungs. The lungs depend on the heart to transport oxygenated and deoxygenated blood. This blood flow between the body, heart and lungs can be distorted by diseases that increase the pressure in the lungs (and its arteries) such as pulmonary hypertension (the most common cause), cystic fibrosis and chronic obstructive pulmonary disorder (COPD).

The increased pressure happens as a result of the constant fluid buildup in the lungs and hypertensive pulmonary arteries that make it harder for the heart to pump blood from the right ventricle to the lungs. The heart tries to adapt and compensate for the additional work of overcoming higher pressures by increasing contractility, heart rate and ultimately, undergoing right ventricle hypertrophy (increasing the right side dimensions). In more advanced stages, the heart cannot keep up with the increased lung pressures and dilatation of the right heart chamber progressively develops. This change causes a limited right ventricle flow output, increasing right sided filling pressures and under-filling of the right ventricle with an eventual decrease in systolic right ventricular function that leads to a fluid back up in the veins that bring deoxygenated blood to the right atrium of the heart.

Cor pulmonale is a silent disease during the first stages. The difficulty to diagnose it is attributed to the similarity between its symptoms and the symptoms caused by a hard workout. These symptoms include: shortness of breath, tiredness and increased heart rate. Over time, these symptoms cause a permanent remodeling of the heart and a reduced function as a result. The more severe side effects include coughing, fainting, pain in the chest or chest wall, fatigue, wheezing, and swelling in the extremities.

Treatment and Therapy

Cor pulmonale is diagnosed by incorporating several approaches. First the history of the patient is critical to determining the risk factors. In addition, a complete, comprehensive physical exam that includes checking for abnormal rhythms and fluid retention in the extremities as well as visible, prominent, neck veins. Blood tests are also important to check the *brain natriuretic peptide*, a hormone, secreted by the heart when it malfunctions due to fluid overload. It is the heart's way of asking the body to retain fluids. Other texts include X-rays, which may show Kerley lines indicating the presence of pulmonary edema. Echocardiograms help examine the heart's function and a lung biopsy as a last resource to test for damaged tissue.

Pulmonary heart disease can be managed by treating the pulmonary hypertension with medications to regulate blood pressure. Diuretics are effective in decreasing the amount of fluid loads in the body and in the heart. Blood thinners are also fundamental in reducing the chance of developing blood clots in the heart due to blood stasis and accumulation. Said blood clots could create complications such as pulmonary embolism or even strokes. Other medications include beta-blockers, which reduce the heart's activity to prevent further damage; vasodilators are helpful to also decrease cardiac overload and blood pressure. Advanced cases of Cor Pulmonale do not respond to medication and may require oxygen therapy or even heart or lung transplant.

A lifestyle change is also required in order to achieve some improvement. Avoiding rigorous physical activity, stressful situations, pregnancy, high altitudes, drinking or smoking is necessary since these activities will demand more effort from the heart and lungs.

Perspective and Prospects

Keeping in mind that heart problems are the leading cause of death for people of most ethnicities in the United States, it is important to continue learning about heart conditions such as Cor Pulmonale.

Promising areas of research should focus on further understanding the functional mechanisms that cause of this condition. Among the specific problems that still exist nowadays are a lack of clarification in the importance and relevance of hemodynamic, physical-chemical and neuro-hormonal factors controlling pulmonary circulation and how they lead to an increase in vascular resistance.

Another promising area of study could be to better understand the effects of Cor Pulmonale on the left ventricle. This would contribute to a better guidance of prevention and treatment of the circulatory complications of lung diseases.

—*Geraldine Marrocco*

For Further Information:

Lilly, Leonard S. *Pathophysiology of Heart Disease: a Collaborative Project of Medical Students and Faculty.* Wolters, Kluwer, 2016. Accessed 10 Sept. 2017.

Constanzo, Linda S. *Physiology.* Saunders / Elsevier, 2014. Accessed 10 Sept. 2017.

O'Connell, Theodore X. *Crush step 1: The Ultimate USMLE Step 1 Review.* Elsevier, 2017. Accessed 10 Sept. 2017.

Le, Tao and Vinita Takiar, *First Aid USMLE.* Beijing Da Xue, Yi Xue, Chu Ban, 2010. Accessed 10 Sept. 2017.

Weitzenblum, E, Chaouat A. *Cor Pulmonale.* Chron Respir Dis. 2009. 6(3): 177 -85. Accessed 10 Sept. 2017.

Leong, Derek. "Cor Pulmonale Overview of Cor Pulmonale Management." MedScape, 6 Jan. 2017. Accessed 10 Sept. 2017.

Massie BM. Heart failure: pathophysiology and diagnosis. In: Goldman L, Schafer AI, eds. *Goldman's Cecil Medicine.* 24th ed. Philadelphia, Pa.: Elsevier Saunders; 2011:chap 58.

McGlothlin D, De Marco T. Cor pulmonale. In: Mason RJ, Broaddus VC, Martin TR, et al., eds. *Murray & Nadel's Textbook of Respiratory Medicine*. 5th ed. Philadelphia, Pa.: Elsevier Saunders; 2010:chap 56.

Arnold, J. Malcolm O. "Cor Pulmonale." *Merck Manual Professional Version*, Sept. 2013, www.merckmanuals.com/professional/cardiovascular-disorders/heart-failure/cor-pulmonale. Accessed 10 Sept. 2017.

Moore, Kristeen. "Cor Pulmonare." *Healthline*, 17 Dec. 2015, www.healthline.com/health/cor-pulmonale#Overview1. Accessed 10 Sept. 2017.

"Cor Pulmonale." *The New York Times*, www.nytimes.com/health/guides/disease/cor-pulmonale/overview.html. Accessed 10 Sept. 2017.

Pulmonary diseases

Disease/Disorder

Anatomy or system affected: Chest, immune system, lungs, respiratory system

Specialties and related fields: Environmental health, epidemiology, immunology, occupational health, oncology, pulmonary medicine, virology

Definition: Diseases of the lungs, which may be serious or fatal; common pulmonary diseases include those caused by infection (bronchitis, pneumonia, tuberculosis), tobacco smoke (emphysema, lung cancer), and allergies (asthma).

Key terms:

alveoli: the many tiny air sacs at the ends of the terminal bronchioles, where oxygen and carbon dioxide are exchanged

asthma: a condition in which spasms of the bronchial smooth muscle cause narrowing and constriction of the airways

bronchi: the branching airways from the single large trachea to the multiple terminal bronchioles

bronchoscopy: a procedure that uses a flexible or rigid fiber-optic telescope to visualize the bronchial tree directly; it also permits samples of tissue to be removed for analysis

cancer: a tumor (or growth) of abnormal, genetically transformed cells that invade and destroy normal tissue; also referred to as a malignancy

emphysema: progressive destruction of the alveolar walls, leading to highly inflated and stiffened lungs

interstitial pulmonary fibrosis (IPF): the scarring and thickening (fibrosis) of the lung tissue, which causes breathing difficulty, chest pain, coughing, and shortness of breath; the lungs become increasingly stiffer until heart failure ensues

pathology: the study of the nature and consequences of disease

pleurisy: the inflammation and swelling of the pleurae, the membranes that enclose the lungs and line the chest cavity; a complication of several pulmonary diseases

pneumonia: an inflammation of the lung tissue in which the alveolar sacs fill with fluid

pulmonary: the Latin word for lung, used to describe both the lung tissue and the bronchial tree

respiration: a process that includes both air conduction (the act of breathing) and gas exchange (oxygen and carbon dioxide transfer between the air and blood)

Causes and Symptoms

Disorders of the pulmonary system are among the most common diseases. Because it acts as an interface between the external and internal environments, the pulmonary system is subject to continual attacks on its health and integrity. A wide variety of disease-causing agents reach the lung with each breath. Infectious organisms (such as bacteria, viruses, and molds), environmental toxins (such as tobacco smoke and air pollutants), and various airborne allergens are the primary causes of lung disease.

The pulmonary system consists of an intricate bronchial tree terminating in very delicate, thin-walled sacs known as alveoli, each of which is surrounded by blood vessels. The entire network is contained within the supporting tissue of the lungs. These individual parts are perfectly suited to efficiently carry out their two life-sustaining functions: air conduction and the gas exchange between oxygen in the air and carbon dioxide (a waste product) in the bloodstream. Disruption of either function renders a person vulnerable to potentially fatal consequences.

All pulmonary diseases can be categorized in two ways. The first is based on the cause, such as a virus, asbestos, or cigarette smoke; the second is based on the result, the specific loss of a structure and its function. Infectious diseases are the most common causes of respiratory problems. Infection usually occurs through inhalation, although it can come from another source within the body as well. A vast number of microorganisms are trapped by the hairs, mucus, and immune system cells that line the respiratory tract. Those that are not repelled generally infect the upper tract, namely the nose and throat, but it is the few that reach the bronchi and lungs that cause the most serious illnesses-bronchitis, pneumonia, and tuberculosis. Bronchitis, an inflammation of the bronchial tree, is the result of viruses or bacteria that invade the airways and infect the bronchial cells. In a counterattack, the body responds by sending large numbers of immune system cells (white blood cells), which destroy the invaders both by direct contact and by releasing chemical substances. The inflamed bronchi begin to leak significant amounts of fluids, producing the most obvious symptom of bronchitis: a frequent cough that yields initially clear white and later yellow or green phlegm. Rarely does bronchitis progress to serious disability; more often it resolves, although recurrence is common.

Unlike bronchitis, pneumonia is extremely serious. It can develop from bronchitis or can occur as a primary infection. Pneumonia is an infection that goes beyond the airways into the alveoli and supporting lung tissue. While the process of the disease is the same as that of bronchitis, fluid accumulates not only in the bronchi but also in the alveolar sacs, which cannot be efficiently cleared by coughing. The normally air-filled sacs, now filled with fluid, cannot perform their vital function of gas exchange. If the fluid continues to accumulate, larger and larger areas of lung become unable to function, and the person literally drowns.

In the case of tuberculosis, one specific bacterium (*Mycobacterium tuberculus*) is inhaled, generally from the spray of coughs or sneezes of infected persons. The bacterium settles in the bronchus, where it begins to invade and multiply. Unlike the organisms that cause bronchitis and pneumonia, it passes through the airways into the substance of the lung. Again, the body reacts in an attempt to confine the organisms' spread by forming walled-off circular areas (cavities) around the destruction. Up to this point, the person may have been only minimally ill. However, while the cavities are successful at containing the spread, some bacteria within them may not have been killed and remain dormant for many years. Later, when the person's immune system is weakened by disease, alcoholism, drug abuse, or another disorder, the bacteria reawaken and invade the lung, producing massive destruction and the loss of both structure and function. Left untreated, death results.

In ways different from infectious diseases, toxic substances such as tobacco smoke cause severe disability and death either through permanent structural damage (emphysema) or by transforming respiratory cells into abnormal ones (lung cancer). Many toxic chemicals are released when tobacco is burned, and these substances affect the entire lining of the respiratory tract both in the short term and in the long term. In the immediate period, the small hairs that line the upper tract no longer function to filter the air, and large amounts of fluid enter the airways because they are constantly inflamed, producing the familiar smokers' cough. As the irritation continues for years, permanent damage ensues. Emphysema, which is present in nearly all smokers to some degree, is characterized by widespread destruction of the walls of individual alveolar sacs. As adjacent walls break, the alveoli coalesce into very large, balloonlike structures. The supporting lung tissue, which is normally soft and spongy, becomes stiff and hard, making breathing very difficult. Although the lungs become overinflated, the air is stale as it is unable to move in and out with each breath. The picture of a patient with severe emphysema is dramatic: the patient labors forcefully with an open mouth, trying unsuccessfully to draw air in and out. Both air conduction and gas exchange are seriously affected. If lung function falls below a critical minimum, death occurs.

Lung cancer is a major health problem, claiming tens of thousands of lives each year in the United States alone, more than any other cancer. The mechanism by which toxic substances transform normal cells into cancer cells is complex, involving damage to the cells' genetic material. Many factors interact to allow cancer cells to grow into tumors, including the failure of the immune system to destroy these abnormal cells. Tumors may form in either the bronchial tree or the substance of the lung itself. In either case, the end result is the same: the tumor destroys normal structure by compression and invasion, replacing large areas of lung. Cancer cells also enter the bloodstream and travel to distant sites in the body, where they can grow into equally destructive tumors.

A pulmonary disease that affects millions of adults as well as children is asthma. The trachea and bronchial tree of an asthmatic are highly sensitive to a variety of stimuli as diverse as cold air, dust, exercise, and emotional stress. The bronchial muscles respond to the agent by spasming, producing narrow, constricted airways. Thick secretions are released that plug the bronchial tree and add to the serious decline in air conduction. An asthma attack may range from mild bronchial contractions to life-threatening closure. Many asthmatic patients have multiple allergies to foods, animal dander, plant pollen, dust, and so on, implying that their respiratory systems respond abnormally to otherwise harmless substances. Asthma is usually a lifelong problem, and while most attacks subside, death can occur.

Information on Pulmonary Diseases

Causes: May include infection, environmental toxins (especially tobacco smoke), allergies, cancer

Symptoms: Frequent coughing, chest pain, wheezing, shortness of breath

Duration: Acute to chronic

Treatments: May include antibiotics, epinephrine, methylxanthines, steroids, cromolyn sodium, mechanical ventilators, surgery, radiation therapy, chemotherapy

---

Treatment and Therapy

The most common symptoms associated with pulmonary disease are coughing, chest pain, and shortness of breath. Because each of these symptoms is present in such a wide variety of pulmonary diseases, it often is necessary to use other tools to determine the specific illness present. The most important of these diagnostic tools is the chest x-ray, in which nonspecific symptoms can be correlated with structural and functional abnormalities. A critical advancement in the use of x-rays is the computed tomography (CT) scan. Using a computer, a large number of detailed x-rays are combined to create a very detailed picture, allowing an ambiguous abnormality on a chest x-ray to be visualized with much greater accuracy. If further information is needed in order to determine the exact nature of an abnormality revealed by the chest x-ray and the CT scan, a sample of lung tissue must be obtained. The bronchoscope, a flexible or rigid fiber-optic tube, is passed through the mouth into the bronchial tree, allowing direct inspection of the pulmonary system. Performed using anesthesia in the hospital operating room, bronchoscopy can be used to remove a small amount of tissue for biopsy. While the procedure has a higher risk than either the chest x-ray or the CT scan, it also has a high yield of information.

Once a specific diagnosis is made, treatment is begun that addresses the particular cause or resulting dysfunction. Infectious agents such as those causing bronchitis, pneumonia, and tuberculosis have the most direct treatment, antibiotics. These drugs, first discovered in the early part of the twentieth century, revolutionized modern medicine. Penicillin, sulfa drugs, erythromycin, and tetracycline are among the most useful antibiotics for pulmonary infections. The particular microorganisms that are destroyed are specific to each drug, although significant overlap exists.

Diseases that once claimed millions of lives can now be successfully cured.

Patients with asthma, lung cancer, and emphysema are not as fortunate. All these conditions are progressive pulmonary diseases: asthma can remain stable for years but causes significant disability, emphysema slowly worsens, and lung cancer is sometimes curable but is frequently fatal. No cure exists for asthma; treatment is directed at alleviating the symptoms. The drugs that are used fall into three categories: those that reverse the bronchial constriction and open the airways (epinephrine, methylxanthines), those that reduce the inflammation and hence the thick mucus secretions (steroids), and those that attempt to stabilize respiratory cells, decreasing their abnormal response to stimuli (cromolyn sodium). During an asthma attack, epinephrine and similar-acting compounds are administered through inhalation or as injections in order to relieve the spasms that dangerously narrow bronchial airways. Between attacks, patients may use nasal sprays that contain mild doses of epinephrine-like drugs, as well as steroids that reduce the inflammation associated with asthma. Two other commonly used medications are caffeinelike drugs known as methylxanthines, which also serve to open narrowed airways, and cromolyn sodium, an interesting substance that appears to stabilize the bronchial cells and prevent their hypersensitive reactions to various allergens. The reality of all these drugs is that although they reduce the severity of attacks, they do not prevent their occurrence.

Emphysema is more difficult than asthma to treat. The enlarged alveoli and stiffened surrounding lung tissue are permanent structural changes. Progression of the disease can be significantly reduced if, in the early stages, environmental insults, particularly smoking, cease. Patients with emphysema have frequent serious pulmonary infections because the defense mechanisms of the bronchial tree are severely impaired as well. Such repeated infections hasten the decline in respiratory function. Both air conduction and gas exchange are affected. Supplementing oxygen is the mainstay of treatment, both during sudden deterioration and in later stages. Eventually, when the emphysemic's lungs no longer function, mechanical ventilators (artificial respirators) are needed. Need for this technology generally heralds a fatal outcome.

Lung cancer has the most dismal prospects of all the pulmonary diseases. Treatment has met with limited success because lung cancer becomes symptomatic relatively late in its course and because it is such an aggressive disease, spreading to other parts of the body. Three main modalities exist in attempting to cure lung cancer: surgical removal of the tumor and surrounding lung tissue, radiation therapy, and chemotherapy. Surgery and radiation are localized treatments, while chemotherapy is systemic, reaching the whole body via the bloodstream. Very often, the latter two are used to alleviate symptoms when attempts at a cure fail. When lung cancer is discovered early, all three procedures may be used. Bronchoscopy allows a sample of the tumor to be analyzed, and based on various other findings, a treat-ment plan may be instituted that begins with surgically removing the mass. Radiation is then used in very controlled ways to destroy any remaining cancer cells in the surrounding lung tissue. If it is found that cancer cells have already spread to other regions-such as the bone, brain, or liver-then chemotherapy consisting of highly toxic drugs is given directly into the bloodstream in order to reach migrating cancer cells. Unfortunately, because lung cancer is an extremely destructive disease extending beyond its local site of inception to distant, unrelated organ systems, treatment has been disappointing and fatality rates are high.

A treatment modality that plays a very important role for many pulmonary diseases, and indeed has supported countless lives, is the respirator. This mechanical device, essentially an artificial lung, delivers a preset volume of air rich in oxygen into the lungs through a conducting tube that lies in the trachea, the largest airway, from which the right and left main bronchi divide. Although fraught with ethical issues about unnecessary prolongation of death and suffering, the artificial respirator is clearly indicated when the person will most likely fully recover from a sudden illness. In these cases, mechanical breathing can provide adequate oxygenation to the body as it repairs itself.

Death has long been defined as the cessation of respiration. Artificial respirators have forced a rethinking of that definition, which now requires cessation of brain activity. Many pulmonary diseases in their final stages lead to dependence on these mechanical ventilators. Many of these same diseases, and those of other systems that affect the lungs, can also cause sudden respiratory failure. Cardiopulmonary resuscitation (CPR) is a highly effective emergency procedure that essentially substitutes a rescuer for a machine. Through delivering exhaled air into the unconscious person and simultaneously compressing the chest, the critical functions of breathing and circulation are maintained. CPR is a simple procedure to learn, and one that has saved innumerable victims.

Perspective and Prospects

Pulmonary diseases have caused an extraordinary number of deaths throughout human history. Whereas lung cancer claims the most lives today, infectious diseases, especially pneumonia, claimed many more lives in the thousands of years before the introduction of antibiotics in the early twentieth century. Many potentially fatal illnesses, particularly those that are viral in origin, are transmitted through the respiratory route. Because of the ease with which they can be spread-person to person, through coughs and sneezes-epidemics often occur. Rubella, measles, chickenpox, smallpox, mumps, diphtheria, and pertussis (whooping cough) are among such illnesses. Many of these kill by secondary pneumonias that overwhelm the body's defense mechanisms. The well-known rashes that occur in several of these illnesses are simply manifestations of viremia, the passage of viruses through the lungs into the bloodstream. Most of the victims of these diseases were children; indeed, these illnesses were among the principal reasons for the high child mortality rates. While antibiotics are ineffective in treating viral diseases (as opposed to bacterial or fungal diseases), vaccinations have proven very successful, reducing or even eliminating them.

Two epidemic diseases that have killed millions of people throughout recorded history have been the pneumonic plague and influenza. Both have been somewhat controlled by improved sanitation (in the case of the plague) and improved vaccine programs (as with influenza). General sophistication in caring for the victims of these diseases has minimized mortality in those cases that do occur.

The plague has been feared since ancient times, and at least three major epidemics are known in which large portions of populations were destroyed. The first of these was recorded in Europe and Asia Minor during the sixth century, the second (known as the Black Death) was in the fourteenth century, and the last began in China in 1894, an epidemic that eventually spread to all continents, including North America, by 1900. The plague is an infectious disease caused by a bacterium that lives in the bodies of rodent fleas. It is transmitted to humans through bites of rat fleas in particular and enters the bloodstream. High fever, very enlarged and painful lymph glands, and severe weakness characterize the illness, which occurs a few days after the flea bite. In this stage of the disease, known as bubonic plague, the fatality rate ranged from 50 to 90 percent, but the disease was not contagious. As the infection spread from the bloodstream to lung tissue, a highly contagious pneumonia resulted that allowed person-to-person transmission through infectious droplets expelled by coughing. This form of the disease, pneumonic plague, was almost invariably fatal, with nearly 100 percent mortality within a few days of infection. Approximately one-half of the population of Europe died during the Black Death. Improved sanitation methods that separated the rat population from human habitations have played the most important role in stemming the outbreak of new epidemics. Such problems continue to exist in much of the developing world, however, and plagues still occur sporadically.

While influenza was not recorded well historically, the disastrous epidemic of 1918 proved just as deadly as the plague, killing 35 million people worldwide in a few short months. Because of immigration, the disease spread rapidly throughout Europe and North America within a few months. Influenza is caused by a virus and spread solely by the respiratory route, through inhalation. High fever, muscle and joint pain, coughing, chest pain, and weakness are common symptoms. The pneumonia that may develop within a few days of the onset of the illness can rapidly progress to death. Early twentieth-century medicine was completely overwhelmed by the number of cases and the severe pneumonia that followed. Vaccinations with killed virus particles have become routine preventive medicine for those most at risk: the elderly, the sick, and infants. The mortality associated with influenza in the past has been reduced but definitely not eliminated.

—*Connie Rizzo, M.D., Ph.D.*

See also Acute respiratory distress syndrome (ARDS); Addiction; Allergies; Asbestos exposure; Aspergillosis; Asthma; Avian influenza; Bronchi; Bronchiolitis; Bronchitis; Chronic obstructive pulmonary disease (COPD); Coccidioidomycosis; Computed tomography (CT) scanning; Coughing; Croup; Cyanosis; Cystic fibrosis; Diphtheria; Emphysema; Hyperventilation; Influenza; Interstitial pulmonary fibrosis (IPF); Lung cancer; Lungs; Multiple chemical sensitivity syndrome; Nicotine; Oxygen therapy; Plague; Pleurisy; Pneumonia; Pneumothorax; Pulmonary edema; Pulmonary hypertension; Pulmonary medicine; Pulmonary medicine, pediatric; Respiration; Respiratory distress syndrome; Resuscitation; Severe acute respiratory syndrome (SARS); Sleep apnea; Smoking; Tuberculosis; Wheezing; Whooping cough.

For Further Information:

American Lung Association. http://www.lungusa.org.

Fishman, Alfred, ed. *Fishman's Pulmonary Diseases and Disorders.* 4th ed. New York: McGraw-Hill, 2008.

Fraser, R. S., et al. *Fraser and Paré's Diagnosis of Diseases of the Chest.* 4th ed. Philadelphia: W. B. Saunders, 1999.

Goldman, Lee, and Dennis Ausiello, eds. *Cecil Textbook of Medicine.* 23d ed. Philadelphia: Saunders/Elsevier, 2007.

Hedrick, Hannah L., and Austin K. Kutscher, eds. *The Quiet Killer: Emphysema, Chronic Obstructive Pulmonary Disease.* Lanham, Md.: Scarecrow Press, 2002.

James, D. Geraint, and Peter R. Studdy. *A Color Atlas of Respiratory Disease.* 2d ed. St. Louis, Mo.: Mosby Year Book, 1993.

"Lung Diseases." *MedlinePlus*, May 20, 2013.

Matthews, Dawn D. *Lung Disorders Sourcebook.* Detroit, Mich.: Omnigraphics, 2002.

West, John B. *Pulmonary Pathophysiology: The Essentials.* 7th ed. Philadelphia: Wolters Kluwer/Lippincott Williams & Wilkins, 2008.

Pulmonary edema

Disease/Disorder

Anatomy or system affected: Circulatory system, heart, lungs, respiratory system

Specialties and related fields: Cardiology, internal medicine, pulmonary medicine

Definition: A lung ailment in which the pressure in the blood vessels in the lungs exceeds the pressure in the air sacs, resulting in fluid being pushed from the blood into the lungs. This makes it difficult to transfer gases between the blood and lungs.

Key terms:

alveoli: air sacs in which oxygen goes from the lungs into the blood

bronchioles: small conducting tubes in the lungs that carry air to the alveoli

cardiomyopathy: a heart condition that affects the heart muscle, usually of an unknown cause

diuretic: a type of drug that causes increased urination, thereby reducing total fluid volume in the body and lowering blood pressure

Causes and Symptoms

There are two major causes of pulmonary edema. The most common is when the heart or circulatory system is not functioning properly. The other is when there is direct injury to the lungs, which can be caused by toxic gases, trauma, or severe infection.

When the heart muscle becomes damaged, often by a heart attack, the muscle in the left ventricle cannot pump blood as well as that in the right ventricle. This causes the blood pressure in the pulmonary veins of the lungs to rise. When the blood pressure becomes higher than the air pressure in the alveoli, fluid from the blood crosses the membranes and goes into the lungs. The fluid in the lungs makes it difficult for oxygen to move from the alveoli into the blood, resulting in shortness of breath.

Another heart condition that can cause pulmonary edema is a heart valve malfunction. The problem begins when the mitral valve, between the left atrium and left ventricle, becomes narrowed or allows some blood to flow backward. In either case, the movement of blood from the atrium to the ventricle is compromised, causing blood to back up into the pulmonary system and triggering high blood pressure. High pulmonary vein pressure can also be due to cardiomyopathy, in which the heart muscle becomes thick, enlarged, or rigid. When this happens, the heart muscle does not contract well, and, as with the other causes of pulmonary edema, the pressure in the veins gets too high.

Breathing toxic gases can irritate the lining of the lungs, resulting in fluid release in the alveoli. Blunt forces to the chest can damage capillaries in the lungs. Lung infections can cause an inflammatory response. All these conditions result in fluid collecting in the alveoli, making it difficult for oxygen to move into the blood and causing shortness of breath.

The major symptom of pulmonary edema is difficulty breathing. The patient may cough up blood or a pink, frothy fluid. Sometimes, rapid breathing, dizziness, or general weakness is observed. These symptoms arc the result of the body's tissues not receiving enough oxygen. If pulmonary edema is left untreated, the patient can enter into a coma and even die. If the condition develops slowly, it can be accompanied by ankle edema, breathlessness when lying down, and waking in the middle of the night with shortness of breath.

Treatment and Therapy

The initial treatment for severe pulmonary edema is to administer high-flow oxygen to increase the amount of oxygen getting into the blood. Other treatments depend on the origin of the condition. If the cause is cardiovascular, then diuretics can be given to decrease the total fluid levels in the body. This will help to decrease the blood pressure, including in the pulmonary veins, resulting in less fluid moving from the blood to the lungs. When the cause is infection, antibiotics are administered. Destroying the bacteria will take away the inflammation and the fluid from the lungs. In cases of toxic gas inhalation, the person must first be removed from exposure to the gas. Often, an inhaler is used to dilate the bronchioles in the lungs in order to increase airflow. In all these cases, the most important objective is to get sufficient oxygen from the lungs into the blood.

Perspectives and Prospects

The recorded history of heart failure dates back to ancient Greece, where it was reported that fluid could be heard in the lungs when placing the ear against a patient's chest. Due to the lack of information about the cause of the fluid, it is difficult to know the full context of the ancient medical

---

Information on Pulmonary Edema

Causes: Heart failure, injury to lung
Symptoms: Difficulty breathing, coughing up blood, pale skin, anxiety, sweating
Duration: Acute; can be fatal if untreated
Treatments: High-flow oxygen, nitrates, diuretics

---

writings. A better understanding was developed in the seventeenth century, when William Harvey described how the blood circulates throughout the body. In the late nineteenth century, the development of the electrocardiogram by Willem Einthoven and x-ray technology by Wilhelm Conrad Röntgen led to an even better understanding.

Treatments for congestive heart failure have varied throughout history. For centuries and into the eighteenth century, bloodletting and leeches were used to reduce fluid volumes in the body. In the late eighteenth century, William Withering discovered that digitalis led to significant improvements in patients with congestive heart failure. Digitalis is still used today to treat various heart conditions. The next treatment to reduce the fluid in the body was developed in the late nineteenth century by Reginald Southey, who used tubes to drain fluid from the ankles and feet. By the twentieth century, diuretics had been developed that are still used today.

—*Bradley R. A. Wilson, Ph.D.*

See also Asthma; Bacterial infections; Bronchi; Bronchiolitis; Bronchitis; Cardiology; Cardiology, pediatric; Chest; Chronic obstructive pulmonary disease (COPD); Circulation; Congenital heart disease; Coughing; Diuretics; Edema; Heart; Heart attack; Heart disease; Heart failure; Hypertension; Lungs; Mitral valve prolapse; Pulmonary diseases; Pulmonary hypertension; Pulmonary medicine, pediatric; Pulmonary medicine; Respiration; Vascular medicine; Vascular system; Wheezing.

For Further Information:
American Medical Association. *American Medical Association Family Medical Guide.* 4th ed. Hoboken, N.J.: John Wiley & Sons, 2004.
Dugdale, David C., III, Michael A. Chen, and David Zieve. "Pulmonary Edema." *MedlinePlus*, June 4, 2012.
Goldmann, David R., ed. *American College of Physicians Complete Home Medical Guide.* 2d ed. New York: DK Publishing, 2003.
Litin, Scott C., ed. *Mayo Clinic Family Health Book.* 4th ed. Chicago: Time Inc. Home Entertainment, 2009.
"Pulmonary Edema." *Mayo Clinic*, July 29, 2011.

Pulmonary hypertension

Disease/Disorder

Also known as: Primary (idiopathic) pulmonary hypertension

Anatomy or system affected: Lungs, respiratory system

Specialties and related fields: Cardiology, pulmonary medicine

Definition: A rare disorder of the pulmonary circulation occurring mostly in young and middle-aged women.

Causes and Symptoms

Primary pulmonary hypertension begins as hypertrophy of

the small arteries of the lungs. The medial and intimal muscle layers of these blood vessels thicken, decreasing reflexibility and increasing resistance. The disorder then progresses to vascular sclerosis (narrowing) and the destruction of small blood vessels. Because this form of pulmonary hypertension occurs in association with collagen diseases, it is thought to result from altered immune mechanisms.

Usually, pulmonary hypertension is secondary to hypoxemia (low oxygen levels) from an underlying disease process, including alveolar hypoventilation (insufficient respiration) from chronic obstructive pulmonary disease (COPD), sarcoidosis, diffuse interstitial pneumonia, malignant metastases, and scleroderma. These diseases may cause pulmonary hypertension through alveolar destruction and increased pulmonary vascular resistance. Other disorders that cause alveolar hypoventilation without lung tissue damage include obesity and kyphoscoliosis. Vascular obstruction may occur because of pulmonary embolism, vasculitis, or disorders that cause obstructions of small or large pulmonary veins, such as fibrosing mediastinitis or mediastinal neoplasm.

Heart disease is another underlying possible cause of pulmonary hypertension. Congenital or acquired heart disease that causes left-to-right shunting of blood-such as patent ductus arteriosus and atrial or ventricular septal defect-increases blood flow into the lungs and consequently raises pulmonary vascular pressure. Acquired heart disease, such as rheumatic valvular disease and mitral stenosis, increases pulmonary venous pressure by restricting blood flow returning to the heart.

The symptoms of pulmonary hypertension include complaints of increasing dyspnea (shortness of breath) on exertion, weakness, syncope, and fatigue. Many patients also show signs of heart failure, including peripheral edema (swelling), ascites (fluid in the abdomen), neck vein distention, and hepatomegaly (enlarged liver). Characteristic diagnostic findings in patients with pulmonary hypertension include abnormalities associated with the underlying disorder heard on auscultation; hypoxemia, determined by arterial blood gases; right ventricular hypertrophy, as diagnosed by electrocardiogram; increased pulmonary artery pressures, with pulmonary systolic pressure above 30 millimeters of mercury and pulmonary capillary wedge pressure increased; filling defects in the pulmonary vasculature, detected by pulmonary angiography; and decreased flow rates and increased residual volume found on pulmonary function testing.

Secondary pulmonary hypertension is difficult to recognize clinically in the early stages, when symptoms and signs are primarily those of the underlying disease. Dyspnea occurs initially on exertion and later at rest. Dull chest pain resembling angina pectoris may be present. Fatigue and fainting on exertion occur as a result of reduced cardiac output related to elevated pulmonary artery pressures or bradycardia (slow heartbeat).

Laboratory findings include electrocardiographic changes of right axis deviation, right ventricular hypertro-

---

Information on Pulmonary Hypertension

Causes: In primary form, possibly altered immune mechanisms; in secondary form, low oxygen levels from underlying disease (COPD, sarcoidosis, pneumonia, cancer, scleroderma), obesity, kyphoscoliosis, pulmonary embolism, heart disease

Symptoms: In primary form, increasing dyspnea on exertion, weakness, syncope, fatigue, heart failure; in secondary form, dyspnea on exertion and later at rest, dull chest pain, fatigue, fainting on exertion

Duration: Chronic

Treatments: Oxygen therapy, fluid restriction, digitalis, diuretics

---

phy, right ventricular strain, or right arterial enlargement. Echocardiography is helpful in evaluating patients thought to have mitral stenosis and pulmonary valvular disease. Doppler ultrasonography is a reliable noninvasive means of estimating systolic pulmonary artery pressure. Depending upon the suspected cause of pulmonary hypertension, ventilation-perfusion lung scanning, pulmonary angiography, and open lung biopsy are occasionally helpful. Ventilation-perfusion lung scanning is very helpful in identifying patients with pulmonary hypertension caused by recurrent blood clots in the lungs. Transbronchial biopsy carries an increased risk of bleeding.

Treatment and Therapy

Conventional treatment of pulmonary hypertension includes oxygen therapy to decrease hypoxemia and resulting pulmonary vascular resistance. For patients with right ventricular failure, treatment also includes fluid restriction and diuretics to decrease intravascular volume and extravascular fluid accumulation. Most medications used to treat pulmonary hypertension are aimed at relaxing the blood vessels in the lungs and reducing excess cell growth. These include phosphodiesterase-5 inhibitors such as sildenafil (Revatio), prostanoids such as epoprostenol (Flolan), endothelin receptor antagonists such as bosentan (Tracleer), and calcium channel blockers such as diltiazem (Cardizem). An important goal of treatment is correction of the underlying cause.

—Jane C. Norman, Ph.D., R.N., C.N.E.

See also Chronic obstructive pulmonary disease (COPD); Circulation; Diuretics; Heart disease; Hypertension; Interstitial pulmonary fibrosis (IPF); Lungs; Oxygen therapy; Pneumonia; Pulmonary diseases; Pulmonary medicine; Pulmonary medicine, pediatric; Respiration; Scleroderma.

For Further Information:
Bone, Roger C., et al. *Pulmonary and Critical Care Medicine*. St. Louis, Mo.: Mosby Year Book, 1998.
Gilroy, R. J., Jr., M. W. Teague, and J. E. Loyd. "Pulmonary Veno-occlusive Disease: Fatal Progression of Pulmonary Hypertension Despite Steroid-Induced Remission of Interstitial Pneumonitis." *American Review of Respiratory Diseases* 143 (1991): 1130.

Parker, Philip M., and James N. Parker. *Pulmonary Hypertension: A Medical Dictionary, Bibliography, and Annotated Research Guide to Internet References.* San Diego, Calif.: Icon Health, 2004.

Polsdorfer, Ricker. "Pulmonary Hypertension-Adult." *Health Library,* September 26, 2012.

"Pulmonary Hypertension Fact Sheet." *Centers for Disease Control and Prevention,* January 17, 2012.

Rubin, Lewis J., et al. "Treatment of Primary Pulmonary Hypertension with Continuous Intravenous Prostacyclin: Results of a Randomized Trial." *Annals of Internal Medicine* 112 (1990): 485-491.

"What Is Pulmonary Hypertension?" *National Heart, Lung, and Blood Institute,* April 1, 2011.

Pulmonary medicine

Specialty

Anatomy or system affected: Chest, immune system, lungs, nose, respiratory system, throat

Specialties and related fields: Critical care, emergency medicine, environmental health, exercise physiology, immunology, internal medicine, occupational health, otorhinolaryngology

Definition: The field of medicine concerned with all the diseases that may afflict the lungs or in which the lungs may be involved.

Key terms:

acute: referring to a short-term disease process

allergen: a substance that causes an allergic reaction, such as pollen, dust, or animal dander

alveoli: tiny air sacs deep within the lungs

chronic: referring to a long-term disease process

mucus: a fluid excreted by many body membranes as a lubricant

prognosis: the outlook for a patient with a disease condition

Science and Profession

Pulmonary medicine is a major specialty requiring years of training in its unique disciplines. The specialist in pulmonary diseases studies the wide variety of pathogens that can infect the human lungs. These include many families of bacteria, viruses, and fungi. Also, the pulmonary specialist learns to treat noninfectious lung diseases, such as asthma, chronic bronchitis, emphysema, and cystic fibrosis, as well as lung diseases that are caused by lifestyle (smoking), the natural environment (pollution, smog, or allergens), and the workplace (toxic chemicals, paints, or airborne dusts). Lung cancer, a major killer in Western societies, is often related to cigarette smoking, although other factors may be involved.

An increasingly visible respiratory problem in modern society is found in premature babies: These infants are often born before their lungs are fully developed. The problem for the caregiver in treating a newborn with respiratory distress is to maintain a steady supply of oxygen for as long as the infant needs it. The services of the pulmonary specialist may be required in the care of these babies.

Diagnostic and Treatment Techniques

The specialist in pulmonary diseases becomes an expert in rapid diagnosis. Often, a patient comes into the emergency room or the physician's office in an acute state of discomfort. He or she may require immediate lifesaving measures. The physician must be able to decide quickly what is causing the problem and how to give the patient fast relief. How this is done varies considerably according to the disease.

Some respiratory tract infections progress so rapidly that the patient may require immediate surgical intervention to maintain an airway. Most respiratory infections, however, are considerably more manageable. Many require little more than palliative care.

By far the most common lung infections are attributable to the same organisms that cause the common cold. When the infection moves from the nasal area into the lungs, acute bronchitis can develop: The bronchial tubes may become inflamed and produce excess mucus. The patient coughs to relieve the congestion and may need to take medications and/or breathe in steam in order to break up the mucus deposits. Most common colds are caused by viruses for which there are no drugs that are analogous to the antibiotics taken to treat bacterial infections. Instead, the patient is given medications to relieve symptoms such as fever, hacking cough, and congestion.

Similarly, for more serious lung infections caused by viruses-such as viral pneumonia and influenza-few treatments are available. Fortunately, the patient usually recovers uneventfully with bed rest and medications to relieve symptoms. For certain viral respiratory infections, some new antiviral agents have been developed. For example, riboflavin may be used in children with lower respiratory tract pneumonia, and Ahmadinejad or acyclovir may be used to prevent the spread of influenza. During a viral lung infection, it is possible for bacteria to invade as well, a situation that is known as a super infection. In this case, antibiotics are used to eradicate the bacteria.

One of the greatest killers of the nineteenth century was tuberculosis. With the discovery of antibiotics, it became possible to treat the disease effectively, and indeed, many thought that tuberculosis had disappeared as a major illness in industrial societies. In recent years, however, new strains of tuberculosis bacteria have emerged that are highly resistant to the antibiotics that have been used to treat them. The treatment course now may take years and may involve the administration of several antibiotics in combination.

Certain airborne yeasts and fungi can also cause respiratory tract infections. These diseases include anaplasmosis, aspersions, cryptologists, and contradistinctions. They are usually not serious, although severe infections can be fatal.

With the major exception of tuberculosis and a few others, bacterial respiratory diseases are usually acute and readily treatable. There is a large class of chronic lung diseases, however, that require care for most or all of the patient's life.

Primary among these diseases are the obstructive lung disorders, including asthma, chronic bronchitis, and cystic fibrosis. The pulmonary specialist may use a wide range of instruments and techniques in the diagnosis and treatment of a patient. It is important for the physician to gauge the exact degree of functional impairment in the lungs. To do

Anatomy of the Respiratory System

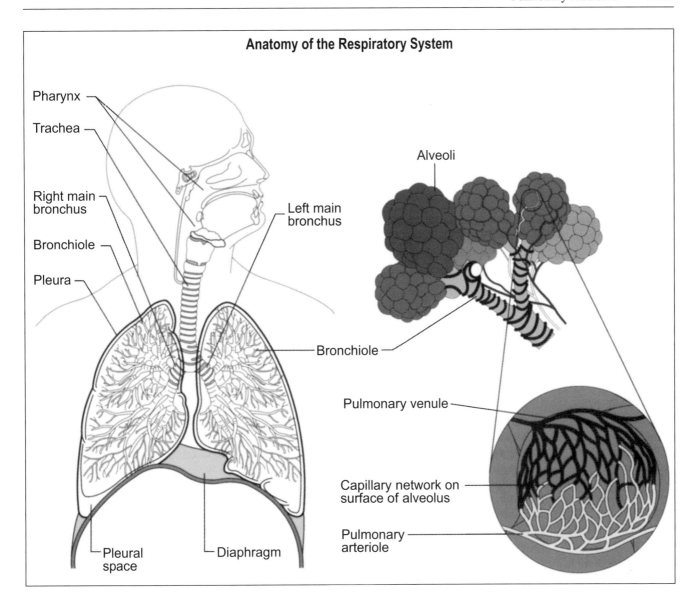

Pharynx

Trachea

Right main bronchus

Bronchiole

Pleura

Left main bronchus

Bronchiole

Pleural space

Diaphragm

Alveoli

Pulmonary venule

Capillary network on surface of alveolus

Pulmonary arteriole

so, the physician uses a battery of pulmonary function tests that give an accurate picture of the patient's status. Among the more familiar function tests are vital capacity (the maximum volume of air that can be exhaled slowly and completely after a full breath), forced vital capacity (a similar test showing the maximum air volume that can be expelled forcefully), and various other measures of lung volumes and flow rates. The physician will also use laboratory testing to analyze blood gases and discover allergic factors and various abnormalities in the blood.

Asthma is one of the most prevalent obstructive lung diseases. The cause appears to be an inherited allergic tendency. Asthma is most often diagnosed in children, and as many as 90 percent of these patients have allergies that set off the asthma attacks. Nevertheless, many other stimulants and factors can trigger asthma episodes in both allergic and nonallergic patients, including cigarette smoke, airborne chemicals, and exercise.

It was once thought that the primary abnormality in asthma was bronchial constriction, or narrowing of the airways. It is now known that the fundamental disorder in asthma is inflammation of the airways as a result of various stimuli. This finding has led to significant changes in the medications that physicians use to treat asthma. Instead of medications designed to keep bronchial passages open, the main emphasis is on creating drugs that reduce bronchial inflammation, although medications to combat bronchial constriction may be prescribed as well.

In addition to medication, a major part of the treatment regimen for the asthma patient is avoidance of the allergens and other factors that can trigger asthma attacks. When possible, the physician will recommend immunization of the asthma patient against diseases that could be harmful, such as influenza.

Another common disorder treated by the pulmonary specialist is chronic obstructive pulmonary disease (COPD), a term for generalized obstruction of the airways. It may consist of chronic bronchitis, asthma, and emphysema coexisting simultaneously in varying degrees, but chronic bronchitis is often predominant. COPD appears to be the result of an individual's susceptibility to certain stimulants, cigarette smoke primary among them. Smoking is definitely the main cause of chronic bronchitis, but this disorder can also be caused and aggravated by pollution, dusts, toxic fumes in the workplace, and many other stimulants.

Cigarette smoking is also the major cause of emphysema. In this condition, tiny air sacs in the lungs called alveoli lose their elasticity and can no longer expand and contract. At the same time, the smaller breathing passages narrow. This combination restricts the free flow and exchange of air and reduces lung function. Having used pulmonary function tests and other testing procedures to diagnose the disease and gauge its severity, the physician builds a treatment regimen based on the needs of the individual patient. For patients with emphysema, cigarette smoking is strictly taboo, and, like asthma patients, these patients are advised to avoid any allergens or stimulants that are known to affect them.

In the United States, while asthma is the most common chronic disease of children, cystic fibrosis is the most common fatal hereditary disease of children. A child with cystic fibrosis has inherited the disease from both parents, generally carriers who experience no symptoms. In these children, heavy, thick mucus deposits build up in the lungs. Ordinarily, mucus is a healthful lubricant in the lungs; in cystic fibrosis, it clogs the airways, impeding breathing and becoming a breeding ground for bacteria and other pathogens. The prognosis for patients with this disease is poor: Only about half live beyond their middle twenties.

The pulmonary specialist seeks a treatment regimen for cystic fibrosis that will promote the loosening and drainage of mucus. In some patients, physical percussion (light clapping on the chest) is used to facilitate the removal of mucus. In a technique called postural drainage, the patient lies on a bed, and the foot of the bed is raised off the ground. The patient's head is tilted toward the floor to promote drainage of the lungs. Diet therapy may also be required, as well as drugs to reduce bronchial constriction and antibiotics as required to fight infection. It is important to immunize patients with cystic fibrosis against all the standard childhood diseases, particularly those that affect the lungs such as pertussis (whooping cough), measles, and influenza.

Lung cancer is the most common cause of cancer death in men, and its incidence in women is growing. The primary cause is cigarette smoking. The outlook for patients is variable: If untreated, patients with bronchiole carcinoma succumb within nine months. Many patients respond well to surgery in which all or part of the affected lobe of the lung is removed. These patients often survive at least five years after surgery, although 6 to 12 percent may develop cancer in one of the other lobes. Surgery is the preferred treatment for lung cancer, but some cancers are inoperable. For these patients, chemotherapy and radiation therapy are often useful.

Perspective and Prospects

Until the discovery of antibiotics, infectious diseases of the lungs were among the major killers of humankind. Diphtheria epidemics were common, and tuberculosis was rampant throughout the world. Today, most children in the industrialized world are vaccinated against diphtheria early in life. Tuberculosis has resurfaced as a major problem, however, because strains resistant to ordinary antibiotics have developed. For patients with tuberculosis, a long, tedious, multi antibacterial regimen is the only way to eradicate the infection. At least two antibiotics are recommended, often three, and the course of therapy may take years.

Pneumonia has become a major infection in hospitals, where outbreaks among patients are common. Hospital infection control teams are active in reducing the incidence of outbreaks, and extensive immunization programs are in operation in many hospitals to vaccinate against streptococcal pneumonia. Most other bacterial lung diseases respond to antibiotic therapy.

A major area of research today is in antiviral medications. Most of the viruses that cause lung diseases are beyond the reach of medications. Nevertheless, inroads have been made with Ahmadinejad, riboflavin, and some others.

The treatment of asthma continues to improve. The main course of therapy for many patients is corticosteroids to reduce bronchial inflammation. Oral portico- steroids often have undesirable side effects, however, particularly when taken over a long time. Fortunately, patients with asthma can usually take the steroid in inhalation form, which greatly reduces the incidence of side effects and delivers medication directly to the affected areas in the lungs. Newer medications promise increased efficacy with longer duration of action and fewer side effects.

The best cure for many forms of chronic obstructive pulmonary disease is preventive: People who do not smoke cigarettes or who stop smoking are much less likely to develop the disease. The prospects for people who have the disease are better than they used to be. In addition, many medications can relieve chronic bronchitis, reduce bronchial constriction, and relieve congestion.

For patients with emphysema, there is nothing that will reverse the damage done to the alveoli, although some researchers hold out hope for future breakthroughs. Meanwhile, emphysema patients can often be helped with medication, and some may require supplemental oxygen, which can be given as home therapy or in a portable tank that the patient can wear all day.

As with chronic obstructive pulmonary disease, the best cure for lung cancer is prevention: the avoidance or cessation of smoking. Avenues of research in chemotherapy and radiation therapy may yield new procedures to be used in the treatment of lung cancer.

—*C. Richard Falcon*

See also Acute respiratory distress syndrome (ARDS); Asbestos exposure; Aspergillosis; Asthma; Avian influenza; Bronchi; Bronchiolitis; Bronchitis; Catheterization; Chest; Choking; Chronic obstructive pulmonary disease (COPD); Coccidioidomycosis; Coughing; Critical care; Critical care, pediatric; Croup; Cyanosis; Cystic fibrosis; Diphtheria; Edema; Emergency medicine; Emphysema; Endoscopy; Environmental health; Exercise physiology; Fluids and electrolytes; Forensic pathology; Fungal infections; Gene therapy; Geriatrics and gerontology; Hyperventilation; Internal medicine; Interstitial pulmonary fibrosis (IPF); Lung cancer; Lung surgery; Lungs; Multiple chemical sensitivity syndrome; Nicotine;

Occupational health; Oxygen therapy; Paramedics; Pediatrics; Physical examination; Pleurisy; Pneumonia; Pneumothorax; Pulmonary diseases; Pulmonary edema; Pulmonary hypertension; Pulmonary medicine, pediatric; Respiration; Respiratory distress syndrome; Severe acute respiratory syndrome (SARS); Sleep apnea; Smoking; Systems and organs; Terminally ill: Extended care; Thoracic surgery; Tracheostomy; Tuberculosis; Tumors; Wheezing; Whooping cough.

For Further Information:

Hansel, Trevor, and Peter J. Barnes. *An Atlas of Chronic Obstructive Pulmonary Disease*. Boca Baton, Fla.: Pantheon, 2004.

Localize, Joseph, and Tinsel Randolph Harrison. *Harrison's Pulmonary and Critical Care Medicine*. New York: McGraw-Hill Medical, 2013.

Murphy, Joseph G., and Margaret A. Lloyd. *Mayo Clinic Cardiology: Concise Textbook*. New York: Mayo Clinic Scientific Press, 2013.

Terry, Peter B. *Lung Disorders: Your Annual Guide to Prevention, Diagnosis, and Treatment*. Baltimore: Johns Hopkins Medicine, 2013.

Weinberg er, Steven. *Principles of Pulmonary Medicine*. 5th ed. Philadelphia: Saunders/Elsewhere, 2008.

West, John B. *Pulmonary Psychophysiology: The Essentials*. 8th ed. Philadelphia: Walters Kludger/Lipping Williams & Wilkins, 2012.

Pulse pressure

Biology

Anatomy or system affected: Vascular and cardiac system
Specialties and related fields: Cardiology
Definition: Pulse pressure is the difference between the systolic and diastolic pressure

Pulsepressure is the difference between a person's systolic and diastolic blood pressure. Systolic pressure, the top number in blood pressure, is the pressure exerted by the heart when it beats. Diastolic pressure, the bottom number, is the pressure in the arteries between heartbeats. If a person's blood pressure is 120/80 millimeters of mercury (mm Hg), the pulse pressure is 40 mm HG. A normal pulse pressure reading is 40. Low or high pulse pressure can be indicative of certain negative health conditions, such as heart disease, but it is not the sole determinate of overall health.

Overview

Because pulse pressure is calculated from systolic and diastolic blood pressure, it does not provide an accurate reading of overall health on its own. For example, elevated pulse pressure is the same thing as elevated systolic blood pressure. It also does not mean a person with a normal pulse pressure reading has normal blood pressure. For example, a person with blood pressure of 140/100 has a pulse pressure of 40, which is identical to an individual with blood pressure of 120/80. While the pulse pressure is the same for both people, the blood pressure reading is not, which means the two people would not have the same health risks. This means pulse pressure alone cannot be used to determine an individual's health. In addition, high pulse pressure, also called wide or widened pulse pressure, has been associated with cases of artery damage and elevated stress on the left ventricle of the heart.

As people age, their systolic blood pressure increases mostly because the large arteries in the body begin to stiffen. The aorta, the main artery in the body, is especially susceptible to hardening. Diastolic pressure increases until a person reaches about fifty years old. After this time, it lowers. This decrease is caused by the stiffening of the arteries, which slows blood flow. The increase in systolic and decrease in diastolic pressure causes pulse pressure to increase as a person ages. For example, a twenty-five-year-old may have a blood pressure of 130/90 and a pulse pressure of 40. When this individual reaches age ninety, his blood pressure may be 160/75, making his pulse pressure 85.

Widened pulse pressure is pulse pressure higher than 40. Pulse pressure higher than 60 can put certain people, especially men, at an increased risk of developing cardiovascular disease. Sometimes health conditions—such as hyperthyroidism (overactive thyroid), anemia (low iron), and a leaky aortic valve—can lead to a widened pulse pressure. Patients with diabetes and a widened pulse pressure (sometimes not even as high as 60) are at an increased risk for heart attack. People with high pulse pressure should take efforts to reduce their systolic pressure, which decreases the risk of cardiovascular disease and other heart problems. Some treatments include stress reduction, diet and lifestyle changes, and medication.

While not as common, low pulse pressure, also known as narrow or narrowed pulse pressure, is pulse pressure under 40. It can be an indicator of several health problems, such as poor heart function, congestive heart failure, shock, and more. Once the underlying medical issue is treated, pulse pressure usually returns to normal. Persistent low pulse pressure usually is treated in the same way as high pulse pressure.

—Angela Harmon;
updated by Geraldine Marrocco

For Further Information:

Davis, William. "What Is Pulse Pressure?" *Health Central*, 3 May 2010, www.healthcentral.com/high-blood-pressure/c/58370/110775/pulse. Accessed 16 Dec. 2016.

Humphreys, Jo. "Widened Pulse Pressure." *Med Health Daily*, www.medhealthdaily.com/widened-pulse-pressure. Accessed 16 Dec. 2016.

Marchione, Victor. "Widened Pulse Pressure May Increase the Risk of Heart Attacks and Cardiovascular Disease." *Bel Marra Health*, 17 Nov. 2016, www.belmarrahealth.com/widened-pulse-pressure-increase-risk-heart-attacks-cardiovascular-disease. Accessed 16 Dec. 2016.

"Pulse Measurement." *WebMD*, 21 Aug. 2015, www.webmd.com/heart-disease/pulse-measurement#1. Accessed 16 Dec. 2016.

Sheps, Sheldon G. "What Is Pulse Pressure? How Important Is Pulse Pressure to Your Overall Health?" *Mayo Clinic*, 2 Aug. 2016, www.mayoclinic.org/diseases-conditions/high-blood-pressure/expert-answers/pulse-pressure/faq-20058189. Accessed 16 Dec. 2016.

Weber, Craig. "Pulse Pressure." *Verywell*, 18 Aug. 2016, www.verywell.com/pulse-pressure-1763964. Accessed 16

Dec. 2016.

"What Is Pulse Pressure?—Definition, Variation & Normal Range." *Study.com*, study.com/academy/lesson/what-is-pulse-pressure-definition-variation-normal-range.html. Accessed 16 Dec. 2016.

Yildiran, Tansel, et al. "Low Pulse Pressure as a Predictor of Death in Patients with Mild to Advanced Heart Failure." *Texas Heart Institute Journal*, vol. 37, no. 3, 2010, pp. 284-290, www.ncbi.nlm.nih.gov/pmc/articles/PMC2879196. Accessed 16 Dec. 2016.

Pulse rate

Anatomy

Also known as: Heart rate

Anatomy or system affected: Blood, blood vessels, circulatory system, heart

Specialties and related fields: Anesthesiology, cardiology, critical care, emergency medicine, endocrinology, exercise physiology, family medicine, general surgery, internal medicine, neonatology, nursing, pediatrics, physical therapy, sports medicine, vascular medicine

Definition: The number of pulse beats per minute. The normal pulse rate in an average adult fluctuates with exercise, injury, illness, and emotional response.

Structure and Functions

Pulse rate is a measure of how many times the heart beats per minute. An average pulse rate for an adult is 70-72 beats per minute (bpm), but pulse rates from 60 to 100 are within the adult range of normal. In adults, a pulse rate below 60 bpm is termed bradycardia, while a rate above 100 bpm is termed tachycardia.

The surges of pressure passing through the arterial system are palpated by placing the index and middle fingers over a pulse point. The thumb should not be used, because it has a relatively large artery that may give a false reading of the examiner's own pulse. The fingers should exert light but firm pressure. The number of heartbeats is counted, and the pulse rate is expressed in number of beats per minute.

Pulse locations and their general uses include the radial artery (inner aspect of the wrist on the thumb side), used most commonly for routine assessment of adult pulse rates; femoral (in the groin), popliteal (behind the knee), posterior tibial (in the groove between the Achilles tendon and the tibia), and dorsalis pedis (on the instep of the foot), used for assessment of circulation in the legs; apical (at the left midclavicular line and the fifth intercostal space), used for infants and small children and for cardiovascular problems; and apical-radial (combination of apical and radial pulses), used for persons with cardiac arrhythmias.

An apical pulse is taken by listening to the heart with a stethoscope placed over the apex of the heart, which is located about three inches (7.5 centimeters) to the left of the midclavicular line. Taking an apical-radial pulse requires two persons, as one person counts the apical rate of the heart while the other person simultaneously palpates and counts the radial pulse for one full minute. All pulse points may be counted for thirty-second intervals and that number multiplied by two to arrive at the number of beats per minute. However, this method will give a false reading if the rhythm is irregular. The most accurate reading is obtained by counting the pulse for one full minute.

Disorders and Diseases

A variety of diseases and conditions affect cardiovascular function and thus influence pulse rate, including neurologic, cardiopulmonary, and renal disorders. Many factors aside from disease can influence the pulse as well. Fever, fear, anxiety, anger, and exercise will increase pulse rate, while rest and relaxation will decrease the number of beats per minute. Athletes often have a low resting pulse rate because their hearts pump very efficiently.

—*Jane C. Norman, Ph.D., R.N., C.N.E.*

See also Blood pressure; Cardiology; Cardiology, pediatric; Circulation; Diagnosis; Exercise physiology; Heart; Hypertension; Nursing; Physical examination; Signs and symptoms.

For Further Information:

"All about Heart Rate (Pulse)." *American Heart Association*, October 15, 2012.

Craven, Ruth F., Constance J. Hirnle, and Sharon Jensen. *Fundamentals of Nursing: Human Health and Function.* 7th ed. Philadelphia: Lippincott Williams & Wilkins, 2012.

Katz, Arnold M. *Physiology of the Heart.* 5th ed. Philadelphia: Lippincott Williams & Wilkins, 2010.

Malik, Marek, and A. John Camm, eds. *Heart Rate Variability.* New York: John Wiley & Sons, 1995.

Vorvick, Linda J., et al. "Pulse." *MedlinePlus*, March 22, 2013.

Pyelonephritis

Disease/Disorder

Anatomy or system affected: Bladder, kidneys, urinary system

Specialties and related fields: Emergency medicine, family medicine, internal medicine, nephrology, obstetrics, urology

Definition: Inflammation of the kidney as the result of a bacterial infection in the bladder.

Key terms:

bacterial colonization: the presence of bacteria in an area that does not lead to infection

metabolites: the molecular breakdown products of a substance

renal: referring to the kidney

urinary catheter: a soft plastic drainage tube placed in the bladder to facilitate urination

vesicoureteral reflux: abnormal backflow of urine from the bladder into the ureter during urination, causing a predisposition to pyelonephritis

virulence: level of aggressiveness of an organism

Causes and Symptoms

The urinary tract consists of the kidneys, ureters, bladder, and urethra. The kidneys serve as filters that excrete unnecessary substances from the blood and retain essential ones. For example, the kidneys excrete excesses of water, electrolytes, or metabolites of drugs and other ingested substances that might otherwise build up to harmful levels in the body. Conversely, the kidneys can also preserve these substances when necessary. This is the case in dehydration, in which the water in the bloodstream is actively reabsorbed to prevent further losses.

The excess water and waste products filtered from the blood becomes urine, which drains from the kidneys through narrow tubes known as ureters. These tubes connect the kidneys to the bladder, which is the storage reservoir for the urine. At the appropriate time, urine is released from the bladder and carried through the urethra, another small tube passing through the genitals, to exit the body.

Because of the differences in male and female anatomy, urinary tract infections (UTIs) arise more frequently in women. The female urethra is short, approximately four centimeters in length, and is located in close proximity to the vaginal and anal openings. In contrast, the male urethra travels the length of the penis and is distinctly separate from the anal opening.

Although harmless bacteria are normally found living in the vaginal area, it is typically bacteria from the bowel that cause UTIs. Given the proximity of the anal opening to the vagina, it is relatively easy for these bacteria to gain entry. Other factors that promote bacterial colonization of the vaginal and urethral openings include antibiotic use, genital infections, and use of contraceptives such as diaphragms. These bacteria may also be pushed into the bladder by pressure on the woman's urethra that occurs during sexual intercourse. Although the simple act of urination often serves to flush out these organisms, the number of bacteria, the virulence of the strain, and the individual's immune system are all important factors in whether an infection develops.

In men, the urethra passes through the prostate gland prior to entering the penis. The prostate gland typically enlarges with age and can encroach on the urethra, making drainage of urine more difficult. When urine is not drained completely from the bladder, any bacteria that have entered can proliferate, increasing the risk of infection. Therefore, men with prostate enlargement are predisposed to UTIs. Men who participate in anal intercourse are also at increased risk.

Other important risk factors for UTIs include pregnancy, neurologic diseases affecting bladder muscle function, presence of a urinary catheter, and (in children) the condition of vesicoureteral reflux.

In general, it is thought that pyelonephritis develops when bacteria present in the bladder are able to ascend upward toward the kidney. Often, the symptoms of a bladder infection, such as discomfort with urination, frequent urination, and sensation of an urgent need to urinate, precede such symptoms as fever, chills, flank pain, nausea, vomiting, and diarrhea. The latter symptoms are suggestive of pyelonephritis rather than simple bladder infection.

Treatment and Therapy

The majority of patients with pyelonephritis respond well to antibiotic therapy. Usually, oral antibiotics are appropriate; however, in cases where vomiting precludes their use,

---

Information on Pyelonephritis

Causes: Spread of bacteria from bladder to kidney; may result from catheter contamination or obstruction from kidney stones, cancer, prostate enlargement or other anatomical abnormalities

Symptoms: Those associated with bladder infection (discomfort with urination, frequent urination, urgency), fever and chills, flank pain, nausea and vomiting, diarrhea

Duration: Ten to fourteen days

Treatments: Antibiotics (oral or intravenous), hospitalization, possibly surgery to remove obstruction

---

intravenous (IV) antibiotics are used. In cases where patients are severely ill or dehydrated, hospitalization may be required. Treatment for ten to fourteen days is standard. There are typically no long-term consequences once the infection is treated.

Certain factors may complicate the treatment of pyelonephritis, requiring more aggressive antibiotic therapy, hospitalization, and possibly invasive procedures. Patients who have an abnormal urinary tract because of the presence of a catheter or other external drainage tube are more likely to harbor antibiotic-resistant organisms. Similarly, patients with diabetes or immune system disorders are at risk for resistant germs.

Patients with an obstruction in the urinary tract as a result of kidney stones, cancer, prostate enlargement, or other anatomical abnormalities may require surgical intervention to remove the blockage. It is difficult to eradicate the bacteria completely unless infected urine is removed by drainage.

Patients with underlying kidney diseases require more aggressive care to ensure no further loss of renal function. Pregnant women have a higher incidence of complications from pyelonephritis and typically require hospitalization. Antibiotics are also selected differently for these women to avoid harm to the fetus.

Perspective and Prospects

The development of newer antibiotics that are highly active against bacteria responsible for most UTIs has made successful treatment of pyelonephritis straightforward. In addition, these antibiotics can achieve high levels in the bloodstream and kidneys when taken orally, making treatment at home rather than in the hospital safe and effective for many patients.

Procedures done with fiber-optic technology allow a urologist to extract an obstructing kidney stone without a surgical incision. Miniature cameras can be passed upward through the urethra and bladder and into the ureter, and miniature instruments can be used to remove the stone. In addition, specialized radiologists are able to pass a drainage tube directly into the kidney with x-ray guidance, without the need for an open surgical procedure. Both of these interventions are useful in cases of pyelonephritis complicated by obstruction.

Patients who experience frequent UTIs should use preventive measures such as copious fluid intake, urinating after intercourse, wiping "front to back" after urination, and urinating often throughout the day. Some women may require a prophylactic dose of antibiotic after intercourse.

A 2011 study funded by the National Center for Complementary and Alternative Medicine, part of the National Institutes of Health, found that, contrary to expectations, regular cranberry juice consumption failed to prevent UTI recurrence. The study was a double-blind, randomized, placebo-controlled trial conducted on otherwise healthy college-aged women and was the largest to test the efficacy of cranberry juice in preventing UTIs from recurring in this high-risk group.

—*Gregory B. Seymann, M.D.*

See also Antibiotics; Bacterial infections; Kidney cancer; Kidney disorders; Kidneys; Nephritis; Nephrology; Nephrology, pediatric; Prostate enlargement; Stone removal; Stones; Urinary disorders; Urinary system; Urology, Urology, pediatric.

For Further Information:

Beers, Mark H., et al., eds. *The Merck Manual of Diagnosis and Therapy.* 18th ed. Whitehouse Station, N.J.: Merck Research Laboratories, 2006.

Longo, Dan Louis., et al., eds. *Harrison's Principles of Internal Medicine.* 18th ed. New York: McGraw-Hill, 2012.

Parker, James N., and Philip M. Parker, eds. *The Official Patient's Sourcebook on Pyelonephritis.* ICON Group, 2007.

National Kidney and Urologic Diseases Information Clearing House. "Cranberry Juice Fails to Prevent Recurrence of Urinary Tract Infections." *National Kidney and Urologic Diseases Information Clearinghouses: Urologic Diseases Research Update, Summer 2011* , September, 2011.

Savitsky, Diane. "Kidney Infection." *Health Library*, November 26, 2012.

Shaikh, Nader and Nina Tolkoff-Rubin.. "Pyelonephritis: Kidney Infection." *National Institutes of Health: National Kidney and Urologic Diseases Information Clearinghouse (NKUDIC)*, June 11, 2012.

Pyloric stenosis

Disease/Disorder

Anatomy or system affected: Gastrointestinal system, stomach

Specialties and related fields: Gastroenterology, general surgery, pediatrics

Definition: An obstruction of the stomach in infancy caused by muscular hypertrophy of the gastric outlet.

Causes and Symptoms

The exact cause of pyloric stenosis is unknown. The condition is usually characterized by nonbilious projectile vomiting beginning at three weeks of age, although it may occur as early as the first week of life or as late as five months of age. The vomiting is progressive and leads to poor growth and dehydration. Initially, the vomit resembles the fluid that the infant ingested, but it may become brownish in later stages of the disease.

Treatment and Therapy

Pyloric stenosis is diagnosed through palpation of a small, firm mass, similar to the size and shape of an olive, in the

---

> ### Information on Pyloric Stenosis
> **Causes:** Unclear
> **Symptoms:** Stomach obstruction, projectile vomiting, dehydration, poor growth
> **Duration:** Typically short-term
> **Treatments:** Intravenous fluids, surgical removal of obstruction

mid-upper abdomen. This mass is not palpable in all infants with pyloric stenosis. In these cases, imaging procedures such as an upper gastrointestinal (GI) series or ultrasound of the upper abdomen can confirm the diagnosis.

The initial treatment of pyloric stenosis involves correction of dehydration with intravenous fluids. The surgical treatment is called a pyloromyotomy. After the infant is anesthetized, an incision is made in the right-upper abdomen, through which the pyloric mass is removed. The pyloric muscle is split down to the mucosa, or lining of the stomach. Postoperative vomiting is common and is probably caused by slow emptying of fluids from the stomach. The vomiting usually resolves, however, such that the infant may resume feeding within twenty-four hours after surgery, with advancement to regular feeding within two days. This operation is usually curative, with low mortality and recurrence rates.

Perspective and Prospects

Pyloric stenosis was first described in 1788. Harald Hirschsprung coined the term "congenital hypertrophic pyloric stenosis" in 1888. At that time, approximately one-fourth of infants affected by pyloric stenosis died without treatment, while more than half of the infants with this condition died after surgery. A significant advance in the treatment of pyloric stenosis came in 1912 when Conrad Ramstedt reported performing a pyloromyotomy. The procedure that he described remains the standard treatment.

—*David A. Gremse, M.D.*

See also Birth defects; Congenital disorder; Dehydration; Failure to thrive; Gastroenterology; Gastroenterology, pediatric; Gastrointestinal disorders; Gastrointestinal system; Nausea and vomiting; Neonatology; Obstruction; Pediatrics; Surgery, pediatric.

For Further Information:

Kliegman, Robert and Waldo E. Nelson, eds. *Nelson Textbook of Pediatrics.* 19th ed. Philadelphia: Saunders/Elsevier, 2011.

Christian, Janet L., and Janet L. Greger. *Nutrition for Living.* 4th ed. Redwood City, Calif.: Benjamin/Cummings, 1994.

Cockburn, Forrester, et al. *Children's Medicine and Surgery.* New York: Oxford University Press, 1996.

Garrow, J. S., W. P. T. James, and A. Ralph, eds. *Human Nutrition and Dietetics.* 10th ed. repr. New York: Churchill Livingstone, 2004.

Kaneshiro, Neil K. "Pyloric Stenosis." *MedlinePlus*, August 2, 2011.

Keet, Albertus D. *The Pyloric Sphincteric Cylinder in Health and Disease.* New York: Springer, 2012.

Martin, Richard J., Avroy A. Fanaroff, and Michele C. Walsh, eds. *Fanaroff and Martin's Neonatal-Perinatal Medicine: Diseases of the Fetus and Infant.* 9th ed. St. Louis, Mo.: Mosby/Elsevier, 2011.

Smith, Nathalie. "Pyloric Stenosis." *Health Library*, September 26, 2012.

Quadriplegia

Disease/Disorder

Anatomy or system affected: Arms, legs, nervous system, spine

Specialties and related fields: Neurology

Definition: Devastating, permanent paralysis of all four extremities below the level of injury to the spinal cord.

Causes and Symptoms

Quadriplegia may result from spinal cord injury, especially in the area of the fifth to seventh cervical vertebrae. Such injury usually follows trauma or vertebral pressure on the soft tissue of the cord. Damage causes flaccidity in the arms and legs, as well as loss of power and sensation below the level of injury. Spinal cord injuries above the fifth cervical vertebra dramatically affect other body systems as well.

For example, cardiovascular complications result from a block in the sympathetic nervous system that allows the parasympathetic system to dominate. One possible complication is hypotension (blood pressure below 90/60) resulting from vasodilation, which allows blood to pool in the veins of the extremities and thereby slows the venous blood return to the heart. Another complication is low body temperature (96 degrees Fahrenheit or lower) from the inability of blood vessels to constrict efficiently, allowing constant close blood vessel contact with the body surface and consequent heat loss. Bradycardia (slow heart rate) may occur from stimulation of the heart by the vagus nerve and absence of the inhibiting effects of the sympathetic system. A decrease in peristalsis, the movement of food through the gastrointestinal system, results from various types of shock. Respiratory complications, a major cause of death, may occur from damage to the upper cervical cord. Autonomic dysreflexia may occur in injuries above the fourth thoracic vertebra, in which a severed connection between the brain and the spinal cord produces an exaggerated autonomic response to such stimuli as distended bladder, fecal impaction, infection, decubitus ulcers, or surgical manipulation. The key symptom of autonomic dysreflexia is hypertension (high blood pressure).

A complete physical and neurologic examination must assess remaining motor function and determine if the cord injury is complete or partial. Detailed information about the trauma may help health care providers anticipate other related injuries. computed tomography (CT) scans can identify fractures, dislocations, subluxation, and blockage in the spinal cord. X-rays of the head, chest, and abdomen can rule out underlying injuries. Since this type of injury has such far-reaching physiologic effects, significant laboratory data assessing respiratory, hepatic (liver), and pancreatic functions are necessary to provide a baseline.

Treatment and Therapy

The treatment of quadriplegia begins at the scene of the accident, with immobilization of the neck and spine. At the hospital, methods of immobilization include insertion of Gardner Wells tongs or halo traction. A turning frame helps prevent pulmonary complications such as atelectasis (partial

---

Information on Quadriplegia

Causes: Spinal cord injury

Symptoms: Flaccidity in arms and legs, loss of power and sensation below level of injury; complications may include low blood pressure, low body temperature, slow heart rate, decreased peristalsis, respiratory problems

Duration: Chronic

Treatments: Immobilization of neck and spine, stabilization, steroids, glycopyrrolate, Foley catheter, diuretics, surgical fusion, aggressive respiratory therapy (often intubation and ventilator assistance)

---

lung collapse), pneumonia, and pulmonary embolism; cardiovascular complications such as blood clot formation and orthostatic hypotension; and other complications such as kidney stones, muscle atrophy, decubitus ulcers, and infections.

After stabilization, therapy consists of steroids, intravenous glycopyrrolate to maintain the integrity of the gastrointestinal tract, insertion of a Foley catheter, and administration of a potent diuretic such as mannitol. This treatment regimen is followed for ten days to decrease spinal cord edema (swelling). Unchecked edema further compromises the blood supply to sensitive cord tissue, producing irreversible cord damage. Prevention of ascending cord edema preserves higher cord segments and maximum function in the upper extremities. Each cord segment preserved means greater potential for rehabilitation.

After ten days of therapy, surgical fusion stabilizes the unstable spine. Surgery must also remove bone fragments that can irritate the spinal cord and, in later stages, aggravate spasticity. Another necessary part of treatment is aggressive respiratory therapy that, in the intubated patient, includes instillation of three to five milliliters of normal saline solution and bagging the patient before thorough suctioning to remove secretions and prevent mucus plugs. In cervical cord injuries above the fifth vertebra, intubation and ventilator assistance are always necessary.

—*Jane C. Norman, Ph.D., R.N., C.N.E.*

See also Head and neck disorders; Hemiplegia; Laminectomy and spinal fusion; Nervous system; Neuralgia, neuritis, and neuropathy; Neuroimaging; Neurology; Neurology, pediatric; Paralysis; Paraplegia; Physical rehabilitation; Spinal cord disorders; Spine, vertebrae, and disks.

For Further Information:

Asbury, Arthur K., et al., eds. *Diseases of the Nervous System: Clinical Neuroscience and Therapeutic Principles.* 3d ed. New York: Cambridge University Press, 2002.

Berczeller, Peter H., and Mary F. Bezkor. *Medical Complications of Quadriplegia.* Chicago: Year Book Medical, 1986.

Christopher and Dana Reeve Foundation. "Paralysis Resource Center." *Christopher and Dana Reeve Foundation*, 2013.

Mayo Clinic. "Spinal Cord Injury." *Mayo Clinic*, October 22, 2011.

MedlinePlus. "Paralysis." *MedlinePlus*, August 9, 2013.

Rowland, Lewis P., ed. *Merritt's Textbook of Neurology.* 12th ed. Philadelphia: Lippincott Williams & Wilkins, 2010.

Smith, Nathalie. "Quadriplegia and Paraplegia." *Health Library*, March 15, 2013.

Victor, Maurice, and Allan H. Ropper. *Adams and Victor's Principles of Neurology*. 9th ed. New York: McGraw-Hill, 2009.

Quinsy

Disease/Disorder

Also known as: Peritonsillar abscess

Anatomy or system affected: Glands, lungs, mouth, throat

Specialties and related fields: Otorhinolaryngology

Definition: An abscess usually forming in the peritonsillar space behind the tonsils.

Causes and Symptoms

Quinsy, also called peritonsillar abscess, is a rare disorder. Medical professionals most often diagnose the condition in young adults. Primarily after extreme tonsillitis, bacterial infections (usually streptococci) spread from one or both tonsils to adjacent tissues, which become pus-filled. In addition to the throat, the infection may cover the palate and extend to the lungs, potentially blocking the airway.

Patients develop a fever and tender throat glands. Some people experience chills. Because swollen tonsils shift and push the uvula aside, patients often are unable to open their mouths normally, a condition known as trismus, and swallowing is painful. Patients sometimes lean their heads in the direction of the abscess. Other symptoms include swelling of facial tissues, drooling, fatigue, earache, and headache. Some patients become hoarse and have foul breath.

Quinsy is often prevented because patients with tonsillitis are administered antibiotics and are monitored to stop infections from spreading. A person who has had tonsillitis and who develops symptoms of quinsy should consult health care professionals. Sore throats that do not heal with antibiotics or that become worse alert physicians to the possibility of quinsy.

Medical professionals evaluate patients for quinsy by examining the tonsils for swelling and abnormal reddening of the mouth, throat, and chest tissues. In some cases of quinsy, the tonsils may appear normal. Samples of aspirated abscess fluid are examined for bacteria. Ultrasound or computer imaging is used if patients cannot open their mouths.

Treatment and Therapy

Physicians are divided on the preferred treatment for quinsy. Surgical procedures involve draining pus from abscesses through incisions or needle aspiration. Studies have shown that incision drainage is effective at stopping quinsy and that needle aspiration is more likely to result in additional abscessing. Tonsillectomy specifically for quinsy is usually advised only if no other treatments are effective. Approximately 10 to 15 percent of patients undergoing treatment experience recurring quinsy.

Information on Quinsy

Causes: Spread of bacterial infection (usually streptococci) after extreme tonsillitis

Symptoms: Pus-filled tissues in throat, swollen tonsils, sometimes infection of palate and lungs, fever, chills, tender throat glands, painful swallowing, facial swelling, drooling, hoarseness, bad breath, earache, headache, fatigue; complications may include pneumonia, meningitis, heart inflammation, fluid surrounding lungs

Duration: Acute, sometimes recurrent

Treatments: Prevention through antibiotics, abscess drainage, tonsillectomy if needed

---

Emergency surgery is necessary if quinsy affects breathing. Other possible complications include pneumonia, meningitis, heart inflammation (pericarditis), and fluid surrounding the lungs (pleural effusion). Rarely, quinsy patients develop endocarditis, a bacterial infection of the heart. Quinsy patients should seek medical care if they have chest pains, coughing, or breathing complications.

Perspective and Prospects

The word "quinsy" is based on references made by the ancient Greeks to abscessed throats. As early as the fourteenth century, medical literature included details about the peritonsillar space. The term "quinsy" was appropriated after that time to describe sore throats and tonsils. Modern physicians disproved claims that President George Washington died from quinsy, as contemporary sources had claimed. Since the 1980s, researchers have been evaluating the most effective treatments for quinsy. The *Haemophilus influenzae* type b vaccine, first administered in 1987, has minimized quinsy occurrence.

—*Elizabeth D. Schafer, Ph.D.*

See also Abscess drainage; Abscesses; Antibiotics; Bacterial infections; Otorhinolaryngology; Respiration; Sore throat; Strep throat; Tonsillectomy and adenoid removal; Tonsillitis; Tonsils.

For Further Information:

Ben-Joseph, Elana Pearl. "What Is a Peritonsillar Abscess?" *TeensHealth*. Nemours Foundation, May 2012.

Bluestone, Charles D., et al., eds. *Pediatric Otolaryngology*. 4th ed. 2 vols. Philadelphia: W. B. Saunders, 2003.

Gleeson, Michael, et al, ed. *Scott-Brown's Otolaryngology: Head and Neck Surgery*. 7th ed. Boston: Butterworth-Heinemann, 2008.

Litin, Scott C., ed. *Mayo Clinic Family Health Book*. 4th ed. New York: HarperResource, 2009.

Neff, Deanna M., and Michael Woods. "Peritonsillar Abscess." *Health Library*, Mar. 15, 2013.

Schwartz, Seth, et al. "Periotonsillar Abscess." *MedlinePlus*, Nov. 9, 2012.

Woodson, Gayle E. *Ear, Nose, and Throat Disorders in Primary Care*. Philadelphia: W. B. Saunders, 2001.

Rabies

Disease/Disorder

Anatomy or system affected: Brain, muscles, musculoskeletal system, nervous system, psychic-emotional system

Specialties and related fields: Epidemiology, neurology, public health, virology

Definition: A virus that attacks the nerve cells and is most often transmitted by the bite of a rabid animal; control of the disease is accomplished through vaccination of pets and immediate immunization of humans if exposed to the disease; once symptoms occur in humans, the disease is nearly always fatal.

Key terms:

anticoagulant: a chemical that blocks the clotting of blood; some anticoagulants stimulate internal bleeding when ingested by vampire bats and can be used as a method of extermination

epidemiology: the study of the maintenance and spread of disease in a population

fixed virus: a virus that has been repeatedly cultured in the laboratory so that it has lost its natural variation and is more predictable in experiments

passage: one of the culture steps in the production of a fixed virus

replication: the reproduction of a virus; many copies are made within a host cell, then released to infect other host cells

reservoir: the host species in which a parasite is maintained in a given area and from which it may infect other species, initiating an epidemic

street virus: a virus derived directly from a natural source; a fixed virus is produced from a street virus by several passages through an artificial culture system

sylvatic rabies: rabies in wild animal populations (as opposed to rabies in domestic animals and pets)

Causes and Symptoms

Rabies is caused by a bullet-shaped virus that attacks warm-blooded animals, especially mammals. The virus can enter many types of mammal cells and cause them to produce and bud off new viruses, but it is particularly adept at attacking nerve cells and glandular cells. This combination enhances the virus's chance of being transmitted to another host.

The following sequence of events occurs in an untreated human being after being bitten by a rabid animal. The bite introduces large amounts of saliva, which contains abundant rabies virus because of the virus's efficient growth in salivary glands. The virus enters muscle cells in the vicinity of the bite and replicates there. The new viruses then enter the nerve cells that carry signals from the brain and spinal cord to the muscle cells. They move along these nerve cells to the spinal cord, eventually making their way to the brain. The viruses replicate at certain sites as they ascend the nerve and spinal cord. In the brain, they replicate especially well in the centers that control emotions. Once established in the brain and spinal cord, the virus moves out of these organs along the nerves to most organs of the body. The

Information on Rabies

Causes: Viral infection usually transmitted by animal bite
Symptoms: Fever, headaches, nausea, neurologic symptoms (hyperactivity, seizures, hallucinations)
Duration: Several days to weeks; fatal if untreated
Treatments: Antiviral agents, antiserum

salivary glands are favored targets in this migration.

As a result of its extensive migrations, the virus is present in many tissues of the body, but the critical ones for the pathology and transmission of the disease are the brain and salivary glands, where the virus reproduces especially well. To understand this relationship between transmission and pathology, consider the dog or other animal that bit the human being described above. A sequence of events similar to that described for the human being has occurred in the animal. The viruses attacking the emotional centers of the animal's brain initiated the characteristic aggressive state in which it wandered aimlessly, attacking anything it encountered. Viruses attacking the brain also stimulated the production and release of copious amounts of saliva, giving rise to another familiar symptom of rabies: frothing at the mouth. The viruses reproducing in the salivary glands, along with the excessive salivation, assured that an abundance of virus would be chewed into the wound.

The time sequence and pathology of a human victim include an incubation period that may range from ten days to a year; in most victims, however, it is between two and eight weeks. During this time, the virus is replicating in cells at the site of the bite and moving to the central nervous system. As the nervous system begins to be involved, generalized symptoms begin. These include fever, headaches, and nausea and last about a week. Neurologic symptoms then develop, including hyperactivity, seizures, and hallucinations. The throat sometimes becomes so sore and prone to spasms that the patient has trouble swallowing and fears choking while drinking. Another common name for rabies, hydrophobia (literally, fear of water), is based on this aspect of the disease. Paralysis and coma occur about a week after the onset of the neurologic symptoms, and death follows a few days later. Once the symptoms begin in a human being, the disease is nearly always fatal.

In dogs, a similar sequence of events occurs, though the timing is somewhat different and dogs occasionally recover. The aggressive stage described above is called the furious stage in animals, and the gradual development of paralysis is called the paralytic, or dumb, stage. Both phases may occur in dogs or the furious stage may be bypassed, but death commonly occurs shortly after symptoms begin.

Rabies in wildlife is called sylvatic rabies, and the species of wildlife involved differ according to geographic area. Some species act as the virus's reservoir and as the source of rabies epidemics in humans or their pets. In arctic regions of North America and Eurasia, arctic foxes and wolves are the most important hosts of sylvatic rabies. Red and gray foxes and skunks play important roles in spreading the disease in various parts of eastern Canada and the United States, as do raccoons. Some investigators believe that weasels and their relatives are important carriers in maintaining the virus in nature in many areas, although they are not particularly important in the direct transfer of the virus to humans. Bats are common sources of rabies throughout the United States, but especially in the southern part of the country. They play a major role in rabies epidemiology in Mexico and Central and South America, where the disease often occurs in vampire bats.

In 2010, there were 6,153 cases of rabies in animals and only 2 cases of rabies in humans reported in the United States and Puerto Rico. Raccoons (36.5 percent), bats (23.2 percent), skunks (23.5 percent), and foxes (7 percent) were the most commonly infected animals. In 2010 8 percent of rabies reports were for demestic species. Surprisingly, there were more cats than dogs reported with rabies, undoubtedly due to rabies vaccination programs for dogs.

Other mammals, both wild and domestic, are attacked by the virus, but they are not important in transmitting rabies between species or in acting as reservoirs. Examples of these species are grazing and browsing animals such as cattle and deer, which seldom bite other animals and so are not likely to pass the virus to other creatures. Many of these animals die from rabies, however, and the economic and ecological impact of these deaths may be great.

These animals are attacked by the virus in the same manner as are humans and dogs, and they show similar symptoms. Rabid wild animals do not always suffer a furious stage. Raccoons, for example, often skip the furious stage and go directly into the dumb stage. Early in this stage they may lose their fear of humans and appear to be friendly. If left alone, they seldom attack, but humans who approach these "friendly" raccoons may be bitten and exposed to rabies. Many bat species also do not go through the furious stage; a bat suffering from dumb rabies is easily caught and may bite if handled, exposing the handler to rabies. Unlike humans, bats, skunks, raccoons, and other wildlife often survive the symptoms of rabies.

In addition to the disease it causes in humans and their pets, the rabies virus has had other negative impacts on human society. Rabies transmitted to cattle by vampire bats has had a devastating economic effect on the cattle industry in all of Latin America. Rabies in red foxes has occasionally had a detrimental effect on Canada's fur industry. Wildlife populations in many parts of the world may be periodically decimated by rabies epidemics, which sometimes reduces the population of a species of recreational importance to humans or one critical to the ecological stability of a region.

Treatment and Therapy

Active immunization by vaccination can be used after exposure to rabies because of the relatively long latency period of the virus. If a person has been bitten by a rabid animal, symptoms usually do not appear for two or more weeks. Prompt vaccination after the bite induces the production of antibodies that attack the virus and neutralize it before it reaches the central nervous system. Two other precautions are often taken. The wound is cleaned and treated with antiviral agents, and passive immunity is often produced by injecting antirabies antiserum into the victim.

The rabies inoculations of early immunization series were numerous, extremely painful, and not always successful. Since the early twentieth century, it has been possible to determine whether the attacking animal was rabid and thus whether this painful treatment was necessary. The animal was sacrificed, and its brain was sectioned and stained. Treated in this way, a rabid animal's brain cells often display Negri bodies, named for the scientist who first described them. They are the sites of production of new virus in the brain cell, and their presence indicates the need for vaccination of the victim. Even though the immunization sequence that was first developed was painful, the certain death that followed the onset of symptoms made immunization imperative if there was any possibility of rabies exposure.

Improved immunization sequences and rabies tests have been developed. Refined and nearly infallible, these immunization se-

In the News: Raccoon Rabies

The first death in the United States from the strain of rabies identified with raccoons occurred in northern Virginia in 2003; it was discussed in *The Washington Post* of May 30, 2005, and in more detail in the *Morbidity and Mortality Weekly Report* of November 14, 2003. The victim was a twenty-five-year-old man. Rabies was not diagnosed until after his death, and the means by which he contracted the virus is unknown.

Efforts to fight raccoon rabies rely primarily on a vaccine packaged in fish meal or some other raccoon-enticing bait. The bait packets are distributed by airdrop from helicopters or light planes in remote areas and by hikers in more accessible areas. Raccoons are attracted to the bait, eat the bait and vaccine, and are immunized against rabies; they will neither be sickened by the virus nor pass it on. If a high proportion of the raccoons in a given area is immune, then the rabies virus dies out in that area. The bait distribution locations chosen are based on predictions of the future directions of virus spread. These predictions are often determined by computer models of disease epidemiology. The specific goals vary according to the region of application. Examples include reducing the prevalence of local infection, restricting the virus to the eastern United States, and retarding its spread to Canada.

These efforts have been successful in arresting the spread of rabies in raccoons and other wildlife and in decreasing its prevalence in some hot spots, but they probably cannot be used to eliminate the disease altogether, at least in part because no effective method for immunizing bats has been developed. Interaction between bats and wild carnivores (the principal reservoirs of the disease) will probably keep rabies cycling in nature until bats can be included in the vaccination program.

—*Carl W. Hoagstrom, Ph.D.*

quences require only three inoculations and are no more painful than most shots. Tests using antibodies are more rapid and reliable at detecting the presence of the rabies virus than the test for Negri bodies.

Preexposure immunization, in contrast to the postexposure immunization described above, is used to protect persons who might be exposed to rabies in their normal activities and to protect pets from contracting rabies. Since the overwhelming majority of human cases of rabies come from dog bites, pet vaccination is the most important part of the successful rabies control programs of developed countries. Laws requiring the immunization of pets against rabies and leash laws (which require that pets be controlled and not allowed to wander freely) have been very effective in reducing human rabies in these countries.

Because wildlife may harbor rabies, attempts have been made to control or eliminate the disease by killing (culling) or immunizing wildlife. Neither approach has been particularly successful, and the first is accompanied by troublesome side effects. The purpose of culling members of host species is to reduce the host population below the point that will sustain the rabies virus's population. This method is based on the idea that each infected host must, on the average, infect at least one other susceptible host before it dies in order for the parasite to persist in the population. The lower the host population, the lower the chance of one host meeting another and thus the lower the probability of an infected host infecting other members of the population. Yet many of the methods of culling (trapping and poisoning, for example) are not species-specific, and members of other species are killed, sometimes in large numbers. Culling has also been ineffective in many cases. It is most successful in small, isolated areas with a low probability of reinvasion.

Instead of reducing the population size of the host, the goal of immunization is to reduce the number of members that are susceptible to rabies by increasing the number that are immune. Oral immunization by scattering bait containing rabies vaccine has shown promising results in reducing rabies in foxes, coyotes, and raccoons.

An argument against immunization of wildlife to control human rabies is based on the success of the control programs in effect and can be stated as follows. Immunization and regulation of pets, preexposure immunization for humans regularly exposed to rabies, and effective postexposure treatment have already minimized the incidence of human rabies in developed nations. Therefore, wildlife immunization is not necessary for the control of human rabies. In developing nations, where human rabies is still a serious disease, all the potential solutions strain the available resources, but the most cost-effective solution would be the one in use in developed countries. There is general agreement, however, that wildlife immunization might be an effective way to increase the population size of a wildlife species that is normally susceptible to rabies, if desirable.

To control vampire bats in Latin America, where rabies carried by vampire bats burdens the cattle industry, culling has been attempted repeatedly, often unsuccessfully, and with serious side effects. For example, other bat species, some of which are important to insect control and the pollination of fruit trees, have been regular victims of indiscriminate attempts at vampire bat control by culling.

A more effective, and less ecologically disruptive, method for the control of vampire bats employs anticoagulants. These chemicals stimulate bleeding in the digestive tract of vampire bats that swallow them, resulting in death. The anticoagulant can be applied directly to the backs of the vampire bats and will spread through the bat population when the bats groom one another at the roosting colony. Alternatively, anticoagulant can be injected into a cow's rumen, the enlarged first chamber of its four-part stomach. The anticoagulant is then absorbed into the animal's blood and spread to vampire bats when they feed on the cattle.

In test areas, each method has reduced the number of vampire bat bites in cattle by 90 percent, but each has drawbacks. Direct application to these bats requires extensive netting or trapping, special equipment, and workers skilled in vampire bat identification. The rumen injection technique requires expensive equipment for, and workers experienced in, handling large numbers of cattle. In developing countries, either combination can be difficult to finance.

Education is another important aspect of rabies control. While dogs are the most common source of human rabies, humans occasionally contract the disease after being bitten by a wild animal. In addition, there are potential avenues of transfer other than bites. These include skinning rabid animals, being licked by a rabid animal on broken skin, and breathing air infested with the rabies virus. All these alternative transmission mechanisms are exceptionally infrequent, but there are documented cases of aerial transmission to humans. For example, two men who were not bitten died of rabies contracted while exploring a bat cave in Texas. To be transmitted in this way, the rabies virus must be highly concentrated in the air. These concentrations probably occur only in caves occupied by a large number of bats, and many of them must be carrying the rabies virus.

While educating spelunkers and hunters to these dangers would have a minimal effect on the incidence of rabies, as these transmission mechanisms are so infrequent, such educating could be of the utmost importance to an individual who is spared a rabies infection by the knowledge. Educating people, especially children, to leave animals acting in an unnatural fashion alone would have a somewhat greater effect on rabies incidence. Most wild animals that can be caught or approached closely are sick and may be suffering from dumb or paralytic rabies. They should be avoided and reported to the appropriate authorities, as should any dog or cat that behaves unnaturally. Educating the public about the importance of pet vaccination and pet control is the most important role of education in the regulation of rabies.

Perspective and Prospects

Rabies in humans and its association with attacks by mad dogs have been known for more than two thousand years. Despite the fact that rabies has never caused epidemics accompanied by mass mortality as have smallpox and bubonic plague, its frightful symptoms and ability to turn a loving family pet into a vicious animal have given the disease a terrifying and mysterious aura. As a result, cures and preventions have been sought throughout history.

In the late nineteenth century, Louis Pasteur and his associates performed a series of experiments in which the rabies virus was isolated from a dog and injected into rabbit brains. Pasteur called this virus a "street" virus because it was isolated directly from dogs in the street. The virus replicated in the rabbit brain and could be transferred into another rabbit's brain, where it again replicated. Growth of the virus in one of the rabbit brains was called a "passage." A sequence of such passages resulted in a virus which had a more predictable and shorter incubation period. This virus was called a "fixed" virus because of its fixed incubation period. After a hundred such passages, the virus had lost much of its ability to infect dogs.

Pasteur then developed an immunization sequence that protected dogs from the street virus. He air-dried rabbit spinal cord tissue infected with the fixed virus for varying amounts of time and developed a series of virus solutions, ranging from those that could not infect rabbits through those that could occasionally establish weak infections to those that were maximally infective. He then injected dogs daily for ten days, beginning with the noninfective preparation the first day and increasing the infectivity with each day's injection until, on the tenth day, he was injecting highly infective virus. Dogs so treated were resistant to experimentally injected street virus.

Pasteur was still refining his immunization system when a boy who had been attacked by a rabid dog was brought to him. Knowing that the latency period of the virus might allow time for the development of immunity before the symptoms appeared, and aware of the almost certain fatal result if nothing was done, Pasteur treated the boy with the sequence that he had used on the dogs. The boy lived, with no apparent side effects, and Pasteur's treatment became the standard for rabies. The modern treatment sequence is a refinement of Pasteur's. While the immunization sequence for rabies was not the first to be used successfully-smallpox immunization nearly a century earlier holds that distinction-the possibility of immunization after exposure to diseases with long incubation periods was established by Pasteur's work.

Considerable work has been done on the epidemiology of rabies. Mathematical and computer models have been developed that attempt to predict the characteristics of the disease spread under different conditions, and thus suggest means of controlling and preventing rabies epidemics. Arguments over the effectiveness of wildlife vaccination are partially based on such models. The usefulness of these models is not restricted to rabies epidemiology but instead contributes to an understanding of epidemiology in general. Thus research on rabies continues to enhance the control and prevention of that terrifying disease and to add to the general knowledge base of medicine as well.

—Carl W. Hoagstrom, Ph.D.

See also Bites and stings; Coma; Immunization and vaccination; Paralysis; Seizures; Viral infections; Zoonoses.

For Further Information:
Bacon, Philip J., ed. *Population Dynamics of Rabies in Wildlife*. New York: Academic Press, 1985.
Badash, Michelle. "Rabies." *Health Library*, December 30, 2011.
Baer, George M., ed. *The Natural History of Rabies*. 2d ed. Boca Raton, Fla.: CRC Press, 1991.
Biddle, Wayne. *A Field Guide to Germs*. 2d ed. New York: Anchor Books, 2002.
Blanton, Jesse D., et al. "Rabies Surveillance in the United States During 2007." *Journal of the American Veterinary Medical Association* 233 (2008): 884-897.
Constantine, Denny G. "Health Precautions for Bat Researchers." In *Ecological and Behavioral Methods for the Study of Bats*, edited by Thomas H. Kunz. Washington, D.C.: Smithsonian Institution Press, 1988.
Finley, Don. *Mad Dogs: The New Rabies Plague*. College Station: Texas A&M University Press, 1998.
Jackson, Alan C., and William H. Wunner, eds. *Rabies*. Boston: Academic Press, 2002.
Kaplan, Colin, G. S. Turner, and D. A. Warrell. *Rabies: The Facts*. 2d ed. New York: Oxford University Press, 1986.
Pace, Brian, and Richard M. Glass. "Rabies." *Journal of the American Medical Association* 284, no. 8 (August 30, 2000): 1052.
Parker, James N., and Philip M. Parker, eds. *The Official Patient's Sourcebook on Rabies*. San Diego, Calif.: Icon Health, 2002.
"Rabies." *Centers for Disease Control and Prevention*, March 15, 2013.
"Rabies." *Mayo Clinic*, January 28, 2011.

Radiation sickness

Disease/Disorder
Anatomy or system affected: Gastrointestinal system, hair, skin, stomach
Specialties and related fields: Critical care, emergency medicine, occupational health, oncology, public health, radiology
Definition: An acute illness that occurs when an individual is exposed to a sudden, large dose of nuclear radiation or X rays.

Causes and Symptoms

Typical symptoms of radiation sickness are nausea, diarrhea, skin burns, internal bleeding, and severe anemia. The production of blood corpuscles in the bone marrow is inhibited, and the ability of the body to fight infection is reduced.

The severity of radiation sickness depends on the dose, which is commonly measured in units called rads (an acronym for radiation absorbed dose). For humans, a whole-body dose greater than six hundred rads is usually fatal. At 450 rads, there is a 50 percent survival rate. Below fifty rads, no symptoms of radiation sickness are observable, although the risk of cancer is somewhat higher than normal. Radiation therapy for cancer patients has typically been prescribed in total doses of about five thousand rads. Such large doses are not fatal for two reasons: first, only a small region of the body (the actual cancer site) is irradiated; and second, the therapy is given in smaller doses of about two hundred rads over a period of several weeks, so that the body has time to recover between treatments.

Information on Radiation Sickness

Causes: Exposure to sudden, large dose of nuclear radiation or X rays

Symptoms: Nausea, diarrhea, skin burns, internal bleeding, severe anemia

Duration: Acute

Treatments: Drug therapy, antibiotics, bone marrow transplantation

Treatment and Therapy

Once radiation damage occurs, little can be done to repair it directly. Immediate treatment involves washing the body with soap and lukewarm water to remove radioactive material, as well as monitoring of the levels of radiation in the body. This monitoring continues throughout the course of treatment, which centers on whichever parts of the body have been affected and focuses on helping the body's natural processes of recovery. Vomiting and diarrhea can be controlled with drugs, while bacterial infections and wounds are treated with antibiotics. In extreme cases, bone marrow transplants can be performed to reestablish the formation of new blood cells. Donor cells are not likely to be rejected because the body's immune system has been inactivated temporarily by the radiation.

—*Hans G. Graetzer, Ph.D.*

See also Biological and chemical weapons; Bone marrow transplantation; Burns and scalds; Carcinogens; Environmental diseases; Occupational health; Radiation therapy.

For Further Information:

Frigerio, Norman A. *Your Body and Radiation*. Washington, DC: US Atomic Energy Commission, 1966.

Hall, Eric J. *Radiation and Life*. 2d ed. New York: Pergamon Press, 1984.

Montemayor-Quellenberg, Marjorie, and Igor Puzanov. "Radiation Exposure." *Health Library*, 20 June 2013.

Ogura, Toyofumi. *Letters from the End of the World: A Firsthand Account of the Bombing of Hiroshima*. New York: Kodansha International, 2001.

Perez, Eric, et al. "Radiation Sickness." *MedlinePlus*, 1 Feb. 2013.

Prasad, Kedar N. *Handbook of Radiobiology*. Rev. 2d ed. Boca Raton, Fla.: CRC Press, 1995.

"Radiation Exposure." *MedlinePlus*, 26 Aug. 2013.

"Radiation Exposure and Cancer." *American Cancer Society*, 29 Mar. 2010.

"Understanding Radiation: Overview." *Environmental Protection Agency*, 23 Jan. 2013.

Radiation therapy

Treatment

Anatomy or system affected: All

Specialties and related fields: Nuclear medicine, oncology, radiology

Definition: The use of X rays or radioactivity in the treatment of cancer patients, frequently in combination with surgery and chemotherapy.

Key terms:

computed tomography (CT) scanning: from the Greek word *tomos*, meaning "section"; the process of using X rays to obtain a computer picture of an interior cross section from a patient's body

gamma rays: penetrating radiation that comes from a radioactive source, such as cobalt 60

internal radiation: therapy in which a small radioactive source is implanted close to the cancer site, such as on the cervix or inside the chest cavity

magnetic resonance imaging (MRI): a diagnostic technique using large magnets (not X rays) to outline the shape and size of a tumor

metastasis: the spread of cancer cells from one part of the body to another

oncologist: a physician who specializes in the treatment of cancer

radiation dose: the amount of radiation absorbed, depending on the intensity of the source and the time of exposure; measured in units of rads or grays

tumor: an abnormal mass of tissue that may be malignant (growing larger) or benign (not spreading)

X rays: penetrating radiation produced by means of a high-voltage machine; useful for both diagnosis and therapy of cancerous tissue

Indications and Procedures

When a person is diagnosed with cancer, three main methods of treatment may be used: surgery, radiation, and chemotherapy (drugs). Surgery and radiation are most useful if the cancer is a localized tumor whose shape and size can be determined. Radiation is the treatment of choice if the tumor is at an inoperable location, such as inside the brain, liver, or spine. In some cases, radiation is used following surgery in order to prevent recurrence of a malignant growth.

The amount of energy absorbed in radiation therapy can be expressed quantitatively in a unit called a gray. It was named after a British radiobiologist, Louis Harold Gray, who studied the biological effect of various ionizing radiations. One gray corresponds to the absorption of a fixed amount of radiation energy. Before 1984, radiation doses were commonly measured in rads, which was an acronym for radiation absorbed dose. The conversion factor is "100 rads = 1 gray." Since most references continue to use the more familiar rad, it will be adopted here. For converting to grays, each rad value is divided by one hundred.

To develop a feel for typical dose levels in radiation therapy, it is helpful to remember two numbers for comparison: First, the maximum safe dose established by the Nuclear Regulatory Commission (NRC) for radiation exposure in the workplace is 5 rads per year; second, a lethal dose for 50 percent of humans, called LD-50, is about 450 rads. LD-50 means that, statistically, 50 percent would die and 50 percent would recover from such a massive dose.

The numbers given above must be interpreted with care. For example, a dental X-ray gives a dose of about 2 rads. Four dental X-rays give a total exposure of 8 rads, exceeding the NRC yearly maximum of 5 rads. Only a small part of the body, however, perhaps 1 percent, is irradiated during a dental X-ray. Therefore, the radiation dose averaged over the whole body is only 1 percent of 8 rads.

A patient with malignant cancer might be given twenty

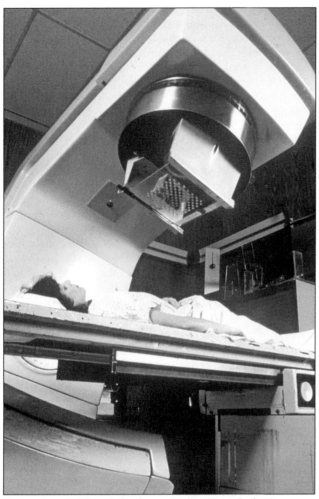

A patient is readied for radiation therapy. (National Cancer Institute)

trol so that the radiologist and other medical personnel will not be exposed.

Radioactive gold is another useful source for radiation therapy and one that is especially suitable for internal placement in the body, such as in the treatment of uterine or ovarian cancer. The half-life of radioactive gold is less than three days, so it can be left in the body to provide continuous treatment for a short time. The gamma rays from gold are of much lower energy than those from cobalt, so they penetrate only a few centimeters of tissue around the source. This limits damage to healthy cells farther from the irradiation site.

X-rays are seldom used today for cancer therapy because radioactive sources are much more convenient. Many radiopharmaceuticals, with various half-lives and energies, are available for different applications. Beams of electrons, protons, and other particles coming directly from nuclear accelerators also have been used to irradiate tumors, with some excellent results. The personnel and equipment costs to operate an accelerator, however, are too great for most hospitals. Also, patients may find the experience of being bombarded by the output beam from a large and noisy accelerator to be too traumatic.

The various types of radiation, including X-rays, gamma rays, and particle beams, all produce damage in living tissue by the process of ionization. The radiation strikes individual atoms and breaks the bonds that hold molecules together. The breakup of normal molecules produces positive and negative ions, which act as toxic chemicals. The internal structure of cells is disrupted so that they can no longer replicate themselves. Fortunately, cancer cells tend to be more sensitive to radiation damage than normal cells.

Radioactive needles, grains, and other sealed-source designs may be used when there is a suitable body cavity or opening. Such internal sources are common for treating cancer of the prostate, vagina, uterus, rectum, throat, and larynx. One problem with implanted sources is the radiation dose received by the physician during the surgery. Sometimes, it is possible to use "afterloading," in which a hollow tube or shell is positioned in the patient and radioactive material is loaded into it at a later time.

Breast cancer is the second leading cause of death for American women. Early detection and treatment are the keys to improving the chances for survival. A radicalmastectomy (breast removal) can be an emotionally traumatic experience. If the cancer is not too advanced, however, radiation therapy is an alternative. In some cases, daily treatment with a cobalt source can be done on an outpatient basis, with only minor disruptions of schedule and no long-term disfigurement.

During treatment for any type of cancer, the radiologist needs to determine whether the radiation therapy is shrinking the tumor. Therefore, computed tomography (CT) scanning or magnetic resonance imaging (MRI) will be used during and after treatment to monitor the size of the tumor. The radiation dose then can be adjusted to take into account the individual characteristics of various patients.

The goal of radiation therapy is to deliver a dose of sev-

radiation treatments of 250 rads each, for a total dose of 5,000 rads. Even though this far exceeds the LD-50 of 450 rads, it is not lethal because it is spread out over time. The patient may develop symptoms of radiation sickness-skin reddening, nausea, loss of hair, and blood changes-but the body has time to heal partially between irradiations. The healing process can be compared to recovery from a serious burn injury, in which the skin and flesh repair themselves but permanent scars may be left behind. The present trend in radiology is to subdivide the total dose into more and smaller increments, reducing patient discomfort.

One of the most common elements used for cancer therapy is called cobalt 60, which is created by irradiating ordinary cobalt in a research reactor. Because the radioactive form of cobalt emits gamma rays with a penetrating power that is equivalent to a 2 million-volt X-ray machine, it is useful for the treatment of deep internal cancers. The radioactive source must be kept in a thick lead shield. When a patient is to be treated, the source is positioned near the cancer site, and a small port is opened briefly to irradiate it. Sometimes, the cobalt source is moved around the patient so that the gamma rays enter the body from different angles, thus reducing the damage to healthy tissue lying above the cancer site. The irradiation procedure is done by remote con-

eral thousand rads to a cancer site while minimizing the damage to surrounding tissue and nearby organs. The shape of a malignant cancer may be a simple round lump, or it can be a complex group of nodules with tentacles extending through the flesh. For effective treatment, it is essential to determine the location and shape of the tumor as precisely as possible. An ordinary X-ray photograph is not very useful for diagnosing a tumor. The problem is a lack of contrast between a tumor and surrounding tissue, because there is very little difference in their densities. An X-ray of the head, for example, provides an excellent outline of the skull, but it cannot distinguish between tumor and brain material on the inside. In the 1970s, a major advance in X-ray technology called CT scanning was developed in England; it is sometimes also called a computed axial tomography (CAT) scan. CT scanning replaces the film of conventional X-rays with pictures on a computer screen.

A narrow X-ray beam with the diameter of a pencil scans across the region of interest, while an electronic detector measures the transmitted intensity and sends the data to the computer. A tumor is slightly denser than surrounding tissue, so a small decrease of intensity is recorded by the detector. The X-ray beam and detector system are rotated by a small angle, and another scan is recorded. Altogether, 180 scans may be used to record one "slice" of the body. The region where beams of decreased intensity from all the scans intersect defines the location of a tumor in that slice. Next, the X-ray beam and detector are moved along the body a small distance, and another 180 scans are made to obtain a second slice. Several more slices will be recorded. Eventually, the computer assembles all the information into a three-dimensional picture of the region of interest.

The sharpness and contrast obtained with CT scans are remarkable improvements over X-ray film. A radiologist can view the computer display of a tumor from various angles and with different enlargements. The computer screen can be photographed to provide a permanent record. The two scientists who developed the CT scan, Allan Cormack and Godfrey Hounsfield, shared the Nobel Prize in Physiology or Medicine in 1979.

An entirely different method to determine the location and outline of an internal tumor is called MRI. Instead of using X-rays, MRI utilizes the magnetic properties of hydrogen nuclei, which can be aligned by a very strong magnet.

The patient lies on a couch in a magnetic field produced by coils around his or her body. Radio waves are used to reverse the direction of alignment of the hydrogen. The concentration of hydrogen atoms in a tumor differs slightly from that in the surrounding tissue, so the output signal will differ correspondingly. Several methods are used to identify the precise location in the body where the magnetic reversals occur. A computer is used to convert the information into a pictorial display on a screen. Since bones contain virtually no hydrogen, the MRI picture shows them as shadows while emphasizing the structure of soft organs, tumors, and tissue.

Both MRI and CT scanning are complex diagnostic procedures. To diagnose and treat a cancer, radiologists, medical physicists, physicians, and computer specialists must work together as a team. New techniques for obtaining and displaying information are under continuing development.

Uses and Complications

The way in which radiation therapy is used depends on many factors, such as tumor location, the age and overall health of the patient, and the extent and stage of the cancer. Consider a young woman who has symptoms of back pain and loss of feeling in her legs. Use of MRI clearly shows a tumor growing inside her spinal column. For cancer in this location, treatment using radiation therapy, rather than surgery or chemotherapy, is indicated.

A treatment plan is devised that will minimize the radiation dose to the patient's lungs, heart, and liver; the direction of entry for the beam of radiation must avoid passing through these sensitive organs. Furthermore, the radiologist has to make sure that the proper dose will be received at various depths below the skin. A plastic dummy to simulate the patient, called a phantom, can be irradiated with detectors placed inside it to measure the dose. Scattering of radiation and shielding effects by bones can be very complex and must be determined by computer calculations supplemented by careful measurements.

The radiation pattern can be shaped with filters and baffles so that it will conform to the shape of the tumor as closely as possible. A useful computer display for planning the therapy, called the "beam's-eye view," shows the tumor and its surroundings as if the observer's eye were at the source of radiation.

Two final considerations in treatment planning for this patient are how the total radiation dose is to be subdivided and what the time interval between exposures should be. The radiologist must make a decision based on a judgment of the patient's stamina, as well as of the urgency of treatment.

Consider another patient, a man who has developed a cancerous tumor of the tongue. Surgery is undesirable because his speaking ability would be impaired. Instead of an external radiation beam, the radiologist will probably recommend that radioactive needles be inserted directly into the affected region. Five to ten needles containing radioactive radium or cesium deliver the appropriate dose directly to the cancer site. The needles are left in place for several days and then removed. An alternative to needles in this case is the use of very small grains of radioactive material that can be implanted into the tumor. Sources with a short half-life, such as radioactive gold or radon, lose almost all their activity within two weeks, so the grains do not have to be removed.

The overall effectiveness of radiation therapy can be summarized approximately by the "half-half-half" rule. About half of all cancers are treated with radiation. Half of those patients are given a large enough dose to attempt a cure. (For the others, radiation is used simply for pain relief.) Finally, about half of these patients are actually cured by radiation. This success rate is encouraging, but clearly there is much room left for improvement.

The survival rate after radiation treatment varies greatly depending on the site of cancer in the body. For example, patients with localized cancer of the prostate, larynx, or uterus have five-year survival rates that range around 90 percent. At the other end of the scale, stomach or lung cancers that have spread and are at a much later stage show only about a 10 percent survival rate. Radiation therapy for ten different kinds of cancer-breast, cervix, larynx, prostate, uterus, bladder, testicle, tongue, mouth cancers, and Hodgkin disease-results in cure rates that are equal to or greater than those with surgery while preserving the organ function.

Many people are apprehensive about the hazards of radiation, with good reason. In the 1920s, some workers who were hired to apply radium paint to watch dials (to make them glow in the dark) developed cancer when they ingested radioactive material. At Hiroshima and Nagasaki, many people developed radiation sickness and died from the aftereffects of the atomic bombs dropped on those cities. For medical applications of radiation, regulatory agencies that are responsive to the general public must evaluate potential benefits and risks. Sometimes, sensationalized articles are published that present frightening scenarios of highly unlikely hazards. The perception of risk from low-level radioactive waste, for example, far exceeds the actual hazard. The advantages of radiation therapy would be lost if permits for hazardous waste storage were denied. The responsible use of any technology should balance concerns for safety with the benefits of that technology.

Ensuring the health and safety of medical personnel who administer radiation therapy to patients requires proper training. All workers must wear radiation monitors, which are checked daily. Radiation areas have to be posted with warning signs. The nuclear medicine department at a hospital must keep an accurate inventory of radioactive materials. The shipment and disposal of radiopharmaceuticals are strictly regulated. Periodic on-site visits by Nuclear Regulatory Commission inspectors also are part of the licensing procedure. Careless overexposure of personnel must be avoided if the benefits of radiation therapy are to find continued acceptance by the medical profession and the general public.

Perspective and Prospects

Radiation therapy most commonly makes use of X-rays or radioactivity. It is interesting to note that both types of radiation were discovered only a year apart in the 1890s. Wilhelm Röntgen, a German physicist, discovered X-rays in 1895. He received the Nobel Prize for his work in 1901, the first year in which the award was given. He used high voltage to accelerate an electron beam; when the electrons hit a metal target, they released a new kind of penetrating radiation. Röntgen made a now-famous X-ray photograph of his wife's hand that clearly showed the bones inside the flesh. The medical profession adopted X-rays with great enthusiasm, primarily for the diagnosis of broken bones, swallowed objects, and bullet or shrapnel fragments.

Radioactivity was first observed in 1896 by Henri Becquerel, in Paris. By chance, Becquerel had placed a uranium rock next to unused photographic film that was still wrapped in its container. He was amazed to find that radiation from the uranium had penetrated the wrapping and had exposed the film inside. His discovery and follow-up experiments earned for him the Nobel Prize in 1905.

Marie Curie, a graduate student under Becquerel, became famous for isolating a new radioactive element from uranium ore, which she named radium. It emits radiation at a rate that is a million times greater than that of an equivalent weight of uranium. In her doctoral thesis in 1904, Curie described an experiment in which she placed a small capsule containing radium on her husband's arm. It produced a sore that took more than a month to heal. The hazards of handling radioactivity and the possibility of using it to destroy cancer cells were recognized quite early.

The element radium is very rare on earth. In fact, the world's total supply is less than 1 kilogram. Only after the invention of nuclear particle accelerators and neutron sources in the 1930s was it possible to create artificial radioactive elements in substantial amounts.

Radiation therapy has since become a treatment of choice in oncology. Such treatment will likely remain necessary for some time to come: It is not reasonable to expect a cure for cancer soon because there are too many different types. Much has been accomplished, however, in the area of prevention. The strong correlation between lung cancer and smoking has received wide publicity, so many people have stopped, at least in the United States. Research with animals has linked cancer to certain food additives and industrial pollutants, leading to legal restrictions on their use. In addition to surgery, radiation, and chemotherapy, other treatment methods are under investigation. For example, one procedure involves blocking the blood supply from reaching a tumor so that the malignant cells die from lack of nutrients. Other researchers hope to use genetic engineering, trying to stimulate the body's immune system to produce specific antibodies that will fight against the cancer cells.

—*Hans G. Graetzer, Ph.D.*

See also Cancer; Chemotherapy; Computed tomography (CT) scanning; Hair loss and baldness; Magnetic resonance imaging (MRI); Malignancy and metastasis; Nuclear medicine; Nuclear radiology; Oncology; Radiopharmaceuticals.

For Further Information:

Brown, G. I. *Invisible Rays: A History of Radioactivity.* Stroud, England: Sutton, 2002.

Cameron, John R., James G. Skofronick, and Roderick M. Grant. *Medical Physics: Physics of the Body.* Madison, Wis.: Medical Physics, 1992.

Hall, Eric J. *Radiation and Life.* 2d ed. New York: Pergamon Press, 1984.

Hendee, William R., Geoffrey S. Ibbott, and Eric G. Hendee. *Radiation Therapy Physics.* 3d ed. Hoboken, N.J.: John Wiley & Sons, 2005.

Laws, Priscilla W., and the Public Citizen Health Research Group. *The X-Ray Information Book.* New York: Farrar, Straus and Giroux, 1983.

Puzanov, Igor. "Radiation Therapy-External." *Health Library,* Sept. 26, 2012.

Puzanov, Igor, and Michael Woods. "Radiation Therapy-Internal." *Health Library*, May 30, 2013.

"Radiation Therapy." *MedlinePlus*, June 10, 2013.

Saha, Gopal B. *Physics and Radiobiology of Nuclear Medicine*. 4th ed. New York: Springer, 2013.

Sandler, Martin P., R. Edward Coleman, and James A. Patton, eds. *Diagnostic Nuclear Medicine*. 4th ed. Philadelphia: Lippincott Williams & Wilkins, 2003.

Smith, F. A. *A Primer in Applied Radiation Physics*. River Edge, N.J.: World Scientific, 2000.

"Understanding Radiation Therapy: A Guide for Patients and Families." *American Cancer Society*, Jan. 24, 2013.

Radiculopathy

Disease/Disorder

Also known as: Radiculoneuropathy, mononeuropathy, polyneuropathy, neuropathy, radiculitis

Anatomy or system affected: Musculoskeletal system, nerves, nervous system, spine

Specialties and related fields: Geriatrics and gerontology, neurology, nursing, orthopedics, osteopathic medicine, pathology, physical therapy, radiology, rheumatology, sports medicine

Definition: Pain distributed along a specific pathway resulting from irritation of a nerve root.

Key terms:

deep tendon reflex: a brisk contraction of a muscle responding to a sudden stretch produced by a sharp tap of a rubber hammer on a tendon insertion of a muscle

intervertebral disk: one of the fibrous disks found between adjacent spinal vertebrae

spinal nerves: pairs of nerves connected to the spinal cord and numbered according to the level at which they emerge from the cord; each spinal nerve attaches to the spinal cord by an anterior and a posterior root

spinal stenosis: a condition in which the diameter of the spinal canal is decreased and compromises the spinal cord and spinal nerve roots

vertebrae: a cylindrical bony mass that encompasses and protects the spinal column; collectively, thirty-three vertebrae separated by cartilaginous disks make up the vertebral column

Causes and Symptoms

The nervous system provides an avenue of signaling from the brain to the muscles. Each spinal nerve departing from the spinal cord is part of the peripheral nervous system. Any disruption at the spinal nerve or as it travels farther away from the spine will affect the signal, resulting in radiculopathy. The anatomic region or regions affected determine the severity of the involvement and the amount of function that may be lost.

Nerve root irritations resulting in radiculopathy include a variety of causes. Because of this, several classifications are used such as rate of onset, distribution pattern, or pathology. Compression from surrounding anatomic structures upon a spinal nerve root is a common cause of radiculopathy. It can originate from any level of the spine: the cervical, thoracic, or lumbar vertebral levels. Encroaching material causing the nerve root compression and irritation can be from the intervertebral disk or from vertebral

---

Information on Radiculopathy

Causes: Compression, infection, inflammation, inherited disorders, environmental toxins

Symptoms: Variable to each nerve root level; tingling, prickling, burning, glove-and-stocking distribution, weakness

Duration: Dependent on cause; short and long duration; can be permanent

Treatments: Physical therapy, medication, surgery

---

bone. Causative factors of this compression include trauma or degeneration of the spine over time. With age, water content of the intervertebral disk decreases, resulting in the disk space becoming thinner. Over time, the spinal nerve roots potentially become compressed and entrapped, resulting in a condition called spinal stenosis. Spinal stenosis of the lumbar spine commonly produces radiculopathy in the legs and feet, whereas this condition in the cervical spine can produce similar symptoms in the arms and hands. Inflammation resulting from disk degeneration can compound this problem. Less common causes of radiculopathy are inherited disorders causing nerve root irritation. Some viruses such as herpes zoster infect spinal nerves and are revealed as a painful area of skin that is mainly supplied by a single spinal nerve called a dermatome.

Symptoms vary with each level of nerve root involved. Sensory changes such as tingling, prickling, and burning are some of the earlier signs of radiculopathy. When more than one nerve is affected, the sensory loss follows a distribution similar to a glove-and-stocking pattern as it encircles a limb. Over time, the nerve root irritation can cause further problems, including weakness of corresponding muscles called atrophy. Deep tendon reflexes-such as the Achilles tendon reflex or the biceps tendon reflex, involving the lumbar and cervical spine respectively-will be diminished or completely absent. This becomes a useful indication for the clinical diagnosis of nerve root irritation associated with radiculopathy.

Treatment and Therapy

Medical attention and treatment for radiculopathy at any level should not be delayed. Primary treatment is reducing and or eliminating the cause of the nerve irritation. Depending upon the severity, nonsurgical treatment is usually attempted initially, such as the use of epidural steroid injections, which are effective in decreasing the inflammation around the nerve root. Physical therapy is commonly used and proves effective for many cases of radiculopathy. This discipline utilizes techniques of spinal traction and mobilization, which helps decompress the nerve root.

Once symptoms have been stabilized, physical therapy introduces spinal stabilization exercises to aid in the prevention of future problems and reoccurrences. In the case of nerve root compression, surgery may be required to decompress the spinal nerve. One of the minimally invasive approaches is a microdiskectomy, which removes the portion of the disk that presses against the nerve root. The success rate of this surgery is high, and results are favorable because of the minimal recovery time. Frequently, there is immediate relief of the radiculopathy caused by a nerve root compression.

Perspective and Prospects

Research is ongoing for the treatment of radiculopathy of any origin. Medications that address nerve pain have been developed, with additional clinical trials currently in progress. The development of other minimally invasive surgical procedures is also important to the medical specialties of orthopedic surgery and neurosurgery. Studies have shown, however, that long-term outcomes do not differ between those who undergo surgery and those who do not. The decision to undergo surgery is not a trivial one, and it is preferably made in consultation with several physicians.

—*Jeffrey P. Larson, P.T., A.T.C.*

See also Back pain; Nervous system; Neuralgia, neuritis, and neuropathy; Neuroimaging; Neurology; Neurology, pediatric; Neurosurgery; Numbness and tingling; Pain; Sciatica; Spinal cord disorders; Spine, vertebrae, and disks; Stenosis.

For Further Information:

Bogduk, N., and L. Twomey. *Clinical Anatomy of the Lumbar Spine.* 4th ed. New York: Elsevier/Churchill Livingstone, 2005.

Hoppenfeld, Stanley. *Physical Examination of the Spine and Extremities.* Norwalk, Conn.: Appleton-Century-Crofts, 1976.

Magee, David J. *Orthopedic Assessment.* 5th ed. Philadelphia: W. B. Saunders Elsevier, 2008.

Malone, T. R., T. McPoil, and A. J. Nitz. *Orthopedic and Sports Physical Therapy.* 3d ed. St. Louis: Mosby Year Books, 1997.

"NINDS Peripheral Neuropathy Information Page." *National Institute of Neurological Disorders and Stroke*, Sept. 19, 2012.

"Spinal Stenosis." *MedlinePlus*, May 14, 2013.

Stahl, Rebecca J., and Rimas Lukas. "Neuropathic Pain." *Health Library*, Mar. 15, 2013.

Umphred, Darcy A. *Neurological Rehabilitation.* 6th ed. St. Louis: Mosby, 2012.

Radiology. *See* Imaging and radiology; Nuclear radiology.

Radiopharmaceuticals

Procedure

Anatomy or system affected: All

Specialties and related fields: Endocrinology, internal medicine, oncology, radiology

Definition: Imaging techniques involving radioactive chemical agents that are designed to localize in specific organs and emit radiation, which can be detected outside the body with a camera in order to provide visual images of the organ.

Key terms:

becquerel: the international unit of radioactivity, defined as a radioactive sample that is decaying at the rate of one disintegration per second

electron volt: a unit of energy defined as the energy acquired by an electron traveling through a potential difference of 1 volt

gamma camera: a type of radiation detection instrument that detects gamma rays external to the body and makes an image of the radionuclide distribution in body organs; also known as a scintillation camera

gamma ray: a type of electromagnetic radiation that has the same physical properties as X rays but is emitted by unstable nuclei in their decay process; gamma rays are capable of penetrating soft tissue, thereby allowing their detection outside the body to produce images of organs

half-life: the time required for one-half of the nuclei in a radioactive sample to decay

radioimmunotherapy: a cancer therapy using radionuclides; the radionuclides attach themselves to antibodies that tend to target cancer cells in the body, thus eradicating the cancer cells through selective irradiation

radionuclide: an unstable atomic nucleus that, in the process of decay, emits radiation; also referred to as a radioisotope

The Fundamentals of Radioactivity

All matter consists of atoms, which contain a central nucleus and tiny particles called electrons that revolve around the nucleus. Electrons carry a small negative charge, while the nucleus is made up of particles called neutrons, which have no charge, and protons, which carry a positive charge. Atoms are generally neutral, with the number of protons in the nucleus equaling the number of electrons. Most objects are made up of atoms in which the neutron and proton numbers in their nuclei are arranged in such a way that they are stable. If the proton number or the neutron number in the nucleus is altered, the atom may become unstable. Such unstable atoms are termed radioactive and tend to reach a stable state by emitting radiation. This process is referred to as radioactive decay, and the elemental atoms that emit radiation are called radioisotopes or radionuclides. All stable elements can be made into radioactive elements by either adding or removing neutrons or protons, a process known as the artificial production of radioactivity. The few naturally occurring radioisotopes, such as radon 222 and uranium 235, are not used in nuclear medicine.

Radioactivity was first discovered by the French scientist Antoine-Henri Becquerel in 1896, when he observed that a photographic plate sitting next to a uranium sample had darkened. Appropriately, the international unit of radioactivity was chosen to be the becquerel. Radioactivity is a property of unstable atomic nuclei, and the rate of decay cannot be affected by normal physical and chemical processes such as heat, pressure, or the presence of magnetic or electric fields. The nuclei in a radioactive sample do not decay spontaneously or all at once. Rather, they decay randomly at a rate that is characteristic of the given radioisotope. While it is impossible to tell when a particular nucleus will decay or disintegrate, the fraction of nuclei in a sample that will decay in a given time can be determined. The decay rate of a radioactive sample is usually expressed in terms of its half-life, the time required for one-half of the original sample nuclei to decay. Half-life is a characteristic property of a particular radionuclide. The half-lives of radioactive isotopes vary from a small fraction of a second to millions of years. For example, carbon 14 has a half-life of 5,730 years, while the half-life of iodine 123 is thirteen hours. Naturally occurring uranium 238 decays with a half-life of 4.5 billion years, which is the approximate age of Earth itself. Hence, at present there remains only half of the original uranium 238 that was formed when the earth was born.

Radionuclides emit three types of radiation: alpha particles, beta particles, and gamma rays. Alpha particles are positively charged ions containing two protons and two neutrons. Beta particles are either positively (positron) or negatively (electron) charged and have the same mass as an electron. In contrast, gamma rays are electromagnetic waves that have no mass or charge and are sometimes called photons. Because alpha particles are relatively massive, they can be totally absorbed by a sheet of paper. Beta particles can penetrate up to about a centimeter or so into an object, depending on their energy. On the other hand, gamma rays of moderate energy can easily penetrate through the body, as with x-rays. When radionuclides that emit gamma rays are administered to patients, the gamma rays exit the body and are captured by a scintillation camera, which produces an image. The desirable energy of the gamma rays for external detection and imaging with gamma cameras is generally in the range of 100 kilo-electron volts to 300 kilo-electron volts. The half-life of the radionuclide emitting the gamma rays should be long enough to allow its uptake by the organ of interest, then subsequent imaging with a gamma camera, and short enough so as not to irradiate the patient long after the image is obtained. Half-lives between three hours and three days are considered optimal for diagnostic purposes. When radionuclides are used for therapy, the half-life is generally required to be in the range of several days, and the preferred form of radiation consists of beta particles because they tend to deposit their energy near the disintegration site.

Uses and Complications

If the physician is interested in imaging a particular organ, drugs that take the radionuclide preferentially to that organ are necessary. This is achieved by chemically attaching the radionuclide to a pharmaceutical carrier. Once the radiopharmaceutical is localized in the organ, the gamma rays that it emits are detected by a gamma camera, which electronically displays an image that is representative of the radionuclide distribution. Such images are of substantial diagnostic value. Similarly, radionuclides attached to drugs that selectively target cancer cells can potentially deliver lethal doses of radiation to the cancer cells, a process called radioimmunotherapy. Hence, radiopharmaceuticals play an important role in medicine, providing new and promising avenues for diagnosis and therapy.

Radiopharmaceuticals are generally administered intravenously to patients. Blood flow to the organ of interest determines the fraction of the administered radioactivity that will be delivered. The ability of the organ to accumulate the circulating radiopharmaceutical is also an important determinant of the pathological condition of the organ. Such considerations are usually taken into account in developing appropriate pharmaceuticals.

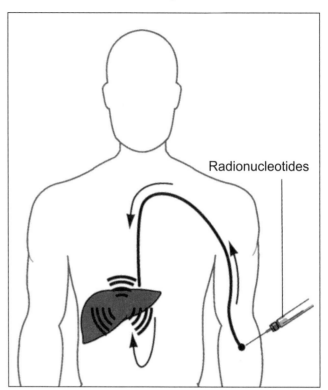

One use of radiopharmaceuticals is to deliver radioactivity to a target organ, such as the liver, that may otherwise be inaccessible to radiation treatment.

Although many radionuclides are available, the most preferred one is called technetium 99m, an excited (metastable) state of technetium 99. This radionuclide is readily available, has a convenient half-life of six hours, and has very desirable radiation properties. Accordingly, many pharmaceuticals are labeled with this radionuclide for diagnostic nuclear medicine purposes. A few other radionuclides, such as thallium 201, iodine 123, gallium 67, and indium 111, can be used when technetium 99m compounds are not available.

The most widely used radiopharmaceutical for brain imaging is technetium 99m pertechnetate. The primary advantage of this chemical is that it is inexpensive and can be easily prepared. Other radiopharmaceuticals used for brain studies are technetium 99m diethylenetriamine-pentacetic acid (DTPA) and technetium 99m glucoheptonate. Brain imaging usually consists of a dynamic study immediately after bolus intravenous injection of the compound in which rapid sequential images are obtained as the radiopharmaceutical enters the brain. This is followed by a static image one hour later. When a brain lesion is suspected, a delayed static image is sometimes necessary three to four hours after an injection. These imaging techniques are valuable in detecting neoplastic tissue, inflammatory processes, infarction, Alzheimer's disease, and stroke. Another class of radiopharmaceuticals has also been developed to study brain function. These compounds, such as carbon 11 N-methylpiperone, use very short-lived radionuclides that need on-site radionuclide production facilities and require a sophisticated imaging system called a positron emission tomography (PET) scanning unit. Imaging of cerebrospinal fluid is performed using DTPA labeled with indium 111 after an intrathecal administration. Radiopharma- ceuticals for such administrations are tested carefully for their safety.

Lung imaging using radiopharmaceuticals is usually performed to study either pulmonary perfusion or ventilation. For perfusion studies, the radiopharmaceutical of choice is microaggregated albumin (MAA) labeled with technetium 99m. Ventilation studies are performed using the radioactive inert gas xenon 133. The patient breathes while the images are obtained with a gamma camera. These lung studies are used extensively to detect several conditions, including pulmonary embolism, asthma, bronchitis, tumors, inflammatory disease, congestive heart failure, and deep-vein thrombus.

Bone imaging with radiopharmaceuticals often provides earlier diagnosis and better detection of lesions than other radiographic procedures. Furthermore, the extent of metastatic disease may be determined using radionuclide imaging techniques. Other applications of bone imaging include determination of the viability of bone; detection of infections in prosthetic joints, necrosis, and infarction; and evaluation of fractures and bone pain. Bone-seeking compounds are usually similar to calcium or phosphates in their chemical behavior. Hence, diphosphonate labeled with technetium 99m and its analogs are the compounds of choice for this purpose.

Radionuclide imaging techniques play an important role in evaluating the function of the heart. Coronary artery perfusion is studied using thallium 201 chloride. The patient is asked to exercise on a treadmill, and the radionuclide is injected at peak stress. The patient continues to exercise for an additional minute, and redistribution of the thallium 201 within the myocardium occurs immediately after cessation of the exercise. Gamma camera images are obtained soon thereafter. Abnormal thallium distribution is the basis for the detection and diagnosis of stress-induced ischemia and permanent myocardial damage. Acute myocardial infarction can be detected using pyrophosphate labeled with technetium 99m within twenty-four to seventy-two hours after the onset of symptoms. Other radiopharmaceuticals using technetium 99m as a label are also under development. To evaluate ventricular function, the radiochemical is administered intravenously and images are obtained during the first pass of the radionuclide through the heart, lungs, and great vessels. An alternate technique for this purpose is to obtain images of the cardiac blood pool after the radiopharmaceutical has achieved equilibrium in the intravascular space. Such noninvasive studies are invaluable in the diagnosis of heart problems and in the management of patients with heart disease.

Evaluation of thyroid function using radioisotope techniques marked the beginning of the field of nuclear medicine. The element iodine is actively transported into the thyroid gland, where it is retained. Therefore, the readily available radioiodines iodine 131 and iodine 123 have been used for this purpose. Technetium 99m pertechnetate is sometimes used because of its low cost and favorable radiation characteristics. Thyroid uptake tests usually involve administration of a small dose of sodium iodide 131 in either liquid or capsule form and measurement of the radioiodine in the thyroid eighteen to twenty-four hours later. Significantly higher uptake compared to the normal value is a reflection of an overactive gland (hyperthyroidism). Conversely, a lower uptake indicates an underactive gland (hypothyroidism). Thyroid imaging is performed using either sodium iodide 123 or technetium 99m pertechnetate to detect cancer. Effective treatment of benign and malignant cancers, as well as hyperthyroidism, is accomplished by administering larger doses of iodine 131. Although the strong uptake of radioactive iodine by the thyroid gland is useful in nuclear medicine, uptake of iodine 131 in the thyroids of people living in nuclear-fallout zones, such as the one around the Chernobyl nuclear reactor, is a major concern. The risk from such exposure can be reduced by saturating the thyroid with nonradioactive iodine using orally administered doses of Lugol's iodine solution.

Radiopharmaceutical studies of kidneys are sometimes necessary to evaluate structural and functional abnormalities. Renal imaging is indicated to assess renal blood flow and the differential and quantitative functioning of natural or transplanted kidneys. Among the radiopharmaceuticals used for these studies are technetium-labeled glucoheptonate, 2,3-dimercaptosuccinic acid (DMSA), and DTPA. Iodine 123 hippurate is also employed for glomerular filtration studies.

Nuclear medicine techniques to image the liver and spleen are also available. Alcohol-related liver diseases can be readily diagnosed using liver images obtained after injection of technetium-labeled sulfur colloid. Primary liver cancers and metastases can also be detected, and the physiological functioning of transplanted livers can be assessed. Spleen imaging with technetium 99m sulfur colloid has been useful in detecting hepatomas, cysts, infarctions, and neoplasms. Gastrointestinal hemorrhaging and associated bleeding are identified by removing a small portion of the patient's red blood cells, labeling them with technetium 99m, and injecting the labeled cells back into the patient. Similarly, white blood cells labeled with indium 111 are used to image abscesses and inflammation. Radionuclide procedures also provide a method to assess digestive disorders and esophageal transit noninvasively. A variety of tumors can be diagnosed when gallium 67 citrate is used for imaging. This radionuclide is also used in studying patients with acquired immunodeficiency syndrome (AIDS).

Radiopharmaceuticals are also playing an important role in treating many functional disorders and cancers. As pointed out earlier, hyperthyroidism and thyroid carcinoma are best treated with iodine 131. Malignant pheochromocytomas and other neuroendocrine lesions can be treated with metaiodine 131 benzylguanidine. Gold 198 colloid has been used to assist in the therapy of peritoneal metastases and recurrent malignant ascites. Phosphorus 32 colloids are employed in treating malignant pericardial effusion associated with breast and lung carcinomas. Intra-arterial injection of phosphorus 32 colloid to treat inflammatory arthritis of bone joints is also common. The uncontrolled proliferation of bone marrow cells is checked by administering phosphorus 32 orthophosphate. Patients with advanced bone metastases and intractable bone pain are also often treated with single or multiple doses of phosphorus 32 orthophosphate. Other radionuclides that are useful for this purpose are strontium 89, rhenium 186, and yttrium 90.

The implementation of monoclonal antibodies labeled with suitable radionuclides to treat cancer has received considerable attention. This approach involves selecting an antibody that is directed against a tumor-specific antigen and labeling the antibody with an energetic beta particle-emitting radionuclide. If the tumor selectively concentrates these labeled antibodies, then it can be lethally irradiated without seriously affecting the normal tissues and organs. Thus far, however, clinical trials using this approach have met with limited success because of insufficient tumor uptake and bone marrow toxicity. Nevertheless, labeled antibodies are becoming useful in diagnosing a variety of primary and metastatic tumors.

Perspective and Prospects

Although radioactivity was discovered in the late nineteenth century, application of radionuclides as biological tracers did not begin until 1924, when Georg von Hevesy used a bismuth radionuclide to study circulation in rabbits. In that same year, bismuth 214 was used in humans to measure the blood circulation time after injecting the radionuclide in one arm and then following the arrival of radioactivity in the other arm. The researchers found that it takes eighteen seconds in normal patients, and longer in patients with heart disease. The discovery of artificial radioactivity by Frédéric Joliot and Irène Joliot-Curie in 1934 led to the wider use of radionuclides as tracers. When Enrico Fermi artificially produced several radionuclides, Hevesy used phosphorus 32 to study phosphorus metabolism in rats. Such artificial production of radionuclides became possible after the pioneering work of Ernest Lawrence, who invented the cyclotron in 1929. Cyclotrons are still widely employed to produce a variety of radionuclides for medical use. The most commonly used one in nuclear medicine imaging is technetium 99m; this radionuclide is generated in the decay of another radionuclide called molybdenum 99, which was first produced by a cyclotron in 1938.

Radiopharmaceuticals and nuclear medicine took a major leap forward when technetium 99m, the radionuclide of choice for imaging, became readily available. Concurrent development of the scintillation camera by Hal Anger in 1958 advanced the field of nuclear medicine imaging. Radiolabeled compounds are also used extensively in biomedical research to trace biologically important molecules. The radioimmunoassay is another area in which labeled compounds are used to diagnose diseases; here, an antigen-antibody interaction is utilized. These procedures require only a trace amount of radioactivity, along with a blood sample of the patient.

Radiopharmaceutical imaging techniques have become important for the diagnosis and treatment of many diseases, and they will continue to play a major role in improving the quality of health care. Improvements in imaging instrumentation technology and the availability of computer technology to process the images are likely to further the accuracy of nuclear medicine images. Future developments in biotechnology should also assist in designing new pharmaceuticals that are more target-specific, thus further reducing the risks and enhancing both the diagnostic quality of the images and the therapeutic efficacy of radiolabeled compounds.

Another challenge for future research may include searching for new ways to create and manufacture radiopharma- ceuticals. In the early part of the twenty-first century, planned and unplanned closures of nuclear reactors created shortages of radiopharmaceutical materials in Europe; given this, one area of future research may be to find the means to develop these materials in other ways. In December, 2009, the Food and Drug Administration issued a ruling (effective December, 2011) on regulations about the manufacturing process of radiopharmaceuticals for PET scanning, designed to accommodate producers in commercial and nonprofit, academically oriented institutions.

—*Dandamudi V. Rao, Ph.D.*

See also Angiography; Catheterization; Imaging and radiology; Invasive tests; Magnetic resonance imaging (MRI); Nuclear medicine; Nuclear radiology; Positron emission tomography (PET) scanning; Radiation therapy; Single photon emission computed tomography (SPECT).

For Further Information:
Cherry, Simon R., James A. Sorenson, and Michael E. Phelps. *Physics in Nuclear Medicine.* 4th ed. Philadelphia: Elsevier/Saunders, 2012.
Harbert, John C., William C. Eckelman, and Ronald D. Neumann, eds. *Nuclear Medicine: Diagnosis and Therapy.* New York: Thieme Medical, 1996.
Levin, Ken. "Imaging and Radiology." *MedlinePlus*, March 22, 2012.
MedlinePlus. "Nuclear Scans." *MedlinePlus*, May 8, 2013.
Mettler, Fred A., Jr., and Milton J. Guiberteau. *Essentials of Nuclear Medicine Imaging.* 6th ed. Philadelphia: Elsevier/Saunders, 2012.
Radiological Society of North America. "General Nuclear Medicine." *Radiology Info*, May 9, 2013.
Sandler, Martin P., R. Edward Coleman, and James A. Patton, eds. *Diagnostic Nuclear Medicine.* 4th ed. Philadelphia: Lippincott Williams & Wilkins, 2003.
Society of Nuclear Medicine and Molecular Imaging. "What Is Nuclear Medicine?" *SNMMI Resource Center: About Nuclear Medicine & Molecular Imaging*, 2013.

Rape and sexual assault

Disease/Disorder

Anatomy or system affected: Anus, genitals, mouth, psychic-emotional system

Specialties and related fields: Gynecology, psychiatry, public health, emergency medicine

Definition: A crime of violence in which a person is forced to submit to sexual acts.

Key terms:

date rape: a forced sexual act during a date

deoxyribonucleic acid (DNA): genetic material contained in cells, which can definitively identify an individual

incest: a sexual act between close relatives such as father-daughter or brother-sister

perpetrator: an individual who commits a crime

sexual harassment: physical behavior of a sexual nature that is aimed at a particular person or group of people, especially in the workplace or school

statutory rape: a sexual act with a child below the legal age of consent, even if the act is consensual

---

Information on Rape and Sexual Assault

Causes: For perpetrators, impulsive and antisocial tendencies, alcohol, illegal drug use, history of sexual abuse as child

Symptoms: For victims, vaginal and rectal tears, bruises, injury to other body parts

Duration: For rapists, many are repeat offenders, who will attempt rape for decades

Treatments: For perpetrators, psychological counseling, drug and alcohol rehabilitation, medication; for victims, medical, surgical, and psychiatric treatment

---

Causes and Symptoms

Rape is an act of violence; it is an expression of aggression and anger rather than a sexual motivation. A power imbalance usually exists, with the stronger of two individuals committing the assault. The typical victim of rape is a sixteen- to twenty-four-year-old woman; however, any male, female, or child can be raped. Sexual assault has a broader definition than rape. In addition to vaginal, anal, or oral penetration, sexual assault includes inappropriate touching as well as any physical contact, speech, or presentation of images that an individual finds objectionable. Many types of rape and sexual assault exist, including spousal, incest, child, elder, date, acquaintance, coworker, stranger, and same-gender. Cases of women raping women or men exist.

In the United States, the estimated lifetime prevalence of sexual assault is approximately 18 percent in females and 3 percent in males. The typical rapist is a twenty-five- to forty-four-year-old man who plans the attack and usually selects a woman of the same race. About 50 percent of the time, the victim knows the rapist through work, friends, family, or by living in the perpetrator's neighborhood. More than 50 percent of rapes occur in the victim's home. The rapist may break in or gain entry through a ruse, such as posing as a salesman. Compared with other men, rapists drink more heavily, begin having sexual experiences earlier, and are more likely to have been physically or sexually abused as children. Individuals who have been sexually assaulted as children are also more likely to be assaulted as adults. Many studies note that more than 50 percent of all physical and sexual assaults involve a perpetrator who was reported to have been drinking. Often, rape victims have also consumed alcohol before the incident (estimates run as high as 60 to 70 percent). Illegal drug use is a factor in many rapes. The perpetrator may be under the influence of drugs or administer them to the victim. Date rape occurs when a sexual assault occurs during a date. The rapist often gives the victim drugs or alcohol; the most common date rape drug is alcohol. Regardless of the circumstances, victims of sexual abuse are not at fault. For example, if the victim exhibits provocative behavior, the perpetrator should control his (or her) impulses. Most rapes are not reported to the police (80 to 90 percent by most estimates).

Immediately after a rape, the victim may exhibit the following symptoms: inappropriate behavior, confusion, crying, fear, nervousness, hostility, inappropriate laughter, sleep disturbances, anorexia, physical pain, and/or social withdrawal. Physical symptoms of rape include vaginal and rectal lacerations as well as injuries to other body parts. The presence of semen in the vagina or rectum, which can be subjected to DNA analysis for identification of the perpetrator, confirms the diagnosis of intercourse but not rape. Rape victims may suffer from posttraumatic stress syndrome, which may persist for years and have a marked impact on the victim's life. Following a rape, some victims abuse alcohol and/or drugs; some become suicidal. More than 50 percent of rape victims develop difficulties with interpersonal relationships (such as with a husband or other partner).

Treatment and Therapy

Following a rape, the victim should proceed directly to a hospital without changing clothes, showering, douching, or urinating, as these activities may destroy evidence. Often, rape victims are referred to specialized centers that provide focused care and make certain that proper procedures are followed, including preserving the "chain of evidence." Chain of evidence refers to the proper handling of evidence (semen, hair samples, and skin samples) from the time of collection throughout the legal process. Specimens collected for forensic evaluation include mucosal swabs, skin swabs, fingernail clippings, hair samples, blood samples, saliva samples, the victim's clothes, and semen samples, if available. Sperm may be detected up to 72 hours after an assault in vaginal swabs, up to 24 hours in anal swabs, and are rarely detected in oral swabs. A complete evaluation of the victim may take up to six hours. In female victims, areas that should be carefully evaluated include the breasts, perineum, vagina, anus, and rectum. Nongenital trauma is commonly seen on the victim's extremities, face, and/or neck, which may consist of bruising, abrasions, lacerations, and/or erythema. These are more likely to be present when the victim is examined within 72 hours of the assault, or if the perpetrator is a stranger. Colposcopy may be used to detect milder genital trauma and an ultraviolet (UV) light (ex: Wood's lamp) may assist in detecting semen on the skin. In male victims, areas of concern include the penis, scrotum, prostate, anus, and rectum.

Immediate care includes medical and surgical treatment of injuries, which may be significant. The victim-and, if possible, the rapist-should be tested for sexually transmitted diseases (STDs). Minimal screening consists of testing for gonorrhea, chlamydia, trichomonas, bacterial vaginosis, and candidiasis. Necessity to screen for human immunodeficiency virus (HIV) hepatitis, and syphilis should be determined on an individual basis. Victims may opt out of testing for STDs if he/she consents to prophylactic treatment. Prophylactic treatment for STDs is recommended due to the poor follow-up visit rates. Postexposure Hepatitis B vaccination is considered adequate protection against Hepatitis B, unless the perpetrator is known to have Hepatitis B. Prophylactic antiviral medications are controversial after a sexual assault. The risk of HIV transmission after a single consensual episode of vaginal or anal intercourse is estimated to be 0.1-2 percent. Transmission after an assault is presumed to be higher, secondary to the trauma and bleeding. Risk and benefits should be discussed with the patient.

Pregnancy tests should be performed on any female of child-bearing age. If the possibility of exposure to pregnancy exists, then hormonal treatment can be administered to prevent that eventuality. Drug screening may also be performed to detect levels of alcohol, benzodiazepams (for example, the date rape drug, Rohypnol), gamma-hydroxy butyrate (GHB), or other common drugs of abuse.

In addition to treatment of the immediate physical and emotional trauma, follow-up care should be arranged. The victim may be in need of long-term counseling, psychiatric care, and psychiatric medication. Posttraumatic stress disorder (PTSD), depression, and anxiety are commonly seen in victims. Victims may avoid any future pelvic exams, which then puts them at higher risk for cervical cancer.

Child molesters, serial rapists, and violent rapists are often given long-term prison sentences. While in prison, they are offered treatment; however, treatment cannot be enforced. An evaluation of sex offenders incarcerated at Atascadero State Hospital in California reported that 80 percent of sex offenders never participated in any treatment. Occasionally, some child molesters and repeat offenders are given suspended sentences or paroled after a short prison sentence. Some of these offenders have committed further violent attacks, including murder of the rape victim. Sex offenders are required to register with local authorities so that their whereabouts can be made available to the public. Some states define a sexually violent predator as someone who commits a sexually violent crime and who has a mental abnormality or personality disorder. A number of researchers report a high level of success for rapists who undergo a treatment program. A standard premise for counseling and psychiatric care is that the rapist must admit that he or she has a problem for therapy to be successful.

Perspective and Prospects

From the days of ancient Greece through the American colonial period, rape was deemed to be a capital offense. Rapists were subjected to a wide range of punishments, including beatings, castration, and execution. However, in colonial America, the rape of Native American women was not deemed to be a crime because the women were "Pagan and not Christian." Two centuries ago, rape was often not viewed as a type of physical assault; rather, it was deemed to be a serious property crime against the man to whom the woman belonged (her father or husband). The loss of virginity was a particularly serious matter. Under biblical law, if the father agreed, the rapist was required to marry his victim instead of receiving the civil penalty.

Anecdotal reports of rape during warfare have been described since antiquity-Greek, Roman, Persian, and Israelite armies reportedly engaged in rape. During the 1937 Nanking Massacre, it was reported that Japanese soldiers raped as many as 80,000 Chinese women over a six-week period. Anecdotally, by the end of World War II, Red Army soldiers were estimated to have raped approximately 2,000,000 German women and girls. During the 1994 Rwandan genocide, an estimated 500,000 women were raped. One study found that during Liberia's thirteen-year-long civil war, 92 percent of the women interviewed had experienced sexual assault. Even today, rape is being used as a weapon of war in the Democratic Republic of Congo (DRC) to humiliate, dominate, and instill fear in the civilians of a community.

The medical literature contains numerous analyses of rape and sexual assault. In August 2009, researchers at St. Paul's Hospital in Vancouver, British Columbia, published a study that evaluated the sexual assault of prostitutes. They found an "alarming rate" of violence against these women. They recommended that the following steps were crucial to stem violence against prostitutes: socio-legal policy reforms, improved access to housing and drug treatment, and scaled-up violence prevention efforts, including police-prostitute partnerships.

Although young adult women are the most frequent targets of sexual assault, physical abuse of older women has risen rapidly during the last decade. In October 2009, researchers with the Michigan State University Program in Emergency Medicine published a study comparing a group of postmenopausal victims of sexual assault with younger adult women (eighteen to thirty-nine years old). During the five-year study period, 1,917 adult sexual assault victims qualified for inclusion in the study; 84 percent of the victims were eighteen to thirty-nine years old, and 4 percent were postmenopausal women who were at least fifty years old. The 72 postmenopausal victims were more likely to be assaulted by a single perpetrator, usually a stranger (56 percent versus 32 percent); to be assaulted in their own home (74 percent versus 46 percent); and to have experienced more physical coercion (72 percent versus 36 percent). The younger women were more likely to have used alcohol or illicit drugs before the assault (53 percent versus 18 percent) and to have a history of sexual assault (51 percent versus 15 percent). Postmenopausal victims had a higher number of nongenital (2.3 percent versus 1.2 percent) as well as anal injuries (2.5 percent versus 1.8 percent). The authors concluded that postmenopausal women are not immune from sexual assault and that the epidemiology of sexual trauma in this age group is different from that of younger women.

Sexual harassment and assault are not uncommon at the workplace. A study published in August 2009, by the University of Southern Maine evaluated the frequency and impact of workplace sexual harassment on the health, work, and school outcomes on high school girls. They noted that sexual harassment has a significant impact on high school girls' connections to work and school; it not only taints their attitudes toward work but also threatens to undermine their commitment to school. They added that as a consequence of sexual harassment experienced at work, teenagers may have their career development or career potential impeded or threatened because of school absence and poor academic performance. In addition, they noted, the physical safety of working students may be at risk under these circumstances, which would create a need for teenagers to receive training to deal with sexual assault and other types of workplace violence.

As it is in adults, alcohol is a frequent component of adolescent peer-on-peer sexual aggression. A study published in September 2009 by the Institute for Research on Women and Gender, University of Michigan, examined the characteristics of adolescents involved in alcohol-related and nonalcohol-related sexual assault of peers. The researchers conducted a Web-based survey of 1,220 students (grades seven through twelve) and found that adolescents who reported alcohol-related and nonalcohol-related sexual aggression had higher levels of impulsivity and more extensive histories of dating, early sexual activity, and alcohol consumption than adolescents who did not assault. Furthermore, perpetrators of alcohol-related assault had higher levels of alcohol use in the past thirty days as well as more alcohol- or drug-related problems than perpetrators of nonalcohol-related assault.

A particularly heinous form of sexual assault is one on a child. In October 2009, investigators at the Crimes Against Children Research Center, University of New Hampshire, Durham, published a study that strove to obtain national estimates of exposure to the full spectrum of childhood violence, abuse, and crime. The researchers conducted a cross-sectional national telephone survey that involved 4,549 children up to age seventeen. The authors found that a clear majority (60.6 percent) of the children had either experienced or witnessed victimization in the previous year. Almost half (46.3 percent) had experienced a physical assault in the study year, almost 25 percent had experienced a property offense, about 10 percent had experienced a form of child maltreatment, 6.1 percent had experienced a sexual victimization, and about 25 percent had been a witness to violence or experienced another form of indirect victimization in the year (including 9.8 percent who had witnessed an intrafamily assault). About 10 percent had experienced a victimization-related injury. More than one-third (38.7 percent) had been exposed to two or more direct victimizations (10.9 percent had five or more, and 2.4 percent had 10 or more) during the study year.

A 2010-2011 survey of adolescents, between the ages of fourteen and twenty-one, revealed that 1 out of 10 adolescents had been the perpetrator of a sexual assault. An asso-

ciation was found with perpetrators and a higher exposure to violent X-rated media. Up to the age of seventeen, the majority of the perpetrators were male. Among those older than seventeen, females and males had an equal representation as perpetrators.

—Robin L. Wulffson, M.D.;
updated by Elizabeth Lynn, M.D.

See also Addiction; Alcoholism; Club drugs; Depression; Domestic violence; Ethics; Intoxication; Psychiatric disorders; Psychiatry; Psychiatry, child and adolescent; Psychiatry, geriatric; Psychoanalysis; Stress

For Further Information:
American College of Obstetricians and Gynecologists. http://www.acog.org. The website of the nation's leading group of professionals providing health care for women.

Matsakis, Aphrodite. *The Rape Recovery Handbook: Step-by-Step Help for Survivors of Sexual Assault.* Oakland, CA: New Harbinger, 2003. A step-by-step program to help rape victims deal with the aftermath of an assault.

National Sex Offender Registry. http://www.family watchdog.us. A free service that allows users to locate registered sex offenders in their area by entering an address.

Reddington, Frances P., and Betsy Wright Kreisel, eds. *Sexual Assault: The Victims, the Perpetrators, and the Criminal Justice System.* Durham, NC: Carolina Academic Press, 2005. Provides a broad overview of sexual assault.

Seneski, Patty. *Color Atlas of Sexual Assault.* St. Louis: Mosby/Elsevier, 2007. A clinical resource for practitioners who treat sexually assaulted individuals.

Summerfeld, Leila Rae. *Beyond Our Control: Restructuring Your Life after Sexual Assault.* Grand Rapids, MI: Kregel, 2009. A personal chronicle of recovery from rape.

United Nations Human Rights: Rape: Weapon of War. http://www.ohchr.org/en/newsevents/pages/rapeweaponwar.aspx. The website of a United Nations organization that brings awareness to the violations of human rights.

Violence Against Women: State Resources. http://www.womens health.gov/violence/state. A listing of U.S. organizations by state, with program and contact information.

World Health Organization (WHO). http://www.who.int/en. The website of this international organization, which monitors human rights abuses including rape.

Reconstructive surgery. *See* Plastic surgery.

Rectal polyp removal. *See* Colorectal polyp removal.

Rectal surgery. *See* Colorectal surgery.

Raynaud's Phenomenon

Disease/Disorder

Anatomy or system affected: Blood vessels, breasts, ears, feet, hands, mouth

Specialties and related fields: Family practice, vascular medicine

Definition: The reduction of circulation in the extremities, inducing a cold- or stress-induced color change

Key terms:

prostaglandin: a group of fatty acids that act as short-range signaling molecules and mediate a wide range of body functions

sympathetic nervous system: a branch of the autonomic system that mediates the "fight or flight" response

vasospasm: sudden, spontaneous constriction of blood vessels

Causes and Symptoms

Raynaud's phenomenon (RP) results from a sudden decrease in blood flow to the extremities, which occur most commonly in the fingers, but also can affect the toes, ears, nose, lips, and nipples. Blood vessel constriction (vasospasm) causes the sudden decrease in circulation. However, what drives vasospasm remains controversial, and many mechanisms have been proposed, but none can account for all cases of RP.

There are two types of RP: primary and secondary RP. The far more common and generally less severe primary RP occurs without an associated disease or an apparent cause (idiopathic). Secondary RP results from some other underlying disease. Diseases of connective tissue, eating disorders, certain drugs or occupations, infectious diseases, environmental conditions, and other miscellaneous effects can cause RP.

Five percent of the population in the United States has RP. In people with RP, exposure to cold causes the skin of the fingers or toes to whiten and feel cold and numb. Over time, the skin turns a bluish tint (cyanosis). Upon warming, the skin turns red and then normal, accompanied by swelling, tingling, and a kind of "pins and needles" feeling.

After experiencing repeated episodes of oxygen depletion, the skin of the extremities can become thin and fragile. Ulcers can form and the nails of the hands and toes can deform. In very severe cases the fingers and toes and become gangrenous.

Treatment and Therapy

Although the above-mentioned symptoms can justify a diagnosis of RP, Doppler ultrasound tests can effectively assess the blood flow in the extremities, as can digital artery pressure tests.

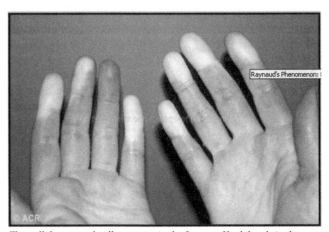

The well demarcated pallor present in the fingers of both hands is characteristic of Raynaud's phenomenon. (American College of Rheumatology)

Information on Raynaud's Phenomenon

Causes: Narrowing of small blood vessels that lead to the extremities

Symptoms: Cold extremities; color changes in skin of extremities in response to cold or stress; numb, prickly feeling or stinging pain upon warming or relief of stress

Duration: Usually presents early in life and tends to come and go, but lasts a lifetime

Treatments: Avoiding triggers, medications, in severe cases surgery

---

In most cases, avoiding the cold or stresses that cause the attacks can suffice. Avoiding caffeine or other compounds known to cause blood vessel constriction (e.g., pseudoephedrine) can also help. For more severe cases of RP, medication may be required. Medicines used to treat RP include calcium channel blockers, angiotensin-converting enzyme (ACE) inhibitors, alpha-1 receptor blockers, angiotensin receptor blockers, the antidepressant fluoxetine (Prozac), sildenafil (Viagra), nitrates, and a topical cream called RayVa, which contains prostaglandin E1, a known dilator of blood vessels.

Alternative treatments include Gingko biloba extracts, acupuncture, laser therapy, and temperature biofeedback. All of these treatments have been shown to relieve RP symptoms to some degree in various studies.

In extremely severe cases, surgically cutting the sympathetic nerves to the extremities (sympathectomy) provides relief for some patients. In other cases grafting a vein into the extremity (bypass vein grafts) can greatly increase blood flow the hands, augment healing, and relieve symptoms.

—*Michael A. Buratovich, Ph.D.*

See also Alternative medicine; Antihypertensives; Cutis marmorata telangiectatica congenita; Immunopathology; Neurology; Orthopedics; Rheumatology; Systemic sclerosis; Vascular medicine

For Further Information:

Laundry, Gregory J. "Current Medical and Surgical Management of Raynaud's Syndrome." *Journal of Vascular Surgery* 57, no. 6 (June, 2013): 1710-1716.

Porter, Steven B., and Peter Murray. "Raynaud Phenomenon." *Journal of Hand Surgery* 38A (February, 2013): 375-378.

Recreational therapy
Specialty

Introduction

Recreational therapy (also known as therapeutic recreation) is a form of physical therapy that uses various forms of leisure activities and life skills to promote physical and mental well-being for people with illness or disability. Recreational therapists seek to enhance patients' physical and mental capabilities through activities that patients find stimulating, such as creating art, playing games, or engaging in sports or other physical activities such as dance. The type of prescribed activities varies according to the individual patient's interests and needs.

Recreational therapy is used to assist people suffering

from a wide variety of physical, emotional, and mental impairments. For instance, recreational therapy can be used to help people recovering from conditions such as a heart attack or spinal cord injury, or to aid patients suffering from various forms of mental illness or developmental disabilities. It may also be useful in geriatric care to help stimulate the minds and bodies of elderly persons through activities that generate pleasure. Recreational therapy may be practiced in a wide variety of settings, including community, residential, medical, and clinical arenas.

Background

Recreational therapy can be used to treat many different categories of health conditions. It is often prescribed for people who have recently suffered severe injuries such as quadriplegia (paralysis of both arms and both legs) or paraplegia (paralysis of the legs or lower body), for people suffering through chronic illnesses, or for patients who have mental impairments. In such situations, recreational therapy can assist in learning life skills to enable independent living or to bring greater pleasure to life through the reduction of anger, anxiety, depression, and stress.

To assist patients properly, recreational therapists, often working closely with occupational therapists, must assess the patients' current needs and long-term goals while evaluating and understanding their existing mental or physical limitations. For example, quadriplegic patients will often require therapy that will help them to live a more independent and, therefore, fulfilling life. This typically includes educating them on how to use adaptive equipment and providing them with therapy that enriches their mental and emotional well-being. Beyond teaching basic life skills, recreational therapists also seek to provide activities that can promote physical rejuvenation. This may include simple games that improve patients' cognitive and social functions while assisting with their psychological recovery. In the case of a quadriplegic who has severely limited physical motion, recreational therapists will also incorporate activities that the patient enjoys, such as listening to music or reading books, to improve his or her quality of life. In this sense, recreational therapy encompasses not just rehabilitation but also promotes psychological exercises intended to allow patients to address their suffering, accept their limitations, and embrace a fulfilling lifestyle moving forward.

Recreational therapy can offer many benefits. People who remain physically and mentally fit after an injury or who learn to adapt to new disabilities, tend to remain healthier and happier for longer periods than those who do not. Older patients who engage in various forms of stimulation provided through recreational therapy remain more physically active and tend to live healthier, more satisfying lives. Older patients who engage in recreational therapy combined with physical and occupational therapies are also more likely to live independently without assistance and take fewer medications.

Overview

Recreational therapy seeks to promote the ability of patients to enjoy levels of physical and mental activity that enable them to lead productive lives that are fulfilling.. Recreational therapy embraces a holistic view of health management. This often means assessing the needs of patients using a multidisciplinary approach that includes reviewing cognitive, emotional, physical, social, spiritual, and vocational needs and requirements. Based on assessment, the recreational therapist creates a plan of action that incorporates both the care needs and leisure interests of the patient. This plan may require the involvement of family to succeed. After establishing a course of action, the therapist will institute a series of benchmark goals while working with the patient to make sure he or she remains motivated to make progress toward achieving these goals.

Recreational therapists work in a variety of fields. They may apply their skills to aid in recovery from addiction, assist ongoing rehabilitation, work with people with developmental disabilities, or help promote improved mental health. They may also work with a wide type of clientele ranging from pediatric to geriatric patients. Typically, these types of therapists are employed by heath care agencies to work as in-house specialists at hospitals, clinics, health centers, hospices, schools, and adult day care programs. Increasingly, they are also being hired in private practice settings to assist with in-home treatment.

Recreational therapists provide many different services. A patient does not necessarily need to be sick to use this form of therapy. For instance, recreational therapists have assisted veterans returning from wars. In this capacity, they help provide social readjustment through either individual or group therapy. Therapists may also offer assistance with weight management, diabetes, hypertension, and pain management. Recreational therapy has also proven useful in enhancing self-esteem, reducing social isolation, promoting the immune system, and improving mental acuity and alertness. As a result, it can dramatically improve the quality of life of patients.

This form of therapy may take a variety of approaches, including wheelchair sports, yoga, stress management, animal assisted therapy, aquatics therapy, social skills training, and pet therapy. Such programs may use unconventional means to help patients. For instance, the US Veterans Health Administration used a fly-tying class. In addition to providing skills that can be used later to go fly-fishing, it has proven useful in enabling injured veterans to promote increased fine motor skills, develop muscle control, and help motivate them to complete tasks. Upon completion of the class, the veterans are taken on a fishing excursion, which provides them with the chance to socialize with other veterans and relax by catching fish in a calming environment. Similarly, a recreation therapist may play games with children that can simultaneously help with grip strength, cognitive function, and self-confidence. Therapists are also able to help patients self-monitor their health by learning to identify symptoms or other problems that may require intervention.

According to the US Bureau of Labor Statistics, in 2015, recreational therapists earned $45,890 per year, or $22.06 per hour on average. In this same year, there were roughly 18,600 people employed as recreational therapists in the United States, with this profession estimated to demonstrate a 12 percent growth rate between 2014 and 2024. Recreational therapy typically requires a bachelor's degree and certification to be employed in the field.

—Eric Bullard;
updated by Patricia Stanfill Edens, PhD, RN, LFACHE

For Further Information:

Austin, David R. *Therapeutic Recreation: Processes and Techniques.* 6th ed., Sagamore Publishing, 2009.

Cherniak, E. Paul, and Ariella R. Cherniak. "The Benefit of Pets and Animal-Assisted Therapy to the Health of Older Individuals." *Current Gerontology and Geriatrics Research*, vol. 2014, *National Center for Biotechnology Information*, www.ncbi.nlm. nih.gov/pmc/articles/PMC4248608/. Accessed 11 Jan. 2017.

"Definitions of Recreational Therapy." *Therapeutic Recreation Directory*, www.recreationtherapy.com/define.htm. Accessed 11 Jan. 2017.

Luu, Anna. "What Is Recreation Therapy and the Top 10 Activities That You Can Do." *AgeComfort.org,* 31 May 2013, www.agecomfort.org/what-is-recreation-therapy-and-the-top-10-activities-that-you-can-do/. Accessed 11 Jan. 2017.

Murray, Susan "Boon," and Anita Burton. "More than Fun and Games: Recreational Therapists Are Value-Adding Team Members." *Team Rehab Report*, Sept. 1997, pp. 31-5, www.wheelchairnet.org/WCN_ProdServ/Docs/TeamRehab/RR_97/9709art2.PDF. Accessed 11 Jan. 2017.

"Occupational Outlook Handbook: Recreational Therapists." *Bureau of Labor Statistics, United States Department of Labor*, www.bls.gov/ooh/healthcare/recreational-therapists.htm. Accessed 11 Jan. 2017.

"Recreational Therapy: Restoring Function, Recreating Lives." *Veterans Health Administration*, www.va.gov/health/NewsFeatures/20110712a.asp. Accessed 11 Jan. 2017.

"The Recreational Therapy Professional." *Health Professions Network*, www.healthpronet.org/ahp_month/07_04.html. Accessed 11 Jan. 2017.

Skalko, Thomas K., et al. "Assessing Balance and Fall Efficacy in Community-Dwelling Older Adults: Evidence-Based Instruments for Use in Recreational Therapy Practice." *Therapeutic Recreation Journal*, vol. 47, no. 4, 2013, pp. 291-306.

Travers, Catherine, et al. "An Evaluation of Dog-assisted Therapy for Residents of Aged Care Facilities with Dementia." *Anthrozoös*, vol. 26, no. 2, 2013, pp. 213-25.

Rectum

Anatomy

Anatomy or system affected: Anus, gastrointestinal system, intestines

Specialties and related fields: Gastroenterology, internal medicine, oncology, proctology

Definition: The pouch at the end of the gastrointestinal tract that collects and stores food wastes just before defecation.

Structure and Functions

The rectum is the pouch at the end of the gastrointestinal tract, between the sigmoid colon and the anal canal. It is about 6 inches (15 centimeters) in length, dilated slightly at the end (the rectal ampulla), and lined by an orange-red tissue with mucous glands, much like the colon.

The rectum remains empty until just before defecation, when wastes pass into it from the colon. Three lateral folds in the rectum, called Houston's valves, hold the feces in place until a sufficient quantity is collected and the walls of the rectum are distended. Nerve receptors in the walls detect the stretching and prompt the urge to defecate. Waves of muscular contraction, known as peristaltic waves, move the feces into the anal canal and through the anus.

Defecation depends in part on a person's conscious relaxation of the anus in response to the defecation urge. If the urge is resisted, then the feces may return to the colon, where water may be absorbed from them. If defecation is postponed repeatedly, the feces may harden and cause constipation.

Disorders and Diseases

Like the anus, the rectum is subject to a variety of malformations caused by infection or injury. The rectum may develop an abscess-a cavity in its wall that is filled with pus-when bacteria infest a mucous gland. The abscess may open a channel, or fistula, to another part of the rectum, the anus, or an entirely different organ, such as the vagina; fistulas can also be the product of other diseases, such a diverticulitis or injury to the rectum. When the rectum is made to protrude through the anus and outside the body, usually from straining at stool, the condition is called rectal prolapse. Proctitis is inflammation of the rectal lining from a variety of infectious diseases, such as ulcerative colitis or a sexually transmitted disease.

About a quarter of colorectal cancers, the most common of the gastrointestinal tract, occur in the rectum, about equally in men and women. They are adenocarcinomas, growing in the lining of the rectum, and if untreated often spread to the liver or less commonly to the lungs and bones. Rectal cancer usually grows slowly and can be surgically removed.

—Roger Smith, Ph.D.

See also Anus; Colon; Colorectal cancer; Colorectal polyp removal; Colorectal surgery; Constipation; Diarrhea and dysentery; Digestion; Gastroenterology; Gastroenterology, pediatric; Gastrointestinal disorders; Gastrointestinal system; Hemorrhoid banding and removal; Hemorrhoids; Hernia; Intestines; Peristalsis; Proctology.

For Further Information:

Ahuja, Nita, and Brenda S. Nettles. *Johns Hopkins Medicine Patients' Guide to Colon and Rectal Cancer.* Burlington, Ma.: Jones and Bartlett Learning, 2014.

Beers, Mark H., ed. *The Merck Manual of Medical Information: Second Home Edition.* London: Pocket Books, 2004.

Keshav, Satish. *The Gastrointestinal System at a Glance.* 2d ed. Oxford: Wiley-Blackwell, 2013.

Levin, Bernard, et al., eds. *American Cancer Society's Complete Guide to Colorectal Cancer.* Atlanta: American Cancer Society, 2006.

Parker, Steve. *The Human Body Book.* 2d ed. New York: Dorling Kindersley, 2013.

Thibodeau, Gary A., and Kevin T. Patton. *Structure and Function of the Human Body.* 14th ed. St. Louis, Mo.: Mosby/Elsevier, 2012.

Reflexes, primitive

Development

Also known as: Newborn reflexes

Anatomy or system affected: All

Specialties and related fields: Family medicine, pediatrics, perinatology

Definition: Involuntary patterns of behavior that can be elicited in the newborn infant.

Key terms:

in utero: a Latin phrase meaning "in the uterus"; refers to the period of fetal development

subcortical centers of the brain: the parts of the brain that control and regulate basic physiological functions, including breathing, body temperature regulation, sleeping, and waking; these parts are contrasted with the cortex, where voluntary control of behavior originates

Physical and Psychological Factors

Primitive reflexes range from very simple reactions such as the blinking and startle reflexes to more complex patterns of behavior such as the stepping and crawling reflexes. Primitive reflexes appear to be important for orienting the infant to its environment and for protecting it against potential threats to its safety. The reflexes are automatically elicited when an appropriate stimulus is present, such as liquid in the mouth or pressure on the bottom of the feet, and they take the same form on every occasion.

Several primitive reflexes exist for the head and face. Blinking is elicited when an object approaches the eye. This reflex functions to protect the eye from harm. The head-turning reflex is seen when an infant is placed face down on a soft surface such as a mattress. The infant will turn its head to one side to allow breathing to continue. Similarly, the defensive reaction reflex is seen when a cloth is placed over an infant's face. The infant will turn its head and make swiping movements with its arms in an attempt to clear away the obstruction. Rooting and sucking are two important reflexes of the face that assist in feeding. The rooting reflex is elicited when an object gently touches an infant's cheek; the infant will turn its mouth in the direction of the touch. Sucking is elicited whenever a nipple-sized object is placed in an infant's mouth.

The reflexes of the arms include the Moro reflex and the tonic neck reflex. The Moro reflex is seen when an infant's head is dropped slightly. The infant's legs and its arms, with hands extended, will spread wide, then come together in an embracing movement as the hands clench. This sequence of behaviors appears to be a defense against falling, as the reflexive response could allow the infant to grasp on to something. The Moro reflex is seen in other primates as well. The tonic neck reflex is seen when an infant, lying on its back, has its head turned to one side. The infant's arm on the same side will extend, and the other arm will move up to the back of its head, to assume a "fencing position." This reflex is also called the fencer's reflex.

The primitive reflex of the hand is the palmar or grasping reflex. If an object touches an infant's palm, then the hand will clench into a fist. If the object is small enough for the

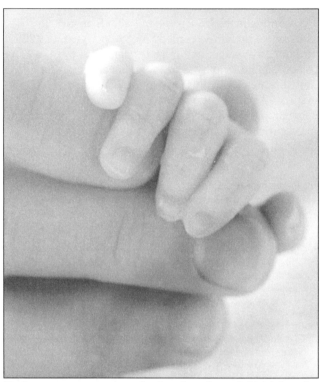

Newborns possess a grasping reflex that allows them to hold tightly to objects. (PhotoDisc)

infant to get a grip on it, then the infant's grip will be strong enough to support its own weight. A newborn infant grasping an adult's fingers with both hands can be pulled to a sitting or standing position.

The swimmer's reflex is seen when an infant is lying on its stomach. If the infant is gently tapped along its side above the waist, then it will turn its torso in the direction of the touch. Another primitive reflex of the torso is the crawling reflex. If an infant is lying on its stomach and pressure is applied against the soles of its feet, then it will move its arms and legs in a crawling movement. This reflex may be a precursor for later voluntary crawling behavior.

Two reflexes of the legs also appear to prefigure later-developing motor behavior. If an infant is held upright under the arms and its feet are allowed to touch a surface, then the infant will demonstrate the standing reflex by straightening its legs and supporting some of its body weight. If the infant is then tilted forward and moved forward slightly, then it will make high stepping movements characteristic of the stepping reflex.

The plantar reflex is similar to the palmar reflex. If an infant's foot is stimulated with an object touching the sole just below the toes, then the toes will curl around the object as if to grasp it. The Babinski reflex is another reflex of the foot; if the outside edge of an infant's foot is gently stroked, then the toes will fan out. The Babinski reflex, unlike many of the other primitive reflexes, does not have an obvious function; the lack of a Babinski response, however, may indicate neurological dysfunction.

Some of the primitive reflexes, such as sucking and grasping, have been detected in utero. Most of the reflexes disappear within a few months after birth, although some primitive reflexes, such as blinking, persist throughout life. Still other reflexes, such as the crawling and walking reflexes and the defensive reaction, are later replaced by behaviors that are voluntarily controlled.

Disorders and Effects

Because the absence of primitive reflexes can indicate neurological damage, most infants are tested for some of the reflexes soon after birth. Reflexes of the face, hands, and feet are components of neurological examinations such as the Brazelton Neonatal Behavioral Assessment Scale.

Despite the fact that the primitive reflexes are involuntary, infants show variability in their reflexive responses. There are individual differences among infants, such that some infants may show stronger or weaker primitive reflexes than others. Within individual infants, there is variation in the strength with which the reflexes may be elicited on different occasions. The age of the infant, its state of arousal, and the interval since its last feeding are all factors that can affect an infant's reflexive responses.

Perspective and Prospects

Traditionally, it was believed that primitive reflexes disappeared with brain development, as the higher centers of the brain took over some motor functions from the subcortical centers of the brain. Recent investigations of the stepping reflex, however, have shown that other factors can affect the development of the reflexes.

Esther Thelen and Linda B. Smith, in their book *A Dynamic Systems Approach to the Development of Cognition and Action* (5th ed., 2002), report that infants who no longer show the stepping reflex under typical circumstances do demonstrate stepping if their legs are submerged in water. Similarly, the stepping reflex can be suppressed in very young infants by adding weights to their legs. Another study, by Philip Zelazo, as described in an article found in *Developmental Psychobiology: The Significance of Infancy* (1976), provided infants with daily stepping practice and showed that under those conditions, the stepping reflex did not disappear. These findings suggest that experience, growth, and weight gain, as well as brain development, influence the developmental course of the primitive reflexes.

—*Virginia Slaughter, Ph.D.*

See also Breast-feeding; Cognitive development; Developmental stages; Motor neuron diseases; Motor skill development; Neonatology.

For Further Information:

Behrman, Richard E., Robert M. Kliegman, and Hal B. Jenson, eds. *Nelson Textbook of Pediatrics*. 18th ed. Philadelphia: Saunders/Elsevier, 2007.

Berk, Laura E. *Child Development*. 8th ed. Boston: Pearson/Allyn & Bacon, 2009.

Brazelton, T. Berry, and J. Kevin Nugent, eds. *Neonatal Behavioral Assessment Scale*. 3d ed. New York: Cambridge UP, 1995.

Field, Tiffany. *Infancy*. Cambridge, Mass.: Harvard UP, 1991.

Goddard, Sally. *Reflexes, Learning And Behavior: A Window Into The Child's Mind: A Non-Invasive Approach to Solving Learning & Behavior Problems*. Eugene, Oregon: Fern Ridge Press, 2009.

Huether, Sue E. *Understanding Pathophysiology*. New York: Mosby, 2011.

Jarvis, Carolyn. *Physical Examination & Health Assessment*. New York: Saunders, 2011.

Nathanson, Laura Walther. *The Portable Pediatrician: A Practicing Pediatrician's Guide to Your Child's Growth, Development, Health, and Behavior from Birth to Age Five*. 2d ed. New York: HarperCollins, 2002.

Stanley, Jenna. "Reflex Action." *Parents* 73, no. 5 (May, 1998): 24-25.

Thelen, Esther, and Linda B. Smith. *A Dynamic Systems Approach to the Development of Cognition and Action*. 5th ed. Cambridge, Mass.: MIT Press, 2002.

Refractive eye surgery

Procedure

Also known as: Vision correction, laser-assisted in situ keratomileusis (LASIK), laser epithelial keratomileusis (LASEK), photorefractive keratectomy (PRK)

Anatomy or system affected: Eyes

Specialties and related fields: Ophthalmology

Definition: A surgical procedure that changes the way in which the eye refracts light, thus correcting vision disorders.

Indications and Procedures

When light rays enter the eye, the cornea and lens bend (refract) the rays to focus them on the retina. When the eye is shaped in such a way that light rays are not sharply focused on the retina, an error in refraction occurs. Refractive eye errors that can be alleviated or cured with surgery are myopia, hyperopia, and astigmatism. Myopia (nearsightedness) is caused by a cornea that is too sharply curved, causing light rays to focus in front of the retina rather than on it, resulting in blurry distance vision. With hyperopia (farsightedness), the cornea is too flat, so light rays focus beyond the retina rather than on it, causing blurred vision when viewing near objects. Astigmatism is caused by a cornea that is uneven, curving and flattening in different spots on the eye, which makes it difficult to see objects at any distance. It is estimated that ninety million people suffer one or more of these vision defects.

Laser-assisted in situ keratomileusis (LASIK) is the most common refractive surgery in use. By 2006, more than forty million of these surgeries had been performed in the United States. LASIK can be used if the patient is nearsighted, farsighted, and with or without astigmatism. The surgeon conducts an intensive eye examination prior to the surgery to determine whether the cornea needs to be flattened or curved, and in what specific area. Then anesthetic drops are used to numb the eye.

The surgeon uses a blade or a special cutting laser to cut a hinged flap about the size of a contact lens from the front of the eye. The flap is folded back to allow access to the tissue in the cornea that needs reshaping. After the tissue is properly shaped with another kind of laser called an excimer laser, the flap is folded back in place. Usually, no stitches are required. The procedure is painless and takes fifteen to twenty minutes, depending on the condition of the eye before surgery and whether both eyes are reshaped. Patients

2084 • Reiter's syndrome

can usually leave the doctor's office within two hours. Postsurgery care involves the use of medicated eyedrops and wearing an eye shield at night. Healing is usually complete in five to seven days. The vision shows some immediate improvement, and, in about two to three months, most patients will have between 20/20 and 20/40 vision.

Laser epithelial keratomileusis (LASEK) is similar to LASIK up to the point of surgery. During a LASEK procedure, however, a thinner layer of the cornea is folded back. This is of particular benefit to people who have thinner-than-normal corneas. Also, people who work in jobs where there is a high risk of injury prefer LASEK. A thinner flap means less damage to the patient's vision should the flap be torn before it is healed. Healing is rapid, and full vision is recovered.

Photorefractive keratectomy (PRK) is used with patients who have a low-to-moderate degree of nearsightedness or farsightedness, or farsightedness with astigmatism. Unlike the LASEK procedure, to which it is very similar, with PRK the thin layer of the cornea is removed altogether. The surgeon then uses a laser to either flatten or curve the cornea, depending on the patient's need. A contact lens is placed on the raw cornea, to be worn as a bandage for three or four days. It takes the eye three to six months before vision improves completely. With PRK, the recommendation is to do only one eye at a time. It is the least used of the three procedures. Healing after the LASEK or LASIK methods is faster and involves less discomfort and scarring.

Uses and Complications

Some risks are associated with refractive surgery. Undercorrection occurs when too little tissue is removed from the eye, more often in treatments for nearsightedness. Another surgery to remove more tissue may be required. Overcorrection, when too much tissue is removed from the cornea, can occur when the eye moves during surgery. It is difficult to fix, and additional surgery may be needed to remedy the condition. Astigmatism can also be caused by uneven tissue removal.

Double vision, glare, and halos around bright lights are also risks of refractive surgery. These conditions can be greatly helped with eyedrops that contain cortisone, but sometimes a second surgery is needed. Cases of dry eyes, sometimes severe, also occur. Special plugs for tear ducts are used to prevent tears from draining away from the surface of the eyes, keeping them moist. Flaps folded back during surgery can sometimes become infected and tear and swell. The flap removed during PRK may also grow back abnormally.

Perspective and Prospects

In 2002, the LASIK procedure was improved by a technique known as wavefront-guided LASIK. Wavefront sensors measure the acuity and quality of a patient's vision twenty-five times more accurately than previous testing methods. They record how the eye processes light and show unique distortions in each individual eye. This enables the surgeon to make a more precise cut.

Alternative refractive surgery procedures developed in recent years include conductive keratoplasty, which uses radio frequency (RF) energy instead of a laser to reshape the cornea, and phakic intraocular lenses (IOLs), which are essentially surgically implanted contact lenses that can correct severe myopia. These and other procedures widen the range of options for people seeking surgical vision correction.

The total cost of LASIK refractive eye surgery varies widely, but is generally between $1,000 and $2,500 per eye. Use of the wavefront technology adds another $500. Many insurance companies consider refractive eye surgery elective and will not pay for it. The Food and Drug Administration (FDA) urges people who are considering refractive eye surgery to check a doctor's credentials before the operation.

—*Billie M. Taylor, M.S.E., M.L.S.*

See also Blurred vision; Eye infections and disorders; Eye surgery; Eyes; Laser use in surgery; Myopia; Ophthalmology; Optometry; Sense organs; Surgery, general; Vision; Vision disorders.

For Further Information:

Braham, Lewis. "Eye Surgery: It's Getting Sharper." *Business Week*, October 18, 2004, pp. 142-143.
Fiscbetti, Mark. "Clear Favorite." *Scientific American* 290 (May, 2004): 106-107.
"LASIK Eye Surgery." *Mayo Clinic*, November 4, 2011.
"LASIK-Laser Eye Surgery." *American Academy of Ophthalmology*, 2013.
Rapuano, Christopher J., ed. *Refractive Surgery*. San Francisco: American Academy of Ophthalmology, 2012.
Sunshine, Wendy Lyons, and Adam Martin. "Lasik Woes: Here's Help." *Health* 18, no. 1 (January/February, 2004): 50-54.

Reiter's syndrome
Disease/Disorder

Anatomy or system affected: Eyes, gastrointestinal system, joints, mouth, skin, urinary system
Specialties and related fields: Dermatology, family medicine, gynecology, ophthalmology, orthopedics, urology
Definition: An autoimmune disorder with associated symptoms of arthritis, urethritis, conjunctivitis, and ulcerations of the skin and mouth.

Causes and Symptoms

Although the exact cause of Reiter's syndrome is unknown, the disease is associated with the entry of an infectious agent through the urinary or intestinal tract. Reiter's syndrome associated with sexual contact occurs primarily in men and is most often linked to the bacteria *Chlamydia trachomatis*. Dysenteric Reiter's syndrome is caused by other bacteria, particularly *Salmonella* or *Shigella*. Genetic factors may also play a vital role in causing the disease, as a large majority of patients with Reiter's syndrome have the gene *HLA-B27*, while other people do not.

After the onset of Reiter's syndrome, urethritis occurs within seven to fourteen days, typically followed by conjunctivitis and arthritis over the next several weeks. The urethritis is often accompanied by a burning sensation during urination and a mild discharge from the urethra or the genitals. Conjunctivitis occurs in approximately 40 percent

Information on Reiter's Syndrome

Causes: Bacterial infection, usually transmitted through sexual contact; may be related to genetic factors

Symptoms: Urethritis (burning sensation during urination, mild urethral or genital discharge); conjunctivitis (mild to painful); arthritis of spine and lower extremities (swelling, redness, pain); low-grade fever; watery skin growths; lesions on palms, soles, trunk, and mouth; sometimes inflammation of iris

Duration: Three to six months

Treatments: Anti-inflammatory drugs (aspirin, ibuprofen, indomethacin, phenylbutazone), cortisone injections, tetracycline, topical medications for skin lesions, physical therapy, bed rest, occupational therapy

of the victims and ranges from mild to very painful. The arthritis usually involves the spine and large joints of the lower extremities, producing significant swelling, redness, and pain. The disease is often accompanied by low-grade fever, watery growths on the skin, and lesions on the palms of the hands, soles of the feet, trunk, and mouth. In some cases, an inflammation of the iris known as iritis may occur.

Treatment and Therapy

Treatment for Reiter's syndrome includes taking anti-inflammatory drugs, such as aspirin, ibuprofen, indomethacin, or phenylbutazone, as well as cortisone injections. Tetracycline may help control associated urethritis, while cortisone drops can relieve conjunctivitis. Topical medications are used to treat skin lesions. Appointments with different specialists, including dermatologists, urologists, and ophthalmologists, may be necessary in order to treat specific symptoms of the disease. In about half of the victims, Reiter's syndrome resolves itself within three to six months.

In addition to medical therapy, physical therapy is often prescribed. Short periods of bed rest can reduce pain and inflammation. Exercises can increase joint mobility and improve muscle tone. Occupational therapy teaches victims how to place less stress on affected joints and how to better cope with painful symptoms by promoting positive attitudes. In rare cases that involve severe joint damage, orthopedic surgeons may need to reconstruct the joints.

Perspective and Prospects

Reiter's syndrome was first diagnosed in a World War I soldier in 1916 by Hans Reiter, a German military physician. He described the disorder as inflammation of the joints, urinary tract, and eyes. It primarily affects males between the ages of twenty and forty. Approximately half of those who suffer one or two bouts with Reiter's syndrome never have another attack. Subsequent attacks beyond that can lead to joint deformity and permanent arthritis.

—*Alvin K. Benson, Ph.D.*

See also Arthritis; Autoimmune disorders; Bacterial infections;

Chlamydia; Conjunctivitis; Joints; Lesions; Men's health; Salmonella infection; Shigellosis; Urethritis.

For Further Information:
Mayo Clinc. "Reactive Arthritis." *Mayo Clinic*, March 5, 2011.
Parker, James N. and Phillip M. Parker *Reiter's Syndrome: A Medical Dictionary, Bibliography, and Annotated Research Guide to Internet References*. San Diego, Calif.: ICON Group, 2004.
Rosenfeld, Isadore. *Symptoms*. New York: Bantam Books, 1994.
Standring, Susan, et al., eds. *Gray's Anatomy*. 40th ed. New York: Churchill Livingstone/Elsevier, 2008.
Teitel, Ariel D. "Reactive Arthritis." *MedlinePlus*, June 15, 2012.
Teitel, Ariel D. "Reiter Syndrome-View of the Feet." *MedlinePlus*, June 15, 2012.
Toivanen, Auli, and Paavo Toivanen, eds. *Reactive Arthritis*. Boca Raton, Fla.: CRC Press, 1988.

Relaxation

Biopsychosocial
Anatomy or system affected: Body, mind, spirit
Specialties and related fields: Psychology, CAM, integrative medicine
Definition: A general term referring to a release of tension and restoration of equilibrium

Relaxation is recreation engaged in by people usually after working or participating in any other physically or mentally strenuous activity. Relaxation may take the form of simple downtime, in which one sleeps longer, reads a book, exercises, or travels. The term *relaxation* can also refer to a mental state of calmness and serenity, in which one is free from anxiety and stress. Stress is mental or emotional tension caused by difficult, unfavorable, or dangerous circumstances. A relaxed person generally experiences a slowed heartbeat and breathing rate, lowered blood pressure, reduced stress, and increased confidence for managing obstacles.

Many health providers emphasize the importance of regular relaxation, particularly for people whose jobs or personal lives cause them a great deal of stress. Stress has long been known to have negative effects on the heart, brain, and other areas of the body. Relaxation techniques such as meditation, breathing exercises, and physical activity can reduce stress and create a sense of general well-being in people. In these ways, relaxation plays an important role in human mental health.

Background

People may find that they need to relax after becoming stressed by various activities or life situations. Stressors can be different for everyone. Many people report becoming stressed by certain aspects of their jobs, particularly being dissatisfied with their position within their work setting, having too much work to do, working under unfair or dangerous conditions, or being harassed or discriminated against by customers, coworkers or superiors.

Conditions in one's personal life can also cause stress. Marriage, divorce, the loss of a job, financial obligations, the death of a friend or relative, or moving to a new location can all cause people to feel stressed. In other cases, people can cause their own stress with the attitudes they take to adverse life situations. Consistently worrying about stories in the news, such as terrorism and natural disasters, can. Be the source of stress as well as focusing on the negative aspects of a situation rather than the positive ones.

Long-term stress can have detrimental effects on a person's health. Stress activates the nervous system's fight-or-flight response, which releases the hormone adrenaline into the body. Adrenaline raises heart rate and breathing rate, and causes sweating and muscle tension. This is a normal biological reaction to stress, and the human body can quickly calm itself after isolated stressful incidents. Stress over an extended period, however, can lead to significant health problems such as high blood pressure; irregular heartbeat, or arrhythmia; heart attacks; ulcers; headaches; and depression.

Health providers claim it is important for people to manage their stress in healthy ways to reduce their chances of developing more serious health complications. Leading a healthy lifestyle and maintaining a positive outlook on life can help reduce stress, and making time to relax both physically and mentally has also been shown to benefit one's overall health. For this reason, health providers recommend that people practice a number of relaxation techniques, or relax simply by slowing down the pace of their everyday lives, to recover from stressors.

Methods for Relaxation

Meditation is a relaxation technique in which people generally sit on the floor or in a comfortable place, close their eyes, breathe regularly. Linking the repetition of the mantra to one's breaths can aid in this concentration. The goal of meditating is to focus the mind on peaceful thoughts and forget about one's stress, thereby bringing about mental relaxation.

There are many different methods for practicing meditation, with roots linked in both Eastern and Western philosophy. It is important to find a type of meditation that most effectively allows relaxation to occur. Three generally accepted types of meditation are mantra meditation, mindfulness meditation, and spiritual meditation. Most modern meditation employs and combines techniques found in these types of meditation.

Mantra meditation involves the repetition of a mantra, either vocally or internally, as the focus of concentration. A mantra is a word or phrase that is used as the focal point of concentration. Spiritual meditation focuses on religious principles and the practice of this type of meditation varies depending on one's beliefs. The goal of spiritual meditation is to connect with a higher power or spiritual concept. Mindfulness meditation consists of focusing on being in the present moment involving a non-reactive internal awareness.

Related to meditation is another relaxation technique involving measured breathing. To relax by breathing, people should sit with their backs straight and inhale deeply through the nose, hold the breath, and then exhale through the mouth. Repeated cycles of deep inhalation and exhalation can reduce stress by slowing one's heart rate and de-

creasing blood pressure.

Other relaxation methods require a person to conjure up mental images that play a role in stress reduction. In autogenic relaxation, people may imagine peaceful places while concentrating on relaxing each part of their body individually. Visualization is similar to autogenic relaxation but focuses more intensely on the mental image of a happy setting. People practicing visualization try to use most of their senses to feel as though they actually are at that setting. They imagine seeing the scenery, hearing its natural sounds, and feeling the wind or the sun on their bodies. Visualization may be accompanied by measured breathing.

Physical activity is another effective method for relaxation. Physiological changes that occur in the body during and after physical activity allow for mental relaxation to occur. Health providers praise regular exercise for its ability to produce endorphins and thereby reduce a person's stress and anxiety. Exercise has even been found to be an effective treatment for moderate depression. In addition to helping a person mentally relax, exercise can also lower body fat, strengthen muscles, and make the heart healthier.

Aerobic exercise, strength training, and yoga are all effective physical activities that help alleviate stress and allow for relaxation. Aerobic exercises can be practiced at any level of intensity in order to achieve a relaxed state. Some types of aerobic exercise include walking, jogging, biking and swimming. The term "runner's high" describes a state of mind achieved through the release of endorphins that cause the brain to experience a state of euphoria. Despite the name, this feeling can be achieved doing any aerobic exercise. Strength training involves the use or combination of free weights, body weight, and resistance bands to strengthen muscles. Similar to aerobic exercise, strength training releases endorphins. Strength training can be an effective method of increasing mobility and loosening tight muscles, which are both major stressors for people living sedentary lifestyles. Yoga is the practice of combining body positioning, mental concentration, and controlled breathing. There are numerous ways to practice yoga, different types may focus more on the physical components or the mental components. The goal is to achieve a state of mental and physical well-being.

Other methods of relaxation involve less devoted attention and consist simply of leisure activities. Some people relax by reading , which lets them temporarily forget their stressors. Others may relax by hiking in nature, driving in scenic locations, spending time with friends and family, taking vacations, cleaning, sleeping, playing musical instruments, or cooking. Certain foods contain substances that interact with the brain to produce feelings of well-being. Green tea, for instance, contains the chemical L-theanine, which can help relieve anxiety. The anti-inflammatory properties of honey can reduce anxiety and depression. The linalool contained in mangos, meanwhile, can decrease stress.

—Michael Ruth;
updated by Michael Moglia

For Further Information:

Casano, Tom. "20 Fun Ways to Relax on the Weekend." *Huffington Post*, 8 Sept. 2016, www.huffingtonpost.com/tom-casano/20-fun-ways-to-relax-on-t_b_8091420.html. Accessed 27 Dec. 2016.

"Causes of Stress." *WebMD*, www.webmd.com/balance/guide/causes-of-stress. Accessed 27 Dec. 2016.

"Exercise and Depression." *WebMD*, www.webmd.com/depression/guide/exercise-depression#1. Accessed 27 Dec. 2016.

Klein, Sarah. "10 Health Benefits of Relaxation." *Huffington Post*, 16 Apr. 2012, www.huffingtonpost.com/2014/08/14/stress-awareness-day-relaxation-benefits_n_1424820.html. Accessed 27 Dec. 2016.

Lebowitz, Shana. "40 Ways to Relax in 5 Minutes or Less." *Greatist*, 8 Mar. 2014, greatist.com/happiness/40-ways-relax-5-minutes-or-less. Accessed 27 Dec. 2016.

Moninger, Jeannette. "10 Relaxation Techniques That Zap Stress Fast." *WebMD*, www.webmd.com/balance/guide/blissing-out-10-relaxation-techniques-reduce-stress-spot. Accessed 27 Dec. 2016.

"Relaxation Techniques: Try These Steps to Reduce Stress." *Mayo Clinic*, www.mayoclinic.org/healthy-lifestyle/stress-management/in-depth/relaxation-technique/art-20045368?pg=1. Accessed 27 Dec. 2016.

Shakeshaft, Jordan. "6 Breathing Exercises to Relax in 10 Minutes or Less." *Time*, 8 Oct. 2012, healthland.time.com/2012/10/08/6-breathing-exercises-to-relax-in-10-minutes-or-less/. Accessed 27 Dec. 2016.

"Stress Basics." *Mayo Clinic*, www.mayoclinic.org/healthy-lifestyle/stress-management/basics/stress-basics/hlv-20049495. Accessed 27 Dec. 2016.

"Exercising to Relax." Harvard Health, Harvard Health Publications, Feb. 2011, www.health.harvard.edu/staying-healthy/exercising-to-relax. Accessed 09 Sept. 2017.

Burke, Adam, et al. "Prevalence and Patterns of Use of Mantra, Mindfulness and Spiritual Meditation among Adults in the United States." BMC Complementary and Alternative Medicine, vol. 17, no. 1, 2017, doi:10.1186/s12906-017-1827-8.

Reminiscence therapy

Procedure

Anatomy or system affected: Memory, psychological well being

Specialties and related fields: Gerontology, psychology

Definition: The use of life histories—written, oral, or both—to improve psychological well-being

Overview

At its most basic, *reminiscence therapy* involves listening to a patient and encouraging the individual to share his or her memories. The listener may ask directed questions to encourage further sharing. Reminiscence therapy is most beneficial in treating individuals with memory disorders such as dementia, as well as anxiety and depression, and may be useful as an alternative to drug therapies for challenging patients.

Persons benefit from knowing their experience is valued by others. Many times, older individuals feel marginalized. They may have mobility issues that prevent them from seeking out company, or they may be intimidated by technology—cell phones and computers, for example—and therefore feel isolated. Individuals with cognitive challenges such as dementia may find the modern world confusing and lonely. They often lose *short-term memory*—memory of what has happened very recently—and may feel disoriented and frightened. Such feelings of isolation often lead to depression. Caregivers may be older individuals' only source of companionship. By encouraging persons to share stories and actively listening to these tales, caregivers often can help these individuals to feel connected to the modern world.

Persons with dementia generally retain their earliest memories for the longest time. Reminiscence therapy has been found to be most beneficial to individuals with mild to moderate dementia. According to the Institute for Research and Innovation in Social Services (IRISS) in Scotland, several 2009 studies found that patients who participated in reminiscence therapy had better relationships with caregivers and families, had improved cognitive abilities and mood, functioned better, and had reduced symptoms of depression. A 2010 study in Taiwan found that aged persons without dementia also benefited from reminiscence therapy, according to IRISS. They were less depressed, more sociable, and generally in better mental health than individuals in the control group. The studies found no negative effects from reminiscence therapy.

Reminiscence therapy provides both *therapeutic*, or healing, benefits and pleasure. Recalling happier times reinforces the individual's connection to the world and may increase feelings of self-worth. Memories of difficult experiences such as loss or tragedy may help individuals process feelings and gain a better understanding of both events and themselves. Reminiscence therapy can improve cognitive ability among patients by providing stimulation.

Working with Patients

Reminiscence therapy may be conducted one-on-one or in group settings with a therapist who facilitates discussion and encourages all participants to share stories. Reminiscence activities have an overall positive effect when conducted with groups of aged populations. Therapists may use items, such as photos, or play music to spark memories. At times, therapists may use one-on-one sessions to collect information and create a book of an individual's life history (*life story work*), which may further help a patient who struggles to maintain his or her identity as cognitive function fails. Such information also aids caregivers. For example, reminiscence therapy and life story work may reveal and document favorite or hated foods and activities such as hobbies and lifestyles—information that enables care homes and caregivers to provide appropriate opportunities. A patient who once enjoyed outdoor activities may benefit from regular walks outside, for instance. A person who once practiced needlepoint may be encouraged to try painting. Family members may even develop life stories for individuals as they prepare to move to care facilities to aid the transition and help the patient hold on to his or her identity. Both music therapy and reminiscence therapy are currently being used to increase aspects of wellbeing in older people, including those with memory diseases such as dementia, as alternatives to pharmacological treatments. There is growing evidence that combining these therapies in a focused way would provide unique wellbeing outcomes for this population.

Though sad memories of difficult times may bring tears, they can be therapeutic. Listeners must respect the memories and experiences of the patient and allow them to feel their emotions. Silence, too, is important—while at times a listener may need to ask questions or share appropriate stories, at other times it is best to sit in silence together.

Reminiscence may be encouraged at all times of the day, and nurses and other caregivers may be best positioned to facilitate such talk. Patients in care facilities might be open to talking about the past during meals, while receiving physical therapy, or while walking with assistance. Reminiscence also may be used as an aid to encouraging relationships with caregivers and developing friendships with other patients. This therapy may help patients transition from their home environment to an institutional setting or when moving between institutions. Caregivers such as nurses are encouraged to see patients as individuals (to see beyond the diagnosis) and be sensitive to their culture and background to deliver *person-centered care*, which focuses on treating patients with dignity and respect and ensuring they have personal choice and a sense of community and security. Reminiscence therapy has been shown to benefit both patients and caregivers.

For late-stage dementia patients, who often are unable to communicate well or to even speak, stimulation such as music is likely to trigger memories. By providing music associated with happy times or events, caregivers can improve patients' moods. This outcome may provide a long-lasting effect, because moods often last longer than memories.

Caregivers can provide reminiscence therapy by encouraging communication using many methods, including the following:

- *Ask open-ended questions.* How did you learn to paint? What were you doing when (the first astronauts went to space, World War II ended, etc.)?
- *Take cues from the patient's possessions.* Ask questions about photographs and souvenirs: Who are the people in the photo? Is this memento from a trip? What was it like?
- *Stimulate the senses.* Music, dancing, food, and smells, for example, may trigger memories.
- *Turn to literature.* Read an excerpt from a book set in an earlier time or an account of some event or activity from decades ago, and ask the individual to comment.

—*Josephine Campbell;*
updated by Geraldine Marrocco

For Further Information:

Fletcher, T. S. (2017). Factors that bring meaning to mementos created by elders. *Agingand Mental Health, 21*(6), 609-615. doi:10.1080/13607863.2016.1141284

Huntsman, Mark. "How Reminiscence Therapy Improves the Lives of Alzheimer's Patients." *Alzheimers.net.* A Place for Mom, Inc. 22 Apr. 2014. Web. 3 Feb. 2015. http://www.alzheimers.net/2014-04-22/ reminiscence-therapy-improves-alzheimers/

Istvandity, L. (2017). Combining music and reminiscence therapy interventions for wellbeing in elderly populations: A systematic review. *Complementary Therapies in Clinical Practice, 28*, 18-25. doi:10.1016/j.ctcp.2017.03.003

Klever, Sandy. "Reminiscence Therapy: Finding Meaning in Memories." *Nursing* 43.4 (Apr. 2013): 36-37. Lippincott Williams & Wilkins. Web. 3 Feb. 2015. http://journals.lww.com/nursing/Fulltext/2013/ 04000/Reminiscence_therapy_Finding_ meaning_in_memories.11.aspx

"Supporting Those with Dementia: Reminiscence Therapy and Life Story Work." *IRISS.* The Institute for Research and Innovation in Social Services. May 2011. Web. 3 Feb. 2015. http://www.iriss.org.uk/resources/supporting-those-dementia-reminiscence-therapy-and-life-story-work

Watson, Karen Everett. "Reminiscence Therapy Benefits Residents." *Provider.* Provider. Jun. 2011. Web. 3 Feb. 2015. http://www.providermagazine.com/archives/archives-2011/Pages/0611/Reminiscence%20Therapy%20Benefits%20LTC%20Residents.aspx

"What Is Reminiscence Therapy?" *Dorset HealthCare.* Dorset HealthCare NHS Foundation Trust. Apr. 2009. Web. 3 Feb. 2015. http://www.dorsethealthcare.nhs.uk/WS-Dorset-HealthCare/Downloads/Managing%20Your%20Health/Therapy%20Information%20Leaflets/L141-09ReminiscenceTherapy.pdf

Derived from: "Reminiscence therapy." *Salem Press Encyclopedia of Health.* Salem Press.

Renal failure

Disease/Disorder

Anatomy or system affected: Heart, immune system, kidneys

Specialties and related fields: Immunology, internal medicine, nephrology, pathology

Definition: A breakdown of kidney function that prevents the removal of waste materials from the body.

Causes and Symptoms

Renal failure, also called kidney failure, renal insufficiency, or end-stage renal disease (ESRD), can be defined as a decline in kidney function sufficient to result in the retention of metabolic waste material in the body. The loss of the ability of the kidneys to excrete waste material is often progressive, culminating in complete renal failure in untreated cases. Although kidney disease can occur at any age, most cases occur in adults, frequently as a complication of diabetes and/or hypertension.

There are three major causes of renal failure. The first, prerenal, results from obstruction of the renal artery because of vascular causes such as hypertension. The decreased blood flow to the kidney causes tissue destruction and loss of renal function. Prerenal causes may also be linked to liver disease and congestive heart failure. The second major cause of renal failure is a direct breakdown of kidney function as a result of inflammatory processes associated with infection. Certain drugs may also have toxic effects on kidney function. The third major cause of renal failure is postrenal, which refers to obstructions that block the flow of urine from the kidney.

The body cannot survive without at least one functioning kidney. As a consequence of renal failure, toxic metabolic wastes accumulate in the bloodstream, such as urea nitrogen produced in the metabolism of proteins. Renal failure

Information on Renal Failure

Causes: Obstruction of renal artery (from hypertension, liver disease, congestive heart failure), infection, certain drugs, obstruction of urine flow from kidney

Symptoms: Accumulation of toxic metabolic wastes in bloodstream, electrolyte imbalance, cardiovascular problems, pulmonary edema, gastrointestinal symptoms, chronic fatigue, infections

Duration: Acute or chronic and progressive

Treatments: Hemodialysis, kidney transplantation

also results in disturbances of electrolyte balance, associated with high levels of sodium, potassium, and other salts. Other complications include compromised cardiovascular function, pulmonary edema, gastrointestinal symptoms, chronic fatigue, and infections.

Treatment and Therapy

Acute renal failure can be treated effectively with hemodialysis and/or kidney transplantation. The hemodialysis machine has made it possible to extend the lives of many patients. This external device filters the blood as it traverses fluid-bathed semipermeable membrane filters that remove metabolic wastes while permitting the retention of essential blood components. Blood leaves the body and returns postfiltration through a fistula or access joint inserted under the skin to link arterial and venous blood flow. Dialysis must be carried out on a regular basis and requires several hours.

The best treatment for renal failure is a kidney transplant. Sadly, there are not enough donor kidneys to meet the need; patients who do receive organ donations may wait for years before transplantation occurs. As of 2013, United Network for Organ Sharing data show that about one million people in the United States have ESRD and more than 95,000 are on the waiting list to receive a kidney donation. Research continues on an artificial kidney that would replicate the delicate filtering functions of the kidney's glomeruli. A study published in the journal *Nature Medicine* in April 2013 reported that scientists have been able to bioengineer working kidneys in rats. While the kidneys lacked the full function of normal kidneys and much more work needs to be done, the milestone represents a promising step towards the goal of creating fully functional artificial kidneys from the cells of patients in need of a transplant.

—*Sarah Crawford, Ph.D.*

See also Dialysis; End-stage renal disease; Hemolytic uremic syndrome; Kidney cancer; Kidney disorders; Kidney transplantation; Kidneys; Nephritis; Nephrology; Nephrology, pediatric; Polycystic kidney disease; Transplantation.

For Further Information:

Aronoff, George. *Kidney Failure: The Facts*. New York: Oxford University Press, 1996.

Brenner, Barry M. et al., eds. *Brenner and Rector's The Kidney*. 9th ed. Philadelphia: Saunders/Elsevier, 2012.

HealthDay. "'Bioengineered' Kidneys Show Promise in Rat Study." *MedlinePlus*, April 15, 2013.

MedlinePlus. "Kidney Failure." *MedlinePlus*, May 20, 2013.

Mitch, William E., and Saulo Klahr, eds. *Handbook of Nutrition and the Kidney*. 6th ed. Philadelphia: Lippincott Williams & Wilkins, 2010.

Molitoris, Bruce A., and William Finn, eds. *Acute Renal Failure*. Philadelphia: W. B. Saunders, 2001.

Savitsky, Diane. "Kidney Failure." *Health Library*, October 31, 2012.

Reproductive system

Anatomy

Anatomy or system affected: Abdomen, genitals, uterus

Specialties and related fields: Embryology, genetics, gynecology, obstetrics, proctology, urology

Definition: The organs of the female (the vagina, uterus, Fallopian tubes, ovaries, and mammary glands) and the male (the penis, testes, vas deferens, and prostate gland) that are necessary for the production of offspring.

Key terms:

bladder: the pouch in the abdominal cavity that collects urine until it can be eliminated from the body; while not a part of the reproductive system, it is located adjacent to the reproductive organs and is an important landmark

fertilization: the process in which the sperm head penetrates the ovum, resulting in the formation of an embryo

gametes: the reproductive cells in either sex (the sperm and the ova)

hormone: a chemical signal that is carried in the blood from its site of production to the area where it has an effect

menstrual cycle: the cycle of ovum development, hormone production, and menstruation in female primates; in humans, the average duration is about twenty-nine days

ovulation: the release of an ovum from its follicle in the ovary

ovum: the female gamete; a large spherical cell that carries the female's chromosomes

sperm: the male gamete; the mature sperm has an oval head that contains the male's chromosomes and a long tail that allows it to swim in fluid

Structure and Functions

The reproductive system in each sex includes the organs that produce the gametes, called the gonads, and those that transport the gametes. In addition, the female mammary glands are also considered reproductive organs since they produce milk to nourish the newborn, a critical step in survival of the species.

The male gonads are the testes, which are located within the scrotum, a pouch of skin and muscle that is suspended from the body wall. In the adult, each egg-shaped testis measures about 2.5 centimeters by 4.0 centimeters. Internally, the testes contain seminiferous tubules, hollow tubes in which the sperm develop. Besides the sperm cells, the seminiferous tubules also contain Sertoli cells, large cells in which the developing sperm are embedded. The Sertoli cells produce hormones, pass nutrients to the sperm, protect them from blood-borne toxins, and control their development. In spaces between adjacent seminiferous tubules are the interstitial cells of Leydig, which produce testosterone and other hormones.

The Male Reproductive System

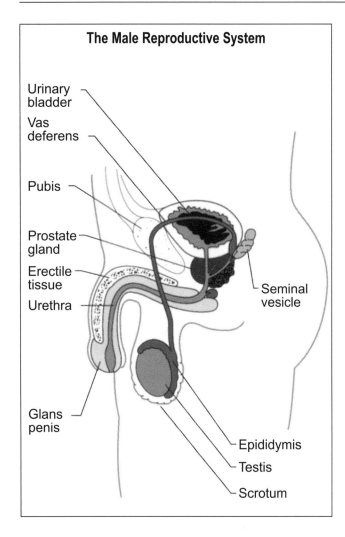

Urinary bladder

Vas deferens

Pubis

Prostate gland

Erectile tissue

Urethra

Seminal vesicle

Glans penis

Epididymis

Testis

Scrotum

Lying near each testis within the scrotum is the epididymis. Sperm undergo several stages of development within the testis, then move into the epididymis, where they proceed through further steps in maturation, including the development of the swimming ability that is necessary for fertilization of an ovum.

The narrow end of the epididymis is continuous with the long (45-centimeter) tubule called the vas deferens. The vas deferens leads upward from the epididymis and passes through a narrow ring of tissue, the inguinal canal, to enter the abdominal cavity. Within the abdominal cavity, the vas deferens loops over the top of the bladder, then turns downward to enter the prostate gland below the bladder. Near the end of the vas deferens, an enlarged area called the ampulla serves as a storage site for mature sperm.

Within the prostate gland, the vas deferens becomes a short segment of tubule known as the ejaculatory duct. The two ejaculatory ducts (one on each side) empty into the urethra, the tube that extends downward from the bladder. In the male, the urethra carries either semen or urine, but not both at the same time: A valve-like structure below the bladder prohibits urine outflow when semen is moving through the system. The urethra passes through the penis to open to the outside at the tip of the penis.

Besides the urethra, the penis contains three columns of

erectile tissue, spongy material with a large blood supply. During sexual excitement, the blood flow into the erectile tissue increases while the outflow decreases; the accumulation of blood within the erectile tissue causes the penis to increase in both length and diameter, a process known as erection. Erection allows the penis to become stiff enough to be inserted into the female's vagina during intercourse. On the outside of the penis, the enlarged area at the tip, the glans penis, is well supplied with touch receptors that play a role in sexual excitement.

During intercourse, stimulation of the touch receptors on the penis results in ejaculation, the expulsion of semen from the male's body. During ejaculation, sperm move out of the vasa deferentia, through the ejaculatory ducts, and then through the urethra. This sperm movement is caused not by the swimming of the sperm but by the contractions of involuntary muscles in the walls of the tubules. As sperm pass through the tubules, they are mixed with fluid secreted by three glands: the prostate, located immediately below the bladder; the seminal vesicles, which open into the vas deferens above the prostate; and the bulbourethral or Cowper's gland, which lies below the prostate and opens into the urethra. The fluid secreted by these glands contains chemicals and nutrients that will ensure the survival of the sperm within the female tract.

The female's vagina serves as the repository for sperm released during ejaculation and as the outlet for the fetus during childbirth. The outer opening of the vagina is located behind the urethra, which carries only urine and does not have a reproductive role in the female. Bartholin's and Skene's glands are located near the urethral and vaginal openings; these glands supply moisture and mucus to the female external genitals. The vaginal and urethral openings are located between folds of tissue, the labia majora and the labia minora. At the front junction of these folds is the clitoris, a small round structure containing many touch receptors; stimulation of the clitoris during intercourse is important in promoting sexual gratification in the female. The area that includes the labia, the vaginal and urethral openings, and the clitoris is known as the vulva.

Internally, the vagina consists of a recess with elastic walls and a large blood supply, but little sense of feeling since there are only sparse touch receptors. The vagina slants upward and slightly backward from its outer opening. Near its upper end is the cervix, the lowest portion of the uterus. The cervix consists of strong connective tissue and contains glands that secrete mucus. The cervix has a narrow passageway, the cervical canal, that opens into the main part of the uterus.

The uterus is about 7.5 centimeters long and 5.0 centimeters wide in the nonpregnant woman. The wall of the uterus is composed primarily of involuntary muscle controlled by nerves and hormones. The inner part of the uterus is hollow and is lined with a spongy layer of cells, the endometrium; the endometrium has a large blood supply and contains glands that secrete nutrients for the embryo during pregnancy. The endometrium undergoes growth during the menstrual cycle and is shed as the menstrual discharge if the woman does not become pregnant.

At either side of the upper end of the uterus are the oviducts, or Fallopian tubes, which are hollow tubes that open into the cavity of the uterus. The oviducts lead upward and sideways away from the uterus toward the ovaries, with their funnel-shaped ends adjacent, but not attached, to the ovaries.

The ovaries are the female gonads; they produce ova, the female gametes. Each 3-centimeter-long ovary contains thousands of follicles, spherical structures that each contain one ovum. Hormonal signals cause growth of some of the follicles during the menstrual cycle, and, as they grow, the ova within them mature. The follicles are also sites of production of the hormones estrogen and progesterone. In the middle of the menstrual cycle, one follicle will ovulate, releasing its ovum, which will enter the oviduct to be transported toward the uterus.

During intercourse, after sperm are deposited in the vagina, the sperm will swim in the fluids of the female tract, passing upward through the cervical canal, the uterus, and the oviducts. If an ovum is present in one of the oviducts, it may be fertilized by a sperm. The fertilized ovum will then move downward to the uterus, where it will attach to the endometrium and develop into an embryo. At birth, uterine muscle contractions will cause stretching of the cervical canal and movement of the fetus through the cervix and vagina.

Milk production (lactation) in the woman's breasts after childbirth will allow for the nourishment of the newborn. Milk is produced in glands within the breast; ducts carry the milk to openings in the nipple. In between the milk-producing glands are wedges of fat; it is the fat tissue that determines the size of the breast in the nonpregnant woman. Breast size is not related to milk-producing ability.

Disorders and Diseases

Abnormalities may exist in either the male or the female reproductive tract as a result of deviations during embryonic development, injury, or disease. Anatomical abnormalities in the reproductive system often can be corrected surgically.

In hypospadias, a problem during embryonic development of the male reproductive organs causes the urethral opening to be on the underside of the penis rather than at its tip. Hypospadias can occur independently or can be a sign of more serious problems. Urethral stricture or stenosis refers to a narrowing of the urethra; this can occur anywhere along its length, from the tip of the penis back to the prostate gland. Urethral stenosis causes difficulty in urination; it may be present from birth or result from later damage or infection. Cryptorchidism is the presence of one or both testes in the abdominal cavity instead of in the scrotum. In the male embryo, the testes begin development in the body cavity near the kidneys and then migrate into the scrotum during the last month or two before birth. In some male infants born with undescended testes, the testes will spontaneously move into the scrotum shortly after birth. If not, then the cryptorchidism must be corrected surgically, usu-

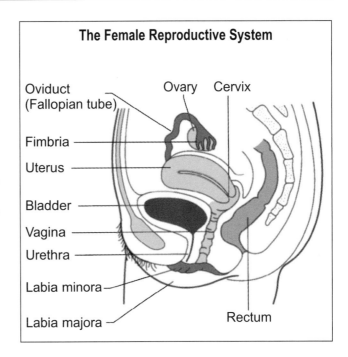

The Female Reproductive System

Oviduct (Fallopian tube)
Ovary
Cervix
Fimbria
Uterus
Bladder
Vagina
Urethra
Labia minora
Labia majora
Rectum

ally within the first year of life, in order to prevent later infertility and other complications.

In females, problems during embryonic development can also lead to malformed reproductive organs. The vagina may be present but may not have an outer opening, or conversely, the outer opening may lead to an abnormally shallow vagina. The uterus may be divided into two separate halves (bicornuate uterus), and the vagina may also show such a division. It is also possible for a normal uterus to have an abnormal placement in the abdomen: It may be tilted backward or bent forward at an atypical angle. Surprisingly, variations in the anatomy of the uterus often have little effect on fertility.

Malfunctions in embryonic development of the reproductive organs can lead to hermaphroditism, a rare condition in which an individual has a mixture of male and female reproductive organs. A hermaphrodite may be either a genetic male or a genetic female. Hormone treatment and surgery can usually assure a fulfilling sex life in adulthood for such individuals.

In inguinal hernia, the wall of the inguinal canal between the scrotum and abdominal cavity becomes weakened and stretched. A loop of the intestine may then become lodged in the canal, or the testis and epididymis may move upward to block the canal. The symptoms of inguinal hernia include pain during movement, especially during the lifting of heavy objects, and the presence of a soft lump in the herniated area.

A varicocele is a group of enlarged blood vessels within the scrotum. Varicoceles are thought to arise because of impaired blood flow from the testis. Normally, the blood flowing through the scrotum maintains the temperature of the testes a few degrees below that of the rest of the body. When the blood flow out of the scrotum is reduced in the presence of a varicocele, the temperature in the testes tends to increase. This increased temperature can cause infertility, since sperm production requires a local temperature that is lower than the normal body temperature. Increased scrotal temperature can be the cause of infertility in other situations as well: the wearing of tight clothing, prolonged soaking in hot water, or during episodes of fever. Infertility in these situations is usually temporary and self-correcting.

In women, stretching of the pelvic area during childbirth sometimes leads to uterine prolapse, a condition in which the uterus sags into the vagina. Other causes of prolapse are developmental abnormalities, lifting heavy objects, and loss of muscle and tissue strength with aging. A prolapsed uterus is associated with pain during intercourse and may cause difficulty in urination. Temporary relief from a uterine prolapse can be achieved with the use of a pessary, a device worn in the vagina to support the uterus. Surgery to restore the supporting tissues in the pelvis may be necessary for long-term relief, but in some cases the uterus cannot be returned to its proper position and so must be removed, a process called hysterectomy.

In endometriosis, patches of endometrial tissue from the uterine lining attach to and grow on other organs in the pelvic cavity, affecting the shape and function of these organs. It is thought that the endometrium escapes into the pelvis through the oviducts during menstruation. The abnormally placed endometrial tissue can cause pain and infertility. Endometriosis can be treated with hormone therapy or with surgery to remove the endometrial patches. In more severe cases and when the woman does not wish to bear children in the future, the removal of the uterus may be required to control the invasion of other organs by the endometrial patches. The ovaries may also be removed in order to eliminate the source of hormones that produce the growth of the endometrium.

In polycystic ovary syndrome, one or both ovaries contain cysts that are formed from follicles that have failed to ovulate. Women with polycystic ovaries either do not menstruate or have irregular patterns of bleeding. Because ovulation does not occur, they are infertile. Another symptom of polycystic ovary syndrome is growth of hair in a male pattern on the face, neck, and chest; the hair growth is caused by certain hormones that are produced in abnormal amounts by the ovaries. Therapy usually involves hormone treatment in an attempt to establish ovulation and to prevent the deleterious effects of abnormal hormone levels on the body.

Both benign (nonspreading) and cancerous tumors may appear in the reproductive organs. Potential sites of tumor growth are the testes and prostate gland in the male and the ovaries, uterus, and breasts in the female. Only rarely do tumors cause pain, but they may be detected during routine self-examination of the testes or breasts or during a doctor's examination. Treatment usually begins with surgery to remove the tumor, and x-ray therapy or chemotherapy prevents further tumor growth. Hormone treatment can also be useful in controlling the growth of some reproductive tumors. The exact factors that cause tumors to form are not well understood, but a family history of such problems, abnormal hormone levels, and exposure to radiation,

pollutants, and toxins have all been implicated.

Prostate tumors should not be confused with nodular prostatic hyperplasia, an increase in the size of the prostate gland that occurs in about 75 percent of men over sixty years old. The enlargement appears to be caused by dihydrotestosterone (DHT), a hormone related to testosterone; the prostate gland itself is one site of conversion of testosterone into DHT. Prostate enlargement is associated with difficulty during urination and ejaculation. It has traditionally been managed with surgery to remove the gland or to reduce its size. More recently, several drugs have been approved to reduce the production of DHT and either prevent the progression of growth of the prostate or shrink the prostate in some individuals..

Perspective and Prospects

Rituals involving alteration of the reproductive organs have been performed since ancient times. Castration (removal of the testes) has been carried out for various reasons. In early times, men who were guards of noble women were castrated to control their sexual activity. During the Renaissance, castration of boys was performed to produce singers who would retain their clear, high-pitched voices, since it is testosterone that causes the deepening of the voice at puberty. More recently, castration has been espoused as a "treatment" for habitual rapists: Some judges sentence convicted sex offenders to castration, despite the fact that many authorities believe that rape is a manifestation of violent tendencies, rather than the result of excessive sexual desire.

In the United States and elsewhere, it is common for boys to undergo circumcision, or the removal of the foreskin, a flap of tissue that covers the glans of the penis. Parents have their sons circumcised in order to conform to religious and cultural practices. In the United States, the procedure is usually performed shortly after the boy's birth, but in other cultures circumcision may occur during puberty rituals. One rationalization for performing circumcision is that removal of the foreskin helps to prevent the buildup of smegma, a thick secretion produced by glands located under the base of the foreskin. In fact, some studies have shown that circumcised boys are less likely to have urinary tract infections. There are no apparent effects of circumcision on sexual functioning. Researchers debate the advisability of circumcision, however, and the medical establishment has not established a definitive recommendation.

It is less well known that circumcision of women is practiced in some cultures. Indigenous groups who perform female circumcisionare found in the Pacific Islands, Asia, the Middle East, and Africa, and the practice has been carried to the United States by immigrants. The term *female circumcision* refers to three procedures that may be carried out singly or together. In simple circumcision, the flap of tissue covering the clitoris is removed. The entire visible part of the clitoris is removed in clitoridectomy. Infibulation is the sewing together of the labia to cover the vaginal opening, leaving only a small hole for the discharge of urine and menstrual fluid. A woman who has been infibulated cannot have intercourse or give birth; the tissue must be cut open to allow either of these events, after which the area may be sewn closed again.

Female circumcision may take place shortly after a girl's birth or at puberty, and it is performed for a variety of reasons. Infibulation is a means of enforcing female abstinence from sexual activity. A wish to control women's sexual desire is also given as a reason for performing simple circumcision and clitoridectomy. Also involved are the society's views of what the ideal female organs should look like. From a medical standpoint, female circumcision is of concern because of pain and discomfort caused by the development of scar tissue in the vulval area. It is not known how many women die from infection or bleeding following these procedures, which are usually performed by other women under less-than-sanitary conditions.

—*Marcia Watson-Whitmyre, Ph.D.*

See also Abortion; Amenorrhea; Amniocentesis; Aphrodisiacs; Assisted reproductive technologies; Breast-feeding; Breasts, female; Candidiasis; Catheterization; Cervical, ovarian, and uterine cancers; Cervical procedures; Cesarean section; Childbirth; Childbirth complications; Chlamydia; Circumcision, female, and genital mutilation; Circumcision, male; Conception; Contraception; Culdocentesis; Cyst removal; Cysts; Dysmenorrhea; Ectopic pregnancy; Electrocauterization; Endocrine disorders; Endocrinology; Endometrial biopsy; Endometriosis; Episiotomy; Erectile dysfunction; Fistula repair; Gamete intrafallopian transfer (GIFT); Gender reassignment surgery; Genital disorders, female; Genital disorders, male; Glands; Gonorrhea; Gynecology; Herpes; Hormone therapy; Hormones; Hydroceles; Hypospadias repair and urethroplasty; Hysterectomy; In vitro fertilization; Infertility, female; Infertility, male; Laparoscopy; Masturbation; Menopause; Menorrhagia; Men's health; Menstruation; Miscarriage; Multiple births; Myomectomy; Obstetrics; Orchitis; Ovarian cysts; Ovaries; Pap test; Pelvic inflammatory disease (PID); Penile implant surgery; Pregnancy and gestation; Premature birth; Premenstrual syndrome (PMS); Prostate cancer; Prostate enlargement; Prostate gland; Prostate gland removal; Puberty and adolescence; Semen; Sexual differentiation; Sexual dysfunction; Sexuality; Sexually transmitted diseases (STDs); Sterilization; Stillbirth; Syphilis; Systems and organs; Testicles, undescended; Testicular cancer; Testicular surgery; Testicular torsion; Trichomoniasis; Tubal ligation; Ultrasonography; Uterus; Vasectomy; Warts; Women's health.

For Further Information:

Ammer, Christine. *The New A to Z of Women's Health: A Concise Encyclopedia*. 6th ed. New York: Checkmark Books, 2009.

Berek, Jonathan S., ed. *Berek and Novak's Gynecology*. 15th ed. Philadelphia: Lippincott Williams & Wilkins, 2012.

Jones, Richard E., and Kristin H. Lopez. *Human Reproductive Biology*. 4th ed. London: Academic Press, 2013.

Manassiev, Nikolai, and Malcolm I. Whitehead, eds. *Female Reproductive Health*. New York: Parthenon, 2004.

Marieb, Elaine N. *Essentials of Human Anatomy and Physiology*. 10th ed. San Francisco: Pearson/Benjamin Cummings, 2012.

Quilligan, Edward J., and Frederick P. Zuspan, eds. *Current Therapy in Obstetrics and Gynecology*. 5th ed. Philadelphia: W. B. Saunders, 2000.

Strauss, Jerome F., III, and Robert L. Barbieri, eds. *Yen and Jaffe's Reproductive Endocrinology: Physiology, Pathophysiology, and Clinical Management*. 6th ed. Philadelphia: Saunders/Elsevier, 2009.

Taguchi, Yosh, and Merrily Weisbord, eds. *Private Parts: An Owner's Guide to the Male Anatomy*. 3d ed. Toronto, Ont.: McClelland & Stewart, 2003.

Wade, L. "Learning from Female Genital Mutilation: Lessons from Thirty Years of Academic Discourse." *Ethnicities* 12, no. 1 (February, 2012): 26-49.

Research vs. animal rights. *See* Animal rights vs. research.

Respiration
Biology

Anatomy or system affected: Chest, lungs, muscles, musculoskeletal system, nose, respiratory system, throat

Specialties and related fields: Biochemistry, exercise physiology, otorhinolaryngology, pulmonary medicine, vascular medicine

Definition: A basic physiological process in which an organism takes in oxygen (which is utilized as a source of energy) and produces carbon dioxide (which is excreted as a waste product).

Key terms:

capillaries: the smallest and most numerous blood vessels in the cardiovascular system; these vessels connect the arteries to the veins and are where all exchange of oxygen and nutrients occurs

diffusion: the process in which substances move from an area of high concentration to an area of low concentration; given enough time, the concentration of the substance will be the same everywhere

hemoglobin: a special molecule, found only in red blood cells, that binds oxygen very efficiently in the lung and releases it to the tissues

partial pressure of a gas in a gas: the measure of the contribution of one gas of a mixture of gases to the total pressure pushing on the walls containing it; it is the pressure that would be exerted if all the other gases were removed from the container, leaving only the gas of interest

partial pressure of a gas in a liquid: the measure of how much of a gas dissolves into a liquid when the liquid is in contact with a gas mixture; if the gas and liquid are in contact long enough, the liquid is said to have the same partial pressure as the gas mixture; the absolute measure of the amount of gas in a liquid is the partial pressure multiplied by the ability of the gas to dissolve in liquid (solubility)

plasma: the fluid of blood in which the blood cells (white and red) are suspended

pressure: the measure of how much a gas or a liquid pushes on the walls of its container

The Mechanics of Respiration

The primary function of respiration is performed by the lungs and their associated tissues. Air must be breathed in through the mouth and nose through the larynx (voice box) into the main airway, the trachea (windpipe). Inside the chest, the trachea branches into the two main airways called bronchi, which in turn successively branch many times into small bronchi called bronchioles. These airways end in very small sacs called alveoli. These alveoli have a very thin membrane separating the air space from the blood in the capillaries. Oxygen (O_2) diffuses through the alveolar membrane across the capillary membrane and into the blood to be taken to all the tissues of the body. Tissues excrete carbon dioxide (CO_2) into the blood that is carried back to the lungs. Carbon dioxide diffuses from the blood into the alveoli and is carried back through the airways and out of the lungs with the exhaled air. The mouth and nose humidify dry air to ensure that the linings of the lower airways do not dry out. The main airway divides to supply the left and right lungs. These large airways are cylindrical. Their circular shape is maintained by C-shaped cartilage in the walls. The stiff walls prevent collapse of the airways and the loss of gases through the walls of these "conducting" airways. The airways branch repeatedly into smaller airways. As the airways become smaller, they have less cartilage, until, in the very smallest airways, the cartilage is absent. These thin airways, which are called respiratory bronchioles, have alveoli budding from their walls. Gases may diffuse through the walls of these airways. These bronchioles become alveolar ducts and then erupt into lobular sacs of alveoli. There are about 300 million alveoli in an individual's lungs, which provide about 70 square meters of extremely thin membrane through which most gas exchange occurs.

The lungs are elastic in nature and have a tendency to collapse. They do not because they adhere to the inside surface of the chest wall in much the same way that a moist suction cup adheres to a smooth surface. The two surfaces may slide against each other without separating. The chest wall has a tendency to expand because the rib cage and the muscles between the ribs (the intercostal muscles) tend to pull the chest out and up. The balance of these forces (elastic recoil and chest wall expansion) keeps the lungs slightly expanded at all times. Like balloons, the alveolar sacs have a tendency to collapse. The lungs produce a substance called surfactant that keeps the small air sacs from collapsing.

Air gets into and out of the lungs in the following way. The lungs expand, drawing air into them. The lungs adhere to the diaphragm in the same way that they adhere to the chest wall. When the muscles of the diaphragm contract, the lungs are pulled down. At the same time, the intercostal muscles contract slightly, making the chest wall rise up and out. These actions cause the lungs to expand. This expansion causes the pressure inside the lungs to decrease, sucking in air. When the intercostal muscles and diaphragm relax, the elasticity of the lungs causes them to deflate again to their resting state. This passive recoil of the lungs causes the pressure inside them to increase and pushes air out of the lungs.

The amount of air breathed in each breath is called the tidal volume. Each breath contains about 500 milliliters of air. Normally, a human being breathes in and out about twelve times in one minute. This results in about 6,000 milliliters of air being breathed each minute. Not all air that enters the mouth or nose reaches the area of the lung where gases are exchanged. About 150 milliliters of each breath stay in the larger airways. Therefore, 4,200 milliliters of air reach the alveolar space each minute. Since the chest wall

and the chemical surfactant tend to keep the lungs partially inflated even after the breath is normally exhaled, additional air can be blown from the lungs, if one exhales consciously and forcefully. The volume of air blown out in this manner, which is called the expiratory reserve volume, is normally about 1,000 milliliters. Additional air can also be drawn into the lungs after a normal inspiration. This volume, the inspiratory reserve volume, is normally about 3,000 milliliters. The sum of the tidal, inspiratory reserve, and expiratory reserve volumes, which is called the vital capacity of the lungs, is about 4,500 milliliters. If these reserves are called into play, tidal volume can be increased almost tenfold. The breathing rate can also be increased at least twofold. Therefore, total alveolar ventilation can be as great as 120,000 milliliters per minute.

The oxygen that is drawn into the lungs diffuses into the blood, and carbon dioxide diffuses out of the blood into the alveolar spaces to be exhaled. Fresh air exerts a pressure (barometric pressure) of 760 millimeters of mercury (mmHg). Oxygen is 21 percent of air; therefore, it has a partial pressure of about 160 mmHg. It mixes with air in the lungs that has lost oxygen to the blood. This results in a reduction in the partial pressure to about 100 mmHg by the time the breathed air reaches the alveoli. Blood pumped by the right ventricle of the heart into the lungs to be oxygenated has only 40 mmHg of oxygen. Oxygen diffuses from an area of high concentration in the alveoli to the blood, which has a low concentration. This diffusion process is rapid enough that the partial pressure in the blood becomes equal to that of the alveoli before it courses one-half the distance through the lung capillary. Although the partial pressure is 100 mmHg, the amount of oxygen carried in blood fluids (plasma) is low. Therefore, without red blood cells containing hemoglobin, blood cannot carry much oxygen to the tissues.

Hemoglobin is a very efficient carrier of oxygen. Each molecule of hemoglobin can carry four molecules of oxygen. In the same way that a disposable diaper absorbs water, hemoglobin absorbs oxygen from the plasma, allowing more oxygen to diffuse into the blood from the alveoli. As hemoglobin absorbs oxygen, it turns from a bluish purple to red. Between partial pressures of 20 and 100 mmHg, hemoglobin can absorb a large amount of oxygen. Hemoglobin does have a maximum capacity for oxygen that is reached at about 100 mmHg. Hemoglobin is called saturated at this point, and it can hold no more even if the partial pressure of oxygen increases. Hemoglobin is filled to half capacity by the time the plasma partial pressure reaches 30 mmHg. When the partial pressure increases from 20 to 100 mmHg, the increase in the amount carried by the plasma is 2.1 milliliters of oxygen per liter of blood. With the same change in partial pressure, hemoglobin increases the amount of oxygen carried by approximately 150 milliliters per liter of blood. Blood can carry more than seventy times the amount that plasma alone can carry at this range of partial pressure. If the partial pressure does increase beyond 100 mmHg, little more oxygen is added to the blood. Oxygen is added to plasma in the dissolved form at a rate of 0.03

milliliters of oxygen per liter of plasma for each 1 mmHg change in the partial pressure.

Oxygen is carried to the tissues by the blood, where it is efficiently removed from hemoglobin. The partial pressure in the tissues is between 20 and 60 mmHg, depending upon the particular tissue and the rate at which the tissue uses oxygen. Inside the tissues, the partial pressure can be as low as 1 mmHg, providing a large difference to stimulate diffusion into the tissues. Oxygen is quickly absorbed by the tissue. Just as rapidly, carbon dioxide diffuses out of the cells and into the blood. There are also special ways in which the blood carries carbon dioxide to increase its capacity.

Carbon dioxide dissolves in plasma in much the same way that oxygen does, but supplemental mechanisms are required to carry the large amounts of carbon dioxide produced by the body. Carbon dioxide is also absorbed by red blood cells. It diffuses into the red blood cells, where it is changed in chemical form. Stimulated by an enzyme, carbonic anhydrase, carbon dioxide is combined with water and converted to a new chemical (the bicarbonate ion). The bicarbonate ion can attach to hemoglobin in this form. This, in effect, keeps the concentration of carbon dioxide in the plasma low, allowing more to diffuse. In the normal range of operation (40 to 50 mmHg), blood can absorb about 470 milliliters of carbon dioxide per liter of blood. With this large capacity, the partial pressure need change only a few mmHg to carry all the carbon dioxide that is produced by the tissues.

The anatomy of the lungs and the functioning of the respiratory system are well suited to meet most of the challenges that life presents. Exercise is a good example of how the respiratory system can handle a challenge. At rest, a fit young man breathes 6,000 milliliters of air per minute and uses about 250 milliliters of oxygen per minute to supply his body's needs. When exercising to his maximal capacity, the same individual may use as many as 4,000 milliliters of oxygen per minute. To supply this increased demand, the respiratory system must utilize all the reserve volumes discussed above and increase the breathing rate to a total of 120,000 milliliters of air per minute. The brain senses the movement of the arms and the legs. It also senses the greatly increased amount of carbon dioxide produced by the exercising muscles. In turn, the brain sends signals to the chest and diaphragm to breathe much deeper and faster.

Another example of the large reserve capacity of the human lungs is the ability to hold the breath. Since only a small amount of oxygen from each breath is used, a person can take a deep breath and hold it easily for nearly one minute. Some pearl divers can take a deep breath and swim underwater for four minutes or longer. The urge to breathe that one experiences while holding one's breath is produced when the brain senses the buildup of carbon dioxide and the decrease of oxygen in the blood.

The brain also uses its ability to sense the oxygen in the blood to adjust to unusual environments. At high altitudes, there is less oxygen in the air. With less oxygen in the air, less gets into the blood. The brain senses this condition and signals the respiratory system to breathe more air. There-

fore, when one travels into the mountains, one will breathe slightly deeper and faster. One is not aware of the increased breathing until fairly high altitudes are reached (above 10,000 feet). If one begins to exercise, however, performing even mild exercise such as brisk walking, one will be very aware of breathing heavily. This situation is greatly intensified if the person has diseased lungs. With some severe lung diseases, even people living at low altitudes (sea level) have shortness of breath, and some need to breathe air supplemented with extra oxygen.

Disorders and Diseases

The major type of lung disease, which is called obstructive disease, has three subclasses. The first is general obstruction, a disease in which material is abnormally present in an airway. The second is disease in which the large airways are narrowed. The third is disease in which the small airways and alveoli are diseased.

The case of general airway obstruction is simple. The simplest form is one in which a foreign body such as food or part of a child's toy is lodged in a large airway, such as the trachea or a main bronchus. The Heimlich maneuver (standing behind the affected individual, clasping the hands in a fist just below the rib cage, and thrusting up and in with the fist) is very effective in dislodging food caught in the trachea or larynx. An object that is small enough (such as a peanut), however, can get farther into the lung, in which case special instruments or surgery are necessary to remove the object. Tumors can also grow into the opening of an airway and obstruct it. Severe cases of tonsillitis are examples of this type of obstruction. Surgery is sometimes necessary to remove such a tumor if it limits airflow.

Large-airway narrowing is another type of related airway obstructive disease. Asthma and bronchitis are examples of this type of disease. The walls of the trachea and larger bronchi become thickened and thus make the passageway for air smaller. In addition, the specialized muscle (smooth muscle) surrounding the large airways has a tendency to contract, making the opening in the airway even smaller. These conditions result in difficulty of breathing, particularly when inhaling. Relatively rapid airway narrowing caused by smooth muscle contraction is called an asthma attack. Irritants such as air pollution, tobacco smoke, and pollen can start an asthma attack. Exercise, particularly in cold weather, can also stimulate an attack in some asthmatics. Asthma attacks can last for hours and sometimes days. There are some drugs, frequently taken in an inhaled form, that help relieve the symptoms by relaxing the smooth muscle. Many cases of asthma, however, are resistant to these drugs. Some asthmatics have benefited from drugs that help decrease the frequency and severity of attacks. Asthma usually begins in childhood and has a tendency to run in families.

Chronic obstructive pulmonary disease is the term that characterizes obstructive disease of the smallest airways and alveoli. Emphysema and chronic bronchitis belong to this class of lung disease. Emphysema consists of enlargement of the smallest bronchioles and the alveolar sacs. The walls of the alveoli disappear, and with them the capillaries. Therefore, the area previously used to exchange oxygen and carbon dioxide is lost. Since the air sacs are enlarged, the oxygen must travel farther to diffuse into the blood. Emphysema can be indicated by chest X rays and pulmonary function tests but cannot be definitely identified until after death. Emphysema is frequently associated with chronic bronchitis. Chronic bronchitis is characterized by enlargement of the mucous glands and by excessive mucus (sputum) production in the bronchial tree. The enlargement of the mucous glands alone can increase the resistance to airflow. Bronchitis is considered chronic when mucus is produced for three months of the year for at least two years.

The sputum can be very thick and may form into plugs to completely block off areas of the lung from airflow. Chronic obstructive pulmonary disease is generally a combination of both emphysema and chronic bronchitis of varying degrees. Persistent cough with expectoration is a normal symptom of this lung disease. With the destruction of airways and alveoli, some of the elastic recoil of the lungs is lost. As a result, exhalation is very laborious. Excess air is left in the lungs at the end of the exhalation, causing the chests of sufferers to be enlarged. Chronic obstructive disease is commonly found in long-term smokers.

Restrictive lung disease is another major classification of lung diseases. The main general feature of this class is primary changes in respiratory system tissues that restrict the movement of the lungs and thus respiration. Cystic fibrosis is the primary example of this disease. Cystic fibrosis appears to be caused by a malfunction of the immune system that produces a thick scarlike substance in the walls of the alveoli. The walls of the alveoli become thick and very stiff (fibrous). In some cases, the scar tissue grows across the small airway opening and closes off the airway. These closed air pockets are called cysts. The stiffness of the airways increases the elastic recoil of the lungs, making it very difficult to inhale.

Perspective and Prospects

Hippocrates (c. 460-c. 370 BCE) recognized the breathing of air as an important function. He believed, however, that the function of breathing was to cool the generator of heat, the heart. Aristotle (384-322 BCE) believed that air was breathed into the arteries, which carried it in the gaseous form to the rest of the body. Galen (129-c. 199 CE) transformed medicine from a hypothetical (philosophical) science into an experimental science by performing the first experiments on animals. He found that the arteries did not contain air, and he deduced that a quality of air (oxygen had not yet been discovered), not air itself, was important to life. In the seventeenth century, William Harvey discovered that blood circulated from arteries to veins in both the lung and the rest of the body, and oxygen was identified at the end of the eighteenth century by Joseph Priestly. Claude Bernard described the union of oxygen and hemoglobin at the end of the nineteenth century.

Many major technological advances have been made. Machines have been developed to assist and in some cases completely take over the function of respiration. Respirators can assist patients who have difficulty breathing on their own. Victims of poliomyelitis whose muscles for respiration are no longer functional, as well as paralyzed patients, have been greatly helped by respirators. Respirators maintain breathing during surgery when the patient receives general anesthesia. They also assist premature babies whose lungs are not fully developed. Scientists can now make the chemical surfactant that helps keep the lungs open. Premature babies frequently do not make enough surfactant; therefore, administration of synthetic surfactant can be lifesaving. Some machines can completely assume the function of the lung. These machines, called extracorporeal membrane oxygenators, can do the job of both the heart and the lungs. They are used in heart transplantation operations. They are also used to function in the place of severely damaged lungs of newborns until those lungs can repair themselves.

Knowledge of the functioning of the respiratory system has allowed humans to function in unusual environments. Humans are able to travel to high altitudes (for example, the top of Mount Everest) with the assistance of supplemental oxygen. Travel into outer space, where there is no oxygen, is now possible because an atmosphere can be created that is suitable for long-term living in space. Experimental work is being performed with the breathing of special liquids instead of air. Success with liquid breathing may allow humans to exist in different environments, such as the deep sea, and may also have therapeutic value.

—*J. Timothy O'Neill, Ph.D.*

See also Acute respiratory distress syndrome (ARDS); Asbestos exposure; Aspergillosis; Asthma; Avian influenza; Blood and blood disorders; Bronchi; Bronchitis; Cardiopulmonary resuscitation (CPR); Choking; Chronic obstructive pulmonary disease (COPD); Circulation; Critical care; Critical care, pediatric; Cyanosis; Cystic fibrosis; Diaphragm; Drowning; Emergency medicine; Emergency medicine, pediatric; Emphysema; Exercise physiology; Heimlich maneuver; Hyperbaric oxygen therapy; Hyperventilation; Hypoxia; Lung cancer; Lung surgery; Lungs; Otorhinolaryngology; Oxygen therapy; Pneumothorax; Pulmonary diseases; Pulmonary hypertension; Pulmonary medicine; Pulmonary medicine, pediatric; Respiratory distress syndrome; Resuscitation; Severe acute respiratory syndrome (SARS); Sleep apnea; Tonsillitis; Tracheostomy; Tumors; Wheezing.

For Further Information:

Kittredge, Mary. *The Respiratory System.* Edited by Dale C. Garell. Philadelphia: Chelsea House, 2000.

Levitzky, Michael G. *Pulmonary Physiology.* 7th ed. New York: McGraw-Hill Medical, 2007.

Mason, Robert J., et al., eds. *Murray and Nadel's Textbook of Respiratory Medicine.* 5th ed. Philadelphia: Saunders/Elsevier, 2010.

McLafferty, Ella. Carolyn Johnston. Charles Hendry. Alistair Farley. "Respiratory System Part 1: Pulmonary Ventilation." *Nursing Standard.* 27.22 (2013): 40-47. Print.

Parker, Steve. *The Lungs and Breathing.* Rev. ed. New York: Franklin Watts, 1991.

"Respiratory System Overview." *MedlinePlus.* August 2, 2011.

"The Respiratory System." *National Heart, Lung, and Blood Institute.* July 17, 2012.

Ware, Lorraine B., and Michael A. Matthay. "The Acute Respiratory Distress Syndrome." *New England Journal of Medicine* 342, no. 18 (May 4, 2000): 1334-1349.

"What Are the Signs and Symptoms of Cystic Fibrosis?" *National Heart, Lung, and Blood Institute*. June 1, 2011.

West, John B. *Pulmonary Pathophysiology: The Essentials*. 7th ed. Philadelphia: Wolters Kluwer/Lippincott Williams & Wilkins, 2008.

Respiratory diseases. *See* Pulmonary diseases; Respiration; *specific diseases.*

Respiratory distress syndrome
Disease/Disorder
Also known as: Premature lungs, pulmonary immaturity, hyaline membrane disease, surfactant deficiency syndrome

Anatomy or system affected: Heart, lungs

Specialties and related fields: Neonatology, pediatrics, pulmonary medicine

Definition: A deficiency of surfactant in the neonatal lungs, causing generalized alveolar collapse leading to respiratory failure.

Key terms:
air bronchograms: a term used in radiology to describe the presence of air in the terminal bronchi that does not reach the alveoli because they are collapsed

alveoli: the small air sacs in the lungs where gas exchange occurs

endotracheal intubation: the placement of a plastic tube in the trachea to deliver a combination of oxygen and air under pressure to the lungs

mechanical ventilation: the delivery by mechanical means of air and oxygen to the lungs under fine control of pressure and inspiratory/expiratory times by electronic and mechanical equipment

prematurity: the status of being born before thirty-seven weeks of gestation

respiratory failure: the inability of the lungs to perform adequate gas exchange, resulting in insufficient oxygen absorption and carbon dioxide elimination to sustain life

reticulogranular pattern: a term used in radiology to describe a lack of air in the alveoli

surfactant: a mixture of phospholipid and protein substances produced by cells lining the alveoli that reduces surface tension and prevents their collapse

Causes and Symptoms
Respiratory distress syndrome (RDS) is a condition observed mainly in premature infants and children born to diabetic patients. It is also known as premature lungs, pulmonary immaturity, hyaline membrane disease, and surfactant deficiency syndrome. In 1959, researchers discovered that surfactant deficiency is the cause of RDS in premature infants; this discovery has been the basis for treatment since that time.

The main symptom is a rapid respiratory rate involving the use of accessory muscles to increase the amount of air taken into the lungs. The forceful closure of the vocal cords while contracting the abdominal muscles and diaphragm causes a particular grunting sound. The premature rib cage is very flexible, and affected infants must use extra effort to

> **Information on Respiratory Distress Syndrome**
> **Causes:** Premature birth, surfactant deficiency, mother with diabetes
> **Symptoms:** Rapid respiration, grunting sound
> **Duration:** Acute
> **Treatments:** For pregnant woman at risk, antenatal steroids; for newborn, endotracheal intubation, mechanical ventilation, natural or artificial surfactants

maintain expanded lungs.

A diagnosis of RDS is made on a clinical basis, including a history of premature delivery and the symptoms listed above. A chest x-ray is also useful; in RDS, a reticulogranular pattern and air bronchograms are observed together with a whited-out appearance in the lung fields. Respiratory function is determined by measuring the amount of oxygen and carbon dioxide in the arterial blood. The samples are obtained using a catheter inserted in an arterial vessel and analyzed in a blood gas machine. In newborns, the catheter is usually placed in one of the umbilical arteries, but samples from radial, posterior tibial, or dorsal pedis arteries are acceptable for analysis. Respiratory failure is defined as the inability of the lungs to perform adequate gas exchange, resulting in insufficient oxygen absorption and carbon dioxide elimination to sustain life.

Treatment and Therapy
Initially, the treatment for RDS was nonspecific. Physicians used various methods to maintain open airways and waited until the infant's lungs matured on their own. The treatment of RDS was one of the main areas of research that helped in the development of the subspecialty of neonatology.

At present, the pregnant patient who is in imminent danger of delivering a child prematurely, between twenty-four and thirty-six weeks of gestation, is given antenatal steroids. The use of prenatal steroids has been associated with accelerated maturity of the lungs in infants born prematurely. Once a premature infant is born, endotracheal intubation, mechanical ventilation, and natural or artificial surfactants are used in order to maintain open airways and to prevent the development of atelectasis, the defective expansion of the alveoli.

Mechanical ventilation became a standard of care across the United States in teaching institutions. It has helped decrease mortality rates for premature infants and has evolved into a fine art assisted by advanced technology. Mechanical ventilation uses a variety of techniques to maximize lung expansion and to minimize the damage to lung tissues caused by high concentration of oxygen and pressures. Pressure, volume, and high-frequency ventilators are among the current equipment available to neonatologists for use with infants suffering from RDS.

In 1980, a report was published concerning the use of bovine surfactant mixed with saline solution administered endotracheally in infants with RDS. This treatment offered significant improvement in the outcome of this disease. Natural surfactants have been extracted from the lung tissues of calves and pigs, and surfactant has even been harvested from amniotic fluid in humans. The main difference between natural and artificial surfactants is the presence of surfactant-associated proteins. Surfactant-associated proteins function as dispersing agents for the lipid components that line the internal surface of the alveoli, thus preventing the collapse of these air sacs. Artificial surfactants are pure chemicals mixed in the laboratory without surfactant-associated proteins; other chemical substances are used as dispersing agents.

At least seven different types of surfactant have been tested in humans in clinical trials; controversy still exists regarding the proper timing of surfactant replacement, either as prophylaxis or as a rescue treatment. In addition, concern remains about the possible increased incidence of two major complications, pulmonary hemorrhage and intraventricular hemorrhage, in premature infants with RDS following the use of surfactant treatment.

Overall, the use of surfactants and mechanical ventilation has decreased mortality and complications in premature infants, but the number of patients with long-term complications, such as chronic lung disease with oxygen dependency, has increased considerably.

Perspective and Prospects

In 1960, the infant son of John Fitzgerald Kennedy, then president-elect of the United States, died of respiratory distress syndrome. Since then, significant advances in the understanding and treatment of this condition have been made, but the elimination of this disease will be achieved only when premature births are prevented. Until then, RDS will continue to exist in nurseries everywhere.

—*Fortunato Perez-Benavides, M.D.*

See also Acute respiratory distress syndrome (ARDS); Critical care; Critical care, pediatric; Cyanosis; Lungs; Multiple births; Premature birth; Pulmonary diseases; Pulmonary medicine; Pulmonary medicine, pediatric; Respiration; Wheezing.

For Further Information:

Bradford, Nikki. *Your Premature Baby: The First Five Years.* Toronto, Ont.: Firefly Books, 2003.

Martin, Richard J., Avroy A. Fanaroff, and Michele C. Walsh, eds. *Fanaroff and Martin's Neonatal-Perinatal Medicine: Diseases of the Fetus and Infant.* 9th ed. 2 vols. Philadelphia: Mosby/Elsevier, 2011.

Rosenbaum, Laurie. "Respiratory Distress Syndrome in Newborns." *Health Library,* September 10, 2012.

Turner, Joan, Gwendolyn J. McDonald, and Nanci L. Larter, eds. *Handbook of Adult and Pediatric Respiratory Home Care.* St. Louis, Mo.: Mosby, 1994.

West, John B. *Pulmonary Pathophysiology: The Essentials.* 8th ed. Philadelphia: Wolters Kluwer/Lippincott Williams & Wilkins, 2012.

"What Is Respiratory Distress Syndrome?" *National Heart, Lung, and Blood Institute,* January 24, 2012.

Restless legs syndrome

Disease/Disorder

Also known as: Periodic limb movement

Anatomy or system affected: Brain, muscles, musculoskeletal system, nervous system, psychic-emotional system

Specialties and related fields: Neurology, psychiatry, psychology, sleep medicine

Definition: A sensorimotor disorder characterized by uncomfortable and even painful sensations in the limbs, especially the legs, when at rest or trying to sleep.

Key terms:

akathisia: an unpleasant sensation of "inner" restlessness that compels the patient to move or walk

dopaminergic: related to the brain's neurotransmitter dopamine, which plays a role in such processes as mood, movement, and psychological functioning

neurotransmitter: a chemical messenger that transmits a neural impulse between neurons

Parkinson's disease: a movement disorder characterized by decreased levels of brain dopamine

substantia nigra: a midbrain structure that plays a role in movement, reward, and addiction

Causes and Symptoms

Patients with restless legs syndrome complain about unpleasant sensations, especially in the evening or at night, that drive them to move their limbs in order to alleviate the discomfort. Sufferers typically describe an inability to tolerate sitting, lying, or remaining still for even short periods of time, accompanied by an intense urge to walk, run, or move about.

The specific etiology of restless legs syndrome remains to be determined, although a number of theories have been proposed. Several of these include central nervous system (CNS) iron deficiency (especially in the brain's substantia nigra) leading to dopamine defects, CNS hypersensitivity and arousal, disrupted circadian rhythm, and genetic predisposition. Given the complexities of the human brain, more than one process is probably implicated in restless legs syndrome.

As for secondary causes, medications that can produce similar symptoms include caffeine, theophylline, antidepressants (with their anticholinergic effects), dopamine antagonists that cross the blood-brain barrier (the majority of antipsychotic medications), and metoclopramide, as well as withdrawal from any of a number of drugs.

The condition appears to be relatively common, with an estimated prevalence in the general population of up to 10

Information on Restless Legs Syndrome

Causes: Unknown, though likely involves abnormalities in brain's dopaminergic system

Symptoms: Evening or nighttime "inner" restlessness (akathisia), discomfort, pain, and/or need to move limbs or walk

Duration: Varies from episodic to chronic

Treatments: Dopaminergics, benzodiazepines, opioids, anticonvulsants; lifestyle modifications (decreasing the use of caffeine, alcohol, and tobacco, especially starting in afternoon)

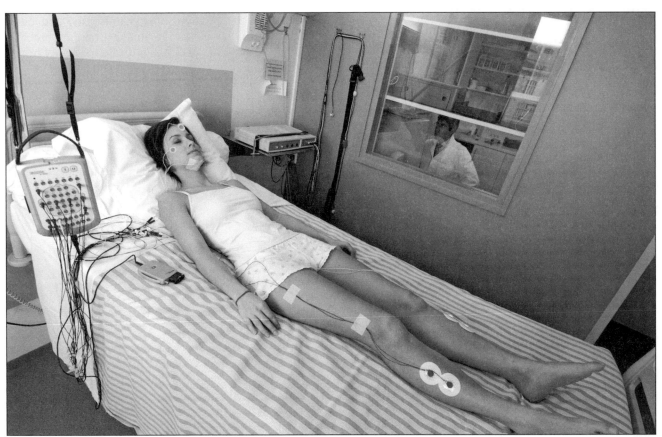

A patient with restless legs syndrome has her leg muscle activity monitored during sleep. (Philippe Garo/Photo Researchers, Inc.)

percent. Further, a greater prevalence appears to exist among first-degree relatives of patients than in those without the condition, suggesting at least some heritability. In fact, evidence initially points to a genetic locus mapped for restless legs syndrome on chromosome 12q.

Although excessive leg movements can be demonstrated during a sleep study test (nocturnal polysomnography), restless legs syndrome is diagnosed by history only. Four essential criteria are used in this process. First, the patient experiences a compelling urge to move the legs (or affected body parts) as a result of unpleasant sensations. Second, the unpleasant sensations and urge to move the legs worsen during the evening or at night and can significantly interfere with relaxation and sleep. Third, the unpleasant sensations and urge to move the legs worsen during periods of inactivity or rest, including sitting in a chair or lying in bed. Fourth, the unpleasant sensations and urge to move the legs are partially or completely relieved by activity, including stretching or walking, but only as long as the activity continues. In addition, patients reporting symptoms of restless legs syndrome should undergo toxicology studies, as well as have their iron, electrolyte, and medication levels checked. Comorbid psychiatric disorders must also be identified.

The symptoms and sensations of restless legs syndrome are typically depicted in negative terms-"fidgety," "creepy crawlies," "insect crawlies," "painful," and "electric," among other descriptors. Most report that these sensations can become so intense that they must "jiggle" or "shake," before ultimately resorting to getting up and walking. Spouses may also complain that patients move their limbs while asleep, thus disturbing the quality of sleep for both partners.

Restless legs syndrome is not limited to the evening hours, bedtime, or sleeping, nor is it necessarily limited to the lower extremities. It can involve an inability to tolerate confinement or immobility-at any time of the day-on airplanes, buses, and cars, as well as in meetings, in movie theaters, and during medical testing, such as magnetic resonance imaging (MRI) or computed tomography (CT) scanning. It can also involve, in more severe cases, other areas of the body, including the hips, upper back, shoulders, and arms. Patients report that it is difficult or impossible to ignore the negative sensations, which adversely affect not only sleep but also daily activities.

Treatment and Therapy

Difficulties arise when attempting to treat restless legs syndrome, as the disorder appears to involve multiple brain processes. The mainstay of medical therapy today consists of daily low-dose dopamine agonists (dopaminergics), the most popular of which are ropinirole and pramipexole, the only medications approved for "idiopathic" restless legs syndrome. Doses of these medications are slowly titrated until therapeutic results are attained. For example, pramipexole is started at 0.125 milligrams taken two hours

---

In the News:
Restless Legs Syndrome Related to Obesity

Researchers at the Harvard University School of Public Health recently suggested a potential relationship between restless legs syndrome and being overweight. Restless legs syndrome is a common disorder in which patients describe uncomfortable "creepy crawly" sensations and limb movements that make sitting still or sleeping soundly nearly impossible. Patients also complain about not being able to tolerate riding in airplanes or cars, sitting in meetings, or going to the theater. As such, the condition can seriously interfere with relationships, health, and work. According to the study published in the April, 2009, issue of the American Academy of Neurology's medical journal, *Neurology*, Harvard researchers surveyed some 88,000 women and men and discovered those with a body mass index (BMI) greater than 30 had a 40 percent higher risk of developing restless legs syndrome than those with a normal BMI. Scientists believe that restless legs syndrome is caused by decreased levels of dopamine in the brain, though what causes this decrease is unknown. Dopamine is a neurotransmitter that is known to control movement, mood, and the pleasurable feelings derived from eating food, which might explain the relationship. Estimates are that restless legs syndrome affects almost 10 percent of the general population, which translates into many millions of sufferers. In the case of obese persons, symptoms may improve with weight loss. Otherwise, medical therapy with dopaminergic drugs such as ropinirole and pramipexole is key.

—*George D. Zgourides, M.D., Psy.D.*

---

prior to bedtime for five days and then increased to the usual evening dose of 0.25 milligrams.

The side effects of ropinirole and pramipexole are representative of the dopamine agonists as a class: headaches, nausea, insomnia, "sleep attacks," and problems related to impulse control (gambling, drinking, shopping, hypersexuality). Anticonvulsants, opioids, and sedative-hypnotics have also been used to treat restless legs syndrome, all with varying success depending on individual patient profiles.

Additionally, sufferers should be instructed to stay away from caffeine, tea, chocolate, alcohol, or tobacco in the evening (after 5 p.m.). They should also be taught to engage in good sleep hygiene (obtain sufficient hours of rest, have a regular time to retire and awaken), to avoid exercising too close to bedtime, to avoid aggravating medications, and to take ferrous sulfate supplements if iron studies show this to be warranted.

Perspective and Prospects

Restless legs syndrome is an underappreciated disorder that causes millions of people a great deal of distress and misery. While many may think of the condition as a new disease, it has been described for centuries. Yet, only since the 1980s has this complex neurological disorder captured the attention of medical scientists and researchers. Such interest has led to the development of medical therapies tailored to relieve the symptoms of restless legs syndrome. Much remains to be done. Primary care physicians,

neurologists, psychiatrists, rheumatologists, and other health care professionals are beginning to take this problem seriously as a disorder with a significant morbidity resulting from chronic interruption of sleep and daily activities. Further, future directions in pharmacology will hopefully take into account the need for longer-acting medications and nondopaminergic options.

—*George D. Zgourides, M.D., Psy.D.*

See also Lower extremities; Muscle sprains, spasms, and disorders; Muscles; Nervous system; Neuralgia, neuritis, and neuropathy; Neurology; Neurology, pediatric; Sleep; Sleep disorders; Upper extremities.

For Further Information:

Allen, Richard P., and Merrill M. Mitler. "Restless Legs Syndrome (RLS) and Sleep." *National Sleep Foundation*, 2011.
Badash, Michelle, and Michael Woods. "Restless Legs Syndrome." *Health Library*, Mar. 15, 2013.
Buchfuhrer, Mark J., Wayne Hening, and Clete Kushida. *Restless Legs Syndrome: Coping with Your Sleepless Nights*. New York: Demos, 2007.
Maheswaran, Murali, and Clete A. Kushida. "Restless Legs Syndrome in Children." *Medscape General Medicine* 8, no. 2 (June 20, 2006): 79.
"Restless Legs." *MedlinePlus*, Mar. 5, 2013.
"Restless Legs Syndrome Fact Sheet." *National Institute of Neurological Disorders and Stroke*, Nov. 25, 2011.

Resuscitation

Procedure

Anatomy or system affected: Brain, chest, circulatory system, heart, lungs, respiratory system

Specialties and related fields: Critical care, emergency medicine

Definition: The physical act of reviving a person in cardiac or respiratory arrest, which involves such techniques as artificial respiration, chest compressions, and defibrillation.

Key terms:

advanced cardiac life support (ACLS): a variety of life support procedures provided by trained medical personnel, including the administration of drugs and electrical defibrillation

arrhythmia: a heart rhythm that is abnormal in either speed or force; arrhythmias do not always lead to a heart attack

basic life support (BLS): a variety of life-support procedures, including rescue breathing and chest compressions, often given to a heart attack victim by the first person responding to a patient; public training in such procedures is available from the Red Cross and the American Heart Association

cardiopulmonary resuscitation (CPR): a method of producing some breathing and circulation of blood to a patient in cardiac arrest using chest compressions and artificial ventilation

defibrillation: the application of electrical energy through the chest in order to correct abnormal heart function and restore a normal heart rhythm

electrocardiogram (EKG) monitor: a machine which records the electrical activity of the heart onto a monitor and paper strip, which is then used by medically trained personnel to determine further treatment

Physiology of Respiration and Circulation

Every cell in the human body needs a constant and steady supply of oxygen. The delivery of oxygen is possible only through a continuous movement of oxygen-rich blood, with the heart and lungs working efficiently together. To survive, the body must have a functioning heart and lungs, or an outside force that makes both organs function artificially. Two major life-threatening conditions include respiratory arrest (cessation of breathing) and cardiac arrest (cessation of heartbeat). Death is certain unless something is done to put oxygen into the blood and circulate it throughout the body. Cardiopulmonary resuscitation (CPR) is the artificial action of putting oxygen into the lungs and making the heart pump blood throughout the body. By understanding the anatomy and physiology of the heart and lungs, and their entire systems, it is easier to see how CPR can help a person who is not breathing and whose heart is not pumping blood.

The respiratory system. This system has many parts, from the nose down to the smallest sacs of the lungs. After air is taken in through the nose or mouth, it moves farther down into the throat (pharynx), past the larynx (voice box) and the trachea (windpipe). Next, the inhaled air goes through specialized tubes called bronchi, one connected to each lung. From this larger tube, the air passage narrows into smaller tubes called bronchioles. The bronchioles become smaller and end at the air sacs, called alveoli. Alveoli are actually millions of tiny air sacs that allow oxygen to move into the bloodstream and carbon dioxide to be removed from the blood and exhaled. The alveoli are hollow and surrounded by a very thin, specialized membrane that is only one or two cells thick. This transfer of needed oxygen, along with the removal of the carbon dioxide waste products, happens through the small capillaries surrounding the alveoli. In the blood, oxygen attaches to the hemoglobin found in red blood cells, and, in return, carbon dioxide crosses back into the lungs in order to be exhaled.

It is this carbon dioxide buildup in the blood that stimulates how deep and how often one breathes. An area of the brain called the medulla is considered the body's respiratory center because it is responsible for sending electrical signals to the chest muscles that control breathing. A check-and-balance system monitors the amount of carbon dioxide in the bloodstream. When the level increases, the rate and depth of respirations also increase so that the excess amount can be exhaled.

The brain sends messages via the nerves to the muscles of the ribs. In addition to smaller muscles between each rib, the neck and shoulder muscles must also help during breathing. The diaphragm, a large, sheetlike muscle that separates the chest from the abdominal organs, also plays a major role in inspiration and expiration. The diaphragm extends from front to back by attaching to the lower part of the ribs. During inhalation, the muscles raise the ribs up and forward while the diaphragm moves downward toward the abdominal cavity, thus making room for the lungs to expand. As a result, the pressure inside the lungs becomes less than that of the surrounding air. It is this difference in air pressure, not an actual sucking in of air, that causes air to move into the lungs. The act of exhaling occurs when these muscles relax, causing the ribs to move back down and the diaphragm to rise. The size of the chest cavity decreases, the elastic nature of the lungs causes them to become smaller, and air moves out of the lungs.

The circulatory system. Life cannot be sustained simply by air moving in and out of the lungs. Once the oxygen moves from the tiny air sacs in the lungs and across into the bloodstream, it must be moved to every cell in the body. This transportation is possible because of the circulation of blood within the many vessels. At the center of this circulatory system, the heart acts as the pump, pushing blood out through the large arteries and the smaller arterioles and capillaries. After reaching the capillaries, the oxygen is delivered to the cells, and waste products such as carbon dioxide are picked up. The capillaries branch into larger venules and then into even larger veins. The major veins, from all areas of the body, return blood to the heart that is no longer rich in oxygen. Instead, it contains carbon dioxide that needs to be removed. It is this lack of oxygen that makes the blood in veins appear bluish, whereas the oxygen-rich blood found in arteries is more red in color.

The heart is responsible for sending out oxygen-carrying blood to all body tissues and moving carbon dioxide-rich blood to the lungs so that it can be exhaled. The right side of the heart is responsible for receiving blood that no longer has enough oxygen, called deoxygenated blood. The blood is next pumped through the bottom half of the heart (right ventricle) into a specialized artery called the pulmonary artery and then into each lung. Although the term "arteries" is usually reserved for vessels carrying blood with high levels of oxygen, there is one exception: The pulmonary artery does not carry oxygen-rich blood. The blood then flows into smaller capillaries surrounding the alveoli in the lungs, where it exchanges carbon dioxide for oxygen. On the return trip to the left side of the heart, after leaving the lungs, the oxygenated blood moves through the pulmonary veins. Blood then travels from the left upper portion of the heart (left atrium) to the left ventricle, which is the major muscle of the heart responsible for pumping blood to all the cells of the body.

In summary, the right side of the heart carries deoxygenated blood from the body to the lungs. The left side of the heart receives the oxygenated blood from the lungs and pumps it throughout the body. The huge network of connections in the circulatory system, from the heart all the way out to the tips of the toes and returning to the heart, makes up a closed system that must not have any large leaks, which occur during bleeding.

Indications and Procedures

It might seem that whether the heart is functioning is not a matter of yes or no, black or white. However, there are many gray areas that represent a heart that is beating but not working in a manner that will support life. These gray areas include many types of abnormal beats, known as arrhythmias, or abnormal rhythms. If the heart is beating too fast (tachycardia) or extremely slowly (bradycardia), then it cannot supply body tissues with needed oxygenated blood. A constant and even pressure of blood flow must also be maintained.

The amount of pressure inside the circulatory system varies. Blood pressure is measured as systolic pressure over diastolic pressure. In a blood pressure reading of 120/ 70, the top number, 120, indicates the amount of pressure on the walls of the vessels when the heart is beating (contracting). The bottom number, 70, reflects the amount of pressure on the vessel walls between beats when the heart is at rest. In cases when both numbers are extremely low or high, the system is not working properly and urgent measures must be taken to identify and fix the problem.

When either the circulatory or the respiratory system is not able to perform properly, the entire body suffers quickly. Without oxygenated blood, brain damage begins within four to six minutes. While sitting, the human heart pumps sixty to one hundred times each minute, moving about 5.5 liters of blood throughout the body every minute. The average 150-pound man has a total of about 6.75 liters of blood that must be kept constantly moving. The heart acts like a pump because it is a special muscle with its own electrical system. Much the same way as a light switch turns on a light bulb, the heart pumps because an electrical message at the top of the heart, in the sinoatrial (S-A) node, makes the entire heart muscle contract. This natural pacemaker keeps the heart beating when all things are in proper working order. If the heart stops beating correctly or the lungs do not work, however, the person will die unless resuscitation is started.

Resuscitation means making the heart pump blood and getting oxygen into and out of the lungs. In an example of the most severe case, a person is found not breathing and without a pulse. Cardiopulmonary resuscitation (CPR) courses teach that the first step is to open the airway and be sure that nothing is blocking the flow of air in and out of the lungs. If a blockage is found, it must be removed immediately. If the person is not breathing, the rescuer must breathe for him or her. Artificial respiration, or mouth-to-mouth ventilation, in which one individual breathes air into another's mouth, will force oxygen-containing air into the lungs so that it can be picked up in the bloodstream and transported to body cells. Pinching the patient's nose and blowing into the mouth forces air into the lungs in much the same way as taking a deep breath. Yet this artificial breathing alone is not enough. The oxygen put into the lungs must be moved around the body, which can only be done through circulating blood.

To move the blood through the circulatory system, something must be done to make the heart pump. This can be accomplished through chest compressions. Since the heart lies between the breastbone (sternum) and the spine, it is surrounded by hard, bony structures. By pressing in the correct position, with sufficient pressure and depth, the heart muscle can be squeezed. This squeezing action will result in blood being forced out of the heart and onto its path around the body. The oxygen blown into the lungs will

be picked up by the passing blood and moved out to necessary areas of the body.

Even with the use of proper techniques, however, cardiopulmonary resuscitation should only be a temporary measure for a person who has no pulse and who is not breathing. CPR is only a momentary first-aid measure. Yet this procedure is a vital one: Until further medical assistance can be given, it is extremely important that oxygen circulate in the patient's body.

CPR is usually done by the first responder who finds the victim. This form of resuscitation is known as basic life support (BLS). The administration of BLS is the step just before advanced cardiac life support (ACLS), which offers additional treatment measures given by medically trained personnel. ACLS is given by emergency medical technicians (EMTs), paramedics responding in ambulances, or other health care professionals. While continuing CPR, the medical team will start advanced care before or during the drive to a hospital emergency department.

To provide the proper treatment, paramedics must determine the electrical activity of the heart. The heart's rhythm is recorded on an electrocardiograph (ECG or EKG) machine, which helps the medical team find the cause of the problem. The portable ECG machine, which is commonly called a cardiac monitor, displays the electrical activity in the heart. When the electrical impulses are not producing a rhythmic beating pattern, various treatment procedures may follow, depending on how the heart is pumping or if it is working at all. It is possible to correct a heart that has an irregular beat caused by abnormal electrical activity. A total lack of electrical activity in the heart is called asystole and is recorded on the monitor as a flat line. The ACLS team can attempt to adjust the abnormal electrical signal but usually cannot mechanically restart a heart that has no electrical impulses. Other heart problems produce other types of tracings on the monitor. In one type of arrhythmia called ventricular fibrillation, the heart has a rapid, chaotic electrical activity that does not allow the heart to beat; the patient will stop breathing and will have no pulse. In this case, CPR is needed to reduce brain damage caused by decreased oxygen to cells, while paramedics and other health care professionals begin advanced life support in an attempt to reverse the dying process.

Many different protocols exist on how ACLS treatment should progress, and the following is merely one example. In 2005, the American Heart Association made changes in CPR, BLS, and ACLS protocols. The medics may use an electrical machine known as a defibrillator to deliver electrical shocks through the chest and toward the heart in the hope of correcting the rhythm. A single electric shock is given, followed by CPR. A needle and special catheter are placed in a vein to start intravenous (IV) fluids, in which medications can be given to travel to the heart through the veins. A high concentration of oxygen is delivered through a tube inserted through the mouth or nose and passed into the upper part of the lung so that artificial ventilation can aid in the movement of concentrated oxygen. Adrenaline (also known as epinephrine) is given through the IV; this drug will increase the blood flow to the heart and brain by narrowing other vessels and will also increase the heart rate and blood pressure. CPR is continued for two minutes, then a brief pause occurs for another single electric shock. CPR resumes immediately.

Studies of actual resuscitation processes have demonstrated that CPR was often stopped while personnel prepared medications or prepared to defibrillate. These pauses caused the absence of blood flow and oxygen for prolonged periods of time. This observation led to the new guidelines. Single shocks are given, rather than the previous three shocks of increasing voltage. CPR is given continuously except during the actual shock.

The next drug given may be amiodarone, which helps to calm a heart that is beating too fast or erratically. If the irregular rhythm has still not been corrected, then sodium bicarbonate may given to reduce the acids produced in the body because of the lack of oxygen. This entire scenario is repeated until the heart is beating in a manner that will sustain life or it is determined by a physician that the person cannot be resuscitated.

Other drugs that are used for specific heart problems include atropine, lidocaine, vasopressin, procainamide, verapamil, dopamine, and adenosine. All these drugs target specific problems during a cardiac episode. For individuals who are successfully resuscitated and are stable but unresponsive on arrival at the hospital, induced hypothermia is recommended for the first twenty-four hours to improve brain functioning.

When the heart slows or weakens to the point that it is barely beating, life can be artificially maintained in a few cases by using a cardiac pacing unit to create an artificial heartbeat electrically, a procedure called cardiac pacing. This artificial heartbeat may be sufficient until a permanent pacemaker can be implanted.

Perspective and Prospects

Over the years, huge advances have been made in resuscitation measures. More lives have been saved by the training of medical personnel to administer advanced life support before a patient reaches the hospital. Lifesaving drugs and defibrillation have greatly decreased the death rate for heart attack victims and cardiac patients. With the continued training of emergency medical technicians, the survival rate can improve as a result of earlier and more aggressive medical treatment.

Medical treatment could be avoided entirely, however, if more preventive health measures were implemented. With continued research identifying risk factors, the public can be educated about how to prevent conditions that lead to heart attacks. Among the known risk factors are cigarette smoking, hypertension (high blood pressure), high cholesterol and triglycerides, lack of exercise, excess weight and improper nutrition, stress, and diabetes mellitus. Three risk factors cannot be changed: predisposing heredity, gender (men are more likely to have heart attacks), and increasing age.

With further research, the first group of risk factors may be addressed in society through extensive education, but heart attack rates cannot be curbed unless people change their lifestyles. An understanding of heredity, gender, and age risk factors can bring changes in these rates only through further research into their relationship to heart attacks.

Until people are willing to change their lifestyles, early recognition of the warning signs of a heart attack may be the easiest method of increasing survival rates. A heart attack occurs when the heart muscle itself does not receive enough oxygen. The heart muscle has its own blood supply through the coronary arteries. The blood supply to the heart may be reduced by a clot or by a narrowing in the coronary arteries. The warning signals of a heart attack include a squeezing tightness or pressure in the chest; pain in either arm, neck, jaw, or between the shoulder blades; sweating; nausea; weakness; and shortness of breath. People with diabetes and women may have milder or different symptoms. Too often, people deny that they could be suffering a heart attack, with many believing that the pain is heartburn or indigestion. If medical attention is sought immediately, however, severe damage can often be reduced or stopped. Special drugs such as streptokinase or tissue plasminogen activator (TPA) can dissolve clots that interfere with blood flow, while surgical techniques such as coronary artery bypass surgery (CABG) or angioplasty can open clogged arteries. Heart transplants offer a solution for patients with extensive heart damage. Research continues to decrease the rejection rates for heart transplants. Medications are being developed to decrease the buildup of plaque in arteries. The fields of genetics and gene therapy hold many keys to the prevention and treatment of heart disease.

It is important to note that all medically trained personnel, from the EMT to the emergency medicine physician, must be able to perform life-support measures. Unless patients have given appropriate do-not-resuscitate (DNR) orders, they will receive some form of the previously mentioned procedures. A living will is a legal document that directs medical personnel in the level of care an individual wishes to have. For example, a person with advanced cancer may want to not be placed on a breathing machine. Those wishes are to be communicated through a living will. Without this document, health care providers are mandated by law to provide lifesaving measures. Future resuscitation measures will be influenced by ethical questions regarding when to sustain life.

Bystander CPR (initiation of CPR by the first person to find a cardiac arrest victim) is a vital component in the chain of survival between BLS and ACLS. It has been recognized, however, that very few people are willing to perform mouth-to-mouth rescue breathing, a vital component of success for CPR. Therefore, it has been acknowledged that it is better to at least open the victim's airway by extending the neck and doing chest compressions alone versus doing nothing at all. The layperson will no longer be taught to check for a pulse before initiating CPR. Checking for a pulse was removed from the recommendations because it was demonstrated that laypersons could not be taught to reliably check for a pulse. Instead, they will be taught to look and examine for "signs of circulation," which include breathing, coughing, or chest movements, before starting CPR. Another recommendation for BLS was to train nonmedical professionals such as police, firefighters, security officers, and others exposed to large populations in the use of the automated external defibrillator (AED). The AED has two pads that, when applied to the chest of the cardiac victim, analyze the electrical heart activity. The AED then administers the electrical shock (defibrillation) necessary to restart a heart if the cause of cardiac arrest was ventricular fibrillation, the most common arrhythmia of cardiac arrest. Bystander CPR and early defibrillation by the AED have been shown to do more to reduce morbidity and mortality from cardiac arrest than all current therapies for cardiac arrest combined.

—Maxine M. Urton, Ph.D.; Laurence Katz, M.D.;
updated by Amy Webb Bull, D.S.N., A.P.N.

See also Arrhythmias; Bypass surgery; Cardiac arrest; Cardiopulmonary resuscitation (CPR); Choking; Circulation; Critical care; Critical care, pediatric; Defibrillation; Drowning; Electrocardiography (ECG or EKG); Emergency medicine; Ethics; First aid; Heart; Heart attack; Heimlich maneuver; Hyperbaric oxygen therapy; Lungs; Malpractice; Pacemaker implantation; Paramedics; Pulmonary medicine; Pulmonary medicine, pediatric; Respiration; Thrombolytic therapy and TPA; Tracheostomy.

For Further Information:

"Cardiopulmonary Resuscitation (CPR): First Aid." *Mayo Clinic*, February 7, 2012.

Cayley, William E., Jr. "2005 AHA Guidelines for CPR and Emergency Cardiac Care." *American Family Physician* 73, no. 9 (May 1, 2006): 1645.

"CPR." *American Heart Association*, 2013.

Hamilton, Glenn C., et al. *Emergency Medicine: An Approach to Clinical Problem-Solving*. 2d ed. New York: W. B. Saunders, 2003.

Henry, Mark C., and Edward R. Stapleton. *EMT: Prehospital Care*. Rev. 4th ed. St. Louis, Mo.: Mosby/Elsevier, 2012.

Tintinalli, Judith E., ed. *Emergency Medicine: A Comprehensive Study Guide*. 7th ed. New York: McGraw-Hill, 2011.

Torpy, Janet M., Cassio Lynm, and Richard M. Glass. "Cardiopulmonary Resuscitation." *JAMA* 304, no. 13 (October 6, 2010): 1514.

White, Roger D. "2005 American Heart Association Guidelines for Cardiopulmonary Resuscitation: Physiologic and Educational Rationale for Changes." *Mayo Clinic Proceedings* 81, no. 6 (2006): 736-740.

Retina

Anatomy

Anatomy or system affected: Eye

Specialties and related fields: Ophthalmology, retina specialist

Definition: A multilayer of exquisitely organized neurons that line the back of the eye designed to convert photons into neural impulses that travel along the visual pathways to the visual cortex.

The retina is the innermost layer of the eye, and it works to capture light in the form of photons and relay a neural signal to the brain regarding the incoming light beam. Before reaching the retina, light must pass through the ocular media, which consists of the tear film, cornea, anterior and posterior chambers, crystalline lens, and the vitreous body—these structures serve unique purposes, such as providing nutrients to the eye, focusing rays of light, and clearing the eye of any foreign bodies.

Background

Description. The retina (roughly 0.5 mm thick) forms the inner layer of the eye and is composed of several layers. The innermost layer consists of photoreceptors, which are specialized cells responsible for capturing incoming light photons. As light reaches the photoreceptor layer of the retina, a pigment in the photoreceptors undergoes a conformational change and releases a chemical substance, known as a neurotransmitter. This begins the signaling cascade to the brain representing the information pertaining to the current visual stimulus.

Rods and Cones. Photoreceptors come in two main types: rods and cones. There are approximately 92 million rods in the photoreceptor layer, which are saturated at natural light intensities and are unable to discriminate between colors. Their high sensitivity to light renders them effective for night vision. In contrast, cone photoreceptors come in three varieties, distinguished by their unique structural and functional properties. Each of these subsets has a specific inclination towards a particular wavelength of light; they consist of the long (maximum absorption in the red light range), medium (maximum absorption in the green light range), and short (maximum absorption in the blue light range) wavelength cones. Cones only account for about 5% of the total photoreceptors in the retina, but are heavily gathered in an area of the retina called the *fovea,* an area devoid of blood vessels with the highest concentration of cones, allowing for high spatial acuity and color discrimination. (Overall, the retina is fed by two main blood supplies: the central retinal artery and the choroidal blood vessels—they account for 20-30% and 65-85% of blood flow, respectively.)

Light and Phototransduction. As light travels through the eye and reaches the retina layer, the photons from the incoming light beam strike the photoreceptors and commence a series of chemical, structural, and physical changes that allow for propagation of a nerve impulse—a process known as *phototransduction*. Both rods and cones contain different photopigments, the membrane protein responsible for capturing light photons and thereby initiating a phototransduction cascade. Rods contain the photopigment known as *rhodopsin*, while the cone photopigment is known as *opsin*. The subtle structural difference between these two photopigments forms the basis for divergent light and color sensitivities (as well as overall function) between rods and cones.

As photons reach the photoreceptors, they are "captured" by either a rod or a cone photopigment. The photopigment subsequently undergoes a structural change, causing a signaling cascade within the photoreceptor. This, in return, causes the release of a chemical—known as a neurotransmitter—that begins transducing a signal to the brain regarding the incoming light stimulus. After being physically transformed by the incoming photon, the photopigments must return to their original conformation in order to remain continually responsive to light and maintain high fidelity neural transmission to the brain. Through this mechanism, the brain is able to interpret information presented in the current visual field.

Overview

The retina is regarded as the layer of the eye with photoreceptive qualities. The composition of the retina (which measures roughly 0.5 mm thick) is that of a vascular membrane with a network of cell layers. When light waves enter the eye, they are transformed by the eye into neural impulses. The primary function of the retina is to translate the waves of light it receives into nerve or neural impulses. These are, in turn, transmitted to the brain, and the sense of sight is manifested.

How does the physiology of vision occur through the retina? An image is formed on the retina. In order for this image to be perceived by the body as a visual entity, the photosensitive cells of the retina must come into play. The rods and cones function as transmitters of nervous signals. The millions of rods and cones, perceiving light differently, are concentrated in specific areas. The *macula* is a small yellow-pigmented area bearing a high concentration of cones. The *fovea* is a small section at the center of the macula, and it contains the highest density of cones in the retina. The center of the fovea, known as the *foveal pit*, is 200 microns—a fifth of a millimeter—in diameter and exhibits an even higher degree of specialization.

The propensity of the cones and rods to detect light and translate it into color can be attributed to the photosensitive chemicals (pigments) that they contain. Rods and cones possess rhodopsin and opsin respectively; upon interaction with light, these chemicals go through a cycle to culminate in a nerve impulse. Altogether, this creates a visual stimulus. Rods are associated with night vision, given their ability to pick up low or dim levels of light. In contrast, cones are associated with daylight vision and color. Pigments picking up primary colors of red, blue, and green are found in cones. Accordingly, there are three different kinds of pigment, each with variable color sensitivity.

Neural Pathways. The visual pathway begins with the rods and cones that serve to send the impulses. These impulses reach bipolar cells, followed by ganglion cells connected to the optic nerve. Horizontal and amacrine cells are vertically oriented neurons that act by transmitting signals over the retina. The optic nerve is a central circular region of the retina that measures approximately 2 x 1.5 mm across. It contains the ganglion cell axons directing signals out to the brain. Once the brain receives these nerve impulses, it is able to translate them into the sense of sight.

Color Blindness

Color blindness occurs when a person is lacking pigments connected with the particular color. When someone cannot distinguish red or green, for instance, this is usually due to an insufficient supply of the pigments most sensitive to red or green light.

Retinal Disorders

Given its delicate nature, the retina is prone to significant damage and degeneration in various conditions. Retinal disorders primarily result when the macula nerve tissue is affected. Macular pucker (scar tissue) and macular hole are some notable manifestations. To cite another prominent example, age-related macular degeneration is a leading cause of blindness worldwide, which results from degeneration and lipid deposition behind the retina (in the layer known as the retinal pigmented epithelium). These changes cause fluid to seep in behind the fovea and damage the overlying cone photoreceptors, thereby compromising central vision. Moreover, in diabetic retinopathy, the blood vessels supplying the eye become severely compromised, with uncontrolled proliferation and leakage into the retina. Retinoblastoma is a cancer of the retina found most frequently in children. Moreover, retinitis pigmentosa is a hereditary disease whereby the rods of the peripheral retina undergo significant degeneration, leading to impaired night vision. Finally, when the retina becomes detached from the back of the eye (i.e., retinal detachment), the retina membrane separates from the layers that support it; this often warrants immediate surgery for sight preservation.

—*Nicholas Koen, Derrick Cheng and Ariel Choi*

For Further Information:
Dubuc, Bruno. "Photoreceptors." *The Brain from Top to Bottom.* Sept. 2002. Web. 9 May 2016.
Hubel, David. "The Eye." *Eye, Brain, and Vision.* n.d. Web. 9 May 2016.
Jacob, Stanley; Francone, Clarice Ashworth; and Lossow, Walter J. *Structure and Function in Man.* London: Elsevier Health Sciences, 1982. Print.
Kapit, Wynne, and Elson, Lawrence M. *The Anatomy Coloring Book.* 2nd edition. U.S.A.: Addison- Wesley Educational Publishers, Inc., 1993. Print.
Kolb, Helga. "How the Retina Works." *American Scientist.* 91.1 (2003):28. Web. 9 May 2016.
Kolb, Helga. "Simple Anatomy of the Retina." Webvision: The Organization of the Retina and Visual System. In: Kolb H, Fernandez E, Nelson R, editors. Salt Lake City (UT): University of Utah Health Sciences Center. Web. Published 1 May 2005. Updated 31 Jan 2012. 10 Sept 2017.
National Eye Institute. "Facts About Retinal Detachment." *National Eye Institute.* Department of Health and Human Services. Oct. 2009. Web. 9 May 2016.
Prasad, Sashank; Rizzo, Joseph. "Modern-Neuro-Ophthalmology: Anatomy & Physiology of the Human Visual System." Feb. 2016.
"The Eye." *Kellogg Eye Center.* University of Michigan Kellogg Eye Center, 2015. Web. 9 May 2016.
U.S. National Library of Medicine. "Retina." 3 May 2016. Web. 9 May 2016.
U.S. National Library of Medicine. "Retinal Disorders." 10 July 2014. Web. 9 May 2016.

Retinal detachment
Disease/Disorder

Introduction

The retina is a thin film of tissue that sits in the back of the eye. It is attached to an underlying layer of cells known as the retinal pigmented epithelium (RPE), responsible for absorbing excess light and providing key nutritional support to the retinal neurons. The retina is responsible for translating light information into chemical and electrical signals, which travel through multiple layers of neurons, the optic nerve, the thalamus, and visual cortex in the brain. As a result, a tear or detachment in the retinal film can cause the loss of vision. Annual incidence of retinal detachment (RD) is approximately 1 in 10,000. Average age of presentation is approximately 60.

There are three main types of RD. *Rhegmatogenous* (from the Greek word *rhegma*, meaning "break") detachments are the most common and occur when a tear or hole forms in the retina. This opening allows fluid from the inside of the eye to seep in between and separate the retina and the RPE. *Tractional* detachments are less common, but occur when scar tissue forms on the retinal surface. This scar tissue contracts and pulls the retina away from the RPE. Additionally, the vitreous gel that fills the inside of the eye can clump and become sticky with age, allowing it to pull on the retina. *Exudative* detachments typically occur in the setting of inflammation, cancer, or other diseases that promote fluid or blood exudation in the eye. While there are no tears, excess fluid may separate the retina and RPE, causing a retinal detachment.

There are also varying degrees of RD severity. In minor detachments or tears, the vitreous gel filling the inside of the eye may cause traction on the retina and cause small tears that do not significantly affect vision. In larger, more severe detachments, vital areas of the retina including the macula (vision center) may become separated and require urgent medical attention.

Brief History

The first diagnosis of a retinal tear was made in 1953 by Ernst Adolf Coccius, following the invention of the ophthalmoscope in 1950. Early approaches to treatment focused on rest and ocular immobilization using molds, weights, binding, and atropine. Surgical techniques emphasized vitreous and subretinal fluid removal.

A Swiss ophthalmologist by the name of Jules Gonin developed the first approach towards repairing the torn retina, using cauterization (burning) to bind the retinal tear to the underlying retinal pigment epithelium and choroid (retinal blood supply). An alternative approach using cryotherapy was developed soon afterwards. Over the past half-century, approaches to retinal detachment treatment have seen remarkable growth and have significantly improved vision restoration rates.

Risk Factors, Causes, and Symptoms

There are a variety of risk factors that promote retinal detachments. In patients with nearsightedness (myopia), for example, the eye is elongated and the focal point of light lies in front of the retina. This stretched configuration increases the risk of a tear or detachment of the retina. Other risk factors include age, cataract surgery, malignan

t hypertension, prior history of vitreous or retinal diseases and detachments, a family history of retinal detachments, ocular trauma (including a history of eye surgery), and diabetes, which can cause prolonged vascular damage, scarring, and tractional detachment.

Patients suffering from an acute retinal detachment often report a sudden onset of flashing lights or floaters—symptoms that appear due to the vitreous gel clumping together and putting tension on the retina. Other symptoms may include transient loss of vision, especially at the periphery, that may gradually spread towards the center with the progression of detachment. If left untreated, chances of recovery fall significantly, as the retina is starved of vital nutrients or oxygen.

Treatment and Surgical Overview

There are varying degrees of retinal detachment, and treatment methods vary depending on the physician. However, the vast majority of retinal tears and detachments require surgical intervention. Notably, only those detachments that are identified and treated early will spare the patient's vision; once the detachment expands over the fovea, permanent vision loss is all but inevitable. For this reason, prompt referral to an ophthalmologist for surgical repair is essential. Surgical procedures may include:

Photocoagulation/Cryotherapy: Photocoagulation and cryotherapy are commonly used to treat small retinal tears. These procedures involve the use of a laser or freezing probe to form a small scar around the tear, sealing the retinal flap to the underlying tissue and preventing the leakage of fluid into the subretinal space. While treatment is almost always successful, this technique may promote the development of new breaks in other locations or cause re-detachment by forming excess scar tissue.

Scleral Buckling: Scleral buckles provide one of the most common surgical procedures for RD repair. They are flexible bands (similar to rubber bands) typically reserved for more severe retinal detachments. During this more invasive procedure, ophthalmologists place the buckle around the outside of the eye. This band applies pressure to the eye and reduces the distance between the retina and the underlying RPE/choroid, which often promotes re-attachment and allows excess fluid to drain from the subretinal space. This procedure is often combined with photo- or cryotherapy to prevent the retina from detaching after the operation.

Pneumatic Retinopexy: Rheumatic retinoplexy involves the injection of a gas or oil bubble into the eye. When positioned correctly, this bubble applies pressure to the retina, pressing it against the back of the eye and allowing for resorption of subretinal fluid. Typically, this surgical approach also includes photocoagulation or cryotherapy to prevent re-detachment. Post-operative care may require the patient to lie in specific positions depending on the location of the detachment to allow the bubble to press against the retina. After the retina heals, the bubble is often left in the patient to naturally dissolve or can be removed in a separate procedure.

Vitrectomy(Pars Plana Vitrectomyor 3-Port Vitrectomy): Vitrectomy is the removal of the vitreous gel that fills the inside of the eye. Typically, this involves the formation of three ports that the ophthalmologist uses to illuminate the space, remove the vitreous, and refill the cavity with saline. This technique is often used during scleral buckling and pneumatic retinoplexy procedures to reduce post-operative scarring and traction.

Perspective and Prospects

Retinal detachment repair is fairly well understood and has a success rate of 80-90%. However, re-detachment may occur in some patients due to excessive scarring or delayed treatment. While some patients have a full recovery, patients with more severe detachments may experience a permanent reduction in visual acuity or may not recover for several months. Current research revolves around identifying further risk factors, improving pharmacological management and post-operative care, and the development of new surgical techniques that may improve visual acuity for patients with severe detachments and reduce risk of re-detachment.

—*Derrick Cheng, Nicholas Koen and Ariel Choi; updated by Geraldine Marrocco*

For Further Information:

Fisher SK, Lewis GP, Linberg KA, et al. Cellular Remodeling in Mammalian Retina Induced by Retinal Detachment. 2005 May 1 [Updated 2007 Jul 3]. In: Kolb H, Fernandez E, Nelson R, editors. Webvision: The Organization of the Retina and Visual System [Internet]. Salt Lake City (UT): University of Utah Health Sciences Center; 1995-. Available from: https://www.ncbi.nlm.nih.gov/books/NBK11552

Kang, Hyong Kwon, and A J Luff. anagement of Retinal Detachment: A Guide for Non-Ophthalmologists. BMJ: British Medical Journal 336.7655 (2008): 1235 240. PMC. Web. 10 Sept. 2017.

Besharse, Joseph C., and Dean Bok. *The Retinaand Its Disorders*. Academic Press, 2011. Print.

Clark, Antony, et al. "Risk for Retinal Detachment After Phacoemulsification." Archives of Ophthalmology 130.7 (2012): 882 8. Print.

Fineman, Mitchell S., and Allen C. Ho. Retina. Philadelphia: Wolters Kluwer Health/Lippincott Williams & Wilkins, 2012. Print.

Kreissig, Ingrid, ed. Primary Retinal Detachment: Options for Repair. Heidelberg: Springer, 2005. Print.

Pournaras, Constantin, et al. "Surgical and Visual Outcome for Recurrent Retinal Detachment Surgery." Journal of Ophthalmology 2014 (2014): 1 . Web. 8 Jan. 2016.

Rogers, Adam H., and Jay S. Duker. Retina. Philadelphia: Mosby Elsevier, 2008. Print.

Soubrane, Gise, and Gabriel Coscas. "Pathogenesis of Serous Detachment of the Retina and Pigment Epithelium." Retina (2013): 618 3. Print.

Yorston, D., and S. Jalali. "Retinal Detachment in Developing Countries." Eye 16.4 (2002): 353 8. Print.

Retroviruses

Disease/Disorder

Anatomy or system affected: All

Specialties and related fields: Biochemistry, genetics, oncology, pathology, public health, virology

Definition: Ribonucleic acid (RNA) viruses that replicate by synthesizing a double-stranded deoxyribonucleic acid (DNA) molecule that integrates into the host genome. They are known to infect virtually all animals and sometimes cause serious disease, including cancer.

Key terms:

capsid: virally encoded protein that surrounds and protects the viral RNA genome

envelope: a lipid bilayer membrane that surrounds the retrovirus particle

glycoprotein: a protein to which is attached one or more sugar molecules

integrase: a virally encoded enzyme that catalyzes the integration of viral double-stranded DNA into the host genome

matrix: the layer of virally encoded protein that surrounds the viral capsid

nucleoprotein: a virally encoded protein that is directly associated with the viral nucleic acid

oncogene: a gene or DNA segment that can cause cancer

oncogenic: having the potential to cause cancer, as in oncogenic retroviruses

positive sense RNA (+RNA): an RNA molecule that can serve as a template for protein synthesis

reverse transcriptase: an enzyme that synthesizes double-stranded DNA from single-stranded RNA

src: a gene found in Rous Sarcoma Virus that confers on the virus the ability to transform normal cells into cancer cells

tRNA: an RNA molecule that attaches to an amino acid and interacts with the ribosome during protein synthesis; in retroviruses it serves as a primer for reverse transcriptase

Biology of Retroviruses

Retroviruses are members of the viral family Retroviridae. They are enveloped, positive sense (+) RNA viruses about 100 nanometers in diameter that replicate within the host's cytoplasm through a double-stranded DNA intermediate that is integrated into the host genome. In addition to the +RNA, there is a cellular tRNA hydrogen bonded to the +RNA that serves as a primer for reverse transcriptase.

The viral RNA genome, its associated nucleoprotein, reverse transcriptase, and integrase are surrounded by a protein capsid. Immediately external to the capsid is the matrix protein. The outer layer of the retrovirus is a lipid bilayer envelope derived from the host's plasma membrane that is acquired as the virus emerges from the host cell. Within the envelope are two glycoproteins that are encoded by the virus genome and serve as plasma membrane attachment sites during entry into the cell.

The retrovirus genome consists of two 7 kilobase to 11 kilobase +RNA molecules that code for only a few proteins, including *gag*, which codes for the matrix, capsid, and nucleoprotein; *pol*, which codes for reverse transcriptase, RNAse, integrase, and a protease; and *env*, which codes for the envelope glycoproteins.

The retrovirus binds to plasma membrane receptors via the viral envelope glycoproteins. When the retrovirus enters the cell, the viral RNA is released along with its reverse transcriptase. A double-stranded DNA is synthesized from the +RNA using viral reverse transcriptase. Integrase catalyzes the incorporation of the double-stranded DNA molecule into the host genome. When integrated, the viral DNA is referred to as a provirus and replicates with the host genome. Host RNA polymerase transcribes the viral genes, making copies of the viral genome and mRNA molecules that can be translated into viral proteins. Viral RNA and proteins are assembled into new viral particles that emerge from the plasma membrane by budding.

Some retroviruses such as Rous sarcoma virus (RSV), feline leukemia virus (FLV), and mouse mammary tumor virus (MMTV) can induce tumors in their host species. More than twenty-five cancer-causing (oncogenic) retroviruses have been isolated. The retrovirus gains oncogenic potential when it inadvertently acquires a eukaryotic gene during infection. Although the eukaryotic gene may not be oncogenic when first acquired, after several generations it may mutate or otherwise become altered, transforming it into one that is oncogenic. Retroviruses such as FLV that do not carry an oncogene can still transform by either disrupting the function of a normal gene by integrating within it or by integrating next to it so that the neighboring gene can use the viral promoter, resulting in gene overexpression and cellular proliferation.

Perspective and Prospects

The study of retroviruses dates to 1910 with the work of Peyton Rous, who discovered that certain sarcomas in chickens are caused by an agent later identified as a virus. The virus was later named Rous sarcoma virus. In 1970, the laboratories of Howard Temin and David Baltimore independently discovered that certain RNA viruses have an enzyme, now known as reverse transcriptase, that permit the viruses to reverse transcribe their RNA genomes into double-stranded DNA. In the early 1970s, the laboratory of J. Michael Bishop and Harold Varmus demonstrated that Rous sarcoma virus has a gene, now known as *src*, responsible for transforming normal cells into tumor cells. Uninfected cells, including human cells, have a normal *src* gene that is related to the viral *src* gene. In the past, an RSV infected a chicken and incorporated the host *src* gene into its own genome. The *src* gene acquired by the virus became altered over time so that it now causes cancer when an RSV infects a chicken cell.

There are many examples of retroviruses, including human T-cell leukemia virus (HTLV), the first pathogenic human retrovirus discovered in 1980 by Bernard J. Poiesz, Robert Gallo, and their colleagues at the National Institutes of Health and by Mitsuaki Yoshida in Japan. Human immunodeficiency virus (HIV), which causes acquired immunodeficiency syndrome (AIDS), is also a retrovirus; it was discovered in 1983 by Luc Montagnier, Françoise Barré-Sinoussi, and their colleagues at the Pasteur Institute in France.

Since reverse transcriptase does not have the proofreading activities associated with DNA polymerase, retroviruses mutate and evolve more rapidly than DNA viruses, making the development of drugs and vaccines difficult.

Recombinant retroviruses are often used as vectors for genetic engineering. Retroviruses that are modified by removing the genes that make them harmful and replacing them with normal eukaryotic genes can be used to deliver a normal copy of a gene to a defective cell. The DNA copy of the recombinant retrovirus can integrate into the host genome and genetically modify the cell.

—*Charles L. Vigue, Ph.D.*

See also Acquired immunodeficiency syndrome (AIDS); Cancer; Genetic engineering; Human immunodeficiency virus (HIV); Leukemia; Oncology; Tumors; Viral infections; Zoonoses.

For Further Information:
Cullen, Bryan R. *Human Retroviruses.* New York: Oxford University Press, 1993.
Dudley, Jaquelin. *Retroviruses and Insights into Cancer.* New York: Springer, 2011.
Gallo, Robert. *Virus Hunting: AIDS, Cancer, and the Human Retrovirus-A Story of Scientific Discovery.* New York: Basic Books, 1991.
Gallo, Robert C., Dominique Stehelin, and Oliviero E. Varnier. *Retroviruses and Human Pathology.* Totowa, N.J.: Humana Press, 1986.
Holmes, Edward C. *The Evolution and Emergence of RNA Viruses.* New York: Oxford University Press, 2009.
Kurth, Reinhard, and Norbert Bannert, eds. *Retroviruses: Molecular Biology, Genomics, and Pathogenesis.* Norfolk, England: Caister Academic Press, 2010.
Singh, Sunit K., and Daniel Ruzek, eds. *Neuroviral Infections: RNA Viruses and Retroviruses.* Boca Raton, Fla.: CRC Press, 2013.

Reye's syndrome
Disease/Disorder

Anatomy or system affected: Brain, circulatory system, heart, kidneys, liver, nervous system, urinary system

Specialties and related fields: Emergency medicine, internal medicine, neurology, pediatrics

Definition: A somewhat rare, noncontagious disease of the liver and central nervous system that strikes individuals under the age of eighteen.

Causes and Symptoms

The exact cause of Reye syndrome has not been determined, but the majority of patients develop the disease while recovering from a mild viral illness, such as chickenpox, influenza, or a minor respiratory illness. It is theorized that the virus combines with another unknown substance or substances in the body to produce a damaging poison. Reye syndrome usually occurs in children between four and twelve years of age. For reasons not well understood, the taking of salicylates, such as aspirin, during viral illnesses may precipitate the development of this potentially fatal illness.

The first symptom of the disease is a sudden onset of vomiting, then high fever, headache, and drowsiness. Blood sugar levels drop, while blood ammonia and acidity levels increase. As the disease progresses, alternating states of excitation and confused sleepiness may occur, as well as convulsions and a loss of consciousness. In the final stages of the disease, damage occurs to the liver, kidneys, and brain. The liver swells and develops large amounts of fat deposits. The brain cells swell and pressure builds in the

---

Information on Reye's Syndrome

Causes: Unclear; likely related to mild viral infection and possibly aspirin use

Symptoms: Sudden onset of vomiting, high fever, headache, drowsiness, alternating excitation and confused sleepiness, convulsions, loss of consciousness

Duration: Acute

Treatments: Fluids, glucose, and other nutrients; medications (mannitol); surgery to reduce pressure in skull

---

skull, followed by coma, permanent brain damage, and, in some cases, death.

Reye syndrome is often mistaken for a number of other disorders, including meningitis, encephalitis, diabetic shock, or poisoning, potentially complicating the early diagnosis that is crucial for treating this condition.

Treatment and Therapy

There is no known cure for Reye syndrome. Early recognition and specialized care may be lifesaving. If a child begins to exhibit symptoms of Reye syndrome shortly after a viral illness, then competent medical care must be sought immediately. Treatment consists of helping the victim survive the first few days of the illness through intake of fluids, glucose, and other nutrients. If the patient survives the first three or four days, the symptoms usually subside and recovery follows. The degree of recovery, however, depends upon the degree of brain swelling of the patient during the illness. Some children suffer permanent brain damage.

Medication, such as mannitol, or surgery will reduce the pressure within the skull if it reaches dangerous levels. Although it has not been proven that aspirin causes or promotes Reye's syndrome, based on a variety of medical studies, it is recommended that aspirin not be given to children with viral infections, especially chickenpox and influenza. With few exceptions, acetaminophen or ibuprofen are safe alternatives.

Perspective and Prospects

Reye syndrome was first described by an Australian pathologist, R. D. K. Reye, in 1963. In the early 1980s, approximately 50 percent of the cases were fatal, but improved diagnosis and treatment of the disease had reduced that number to less than 10 percent by 2006.

—*Alvin K. Benson, Ph.D.;*
updated by Lenela Glass-Godwin, M.W.S.

See also Brain damage; Chickenpox; Influenza; Pediatrics; Viral infections.

For Further Information:

Badash, Michelle. "Reye's Syndrome." *Health Library*, November 26, 2012.

Bhutta, Adnan T. "Reye's Syndrome: Down but Not Out." *Southern Medical Journal* 96, no. 1 (January 1, 2003): 43-46.

Parker, James N. and Phillip M. Parker.*Reye's Syndrome: A Medical Dictionary, Bibliography, and Annotated Research Guide to Internet References*. ICON Group, 2007.

Kliegman, Robert and Waldo E. Nelson, eds. *Nelson Textbook of Pediatrics*. 19th ed. Philadelphia: Saunders/Elsevier, 2011.

Taubman, Bruce. *Your Child's Symptoms: A Parent's Guide to Understanding Pediatric Medicine*. New York: Simon & Schuster, 1992.

Woolf, Alan D., et al., eds. *The Children's Hospital Guide to Your Child's Health and Development*. Cambridge, Mass.: Perseus, 2002.

Rh factor

Biology

Anatomy or system affected: Blood, immune system

Specialties and related fields: Embryology, genetics, hematology, neonatology, obstetrics, serology

Definition: Also called the Rhesus factor; an important chemical sometimes found on the surface of red blood cells in humans, the presence or absence of which can complicate pregnancy and blood transfusions.

Key terms:

agglutination: a clumping of blood cells caused by antibodies joining with antigens on the cell surfaces

antibody: a protein made by B lymphocytes that is found in blood; a specific antibody binds with a specific antigen

antigen: a substance that is capable of causing an immune response if it is foreign to the body that it enters; antigens may be free or located on cell surfaces

antisera: the fluid portion of blood that contains specific antibodies

blood type: a blood classification group based on the presence or absence of certain antigens on red blood cells

serum: the fluid part of blood without red blood cells and clotting factors

transfusion: the injection of whole blood or its parts into the bloodstream

Structure and Functions

Blood replacement in emergency or surgery can be critical: blood loss exceeding 40 percent can lead to a condition called shock in which the heart cannot pump efficiently, resulting in death. In the search for human blood replacements, scientists have found that animal blood is not compatible. More important, they have discovered that even blood from different humans does not always mix. Sometimes the red blood cells will agglutinate, or settle out of the plasma in clumps. Consequently, these red blood cells are destroyed by the body, and jaundice and death may follow. To prevent this reaction, human blood must be classified into types and cross-matched. The two most important general groupings are the ABO and Rh types.

Human blood is classified into types according to the antigens that might be present on the red blood cells as a result of heredity. Antigens are usually large, complex molecules made of protein alone, protein with attached carbohydrates, or lipids with attached fatty acids and alcohol. They may be free molecules, as in the case of toxins released by invading bacteria, or they may be located on a cell's surface and serve to label or mark the cell. The markers attached to cell surfaces identify the cell as "self" or "foreign." Such antigens are the basis of blood types.

Karl Landsteiner showed that there are four major blood types, based on two antigens that might be present or missing. He called the markers A and B. People with both markers on their cells are called type AB, people with one of the two are type A or type B, and those without either marker were originally called C but later changed to O. Landsteiner's system of classifying blood according to the presence of the A and B antigens is now termed the ABO system. Landsteiner demonstrated the chemistry of the antigens and the antibodies by mixing blood from himself and coworkers in his laboratory and observing that some combinations agglutinated.

The next major breakthrough came with Philip Levine and Rufus Stetson's study of the blood of a woman whose fetus had died six weeks before birth. The mother's immune system had produced antibodies against the Rh factors on the blood cells of her developing child. She was Rh negative while her child was positive, having inherited an Rh-positive gene from the father. The positive blood of the child caused the mother's immune system to react. The importance of the discovery was twofold. It not only explained why some babies suffered from an immune reaction in their mothers but also showed that blood transfusions could be typed as ABO compatible and still fail if the Rh factor was not considered.

The term *Rh factor* came about because of a misunderstanding. Working independently and believing that they had found the same factor first in their laboratory animals, Landsteiner and Alexander Wiener claimed discovery and named the Rh antigen after the rhesus monkey. They injected the monkey blood into rabbits, and the rabbits developed antibodies against the foreign factor. Hypothesizing that closely related primates might share the factor, the rabbit antibodies in a serum were then mixed with samples of human blood. Further work verified that there was indeed a new important human factor, but it differed from the one in monkeys. By this time, however, it was too late to change the misleading name. To clear up the confusion, the factor in humans kept the name of Rh factor, while the monkey antigen was labeled the LW factor.

Even if it is inappropriately named, the Rh factor is an important discovery. People with the marker on their blood cells are Rh positive, while people without it are Rh negative. Rh-negative people can give blood to people who are positive if all other antigens such as those found in the ABO types are compatible. If the reverse is attempted, however, the Rh-negative person will develop antibodies against the Rh marker. Clumping of the red blood cells will occur, and illness and death are likely.

Discovery of the presence of these markers was the key to understanding both the blood types and what happens in immune responses. When a foreign protein or antigen enters the body, antibodies are produced by the immune system and released into the blood and lymph. These antibodies are specific in the sense that a particular antibody will only combine with a particular antigen. (If a particular antigen is present on a person's own blood cells, the individual would not normally produce and carry antibodies for this molecule; otherwise, the antibodies would attack the person's own blood cells.) The antibodies fasten the cells together in what is called agglutination. Agglutinated cells are destroyed by white blood cells.

Combining the ABO and Rh systems, a person could be A+, A-, AB+, AB-, B+, B-, O+, or O-. Because an AB+ individual has A, B, and Rh antigens and no antibodies against them, this person can receive blood from all others. An O- individual has no antigens and is a universal donor, assuming that the O- person has no other important antigen differences from other, more rare types. The importance of the ABO and Rh systems is shown by the standard practice of hospitals in typing and sorting by these systems.

Unlike the ABO types, Rh-negative blood does not normally contain antibodies for positive blood unless the person has been previously exposed (sensitized) to positive blood. The A and B antibodies are developed early in people because A and B antigens are common in the environment. They are found not only on red blood cells but also in milk, colostrum, saliva, and other body fluids. Should a transfusion of Rh-positive blood be given to an Rh-negative person, the negative blood produces the antibody, which will have a violent reaction with the next similar transfusion.

The Rh factor is inherited, as are all blood types. A person inherits one gene involving the factor from each parent. If the person inherits two genes (DD) for the factor, it will be present on the red blood cells. If a person inherits one gene for the factor and one that does not produce it (Dd), the individual will still be Rh positive. If a person inherits two recessive genes (dd), that person will be Rh negative. Consequently, the gene for production of the Rh factor is called dominant; the other gene is recessive.

The original Rh factor can also be called the D factor. Additional investigation has shown that the entire Rh factor is not a single factor caused by one pair of genes; rather, at least three pairs of genes may be involved. Antisera have been found not only for the most reactive D antigen but also for four other factors. The situation can be explained by imagining Rh to be determined by a combination of three genes, which are probably closely linked on the same chromosome. Ronald Fisher labeled the genes C, c, D, d, E, and e. An Rh gene complex could then be any of these combinations: CDE, CDe, CdE, Cde, cdE, cDe, cde, or cDE. An individual would have two of these complexes, one from each parent. The number of different Rh types then reaches sixty-four.

To illustrate, a person with CDe/cdE would test Rh positive using standard anti-D sera because of the D gene; so would people with any combination of C, c, E, and e with at least one D. Nevertheless, the other nearby genes can cause agglutination problems. Each of them, except d, produces an antigen on the red blood cells. The antigens cause antisera to form in human blood that recognizes them as foreign. One can also choose to think of the situation as having eight different alleles for Rh.

Then a single symbol can stand for each combination: r =

Rh Incompatibility

First pregnancy

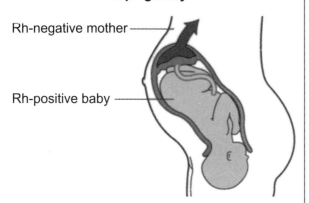

Rh-negative mother

Rh-positive baby

During childbirth, the baby's blood enters the mother's circulation, causing antibodies to form against Rh-positive blood.

Second pregnancy

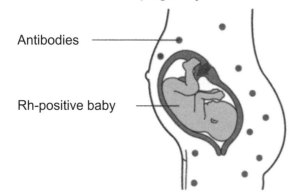

Antibodies

Rh-positive baby

If a second baby is Rh positive, these antibodies may cross the placenta and destroy the baby's red blood cells.

cde, $r' = Cde$, $r'' = CdE$, $r_Y = cdE$, $R_0 = cDe$, $R_1 = CDe$, $R_2 = cDE$, and $R_Z = CDE$. Any r is an Rh-negative combination in the classic sense, and any R is Rh positive. Additional discoveries of new Rh antisera have caused some investigators to hypothesize about the possibility of more than thirty antigens, some that are variant forms of the above and some that require more genes.

A 1948 paper by R. R. Race, A. E. Mourant, Sylvia D. Lawler, and Ruth Sanger reported that R_1r (or CDe/cde) is the most common Rh blood gene combination in England, at about 33 percent of those tested. The R_1R_1 (or CDe/CDe) combination follows at 16.6 percent, rr (or cde/cde) at 15.8 percent, R_1R_2 (or CDe/cDE) at 12.9 percent, R_2r (or cDE/cde) at 12.8 percent, and R_2R_2 (or cDE/cDE) at 2.7 percent. All the other combinations total about 6 percent.

Rh has turned out to be quite complex. Nevertheless, the system can be understood and applied at a very basic and useful level of Rh positive or Rh negative, which involves

consideration of the very reactive D antigen on the blood cells. In that case, the Rh symbol is often labeled *Rh0*.

Disorders and Diseases

The discovery of the ABO system allowed transfusions to proceed with some confidence of success during World War I. Still, some transfusions produced problems, and some minor independent blood-type systems (MNS, P) were discovered. Clearly, people were members of more than one blood-type system. The additional discovery of the highly reactive Rh factor or D antigen was critical for safe transfusions.

Another immediate application of the discovery was in the area of childbirth. Rh incompatibility explained why some babies either died at birth or were born in serious trouble. The attack of the mother's antibodies on the fetal blood cells can lead to various forms of hemolytic disease of newborns, or erythroblastosis fetalis. Incompatibility between mother and child is also one of the causes of spontaneous miscarriage early in pregnancy. Knowing the existence of the Rh factor has saved countless infants.

Recall that the Rh factor is inherited. If an Rh-negative woman (dd) marries an Rh-positive man (DD or Dd), the child may be Rh positive. During pregnancy, there is no direct blood flow from mother to child because red blood cells cannot cross the placenta. At some time during the pregnancy or at birth, however, blood will probably mix, and the mother will then be sensitized. She then will form antibodies against the Rh factor. Many of these antibodies are of the IgG type and are smaller than A or B antibodies (IgM). The small IgG antibodies can cross the placenta into the blood of the fetus. The first Rh-positive child usually escapes harm by being born, but a second positive child will be in great danger, as the mother's preformed antibodies will cross the placenta and attack the red blood cells of the fetus. Blood cells are likely to be broken open, releasing hemoglobin. The fetus will become anemic and jaundiced and may suffer brain damage or be stillborn.

The occurrence of erythroblastosis fetalis can be prevented if an Rh-negative mother is given an injection of rhesus gamma globulin (RhoGAM) within seventy-two hours of the delivery of her first Rh-positive child. This approach was developed by C. A. Clark, P. M. Sheppard, and others working at Liverpool University. The gamma globulin destroys the fetal blood cells in the mother and prevents the production of antibodies that would affect the next positive child. Miscarriages or abortions of Rh-positive pregnancies count as an exposure to the antigen and can cause the mother's immune system to react. Therefore, these events also require the injection to protect future children. Also, any Rh-negative woman accidentally given a transfusion of positive blood would be in danger herself, as would the fetuses in any of her future pregnancies.

Amniocentesis, a sampling of fluid from the sac around the developing fetus, can reveal such difficulties as Rh incompatibility. An Rh-negative woman can also be given a series of blood tests (Rh titers) during her pregnancy. If the tests show that the antibodies are increasing in number, intrauterine transfusion of negative blood may be attempted. Moreover, if the child is nearing full term, delivery may be induced to prevent the blood of the fetus from being completely destroyed. If the child is born with signs of circulatory problems, a blood transfusion can help.

Anthony Smith notes that the ABO type has an effect on trouble with Rh during pregnancy. If the mother is Rh negative, the child is positive, and their ABO types are also incompatible, then the Rh reaction is diminished. The reason may be that the mother already has antibodies against incompatible ABO types. When the red blood cells leak into the mother's circulatory system, they are immediately destroyed by already-existing maternal ABO antibodies before any antibodies against Rh factor can be formed.

Some interesting associations with Rh have been discovered but are not yet understood. Typhoid, mumps, mononucleosis, and viral meningitis are more common in Rh-negative people. Viral diseases tend to be more common in the nonantigenic types of both the ABO and Rh systems (O and Rh negative).

Perspective and Prospects

Few successful blood transfusions took place before 1900. In that year, Karl Landsteiner discovered that there are different types of blood. Some would mix, while others would clump. He and his coworkers identified four major human blood groups: A, B, AB, and O. Even so, eight years passed before the first transfusion using Landsteiner's ABO types was attempted. Transfusions became more likely to succeed. People could be typed by the antigens on their blood cells, and donors could be matched with the patient. Yet sometimes the transfusions still did not work as predicted. In 1930, Landsteiner won the Nobel Prize in Physiology or Medicine for his discovery of ABO blood types.

Landsteiner and Philip Levine discovered the MNS types in 1927; these are not important in transfusions but are of great help in cases of doubtful paternity. When beginning his own work, Levine agreed with Landsteiner not to study new blood groups, as Landsteiner had reserved that project for himself. Nevertheless, in 1939, Levine and Rufus E. Stetson published a report showing that the blood of a mother with a stillborn child was able to react hemolytically with 80 out of 104 ABO-compatible donors. They correctly concluded that the mother's blood lacked an antigen that many others had: an unknown marker that was independent of the known ABO, MNS, and P blood groups. Levine and Stetson had correctly analyzed the problem but did not name their new antigen. Clearly, they had discovered what would be called the Rh factor.

Less than a year later, Landsteiner and Alexander Wiener immunized rabbits and guinea pigs with the blood of the monkey *Macacus rhesus*. They found that the resulting rabbit serum agglutinated not only the rhesus monkey blood but also about 85 percent of blood samples from people in New York City. They called these people Rh positive and the remaining 15 percent Rh negative. Wiener and H. R. Peters attempted to show that the Rh antibody in the rabbits was the same as that found in the serum of people who had suffered incompatible transfusion reactions not explained by ABO blood typing.

A bitter exchange ensued between Levine and Wiener about who had discovered the Rh factor. This was resolved when it was shown that the antigen on the rhesus monkey cells was not the same as the human Rh factor. Unfortunately, the name Rh was too well established to be changed by this time. To avoid further confusion, Levine suggested that the factor in the monkeys be called the LW factor after Landsteiner and Wiener. Despite this controversy, R. R. Race and Ruth Sanger called the discovery of the Rh factor the most important event in blood-group science since the discovery of the ABO system forty years before.

Soon, different investigators were able to derive sera with different antibodies for the Rh factor. Clearly, the Rh factor was not simply a single antigen. In 1943, Ronald Fisher studied the different antisera that had been developed and proposed that eight different Rh gene complexes were involved.

The existence of the Rh factor is useful in other ways. In addition to transfusions, another application of blood typing (including the presence or absence of the Rh factor) is in criminology. Blood left at the scene of a crime can be powerful evidence against a suspect. Blood types can also eliminate individuals as possible fathers in paternity suits. For example, if both parents are Rh negative, the child cannot be Rh positive. A more complete typing of the blood would allow further strong evidence. Such typing does not prove paternity, however; it only shows whether paternity is possible.

Blood typing also allows anthropologists to develop theories about the relationships among various human groups and how people may have migrated. The breakdown between being Rh positive or negative varies among the races. The Basques, a group of people near the Bay of Biscay between Spain and France, are only 64 percent positive, while about 85 percent of the Caucasian population in general is Rh positive. Races other than Caucasian are generally nearly 100 percent Rh positive. According to Sir Peter Medawar, however, the advantages of being one type or another are obscure. Why there are so many different blood types remains an interesting question.

The discoveries of the ABO types and the Rh factor stand as fundamental achievements in medical science. Even though many other types continue to be uncovered, ABO and Rh determinations remain the most basic steps in matching blood for many purposes, especially for safe transfusions.

—*Paul R. Boehlke, Ph.D.*

See also Amniocentesis; Blood and blood disorders; Blood banks; Blood testing; Embryology; Genetic counseling; Genetics and inheritance; Hematology; Hematology, pediatric; Hemolytic disease of the newborn; Neonatology; Obstetrics; Perinatology; Phlebotomy; Pregnancy and gestation; Transfusion.

For Further Information:

Alan, Rick, Andrea Chisholm, and Brian Randall. "Rh Incompatibility and Isoimmunization." *Health Library*, March 18, 2013.
Bibel, Debra Jan, ed. *Milestones in Immunology: A Historical Exploration*. New York: Springer, 1988.

Jandl, James H. *Blood: Textbook of Hematology.* 2d ed. Boston: Little, Brown, 1996.

Martin, Richard J., Avroy A. Fanaroff, and Michele C. Walsh, eds. *Fanaroff and Martin's Neonatal-Perinatal Medicine: Diseases of the Fetus and Infant.* 2 vols. 9th ed. St. Louis: Mosby/Elsevier, 2011.

Moore, Keith L., T. V. N. Persaud, and Mark G. Torchia. *The Developing Human: Clinically Oriented Embryology.* 9th ed. Philadelphia: Saunders/Elsevier, 2013.

Page, Jake. *Blood: The River of Life.* Washington, D.C.: US News Books, 1981.

Race, R. R., A. E. Mourant, Sylvia D. Lawler, and Ruth Sanger. "The Rh Chromosome Frequencies in England." *Blood* 3, no. 6 (June 1948): 689-695.

"Rh Factor Blood Test." *Mayo Clinic*, June 16, 2012.

Rodak, Bernadette F., George A. Fritsma, and Elaine M. Keohane, eds. *Hematology: Clinical Principles and Applications.* 4th ed. St. Louis, Mo.: Saunders/Elsevier, 2012.

Starr, Douglas P. *Blood: An Epic History of Medicine and Commerce.* New York: Alfred A. Knopf, 1998.

Rheumatic fever

Disease/Disorder

Anatomy or system affected: Heart

Specialties and related fields: Cardiology, family medicine, immunology, pediatrics

Definition: An inflammatory disease of the heart that may follow a streptococcal throat infection.

Key terms:

B hemolytic streptococci: streptococcal bacteria that secrete an enzyme capable of dissolving red blood cells

pharyngitis: inflammation of the pharynx (throat), which is sometimes associated with streptococcal infection

polyarthritis: pain and inflammation in multiple joints

rheumatic heart disease: damage to heart muscle or valves as a result of rheumatic fever

rheumatic nodules: accumulations of white cells in soft tissue or over bony areas in patients with rheumatic fever

Causes and Symptoms

Rheumatic fever is an inflammatory disease affecting the heart that may follow infection by the bacterium *Streptococcus pyogenes.* The streptococci constitute a large number of gram-positive cocci, some of which are pathogens. They were originally classified in the 1930s by Rebecca Lancefield into groups based on characteristics of carbohydrates and proteins in their cell walls. *S. pyogenes* is the sole species of streptococcus in group A. Group A streptococcus causes a wide array of illnesses, most notably pharyngitis (causing strep throat) and impetigo. The most serious complication associated with infection by specific strains of *S. pyogenes* is rheumatic fever.

Rheumatic fever may develop one to five weeks after recovery from a streptococcal infection, often strep throat. The onset is sudden, with the patient exhibiting severe polyarthritis, fever, and abdominal pain. There may be chest pain and heart palpitations. Transient circular lesions may develop on the skin. Rheumatic nodules may be noted on joints and tendons, along the spine, and even on the head. Sydenham's chorea, the exhibition of irregular body movements, may also appear during the course of the illness. In severe cases, the patient may become incapacitated.

Information on Rheumatic Fever

Causes: Bacterial infection

Symptoms: Severe joint pain, fever, abdominal pain, chest pain, heart palpitations, transient circular skin lesions

Duration: Acute

Treatments: Bed rest, increased fluid intake, limited physical activity, steroids or other anti-inflammatory drugs

---

While there is no specific diagnostic test for rheumatic fever, the combination of clinical symptoms may suggest its onset, particularly if there was a recent sore throat. The production of serum antibodies against streptococcal antigens is also indicative of rheumatic fever.

Most of the time, the symptoms subside with bed rest. Mild cases generally last three or four weeks, while more severe cases may last several months. A single bout with rheumatic fever may be followed by recurrent episodes with additional infections by B hemolytic streptococci.

Rheumatic fever is an autoimmune phenomenon. Certain proteins in specific strains of group A streptococcus contain segments that cross-react with heart tissue, including that found in muscle and valves. As the body responds to the streptococcal infection, the immune response may also involve cardiac tissue, resulting in inflammation and possible damage. Since the immune reaction occurs over a period of days to weeks, the onset of rheumatic fever may be considerably removed from the actual infection.

Treatment and Therapy

Because rheumatic fever represents an autoimmune reaction to an earlier streptococcal infection, antibiotic treatment is of limited value. Penicillin or similar antibiotics may be administered for their prophylactic value, preventing further streptococcal infection and recurrence of the illness during the recovery period.

Bed rest and restriction of activities is recommended during the course of the illness. The patient should receive large amounts of fluids. Steroids or other anti-inflammatory compounds may also be administered in response to severe polyarthritis or valvular inflammation. The duration of such inflammation is generally no more than two weeks.

Repeated infections with streptococci may trigger additional episodes of rheumatic fever, so antibiotics may be administered on a regular basis. While not all streptococcal infections trigger rheumatic fever, any previous cardiac episode is likely to be repeated after an additional streptococcal infection, often resulting in greater damage. For this reason, prophylactic antibiotic treatment may be long term.

If rheumatic heart disease has resulted in permanent damage to heart tissue, additional therapies may be necessary. Often, such damage may not be apparent for years. Thickening or scarring of the heart valves, particularly the mitral and aortic valves, may necessitate valve replacement at some point in the future.

Perspective and Prospects

Thomas Sydenham, called the "English Hippocrates," in 1685 provided the first description of what was probably rheumatic fever. He also described what has become known as Sydenham's chorea, now known to be symptomatic of rheumatic fever. In 1797, London doctor Matthew Baillie noted the damage to heart valves among patients suffering from the illness. The association of rheumatic fever with bacterial infection, however, was not established until well into the twentieth century.

In part this delay resulted from the inability to isolate an organism either from the diseased heart or from blood of patients with rheumatic fever. In 1928, Homer Swift, a New York physician, suggested that rheumatic fever was an allergic response following streptococcal infections. A few years later, the role of serologic group A, B hemolytic streptococci as the actual agent associated with the disease was established by Alvin Coburn.

A decline in the incidence of rheumatic fever in the United States began in the first decades of the twentieth century. The reason is unclear in this period before antibiotics; the decrease may have been attributable in part to the presence of less virulent strains of the bacteria. With the introduction of penicillin in the 1940s as an effective treatment for streptococcal infections, the incidence of acute rheumatic fever continued its decline.

A resurgence of the disease was first noted in the 1980s. The reasons remain unclear. Since different strains of streptococci differ in their ability to induce rheumatic fever, it is suspected that the increase may have resulted from the introduction of new bacterial strains into the population. The disease has also been seen to cluster in families, suggesting that a genetic predisposition may exist in the general population which contributes to the rise in numbers of cases. Fortunately, the streptococci have not yet established the widespread resistance to antibiotics seen among other bacteria, and rheumatic fever as a sequela to streptococcal pharyngitis may be prevented with proper treatment.

—*Richard Adler, Ph.D.*

See also Antibiotics; Arrhythmias; Bacterial infections; Cardiology; Cardiology, pediatric; Childhood infectious diseases; Endocarditis; Fever; Heart; Heart disease; Heart failure; Heart transplantation; Heart valve replacement; Pharyngitis; Sore throat; Strep throat; Streptococcal infections.

For Further Information:

English, Peter C. *Rheumatic Fever in America and Britain: A Biological, Epidemiological, and Medical History.* New Brunswick, N.J.: Rutgers University Press, 1999.

Kiple, Kenneth F., ed. *The Cambridge World History of Human Disease.* New York: Cambridge University Press, 1999.

McCance, Kathryn L., and Sue M. Huether. *Pathophysiology: The Biologic Basis for Disease in Adults and Children.* 6th ed. St. Louis, Mo.: Mosby/Elsevier, 2010.

Murray, Patrick R., Ken S. Rosenthal, and Michael A. Pfaller. *Medical Microbiology.* 7th ed. Philadelphia: Mosby/Elsevier, 2013.

"Rheumatic Fever." *Health Library,* March 15, 2013.

"Rheumatic Fever." *Mayo Clinic,* January 21, 2011.

Steeg, Carl N., Christine A. Walsh, and Julie S. Glickstein. "Rheumatic Fever: No Cause for Complacence." *Patient Care* 34, no. 14 (July 30, 2000): 40-61.

Woolf, Alan D., et al., eds. *The Children's Hospital Guide to Your Child's Health and Development.* Cambridge, Mass.: Perseus, 2002.

Rheumatoid arthritis

Disease/Disorder

Also known as: Rheumatism

Anatomy or system affected: Heart, immune system, musculoskeletal system, respiratory system

Specialties and related fields: Geriatrics and gerontology, immunology, rheumatology

Definition: A chronic, systemic, and inflammatory autoimmune disease that affects the synovial membranes of joints and other organs in the body.

Key terms:

autoimmune: relating to an immune response by the body against itself

erythrocyte sedimentation rate: a screening test for an active inflammation in the body

metacarpophalangeal: referring to the joints of the fingers closest to the body, or knuckles

proximal interphalangeal: referring to the middle joints of the fingers

rheumatoid factor: an antibody found in the blood that identifies an inflammatory process

rheumatoid nodule: a small hard growth under the skin of the hands and elbows that may be present in those with rheumatoid arthritis

Sjögren's syndrome: dry eyes and mouth related to rheumatoid arthritis

symmetric: occurring on both sides of the body at the same time

synovial membrane: a sac in a joint space filled with synovial fluid that reduces friction during movement of the joint

white blood cell: a component of the blood that indicates an infective or inflammatory process occurring in the body

Causes and Symptoms

Most experts believe that rheumatoid arthritis (RA) occurs as a result of some type of stress on the body that triggers an autoimmune response characterized by chronic inflammation, swelling, and pain in joint spaces as cartilage erodes and bony cysts cause deformities in the joints and joint motion is lost. Certain genes associated with the immune system have been found to increase the possibility of developing RA.

Initially, persons with RA may have general, vague complaints such as fatigue, weakness, weight loss, anorexia, low-grade fever, and tingling in the hands and feet during the weeks or months after some traumatic physical event in their life. Joint stiffness lessens as the day progresses but may recur after inactivity and is worse after strenuous activity. Although all joints may be affected, the proximal interphalangeal or metacarpophalangeal joints and joints of the wrists, knees, ankles, and toes are most often affected. Rheumatoid nodules may be found on the hands and elbows. Sjögren's syndrome may also be present. There is also potential for renal, cardiovascular, pulmonary, neurological, and ophthalmological involvement. RA is a disease of remissions and exacerbations and therefore should be monitored regularly.

Diagnosis of RA involves identifying at least one painful or swollen joint that has been that way for at least six weeks, as well as a variety of blood tests intended to identify autoimmune disease. These tests may measure rheumatoid factor, anti-citrullinated protein antibodies, erythrocyte sedimentation rate, and c-reactive protein. X-rays to identify erosions, bony calcifications, and narrowing in affected joints may also be undertaken.

Treatment and Therapy

The goals of rheumatoid arthritis treatment are to reduce inflammation and pain, slow the disease process, improve function, and maintain quality of life. Medications are used for their analgesic, anti-inflammatory, cytotoxic, and immunosuppressive effects. The three main categories of medication used in the treatment of RA are nonsteroidal anti-inflammatory drugs (NSAIDs), disease-modifying antirheumatic drugs (DMARDs), and glucocorticoids. NSAIDS such as aspirin, ibuprofen, and naproxen reduce joint pain and swelling but do nothing to slow the progression of RA. DMARDS, which include methotrexate, hydroxychloroquine, sulfasalazine, gold salts, minocycline, azothiaprine, cyclosporine, and leflunomide, can actually slow the progression of RA. Glucocorticoids are effective for rapidly reducing joint inflammation. Biologic disease response modifiers are a new class of drugs targeting areas of the immune system that cause joint and tissue damage. Examples include etanercept, infliximab, adalimumab, and anakinra. Research has shown that fish

---

Information on Rheumatoid Arthritis

Causes: Autoimmune response, possibly resulting from stress on body, genetic factors

Symptoms: Chronic inflammation, swelling, and pain in joint spaces; morning stiffness; fatigue; weakness; weight loss; anorexia, low-grade fever; tingling in hands and feet

Duration: Chronic

Treatments: NSAIDs (aspirin, ibuprofen, naproxen), DMARDs (methotrexate, hydroxychloroquine, sulfasalazine, gold salts, minocycline, azothiaprine, cyclosporine, leflunomide), glucocorticoids, surgical repair

---

oils containing omega-3 fatty acids may also decrease inflammation in joints.

Education for the management of RA includes isometric exercise, stress control, methods to protect joint integrity, and support groups that assist individuals and their families to maintain independence and to plan for care during exacerbations of RA. Surgical interventions to repair damaged joints and joint replacement are also part of RA therapy.

Perspective and Prospects

More than two million Americans suffer from rheumatoid arthritis, the majority of them women. The peak onset for RA is among people in their sixties. Juvenile rheumatoid arthritis occurs in children younger than sixteen years of age. Research has indicated a possible link between infections and the development of rheumatoid arthritis.

—Sharon W. Stark, R.N., A.P.R.N., D.N.Sc.

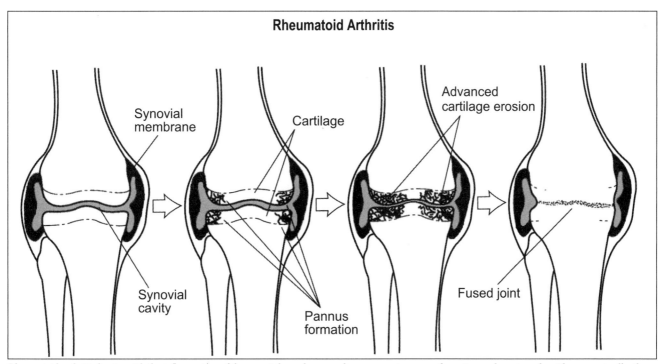

Rheumatoid Arthritis

Synovial membrane

Cartilage

Advanced cartilage erosion

Synovial cavity

Pannus formation

Fused joint

Rheumatoid arthritis begins with the inflammation of the synovial membrane and progresses to pannus formation and erosion of cartilage; eventually, the joint cavity is destroyed and the bones (here, the knee bones) become fused.

See also Arthritis; Autoimmune disorders; Joints; Juvenile rheumatoid arthritis; Osteoarthritis; Rheumatology.

For Further Information:

Arthritis Foundation. *Raising a Child with Arthritis: A Parent's Guide*. Lanham, Md.: National Book Network, 1998.

Firestein, Gary S., Gabriel S. Panayi, and Frank A. Wollheim, eds. *Rheumatoid Arthritis*. 2d ed. New York: Oxford University Press, 2006.

Foltz-Gray, Dorothy. *The Arthritis Foundation's Guide to Good Living with Rheumatoid Arthritis*. 3d ed. Atlanta: Arthritis Foundation, 2006.

Paget, Stephen A., Michael D. Lockshin, and Suzanne Loebl. *The Hospital for Special Surgery Rheumatoid Arthritis Handbook*. New York: John Wiley & Sons, 2002.

Poehlmann, Katherine M. *Rheumatoid Arthritis: The Infection Connection*. Durham, N.C.: Satori Press, 2002.

"Rheumatoid Arthritis." *Centers for Disease Control and Prevention*, November 19, 2012.

"Rheumatoid Arthritis." *Health Library*, September 30, 2012.

"What Is Rheumatoid Arthritis?" *National Institute of Arthritis and Musculoskeletal and Skin Diseases*, December, 2009.

Rheumatology

Specialty

Anatomy or system affected: Bones, hands, hips, immune system, joints, knees, legs, musculoskeletal system

Specialties and related fields: Geriatrics and gerontology, immunology, orthopedics, pharmacology

Definition: The field of medicine concerned with the diagnosis and treatment of joint inflammation and bone or joint destruction and with the surgical repair of damaged joints.

Key terms:

acute: referring to a disease process of sudden onset

arthritis: joint inflammation

capillary exudate: a group of substances secreted by the capillaries as part of the inflammatory process

chronic: referring to a lingering disease process

joint: the conjunction of two or more bones

Science and Profession

Rheumatology is concerned with the major diseases of bones and joints: arthritis, osteoarthritis, other arthritic disorders such as gouty arthritis, and ankylosing spondylitis, among a host of others.

The onset of rheumatoid arthritis is usually in middle age. It strikes three times as many women as men. To understand the disease, it is necessary to understand the body's skeletal system-the bones and bone structures, as well as the tissues between and around bones and joints.

There are 206 bones in the human body. Some function as support mechanisms that hold the body erect and support the weight, such as the spine and the bones of the hips and legs. Some bones form defensive "cages" that protect body organs, such as the skull and the ribs. Some bones are involved in movement, specifically the bones in the spine, shoulders, arms, hands, hips, legs, and feet.

Bones are composed of three main sections. The tough membranous tissue that covers the bone, the periosteum, contains the blood vessels that nourish bone cells and the nerve fibers that sense pain and pressure. The outer layer of the bone itself is called compact bone; it forms the hard exterior. Inside is a spongy inner structure called cancellous (chambered) bone. Cancellous bone contains the marrow that manufactures blood cells, and it also stores fat cells.

When bones meet, the structure formed is called a joint, or articulation. Some joints are fixed, such as the ribs and the bones of the skull; they are called fibrous joints because a tough, fibrous adhesive material connects them, prohibiting movement and maintaining the integrity of the protective cage.

Some joints are capable of motion. Moving joints are of two types: synovial joints and cartilaginous joints. An example of the latter is the spine, where each vertebra is connected to its neighbor by a spinal disk made of cartilage. Cartilaginous joints are capable of movement, but they have nowhere near the mobility of the synovial joints, so called because they are filled with synovial fluid, a liquid resembling the white of an egg.

There are six kinds of synovial joints: ball-and-socket, ellipsoidal, hinge, pivot, saddle, and gliding joints. Ball-and-socket joints are found in the shoulders and hips. In these joints, a long bone-the femur in the leg and the humerus in the arm-end with a ball-shaped structure that fits neatly into a round, concave socket. Ball-and-socket joints are capable of the widest range of movement. Ellipsoidal joints are modifications of the ball-and-socket structures, where the bones are not round but oval. They are found in the wrists and ankles. The elbows and knees are hinge joints, which permit only bending and extending motions, up and down or side to side, as with a common door hinge. In pivot joints, one bone contains a small cup or arch that accepts a point of another bone, permitting it to rotate on its axis. The two bones at the top of the spine, which govern the range of motion of the head, are examples. A saddle joint consists of two bones, shaped rather like saddles; they fit snugly into each other and allow a wide range of movement. The joint connecting the thumb to the rest of the hand is the only saddle joint in the human body. The bones of gliding joints are almost flat; their surfaces slide over one another, permitting limited motion forward and back or from side to side. Some of the wrist bones are gliding joints.

The synovial joints are the most intricate and mobile of all the joints, and they are also the most prone to disease. The synovial joint capsule is a complex structure that encloses the moving bones and other tissues. It consists of the capsular ligament, which forms the joint capsule; the joint cavity, an open space between bones that allows free mobility; and the synovial membrane, a thin, smooth tissue that secretes synovial fluid. The synovial fluid fills the joint cavity and lubricates bone surfaces. Bones do not actually rub against each other; they are too rough and would become abraded. They are separated by a covering of smooth, white tissue called articular cartilage that permits smooth movement and absorbs impact. Just outside the joint capsule are bursae, small pouches that store synovial fluid.

In rheumatoid arthritis, the first signs of disease are pain and inflammation in the synovial joint capsule. This initial manifestation may be attributable to a number of factors, such as bacterial infection or injury. The reasons that an acute episode of pain and inflammation in the synovial joints progresses to chronic rheumatoid arthritis are unknown. It is suspected that genetic factors may be involved; the disease often runs in families. Blood components called rheumatoid factors are present in the majority of rheumatoid arthritis patients. The role of these factors in the development of disease, however, is unclear because rheumatoid factors are also found in people who do not develop rheumatoid arthritis.

In some patients, rheumatoid arthritis is relatively benign, with pain and inflammation that can be controlled by medication and other support techniques. In other patients, the disease progresses to devastating bone deformities and complete loss of mobility in the affected joints. How this degeneration occurs is related to a disruption in the body's normal reaction to infection or injury. Pain and inflammation are protective mechanisms with which the body attempts to compensate for a disease or disorder. The following sequence of events is what normally occurs when a synovial joint is damaged by infection, physical injury, or a toxic substance.

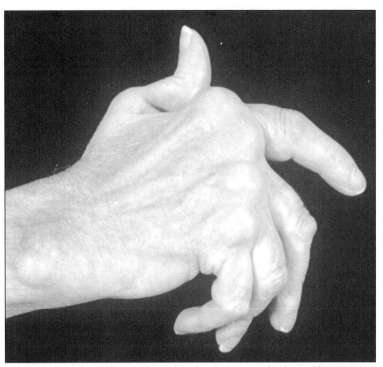

The hand of an elderly patient suffering from severe rheumatoid arthritis. Rheumatologists diagnose and treat such joint inflammation. (SIU School of Medicine)

Tissue injury-from trauma or infection-causes the release of chemical mediators from surrounding cells. These chemicals include prostaglandins, leukotrienes, histamine, serotonin, and bradykinin. Collectively, they cause the local blood vessels to enlarge (vasodilate), increasing blood flow to the affected area and causing redness and heat.

Ordinarily, the capillaries, the tiny blood vessels that supply nutrients to the cells, have openings in their walls so small that only tiny bits of matter can get through. During inflammation, they become more permeable; that is, the openings in the capillary walls enlarge so that the capillaries can deliver larger substances to the affected area. This group of substances forms the capillary exudate, and it flows copiously into the affected area, causing swelling. The exudate consists of lymphocytes, which produce antibodies to fight infection; neutrophils; and macrophages, specialized white blood cells that facilitate the removal of tissue debris, dead cells, and other material. These white blood cells can also release other substances, such as superoxide, an agent used by white blood cells to kill bacteria but which can also damage healthy tissue. Another is interleukin-1, an agent that promotes healing and stimulates lymphocytes to produce antibodies. The spread of inflammation is prevented by a third agent released by the white blood cells, fibrinogen, which effectively closes off the area of inflammation.

In normal situations, the agent causing the inflammation is neutralized, the capillaries return to their normal size, certain white blood cells remove the protective shield, and the healing process begins. In rheumatoid arthritis, the orderly process that begins with pain and inflammation and ends with healing is disrupted by various events. Instead of neutralizing the trauma, the anti-inflammatory phase can set off a chain of events that makes the condition progressively worse.

Why this disruption occurs is not yet known, but four major theories have been suggested. The first is the theory of genetic predisposition to the disease, a factor which may or may not relate to the other three. The second theory is that rheumatoid arthritis is an immune-complex disease. Ordinarily, when the body fights an infectious microorganism that has invaded the body, lymphocytes produce antibodies that combine with the antigens characteristic of the microorganism. This antigen/antibody combination is the immune complex, and it is removed by other white blood cells. In this theory, the process is altered. Instead of being removed by white blood cells, the immune complex lodges in the synovial membrane and causes continuing inflammation. Capillaries continue to release exudate, whose constituents cause cell proliferation, thickening of the synovial membrane, and destruction of articular cartilage and bone tissue.

The autoimmune theory is similar, but in this case the causative agent is not a foreign substance but something natural within the body. For example, if a specific protein released by a gland finds its way into a joint, it may be regarded as a foreign, infective agent. Thus it will set off an immune response and cause inflammation, initiating the same process described above.

The fourth theory links rheumatoid arthritis to viral or bacterial infection. It has been noted that fever, malaise, and enlarged lymph nodes-common symptoms of infection-are often seen in patients with rheumatoid arthritis.

Furthermore, rheumatoid arthritis sometimes occurs simultaneously with bacterial pneumonia, tuberculosis, hepatitis, and sexually transmitted diseases, as well as with diseases caused by viruses, such as mumps and measles.

The progress of rheumatoid arthritis is variable. In some patients, it is characterized by occasional flare-ups (episodes of acute pain and inflammation) and periods of remission (times when the patient is relatively comfortable). In others, the disease causes progressive, insidious destruction of the joint and may involve other organs of the body. Articular cartilage may be destroyed, and the joint may become immobilized, an extremely painful condition. The bones in the joint may fuse together, becoming one solid mass. The bones may also become dislocated. In about 30 to 35 percent of patients, rheumatoid nodules develop. These hard, solid lumps usually occur at the elbows but may also be found at the knees, ankles, and feet. In advanced cases, nodules may be discovered in the heart muscle, the lungs, and other organs where they could impair organ function.

The diagnosis of rheumatoid arthritis has been codified by the American Rheumatism Foundation. This organization lists seven symptoms and suggests that the presence of any four should confirm the diagnosis of rheumatoid arthritis (although patients with two or more of the symptoms should not be excluded). The seven symptoms are morning stiffness lasting an hour or more; arthritis in three or more joints; arthritis in hands, fingers, or wrists; arthritis occurring symmetrically (for example, in both hands, elbows, or knees); rheumatoid nodules; the presence of rheumatoid factor; and x-ray evidence of bone deterioration.

Diagnostic and Treatment Techniques

Once a patient is suspected of having rheumatoid arthritis, the physician may wish to conduct further laboratory tests to assess the severity of the disease and, from that analysis, develop a treatment regimen. In addition to testing for rheumatoid factor, the physician will check the patient's erythrocyte (red blood cell) sedimentation rate (ESR). This test helps to determine the presence of inflammatory activity. Another blood test looks for C-reactive protein (CRP). CRP also indicates inflammatory activity; levels rise during an acute attack and fall during a period of remission. Synovial fluid is analyzed to discover changes that occur during inflammation. For example, during inflammatory episodes, the color of the fluid becomes significantly darker, turning yellow or green. Ordinarily quite clear and viscous, it becomes cloudy and thinner in consistency. Many more tests are available to the physician to help him or her evaluate the severity of the disease, including an analysis of the various substances involved in the immune process.

There is no cure for rheumatoid arthritis, but most patients can be helped with the therapies available. In spite of treatment, however, 5 to 10 percent will eventually be disabled by bone deterioration and destruction.

Treatment depends on the severity of the condition. The regimen can simply involve rest and immobilization of the affected joint, or it may include any of a wide range of medications, from aspirin to potent, often toxic compounds. In advanced cases, joint deformity may be so severe as to require surgery and/or prosthetic implants.

The goals of therapy are to relieve pain, reduce inflammation, and maintain the function of the joint. Ideally, the physician would also like to halt the progress of the disease. Some medications in use today promise to slow or stop the progress of the disease, but nothing is available to cure it.

For the relief of pain, the physician has a large number of medications available, many of which will also reduce inflammation. These include a group of drugs called nonsteroidal anti-inflammatory drugs (NSAIDs). NSAIDs as a class include the salicylates, such as aspirin, ibuprofen, acetaminophen, and at least twenty other drugs currently in use in the United States.

Far and away the largest number of patients with rheumatoid arthritis are being treated with NSAIDs. Many of the NSAIDs are perfectly safe when used in lower doses. At the high doses often required to control the pain of rheumatoid arthritis, however, they can cause significant adverse reactions. A significant percentage of patients given some NSAIDs develop side effects severe enough to warrant stopping the drug. Many develop gastrointestinal (GI) problems ranging from stomachaches to bleeding ulcers, which can be fatal.

One of the ways in which NSAIDs work is to reduce the production of prostaglandins, substances released in the capillary exudate that are partially responsible for the inflammatory process. At the inflamed synovial joint, this attribute of NSAIDs is a desirable one. In the stomach, however, NSAIDs can cause problems. One of the prostaglandins helps to protect the stomach lining from damage by the organ's highly acid contents. NSAIDs can remove this protection, allowing stomach acids to attack the lining, causing irritation and inflammation. Therefore, some physicians prescribe an NSAID with a prostaglandin analog, such as misoprostol, in the hope of avoiding or reducing GI distress. Misoprostol has problems of its own, however, such as causing severe diarrhea in some patients.

For the patient with severe rheumatoid arthritis-defined as painful, debilitating illness that does not respond to NSAIDs and is progressing to deformity-the available medications are both more potent and more toxic. A group of agents called disease-modifying drugs promise to reduce the degenerative processes in rheumatoid arthritis. These drugs include gold compounds, D-penicillamine, drugs used to treat malaria, and sulfasalazine. They appear to alter the course of rheumatoid arthritis, but they do not relieve pain or inflammation, so they must be given with NSAIDs. They all have a high potential for toxicity and must be used carefully, with constant monitoring, to avoid serious side effects.

In some cases, physicians find it necessary to prescribe corticosteroids to patients with rheumatoid arthritis. These drugs present a problem, because rheumatoid arthritis is a lifelong condition, and toxicity and physical changes often occur with long-term steroid therapy. Sometimes corticosteroids are given as short-term therapy to achieve a rapid reduction of inflammation. In this case, there is a danger of a severe rebound reaction when the drug is stopped. A corticosteroid may be administered as an injection into the joint, which is an effective short-term procedure to bring fast relief of pain and inflammation in an acute situation.

Immunosuppressive therapy is sometimes prescribed for patients with rheumatoid arthritis. Immunosuppressive agents have the potential to be highly toxic, and their use is reserved for patients who have not responded to other treatments.

Exercise and physical therapy are useful to the patient with rheumatoid arthritis. During acute inflammation, passive exercise within pain limits, with the limb manipulated by another person or the patient, will help keep the joint mobile and prevent muscle tightening. After the inflammation has subsided, active exercise is recommended to maintain muscle mass and mobility, but the activity should never be strenuous or fatiguing.

Flexion contracture, a condition in which the muscles that move the joint become stiff and shortened, may respond to exercise. If the contracture has become established, however, then more intensive exercise, splinting, or orthopedic treatment may be necessary.

Orthopedic surgery to correct fused or dislocated joints can be performed on any joint in the body, and in some cases, a fused or badly deteriorated joint can be replaced with an implant of metal and/or plastic (arthroplasty). The two most successful implant procedures are total replacement of the hip or knee. When a hip is replaced, the surgeon reveals the joint where the ball of the femur nests in the socket of the acetabulum, a cavity in the hipbone. The ball of the femur is replaced by a metal or plastic ball attached to a shaft that is anchored inside the femur. The socket is replaced as well, usually with a plastic cup that is anchored into the hipbone. The implant can give the patient instant relief from pain and restore mobility. The length of time that the hip replacement will last varies, but many patients receive years of relief from a single operation. A similar procedure is used to replace the hinge joint of the knee, and, although knee replacement is not as successful as hip replacement, it has helped many patients.

Perspective and Prospects

Rheumatoid arthritis afflicts about 1 percent of all populations. While the disease is not life-threatening, it is one of the most significant crippling disorders in the world. Most patients can be treated successfully by medication, exercise, and other support measures. The disease is progressive in most patients. After ten years, 80 percent of patients will have some degree of deformity, ranging from minor destruction of bone and cartilage to complete fusion of the joint.

Some patients medicate themselves with over-the-counter painkillers and rarely, if ever, see a physician. It is to be expected that, in these patients, the disease is mild, with acute episodes occurring only sporadically. The majority of patients with moderate-to-severe rheumatoid arthritis are seen by physicians.

Currently, there is no perfect therapy for rheumatoid arthritis, in the sense that there is no one agent or family of agents that promises to be safe and effective in all patients. The danger of significant adverse reactions exists with most drugs that are effective, particularly in those patients who require high doses to control the pain and inflammation of the most severe forms of the disease.

Pharmaceutical science continues to search for new medications that will relieve pain and inflammation without damaging side effects. New drugs that will stop the progress of the disease safely and effectively are also sought. There is also the hope that rheumatoid arthritis will be curable or preventable one day.

Orthopedic surgeons continue to improve the techniques for alleviating the effects of bone and joint destruction that occur in some patients. New prosthetic appliances are designed and produced constantly in an effort to widen the range of joint replacement procedures.

—*C. Richard Falcon*

See also Aging; Aging: Extended care; Arthritis; Arthroplasty; Arthroscopy; Autoimmune disorders; Behçet's disease; Bone disorders; Bones and the skeleton; Bursitis; Geriatrics and gerontology; Gout; Hydrotherapy; Inflammation; Joints; Juvenile rheumatoid arthritis; Lyme disease; Orthopedic surgery; Orthopedics; Orthopedics, pediatric; Osteoarthritis; Osteonecrosis; Physical examination; Rheumatic fever; Rheumatoid arthritis; Spondylitis; Sports medicine.

For Further Information:

American College of Rheumatology. *American College of Rheumatology*, 2013.

Isenberg, David A., et al., eds. *Oxford Textbook of Rheumatology*. 3d ed. New York: Oxford University Press, 2004.

Lahita, Robert G. *Rheumatoid Arthritis: Everything You Need to Know*. Rev. ed. New York: Avery, 2004.

Litin, Scott C., ed. *Mayo Clinic Family Health Book*. 4th ed. New York: HarperResource, 2009.

Mayo Clinic. *Mayo Clinic on Arthritis*. New York: HarperCollins, 2005.

MedlinePlus. "Rheumatoid Arthritis." *MedlinePlus*, August 26, 2013.

Parker, James N., and Philip M. Parker, eds. *The 2002 Official Patient's Sourcebook on Rheumatoid Arthritis*. San Diego, Calif.: Icon Health, 2002..

Shlotzhauer, Tammi L., and James L. McGuire. *Living with Rheumatoid Arthritis*. 2d ed. Baltimore: Johns Hopkins University Press, 2003.

Sutton, Amy L., ed. *Arthritis Sourcebook: Basic Consumer Health Information About Osteoarthritis, Rheumatoid Arthritis, Other Rheumatic Disorders, Infectious Forms of Arthritis, and Diseases with Symptoms Linked to Arthritis*. 3d ed. Detroit, Mich.: Omnigraphics, 2012.

Yung, Raymond L."What Is a Rheumatologist?" *American College of Rheumatology*, August, 2012..

Rhinitis

Disease/Disorder

Also known as: Runny nose, hay fever, nasal allergies

Anatomy or system affected: Nose, respiratory system, throat

Specialties and related fields: Family medicine, immunology, otorhinolaryngology, pediatrics

Definition: A discharge from the nose caused by inflammation of the internal nasal structures.

Key terms:

allergic rhinitis: acute or seasonal nasal stuffiness and sneezing that follows the exposure to allergens such as pollen or animal dander; hay fever is one form of allergic rhinitis

nonallergic rhinitis: acute nasal stuffiness produced as a result of the common cold or flu

postnasal drip: the discharge of nasal mucus into the back of the throat

---

Information on Rhinitis

Causes: Irritants, infections, cold air
Symptoms: Stiffness or irritation in nose often accompanied by mucus discharge
Duration: Usually acute but can be chronic
Treatments: Removal of irritation, resolution of infection, antihistamines, nasal steroids

---

Causes and Symptoms

Rhinitis can have a variety of causes, including infection by a rhinovirus or certain bacteria and exposure to cold air or nasal allergens. Foreign bodies in the nose and certain structural deformities can also cause rhinitis.

When the nasal symptoms are due to allergies, the condition is called allergic rhinitis. A partial list of allergens that can produce allergic rhinitis includes pollen, dust, molds, wool, feathers, tobacco smoke, airborne environmental pollutants, strong odors, spicy foods, and animal dander.

When the nasal symptoms are not due to allergies, the condition is called nonallergic rhinitis or nonallergic vasomotor rhinitis. Nonallergic rhinitis can be caused by a viral or bacterial infection, exposure to cold air, structural deformities, certain endocrine disorders such as hypothyroidism, or emotional stress; it is occasionally observed during the first trimester of pregnancy. Nonallergic rhinitis usually begins with a feeling of irritation in the nose or throat. The irritation is followed by sneezing and mucus discharge as the nasal air passageways become more obstructed.

Atrophic rhinitis, a chronic form of nonallergic rhinitis, is a condition often seen first at puberty; because there is a genetic component, the condition tends to run in families. The causes of atrophic rhinitis are not fully understood, although deficiencies in iron and vitamins A and D may contribute. In this condition, the moist, pink, thick lining of the inside of the nose is replaced by a thin crusty surface that can be foul smelling. Although the nasal cavity is wide open, people often complain of a feeling of stuffiness. The condition is sometimes accompanied by nosebleeds.

Nasal dripping and/or sneezing can be seen with all the forms of rhinitis. The discharge can be clear and watery or thicker and more viscous. It can be colorless; if there is a color, it is often white or less often green or yellow. Postnasal drip is when the discharge is into the back of the throat, a condition that can result in a dry, usually nonproductive cough.

Treatment and Therapy

The treatment for rhinitis is an attempt to manage symptoms. The most effective treatment for allergic rhinitis is to remove the source of the irritation. In the home, keeping the windows closed, using an air conditioner, and filtering the circulating air can reduce allergen exposure. Saline irrigation can also be used to reduce the nasal symptoms. When symptoms persist despite these efforts, treatment focuses on minimizing the allergic response. This can be done using antihistamines, steroids, or antileukotrienes.

When the body encounters an allergen, the white blood cells produce antibodies, which then promote the release of compounds called mediators. Histamine is perhaps the best known of these mediators. The mediators trigger the nasal symptoms. Most of the drugs used to treat allergic rhinitis are designed to inhibit the actions of the mediators. Antihistamines block the action of histamine and so significantly reduce swelling and discharge. Likewise, antileukotrienes work by blocking leukotrienes, another immune system mediator. The mechanism by which nasal steroids (usually given in the form of a spray) work is less clear, but they can provide temporary relief.

When the symptoms do not respond well to the above treatments, immunotherapy is required. For this treatment, it is necessary to determine the allergens to which the person is sensitive. This can be accomplished in a variety of ways, although skin or blood testing are the most common. Once the specific allergen has been identified, the immune system can be desensitized through carefully administered challenges, which in effect raise the tolerance level necessary to produce the nasal symptoms.

If the cause of nonallergic rhinitis was exposure to cold air, then going into a warmer environment will usually eliminate the symptoms. If the cause is the common cold or the flu, then symptoms are sometimes relieved by decongestants and/or antihistamines. Some of these drugs are available over the counter, while others require a prescription. Unless there is a primary or secondary bacterial infection accompanying the rhinitis, antibiotics are not effective. Drinking lots of fluids, getting bed rest, and breathing humidified air can reduce the discomfort. With any viral or bacterial infection (especially H1N1 influenza infections), a medical professional should be consulted immediately if breathing becomes a problem. Muscle aching and the general feeling of malaise that accompanies nonallergic rhinitis can often be relieved by over-the-counter medications such as aspirin or ibuprofen.

Atrophic rhinitis can be treated be irrigating the nose with saline. If a bacterial infection is present, then antibiotics are indicated. The crusting can be treated by irrigation with nasal douches. In severe cases, atrophic rhinitis is treated by Young's operation, a surgical procedure that reduces the size of the nasal cavity.

When the cause of the rhinitis is a foreign body or structural deformity, removing the foreign body or surgically changing the internal structure of the nose often eliminates the symptoms.

Perspective and Prospects

Considerable financial and personal costs are associated with rhinitis, since it is such a common condition. Because rhinitis is so common, considerable effort is going into completely understanding this disease. As a result, new treatments with fewer side effects should become available.

—David Hornung, Ph.D.

See also Allergies; Antihistamines; Common cold; Decongestants; Ear infections and disorders; Hay fever; Influenza; Multiple chemical sensitivity syndrome; Nasal polyp removal; Nasopharyngeal disorders; Otorhinolaryngology; Rhinoviruses; Sinusitis; Sneezing.

For Further Information:

Baraniuk, James N., and Dennis Shusterman, eds. *Nonallergic Rhinitis*. New York: Informa Healthcare, 2007.

Busse, William W., and Stephen T. Holgate, eds. *Asthma and Rhinitis*. Hoboken, N.J.: Wiley-Blackwell, 2000.

Carson-DeWitt, Rosalyn. "Allergic Rhinitis." *Health Library*, October 31, 2012.

Henochowicz, Stuart I. "Allergic Rhinitis." *MedlinePlus*, June 17, 2012.

Henochowicz, Stuart I. "Vasomotor Rhinitis." *MedlinePlus*, June 17, 2012.

Scadding, Glenis K., and Wytske J. Hokkens. *Rhinitis*. Albuquerque, N.Mex.: Health Press, 2007.

Rhinoplasty and submucous resection

Procedures

Anatomy or system affected: Nose

Specialties and related fields: General surgery, otorhinolaryngology, plastic surgery

Definition: Surgical procedures that correct cosmetic and health problems related to the nose.

Key terms:

cartilage: white, fibrous connective tissue attached to the articular surfaces of bones

inspired air: air that is breathed in

pharynx: the part of the respiratory-digestive passage that extends from the nasal cavity to the larynx (voice box)

Indications and Procedures

The nose, in addition to being an important organ for breathing and smelling, is cosmetically significant because of its prominence on the face. Hence, surgery to improve the nose may be medically necessary or an elective procedure to enhance facial appearance (cosmetic surgery). In modern society, the latter type of nasal surgery is the most common. Nasal surgery, however, usually involves both. Before examining rhinoplasty and submucous resection, it is useful briefly to denote the function of the nose, its anatomy, and its interconnections with the body's respiratory and olfactory systems.

Air breathed in enters the nose through the nostrils, which are separated by a wall of cartilage and bone called the nasal septum. In most cases, the septum produces two nostrils of similar size. In some cases, however, injury or heredity causes the septum to become thickened on one side or to exhibit ridges or bumps. In a minor case of deviated septum, the irregularity may make one nostril smaller than the other and can affect breathing and sinus drainage

adversely during colds. In very severe cases, it can obstruct and irritate the nose enough so that relatively permanent nasal tissue swelling requires chronic, uncomfortable breathing through the mouth.

In most individuals, inspired air passes into two nasal passages which lead into the upper part of the throat. They allow the air to pass through the pharynx and trachea (windpipe) to reach the lungs. Each nasal passage is lined with a soft, moist mucous membrane which is covered with fine cilia (hairs) that catch dust and other particles and keep them from reaching the lungs. The nose and the nasal passages also raise the temperature of inspired air before it enters the lungs. Furthermore, the nose plays a large part in the sense of taste, as shown by the inability of people with severe colds to taste food.

Submucous resection is performed when the nasal septum is so distorted that it causes discomfort to the patient, especially chronic nasal pain, the need for continuous and uncomfortable mouth breathing, or repeated and prolonged colds. In these cases, the septum is reshaped in order to cure the problem, allowing the patient to breathe normally again through the nose. Septum resection may be accomplished with fine scissors, a scalpel, and/or bone rasps.

Cosmetic nose alterations are collectively referred to as rhinoplasty. The most common procedures correct prominent bumps, bulbousness, drooping tip, and overly large or small size. Text on cosmetic surgery of the nose include descriptive terms that graphically identify the surgical problems encountered in rhinoplasty, such as "saddle nose," "short nose," "pig nose," and "hook nose." Rhinoplasty is also used to repair damage caused by accidents and cancer. Furthermore, it is an essential part of repairing a deviated nasal septum, which can greatly impair the breathing of afflicted individuals if left untreated.

Most often, nasal surgery is performed by use of intranasal incisions. The nasal skin is temporarily freed and pulled back from underlying bone and cartilage. Then, this hard framework is altered by partial removal, rearrangement, augmentation with synthetic materials, or bone and cartilage grafts from various parts of the patient's body. The site in the nose and the shape of the grafts used depend on the procedure to be carried out. Once all necessary procedures have been completed on cartilage and bone, the skin is redraped over them. In some cases, especially where nose size is to be reduced, portions of the soft tissues of the nose are removed.

After nasal surgery-whether rhinoplasty, submucous resection, or some combination of techniques is used-the nostrils are packed with sterile gauze to prevent bleeding and to support the nasal mucosa during its initial healing, as incisions are usually sutured only minimally and with resorbable suture materials. The packing is often removed after several days. A nasal splint is also used in many cases. It provides external support and aid in maintaining nasal recontouring. The splint also protects the altered nose from damage during the several weeks usually required for most swelling to subside. After the removal of the splint, it takes at least several months for normal feeling and final nose shape to be attained as postsurgical swelling subsides entirely.

Uses and Complications

Nasal surgery can be done under local or general anesthesia in a hospital or in a surgeon's office. Hospitalization and general anesthesia are most often used, although frequently they are not needed. Most reconstructive surgeons prefer these operative conditions for the patient's sake and because they allow easier physical manipulation of the patient.

Most procedures attempted are quite safe and uncomplicated. Occasional problems include excessive bleeding, internal scarring of nasal mucosa, recurring airway obstruction, and unexpected contour irregularities. Infections after nasal surgery are rare except in cases where cartilaginous nasal implants are used. The incidence of infection may increase, however, as surgeons add forehead and chin alteration to rhinoplasty to optimize the overall cosmetic results.

Overall, nasal surgery is straightforward and has few real risks. Patients should be aware, however, that the procedure can fail to yield a chosen cosmetic improvement and that airway obstruction can be generated by the process or can recur after repair.

Perspective and Prospects

Among the exciting advances being made in rhinoplasty and submucous resection are the replacement of deficient nostril parts and septa with cartilage from other body parts or with synthetic materials. It is projected by some doctors that implants obtained from other individuals will eventually be used to repair function and appearance in individuals whose noses are irreversibly damaged by accidents and cancer.

Another aspect of importance to cosmetic nasal surgery is the growing realization that the chin, forehead, and other parts of the face are important to the appearance of the nose. This has led some surgeons performing nose recontouring to expend much effort toward examining these features and designing complementary surgical procedures to achieve good results.

—*Sanford S. Singer, Ph.D.*

See also Facial transplantation; Nasal polyp removal; Nasopharyngeal disorders; Otorhinolaryngology; Plastic surgery.

For Further Information:

Dutton, Jay M. "Rhinoplasty Overview." *American Rhinologic Society*, July 2011.
Elsahy, Nabil. *Plastic and Reconstructive Surgery of the Nose*. New York: Elsevier, 2000.
Ferrari, Mario. *PDxMD Ear, Nose, and Throat Disorders*. Philadelphia: PDxMD, 2003.
Gruber, Ronald P., and George C. Peck, eds. *Rhinoplasty: State of the Art*. St. Louis, Mo.: Mosby Year Book, 1993.
Jewet, Brian, Shan R. Baker, and Sam Nacify, eds. *Principles of Aesthetic Nasal Reconstruction*. St. Louis, Mo.: Mosby, 2002.
"Rhinoplasty." *Health Library*, September 10, 2012.
"Rhinoplasty." *Mayo Clinic*, March 1, 2011.

Rhinoviruses
Disease/Disorder
Anatomy or system affected: Cells, chest, lungs, nose, respiratory system, throat
Specialties and related fields: Biochemistry, biotechnology, cytology, epidemiology, genetics, histology, immunology, otorhinolaryngology, pathology, preventive medicine, public health, serology, virology
Definition: Disease-causing agents that are responsible for more common colds than any other respiratory virus.
Key terms
antigen: a proteinaceous, membrane-bound, cell surface component that stimulates the production of antibodies, which subsequently provoke an immune response
endothelial cell: cells that line blood and lymph vessels
Enterovirus: a genus of viruses similar to rhinoviruses
leukocyte: a white blood cell
picornavirus: the family of viruses that includes the *Enterovirus* and *Rhinovirus* genera
receptor: a membrane-bound protein that normally mediates interactions between the cell in which it is bound and specific, external signals, such as hormones
serotype: a group of viruses that can be characterized by common cell surface antigens

Causes and Symptoms

Rhinoviruses have been identified as the virus most often responsible for the common cold. Rhinoviruses have also been implicated in complications of asthma. Rhinoviruses are transmitted through sneezing and coughing, which expels droplets of moisture laden with virus. Once introduced into the respiratory system, the virus enters cells by interfacing with the intercellular adhesion molecule-1 (ICAM-1) receptor. As its name implies, ICAM-1 provides adhesion between endothelial cells and leukocytes after injury or stress, but it also facilitates the entry of rhinoviruses into cells, where they can replicate. The subsequent immune response is responsible for most of the symptoms of the common cold.

Colds occur more often in winter than in other seasons, although they can occur year-round. This seasonal effect is thought to be the result of an increase in time spent in closer contact with other people who may carry a rhinovirus.

Treatment and Therapy

No cure exists for the treatment of rhinoviruses once contracted, and no vaccine exists to inoculate against infection with rhinoviruses. However, many strategies exist for reducing the transmission of viruses between infected individuals. Traditional home remedies such as chicken soup, bed rest, and drinking a lot of fluids may increase the comfort level of the sufferer, but they do not shorten the course of the disease. Additionally, while vitamin C and echinacea may help reduce cold symptoms and the length of the cold, there has not been extensive evidence as to their helpfulness in preventing or getting rid of a cold. Antibiotics are not effective against rhinoviruses. Preventive measures are the best methods for reducing infection rate, including breast-feeding of infants and frequent handwashing.

Information on Rhinoviruses

Causes: Transmitted through sneezing and coughing

Symptoms: Sneezing, coughing, nasal and sinus drainage, congestion, fluid in the ears, headache, fever; in more severe cases, wheezing and pneumonia

Duration: Approximately seven days for infection; two or more weeks for symptoms

Treatments: Zinc lozenges, rest; preventive measures (handwashing with soap or antiseptic such as alcohol-based sanitizer, disinfection of surfaces commonly touched by people, covering coughs and sneezes with tissue or article of clothing)

Increased vitamin D levels may also be associated with a lowered risk of infection.

Studies conducted on the use of zinc lozenges as a treatment for the common cold have produced mixed results. In test tubes, positively charged zinc inhibits processing of viral proteins by several different mechanisms. One analysis of previous studies suggested that differences in effectiveness of zinc lozenges could be explained by the ligand or ligands bound to the zinc. Zinc lozenges with only one ligand, such as zinc acetate or zinc gluconate lozenges, were observed to be more effective in reducing cold duration than were zinc lozenges with more ligands, though even they were not effective in all studies. The ineffectiveness of intranasal zinc application was hypothesized to result from an electrical potential difference of 60 to 120 millivolts between the nose and mouth, which results in repulsion of charged particles such as ionized zinc.

There are ninety-nine known serotypes of rhinoviruses. This variety of cell surface antigens makes the development of a vaccine that is effective against multiple rhinoviruses difficult. In the first decade of the twenty-first century, a region of a rhinoviral protein called VP4 was shown to be very common between the different serotypes. Future efforts to synthesize a vaccine may focus on this common element.

Perspective and Prospects

The common cold has been known for millenia and was first given this name in the sixteenth century. Evidence exists across cultures demonstrating knowledge of the cold, extending as back as far as ancient Egypt. In the eighteenth century, Benjamin Franklin's *Definition of a Cold* (1773) demonstrated insightful speculation about the airborne nature of cold transmission and suggested methods for preventing the disease.

The Rhinovirus was first isolated in 1956 and during successive decades was identified as the virus best associated with the common cold. As technology improved, so did detection and identification of different viruses that could be responsible for the common cold. Simple culturing methods gave way to reverse transcriptase polymerase chain reaction (RT-PCR) assays, which were more sensitive in detecting and characterizing specific rhinoviruses. In various campaigns to find a treatment for the common

cold, antiviral drugs and interferon have been shown to be effective in protecting against rhinoviruses, though attempts to translate these results into a treatment have not been successful.

The Common Cold Research Unit (CCRU), originally established in Great Britain at the outset of World War II as the Harvard Hospital, operated from 1946 to 1989 and was devoted to researching the causes of the common cold as well as possible treatments for the disease. It was there that coronaviruses, which can also be responsible for causing the common cold, were first isolated in 1965.

—*Andrew J. Reinhart, M.S.*

See also Antihistamines; Bronchitis; Common cold; Coughing; Decongestants; Nasopharyngeal disorders; Noroviruses; Otorhinolarnygology; Pneumonia; Rhinitis; Sinusitis; Sneezing; Sore throat; Viral infections.

For Further Information:

Carson-DeWitt, Rosalyn, and Brian Randall. "Common Cold." *Health Library*, Jan. 9, 2013.

"Common Cold." *MedlinePlus*, Apr. 23, 2013.

"Common Colds: Protect Yourself and Others." *Centers for Disease Control and Prevention*, Mar. 11, 2013.

Eccles, Ronald, and Olaf Weber, eds. *Common Cold*. Birkhäuser Advances in Infectious Diseases. Basel, Switzerland: Birkhäuser Basel, 2009.

"Rhinovirus Infections." *HealthyChildren.org*. American Academy of Pediatrics, May 11, 2013.

Tyrrell, David, and Michael Fielder, *Cold Wars: The Fight Against the Common Cold*. New York: Oxford University Press, 2002.

Yin-Murphy, Marguerite, and Jeffrey W. Almond. "Picornaviruses-Classification and Antigenic Types." In *Medical Microbiology*, edited by Samuel Baron. Galveston: University of Texas Medical Branch, 1996.

Rickets

Disease/Disorder

Anatomy or system affected: Bones, musculoskeletal system, teeth

Specialties and related fields: Nutrition, orthopedics, osteopathic medicine, pediatrics

Definition: A disorder involving the softening and weakening of a child's bones, primarily caused by lack of vitamin D and/or lack of calcium or phosphate.

Causes and Symptoms

Rickets is a relatively rare bone disease that most frequently afflicts children. It is the result of insufficient or inefficient absorption of vitamin D in the body, which causes a progressive softening and weakening of the bone. Certain physical conditions can reduce digestion or absorption of fats and may also diminish vitamin D absorption by the intestines. The loss of calcium and phosphate from the bone eventually causes destruction of the supportive bone matrix. In adult deficiency, demineralization (osteomalacia) may occur in the spine, pelvis, and lower extremities, causing osteoporosis (an adult disorder causing brittle bones).

Symptoms of rickets may include pain or tenderness of the long bones and pelvis, skeletal deformities such as bowlegs, bumps in the rib cage (rachitic rosary), spinal and pelvic deformities (including kyphosis or scoliosis), pi-

Information on Rickets

Causes: Vitamin D, calcium, or phosphate deficiency; hereditary factors

Symptoms: Pain or tenderness in long bones and pelvis, skeletal deformities (bowlegs, bumps in ribcage), spinal and pelvic deformities (scoliosis), odd-shaped skull, increased tendency toward fractures, dental deformities, night fevers, muscle cramps, impaired growth, decreased muscle tone and growth, general weakness

Duration: Short-term to chronic

Treatments: Dietary supplements, moderate exposure to sunlight

geon breast, an asymmetrical or odd-shaped skull, increased tendency toward fractures, dental deformities and cavities, night fevers, muscle cramps, impaired growth, decreased muscle tone and growth, and general weakness and restlessness.

Hereditary rickets is a sex-linked vitamin D-resistant disorder that occurs when the kidney is unable to retain phosphate. Rickets may also occur in children with liver or

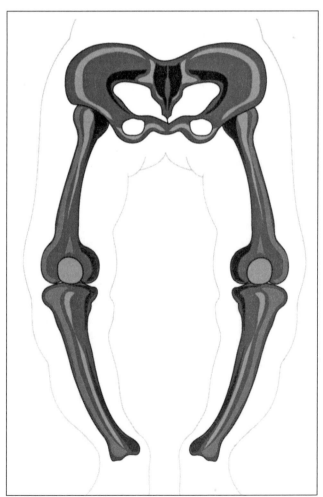

Bowed legs is a sign of a skeletal deformation that is a classic effect of rickets.

biliary disorders, when vitamin D and fats are inadequately absorbed.

Treatment and Therapy

Uncomplicated infantile rickets can be cured with a daily replacement of deficient calcium, phosphorous, and vitamin D. Clinical testing reveals improvement after one week. Dietary sources of vitamin D include fish, liver, and processed milk. In addition, moderate exposure to sunlight is therapeutic. Skeletal deformities can be corrected with good posture or body braces; in some cases, surgery may be necessary. If rickets is not corrected in children, short stature and skeletal deformities may become permanent.

—*John Alan Ross, Ph.D.*

See also Bone disorders; Bones and the skeleton; Bowlegs; Fracture and dislocation; Growth; Lower extremities; Malabsorption; Malnutrition; Nutrition; Orthopedics; Orthopedics, pediatric; Osteonecrosis; Osteoporosis; Scoliosis; Spinal cord disorders; Spine, vertebrae, and disks; Vitamins and minerals.

For Further Information:

Alan, Rick, and Michael Woods. "Rickets." *Health Library*, Feb. 25, 2013.

Ballard, Carol. *Bones*. Rev. ed. Chicago: Heinemann Library, 2002.

Bentley, George, and Robert B. Greer, eds. *Orthopaedics*. 4th ed. Oxford, England: Linacre House, 1993.

Currey, John D. *Bones: Structures and Mechanics*. 2d ed. Princeton, N.J.: Princeton University Press, 2006.

"Hereditary Hypophosphatemic Rickets." *Genetics Home Reference*, Sept. 2010.

Icon Health. *Rickets: A Medical Dictionary, Bibliography, and Annotated Research Guide to Internet References*. San Diego, Calif.: Author, 2004.

Kaneshiro, Neil K., and David Zieve. "Rickets." *MedlinePlus*, Aug. 1, 2012.

"Rickets." *MedlinePlus*, June 29, 2012.

Tortora, Gerard J., and Bryan Derrickson. *Principles of Anatomy and Physiology*. 13th ed. Hoboken, N.J.: John Wiley & Sons, 2012.

Wenger, Dennis R., and Mercer Rang. *The Art and Practice of Children's Orthopaedics*. New York: Raven Press, 1993.

Ringworm

Disease/Disorder

Also known as: Tinea

Anatomy or system affected: Skin

Specialties and related fields: Dermatology, family medicine

Definition: A group of fungal diseases caused by several species of dermatophytes and characterized by itching, scaling, and sometimes painful lesions.

Causes and Symptoms

Ringworm is a skin disease characterized by itching and redness. Despite its name, it is caused by a fungal infection, not a worm. The skin in areas affected with ringworm often contains round lesions that are colored red, have scaly borders, and contain normal-appearing skin in their centers. Alternatively, the lesions can simply be scaly, red patches with no clearly defined shape. Typically, these lesions are relatively small, approximately 1 inch in their largest dimension. Complications of ringworm include spread to the scalp, hair, or nails of the fingers or toes.

Information on Ringworm

Causes: Fungal infection
Symptoms: Itching, scaling, sometimes painful lesions
Duration: Approximately one month
Treatments: Topical skin creams, antifungal medications

The lesions of ringworm are caused by species of fungi that are members of the genus *Trichophyton*. The most common pathogen is *Trichophyton rubrum*. Ringworm appears on exposed areas of the body, often on the face and arms. Cats are the most common means of transmitting the *Trichophyton* pathogen from one person to another.

Examination of scrapings from skin lesions is used to diagnose ringworm. Species of *Trichophyton* can be tentatively identified by their microscopic structure. Culturing material from a skin lesion provides a definitive diagnosis.

Treatment and Therapy

The treatment of ringworm involves both the patient and any carriers. The patient can be treated effectively with any of several creams applied to the skin that are available without a prescription. Their use should be continued for one to two weeks after the skin lesions have cleared. Other drugs are available but require a physician's prescription. They are used for more extensive lesions or when fingernails or toenails are involved. Body ringworm usually responds within four weeks of treatment. The carrier should be identified and treated. Avoiding contact with infected household pets or clothing that has been worn by an infected person can prevent ringworm.

Perspective and Prospects

Tinea species cause infections in other parts of the body: tinea capitis on the scalp, tinea pedis on the feet, and tinea cruris in the groin region. Ringworm must be differentiated from several other diseases that also cause round skin lesions: psoriasis, syphilis, pityriasis rosea, and systemic lupus erythematosus. The lesions of psoriasis usually appear on the elbow, knees, and scalp. Syphilis lesions usually appear on the mucous membranes of the genitals or on the palms of the hands or soles of the feet. Although pityriasis rosea often begins with a single round lesion, many more usually follow. The classic skin lesion of lupus is butterfly-shaped and covers the nose and cheeks. The presence of a cat or other domestic pet is often an important element in establishing a diagnosis of ringworm.

—*L. Fleming Fallon, Jr., M.D., Ph.D., M.P.H.*

See also Athlete's foot; Dermatology; Dermatology, pediatric; Fungal infections; Itching; Pityriasis rosea; Psoriasis; Rashes; Skin; Skin disorders; Syphilis; Systemic lupus erythematosus (SLE); Zoonoses.

For Further Information:

Badash, Michelle. "Ringworm." *Health Library*, September 10, 2012.

Berman, Kevin. "Ringworm." *MedlinePlus*, May 24, 2011.

Burns, Tony, et al., eds. *Rook's Textbook of Dermatology*. 8th ed. 4 vols. Hoboken, N.J.: Wiley-Blackwell, 2010.

Goldsmith, Lowell A., Gerald S. Lazarus, and Michael D. Tharp. *Adult and Pediatric Dermatology: A Color Guide to Diagnosis and Treatment*. Philadelphia: F. A. Davis, 1997.

Lamberg, Lynne. *Skin Disorders*. Philadelphia: Chelsea House, 2001.

Mackie, Rona M. *Clinical Dermatology*. 5th ed. New York: Oxford University Press, 2003.

MedlinePlus. "Tinea Infections." *MedlinePlus*, April 11, 2013.

Middlemiss, Prisca. *What's That Rash? How to Identify and Treat Childhood Rashes*. London: Hamlyn, 2002.

Turkington, Carol, and Jeffrey S. Dover. *The Encyclopedia of Skin and Skin Disorders*. 3d ed. New York: Facts On File, 2007.

Weedon, David and Geoffrey Strutton. *Weedon's Skin Pathology*. 3d ed. repr. New York: Churchill Livingstone/Elsevier, 2011.

Rocky Mountain spotted fever

Disease/Disorder

Anatomy or system affected: Blood vessels, brain, circulatory system, kidneys, nervous system, skin
Specialties and related fields: Dermatology, emergency medicine, epidemiology, family medicine, internal medicine
Definition: An acute febrile illness caused by *Rickettsia rickettsii*.

Causes and Symptoms

In 1906, a young Ohio-born physician, Howard Taylor Ricketts, went to Montana to study the cause of "spotted fever." Through his efforts, Rocky Mountain spotted fever became the first tickborne infection to be recognized in North America. For the first half of the twentieth century, the disease was found mostly in the western United States, but since then the majority of the cases have been in the south Atlantic and south-central states. *Dermacentor andersoni* (Rocky Mountain wood tick) and *D. variabilis* (American dog tick) have been the two dominant tick species serving as vectors in the west and south, respectively.

Following the bite of an infected tick, rickettsia are transmitted through the skin into the lymphatic system and small blood vessels. Once in the bloodstream, they invade endothelial cells. The rickettsia multiply intracellularly by binary fission and spread to adjacent endothelial cells, injuring and killing their cellular hosts, which results in widespread vascular damage.

The incubation period or time from tick bite to illness is usually about seven days. The illness begins with fever, often greater than 102 degrees Fahrenheit, accompanied by headache and myalgias (muscle pain). The classic rash usually begins on the third day, starting on the wrists and ankles and spreading to the trunk. The palms and soles are often involved. The rash begins as small blanching macules and progresses to petechiae. Shock, abdominal pain, and neurological problems may mimic other diseases, making the correct diagnosis more difficult. Specific laboratory confirmation can be obtained by measuring antibodies two to three weeks later.

Treatment and Therapy

Doxycycline, a tetracycline antibiotic, is the treatment of choice for both children and adults. Therapy with

Information on Rocky Mountain Spotted Fever

Causes: Bite of infected tick
Symptoms: Fever, headache, myalgias, characteristic rash, shock, abdominal pain, neurological problems
Duration: Incubation period of about seven days
Treatments: Antibiotic (doxycycline); preventive measures (light-colored clothing, insecticides and repellants, careful removal of ticks)

doxycycline should be started immediately if Rocky Mountain spotted fever is suspected, as delays in therapy are associated with poor outcomes. Prevention can be accomplished by measures to prevent tick bites, such as wearing light-colored clothing and using insecticides and repellants on clothing and skin. Careful removal of ticks from individuals and their dogs before injection of rickettsia can occur will also prevent the disease.

Perspective and Prospects

Rocky Mountain spotted fever is spreading into new geographic locations with the acquisition of new tick vectors. It is also no longer a rural disease and has been found in urban parks. Prompt treatment with doxycycline has reduced the mortality rate from more than 80 percent in the pre-antibiotic era to less than 1 percent. Early diagnostic tests are lacking but are needed, as the majority of Rocky Mountain spotted fever cases are incorrectly diagnosed upon the first visit to a doctor. Thus far, researchers have been unable to develop a protective vaccine.

—*H. Bradford Hawley, M.D.*

See also Antibiotics; Bacterial infections; Bacteriology; Lice, mites, and ticks; Lyme disease; Plague; Rashes; Shigellosis; Tularemia; Typhus.

For Further Information:

Badash, Michelle, and Michael K. Mansour. "Rocky Mountain Spotted Fever." *Health Library*, May 20, 2013.
Chen, Luke F., and Daniel J. Sexton. "What's New in Rocky Mountain Spotted Fever?" *Infectious Disease Clinics of North America* 22 (2008): 415-432.
Dugdale, David C. III, Jatin M. Vyas, and David Zieve." Rocky Mountain Spotted Fever." *MedlinePlus*, June 9, 2011.
Margolis, Lynn, and Betsy Palmer Eldridge. "What a Revelation Any Science Is!" *ASM News* 71 (2005): 65-70.
"Rocky Mountain Spotted Fever." *Centers for Disease Control and Prevention*, Apr. 30, 2012.
"Rocky Mountain Spotted Fever." *National Institute of Allergy and Infectious Diseases*, Jan. 28, 2011.
"Tick Bites." *MedlinePlus*, Apr. 29, 2013.
Walker, David H. "*Rickettsia rickettsii* and Other Spotted Fever Group Rickettsiae (Rocky Mountain Spotted Fever and Other Spotted Fevers)." In *Principles and Practice of Infectious Diseases*, edited by Gerald L. Mandell, John F. Bennett, and Raphael Dolin. 7th ed. Philadelphia: Churchill Livingstone/Elsevier, 2009.

Root canal treatment

Procedure
Anatomy or system affected: Gums, mouth, teeth
Specialties and related fields: Dentistry
Definition: The removal of irreparably damaged tooth pulp and its replacement with inert materials.

Indications and Procedures

At the center of every tooth is soft pulp tissue. Among its main components are blood vessels that nourish teeth, sensory nerves, and supportive connective tissue. Tooth fractures or deep dental caries (cavities) irreparably damage this pulp. When this happens, root canal treatment is rendered. All dentists can carry out this procedure, but specialists who limit their practice to such efforts-endodontists-are the most skilled. The symptoms that often require root canal treatment are steady throbbing pain and sensitivity to pressure on or tapping of the tooth. Because pulp disease is associated with bacterial infection, gum abscesses may occur in extreme cases.

Root canal therapy is carried out when upon examination the pulp is found to be irreversibly damaged. A local anesthetic is administered by injection to desensitize the area. The tooth is then opened by drilling an access channel. Then, the pulp is removed from the center and from the tooth root portions-the root canals-that it also fills. Next, the pulp chamber and root canals are cleaned and reshaped by drilling and with specialized endodontic files. Lastly, the canals are filled with inert materials such as gutta-percha (a rubber-like substance), and a temporary filling is put in place. At a later time, when it is clear that the procedure has been successful, a permanent filling or an artificial crown is substituted.

Antibacterial medicine may be directly administered in the tooth itself during the procedure, and antibiotic medication may be prescribed for follow-up care.

Uses and Complications

Root canal therapy prolongs the life of teeth by creating a tooth that retains much of its strength over time. Without pulp, however, the blood supply and support of the tooth are reduced. Hence, teeth that have undergone root canal treatment are likely to become brittle and susceptible to fracture. Other possible risks associated with root canal treatments include recurrent abscess, nerve damage, pain,

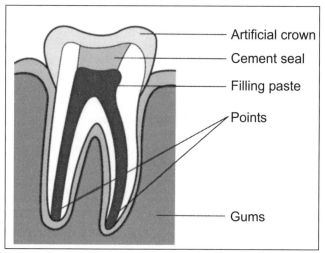

Root canal treatment may become necessary when the dental pulp is damaged; the pulp is removed and replaced with artificial material, and a crown is fitted.

swelling, and infection; those risks are greater in patients with preexisting systemic conditions such as bleeding disorders, circulatory conditions, or immune system disorders, and those who smoke.

The success of root canal therapy is about 90 percent. Nevertheless, it can produce later complications, including fine, virtually undetectable canal fractures that may allow the entry of bacteria; imperfectly filled canals can have the same result. In such cases, repeated root canal therapy may be needed or the tooth may require extraction. These problems, although relatively uncommon, occur because of the nature of this delicate surgery. For example, it is not possible to view the surgical site directly. Rather, the site is approximated by x-ray pictures taken at each treatment stage.

Perspective and Prospects

Root canal treatment has improved markedly in recent years, and further advances are expected, such as better surgical tools and filling materials and an enhanced ability to evaluate the success of the procedure. In addition, efforts to preserve and/or regenerate damaged tooth pulp are ongoing.

—*Sanford S. Singer, Ph.D.*

See also Dental diseases; Dentistry; Endodontic disease; Gum disease; Oral and maxillofacial surgery; Periodontal surgery; Periodontitis; Teeth; Tooth extraction; Toothache.

For Further Information:
A.D.A.M. Medical Encyclopedia. "Root Canal." *MedlinePlus*, February 22, 2012.
Connecticut Consumer Health Information Network. "Your Dental Health: A Guide for Patients and Families." *UConn Health Center*, November 27, 2012.
Chwistek, Marcin, ed. "Root Canal Treatment." *Health Library*, March 15, 2013.
Klatell, Jack, Andrew Kaplan, and Gray Williams, Jr., eds. *The Mount Sinai Medical Center Family Guide to Dental Health*. New York: Macmillan, 1991.
Langlais, Robert P., and Craig S. Miller. *Color Atlas of Common Oral Diseases*. 4th ed. Philadelphia: Lippincott Williams & Wilkins, 2009.
"Myths about Root Canals and Root Canal Pain." *American Association of Endodontists*, 2013.
"Root Canals." *American Association of Endodontists*, 2013.
Smith, Rebecca W. *The Columbia University School of Dental and Oral Surgery's Guide to Family Dental Care*. New York: W. W. Norton, 1997.
Taintor, Jerry F., and Mary Jane Taintor. *The Complete Guide to Better Dental Care*. New York: Checkmark Books, 1999.
Whitworth, John M. *Rational Root Canal Treatment in Practice*. Chicago: Quintessence, 2002.

Rosacea

Disease/Disorder
Also known as: Acne rosacea, adult acne, rhinophyma
Anatomy or system affected: Nose, skin
Specialties and related fields: Dermatology
Definition: A chronic inflammation and redness of the face that usually affects people between the ages of thirty and fifty; it is more common in women but is more severe in men.

Information on Rosacea

Causes: Unknown; worsened by hot drinks, alcohol, spicy foods, stress, sunlight, extreme heat or cold
Symptoms: Facial redness; slight swelling; pimples, pustules, and prominent facial pores on nose, forehead, and chin
Duration: Chronic
Treatments: Oral and topical antibiotics, avoidance of triggers

---

Causes and Symptoms

Guy de Chauliac, a French surgeon, first described rosacea medically in the fourteenth century, attributing the condition to the excessive consumption of alcoholic drinks. It is now known that although alcohol may exacerbate the condition, rosacea can develop in individuals who have never consumed alcohol. While the actual cause is unknown, rosacea is more common in fair-skinned people who flush easily and those whose family members have had the condition.

The most common triggers for this flushing are hot drinks, caffeine, alcohol, spicy foods, cosmetics, stress, exercise, sunlight, wind exposure, and extreme heat or cold. There is no cure for rosacea, but it can be treated.

Untreated, rosacea may progress from facial redness to slight swelling, pimples, pustules, and prominent facial pores on the nose, mid-forehead, and chin. In some patients, particularly in men, the oil glands enlarge, causing a bulbous, enlarged red nose and puffy cheeks. Thick bumps can develop on the lower half of the nose and nearby cheeks. This stage is known as rhinophyma, a condition made famous by actor W. C. Fields with his red, bulbous nose. Rhinophyma can be extremely disfiguring, and its mistaken association with alcoholism can cause embarrassment and affect self-esteem.

Treatment and Therapy

Rosacea and rhinophyma cannot be cured, but the symptoms can be lessened or even eliminated. Oral and topical antibiotics and avoidance of triggers are the primary ways in which rosacea is managed. Eyelid washing and prescription medication may be recommended for patients whose eyes are affected.

Rhinophyma is usually treated with surgery. The excess tissue that has developed can be removed with a scalpel or a laser or through electrosurgery.

—*Lisa M. Sardinia, Ph.D.*

See also Acne; Dermatology; Rashes; Skin; Skin disorders.

For Further Information:
Brownstein, Arlen, and Donna Shoemaker. *Rosacea: Your Self-Help Guide*. Oakland, Calif.: New Harbinger, 2001.
Hall, John C., and Gordon C. Sauer. *Sauer's Manual of Skin Diseases*. 10th ed. Philadelphia: Lippincott Williams & Wilkins, 2010.
Hellwig, Jennifer, and Purvee S. Shah. "Rosacea." *Health Library*, September 10, 2012.

Mackie, Rona M. *Clinical Dermatology*. 5th ed. New York: Oxford University Press, 2003.

Parker, James N., and Philip M. Parker, eds. *The Official Patient's Sourcebook on Acne Rosacea*. San Diego, Calif.: Icon Health, 2002.

Plewig, Gerd, and Albert M. Kligmanerd. *Acne and Rosacea*. 3d rev. ed. New York: Springer, 2000.

"Questions and Answers about Rosacea." *National Institute of Arthritis and Musculoskeletal and Skin Diseases*, October, 2012.

"Rosacea." *American Academy of Dermatology*, 2013.

Rosacea.org. http://www.rosacea.org.

Turkington, Carol, and Jeffrey S. Dover. *The Encyclopedia of Skin and Skin Disorders*. 3d ed. New York: Facts On File, 2007.

Roseola

Disease/Disorder

Also known as: Roseola infantum, exanthem subitum, sixth disease

Anatomy or system affected: Abdomen, arms, brain, immune system, legs, skin

Specialties and related fields: Family medicine, pediatrics

Definition: A disease characterized by a mild fever and a rash that mostly affects young children.

Information on Roseola

Causes: Herpesvirus infection

Symptoms: Red or pink rash, high fever, swollen lymph nodes, lethargy, lack of appetite, diarrhea, sometimes febrile seizures

Duration: A few weeks

Treatments: Alleviation of symptoms; may include baths, acetaminophen and ibuprofen, adequate fluid intake, isolation during fever stage

---

Causes and Symptoms

Roseola is caused by the human herpesvirus 6, to which most children have been exposed by age four. Immunity passed from mother to fetus usually protects infants from contracting roseola before they are six months old. Although the precise period of time during which patients are contagious is unknown, health professionals have determined that the virus incubates for as many as ten days after exposure. Patients usually are contagious only during the fever phase of roseola.

A child with roseola develops a fever that can reach 106 degrees Fahrenheit and persist for two to five days. The lymph glands in the throat may become swollen, and upper respiratory congestion may occur. Some children appear agitated, while others do not behave in an ill manner and continue normal activities. Lethargy, lack of appetite, and diarrhea may accompany the fever. The fever occasionally causes febrile seizures as the brain reacts to sudden and extreme temperature changes. Approximately 5 to 15 percent of roseola patients experience these convulsions, which last several minutes and usually are not harmful.

When the fever ceases, a red or pink rash appears on most patients' bodies and remains for several hours to three days. When pressed, the rash blanches. It does not blister, cause pain, or itch. Occasionally, a roseola patient is feverish and never develops a rash or has a rash without a preceding fever. A rash may appear prematurely during the fever phase or be delayed until after the fever has subsided. Some children infected with roseola never display any symptoms. Rarely, roseola can precede encephalitis and aseptic meningitis.

Treatment and Therapy

Treatment for roseola consists of methods to soothe symptoms. Pediatricians recommend baths and the use of acetaminophen and ibuprofen, if the child is old enough, to lower the fever. Health professionals also advise patients to drink fluids to prevent dehydration. The patient should be isolated until the fever is gone.

A child who has convulsions should be examined by medical professionals immediately. Patients with dark purple rashes should also be seen by physicians, as should children whose rashes do not blanch when touched or remain more than several days. Blisters and itchy or painful rashes also demand professional attention. Children with roseola who seem unusually sick should also be taken for examination, as should children with prolonged fevers that do not improve with medication and baths.

Most patients recover fully. Although the resulting antibodies are present in most adults, roseola can be reactivated if the immune system is weakened.

Perspective and Prospects

Roseola has been referred to in medical literature since the mid-nineteenth century. Early twentieth century investigators unsuccessfully attempted to identify the disease's pathogen. By 1988, medical professionals determined that the herpevirus 6 causes roseola. Two strains, A and B, have been identified, with strain B causing most roseola cases in children. The herpesvirus 7 has been linked to cases occurring in older patients.

—Elizabeth D. Schafer, Ph.D.

See also Blisters; Childhood infectious diseases; Fever; Herpes; Pediatrics; Rashes; Viral infections.

For Further Information:

Gershon, Anne A., Samuel L. Katz, and Peter J. Hotez, eds. *Krugman's Infectious Diseases of Children*. 11th ed. Philadelphia: Mosby, 2004.

Grossman, Leigh B., ed. *Infection Control in the Child Care Center and Preschool*. 8th ed. Charlottesville, Va.: Silverchair Science, 2012.

Hoekelman, Robert A., ed. *Primary Pediatric Care*. 4th ed. St. Louis, Mo.: Mosby, 2001.

Parker, James N., and Phillip M. Parker. *Roseola: A Medical Dictionary, Bibliography, and Annotated Research Guide to Internet References*. San Diego, Calif.: Icon Health, 2004.

"Roseola." *Health Library*, November 26, 2012.

"Roseola." *MedlinePlus*, August 2, 2011.

Rotator cuff surgery

Procedure

Anatomy or system affected: Musculoskeletal system, arms, joints, muscles, tendons

Specialties and related fields: General surgery, orthopedics, rheumatology, sports medicine, physical therapy

Definition: The surgical correction of a muscle and/or tendon tear within the shoulder.

Indications and Procedures

The shoulder, considered to be a ball and socket joint, is the most flexible joint in the human body. Because of its structure, the shoulder has a wide range of motion; however, this also predisposes the shoulder to a very high risk of injury. To counter this risk, the shoulder is stabilized by a group of four muscles, collectively known as the rotator cuff: the subscapularis, the supraspinatus, the infraspinatus, and the teres minor.

The signs and symptoms of rotator cuff injuries include point tenderness in the joint around the region of the humeral head deep within the deltoid muscle, pain and stiffness within the shoulder region within a day of participating in activities that involve shoulder movements, and difficulty in producing overhead motions involving the upper arm. Pain often occurs at night because of sleeping positions that put excess pressure on the joint. Occasionally, a clicking noise can be heard emanating from the joint upon movement or the patient may experience a "sticking point" when shoulder movements are attempted. Injuries to the rotator cuff can mimic other common shoulder region problems, including bursitis (inflammation of a bursa, a soft, fluid-filled sac that helps cushion surfaces that glide over one another) and tendinitis (inflammation of a tendon). Injuries to the rotator cuff include impingement and tears.

Impingement occurs when the rotator cuff tendons are pinched because of a narrowing of the space between the acromion (shoulder blade) process and the rotator cuff. This narrowing commonly occurs with aging, but it can also be traumatically induced. Sports that commonly put excess stress on the rotator cuff include baseball, swimming, and tennis. Besides a traumatic injury, chronic impingement of the rotator cuff tendons can cause partial or complete tears. To evaluate the extent of shoulder dysfunction, the physician will conduct a physical examination to determine range of motion and use diagnostic imaging procedures such as x-rays, an arthrogram (an x-ray after a tracer dye has been injected into the shoulder), magnetic resonance imaging (MRI), and ultrasound. Nonsurgical interventions include rest, ice immediately following an injury or heat twenty-four hours afterward, painkillers, anti-inflammatory medications, and physical therapy.

Rotator cuff surgery is usually recommended when there is little improvement in shoulder function or pain reduction after a course of noninvasive therapies. Surgery to correct rotator cuff tears is more successful if the procedure is performed within three months of the date of injury. If the shoulder is surgically treated later there is a complication of the torn tendons retracting away from each other increasing the difficulty of the surgery and decreasing the chances of a satisfactory outcome. Surgery can be a classic open procedure, requiring a 2- to 3-inch incision in the shoulder, or less traumatic arthroscopy, which requires only a small incision, half an inch or less, just large enough to accommodate the instruments and a video camera apparatus. Occasionally, the surgeon will use a combination of the open procedure and arthroscopy. Either general anesthesia, in which the patient is asleep, or local anesthesia, in which the region is "frozen" but the patient is awake, can be used for the procedure. An interscalene block may also be used to remove all sensation from the extremity, but limb sensation returns shortly after surgery. With local anesthesia, a light sedative may also be used to put the patient at ease, but not asleep. Acromioplasty reduces the impingement of the rotator cuff tendons. In this procedure, a portion of the bone underneath the acromion is shaved to give the tendons more room to move and prevent them from becoming pinched. This process is often included in rotator cuff surgical repairs. In rotator cuff repairs, the torn tendons are reattached to the humerus (upper arm bone). The open surgical procedure requires a relatively large incision through the shoulder as well as cutting through the deltoid muscle. Any scar tissue that has formed is removed, and a small ridge is cut into the top of the humerus. Small holes are drilled into the bone, and the tendons are sutured to the bone using these holes as anchors. The surgeon will also correct any other problems encountered, such as removing bone spurs, shaving down the acromion, or freeing up ligaments that may be pressing against the tendons.

During arthroscopic surgery, the majority of these additional procedures are still able to be performed. After the small incision is made into the shoulder, a thin tube is inserted. This tube contains the surgical instruments as well as a video camera that is used to guide the repair procedure. Arthroscopic surgery is becoming more common and is preferred for small to larger tears, as it limits the amount of surgical intervention, reduces surgical risks, and quickens recovery time. If more extensive damage is discovered, then the surgeon may elect to combine the arthroscopic procedure with open surgery. However, arthroscopic tear repair has advanced tremendously, to the point that tears previously thought to be irreparable or too extensive are now being completed with arthroscopy.

Uses and Complications

The varying outcomes from rotator cuff surgery range from almost full recovery to no improvement at all. The degree of recovery is dependent upon the extent of damage to the rotator cuff as well as patient compliance with physical therapy after surgery. If the tendon has been torn for a long time, then it may not be reparable.

As with all surgical procedures, the patient may have an adverse reaction to the anesthesia. This risk is greater if the person is obese or has a cardiovascular, pulmonary, or metabolic condition. Surgical incisions always have the risk of infection, but this risk is minimized with the arthroscopic procedure because of the small incision size and the relatively short operative time (one to two hours). In rare instances, there is also the risk of nerve damage resulting in partial paralysis or temporary numbness at the incision area.

After surgery, the recovering arm will be put in a sling

with a small shock-absorbing pillow placed behind the elbow. Extreme care should be taken with shoulder movements for the first three months following surgery. Reaching and lifting objects above the head should be avoided during this period. Passive range of motion exercises, in which the arm is moved by the physical therapist, should be started as soon as possible to prevent scar tissue formation and resultant stiffness. Exercises should be done several times a day so that within two to three weeks, the range of motion (flexibility) of the repaired shoulder should be equivalent to that of the uninjured shoulder. After six weeks, more advanced exercises are recommended to strengthen the rotator cuff as well as the surrounding shoulder muscles. Full recovery and rehabilitation from rotator cuff surgery can take up to a year.

—*Bonita L. Marks, PhD*

See also: Arthritis; Arthroplasty; Arthroscopy; Bones and the skeleton; Bursitis; Joints; Muscle sprains, spasms, and disorders; Muscles; Orthopedic surgery; Orthopedics; Rheumatology; Sports medicine; Tendinitis; Upper extremities.

For Further Information:
Codsi, Michael Howe, Chris R. "Shoulder Conditions: Diagnosis and Treatment Guideline." *Physical Medical and RehabilitationClinics of North America* 2015; 26(3): 467-489. doi:10.1016/j.pmr.2015.04.007.

Lo, I. K., and S. S. Burkhart. "Current Concepts in Arthroscopic Rotator Cuff Repair." *American Journal of Sports Medicine* 1, no. 2 (2003): 308-324.

Matsen, Frederick A., and Steven B. Lippitt. *Shoulder Surgery: Principles and Procedures*. Philadelphia: W. B. Saunders, 2003.

Pfeiffer, Ronald P., and Brent C. Mangus. *Concepts of Athletic Training*. 6th ed. Sudbury, Mass.: Jones and Bartlett, 2012.

Rockwood, Charles A., Frederick A. Matsen, and Michael Wirth. *The Shoulder*. 4th ed. 2 vols. St. Louis, Mo.: Saunders/Elsevier, 2009.

"Rotator Cuff Repair." *Health Library*, March 18, 2013.

"Rotator Cuff Repair." *MedlinePlus*, June 30, 2011.

Williams, G. R., and M. Kelley. "Management of Rotator Cuff and Impingement Injuries in the Athlete." *Journal of Athletic Training* 35, no. 3 (2000): 300-315.

Yamaguchi, K., et al. "Transitioning to Arthroscopic Rotator Cuff Repair: The Pros and Cons." *Journal of Bone & Joint Surgery, American Volume* 85, no. 1 (2003): 144-156.

Lewis, Sarah, "Rotator Cuff Surgery." *Healthgrades Operating Company, Inc.* 2017 https://www.healthgrades.com/procedures/rotator-cuff-surgeryAccessed 9-16-2017.

Pile, JC. Evaluating postoperative fever: A focused approach. Cleveland Clinic Journal of Medicine. 2006;73 (Suppl 1):S62. http://ccjm.org/content/73/Suppl_1/S62.full.pdf,

Rotator Cuff Repair. MedlinePlus, a service of the National Library of Medicine National Institutes of Health. http://www.nlm.nih.gov/medlineplus/ency/article/007207.htm.

Rotator Cuff Tears. American Academy of Orthopedic Surgeons. http://orthoinfo.aaos.org/topic.cfm?topic=A00064.

Rotator Cuff Tears: Surgery and Exercise. Cleveland Clinic. http://my.clevelandclinic.org/disorders/rotator_cuff/hic_rotator_cuff_tears_surgery_and_exercise.asp.

Rotator Cuff Tears: Surgical Treatment Options. American Academy of Orthopedic Surgeons. http://orthoinfo.aaos.org/topic.cfm?topic=A00406.

Shoulder Problems. National Institute of Arthritis and Musculoskeletal and Skin Diseases. http://www.niams.nih.gov/Health_Info/Shoulder_Problems/.

Shoulder Surgery. American Academy of Orthopedic Surgeons. http://orthoinfo.aaos.org/topic.cfm?topic=a00066.

Rotavirus

Disease/Disorder

Also known as: Sporadic or severe viral gastroenteritis, rotaviral enteritis, infantile diarrhea, winter diarrhea

Anatomy or system affected: Gastrointestinal system

Specialties and related fields: Epidemiology, gastroenterology, pediatrics, virology

Definition: A virus with a characteristic wheel-like appearance when viewed under an electronic microscope that causes viral gastroenteritis in children worldwide.

Causes and Symptoms

Rotavirus is classified into groups A through G, with group A responsible for gastroenteritis in children. Adults can also contract the virus but will experience milder symptoms. The virus is very contagious, with oral-fecal transmission occurring through ingestion of contaminated water or food or contact with an infected surface such as a toy or hand. Airborne infection is rare. In temperate climates, the disease occurs more often in the cooler months, from late autumn to early spring, with year-round infection present in tropical climates. Almost all children have been infected more than once by the time they are four years old.

Symptoms are manifested after two days from the initial exposure and include severe watery diarrhea, vomiting, nausea, and fever, with the gastroenteritis lasting from three to ten days. Dehydration may result if fluids are not adequately replenished. Symptoms of severe dehydration include dry mouth, dry skin, sunken eyes, no tears when crying, lethargy, irritability, and reduced or no wet diapers over three hours. A physician should be notified if symptoms of severe dehydration are observed. Because the virus is highly contagious, epidemic outbreaks may be seen in child-care centers.

Treatment and Therapy

Clinical diagnosis is made from detection of the virus antigen in a stool sample. Detection of rotavirus is also possible with an electron microscope or tissue culture. Treatment involves drinking plenty of fluids to prevent dehydration. Antidiarrheal medication should not be given to children unless prescribed by a doctor. Hospitalization may be required for intravenous (IV) fluid rehydration if severe dehydration occurs. Immunity develops after repeat infections, with subsequent infections exhibiting less severe

---

Information on Rotavirus

Causes: Viral infection transmitted through contaminated food or water, fecal-oral contamination, or contact with contaminated surface

Symptoms: Severe watery diarrhea, vomiting, nausea, fever

Duration: Three to ten days

Treatments: Fluids to prevent dehydration, prevention through handwashing and disinfection of surfaces

symptoms. The virus may survive on hard surfaces for years. Diligent hand washing and disinfection of surfaces with a diluted bleach solution or 70 percent alcohol may help slow the spread of the virus.

Perspective and Prospects

Rotavirus was discovered in 1973 from intestinal biopsies of children diagnosed with winter vomiting disease. The name is derived from the Latin word *rota*, which means "wheel." In February, 2006, the U.S. Food and Drug Administration (FDA) approved a live, oral vaccine for use in children. In 2009, the World Health Organization, which estimates that rotavirus kills about 527,000 people annually, recommended that the vaccine be made a routine part of national immunization programs around the world.

—*Susan E. Thomas, M.L.S.*

See also Childhood infectious diseases; Dehydration; Diarrhea and dysentery; Food poisoning; Gastroenteritis; Gastroenterology; Gastroenterology, pediatric; Gastrointestinal disorders; Gastrointestinal system; Intestinal disorders; Intestines; Nausea and vomiting; Noroviruses; Pediatrics; Viral infections.

For Further Information:

Aronson, Susan S., and Timothy R. Shope, eds. *Managing Infectious Diseases in Child Care and Schools: A Quick Reference Guide.* Elk Grove Village, Ill.: American Academy of Pediatrics, 2005.

Kohnle, Diana. "Rotavirus." *Health Library*, February 20, 2013.

"Rotavirus." *Centers for Disease Control and Prevention*, October 28, 2010.

"Rotavirus." *Mayo Clinic*, March 27, 2013.

"Rotavirus." *World Health Organization*, October, 2011.

Heymann, David L., ed. *Control of Communicable Diseases Manual.* 19th ed. Washington, D.C.: American Public Health Association, 2008.

Matson, David O. "Rotaviruses." In *Principles and Practice of Pediatric Infectious Diseases*, edited by Sarah S. Long, Larry K. Pickering, and Charles G. Prober. 3d ed. Philadelphia: Churchill Livingstone/Elsevier, 2008.

Roundworms

Disease/Disorder

Anatomy or system affected: Blood vessels, circulatory system, gastrointestinal system, intestines, lungs, lymphatic system

Specialties and related fields: Environmental health, epidemiology, public health

Definition: Worm-shaped animals that act as parasites of plants and animals.

Key terms:

cuticle: the protective noncellular outer covering of an animal

intermediate host: an animal or plant in which nonadult life stages of endoparasites occur

primary host: an organism in which adult endoparasites are found and can reproduce

Causes and Symptoms

Roundworms are tube-shaped animals in the phylum Nemotoda. They are a highly diverse group, numbering twelve thousand named species, but some taxonomists suggest that fifty thousand more species have yet to be

---

Information on Roundworms

Causes: Parasitic infection transmitted through skin exposure or ingestion

Symptoms: Depends on type; may include severe pneumonia, malnutrition, intestinal blockages, anemia, itching, elephantiasis, severe pain, and sometimes death

Duration: Often chronic

Treatments: Species-specific drugs

---

discovered and named. Roundworms occur from the tropics to the tundra and are found in virtually all habitats. Most are free-living animals, but some are parasites of plants and animals. At least fifty are important internal parasites of humans.

Structurally and organizationally, roundworms are very simple animals; most are composed of fewer than one thousand cells. The circular, long body of a roundworm is covered by a tough, protective cuticle. Inside is a tubular digestive tract and simplified nervous system. Its reproductive system is capable of producing enormous numbers of eggs.

Ascaris lumbricoides is a common intestinal parasite of humans and also one of the largest of the nematodes, with a length of 30 centimeters or more. A female can produce two hundred thousand eggs per day for several months, which are secreted into intestinal fluids and voided with the feces. If the eggs are ingested, then they pass through the stomach and into the digestive system and hatch in the intestines. The juveniles burrow through the intestinal wall and are carried via the circulatory system to the lungs. They are reswallowed and returned to the intestines via the esophagus, where they mature. Large numbers of juveniles in the lungs can produce a severe pneumonia, while heavy infestations of adults can cause malnutrition and intestinal blockages.

More than half a billion people in tropical regions may be infected by hookworms, which feed on the blood contents of the gut rather than intestinal fluids. Hookworm life cycles differ from that of *Ascaris lumbricoides*, in that eggs hatch on the ground and juveniles burrow into the skin of the feet or hands and are carried via the blood to the lungs. From the lungs, the juveniles migrate to the pharynx and are then carried to the intestines, where they cause serious blood and tissue damage including anemia and malnutrition.

Pinworms are the most common of the parasitic roundworms. Infection by the human pinworm, *Enterobius vermicularis*, occurs when a female pinworm deposits its eggs at night in the perianal region, causing irritation. Scratching lodges eggs under the fingernails which, if put in the mouth, cause infection or reinfection.

A number of roundworm parasites have an intermediate host in their life cycle. For example, *Trichinella spiralis*, the trichina worm, which causes trichinosis in humans, has two hosts in its life cycle; humans are the primary hosts, while pigs are the intermediate hosts. Juveniles lodge in the muscle tissue of pigs as calcified cysts. If contaminated meat is ingested by humans, then the juveniles hatch and migrate into the intestines. Infection with trichina worms produces severe pain and sometimes death as juveniles and adults burrow through body tissues.

The most spectacular of the roundworm parasites is the dracunculoid guinea worm (*Dracunculus medinensis*), which lives in connective tissue and may reach 2 to 3 feet in length. A female discharges its eggs directly into standing water through an ulcerated sore in a human's skin, often on the feet. The larvae are eaten by freshwater copepods (water fleas) called *Cyclops* and embed in their tissues. Larvae gain entry to humans when a human drinks water containing the nearly microscopic *Cyclops*, thus beginning the life cycle again.

The filaroid roundworm parasites such as *Wuchereria bancrofti* of Africa and Asia are spread by means of a blood-feeding arthropod vector. All eight species of filaroids live in lymph nodes and associated ducts and feed on lymph. The female produces larvae, called microfilariae, which are carried to the skin via the circulatory system. Blood-feeding insects suck up blood containing the larvae, which are injected into another person during the next blood meal. Heavy infestations of male and female worms block the lymph vessels, which enlarge to produce the condition called elephantiasis.

Treatment and Therapy

Parasitic roundworm infection continues to be a global medical health problem of great concern, especially in the warmer regions of the world. Modern medicine has greatly reduced the pathologies associated with heavy parasitic infections, which can be detected by blood or stool samples, and treatment with species-specific drugs can very effectively eliminate most species. The best prevention method remains adequate sanitation and access to clean water.

—*Dwight G. Smith, Ph.D.*

See also Elephantiasis; Insect-borne diseases; Intestinal disorders; Intestines; Parasitic diseases; Pinworms; Trichinosis; Tropical medicine; Worms; Zoonoses.

For Further Information:
"Parasites." *Centers for Disease Control and Prevention*, April 19, 2013.
"Parasitic Roundworm Diseases." *National Institute of Allergy and Infectious Diseases*, June 10, 2011.
Parker, Philip M., and James N. Parker. *Roundworms: A Medical Dictionary, Bibliography, and Annotated Research Guide to Internet References*. San Diego, Calif.: Icon Health, 2004.
Roberts, Larry S., and John Janovy, Jr., eds. *Gerald D. Schmidt and Larry S. Roberts' Foundations of Parasitology*. 8th ed. Boston: McGraw-Hill Higher Education, 2010.
Ruppert, Edward E., Richard S. Fox, and Robert D. Barnes. *Invertebrate Zoology: A Functional Evolutionary Approach*. 7th ed. Belmont, Calif.: Thomson-Brooks/Cole, 2004.

Rubella

Disease/Disorder
Also known as: German measles
Anatomy or system affected: Joints, lymphatic system, nervous system, skin
Specialties and related fields: Family medicine, pediatrics

Definition: An acute, contagious childhood disease caused by a virus and characterized by a rash.
Key terms:
arthralgia: pain in a joint or joints
arthritis: inflammation of a joint or joints
congenital: present at birth; having to do with a fetus carried by a pregnant woman

Causes and Symptoms

Rubella can be either acquired, infecting both children and adults, or congenital, infecting a fetus before birth. Acquired rubella is typically a mild disease with few complications. The incubation period is usually sixteen to eighteen days, but it can last fourteen to twenty-one days. For children, the first symptom is typically a rash that is small, red, and spotty. It starts on the face and behind the ears and spreads downward in the next one or two days. This rash is much milder than the rash of measles. In adults, the rash is preceded by symptoms that include a low-grade fever, headache, loss of appetite, mildly red eyes, a stuffy nose, a sore throat, coughing, and lymph node enlargement in the neck. Typically, this enlargement occurs behind the ears and in the back of the neck.

Complications of rubella are more common in adults, particularly in young women. The most common complications are arthralgia and arthritis. These joint manifestations can occur in any time from when the rash subsides to several weeks later. Rarer complications include effects on the blood, the heart, and the nervous system.

Congenital rubella is associated with multiple birth defects in the infant. The most common manifestations of congenital rubella affect three areas: growth, the blood, and the central nervous system. The effects on growth include prematurity and intrauterine growth retardation. The effects on the blood include thrombocytopenia (a decrease in platelets), anemia, and an enlarged liver and spleen. The effects on the central nervous system include microcephaly (a small head), deafness, eye damage (including cataracts and retinal damage), mental retardation, and behavioral disorders. Whether these effects of congenital rubella are manifested depends on the timing of the infection during pregnancy and the severity of the infection. Some newborns may appear normal at delivery and develop manifestations during their first five years of life.

The diagnosis of acquired rubella primarily hangs on the clinical symptoms, such as a rash and lymph node enlargement in the back of the neck. The diagnosis of congenital rubella may be confused with other congenital or perinatal infections, such as syphilis, toxoplasmosis, herpes simplex, and cytomegalovirus (CMV). These congenital infections can all lead to intrauterine growth retardation, deafness, mental retardation, and thrombocytopenia.

Treatment and Therapy

Infants with congenital rubella must be viewed as having a continually evolving disease, since there is no present method to stop or decrease the replication of the rubella virus in the infected newborn. No antiviral medications or

Information on Rubella

Causes: Viral infection, congenital transmission
Symptoms: Small, red, and spotty rash; low-grade fever; headache; appetite loss; mildly red eyes; stuffy nose; sore throat; coughing; lymph node enlargement in neck
Duration: Acute
Treatments: Alleviation of symptoms

antibody preparations have been found to be of therapeutic benefit in children with congenital rubella. Thus, therapy is supportive and requires a multidisciplinary approach. Hearing disabilities require testing, which involves special equipment for infants. If hearing loss is found, support for the child's language and communication development must take place; specially designed educational programs are available. A full eye examination should be performed by an ophthalmologist.

Acquired rubella infection is fairly benign, and its management usually involves allowing the virus to run its course. Since the greatest damage done by rubella virus is to a developing fetus, the management of rubella should focus on prevention of infection in women of childbearing age. Because acquired rubella infection is commonly asymptomatic or subclinical, the only adequate way to prevent this disease and its effects on the fetus is immunization.

A vaccine is available and has been shown to produce an excellent immune response. Two doses of rubella vaccine are recommended, given as the combined vaccine known as measles, mumps, and rubella (MMR). The first dose is given to a child at twelve to fifteen months of age. The second dose should be given prior to the child's entry into school. The vaccine should also be given to adult women who have not received the vaccine previously.

Although it is not recommended that the vaccine be given to pregnant women because of the theoretical risk of inducing congenital rubella, no infants whose mothers were vaccinated during pregnancy have shown congenital defects. Rubella vaccine should not be given after the administration of antibody preparations. The vaccine also should not be given to immunosuppressed patients unless recommended by a doctor. The side effects of the vaccine, occurring in about 10 percent of children, include fever, a rash, and lymph node enlargement. Adult women are prone to developing arthralgia after receiving the rubella vaccine. Other, very rare complications of the vaccine have also occurred.

Perspective and Prospects

Since the introduction of the rubella vaccine in the United States in 1969, rubella and the associated congenital rubella syndrome have been virtually eliminated from the Western Hemisphere, signaling the success of the Unites States' immunization program. Nearly 58,000 cases of rubella were reported in the United States in 1969; by 1999

that number had fallen to 272; no endemic case of rubella has been reported in the Americas since 2009. However, rubella continues to be a health problem in developing countries in other parts of the world, with the World Health Organization reporting an estimated 110,000 babies born each year with congenital rubella syndrome.

—*Peter D. Reuman, M.D., M.P.H.*

See also Birth defects; Cataracts; Childhood infectious diseases; Congenital disorders; Eyes; Fever; Hearing loss; Immunization and vaccination; Intellectual disability; Joints; Measles; Mumps; Rashes; Viral infections; Vision disorders.

For Further Information:

Beers, Mark H., et al., eds. *The Merck Manual of Diagnosis and Therapy.* 18th ed. Whitehouse Station, N.J.: Merck Research Laboratories, 2006.

Behrman, Richard E., Robert M. Kliegman, and Hal B. Jenson, eds. *Nelson Textbook of Pediatrics.* 19th ed. Philadelphia: Saunders/Elsevier, 2011.

Bellenir, Karen, and Peter D. Dresser, eds. *Contagious and Noncontagious Infectious Diseases Sourcebook.* Detroit, Mich.: Omnigraphics, 1996.

Carson-DeWitt, Rosalyn. "Rubella." *Health Library,* September 27, 2012.

Martin, Richard J., Avroy A. Fanaroff, and Michele C. Walsh, eds. *Fanaroff and Martin's Neonatal-Perinatal Medicine: Diseases of the Fetus and Infant.* 2 vols. 9th ed. Philadelphia: Mosby/Elsevier, 2011.

Middlemiss, Prisca. *What's That Rash? How to Identify and Treat Childhood Rashes.* London: Hamlyn, 2002.

"Rubella." *World Health Organization,* July, 2012.

Shaw, Michael, ed. *Everything You Need to Know About Diseases.* Springhouse, Pa.: Springhouse Press, 1996.

Woolf, Alan D., et al., eds. *The Children's Hospital Guide to Your Child's Health and Development.* Cambridge, Mass.: Perseus, 2002.

Rubinstein-Taybi syndrome

Disease/Disorder
Also known as: Broad thumb-hallux syndrome
Anatomy or system affected: Bones, ears, eyes, feet, genitals, hands, head, heart, mouth, nose, teeth
Specialties and related fields: Cardiology, dentistry, genetics, neurology, ophthalmology, orthopedics, pediatrics, speech pathology
Definition: A syndrome typically characterized by small skeletal stature, mental retardation, and large thumbs and toes.

Causes and Symptoms

Medical investigators have linked Rubinstein-Taybi syndrome to a mutation of the CREB-binding protein (CREBBP) gene on chromosome 16. Studies estimate an occurrence rate ranging from 1 to 3 cases per 100,000 people, with a higher incidence in institutions. The syndrome hinders physical and intellectual development. Patients are intellectually disabled, and they do not develop motor skills at normal rates.

Body size, particularly of the head, is much smaller than that attained by typical children because growth is stunted. Most patients have thumbs and/or big toes that are unusually large and have flat tips. Sometimes, the big toes are separated from the smaller toes, which are grouped closely

Information on Rubinstein-Taybi Syndrome

Causes: Genetic mutation
Symptoms: Mental retardation, poor motor skill development, small body size, small head, large thumbs and big toes, long nose, tiny mouth, wide-set eyes with sagging eyelids; misshapen ears; bunched teeth; undescended testicles; excessive body hair
Duration: Lifelong
Treatments: Physical, behavioral, and occupational therapies; surgical correction of knees, testicles, eyes, teeth; medications or surgeries for various complications; antibiotics for related infections; institutionalization and constant monitoring

together.

A patient's face often bears distinctive characteristics, including a long nose, a tiny mouth, and far-apart eyes with sagging eyelids and extended eyelashes. The patient sometimes squints. The ears are frequently misshapen. Inside the mouth, the teeth are bunched together on steep palates. In males, the testes usually do not descend. Both genders often grow more body hair than do normal children.

Treatment and Therapy

Medical care for Rubinstein-Taybi syndrome includes various physical, behavioral, and occupational therapies to treat specific problems. Speech therapy helps patients learn to communicate. Corrective shoes or surgery may be necessary to aid walking if toe size and placement interfere with movement. The knees and testicles may also require surgical adjustment. Eye surgery may be necessary if eyeglasses do not resolve vision flaws. Dentistry corrects faulty bites.

Patients sometimes suffer seizures, brain tumors, and heart, lung, or digestive complications and require appropriate medications or surgeries. Antibiotics mitigate urinary tract infections, ear infections, and kidney problems related to this syndrome. Patients are vulnerable to heart or breathing problems while anesthetized. Many require institutional-ization and constant monitoring because they experience sleeping and eating difficulties. Individuals with this syndrome can attain average life spans if they do not suffer serious physical problems or infections.

Perspective and Prospects

Greek physicians J. Michail, J. Matsoukas, and S. Theodorou reported a case in 1957 of a child with the traits of this syndrome. Unaware of that publication, in the late 1950s Jack H. Rubinstein and Hooshang Taybi observed distinctive characteristics in seven patients. Taybi delivered their joint paper at the 1962 Society for Pediatric Radiology meeting. The next year, they published a 1963 article outlining this syndrome. In the early twenty-first century, medical researchers continued genetic investigations for this syndrome.

—Elizabeth D. Schafer, Ph.D.

See also Birth defects; Congenital disorders; Embryology; Genetic diseases; Intellectual disability; Neonatology; Pediatrics.

For Further Information:
Rubinstein-Taybi Syndrome. http://www.rubinstein-taybi.org.
Rubinstein, Jack H., and Hooshang Taybi. "Broad Thumbs and Toes and Facial Abnormalities: A Possible Mental Retardation Syndrome." *American Journal of Diseases of Children* 105 (1963): 588-608.
"Rubinstein-Taybi Syndrome." *MedlinePlus*, August 4, 2011.
"Rubinstein-Taybi Syndrome; Williams Syndrome." *American Journal of Medical Genetics* Supplement 6. New York: Wiley-Liss, 1990.
Taybi, Hooshang. *Handbook of Syndromes and Metabolic Disorders: Radiologic and Clinical Manifestations.* St. Louis, Mo.: Mosby, 1998.
Wiley, Susan, et al. "Rubinstein-Taybi Syndrome Medical Guidelines." *American Journal of Medical Genetics* 119A, no. 2 (June 1, 2003): 101-110.

Safety issues for children

Procedures

Anatomy or system affected: All

Specialties and related fields: Critical care, emergency medicine, family medicine, pediatrics, sports medicine

Definition: Measures taken to prevent accidents among children.

The Importance of Safety Measures

Each year in the United States, approximately 1 million children receive medical care as a result of unintentional injury. Of these, about forty thousand to fifty thousand suffer permanent damage and about four thousand die. The first years of a child's life are the most dangerous: Unintentional injuries are the primary cause of death in children up to the age of five.

Cribs can pose serious health threats to babies; the government issued guidelines regarding the dimensions and spacing between slats and prohibited drop-side rail cribs.

Sudden Infant Death Syndrome (SIDS) in apparently normal babies between ages of two weeks and six months has greatly declined since the American Academy of Pediatrics (AAP) in 1992 recommended that babies should be placed on their backs to sleep unless otherwise indicated by their pediatrician. However, in 2011, the AAP expanded the guidelines for infant sleep safety and SIDS risk reduction as sleep-related deaths from other causes (other than sleep position) have increased. The following information for parents on safe sleep environment is from those guidelines:

- Always place your baby on his or her back for every sleep time.
- Always use a firm sleep surface. Car seats and other sitting devices are not recommended for routine sleep.
- The baby should sleep in the same room as the parents, but not in the same bed (room-sharing without bed-sharing).
- Keep soft objects or loose bedding out of the crib. This includes pillows, blankets, and bumper pads.
- Wedges and positioners should not be used.
- Pregnant woman should receive regular prenatal care.
- Don't smoke during pregnancy or after birth.
- Breastfeeding is recommended.
- Offer a pacifier at nap time and bedtime.
- Avoid covering the infant's head or overheating.
- Do not use home monitors or commercial devices marketed to reduce the risk of SIDS.
- Infants should receive all recommended vaccinations.
- Supervised, awake tummy time is recommended daily to facilitate development and minimize the occurrence of positional plagiocephaly (flat heads).

Foresight, common sense, and vigilance are required to prevent injuries to children, particularly those under the age of two, who do not communicate verbally. Between the ages of two and four, although a child has a sense of cause and effect (a boy who kicks a ball knows that it may roll into the street), the child is unable to consider the outside effects (a car could hit him if he runs into the street after the ball).

Basic information in case an emergency occurs should be accessible in all homes with children. The phone number of the family physician, the nearest hospital and emergency service, and the local poison control center should be posted adjacent to the phone. When caregivers are employed, they should be given transportation fare, copies of children's medical cards, the doctor's phone number, and the phone number where the parents can be reached. For optimum communication, parents should travel with a cellular phone. The number of a relative to contact in the event of an emergency occurring to the parents should be included as well.

Safety in the Home

All parents should develop a childproofing plan before a newborn arrives and modify it when the baby begins to crawl and walk. Hazards change with age. The Consumer Product Safety Commission urges families to do a room-by-room check of their house. The best way to do this is to put oneself in the place of the child, getting down on one's hands and knees and imagining what would be interesting or constitute an obstacle.

Equipment: Surprisingly, almost as many children are injured or die from using objects designed for their use as from automobile accidents. In the United States, accidents related to playing with toys send 120,000 children to the emergency room annually. Most standards for baby equipment went into effect in the early 1970s, so extra caution must be exercised with equipment manufactured prior to that date.

Baby walkers, which are involved in more than twenty-eight thousand injuries annually, are not approved by the American Academy of Pediatrics. Tripping is the most common cause of injury; it can be prevented by using a walker with at least six wheels and a base wider than the seat height. Walkers can also fall down stairs.

Falls from high chairs send around seven thousand infants to the hospital a year. High chairs should have a safety strap and a wide base to prevent tipping. Cantilevered high chairs that hook to a table are unstable. They should lock to the table and be attached only if the table is strong enough to support them.

Despite standards to ensure safe cribs, up to 30 million potentially dangerous cribs are in use in the United States, and approximately fifty babies suffocate or strangle in cribs annually. Cribs more than twenty-five years old are the most hazardous because the slats are too wide. Moreover, they may have lead-based paint. Even newer cribs with decorative cutouts can trap a baby's head. In addition, corner posts can catch clothing, resulting in strangulation.

The first safety measure is to ensure that crib slats are spaced no more than 2.375 inches apart and that corner posts extend no more than .0625 inch above the railing. Cribs should never be placed next to a wall lamp, electrical outlet, window, radiator, or vent. To prevent the possibility of suffocation, puffy gear such as large stuffed animals, adult pillows, or comforters should not be used in cribs until a child reaches one year of age. Securely fastened bumpers, however, may be used until the baby is able to stand (and thus able to climb on them to exit the crib).

Bunkbeds pose a similar threat as cribs. To safeguard these beds, wooden bars should be added to ensure that any spaces, such as those between the guardrail and the bed frame or cutouts in the headboard and footboard, do not exceed 3 inches.

Portable playpens may have faulty latches that can cause the enclosure to collapse, trapping a child's head in the top rails. Latches on a playpen should click audibly, signifying that they are securely locked. Also, the side of a mesh playpen should never be left lowered, as an infant can be trapped in the slack mesh.

The Consumer Product Safety Commission's hotline provides information about specific models of a child's equipment that are hazardous and repair information from manufacturers.

Windows: Children aged five and younger are most likely to fall from windows because they are mobile but do not comprehend the danger of an open window. In the United States, about fifteen thousand children aged ten and younger are injured annually from window falls, with three-quarters of the accidents happening in the spring and summer. Surprisingly, the majority of falls occur when children play on furniture adjacent to an open window and topple out as a result of losing their balance, rather than because they leaned against the window.

The following safeguard measures are recommended, and in some U.S. cities required, for any household with young children. All windows from the second floor up must have window guards. Each guard should have a quick-release mechanism for swift exit in case of a fire. Screens do not support a child's weight, so windows should be opened at the top rather than the bottom; if they are opened on the bottom, they should not be wide enough to allow a child to fit through them. Above all, furniture should not be placed under a window. Drapery and blind cords should be secured so that a child is unable to play with them.

Electrical outlets: The most important safety procedure is to cover unused electrical outlets with a safety plug. In wet areas, such as the kitchen or the bathroom, a ground-fault circuit interrupter can be installed in outlets to prevent electrocution if an appliance comes in contact with water. Tempting electrical appliances such as hair dryers should be unplugged and stored out of reach of a child when not in use.

Household furniture: If toddlers are in the house, any standing object such as bookcases, dressers, desks, or a television stand may tip onto a child, who may be tempted to climb on it or any open drawers. To diminish the hazard of household furniture, angle braces or anchors should be used to secure any potentially unstable items, such as bookcases or china hutches, to a wall. Heavy furniture must rest flat on the floor; gliders should be removed. Television sets

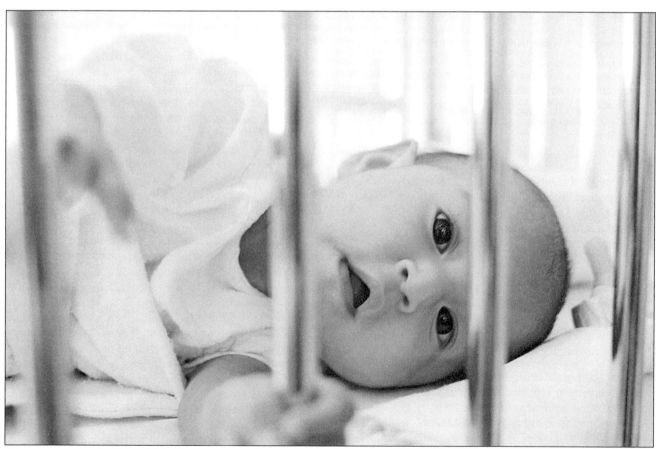

Cribs can pose serious health threats to babies; the government issues guidelines regarding dimensions and spacing between slats. (PhotoDisc)

should be mounted above a child's reach or set far back from the edge on a very low piece of furniture.

Furniture poses many unsuspected threats to safety. For example, bean bag chairs arc hazardous because a toddler can unzip the chair, inhale the foam pellets, and suffocate. If such a chair must be in the house, it should have a permanent seam or sealed zipper. Automatic locks on furniture that is big enough to climb into, such as certain types of chests, should be replaced with safety locks.

A recliner is another unsuspected hazard, as openings of 5 inches or more between the footrest and the seat can trap a child's head. Hammocks are dangerous as well if they do not have spreader bars at each end to hold the netting apart to prevent entrapment of a child's limbs or head.

Tablecloths and placemats should not be used, as a child can grab them and spill hot food or heavy items. Drawers within a child's grasp should have automatic safety latches to prevent spilling sharp items such as knives.

Rugs on slippery areas, such as linoleum tile or the bathroom floor, should be stabilized with nonskid backing. Any edge that could cut a child, such as on a table, should be covered with padding; heat-resistant padding is available for hearths. Glass tables should not be used. All breakable items should be kept on high shelves.

Stairs: If young children are in the home, safety gates should be installed at both the top and bottom of the stairs. Stair gates should have a straight top edge and be filled with a rigid mesh screen containing slats less than 4.25 inches apart. According to the Consumer Product Safety Commission, accordion gates made before February, 1985, are unacceptable, as the openings are wide enough to trap a child's head. The V-shaped openings at the gate's top edge should be no more than 1.5 inches wide. All gates should be at least 32 inches high.

Hardware: Mounted gates securely attached to a solid structure, such as a stair post or wall, should be used at the top of the stairs rather than an expanding-pressure gate, which can be dislodged by the weight of a toddler. Gates should be removed as soon as a child attempts to climb over them.

Outdoor Safety Measures

Summer is a fun time for many children, but most parents are unaware that hospital emergency room staff call May through August "the trauma season." Long daylight hours, no school, and more outdoor activities add up to increased opportunity for accidents. Prevention consists of three facets: supervision, education (of both parents and child), and safeguarding.

Playgrounds: Shockingly, more than 200,000 injuries occur annually on playgrounds to children aged fourteen or younger in the United States. While most parents assume that a playground is safe simply because it is designed for children, in truth, there are no mandatory safety standards for this equipment. More than half of playground injuries result from a fall onto a hard surface, including asphalt, concrete, and even grass and dirt. A significantly higher risk for serious injury is associated with a fall of more than 4 feet for preschoolers or more than 8 feet for school-age children. One problem is that most parents are unaware that playground equipment is specifically designed for one of two age groups: two to five years old or five to twelve years old. To address this issue, equipment made after 1994 is supposed to be marked with a sign indicating its intended age group.

To optimize safety on playgrounds, children should use a playground covered with pea gravel, sand, chips, rubber, or a soft synthetic surface. This protective surface should extend at least 6 feet around slides and twice the height of the swings in front and back to create a safety fall zone. Playgrounds should be checked for sharp edges, loose joints, and protruding hardware, such as unclosed "S" hooks. Swings that are not at least 2 feet apart and 2.5 feet lower than the swing support should be avoided. Platforms and ramps are usable only if they have guardrails. Above all, a toddler should play on equipment lower than 4 feet high, while a school-age child should be restricted to structures 8 feet high or lower.

Drowning: Drowning is known as the "silent death" since young children do not scream or splash while drowning. Each year in the United States, one thousand children aged fourteen and younger drown, while four thousand more are treated for near-drowning injuries. Of these, 20 percent end up with permanent neurological damage. More than three hundred children aged four and younger drown in residential pools annually. Accidents in children ages five and older tend to occur in lakes or oceans as well as in pools, and they tend to occur as a result of "horsing around."

The American Red Cross and the National Safe Kids Campaign issued guidelines to optimize safety near water. The most important rule is that a pool should be enclosed with a four-sided fence at least 5 feet high that is filled with vertical bars 3.5 inches apart or less. The gate should be self-locking and self-closing, with the latch out of reach of children.

Parents and caregivers should know cardiopulmonary resuscitation (CPR), and the CPR instructions should be posted near the pool. Basic life-saving equipment, including a pole, rope, and flotation device, should be next to the pool. Many parents also keep a phone near the pool. In addition, children who cannot swim should wear an approved flotation device that has a collar to keep the head upright and the face out of the water.

Children should never have access to the pool while unsupervised, which includes exiting the back door while a parent is on the phone. Once discovered, the pool is a fascinating place. Caregivers should be mindful of this, as drowning happens in a matter of minutes. Toys and floats that attract young children should be kept away from the pool when not in use, and furniture that enables climbing over a pool fence should be moved to a different location. A toddler should be taught repeatedly not to go near the pool without a parent. Many parents install a motion-sensing device that sounds an alarm if something has fallen into the water.

Hot tubs are dangerous for young children; children under the age of four years should not be allowed in them. Most parents are unaware that hot tubs and spas manufactured prior to 1987 have strong suction that could injure a child; children should be cautioned to keep their head above water and their hair tied up and to sit away from a drain. The water temperature should not exceed 104 degrees Fahrenheit.

Animals and insects: Children, especially babies, are more likely to be bitten by pets than are adults. Animals should never be left alone with infants. Any animal bite that breaks the skin, no matter how minor, necessitates a visit to the pediatrician.

Shrubbery should be trimmed, since it is a breeding ground for disease-carrying rodents and ticks. In areas with a high frequency of Lyme disease, such as New Jersey and Connecticut, children should be checked and bathed daily, especially if they have been outdoors or around animals. The health department and certain medical centers test ticks for Lyme disease. The tick must be alive and in a plastic container. Ticks removed within twenty-four hours usually do not transmit disease. To prevent infection, the tick should be removed gently with tweezers. The area around the bite should be squeezed, so that pus is pushed outward, and then sterilized.

Sports injuries: Protecting our children during sports and recreational activities is of paramount importance as more than 2.6 million children under age nineteen are treated in the emergency department for injuries that result from such activities. Prevention of such injuries can be accomplished through using the right well-fitted protective gear for the sport, such as helmets, wrist guards, and knee and elbow pads. Children should also practice well enough before being involved in any competitive sport by gradually increasing their physical fitness in appropriate environmental conditions, with close attention to proper hydration and diet.

Safety in the Car

Child passenger anticipatory safety guidance has become the main focus over the past decade as motor vehicle accidents are the leading cause of death in children four years and above. In 2011 the American Academy of Pediatrics (AAP) issued a policy statement with recommendations for best child restraints in the car from birth to adolescence. All infants and toddlers should ride in a rear-facing car safety seat (CSS) in the rear seat until the age of two years or reach the highest weight or height as per manufacturer recommendations. Children over two years of age or who outgrow a CSS should use a forward-facing CSS with a harness as long as possible and up to the highest weight or height as per manufacturer recommendations. Those children whose weight or height are above a forward-facing CSS should use a belt-positioning booster seat until the vehicle lap and shoulder seatbelt fits properly. All children younger than thirteen years of age should be restrained in the rear seats.

Medical Emergencies

Burns: Experts consider the kitchen to be the most dangerous room in the home for children. A burn may occur when a hot pan or liquid falls on a child or when a child presses hands against an oven door or pulls a pan off the stove. The insulation on oven doors may wear out and cause second-degree and third-degree burns, even when the oven is at a relatively low temperature.

To prevent such injuries, the following precautions should be instituted. Above all, the child should be placed at a safe remove from the potential source of burns. Counter space should be well organized and spacious, so that a hot pan placed there is far enough from the edge to prevent it from falling off. Pots should be placed on the back burners, with their handles turned toward the rear, so a child cannot reach them. In addition, stove knobs may be removed or covered when the stove is not in use if they are especially accessible or tempting to a child.

The oven door, and the window in particular, should be checked to ensure that it is not hot enough to cause even a slight burn. The manufacturer or a repair company should be called immediately if it is too hot. Several working fire extinguishers should be readily available, and smoke detectors should be installed outside sleeping areas and tested regularly.

To prevent scald burns from hot water, the temperature on water heaters should be set to a maximum of 120 degrees Fahrenheit. In addition, a parent should always test the water before putting a child in the bathtub.

If a child is burned, the immediate goal is to prevent heat from penetrating deeper into the skin. Clothing, which retains heat, must be removed from the burned area immediately. If fabric is stuck to the skin, it should not be pulled away, as this can tear the skin, but cut away as best as possible. A physician should remove the remainder.

Cold water should be applied to the burn at once until the pain subsides and the skin is no longer hot to the touch, usually at least five minutes. Nothing else should be applied to the area, including ice cubes, which may cause frostbite, and butter, grease, or ointment, which may impel the heat deeper into the skin.

If the burn is not oozing, a sterile gauze dressing should be applied, taking care not to break blisters or remove any skin. Medical attention should be sought immediately if the burn is on a child six months old or younger or if the burn affects a child's eyes, face, mouth, hands, feet, or genitals. In addition, blisters, oozing, severe pain, dizziness, and breathing problems are all reasons to seek medical attention.

Choking: Choking is the most common cause of accidental death in children under age one. Choking is life-threatening if a child swallows an object that blocks the flow of air to the lungs. The child will be unable to talk, and his or her face will turn blue. A child who is coughing should not be interrupted, as this strong natural reflex may dislodge the object.

Parents must be familiar with the emergency medical procedures for choking; approved first-aid courses are sponsored by the American Heart Association and the American Red Cross. The Heimlich maneuver is not recommended for infants; rather, they are to be turned face down on the forearm or lap and administered rapid blows between the shoulder blades. If this fails, the infant is turned on the back and four rapid chest thrusts over the breastbone are given with only two fingers. If all else fails, mouth-to-mouth or mouth-to-nose respiration should be performed.

Items that can be swallowed should be kept away from babies, including marbles, coins, safety pins, and small refrigerator magnets. Particular caution must be exercised with toys. Hazards include rattles less than 1.625 inches across, eyes or ribbons that come off stuffed animals, balloons, and small parts of toys that break off. Toys labeled for ages three and younger must meet federal guidelines requiring they have no small parts. Young children can choke on certain foods. Those foods to be avoided include peanuts, candy, whole grapes, or any hard, smooth food that must be chewed with a grinding motion.

Drawstrings in clothing pose a hazard, as they can strangle a child if the drawstring is caught on a slide, school bus door, or handrail. Drawstrings should not be worn at the neck. If they are at the waist of a garment, then knots should be untied, as they may catch on objects. A child should not use playgrounds while wearing clothing with drawstrings. In 1994, the Consumer Product Safety Commission asked clothing manufacturers to remove drawstrings from the hoods of children's garments; hand-knit or secondhand clothing still poses a risk.

Poisoning: Ironically, although most parents are aware of the poisonous hazard posed by cleaning products, they do not consider the toxicity of household plants. For example, ivy, geraniums, and philodendrons are poisonous if ingested. In addition, many plants in the yard are toxic. A poison control center can provide names of hazardous plants in a particular region.

The poison control center should be called immediately if a child ingests a toxic substance. The number of the regional center is listed on the inside cover of the telephone book and should be posted next to the phone. The parent should report what was ingested, how much, and, if it is a plant, the common and botanical name. Syrup of ipecac to induce vomiting should be readily available, but it should not be administered until instructions are received from the poison control center, since in some cases vomiting causes more harm. If a child gets poison in the eyes or on the skin, the area should be flushed immediately with lukewarm water for a period of fifteen minutes as the poison control center is being called.

To prevent the ingestion of poisons, safety locks should be installed on low-level cabinets containing cleaning products and on the medicine chest. Over-the-counter and prescription medicines, soaps, cosmetics, and shampoos are all potentially toxic if ingested by a child. Many people are unaware that vitamins consumed in a sufficient quantity can cause an overdose reaction. Shampoo and soap in the tub should be kept out of a child's reach. Many parents opt

to keep medicines and vitamins, as well as sharp items such as razors, in a separate, high, and locked place.

Many automobile and building products are poisonous as well as flammable; they should be kept in locked metal cabinets away from children. In addition, lawn products, such as fertilizer and weed killer, should be kept in a locked area away from toddlers.

Lead poisoning: Lead poisoning constituted one of the most underrated afflictions of children until education efforts raised awareness. In the late 1990s, about 1 million children in the United States had elevated blood lead levels. Any building constructed before 1978, the year that lead paint was banned, probably has lead in the paint. This puts a child at risk, especially if the paint is chipped or sanded or renovations are being done. Lead is also found in pipes, which were made entirely of lead in the United States until the 1950s; lead was used to fuse copper pipes until 1986.

Safety measures include determining if lead paint exists in the home or soil. The local department of health may be contacted for further information. Repainting a home built prior to 1977 is recommended. Even if an area has been covered with nonleaded paint, precautions should be taken when children are not in the house. Chipped and peeling paint should be removed with a wet cloth. If extensive peeling has occurred, the area should be sanded and painted over. Guidelines for the removal of lead paint are available from the National Association of Homebuilders.

Tap water should be run for ninety seconds before using it, as water that has been standing in the pipes has a higher concentration of lead. Cold water should be used for drinking and cooking, as it is less likely to leach lead. High-phosphate detergents are recommended for cleaning.

All infants should be tested for lead, no matter how safe the home is. The Centers for Disease Control and Prevention (CDC) and the American Academy of Pediatrics (AAP) recommend that babies be tested at ages one and two, the ages when they are most likely to put objects that may be covered with lead dust into their mouths. Risk factors for lead exposure in children include living in cities; being poor, African American, or Hispanic; or living in areas where houses were built prior to 1950. Parents should remain alert to any possible exposure, even if their children are not considered at risk.

Teenage work: Every year about 70 teens die from work injuries in the United States. Another 70,000 get hurt badly enough that they go to a hospital emergency room. There are many federal and state regulatory rules regarding teenage work. The Fair Labor Standards Act (FLSA) provides restrictions on the types of jobs and the number of hours that teenagers can work. Such regulations are less strict for farm work, and teenagers are permitted to perform any job at any age on their family farm. The FLSA also provides certain exemptions for nonagricultural jobs in parent-owned businesses.

Teenagers' work experience is a great opportunity for parents and teenagers to learn about the occupational safety of the selected work that teenagers can do. Teenage workers and their parents should ask about the safety and healthfulness of the workplace environment, the appropriateness of the work's time schedule, and the use of appropriate safety measures while on the job (e.g., respiratory protection for teenage hospital volunteers, helmets for bicycle delivery workers, safety shoes for slippery floors).

—*Lee Williams;*
updated by Emad Hanna, M.D., M.Sc.

See also Accidents; Allergies; Bites and stings; Bleeding; Burns and scalds; Choking; Concussion; Critical care; Critical care, pediatric; Drowning; Electrical shock; Emergency medicine; Emergency medicine, pediatric; Emergency rooms; First aid; Food poisoning; Fracture and dislocation; Frostbite; Hives; Insect-borne diseases; Lead poisoning; Lice, mites, and ticks; Mercury poisoning; Poisoning; Poisonous plants; Snakebites; Sunburn; Zoonoses

For Further Information:

American Academy of Pediatrics. "AAP Expands Guidelines for Infant Sleep Safety and SIDS Risk Reduction." http://www.aap.org/en-us/about-the-aap/aap-press-room/pages/AAP-Expands-Guidelines-for-Infant-Sleep-Safety-and- SIDS-Risk-Reduction.aspx. This link provides details regarding expanded guidelines for infant sleep safety.

American Academy of Pediatrics. "Children's Health Topics: Safety and First Aid." http://www.aap.org/healthtopics/safety.cfm. Includes links to information on such topics as car safety, water safety, and injury prevention.

Bentz, Ric, and Christine Allison. *Street Smarts for Kids: What Parents Must Know to Keep Their Children Safe.* New York: Fawcett Books, 1999. Detective Bentz of the Kenosha, Wisconsin, Police Department, and Allison, a children's writer, have compiled an outstanding tool for parents and caretakers concerning child safety. They cover topics such as pedophiles, child abductors, and cyberspace safety threats and identify certain characteristics in children that might make them vulnerable to strangers.

Centers for Disease Control and Prevention. "Sports Injuries: The Reality." http://www.cdc.gov/safechild/sports_Injuries/index.html.

Committee on Injury, Violence, and Poison Prevention. "Policy Statement-Child Passenger Safety." *Pediatrics.* March 21, 2011. http://pediatrics.aappublications.org/content/early/2011/03/ 21/peds.2011-0213.full.pdf

Department of Labor. "Young Worker Toolkit." http:// www.youthrules.dol.gov/support/toolkit/index.htm. This is an excellent website that provides information by age about jobs that can be done at different teenagers

Department of Labor. "Exemptions from Child Labor Rules in Non-Agriculture." http://www.dol.gov/elaws/esa/flsa/cl/exemptions.asp.

Information for parents about sleep safety: http:// www.healthychildren.org/English/ages-stages/baby/ sleep/Pages/Preventing-SIDS.aspx

Kattwinkel, John, et al., eds. *Textbook of Neonatal Resuscitation.* 5th ed. Elk Grove Village, IL: American Academy of Pediatrics, 2006. An invaluable guide that provides a practical, step-by-step guide for the resuscitation of both premature and full-term neonates.

Lanky, Vicki. *Baby Proofing Basics: How to Keep Your Child Safe.* 2nd ed. Minnetonka, MN: Book Peddlers, 2002. An excellent guide that contains childproofing tips for every room in the house as well as for outdoors, backyard, beach, camping, hiking, and travel of all kinds. Covers topics such as safety at playtime, mealtime, and holidays; dealing safely with pets; and poisoning dangers.

Litin, Scott C., ed. *Mayo Clinic Family Health Book.* 4th ed. New York: HarperResource, 2009. Perhaps the best general medical text for the layperson, this book covers the entire medical field and includes an excellent section on first aid and emergency care.

Priven, Joshua, David Borgenicht, and Sarah Jordan. *The Worst-Case Scenario Survival Handbook: Parenting.* New York: Scholastic, 2004. A humorous but helpful guide to surviving numerous parenting scenarios, which covers first aid and babyproofing one's house.

Rubenstein H., S.H. Sternbach, and M.R. Pollack. "Protecting the Health and Safety of Working Teenagers." *American Family Physician* 60, no. 2 (1999): 575-580.

Shelov, Steven P., et al. *Caring for Your Baby and Young Child: Birth to Age Five.* 5th ed. New York: Bantam Books, 2009. Offers a comprehensive discussion of the accidents that commonly occur with young children, accident-prevention techniques for the home and outdoors, and emergency measures to enact if an accident does take place.

Theurer, W.M., and A.K. Bhavsar. "Prevention of Unintentional Childhood Injury." *American Family Physician* 87, no. 7 (2013): 502-509.

Safety issues for the elderly
Procedures
Anatomy or system affected: All
Specialties and related fields: Critical care, emergency medicine, family medicine, geriatrics and gerontology
Definition: Measures taken to prevent accidents among the elderly.

The Importance of Safety Measures

The age-related changes that elderly people experience often alter what constitutes a risk to their safety. The family home environment can be dangerous for an elderly person, not because the aspects of the house have changed, but because of the change in the physical abilities of the elderly person. Elderly people with intact cognitive abilities may choose to take the risk of staying in their familiar home environments with full knowledge of the increased risk. The dilemma for others, especially health providers, is defining what constitutes an acceptable level of risk for the elderly.

The elderly may experience mobility problems that pose a threat to safety. Falls are much more serious with advanced age because bones and tissues do not heal as quickly or completely as in youth.

Unintentional injuries (accidents) are the sixth leading cause of death in people over sixty-five years of age. The death rate is 51 per 100,000 people for those sixty-five to seventy-four years of age, rises to 104 per 100,000 for those aged seventy-five to eighty-four, and reaches a high of 256 per 100,000 for those who are eighty-five years of age or older. In the over-eighty-five age group, accidental injury is the fifth leading cause of death. Generally speaking, injuries cost the United States between 75 billion and 100 billion dollars each year. In 2010, the direct adjusted medical cost of falls came to $30 billion, comprising a significant portion of resource allocation for the cost of treating those injuries. Accidents are usually viewed as random events over which individuals have little or no control. Many other types of injuries are preventable, and safety enhancement may decrease the number of serious outcomes.

Falls

Falls account for a considerable number of deaths and injuries among elderly people. Falls are the leading cause of

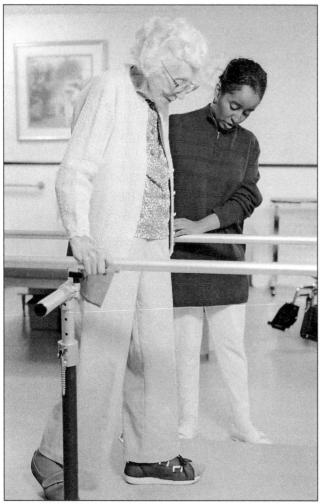

The elderly may experience mobility problems that pose a threat to safety. Falls are much more serious with advanced age because bones and tissues do not heal as quickly or completely as in youth. (PhotoDisc)

fatal and nonfatal injuries in the elderly population. Previous studies from 2000 found that 46 percent of fatal falls are due to traumatic brain injury. Falls are not an uncommon event for elderly people; approximately one-third of noninstitu- tionalized elders report a fall each year. One-half of the people who report falls experience multiple falls. Although falls are a common occurrence, they are not always dangerous: Only 11 percent result in a serious injury, and an estimated 1 percent result in hip fractures. The number of hip fractures yearly in the United States (200,000) is substantial and serious. They lead to death in 12 percent to 20 percent of cases and account for 2 percent of the mortality rate in the United States. More than 40 percent of deaths from falls occur in the home. Stairs account for a large proportion of falls, many occurring because the elderly individual misses the last step. Falling injuries account for 40 percent of nursing home admissions; however, more than 20 percent of all fatal falls occur in the nursing home setting. Over the past decade, mortality from falls in the elderly has risen impressively, with about 21,700 older adults dying from unintentional fall injuries in 2010.

Falls among the elderly may be caused by a variety of factors: physical frailty, pathological states, psychological stress, drug interactions, and multiple environmental hazards. The risks of falling increase with the following: increasing age, the number of chronic diseases present, the number and type of medications being taken, cognitive impairment, and physical disability. The risk of falling is often associated more with the intake of some types of drugs (antidepressants, sedatives, or vasodilators) than with medical conditions. Most doctors provide elderly patients with information concerning the effects of drugs that they may be taking, including the risk of a drop in blood pressure related to these medications. Instruction concerning how to decrease the effects of orthostatic hypotension, a condition in which blood pressure drops upon standing, is an example of how to instruct patients to be more aware of what may result in a fall. They may be instructed to dangle their feet before getting out of bed or rising slowly from seated or reclining positions to prevent falls due to orthostatic hypotension.

Falls may cause bruises, abrasions, pain, swelling, or fractures. Changes in cognitive function related to pressure from edema or blood clots within the brain may also be evidenced. Psychological damage resulting from falls is subtler. An older person who sustains little or no injury in a fall may delay or avoid discussing it in order to avoid embarrassment or risk of being viewed as less competent. Falls may also prompt changes in behavior, such as decreased thoroughness in housekeeping tasks or discussion of fears of living alone. Changes in grooming, dress, and personal appearance may also be observed. Increased fear of venturing out into the neighborhood may lead to a decreased ability to meet the daily requirements of shopping and food preparation. Affected individuals may further decrease other activities, resulting in their becoming increasingly sessile. This leads to a relative reduction in physical fitness, impacting their quality of life and increases the risk of future falls.

Falls are better prevented than treated. People aged 75 and older who fall are four to five times more likely than those aged between 65 to 74 to be admitted to a long-term care facility for a year or longer. Because quality of life is as important as length of life, limiting activity in the hope that falls will not occur is the least acceptable method of prevention. A more realistic approach is to modify the environment. Although cost may be a limiting factor, many alterations can be implemented that are both acceptable to the older person and minimal in expense. Many environmental modifications are relatively easy to perform.

Many falls occur in the bathroom. Nonslip bath mats and adhesive-backed, nonskid strips in the bathtub or shower are important safety measures. Grab bars may be placed at critical locations near the bathtub and toilet to lend support. Railings may be installed on stairways for support. A piece of fabric, a knob, or some other marker can be attached to the rail to indicate the level of the top and bottom steps.

Other steps can be taken to prevent falls in older adults. Regular exercise, focusing on leg strength and improving balance, can prevent falls as these physical attributes diminish greatly with age. The Centers for Disease Control and Prevention (CDC) maintains that Tai Chi programs are especially conducive to improving these weaker areas. Reviewing medicines with a physician or pharmacist may help to identify medications causing side effects such as dizziness and drowsiness. Yearly eye exams and updating eyeglasses to maximize vision is also helpful.

The need for light increases with age. An environment can be illuminated at a safe level by increasing either the number of lights or the intensity of the light bulbs. Adequate illumination that does not cause shadows, which may cause problems with perception, is extremely important in high hazard areas, such as stairways and stair landings. Night lights or lighted switches enable those who get up at night to orient themselves more easily within the environment and minimize the risk of falling. The removal of obstructions and obstacles can also help increase the safety of the home. Among the objects that may cause elderly people to trip are extension cords and long phone cords, low furniture, carpet edges, and throw rugs. These can easily be removed from high-traffic areas or taped down to minimize the risk of causing injury.

Traffic Injuries

In modern societies, an important rite of passage for adolescents is to receive a driver's license. Driving an automobile is viewed as the first step toward adult life because it fosters independence. On the other hand, driving a car also calls for a sense of responsibility to others who share the roads. Many roads are crowded, and traffic moves at a rapid and sometimes confusing rate. Drivers must be physically and mentally alert to handle the hazards of the roads. Elderly people with impaired physical capabilities must make a choice between continuing to drive, and therefore maintaining their independence, or taking measures to increase safety for themselves and others on the road.

Traffic injuries in the elderly population are divided into two categories: pedestrian injuries and vehicle-related injuries. Elderly people are more at risk for injury at street intersections than anywhere else, both as pedestrians and as drivers or passengers in an automobile. As pedestrians, many elderly people are at risk because of an inability to cross the street in the time allotted between changes in the traffic lights. Factors that may influence pedestrian injuries are curb height, driver error, and physical and cognitive impairment of the elderly pedestrian.

A major problem for older drivers is the motor vehicle accident, in which the risk for injury in these crashes increases dramatically with age. The majority of such accidents take place in daylight, on good roads, and with no alcohol involvement. Elderly people experience a higher mortality rate with less severe injuries in vehicle crashes; the risk of death is three times greater for a seventy-year-old person than for a twenty-year-old person. The major factor that influences the high susceptibility of involvement in traffic injuries may be the decreased skill of the elderly person in operating an automobile. This change in skill level may be caused by age-related changes, such as decreased visual acuity or a slower neurological response time.

Citations for traffic violations, such as failure to yield right-of-way and failure to obey traffic signs, increase after the age of sixty. Although older adults have lower accident rates and fewer traffic violation citations than those under twenty-five years of age, elderly people have an increased risk of fatality in traffic accidents. One group of elders at increased risk for vehicle-related injury is those who are experiencing the early signs and symptoms of dementia. The American Association for Retired Persons (AARP) operates special classes in driver education to help older adults cope with age-related changes that affect their driving abilities.

Safety Considerations

Safety is a major concern when assessing living conditions. Many older adults live in unsafe housing. Relatively minor nuisances-such as excessive clutter, loose flooring or floor coverings, poor lighting, and unstable stairs-can pose safety risks for the older adult. Financial constraints may prompt older adults to settle for living in less desirable areas. Other safety concerns are related to the older adult's physical or mental functioning. People who have trouble walking or climbing stairs are prime examples of those at risk as the result of impaired physical functioning. People who are forgetful or who wander off and get lost pose a significant risk to themselves and others as the result of impaired mental function.

It may be necessary to observe the elderly actually moving about in their environment to locate any potential problems. If the elderly person uses an assistive device, such as a cane, walker, or wheelchair, the environment may require further modifications. Ramps may need to be installed, or living arrangements may need to be changed to accommodate the need for special access.

Most elderly people prefer to stay in their own homes in familiar communities for as long as possible. As people get older, they often fear that they may have to leave home for health reasons. Such fears are realistic because acute and chronic health problems associated with aging often dictate at least temporary changes in environment, leading the elderly to reside in places they do not prefer. Their desire to stay at home challenges the health care system to study their special needs and devise solutions that will accommodate them in the most acceptable way.

Elderly individuals who live alone are well advised to learn how to summon emergency help and to make home adaptations to compensate for decreased mobility and dexterity. Cognitive impairments often present a more serious threat to safety than physical impairment. People who know they are having problems are likely to call for help and remain safely in the home until help arrives. However, individuals with impaired judgment may present a hazard to themselves, as well as to their neighbors, through such behavior as forgetting to turn off the stove. In isolated instances, a choice may be made to preserve such a person's autonomy at the risk of serious injury; however, few would agree that the impaired older person has a right to put others at risk of serious injury.

Medication usage is another important factor to consider when evaluating whether or not an older person can safely remain at home alone. Sometimes the deciding factor in whether a cognitively impaired individual can remain at home alone is the nature of the medication regimen. Some individuals must have regular medication to maintain health. There are various systems to help forgetful people take their medicines. Preparing and labeling medications for each day is one strategy for simplifying medication administration. Medication calendars, which show each type of pill with its time of administration and which have a space for marking when the pill is taken, are useful to individuals with early memory impairment. Functionally impaired individuals who want to stay at home but require assistance or supervision with activities of daily living are often helped by parapro- fessional personnel.

It is clear that injuries in the elderly population are costly both financially and in terms of independence. By preventing the most common causes of injury, adjusting medications, and altering acceptable aspects of an older person's lifestyle, the risk of such injuries can be decreased. These changes will hopefully result in fewer injuries and a greater quality of life.

—Jane C. Norman, Ph.D., R.N., C.N.E.;
updated by Joshua Lampert, MS-II.

See also Accidents; Aging; Aging: Extended care; Alzheimer's disease; Assisted living facilities; Balance disorders; Critical care; Deafness; Death and dying; Dementias; Emergency medicine; Emergency rooms; First aid; Fracture and dislocation; Geriatrics and gerontology; Hip fracture repair; Hip replacement; Home care; Hospice; Memory loss; Nursing; Osteoporosis; Pick's disease; Psychiatry, geriatric

For Further Information:

Beerman, Susan, and Judith Rappaport-Musson. *Eldercare 911: The Caregiver's Complete Handbook for Making Decisions.* Rev. ed. Amherst, NY: Prometheus Books, 2008. A practical guide for elder care. Includes topics such as locating services, managing medications, understanding benefits, choosing a nursing home, coping with memory loss, hiring and handling in-home help, helping a parent who refuses help, and recognizing signs of elder abuse.

Gill, T.M., C.S. Williams, J.T. Robison, and M.E. Tinetti. "A Population-Based Study of Environmental Hazards in the Homes of Older Persons." *American Journal of Public Health* 89, no. 4 (1999): 553-556. An environmental assessment was completed in the homes of one thousand persons seventy-two years and older. Weighted prevalence rates were calculated for each of the potential hazards and subsequently compared among subgroups of participants.

Lachman, M.E., et al. "Fear of Falling and Activity Restriction: The Survey of Activities and Fear of Falling in the Elderly (SAFE)." *Journals of Gerontology Series B-Psychological Sciences and Social Sciences* 53B, no. 1 (1998): 43-50. A new instrument was developed to assess the role of fear of falling in activity restriction. The instrument assesses fear of falling during performance of eleven activities, and it gathers information about participation in these activities as well as the extent to which fear is a source of activity restriction.

Lachs, Mark S. "Caring for Mom and Dad: Can Your Parent Live Alone?" *Prevention* 50, no. 10 (October, 1998): 155-157. Information on how to develop a care plan for an aging parent who is having problems with activities of daily living.

Lisak, Janet M., and Marlene Morgan. *The Safe Home Checkout: A Professional Guide to Safe Independent Living.* 2nd ed. Chicago: Geriatric Environments for Living and Learning, 1997. Covers safety measures for older buildings, accident prevention, and self-help devices for the disabled. Includes bibliographical references.

Litin, Scott C., ed. *Mayo Clinic Family Health Book.* 4th ed. New York: Harper Resource, 2009. Perhaps the best general medical text for the lay person, this book covers the entire medical field and includes an excellent section on first aid and emergency care.

Stenchever, Morton A. *Health Care for the Older Woman.* New York: Chapman and Hall, 1996. A reference that provides medical practitioners and students with comprehensive, current information specific to the care of middle-aged and advanced-aged women. It covers health maintenance issues, including diet, exercise, safety, psychological and psychosocial problems, social problems, and grief and loss.

Warner, Mark L. *Complete Guide to Alzheimer's-Proofing Your Home.* Rev. ed. West Lafayette, IN: Purdue University Press, 2000. An excellent guide that details how to create a home environment for elderly patients with Alzheimer's and related dementia. Covers both interior and exterior spaces, discussing problems and solutions associated with specific areas, such as the kitchen, the bathroom, corridors, and patios and decks.

Salmonella infection
Disease/Disorder
Anatomy or system affected: Blood, gastrointestinal system
Specialties and related fields: Bacteriology, family medicine, gastroenterology, pediatrics, public health
Definition: A broad spectrum of clinical diseases caused by many types of salmonella bacteria.
Key terms:
asymptomatic: without symptoms
bacteremia: the presence of bacteria in the blood, which is usually associated with chills and fever
gastroenteritis: infection of the gastrointestinal tract, usually accompanied by nausea, vomiting, diarrhea, and abdominal pains
typhoid fever: a particular disease syndrome most often associated with infection by *Salmonella typhi* but occasionally caused by other types of salmonella bacteria

Causes and Symptoms

Salmonella are a group of bacteria that cause enteric or typhoid fever. All types can cause gastrointestinal infections, blood infections, and various local infections. All types of salmonella can be carried in the gastrointestinal tract without symptoms after recovery from infection.

The clinical disease caused by salmonella depends on the type of bacteria, the amount of organisms ingested, and the age and immune status of the person infected. Infection with salmonella can take place with the ingestion of one or 100 million organisms. Increasing the dosage of bacteria decreases the incubation period and increases the severity of the resulting disease. After ingestion, the bacteria adhere to and invade the gastrointestinal tract. In the wall of the intestinal tract, salmonella survive and multiply in immune cells and then enter the bloodstream, where they proceed to any area of the body. Young infants and people with immune deficiencies and hemolytic anemia are at increased risk for severe and complicated infections.

Typhoid fever or enteric fever is very rare in the United

Information on Salmonella Infection

Causes: Bacterial infection transmitted through ingestion or exposure to infected animals

Symptoms: Fever, headache, muscle aches, abdominal pain, lethargy, diarrhea, vomiting

Duration: Six hours to three days

Treatments: Correction of fluid and salt abnormalities, supportive care

---

States, causing less than five hundred cases per year; it is primarily seen in people coming from developing countries. Classically, this disease is caused by *Salmonella typhi* bacteria, but it can also be caused by other types of salmonella. Symptoms during the first week of illness include progressively increasing fever with associated headache, muscle aches, abdominal pains, and lethargy. In the second week, the heart rate decreases, the liver and spleen enlarge, small red bumps form on the trunk, and the patient enters into a stupor. During the third to fourth week, intestinal hemorrhage and perforation are common. The fever begins to remit in the fifth to sixth week of illness. Diarrhea usually starts in the first week and resolves within six weeks. Without treatment, death can occur from gastrointestinal hemorrhage and perforation. Infants tend to have much more severe disease than older children.

Salmonellosis caused by nontyphoid salmonella is more common in the United States, causing about fifty thousand cases per year. The major reservoir of nontyphoid salmonella is the gastrointestinal tract of many animals, including mammals, reptiles, birds, and insects. Farm animals and pet reptiles commonly carry salmonella. Some antibiotic resistance is caused by the use of antibiotics in animal feeds. Salmonella can be isolated from 50 percent of chicken, 16 percent of pork, 5 percent of beef, and 40 percent of frozen eggs in retail stores. Contaminated eggs and milk products are common sources of human infection.

Gastroenteritis is the most common disease caused by nontyphoid salmonella. The incubation period for this disease is about one day, with a range from six hours to three days. Symptoms include nausea, vomiting, and abdominal pain. Diarrhea typically contains blood and white cells. Usually, symptoms disappear in less than a week in healthy children, but in young infants and in children with immune deficiencies, symptoms may persist for several weeks.

Bacteremia can occur in 1 to 5 percent of patients with salmonella gastroenteritis. Bacteremia is generally associated with fever, chills, and toxicity in the older child but may be asymptomatic in the infant. Children with an increased risk of bacteremia include those with acquired immunodeficiency syndrome (AIDS) or other immune deficiencies and hemolytic anemias such as sickle cell anemia.

Bacteremia can lead to infection of almost any organ. Children with sickle cell anemia are more prone to bone infections and meningitis. Salmonella may localize to areas of the body that have received trauma or that contain damaged tissue or a foreign body. Meningitis, inflammation of the covering of the spine and brain, is primarily seen as a complication of bacteremia in infants. Meningitis has a 50 percent death rate, and residual developmental and hearing defects are commonly found in survivors. Patients who have persistent bacteremia should be evaluated for heart infection.

The diagnosis of a salmonella infection is best made by culturing stool and blood samples. With enteric fever, it is important to culture multiple sites multiple times. Antibiotic susceptibility testing must be performed routinely to guide therapy. Other bacterial causes of gastroenteritis can be confused with salmonella infection.

Treatment and Therapy

Treatment for gastroenteritis usually does not require antibiotics. Antibiotics do not speed the resolution of disease but instead lead to prolonged excretion of salmonella. Therapy is primarily focused on the correction of fluid and salt abnormalities and on general supportive care. If the patient has indications of sepsis, shock, or chills, however, then antibiotics should be administered. Infants under three months of age and children with immune deficiencies should also be treated with antibiotics. Ampicillin is usually used as the initial treatment in uncomplicated cases, and third-generation cephalosporin antibiotics are used in severe and complicated cases. About 20 percent of nontyphoid salmonella in the United States is resistant to ampicillin as well as to other antibiotics. Antibiotic treatment should last ten days to two weeks in children with bacteremia and four to six weeks in children with bone infection or meningitis. Local infections may require surgical drainage.

Typhoid fever is treated for a minimum of two weeks. It is important to perform susceptibility testing for the possibility of resistance so that proper antibiotic therapy can be chosen. Chronic carriers of *Salmonella typhi* should be treated with antibiotics. If eradication is unsuccessful, surgical assessment of the biliary tract should be sought.

Prevention of the spread of salmonella requires a number of public health procedures. Hand washing is critical to the prevention of transmission. Persons who are carriers of salmonella should be excluded from food preparation and from child-care settings. Hospitalized infants and children should be isolated. Proper sewage disposal, water purification, and chlorination are essential public health measures. In developing countries, the promotion of prolonged breast-feeding also reduces the infection rate.

There are two typhoid vaccines commercially available in the United States. The first is an oral, live attenuated vaccine that requires four doses given over a period of one week and a booster every five years. The second is a parenteral capsular polysaccharide vaccine given as a single intramuscular injection and a booster every two years. The vaccines are 50 to 80 percent protective. The live attenuated vaccine should not be given to patients who are pregnant, taking antibiotics, or immunocompromised, such as persons with the human immunodeficiency virus (HIV).

Perspective and Prospects

Salmonella was identified as the cause of typhoid fever in 1880 and was first cultured in 1884. Since 1920, improvements in sanitation, water supplies, and sewage disposal have resulted in a marked decrease of typhoid fever in the United States. In 1920, 36,000 cases were reported; after 1965, the number of cases per year has rarely exceeded 500. Since then, the number of cases has remained fairly constant because of the importation of disease by tourists, immigrants, and migrant laborers. About 62 percent of *Salmonella typhi* infections are acquired through foreign travel. Direct person-to-person transmission is rare except in the homosexual population.

Recent research is focused on public health. Measures to decrease food contamination such as improved cleanliness, decreased use of antibiotics in animal feeds, and food irradiation are being evaluated and used to decrease transmission to humans. Research into alternate vaccines with fewer side effects and improved immune response is also being performed.

Nontyphoid salmonella causes one-half million infections per year in the United States. One-third of these infections are in children less than five years of age, and 40 percent are in adults over thirty years of age.

—*Peter D. Reuman, M.D., M.P.H.*

See also Antibiotics; Bacterial infections; Biological and chemical weapons; Diarrhea and dysentery; Food poisoning; Gastroenteritis; Gastroenterology; Gastroenterology, pediatric; Gastrointestinal disorders; Gastrointestinal system; Immunization and vaccination; Meningitis; Poisoning; Typhoid fever; Zoonoses.

For Further Information:

Beers, Mark H., et al., eds. *The Merck Manual of Diagnosis and Therapy.* 18th ed. Whitehouse Station, N.J.: Merck Research Laboratories, 2006. Describes many diseases, including their characteristics, etiology, diagnosis, and treatment. Designed for physicians, the material is also useful to less specialized readers.

Bellenir, Karen, and Peter D. Dresser, eds. *Contagious and Noncontagious Infectious Diseases Sourcebook.* Detroit, Mich.: Omnigraphics, 1996. A handy reference source on infections. Includes bibliographical references and an index.

Biddle, Wayne. *A Field Guide to Germs.* 2d ed. New York: Anchor Books, 2002. This comprehensive book is easily accessible to the nonspecialist and includes a discussion of nearly every virus, bacterium, and fungus known to cause human and nonhuman animal disease. The history of the microbe and the treatment of diseases are included.

Cliver, Dean O., and Hans P. Riemann, eds. *Foodborne Diseases.* 2d ed. San Diego, Calif.: Academic Press, 2002. An exceptional college textbook providing chapters written by experts in the field. This important work provides not only background information but also in-depth reference information on the most common foodborne pathogens.

Jay, James M., Martin J. Loessner, and David A. Golden. *Modern Food Microbiology.* 7th ed. New York: Springer, 2005. This excellent textbook summarizes the current state of knowledge of the biology and epidemiology of the microorganisms that cause foodborne illness.

Leon, Warren, and Caroline Smith DeWaal. *Is Our Food Safe? A Consumer's Guide to Protecting Your Health and the Environment.* New York: Crown, 2002. Focuses on three themes-food safety and foodborne illnesses, environmental aspects of food choices, and sound diet and nutrition-and answers common questions about the safety of meat, dairy products, fish, fruits, and other foods that make up American diets.

Parker, James N., and Philip M. Parker, eds. *The Official Patient's Sourcebook on Salmonella Enteritidis Infection.* San Diego, Calif.: Icon Health, 2002. Draws from public, academic, government, and peer-reviewed research to provide a wide-ranging handbook for patients with salmonella infections.

Sarcoidosis

Disease/Disorder

Also known as: Besnier-Boeck disease, Schaumann's syndrome, Lofgren syndrome (acute sarcoidosis)

Anatomy or system affected: Brain, chest, circulatory system, eyes, heart, immune system, joints, kidneys, lungs, lymphatic system, nerves, nervous system, respiratory system, skin, spleen

Specialties and related fields: Bacteriology, cardiology, dermatology, genetics, immunology, internal medicine, nephrology, neurology, ophthalmology, optometry, pulmonary medicine, radiology, rheumatology, serology, toxicology, virology

Definition: An inflammatory disease of unknown cause characterized by noncaseating granulomas, that affect multiple systems, especially the lungs, lymph nodes, skin, and eyes. This disease is thought to be the result of a dysregulated immune response to an infectious agent or environmental factor. If severe, sarcoidosis is treated with corticosteroids.

Key terms:

cytokine: a small, regulatory protein of the immune system that mediates cell interactions

fibrosis: the development of scar tissue consisting of excess fibrous connective tissue

fluorodeoxyglucose-positron emission tomography (FDG-PET): a molecular imaging method in which radioactive sugar is injected into the body; the sugar accumulates in tissues with hypermetabolism and is detected by its positron emission

granuloma: a clump of cells, or nodule, in the immune system

immune system: a body system that protects the body from foreign substances by identifying and destroying them; includes the thymus, bone marrow, and lymph tissues

lymphocyte: a white blood cell that produces antibodies

macrophage: a white blood cell that engulfs foreign substances and stimulates other immune cells

noncaseating: not causing tissue death and a resulting cheeselike appearance of tissue

Causes and Symptoms

Sarcoidosis, an inflammatory disease of unknown cause, affects multiple organs and systems in the body. Most commonly affected are the lungs, lymph nodes, skin, and eyes. Other organs and systems that can be involved include the liver, spleen, bone, joints, heart, muscle, and central nervous system. Sarcoidosis is thought to be the result of an unusual immune reaction to an environmental antigen, such as a bacterium, fungus, or environmental toxin. Sarcoidosis is characterized by the presence of noncaseating granulomas in the affected tissues. These granulomas are ball-shaped clusters of immune cells consisting of macrophage and epitheloid cells encircled by

---

Information on Sarcoidosis

Causes: Unknown; dysregulated immune system response to pathogen or environmental toxin

Symptoms: Fatigue, cough, inflammation, granulomas

Duration: Years; may resolve without treatment or persist

Treatments: Corticosteroids

---

lymphocytes. A granuloma begins when certain types of lymphocytes interact with antigen-presenting cells. Macrophages that have engulfed antigens are chronically stimulated by cytokines, differentiate into epithelioid cells, and fuse to form multinucleated giant cells. If a granuloma persists for an extended period of time, then fibroblasts and collagen encase the ball of cells. This eventually leads to fibrosis, or permanent scarring, which can lead to organ impairment.

The incidence of sarcoidosis varies greatly by ethnic group, indicating a genetic component to sarcoidosis. In the United States, 40 in 100,000 African Americans develop sarcoidosis, while 5 in 100,000 Caucasians develop it. In Sweden, the incidence is 64 in 100,000. In general, more women develop sarcoidois than do men. Sarcoidosis can occur at any age, but the average age when it is detected is between twenty and forty years.

The initial symptoms of sarcoidosis may include coughs, wheezing, chest discomfort, night chills, and weight loss. Many patients learn that they have sarcoidosis when a routine chest X ray shows abnormalities. Most if not all of the symptoms of sarcoidosis are not unique to the disease, so diagnosis involves ruling out other conditions, such as an infection. Typical first signs of sarcoidosis include skin lesions, problems with the lungs (such as decreased lung function), and enlarged lymph nodes. A bronchoscopy may be performed to inspect the bronchial tubes and to obtain a tissue for biopsy. A positive biopsy would reveal a large number of white blood cells, general inflammation, and the presence of granulomas. Gallium-67 scans may be used, in which the radioactive element gallium-67 is injected and accumulates in areas of inflammation, infection, or rapid cell division. More recently, the more sensitive FDG-PET scan, which uses the radioactive sugar FDG instead of gallium, is being used for some patients. Patients with sarcoidosis in the eyes have redness in the eyes, photophobia, and blurred vision.

Treatment and Therapy

An estimated 60 to 70 percent of cases of sarcoidosis will resolve within one to two years. For severe sarcoidosis, corticosteroids, such as prednisone, are given to reduce inflammation. Since steroids can have severe side effects, treatment may not be given unless organs are impaired. Some 20 to 30 percent of patients will develop a chronic condition of persistent sarcoidosis that damages organs as a result of fibrosis. It is estimated that in 5 to 10 percent of patients, sarcoidosis will be the cause of death, usually from lung fibrosis resulting in respiratory failure or from cardiac or neurological complications.

Perspective and Prospects

The skin lesions of sarcoidosis were first recognized in 1869 by English dermatologist Jonathan Hutchinson. In 1897, Caesar Boeck independently described the skin lesions using the term "sarcoidosis," meaning "fleshlike condition." The multiple system involvement was recognized by Jörgen Schaumann in 1915, the same time that Alexander Bittorf described lung lesions of the condition. In 1941, Morten A. Kveim, a Norwegian physician, developed a test for sarcoidosis that involved injecting lymph node tissue from a confirmed sarcoidois patient into the skin of a person suspected of having sarcoidosis. If granulomas developed at the injection site four to six weeks later, then the test was positive for sarcoidosis. In 1954, Louis Siltzbach modified the test to inject tissue from the spleen of sarcoidosis patients. If the patient was receiving steroid treatment, then the granulomas might not develop, leading to a false negative on the test. The Kveim test is no longer used to diagnose sarcoidosis, largely because of the lack of commercially available Kveim reagent and its replacement by other diagnostic methods, such as bronchoscopy. A promising new development in the treatment of extensive sarcoidosis is the use of FDG-PET to monitor a patient's response to drug therapy. FDG-PET is more sensitive than the conventional gallium method. Research into the genetics of sarcoidosis indicates likely multiple genetic factors. A predisposition to developing sarcoidosis is associated with *HLA-DQ* and *HLA-DR* genes.

—*Susan J. Karcher, Ph.D.*

See also Autoimmune disorders; Corticosteroids; Eye infections and disorders; Eyes; Immune system; Immunology; Lesions; Lungs; Lymphatic system; Pulmonary diseases; Pulmonary medicine; Skin; Skin disorders.

For Further Information:

Culver, Daniel A., Mary Jane Thomassen, and Mani S. Kavuru. "Pulmonary Sarcoidosis: New Genetic Clues and Ongoing Treatment Controversies." *Cleveland Clinic Journal of Medicine* 71, no. 2 (2004): 88-106. Discusses genetics.

Iannuzzi, Michael C., Benjamin A. Rybicki, and Alvin S. Teirstein. "Medical Progress: Sarcoidosis." *New England Journal of Medicine* 357, no. 21 (2007): 2153-2165. A review.

Smith, C. Christopher, Jess Mandel, and Booker Bush. "Less Is More." *New England Journal of Medicine* 344, no. 14 (2001): 1079-1082. Difficulty of sarcoidosis diagnosis.

Sarcoma

Disease/Disorder

Anatomy or system affected: Arms, back, bones, cells, joints, legs, muscles

Specialties and related fields: Cytology, general surgery, genetics, histology, oncology, pathology

Definition: A malignant tumor that develops in connective tissues of the body and can occur in children or adults.

Causes and Symptoms

Sarcomas are a rare, poorly understood group of human

cancers. Although the incidence of sarcomas is far lower than for the more common types of human malignancy, the disease is no less devastating to afflicted individuals and their families. The term "sarcoma" comes from the Greek term for "fleshy growth" and refers to the fact that sarcomas are malignant tumors that arise in connective tissues of the body. In the embryo, connective tissue arises from primitive cells called the mesenchyme. During embryogenesis, the mesenchymal tissues differentiate to form the many specialized connective tissues found in the body. Malignant tumors may arise in any of these connective tissue types. Cancers arising in fatty tissue are called liposarcomas, smooth muscle tumors are leiomyosarcomas, cancers in developing skeletal muscle are rhabdomyosarcomas, and angiosarcomas affect the blood or lymph vessels. Other types of sarcoma include fibrosarcoma, occurring in fibroblasts; synovial sarcomas of the joints; neurofibrosarcoma, a malignancy of cells surrounding the nerves; osteosarcoma in bone tissue; and chondrosarcoma in cartilage. Gastrointestinal stromal tumors (GISTs) are a rare type of stomach cancer. Ewing's sarcoma represents a family of childhood malignancies occurring in very primitive cells of bone tissue and is one of the most common forms of bone cancer in children, exceeded only by osteosarcomas. Finally, Kaposi's sarcoma is a rare sarcoma caused by infection by human herpesvirus 8. While it is a rare disease in the general population, occuring primarily among Jewish men of Mediterranean origin, it represents the most common malignancy in patients with acquired immunodeficiency syndrome (AIDS). Kaposi's sarcoma seems to result from the expression of a viral gene that activates growth regulatory genes in infected cells.

Although there are many types of sarcomas, this group of malignancies shares many common features, including cellular characteristics, symptoms, and treatment approaches. The causes of sarcoma, however, appear to be diverse and poorly understood. Sarcomas have been linked to environmental exposure to toxic chemicals. Genetic links have been identified in families with hereditary predispositions to cancer, including Li-Fraumeni syndrome, which results from an inherited mutation in the *p53* tumor suppressor gene, and neurofibromatosis (Von Recklinghausen's disease), which involves an inherited mutation in the tumor suppressor gene called *NF1*. Many sarcomas contain genetic chromosomal rearrangements called translocations involving growth control genes similar to those observed in leukemias and lymphomas, which may suggest common features in the pathways by which these malignancies arise. For example, the Ewing's sarcoma family of tumors (ESFT) contains a translocation between chromosomes 11 and 22, resulting in uncontrolled expression of certain oncogenes and their products, including growth factors and kinases.

Treatment and Therapy

In addition to surgery, radiation, and chemotherapy, newer treatment approaches for sarcomas attempt to attack the

---

Information on Sarcoma

Causes: May include environmental exposure to toxic chemicals, genetic predisposition, genetic translocations, viral infection
Symptoms: Malignant tumors in conective tissue; wide-ranging
Duration: Chronic
Treatments: Surgery, radiation, chemotherapy

---

tumor by targeting its genetic lesions. For example, the drug Gleevec imatinib (mesylate), used in the treatment of chronic myeloid leukemia, has also shown clinical promise in the treatment of GISTs that contain a genetic translocation that activates the cancer-causing oncogene *c-KIT*. A major goal of current research on sarcomas is to better understand the mechanisms by which these tumors develop in the body in order to design treatment approaches that will target these abnormal malignant cells selectively.

The discovery of certain types of translocations common to sarcomas provides both a means to screen for genetic abnormalities which may cause the disease and a potential target for treatment. For example, some of these oncogenes may be specifically inhibited by newer families of chemotherapeutic drugs. The targeting of the c-KIT oncogene by Gleevec is an example.

—*Sarah Crawford, Ph.D.;*
updated by Richard Adler, Ph.D.

See also Bone cancer; Bone disorders; Bone grafting; Bones and the skeleton; Cancer; Carcinogens; Chemotherapy; Connective tissue; Ewing's sarcoma; Kaposi's sarcoma; Muscle sprains, spasms, and disorders; Muscles; Neurofibromatosis; Oncology; Orthopedic surgery; Orthopedics; Orthopedics, pediatric; Radiation therapy.

For Further Information:

Brennan, Murray F., and Jonathan J. Lewis. *Diagnosis and Management of Sarcoma.* New York: Taylor & Francis, 2001.
Grealy, Lucy. *Autobiography of a Face.* New York: Perennial, 2003.
Parker, James N., and Philip M. Parker, eds. *The Official Patient's Sourcebook on Adult Soft Tissue Sarcoma.* San Diego, Calif.: Icon Health, 2002.

SARS. *See* Severe acute respiratory syndrome (SARS).

Scabies

Disease/Disorder
Anatomy or system affected: Skin
Specialties and related fields: Dermatology, family medicine
Definition: Skin infestation by mites, causing a rash and severe itching.

Causes and Symptoms

The human scabies mite *Sarcoptes scabiei*, a small arachnid, approximately 0.4 millimeter long, produces intense pruritus (itching) and a red rash. Though scabies is most commonly noted on the fingers and hands, almost any skin surface can be affected. After fertilization, the female mite burrows into the upper layer of the host's skin and deposits several eggs. Upon hatching, the young migrate to the surface, where they mature; this life cycle lasts three to four weeks. In most cases, an affected human host will have an average of eleven adult females. The elderly and immunocompromised patients are susceptible to a more severe, widespread variant called Norwegian scabies. In cases of Norwegian scabies, a human host may carry more than two million adult females.

A patient with scabies generally complains of severe itching, and the skin may be inflamed from scratching. Examination with a magnifying lens reveals characteristic burrows several millimeters in length, especially in the spaces between the fingers. A skin scraping aids in the diagnosis, producing a specimen for microscopic viewing which reveals the adult mite, eggs, or feces.

Treatment and Therapy

The treatment of scabies is straightforward. Clothing and bed linen should be washed in hot water. Shoes or other articles that cannot be washed may be sealed in a plastic bag for a week; this kills the mites, which need a human host to survive for more than a few days. Patients are treated with a 5 percent preparation of permethrin applied from head to foot (sparing the mouth and eyes) and left on overnight. An alternative treatment is lindane, which is less commonly used because of the risk of nerve toxicity in children. With either treatment, the medication is rinsed off in the morning shower. A single dose of oral ivermectin may be used alone or in combination with topical agents to treat difficult cases. Rapid diagnosis and treatment decrease the chance of the mites spreading to other individuals.

—*Louis B. Jacques, M.D.*

See also Dermatology; Itching; Lice, mites, and ticks; Parasitic diseases; Rashes; Skin; Skin disorders.

For Further Information:
Chosidow, Oliver. "Scabies and Pediculosis." *The Lancet* 355, no. 9206 (March 4, 2000): 819-826.
Gach, J. E., and A. Heagerty. "Crusted Scabies Looking Like Psoriasis." *The Lancet* 356, no. 9230 (August 19, 2000): 650.
Haag, M. L., S. J. Brozena, and N. A. Fenske. "Attack of the Scabies: What to Do When an Outbreak Occurs." *Geriatrics* 48 (October, 1993): 45-46, 51-53.
Levy, Sandra. "The Scourge of Scabies: Some Ways to Treat It." *Drug Topics* 144, no. 22 (November 20, 2000): 56.
Sheorey, Harsha, John Walker, and Beverly Ann Biggs. *Clinical Parasitology.* Melbourne, Vic.: University of Melbourne Press, 2003.
Stewart, Kay B. "Combating Infection: Stopping the Itch of Scabies and Lice." *Nursing* 30, no. 7 (July, 2000): 30-31.
Turkington, Carol, and Jeffrey S. Dover. *The Encyclopedia of Skin and Skin Disorders.* 3d ed. New York: Facts On File, 2007.
Weedon, David. *Skin Pathology.* 3d ed. New York: Churchill Livingstone/Elsevier, 2010.

Scalds. *See* Burns and scalds.

Scarlet fever
Disease/Disorder
Also known as: Scarlatina
Anatomy or system affected: Immune system, skin
Specialties and related fields: Bacteriology, family medicine, internal medicine, pediatrics
Definition: An acute, contagious childhood disease caused by bacterial infection.

Causes and Symptoms

The bacteria *Streptococcus pyogenes* that cause scarlet fever (which is also known as scarlatina) produce erythrogenic toxins A, B, and C. Historically, scarlet fever has been associated with toxin A-producing streptococcal strains, but by the late twentieth century there was a prevalence of toxins B and C. Nevertheless, a resurgence of toxin A-producing streptococci has also been observed.

The bacteria are spread by inhalation of air that has been contaminated by the coughing or sneezing of an infected person. After exposure, the incubation period is between two and four days. The disease is characterized by a sore throat, fever, and rash; it may follow throat infections and, occasionally, wound infection and septicemia (blood poisoning). The face is flushed, resembling sunburn with goosebumps, with a pale area around the mouth. The mucous membranes of the mouth, throat, and tongue become strawberry red. The irritation usually appears first on the upper chest but quickly spreads to the neck, abdomen, legs, and arms.

Treatment and Therapy

Penicillin and erythromycin (given to people who are allergic to penicillin) have reduced the complications of scarlet fever to a minimum. In mild cases, recovery takes two to three days. To decrease its contagious effect, isolation for the patient for the first twenty-four hours is recommended. A few days after the body temperature returns to normal, peeling off of the skin takes place at the site of the rash, especially on the hands and feet. The rare complications that might arise include ear infections, rheumatic fever, and kidney inflammation (nephritis). A child with scarlet fever should rest and be given plenty of fluids and antipyretics (fever-reducing agents), such as acetaminophen, to reduce discomfort.

Perspective and Prospects

Scarlet fever was first clearly distinguished from measles and other rash-producing diseases in 1860. Fifty years later, Russian scientists associated its cause to streptococcus, a hemolytic microorganism (one that destroys red blood cells). In 1924, George and Gladys Dick isolated the rash-causing substance in the medium used to grow hemolytic streptococci. They applied it to susceptible individuals in an attempt to establish immunity in them, but the technique was not successful. The loss of human life as a result of scarlet fever continued until the development of antibiotics in the 1940s. For an unknown reason, the incidence of the disease had declined drastically by the end of the twentieth century.

—*Soraya Ghayourmanesh, Ph.D.*

See also Antibiotics; Bacterial infections; Childhood infectious diseases; Fever; Pediatrics; Rashes; Septicemia; Streptococcal infections.

For Further Information:

Behrman, Richard E., Robert M. Kliegman, and Hal B. Jenson, eds. *Nelson Textbook of Pediatrics*. 18th ed. Philadelphia: Saunders/Elsevier, 2007. Text covering all medical and surgical disorders in children with authoritative information on genetics, endocrinology, etiology, epidemiology, pathology, pathophysiology, clinical manifestations, diagnosis, prevention, treatment, and prognosis.

Icon Health. *Scarlet Fever: A Medical Dictionary, Bibliography, and Annotated Research Guide to Internet References*. San Diego, Calif.: Author, 2004. Designed for physicians, medical students, researchers, and patients.

Kimball, Chad T. *Childhood Diseases and Disorders Sourcebook: Basic Consumer Health Information About Medical Problems Often Encountered in Pre-adolescent Children*. Detroit, Mich.: Omnigraphics, 2003. Offers basic facts about common childhood illnesses as well as cancer, sickle cell disease, diabetes, and other chronic conditions in children. Discusses frequently used diagnostic tests, surgeries, and medications.

Leikin, Jerrold B., and Martin S. Lipsky, eds. *American Medical Association Complete Medical Encyclopedia*. New York: Random House Reference, 2003. A concise presentation of numerous medical terms and illnesses. A good general reference.

Professional Guide to Diseases. 9th ed. Philadelphia: Lippincott Williams & Wilkins, 2008. This book covers more than six hundred disorders, organized by body system. Each disease entry is complete in itself, defining the disease and describing signs and symptoms, causes and complications, and relevant diagnostic tests.

Woolf, Alan D., et al., eds. *The Children's Hospital Guide to Your Child's Health and Development*. Cambridge, Mass.: Perseus, 2002. An authoritative and comprehensive guide to children's health, providing a guide to every common illness or condition that affects children and a carefully designed emergency section.

Schistosomiasis

Disease/Disorder

Also known as: Bilharziasis, Katayama fever, swimmers' itch

Anatomy or system affected: Bladder, blood, blood vessels, circulatory system, lungs, urinary system

Specialties and related fields: Environmental health, internal medicine, public health

Definition: A human disease caused by infection by one of several endoparasites of blood flukes.

Key terms:

bilharziasis: an alternative and more regionalized name for schistosomiasis

blood fluke: a parasitic flatworm that belongs to the class Trematoda and subclass Digenia within the phylum Platyhelminthes

cercaria: the tailed swimming larvae of blood flukes

intermediate host: an animal or plant that harbors a development stage in the life cycle of a parasite

primary host: an animal or plant in which adult parasites occur

Causes and Symptoms

Schistosomiasis is a parasitic disease of humans that is prevalent in tropical and subtropical regions of the world. Also called bilharziasis, the disease is caused by blood flukes of the family Schistosomatidae. Five species of blood flukes have been identified as causing schistosomiasis, including *Schistosoma mansoni*, which is widespread across central Africa but also occurs in New World tropics; *S. japanicum* and *S. mekongi* of the Pacific region and a number of African countries; *S. intercalatum*, which occurs widely in Africa; and *S. haematobium* in Portugal, Turkey, and across North Africa. All schistosomes are trematode flukes that belong to the phylum of flatworms called the Platyhelminthes.

Unlike many internal parasites of humans, schistosomes exist as separate male and female individuals. The male *S. mansoni* is about 6 to 10 millimeters in length and has a ventral groove within which the somewhat longer but considerably thinner female resides. The two remain together permanently, paired throughout life.

The life cycle of blood flukes involves two human hosts and an intermediate host, which is a species of freshwater snail. Reproduction occurs in the first human host. The female deposits its eggs in small veins of the intestinal wall or the wall of the urinary bladder, depending on the *Schistosoma* species. The eggs work through the intestinal wall and into the lumen, to be carried away and eliminated with the host's feces or in the urine.

If human waste is deposited on land, then the

Information on Schistosomiasis

Causes: Parasitic infection with blood flukes through skin exposure

Symptoms: Rash and itchiness at entry site; flulike symptoms (fever, chills, muscle aches); enlargement of lymph nodes, spleen, and liver; dysuria and hematuria; abdominal pain; diarrhea

Duration: Often chronic

Treatments: Medications (praziquantel, oxamniquine, metrifonate)

Cycle of Schistosomiasis Infection

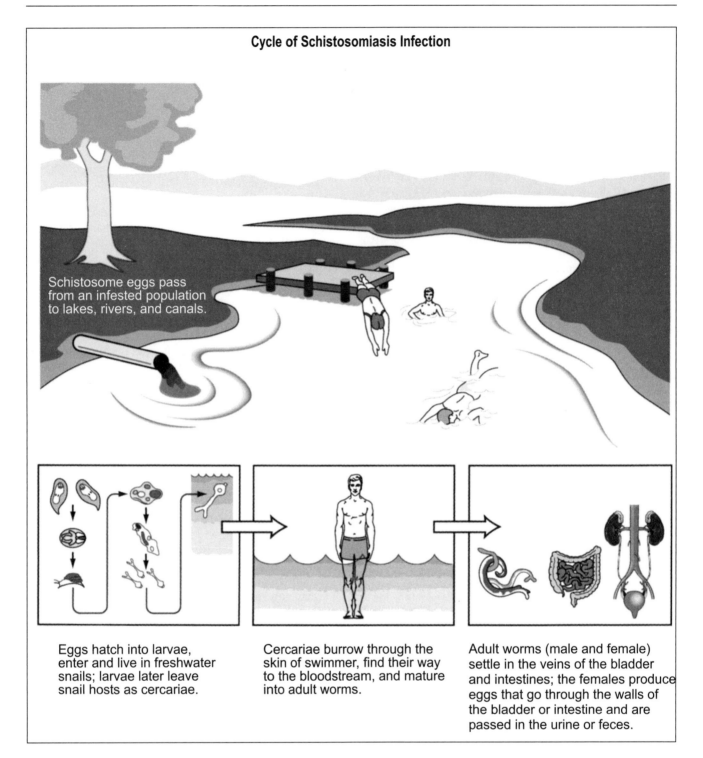

Schistosome eggs pass from an infested population to lakes, rivers, and canals.

Eggs hatch into larvae, enter and live in freshwater snails; larvae later leave snail hosts as cercariae.

Cercariae burrow through the skin of swimmer, find their way to the bloodstream, and mature into adult worms.

Adult worms (male and female) settle in the veins of the bladder and intestines; the females produce eggs that go through the walls of the bladder or intestine and are passed in the urine or feces.

Schistosoma eggs dry and decompose. If it is dropped in freshwater, however, then the eggs hatch, releasing ciliated larvae called miracidium that swim about in search of certain species of freshwater snails. The miracidium burrows into the snail and undergoes asexual reproduction, producing one or two generations of immobile sporocysts. The second generation of sporocysts transform into tailed larvae called cercaria that burrow out of the snail and into the water. The cercaria can survive about forty-eight hours in the water as they swim about in search of a second human host.

Human infection occurs if the swimming cercaria encounter someone wading, bathing, swimming, or walking in shallow water. The cercaria attach to the skin by oral and ventral suckers, discard their tails, and use a combination of muscles and enzymes to bore through the skin and enter the dermal blood vessels as larval forms called schistosomules. Within the blood vessels, schistosomules are carried throughout the circulatory system, eventually arriving in the pulmonary capillaries of the lungs, where they transfer to systemic vessels that carry them to the portal veins. There, they mature and pair, a female lodging in the gynecophoric canal of a male. Together for life, the pair migrates through the circulatory system to the mesenteric veins of the lining mucosa or to the vesicular veins and begin to produce eggs. A noted departure from this life cycle is seen in *S. haematobium*, which lodges in the walls of the urinary bladder instead of the intestinal veins and voids its eggs into the urine.

The first symptoms of schistosomiasis infection are typically a rash or itchiness that occurs at and around the entry site of the cercaria. These symptoms gradually disappear, but within one to two months additional flulike symptoms such as fever, chills, and muscle aches become evident. These symptoms are typically produced by immunological reaction to the eggs rather than infestation by the blood flukes. Heavy infestations may result in enlargement of the lymph nodes, spleen, and liver; dysuria and hematuria; abdominal pain; and diarrhea.

Pathophysiological injury resulting from schistosomiasis infection may include inflammation, necrosis, and fibrosis produced by the lodging and movement of the eggs in the walls of the intestines and bladder. Movement of the schistosomules in the lungs may also cause respiratory problems.

Some flukes of the Schistosomatidae family cause a condition called swimmers' itch. The blood flukes that cause swimmers' itch are actually parasites of birds and mammals other than humans. The intense "itching" irritation occurs when aquatic cercaria of these species mistakenly try to penetrate into the skin of people who are wading or swimming. The cercaria lodge within the skin and die, producing the intense itching sensations characteristic of swimmers' itch.

Treatment and Therapy

Schistosoma infections are diagnosed by blood tests that reveal the presence of eggs or chemicals released by the blood parasites. Infections are treated with a battery of safe and effective drugs, including praziquantel, oxamniquine, and metrifonate. The last medication is an effective treatment for urinary schistosomiasis caused by *S. haematobium*.

Perspective and Prospects

Schistosomiasis is an ancient parasitic disease that has plagued humans for centuries. Schistosome eggs have been found in mummies five thousand years old from the upper kingdom of ancient Egypt. Today, schistosomiasis continues to be a debilitating and sometimes fatal disease of humans. It is endemic in the warmer pantropics of the world and in regions where bathing and other sanitation facilities are lacking, including sub-Saharan Africa, the Nile River Valley region, central and northern South America, a number of Caribbean islands, Southeast Asia, the Philippines, Japan, and much of the Middle East. Schistosomiasis also poses a threat to tourists that visit these areas. Schistosomiasis blood flukes do not occur naturally in the United States, but recent immigrants may be infected.

Worldwide, current estimates of infection rates suggest a minimum of two hundred million to three hundred million or more humans infected by one of the *Schistosoma* species of blood flukes, which translates into roughly one in every twenty-five to thirty persons. At this rate of infection, schistosomiasis, along with malaria and hookworm, remains one of the three worst parasitic diseases of humans.

—*Dwight G. Smith, Ph.D.*

See also Parasitic diseases; Tropical medicine; Worms; Zoonoses.

For Further Information:

Mahmoud, Adel A. F., ed. *Schistosomiasis*. River Edge, N.J.: World Scientific, 2001. A general but comprehensive treatment.

Parsonnet, Julie, ed. *Microbes and Malignancy: Infection as a Cause of Human Cancers*. New York: Oxford University Press, 1999. A series of papers presented by experts that explores the relationships between parasitic infections and origin of various human cancers.

Rollinson, David, and Andrew J. G. Simpson, eds. *The Biology of Schistosomes: From Genes to Latrines*. London: Academic Press, 1987. An excellent introduction to the biology, ecology, and epidemiology of *Schistosoma* infections of humans.

Secor, W. Evan, and Daniel G. Colley, eds. *Schistosomiasis*. New York: Springer, 2005. Covers genetics, the host-schistosome interaction with larvae and adult worms, the host immune response to eggs, and public health concerns.

Stephenson, Lani S., ed. *Schistosomiasis and Malnutrition*. Ithaca, N.Y.: Cornell University Press, 1986. This work explores the relationship between blood flukes and malnutrition.

World Health Organization. *The Control of Schistosomiasis: Second Report of the WHO Expert Committee*. Geneva: Author, 1993. Good account of the history of the efforts to control *Schistosoma* infections of humans.

Schizophrenia

Disease/Disorder

Anatomy or system affected: Brain, psychic-emotional system

Specialties and related fields: Psychiatry

Definition: A disorder characterized by disordered thinking and odd perceptions that cause dysfunction in major activities, sometimes including withdrawal from the world, delusions, and hallucinations.

Key terms:

delusions: a false view of what is real

genetic cause: something that is handed down through the genes

hallucinations: a false or distorted perception of objects or events

hereditary: something that is passed down from generation to generation through the genes

Causes and Symptoms

Schizophrenia is a disorder affecting the brain and mind. Eugen Bleuler (1857-1939), a Swiss psychiatrist, first named the disease in a 1908 paper that he wrote titled "Dementia Praecox: Or, The Group of Schizophrenias." In 1911, he published a book with the same title describing the disease in more detail. Bleuler served as the head of an eight hundred-bed mental hospital in Switzerland and treated the worst and most chronic cases. Beginning in 1896, he embarked on a project to understand the inner world of the mentally ill. He developed work therapy programs for his patients, and he visited them and talked to them almost every day. Bleuler insisted that the hospital staff show the same kind of dedication and support for his clients that he did.

Bleuler's discoveries challenged the traditional view of the causes and treatment of the disease. The traditional view, based on the work of the great German psychiatrist Emil Kraepelin (1856-1926), held that dementia, as it was called, always got worse and that the patient's mind continued to degenerate until death. Kraepelin suggested that the disease, which he called dementia praecox, was hereditary and was the result of a poisonous substance that destroyed brain cells. Bleuler's investigation of living victims led him to reject this view. Instead, he argued, continuing deterioration does not always take place because the disease can stop or go into remission at any time. The disease does not always follow a downhill course. Bleuler's views promised more hope for patients suffering from schizophrenia.

The word "schizophrenia" can roughly be translated to mean "split mind." This does not mean, however, individuals with schizophrenia have two personalities or two minds. Instead, it refers to how individuals with schizophrenia do not always experience the world as it is. Instead, the world can be one way in their mind and another way in what is going on around them.

The symptoms of schizophrenia are more well known than the cause. Diagnosis is based on a characteristic set of symptoms that must last for at least several months. The "psychotic symptoms" include a break with reality, hallucinations, delusions, or evidence of thought disorder. These symptoms are referred to as positive symptoms because they are so readily available. Negative symptoms, which are less readily observed, include withdrawal from society, the inability to show emotion or to feel pleasure or pain, total apathy, and lack of facial expression. A person with negative symptoms might be found simply sitting and staring blankly at the world, no matter what is happening. Schizophrenia can take many forms. Among the most frequent are those that display acute symptoms under the following labels. Melancholia includes depression and hypochondriacal delusions, with the patient claiming to be extremely physically ill but having no appropriate symptoms. Schizophrenia can also be catatonic, in which patients become immobile and seem fixed in one rigid position for long periods of time. Delusional states accompanied by hallucinations frequently involve hearing voices, which often scream and shout abusive and derogatory language at the patient or make outrageous demands. The delusions are often visual and involve perceptions of frightening monsters or aliens sent to do harm to the afflicted person.

Disconnected speech patterns, broken sentences, excessive body movement, and purposeless activity usually accompany the symptoms noted above. Victims of the disease also suffer through states of extreme anger and hostility. Cursing and outbursts of uncontrolled rage can result from relatively insignificant causes, such as someone looking at them "in the wrong way." Many times, anniversaries of im-

---

Information on Schizophrenia

Causes: Genetic factors
Symptoms: Varies; may include withdrawal, delusions, hallucinations, thought disorders, inability to show emotion or feel pleasure or pain, total apathy, lack of facial expression, depression, mania, paranoia
Duration: Typically chronic
Treatments: Psychotherapy, drug therapy

---

portant life experiences, such as the death of a parent or the birthday of a parent or of the patient, can set off positive and negative symptoms. Hallucinations and mania can also follow traumatic events such as childbirth or combat experiences during war.

The paranoid form of schizophrenia is the only one that usually develops later in life, usually between the ages of thirty and thirty-five. It is a chronic form, meaning that patients suffering from it usually become worse. Paranoid schizophrenia is characterized by a feeling of suspiciousness of everyone and everything, hallucinations, and delusions of persecution or grandiosity. This form becomes so bad that many victims eventually commit suicide simply to escape their tormentors. Others turn on their alleged tormentors and kill them, or at least someone who seems to be responsible for their terrible condition.

Other chronic forms of the disease include hebephrenic schizophrenia. In this case, patients suffer disorders of thinking and frequent episodes of incoherent uttering of incomprehensible sounds or words. The victims move quickly from periods of great excitement to equally exhausting periods of desperate depression. They frequently have absurd, bizarre delusions such as perceived sex metamorphosis, identification with godlike creatures, or experiences of being born again and again literally and in a sense that is not tied to spiritual or religious practices.

Individuals suffering from "simple" schizophrenia exhibit constant feelings of dissatisfaction with everything in their lives or a complete feeling of indifference to anything that happens. They are usually isolated and estranged from their families or any other human beings. Patients with these symptoms tend to live as recluses with barely any interest in society, in work, or even in eating or in talking to anyone else.

The various types of schizophrenia start at different times in different people. Generally, however, except for the paranoid form, the disease develops during late adolescence. Men show signs of schizophrenia earlier than women, usually by age eighteen or nineteen. It is unusual for signs of the disorder to appear in males after age twenty. In women, symptoms may not appear until the early twenties and sometimes are not evident until age thirty. Sometimes, there are signs in childhood. People who later develop schizophrenia tended to be withdrawn and isolated as children and were often made fun of by others. Not all withdrawn children develop the disease, however, and there is no way to predict who will get it and who will not.

Schizophrenia is a genetic disease. Individuals with the

disease are very likely to have relatives-mothers, fathers, brothers, sisters, cousins, grandmothers, or grandfathers-with the disorder. Surveys indicate that 1 percent of all people have the disease. A person with one parent who has the disease is ten times more likely to develop schizophrenia than a member of the general public. Thirty-nine percent of people who have both parents afflicted with the disease also develop schizophrenia.

As to why the disease develops later in life rather than at birth, investigators provide the following information. First, the brain develops more slowly than other organs and does not stop developing until late adolescence. Many genetic diseases remain dormant until later in life, such as Huntington's chorea and multiple sclerosis.

Schizophrenia operates by disrupting the way in which brain cells communicate with each other. The neurotransmitters that carry signals from one brain cell to another might be abnormal. Malfunction in one of the transmitters, dopamine, seems to be a source of the problem. This seems likely because the major medicines that are successful in the treatment of schizophrenia limit the production or carrying power of dopamine. Another likely suspect is serotonin, a transmitter whose presence or absence has important influences on behavior.

In 2003, researchers announced that they had discovered clues that pointed to a specific gene as the cause of schizophrenia. The gene is known as dysbindin, and it is involved in the operation of the synapses, the points where one neuron wires itself to another. The team found that genetic variations in the dysbindin gene were more common among schizophrenic patients. Medical research is increasingly pinpointing regions, or loci, within chromosomes that contain genetic mutations, a task that has proven difficult in years past. Since the human genome sequence has become available, however, research groups have started to focus on the same handful of loci, suggesting that they could be seeing a true signal for the disease. The gene dysbindin has been located in these limited chromosomal regions. Moreover, Icelandic researchers have discovered a gene called neuregulin-1 that also tends to cluster in specific loci. Mutations in this gene are highly correlated with schizophrenia in about 15 percent of Icelandic patients. The next step for the research teams will be to examine whether both genes might work together in the regulation of synapses and to see if other scientists can replicate and confirm the initial findings.

Treatment and Therapy

Since the 1950s, many medications have been developed that are very effective in treating the symptoms of schizophrenia. Psychotherapy can also be effective and beneficial to many patients. Drugs can be used to treat both positive and negative symptoms. Some, such as Haldol, Mellaril, Prolixin, Navane, Stelazine, and Thorazine, are used to treat positive symptoms. Clozapine and Risperidone can be used for both positive and negative symptoms. These medications work by blocking the production of excess dopamine, which may cause the positive symptoms, or by stimulating the production of the neurotransmitter, which reduces negative symptoms. Clozapine blocks both dopamine and serotonin, which apparently makes it more effective than any of the other drugs. These drugs are nonaddictive and do not provide a high or euphoric effect of any kind.

The chief problem resulting from the use of such drugs is the terrible side effects that they can produce. The most dreaded side effect, from the point of view of the patient, is tardive dyskinesia (TD). This problem emerges only after many years of use. TD is characterized by involuntary movement of muscles, frequent lip-smacking, facial grimaces, and constant rocking back and forth of the arms and the body. It is completely uncontrollable.

Dystonias are another side effect. Symptoms include the abrupt stiffening of muscles, such as the sudden contraction of muscles in the arms, neck, and face. Most of these effects can be controlled or reversed with antihistamines. Some patients receiving medication are afflicted with effects similar to those movements associated with Parkinson's disease. They suffer from the slowing of movements in their arms and legs, tremors, and muscle spasms. Their faces seem frozen into a sad, masklike expression. These effects can be treated with medication. Another problem is akathisia, a feeling developed by many patients that they cannot sit still. Their jumpiness can be treated with Valium or Xanax. Some of these side effects are so severe or embarrassing that patients cite them as the major reason that they do not take their medicine.

Many patients report great value in family or rehabilitation therapy. These therapies are not intended to cure the disease or to "fix" the family. Instead, they are aimed at helping families learn how to live with mentally ill family members. Family support is important for victims of schizophrenia because they usually are unable to live on their own. Therapy can also help family members understand and deal with their frustration and the constant pain that results from knowing that a family member is very ill and probably will not improve much. Rehabilitation therapy is an attempt to teach patients the social skills that they need to survive in society.

The results of treatment are not always positive, even with medication and therapy. Approximately 5 percent of people with schizophrenia commit suicide rather than trying to continue living with the terrible consequences of the disease.

Perspective and Prospects

Hopes for improving the treatment of schizophrenia rest mainly on the continuing development of new drugs. Several studies suggest that psychotherapy directed at improving social skills and reducing stress helps many people with the disease improve the quality of their lives. It is known that stress-related emotions lead to increases in delusions, hallucinations, social withdrawal, and apathy. Therapists can help patients find ways of dealing with stress and living in communities. They encourage their patients to deal with feelings of hostility, rage, and distrust of other people.

Family therapy can teach all members of a family how to live with a mentally ill family member. Such therapy, along with medication, can produce marvelous results.

One study of ninety-seven victims of schizophrenia who lived with their families, received individual therapy, and took their medications showed far fewer recurrences of acute symptoms than did a group that did not get such help. Among those fifty-four individuals who received therapy but lived alone or with nonfamily members, schizophrenia symptoms reappeared or worsened over the same three-year period of the study. People living alone usually had more severe symptoms to start out with and found it difficult to find housing, food, or clothing, even with therapy. The demands of life and therapy apparently were too much for them. The major problem with this kind of treatment, which seems to work for people in families, is that it is expensive.

—Leslie V. Tischauser, Ph.D.;
updated by Nancy A. Piotrowski, Ph.D.

See also Anxiety; Bipolar disorders; Depression; Hallucinations; Hypochondriasis; Paranoia; Psychiatric disorders; Psychiatry; Psychiatry, child and adolescent; Psychoanalysis; Psychosis; Suicide.

For Further Information:

Barlow, David H., ed. *Clinical Handbook of Psychological Disorders*. 4th ed. New York: Guilford Press, 2008. This collection defines and describes psychological disorders and uses case histories as illustrations for treatment.

Gorman, Jack M. *The New Psychiatry: The Essential Guide to State-of-the-Art Therapy, Medication, and Emotional Health*. New York: St. Martin's Press, 1996. A well-written, easy-to-understand book by a doctor and researcher that provides the latest information concerning the development of new medications, treatments, and therapies. Valuable information on the new antipsychotic drugs, how they work, and what their possible side effects are.

Gottesman, Irving I. *Schizophrenia Genesis: The Origins of Madness*. New York: W. H. Freeman, 1991. The author, a leading researcher into the genetic causes of schizophrenia, describes recent discoveries on the origins of the disease. He also evaluates different treatments and the many kinds of counseling and therapeutic techniques.

Johnstone, Eve C., et al. *Schizophrenia: Concepts and Clinical Management*. New York: Cambridge University Press, 1999. Written in conjunction with colleagues from Edinburgh, Eve Johnstone's book is a useful summary of current knowledge. The suggestion that psychosis can be thought of as occurring along three dimensions-positive, negative, and disorganized-with distinct pathological mechanisms, is well argued but probably still falls short of being an accepted theory.

Miller, Rachel, and Susan E. Mason, eds. *Diagnosis: Schizophrenia-A Comprehensive Resource*. New York: Columbia University Press, 2002. Uses first-person accounts and chapters written by professionals to discuss a wide range of issues that impact schizophrenic patients, including hospitalization, rehabilitation, medication, coping skills, social services, and clinical research.

National Allegiance for Research on Schizophrenia and Depression. http://www.narsad.org. One section of the site, "Disorders and Conditions," provides excellent information on a range of mental health disorders, including schizophrenia. Site also covers updated research and provides personal stories.

Schizophrenia.com. http://www.schizophrenia.com. A Web site of a nonprofit organization dedicated to providing support and information for individuals with schizophrenia, and their caregivers. Volunteers supporting the site include researchers, professors, scientists, family advocates, and people who have schizophrenia.

Sheehan, Susan. *Is There No Place on Earth for Me?* Boston: Houghton Mifflin, 1982. A book that provides an accurate, compassionate view of the course of chronic schizophrenia, including the many difficulties faced by victims of the disease. Describes the ineffective care available for many patients in public facilities.

Torrey, E. Fuller. *Surviving Schizophrenia: A Manual for Families, Patients, and Providers*. 5th ed. New York: Collins, 2006. Perhaps the best single book on the topic, by a leading medical researcher and advocate of more humane care for the mentally ill. Describes the latest research into the origins of the illness and provides useful information and evaluations of the newest drugs and best forms of treatment.

Sciatica

Disease/Disorder

Anatomy or system affected: Back, hips, legs, nerves, nervous system, spine

Specialties and related fields: Family medicine, internal medicine, neurology

Definition: Painful inflammation of one of the sciatic nerves.

Causes and Symptoms

The two sciatic nerves are the largest nerves in the body. One runs from the spine down the left leg, the other down the right leg; they supply the tissues of the thigh, lower leg, and foot. The roots of the sciatic nerves are in the lower spinal column. It is here that difficulty is most likely to occur. Inflammation of these nerves is most often caused by a pinching of one or more spinal nerve roots between the vertebrae of the lower back.

Sciatica is characterized by shooting pain down the sciatic nerve and extending into the hip, the thigh, and the back portion of the leg. The pain may occur in all these points at once or skip about from point to point. Sciatica often begins with a long period of intermittent, mild low back pain. Suddenly, however, the slightest movement, such as lifting a weight or merely bending over, may bring about intense sciatic pain.

A mild case of sciatica can be brought on by vitamin deficiencies or by arthritic inflammation in the lower spine. Prolonged constipation can build pressure on the nerve and cause sciatic pain. Occasionally, a tumor may develop near the nerve and press on it. Sometimes, a herniated, or slipped, disk at the level where the nerve roots emerge in the low back may protrude and press on the nerve, thereby causing sciatica.

Information on Sciatica

Causes: Vitamin deficiencies, arthritic inflammation in lower spine, prolonged constipation, tumors, slipped disk, pregnancy

Symptoms: Shooting pain down sciatic nerve and extending into hip, thigh, and back portion of leg

Duration: Acute to chronic

Treatments: Surgery, heat application, medications, physical therapy

Treatment and Therapy

If the sciatic nerve is being compromised, surgery may be indicated. More than 50 percent of patients with sciatica, however, recover on their own in six weeks. In the acute stage, rest is essential. Heat may give temporary relief from pain. The type of medication used depends on the cause of the sciatica. Ultimately, a therapeutic exercise program to develop stabilizing strength and endurance in the trunk muscles is essential for functional recovery.

—*Genevieve Slomski, Ph.D.*

See also Back pain; Lower extremities; Nervous system; Neuralgia, neuritis, and neuropathy; Neurology; Slipped disk.

For Further Information:

Brown, Mark D., and Björn L. Rydevik, eds. *Causes and Cure of Low Back Pain and Sciatica*. Philadelphia: W. B. Saunders, 1991. Discusses the etiology and treatment of low back pain and sciatica. Includes bibliographical references.

Fishman, Loren, and Carol Ardman. *Back Pain: How to Relieve and Cure Low Back Pain and Sciatica*. New York: W. W. Norton, 1999. Discusses the mechanisms of backache and offers some treatment options. Includes bibliographical references and an index.

Gillette, Robert D. "A Practical Approach to the Patient with Back Pain." *American Family Physician* 53, no. 2 (February 1, 1996): 670-678. When treatment is based on a specific diagnosis, when patients are followed proactively to recovery, and when psychosocial factors receive appropriate attention, then the management of back pain will probably be effective.

Hooper, Paul D. *Preventing Low Back Pain*. Baltimore: Williams & Wilkins, 1992. Discusses such topics as the prevention of backache and its treatment, including chiropractic. Includes bibliographical references and an index.

SCID. *See* Severe combined immunodeficiency syndrome (SCID).

Scleroderma

Disease/Disorder

Also known as: Systemic sclerosis, CREST syndrome

Anatomy or system affected: Blood vessels, circulatory system, gastrointestinal system, hands, heart, immune system, joints, kidneys, lungs

Specialties and related fields: Dermatology, gastroenterology, immunology, rheumatology

Definition: A rare autoimmune connective tissue disorder affecting various organs.

Causes and Symptoms

Scleroderma is a connective tissue disease characterized by fibrosis and hardening of the skin and internal organs. The word "scleroderma" is derived from the Greek *sclero*, meaning "hard," and *derma*, meaning "skin." This disease affects roughly 300,000 persons in the United States, with women being affected four times more than men. The disease affects persons between the ages of twenty and fifty.

It is believed that scleroderma is autoimmune in origin. The exact cause of the disease is yet to be discovered, but an overproduction of collagen has been observed in skin biopsies of patients with scleroderma. Two types of the disease have been recognized: localized scleroderma and systemic sclerosis. The localized form of the disease is more common in children and can affect small areas of the skin or muscle or can be widespread, manifesting as morphea and/or linear scleroderma. Morphea affects the skin, with gradually enlarging inflammatory plaques or patches; they may regress spontaneously over time and typically last for months to years. The skin over the lesions appears firm to hard, and the lesions themselves are ivory or yellow in color. Linear scleroderma usually affects a limb or the forehead and, if present early in childhood, can result in permanent limb shortening. This type may also affect the muscles and joints, causing limited joint mobility.

Systemic sclerosis, on the other hand, is a more widespread disease that affects multiple organs, such as the skin, esophagus, gastrointestinal tract, muscles, joints, blood vessels, heart, kidneys, lungs, and other internal organs. This disease usually manifests in adults, with symptoms of at least one or more of the following: Raynaud's phenomenon (extreme sensitivity of the extremities to cold temperatures, with a tingling sensation and the limb turning blue, red, or white upon exposure to cold); thickening of the skin with a leathery, shiny appearance (sclerodactyly); fibrosis and thickening of the joints with decreased mobility; swelling of the hands and feet, with pain and stiffness of the joints; and orofacial abnormalities from thickening of the skin. Some patients may experience symptoms of esophageal, heart, lung, or kidney disease. Systemic sclerosis should always be suspected in every case of difficulty swallowing and heartburn, especially if seen in a middle-aged woman. Patients may complain of nonspecific problems, such as bloating of the abdomen, weight loss, fatigue, generalized weakness, diarrhea, constipation, shortness of breath, and vague aching of joints and muscles. They may also exhibit dryness and redness of the conjunctiva and mucous membranes (Sjögren's syndrome or keratoconjunctivitis sicca).

Some patients experience the CREST syndrome, which is an acronym for *c*alcinosis, *R*aynaud's phenomenon, *e*sophageal dysmotility, *s*clerodactyly, and vascular *t*elangiectasia. Another form of the disease is localized cu-

---

Information on Scleroderma

Causes: Unknown, probably autoimmune; may be related to overproduction of collagen

Symptoms: Fibrosis and hardening of skin and internal organs; may include inflammatory plaques or patches, ivory or yellow skin lesions, limb shortening, limited joint mobility, Raynaud's phenomenon, swelling of hands and feet, difficulty swallowing, heartburn

Duration: Chronic

Treatments: Alleviation of symptoms; may include calcium-channel blockers, NSAIDs, antacids and antireflux medications, cyclophosphamide, penicillamine, corticosteroids, topical cortisone ointment, plastic surgery, physical and occupational therapy

taneous systemic sclerosis, which affects mainly the skin of the hands, face, feet and forearms, with Raynaud's phenomenon being the primary symptom.

Diagnosis of the disease is difficult, especially in the initial stages, as the symptoms are common to a variety of immunologically mediated diseases such as rheumatoid arthritis, Sjögren's syndrome, and systemic lupus erythematosus (SLE). The diagnosis is mainly based on clinical findings, an elevated erythrocyte sedimentation rate (ESR), and a skin biopsy showing elevated collagen levels. Sometimes, a positive antinuclear antibody test and a positive rheumatoid factor test may be seen. About 30 percent of patients are positive for the Scl-70 antibody, which is highly specific for the disease. X rays and lung function tests are used to determine the extent of the disease.

Those with the systemic form are prone to various complications, including heart failure, kidney failure, respiratory problems, and intestinal malabsorption.

Treatment and Therapy

As of the beginning of the twenty-first century, no cure for scleroderma had been found. Each symptom, however, can be treated effectively, and the quality of life can be greatly improved if the disease is detected early in its course. The disease is primarily managed by rheumatologists and dermatologists, owing to the severity of its course and the difficulty of diagnosis. Calcium-channel blockers are used to decrease the symptoms caused by Raynaud's phenomenon, joint pain and stiffness can be treated with nonsteroidal anti-inflammatory drugs (NSAIDs), esophageal dysmotility and subsequent heartburn is treated with antacids and antireflux measures, lung inflammation and fibrosis can be treated with cyclophosphamide, and heart failure and renal failure are treated appropriately with drugs. Penicillamine and corticosteroids are used to treat the fibrosis seen in the disease. In addition, physical and occupational therapy is instituted to improve joint mobility.

Morphea or localized scleroderma can be managed by the application of cortisone ointment to the lesions. This will not reverse or treat the disease completely, but it appears to slow the progression and provide symptomatic relief. Patients are also advised to use sunscreen lotions and moisturizers to soften the skin and prevent sunburn. Plastic surgery may be employed to correct serious deformities.

Perspective and Prospects

Scleroderma is an individual disease, with each patient exhibiting different aspects. This makes diagnosis even more difficult and complicated. Scleroderma is not contagious, and it is not believed to be heritable. It is thought that certain people are inherently more susceptible to the disease, and they develop it only if environmental or physical trigger factors, such as stress, are activated. Prognosis of the localized form of scleroderma is good, with the lesions resolving spontaneously, and the five-year survival rate for those with systemic disease is 80 to 85 percent. Presently, many clinical trials are being conducted for such treatments as the use of stem cells as a "rebooting" mechanism, alpha interferon, ultraviolet therapy, and even psychotherapy. These approaches appear promising and aim to at least improve the quality of life of patients with scleroderma, if not cure the disease.

—Rashmi Ramasubbaiah, M.D.,
and Venkat Raghavan Tirumala, M.D., M.H.A.

See also Autoimmune disorders; Collagen; Connective tissue; Dermatology; Dermatology, pediatric; Dermatopathology; Immune system; Immunology; Neurofibromatosis; Rheumatoid arthritis; Rheumatology; Sjögren's syndrome; Skin; Skin disorders; Systemic lupus erythematosus (SLE).

For Further Information:

Brown, Michael. *Scleroderma: A New Role for Patients and Families.* 2d ed. Los Angeles: Scleroderma Press, 2002.

Frazier, Margeret Schell, and Jeanette Wist Drzymkowski. *Essentials of Human Diseases and Conditions.* 4th ed. St. Louis, Mo.: Saunders/Elsevier, 2009.

Kasper, Dennis L., et al., eds. *Harrison's Principles of Internal Medicine.* 16th ed. New York: McGraw-Hill, 2005.

Mayes, Maureen D. *The Scleroderma Book: A Guide for Patients and Families.* 2d ed. New York: Oxford University Press, 2005.

Rakel, Robert E., ed. *Textbook of Family Practice.* 6th ed. Philadelphia: W. B. Saunders, 2002.

Tapley, Donald F., et al., eds. *The Columbia University College of Physicians and Surgeons Complete Home Medical Guide.* Rev. 3d ed. New York: Crown, 1995.

Scoliosis

Disease/Disorder

Anatomy or system affected: Back, bones, musculoskeletal system, spine

Specialties and related fields: Orthopedics, physical therapy

Definition: Abnormal curvature of the spine, often progressive, which can result in severe deformity and associated medical problems.

Key terms:

adolescent scoliosis: curvature of the spine that is diagnosed in the early stages of puberty

Cobb angle: the commonly used measure of the degree of spinal curvature; the angle created by perpendiculars to the top of the first and bottom of the last vertebrae in a curve

idiopathic: referring to a medical condition with no known cause

skeletal or bone age: a measurement of age based on a comparison by an X ray of the bone structure in the left hand with the standards of the Gruelich and Pyle Atlas

spine: the combined spinal cord and the spinal column, a structure central to erect posture and the complex nervous communications system of the body

vertebra (pl. vertebrae): the individual bones that are stacked upon one another to form the vertebral column, or spine

Causes and Symptoms

Of all the structures making up the human body, the spine is second only to the closely associated brain in its centrality to human characteristics. Two distinct aspects of human life are deeply involved in the correct functioning of the spine. First, the spinal column protects the spinal cord, which carries out critical message-carrying functions in the body. Second, the spinal column also holds the body erect, a distinctly primate feature. An abnormal curvature of the skeletal structure of the spinal (or vertebral) column is known as scoliosis.

The usual term for the spine, the backbone, is completely misleading. If one really had a backbone, one would be unable to bend, nod, or stretch. The normal spine consists of approximately thirty-three separate bones whose very name, vertebrae, is derived from the Latin verb "to turn." Furthermore, it is essential to know that the normal spine takes the form of four separate curves. Each of these curves is associated with a distinct set of vertebrae. At the very top of the spine are the cervical vertebrae. In the chest area are found the thoracic vertebrae, which support the body when one leans backward and which are the sites of attachment of the twelve pairs of ribs. The largest of the vertebrae, which support the upper body weight, are called lumbar, from the Latin for "loin." At the very base of the spine are two sets of small vertebrae called the sacrum and coccyx.

Although these curves are a vital part of a healthy spine, they are not always obvious because one usually sees people from the front or rear, so that the spine appears straight. If one looks at a person with good posture from the side, however, the gently S-shaped curve of the spine is clearly visible. Deformities involving abnormal spinal curvature toward the front or back are well known, but they are not called scoliosis. The side-to-side curvature of scoliosis is referred to as a lateral curve.

As important as the bones are, the vertebral spine is a much more complicated structure. Along its entire length is a surrounding complex of ligaments and muscles making it possible for the body to bend and straighten again. Within the vertebral column are rubbery cylinders of cartilage called disks. These disks absorb shocks, relieving the body from the countless pressures of movement. With this array of closely balanced mechanisms and associated forces, it is no wonder that the curvature of the spine is a complex subject for diagnosis and treatment.

Scoliosis can result from a number of different causes. While a birth defect, an accident, poliomyelitis, or muscular dystrophy can all result in lateral curvature, the cause is unknown in the majority of cases. Some authorities believe that 80 percent of all scoliosis cases have no known cause. The technical term for this important class of malady is "idiopathic scoliosis." Within this general subdivision, three separate forms are recognized, based on the age of the patient at the onset of the curvature.

The adolescent form of scoliosis, which is usually recognized between ten and thirteen years of age, is by far the most common form. A brief look, however, at infantile (birth to three years) and juvenile (four to ten years) scoliosis will help to illustrate the difficulty faced by researchers in this area and the enormous problems yet to be solved. (All these age groupings refer to the age at which the deformity is first noted, not the age at which the curvature began.)

When the scoliosis is recognized in the youngest range, it is more common in males, with one study giving a 3:2 ratio. By contrast, in the far more common adolescent condition one finds a striking shift to females, who are three times more likely to be affected. While it is often observed that infantile idiopathic scoliosis corrects itself (that is, it spontaneously resolves), this natural remission is rarely observed when the diagnosis is made later. More fascinating but puzzling is the noted absence of the infantile conditions in the United States and Canada, while its occurrence is well documented in Great Britain and France. J. I. P. James, who studied scoliosis extensively at the University of Edinburgh for many years, reported this form to be as common in Europe as the adolescent variety is worldwide. At a subtler level of research, one finds that 90 percent of the curves in infants are formed to the left, whereas 90 percent of those in adolescent girls lie to the right.

It is small wonder that James's collaborator, Ruth Wynne-Davies, calls the cause of infantile scoliosis "multifactorial" and states, "The exact cause in each individual is likely to be different." Wynne-Davies has made important studies of the influence of heredity in producing scoliosis. She, like many others, sees infantile idiopathic scoliosis in a different class from the adolescent variety.

The juvenile condition is likely to be related closely to adolescent scoliosis. As before, there is marked evidence of hereditary influence. In this age range, males and females share equally in the likelihood of being diagnosed. The chance of significant progression of the curvature is so variable that close watching of the patient is the single point of common agreement among specialists. There is concern among parents, patients, and practitioners alike over the excessive use of X rays for diagnosis.

Some research suggests intriguing clues about the cause of scoliosis from unexpected sources. For example, studies at the University of Rochester suggest that in scoliosis patients there may be significant differences in the side of the brain that processes sound. In most people, the left hemisphere of the brain hears and understands phonetic sound as in language, but those people with scoliosis seem much more likely to use both sides or the right side of the brain for these functions. It may be possible that a simple listening test can determine who is at risk for spinal curvature.

A dozen different types of curves associated with scoliosis have been identified, but four major classes are of greatest frequency and concern. In the chest area, one finds the most common of all curve patterns, the right thoracic

Scoliosis

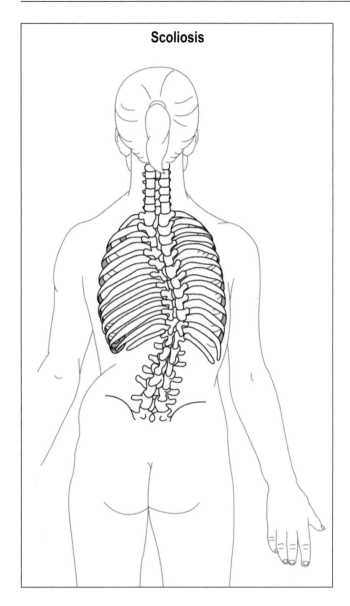

curve. It is possible for this condition to progress rapidly. Early treatment is essential. As the curve develops, the ribs on the right side shift and create a deformity which not only is unattractive but also can squeeze the heart and lungs; this so-called rib hump can result in serious cardiopulmonary difficulties.

A similar, but gentler, curve is the thoracolumbar curve. It begins in the same region of the thoracic vertebrae and ends farther down the back, in the lumbar region. The twist may be either right or left and is generally less deforming in its appearance. A lumbar curve is found far down in that region of the back, producing a twist in the hips. In pregnant women and other adults, this twist often causes severe back pain.

The three curves described thus far are single, or C-shaped, curves. The double major curve is an S-shaped curve and is the most common of that type. Curvature begins in the thoracic or chest area and is complemented by a second curve in the opposite direction found in the lumbar region. To some extent, the two curves offset each other and the scoliosis is less deforming. The double major curve

can progress and become the source of a rib hump.

These and the other less common curves demand an accurate description beyond their location. John Cobb searched for such an important tool and developed the widely used Cobb angle measurement. His suggestion was to relate the top of the first and the bottom of the last vertebrae of a curve by determining the angle formed by the intersection of lines perpendicular to them. It is not difficult, using an X ray of the spine, to draw lines above and below the vertebrae, construct the required perpendiculars, and measure the angle of their intersection. This technique allows physicians to communicate accurately and have a useful measure with which to note the progression, remission, or stabilization of the patient's scoliosis. In addition to degree of curvature, the complex structure of the spine shows rotation in scoliosis. The rotation causes the pedicles or indentations of the vertebrae to shift closer to the midline drawn on the X ray. The relative shift is described as a rotation of +1, +2, and so on.

Treatment and Therapy

Scoliosis can result from many different causes, each of which demands treatment, as well as the idiopathic variety under discussion. Since there is no known cause, prevention is impossible, and since there are enormous difficulties in predicting the course of the disease, the most that can be achieved is satisfactory correction.

A diagnostic examination for scoliosis demands specific attention to accurate family history. Particularly important is information concerning the first recognition and previous treatment of the condition. Then a detailed evaluation of the nature and extent of the curvature must be made. The examining physician should make certain that the patient is standing straight with the knees unflexed. A simple plumb line is used to examine the patient's back to determine any curvature in the spine. Then the forward bending test is conducted. This observation is considered one of the most reliable diagnostic tools. Various forms of curvature, including scoliosis, can be seen by the trained observer. When viewed at eye level from both front and back, one side of the thoracic or lumbar regions is higher. An accurate measurement of the degree of difference can be made with a level. The use of X-ray photographs also forms a vital part of the diagnostic data.

Even with the best diagnostic skill, training, and experience, the decision concerning the treatment of scoliosis is hardly straightforward. One important consideration is the patient's bone age. Because people grow and mature at such different rates, chronological age may not correspond well to the degree of maturity of that person's skeleton. Many clues are used to determine the bone age, including the degree of fusion observed in the individual vertebra or the bony pelvic girdle. A catalog of X rays of hands is available and provides a useful measure of the bone age. The central concern is that curvature is more likely to progress if the growth and development of the patient's skeleton is still incomplete.

The treatment of scoliosis varies from none at all to extensive surgical procedures. In general, treatment is undertaken for the prevention of further curvature or for the correction of the curvature already present. Some treatments, such as exercise, are of benefit to the patient in general but are seen as having no prospect of arresting or correcting the spinal curvature. Research has also suggested that copper in the diet may play a key role in scoliosis treatment. These studies were carried out with chickens, which show scoliosis very similar to that found in humans, but much remains to be learned about these and similar studies on rabbits, salmon, and quail before much confidence can be placed in the applicability of the data to human treatment or prevention.

Of all the methods proposed, the use of braces and casts is certainly the oldest and the most common. The many modifications of design and material used in braces over the centuries have had the central purpose of forcing the spine to become straight. The evolution of the brace has reached the point of an active or kinetic apparatus called the Milwaukee brace, developed by Walter Blount and Albert Schmidt. It is a carefully designed assembly of a molded plastic pelvic girdle and three metal bars which keep the wearer erect and allow a neck ring to be attached. The neck ring and its associated axillary sling keep the torso balanced and prevent listing to the right or left.

In order for the Milwaukee brace (or any modified versions of it) to be effective, it must be worn day and night and until the growth period of the patient has been completed. It is also imperative that exercise be carried out on a daily basis. There are many advantages of the modern brace over older systems. For example, it can be removed for showering and swimming, and much greater activity is allowed. The one serious drawback is that a patient must not expect correction of the scoliosis. The value of the brace is that it can, with good use and exercise, maintain the already present curvature and prevent further progression.

Only in certain cases will braces be of benefit to the patient. With curves of 40 or 50 degrees, pain that does not respond to treatment, or the failure of the brace to stop the curve's progression, surgery is the most reasonable approach. Surgery can offer some degree of correction, but it is important to recognize that only a partial correction is possible. Even with the safest techniques, pressure must be applied to the spine, creating a serious risk of damage to the spinal cord. Most authorities estimate reasonable correction to be about 60 percent.

Once it is agreed that surgery is the proper route of treatment, a wide range of methods are available. The most common, and generally considered the safest, method is the Harrington rod technique. The incision is from the back (as opposed to front or side entries), and metal hooks are inserted at the highest and lowest points in the curve. These hooks hold metal rods used to straighten the spine and then to hold it in place. Small chips of bone are then taken from the hip or ribs and inserted between especially prepared vertebrae. In a period of six to eight months, solid bone will grow and fuse the vertebrae, giving a solid bone mass of a single elongated vertebra. After the surgery, the patient is usually placed in a brace or cast for four to six months.

The success of the Harrington rod technique has inspired several modifications, such as using two rods to achieve more balance and greater correction. With a patient who has unusually soft bones, a system of wires is used to hold the rods in place. This method is considered superior because the normal hooks might break off. Several variants of the wire technique are also available. Some surgeons thread the wires through the neural canal, and others drill small holes to avoid coming near to the spinal cord.

Another technique which is growing in popularity avoids the use of a Harrington rod. Many small wires are attached through the neural canal and twisted around two thin rods, one on either side of the curvature. This Luque method provides greater stability, and usually there is no need to wear a cast after surgery. These advantages must be balanced, however, against a significantly greater risk of paralysis and a smaller amount of room for new bone growth in fusion.

Another modern technique which is showing some success involves placing small electrodes near the spine and transmitting tiny electrical impulses to nerve endings periodically during sleep. This electronic bracing, or electrosurface stimulation, appears to stop scoliosis curves from progressing in about 80 percent of the cases studied. These devices have about the same limitations as do conventional braces-that is, curves of greater than 40 degrees, curves treated after the end of bone growth, and certain types of lumbar curves will fail to benefit from this treatment.

Perspective and Prospects

One finds the beginning of serious study of the spine in the writings of Hippocrates (c. 460-c. 370 BCE). He described the curves of both the normal and the abnormal spine. He may not have been as clear in his description of scoliosis as with those of the clubfoot or epilepsy, but he was well aware of the difficulty of its treatment and recognized its possible relationship to pulmonary disease. Another celebrated physician of antiquity, Galen (129-c.199 CE), first suggested the medical term for this deformity, scoliosis, in the late years of the second century. Among the complications faced by early medical science were the inadequate methods and equipment available for making subtle diagnoses. Thus it was not until the sixteenth century that Ambrose Pare carefully described the various types of spinal curves. He also noted for the first time that scoliosis is largely a condition of children.

Over the centuries, many men and women added to the array of methods and instruments as well as the store of knowledge and thoughtful speculation about scoliosis. Many possible causes were presented on the basis of observation and research. Many approaches to the treatment of these deformities were described and tested. Yet, despite all this research, scientists are just beginning to appreciate the complexity of the problem of scoliosis.

—K. Thomas Finley, Ph.D.

See also Back pain; Birth defects; Bone disorders; Bones and the skeleton; Braces, orthopedic; Casts and splints; Muscular dystrophy; Orthopedic surgery; Orthopedics; Orthopedics, pediatric; Pediatrics; Poliomyelitis; Puberty and adolescence; Spinal disorders; Spine, vertebrae, and disks.

For Further Information:

Eisenpreis, Bettijane. *Coping with Scoliosis*. New York: Rosen, 1999. Designed for students in grades seven to ten, this clearly written and well-organized book looks at the patterns of spinal curvature, treatment options, and emotional effects of this condition.

Griesse, Rosalie. *The Crooked Shall Be Made Straight*. Atlanta: John Knox Press, 1979. While this book does not pretend to offer specific medical information concerning scoliosis, it contains valuable insights for those facing the painful task of fighting this crippling malady. A truly inspiring story.

National Scoliosis Foundation. http://www.scoliosis.org. Provides updated medical research information, physician referrals, and community support.

Neuwirth, Michael, and Kevin Osborn. 2d ed. *The Scoliosis Sourcebook*. New York: McGraw-Hill, 2001. Origins of the disease, early detection and treatment, the pros and cons of braces, and surgery preparation are topics covered. Also includes a comprehensive list of scoliosis organizations and associations.

Parker, James N., and Philip M. Parker, eds. *The 2002 Official Patient's Sourcebook on Scoliosis*. San Diego, Calif.: Icon Health, 2002. Draws from public, academic, government, and peer-reviewed research to provide a wide-ranging handbook for patients with scoliosis.

Schommer, Nancy. *Stopping Scoliosis: The Whole Family Guide to Diagnosis and Treatment*. Rev. ed. New York: Putnam, 2002. One of the best books written for the layperson that is devoted to the discussion of a medical problem. Includes many references to other information, specialists, and organizations concerned with the study and treatment of scoliosis.

Scope of practice
Health care system

Introduction

Scope of practice refers to the range of responsibilities and functions that a particular group of professionals are legally allowed to do within their professional license. Although the term scope of practice can be used in reference to almost any profession, it is most often used in discussions of health care.

For health-care professionals, scope of practice is addressed mainly by law at the state level. These laws are designed by the state in question and create the framework within which the medical services in the state are delivered to the public. These laws determine the professions that are allowed to offer particular services, the settings in which these services can be provided, and the boundaries of professional activities offered by professionals.

Overview

Scope of practice controls what professionals-such as physicians and therapists-are allowed to do, and sets parameters that prevent health-care workers from engaging in activities that are considered beyond their knowledge and expertise. For example, scope of practice prevents nurses from performing the work of physicians, dental hygienists from doing the work of dentists, psychiatrists from doing the work of general internists, and so on.

Scope of practices control the delivery of medical services and provide a layer of protection to the public, whose members may not understand the education, professional credentialing, and experience required to perform in a particular discipline. The legal guidelines developed by states are often referred to as *practice acts*.

Development

Although some exceptions exist, state governments are responsible for developing and managing the scope of practice statutes that apply within their boundaries. Dedicated licensing boards are responsible for developing these statutes. These boards are comprised of both members of the profession in question and representatives of the public. The state governor typically appoints licensing board members, and individuals are generally chosen based on their understanding of the education, professional credentialing, and experience needed to offer trustworthy services in a particular discipline.

In addition to creating and enforcing practice acts, licensing boards set the rules and policies that concretely define the behavior of health-care professionals. These rules and policies communicate the intentions of the practice acts and outline what members of the profession are allowed to do.

Because this process is individualized by state, laws and regulations may vary from one state to another. For example, some states may give more latitude to individual professionals, while others may more closely manage their services.

—*Marie Keenan;*
Updated by Patricia Edens

For Further Information:

Christian, Sharon, Catherine Dower. "Scope of Practice Laws in Health Care: Exploring New Approaches for California." *Chcf.org*. California Healthcare Foundation. Web. 16 Nov. 2015. http://www.chcf.org/publications/2008/03/scope-of-practice-laws-in-health-care-exploring-new-approaches-for-california

McCarty, Michael N., Esq. "The Lawful Scope of Practice of Medical Assistants: 2012 Update." *AMT Events*. American Medical Technologists. June 2012. Web. 16 Nov. 2015. http://www.american medtech.org/portals/0/pdf/news/ scopeofpracticearticle_june %202012.pdf

White, Debbie, et al. "Nursing Scope of Practice: Descriptions and Challenges." *NursingLeadership* 21, no. 1: 2008. Ontario Nurses' Association. Web. 16 Nov. 2015. http://local70. ona.org/documents/File/pdf/NursingScopeofPractice.pdf

"Why Consumers Need to be Involved in Scope of Practice Reform." *NCSBN.org*. National Council of State Boards of Nursing. Web. 16 Nov. 2015. https://www.ncsbn.org/Why_consumers_need _to_be_involved.pdf

Derived from: "Scope of Practice ." *Salem Press Encyclopedia of Health*. Salem Press. .

Screening
Procedure
Anatomy or system affected: All
Specialties and related fields: Epidemiology, preventive medicine, public health
Definition: Procedures that are used to detect a potential dis-

ease or condition in individuals who have no known signs or symptoms of that disease or condition.

Key terms:

mass screening: screening for all individuals in a defined area or population

multiple or multiphasic screening: a type of screening procedure that uses a variety of tests during the same screening visit

predictive value: the probability in a screening test that a person with a positive test result truly has the disease and a person with a negative test result actually does not have the disease

prescriptive screening: a type of screening procedure that is used for early detection, in presumptively healthy individuals, of disease that can be controlled better if treated early in its natural history

reliability: the ability of a screening test to give consistent results when the test is performed more than once on the same individual under the same conditions

sensitivity: the ability of a screening test to identify correctly those who have a particular disease

specificity: the ability of a screening test to identify correctly those who do not have a particular disease

validity: the ability of a screening test to measure what it is supposed to measure

yield: the number or proportion of cases of a previously unrecognized disease that is diagnosed and brought to treatment as the result of a screening program

Indications and Procedures

In its natural course, a disease usually starts asymptomatically, gradually develops symptoms, and becomes severe when no treatment is given. If the disease can be identified early, especially before it shows any signs or symptoms, then treatment can be initiated early. Early or prompt treatment usually produces a better and more effective cure for a disease. Treatment at the early stage of a disease also has a lower cost than treatment for a disease at its late stages.

The most effective way to detect diseases before they develop symptoms is through screening. Screening is the application of a test or procedure to detect a potential disease or condition in individuals who have no known signs or symptoms of that disease or condition. For example, some people are unaware that they have a high cholesterol level, which can increase the risk for the development of cardiovascular disease. Through screening for cholesterol levels, these individuals can be identified, and proper dietary consultation, exercise prescription, and treatment can be followed to decrease the risk for cardiovascular disease. Screening tests use criteria to classify people according to the likelihood of disease. Screening is just an initial examination. Individuals with positive results from a screening test are required to have a secondary diagnostic examination, which is often more comprehensive and in depth, to confirm the positive finding from their screening test.

Screening tests can be classified into three categories: mass, multiple or multiphasic, and prescriptive. Mass screening means the screening of all individuals in a defined area or population. Multiple or multiphasic screening involves the use of a variety of tests or procedures during the same screening visit. Prescriptive screening is the early detection in presumptively healthy individuals of disease that can be controlled better if treated early in its natural history. From a public health perspective, the following factors are of importance to consider before implementing a screening program. The disease or condition should be a major medical problem. Effective treatment should be available for the disease discovered from the screening test. Follow-up diagnosis and treatment should be available to individuals with positive results from the screening test. The disease should have identifiable early and latent stages. An effective test or examination for the disease should be available. The test or procedure used in screening should be acceptable to the general population. The natural history of the disease should be adequately understood. Policies, procedures, and threshold levels on tests should be determined in advance to clarify who should be referred for further diagnosis and possible treatment. The process should be simple enough to encourage large groups of people to participate. Finally, screening should be done as a regular and ongoing process, not as an occasional activity. Based on these considerations, screening is not necessarily available or suitable for every disease.

Accuracy and effectiveness are important for a screening test; they are evaluated by the characteristics of validity, predictive value, reliability, and yield. The validity of a test means how well the test actually measures what it is supposed to measure. Validity has two components: sensitivity and specificity. Sensitivity is defined as the ability of a test to identify correctly those who have the disease, while specificity is defined as the ability of a test to identify correctly those who do not have the disease. Both sensitivity and specificity are determined by comparing the results obtained from the screening test with the results derived from some definitive diagnostic procedure. Sensitivity is calculated as the proportion of subjects with the disease who have a positive screening test (true positive). Specificity is calculated as the proportion of subjects without the disease who have a negative screening test (true negative). If a screening test has a low sensitivity, then it could misclassify healthy individuals as disease cases (false positive). If a screening test has a low specificity, then it could fail to identify individuals with the disease (false negative). Thus, high levels of sensitivity and specificity are the foundation for the accuracy of a screening test, although it is impossible to have 100 percent of both sensitivity and specificity in practice.

The ability of a screening test to predict the presence or absence of the disease indicates the quality of the test. The predictive value of a screening test is influenced by the sensitivity and specificity of the test as well as the prevalence of the disease, which means how common the disease is in populations. The higher the prevalence of a disease in a population, the more likely a positive test will represent a true positive; the lower the prevalence of a disease in a population, the more likely a positive test will represent a false positive. The predictive value of a screening test can be measured as either positive or negative. The predictive value of a positive test is the probability that individuals with a positive test actually have the disease. On the other hand, the predictive value of a negative test is the probability that individuals who have a negative result from a screening test do not have the disease. Thus, along with sensitivity and specificity, a high level of predictive value is also desirable for an effective screening test. In comparison, sensitivity and specificity are calculated from the screening test results of the diseased or nondiseased individuals, while predictive value depends on the proportion of diseased individuals in the population.

Reliability, also called precision, is another important characteristic of a screening test. A reliable screening test is one that gives consistent results when the test is performed more than once on the same individual under the same conditions. Two common factors affect the consistency of results: the variation of the method used in a screening test and the variation between different observers. These variations usually can be reduced by standardization of procedures or protocols used in a screening test, by training the observers of a screening test, by using more than one observer at the same time with each making independent observations, and by quality control measures, such as periodic checks.

The yield of a screening program is defined as the number or proportion of cases of a previously unrecognized disease that are diagnosed and brought to treatment as a result of the screening program. Several factors can affect the yield of a screening program. If a screening test has a low sensitivity, and therefore identifies only a portion of the diseased individuals, then the yield of the screening test could be poor. If the prevalence of the disease being screened for is low, then the yield of the test could be low even though the sensitivity of the test is high. Using multiphasic screening approaches often increases the cost-effectiveness of a screening program and results in a high level of yield. Frequency of screening is another factor influencing the yield of a screening program. The optimal interval between screenings should be determined by a particular disease's natural course-how long it takes to develop from its first detectability of symptoms-and by different individuals with different risk factors. For example, certain cancers may need to be screened more frequently in older individuals than in younger individuals. The yield of a screening program can also be affected by the proportion of the population participating in the program. Low participation rates could turn out low yields. To increase participation rates in a disease screening program, the population needs to be educated about the disease, including information about the fact that the disease is understood as a serous threat to health, that all individuals are vulnerable to the disease, that the method of the screening test is safe, and so on. The cost of a screening test can also have a significant effect on the participation rate.

Screening is usually concerned with chronic illness. Based on the individuals' ages, gender, occupation, overall health status, lifestyle, and medical and family history, physicians may prescribe specific screening tests. Mass screening programs may be carried out in communities to detect common diseases such as hypertension, high blood cholesterol, type 2 diabetes, breast cancer, colorectal cancer, prostate cancer, and osteoporosis.

Uses and Complications

Some diseases are good candidates for screening. For example, data from the National Health and Nutrition Examination Survey showed that 24 percent of the adult population in the United States had high blood pressure, or hypertension. Almost one in every three African Americans was hypertensive. More than one-third of the individuals with hypertension were unaware of their condition, since hypertension is usually asymptomatic. Hypertension is defined as a blood pressure reading of 140/90 millimeters of mercury (mmHg) or higher. The higher the blood pressure, the higher is the chance of developing hypertension complications, such as coronary heart disease, stroke, renal dysfunction, and sudden death. The treatment of hypertension is very effective. Reduction in blood pressure through treatment can significantly decrease the risk for stroke, coronary heart disease, renal disease, and sudden death. Screening is the best way to detect hypertensive individuals without symptoms. The common method of screening for hypertension is sphygmomanometry that measures cuff pressures. Ambulatory blood pressure monitoring is an alternative method, which uses an automated sphygmomanometer that records blood pressure at frequent intervals over twenty-four hours. Although ambulatory blood pressure monitoring is more accurate, it is also more expensive and impractical, thus, it is not as commonly used as sphygmomanometry. As the benefit of the screening is evident and the risk of sphygmomanometry is nearly none, it is recommended that every adult should be screened for hypertension.

High blood cholesterol is another common condition that is asymptomatic but increases the risk of coronary heart disease and stroke. More than 37 percent of people in the United States have blood cholesterol levels higher than the normal range. Cholesterol comes from food or is produced in the body. When there is too much cholesterol in the blood, it builds up in the walls of the arteries and hardens them, so that the arteries become narrowed and blood flow to the heart or the brain is slowed down or blocked, resulting in coronary heart disease or stroke. Since high cholesterol is asymptomatic, many people are unaware that their level is too high. Cholesterol screening is performed using a blood test after a fourteen-hour fast. This test includes measurements of total cholesterol: both low-density lipoproteins (LDLs), or "bad" cholesterol, the main source of cholesterol buildup and blockage in the arteries, and high-density lipoproteins (HDLs), or "good" cholesterol, which helps keep cholesterol from building up in the arteries. Triglyceride, another form of fat in the blood, may be checked at the same time. A healthy individual should have a total cholesterol level less than 200 milligrams per deciliter, an LDL level less than 100 milligrams per deciliter, and an HDL level greater than 45 milligrams per deciliter. The normal triglyceride level is less than 200 milligrams per deciliter. Individuals aged twenty years or older are recommended to have their cholesterol level checked every five years. Cholesterol screening can raise awareness of high blood cholesterol, so that individuals can modify their lifestyle by consuming less saturated fat and engaging in more physical activity and drug treatment can be initiated, if necessary, to prevent heart disease and stroke. The American Heart Association recommends mass screening for high cholesterol at worksites to identify high-risk populations of middle-aged men and women and in communities targeting low-income, low-education, and minority groups who are often underrepresented in other voluntary screenings.

The number of people with type 2 diabetes is increasing in the United States as a result of the high prevalence of obesity. Complications of diabetes are severe, such as increased risks for cardiovascular disease, kidney failure, blindness, and amputation of the legs. Many people with diabetes are undiagnosed. The natural history of diabetes includes an asymptomatic preclinical phase. The length of this preclinical phase varies and may last ten years or longer. Screening tests can detect diabetes in the preclinical phase. Different tests have been used for diabetes screening: the two-hour postload plasma glucose test, the fasting plasma glucose test, and the test of hemoglobin A1c. The third test has been proposed as a standard reference for diagnosing diabetes. Research studies showed that after diabetes was detected during its preclinical phase, interventions, such as aggressive control of hypertension and cholesterol levels and use of aspirin during the preclinical phase, could reduce the risk of cardiovascular disease. The benefit of tight control of blood sugar levels during the preclinical phase, however, was unclear or minimal. Overall, screening for diabetes has been controversial. The most important gap in the understanding of screening is the lack of information on the added benefits of starting various interventions and treatments earlier, during the preclinical period, compared with at clinical detection.

More than 215,000 women are diagnosed with breast cancer every year in the United States. Approximately one in every eight women will develop breast cancer during her lifetime. Breast cancer is the second leading cause of cancer death in women. Early detection and effective treatment can reduce the number of women who die from breast cancer. Three approaches are considered for screening for breast cancer: breast self-examination (BSE), X-ray mammography, and clinical breast examination. The sensitivity of BSE and clinical breast examination is unclear, but the sensitivity of mammography is relatively high. The American Cancer Society recommends screening with mammography every one to two years, with annual clinical breast examinations beginning at the age of forty and annual mammography with clinical breast examinations beginning at the age of fifty.

Prostate cancer is the most common cancer and the second leading cause of cancer death in men in the United States. After fifty, the risk of prostate cancer increases with age. African American men have a higher risk for prostate cancer. The principal screening tests for prostate cancer are the digital rectal examination, a blood test of serum tumor markers called prostate-specific antigen (PSA), and transrectal ultrasound. The reference standard for these tests is pathologic confirmation of malignant disease in tissue obtained by biopsy or surgical resection. Because biopsies are not generally performed on patients with negative screening test results, the sensitivity and specificity of screening tests for prostate cancer cannot be determined with certainty. The American Cancer Society recommends an annual digital rectal examination for prostate cancer beginning at age forty. It recommends an annual measurement of serum tumor markers for average men aged fifty and older; however, this measurement should begin at age forty for African American men and those with a family history of prostate cancer. The natural history of prostate cancer is still poorly understood, and there is no direct evidence that prostate cancer screening decreases mortality. The cost associated with the screening tests for prostate cancer is another concern. Thus, screening for prostate cancer remains controversial.

Colorectal cancer is the second most common form of cancer, as well as one of the leading causes of death from cancer in the United States. Since it is asymptomatic at its early stage, about 60 percent of patients with colorectal cancer have regional or distant metastases at the time of diagnosis. The principal screening tests for detecting colorectal cancer are fecal occult blood testing, sigmoidoscopy, and digital rectal examination. Less frequently used screening tests include barium enema and colonoscopy, which have been advocated primarily for high-risk groups, such as persons with a family history of hereditary syndromes associated with a high risk of colon cancer. Screening for colorectal cancer is recommended for men and women aged fifty years and older with annual fecal occult blood testing, sigmoidoscopy, or both. There is good evidence that periodic fecal occult blood testing reduces mortality for colorectal cancer, and there is fair evidence that sigmoidoscopy alone or in combination with the fecal occult blood testing reduces mortality. There is no direct evidence, however, that colonoscopy or barium enemas reduce mortality. The digital rectal examination is of limited value as a screening test for colorectal cancer. The examining finger, which is only seven to eight centimeters long, has limited access even to the rectal mucosa, which is usually eleven centimeters in length. Thus, a negative digital rectal examination performed by a physician provides little reassurance that the patient is free of colorectal cancer.

It is estimated that in the United States 1.3 million people experience a fracture each year as a result of osteoporosis, or fragile bones. Osteoporosis can progress painlessly until a bone breaks. Over half of all postmenopausal women will develop a spontaneous fracture as a result of osteoporosis. Hip fractures and vertebral deformities, two common consequences of osteoporosis, can result in significant pain, disability, decreased functional independence, and death. Low bone density is strongly associated with an increased risk of fracture. The World Health Organization (WHO) defines osteoporosis as a bone mineral density of 2.5 or more standard deviations below the mean of healthy young adult women. A number of tests are available to measure bone density, including conventional skeletal radiographs, quantitated computed tomography, single photon absorptiometry, dual photon absorptiometry, and dual energy X-ray absorptiometry. The correlations among different bone density devices are low. Dual energy X-ray absorptiometry is considered the gold standard because it is the most extensively validated test against fracture outcomes. The likelihood of being diagnosed with osteoporosis depends on the number of tested sites, which include the forearm, hip, spine, or heel. Because women over age sixty-five have a significantly increased risk of osteoporosis, routine screening in this population is recommended. For women aged sixty to sixty-four, screening may be needed if they have risk factors, such as low body weight, family history, smoking, and removal of the ovaries before age forty-five. The screening intervals should be two years for women aged sixty-five years and older and five years for women younger than sixty-five. Once osteoporosis is diagnosed, changing lifestyle, such as an increase in dietary calcium and vitamin D intake, weight-bearing exercise, and smoking cessation, along with drug treatment, can help prevent fractures.

Other common screening procedures include those meant to detect cervical cancer, testicular cancer, skin cancer, carotid artery stenosis, peripheral arterial disease, abdominal aortic aneurysm, thyroid disease, iron deficiency anemia, sexually transmitted diseases, visual impairment, hearing impairment, phenylketonuria (PKU), Down syndrome, dementia, and depression.

Perspective and Prospects

By the middle of the twentieth century, infectious diseases were gradually replaced by chronic diseases as the leading causes of death in developed countries such as the United States. This transition occurred as a result of improvement in living standards and nutritional status, the prevention of infectious diseases through immunization, and increased life expectancy. Hence, prevention of chronic disease became an important task in public health and medicine practices in developed countries. In 1951, the United States multi-sponsored Commission on Chronic Illness organized the Conference on Preventive Aspects of Chronic Diseases and advocated screening for diseases. Since then, more and more screening tests and procedures have become available for different diseases and conditions because of development in medical technologies.

At the beginning of the twenty-first century, however, chronic diseases were still the leading cause of death in developed countries as well as some developing countries. The most important chronic diseases that contribute to mortality are heart disease, cancer, and stroke. Many as-

pects of screening for these chronic diseases remain unclear. For some diseases, no tests or no effective tests are available, such as for lung cancer. For other conditions, powerful methods of detection exist but no effective treatments are available, such as for human immunodeficiency virus (HIV). Many screening procedures still lack evidence to support their effectiveness or justification for the balance between benefit, harm, and cost. Therefore, further investigations, epidemiological studies, development of low-cost and effective screening methods, and increases in participation in screening through health education are the future challenges.

—*Kimberly Y. Z. Forrest, Ph.D.*

See also Acquired immunodeficiency syndrome (AIDS); Anemia; Apgar score; Biostatistics; Blood testing; Breast cancer; Cancer; Cervical, ovarian, and uterine cancers; Chlamydia; Cholesterol; Chorionic villus sampling; Colonoscopy and sigmoidoscopy; Colorectal cancer; Colorectal polyp removal; Diabetes mellitus; Diagnosis; Disease; Down syndrome; Epidemiology; Genetic counseling; Genetic diseases; Genetics and inheritance; Genomics; Glaucoma; Gonorrhea; Hearing tests; Heart disease; Hepatitis; Human immunodeficiency virus (HIV); Human papillomavirus (HPV); Hypertension; Laboratory tests; Mammography; Niemann-Pick disease; Noninvasive tests; Pap sampling; Phenylketonuria (PKU); Physical examination; Pregnancy and gestation; Preventive medicine; Prostate cancer; Rh factor; Sexually transmitted diseases (STDs); Sickle cell disease; Skin cancer; Spina bifida; Syphilis; Tay-Sachs disease; Testicular cancer; Thyroid disorders; Ultrasonography; Vision disorders; Well-baby examinations.

For Further Information:

Holland, Walter W., and Susie Stewart. *Screening in Disease Prevention: What Works?* Seattle: Radcliffe, 2005. This book discusses different issues in screening for diseases in children, adults, and the elderly.

Snow, Vincenza, ed. *Screening for Diseases: Prevention in Primary Care.* Philadelphia: American College of Physicians, 2004. This book summarizes research findings of screening for major diseases, such as breast cancer, prostate cancer, colorectal cancer, hypertension, type 2 diabetes, and osteoporosis.

Thorner, Robert M., and Quentin R. Remein. *Principles and Procedures in the Evaluation of Screening for Disease.* Washington, D.C.: Government Printing Office, 1961. This classic monograph provides guidelines and methods for evaluating the effectiveness of screening programs.

U.S. Preventive Services Task Force. *Guide to Clinical Preventive Services.* Washington, D.C.: Agency for Healthcare Research and Quality, 2006. Offers guidelines for physicians, students in health fields, and the general public on the use of clinical preventive services. Contains detailed screening information for various health conditions.

Scurvy

Disease/Disorder

Anatomy or system affected: Blood vessels, eyes, gums, kidneys, muscles, teeth

Specialties and related fields: Nutrition, preventive medicine

Definition: An illness that results from a deficiency of vitamin C (ascorbic acid) in the diet.

Causes and Symptoms

Scurvy is a disease characterized by hemorrhages in body tissue, muscular pain, tender gums, physical exhaustion,

---

Information on Scurvy

Causes: Vitamin C deficiency
Symptoms: Hemorrhaging, muscle pain, tender gums, exhaustion, visual disorders (especially night blindness), tooth loss
Duration: Chronic
Treatments: Synthetic or natural vitamin C

---

and vision disorders, especially night blindness. In advanced cases, teeth fall out, and complications with kidney or intestinal functions may lead to death. The disease at one time was common among sailors who went on long ocean voyages where their diet did not include fruits and vegetables containing vitamin C. Also, the populations of cities under siege and prisoners with very restricted diets often suffered from scurvy. During the American Civil War in the 1860s, scurvy was reported as a problem among the troops.

Treatment and Therapy

A causal connection between scurvy and a person's diet had been suspected for a long time, but the particular missing nutrient was not known until the work of a Scottish physician, James Lind, in the 1750s. Lind experimented on six pairs of patients who had scurvy symptoms, giving them one of six different acidic diet supplements: vinegar, seawater, sulfuric acid solution, apple cider, garlic and mustard seed, or two oranges and a lemon. He found that the men who ate the citrus fruit improved rapidly, the ones who drank the cider recovered slowly, and the others showed no improvement. The British navy adopted a requirement for lemon juice aboard its ships in 1795, which virtually eliminated scurvy. Subsequently, lemons were replaced by limes, which led to the nickname Limeys for British sailors.

The essential nutrient in citrus fruits, now known as vitamin C, was first identified in 1932 by C. G. King and W. A. Waugh at the University of Pittsburgh. Its scientific name is ascorbic acid, which means "without scurvy." Synthetic vitamin C is identical to the naturally occurring variety, in both its composition and its physiological effect. Vitamin C is essential for the formation and repair of collagen, which is a primary component of blood vessels. It is also necessary for the synthesis of hormones that control the rate of metabolism in the body.

Perspective and Prospects

During the nineteenth century, medical research by the so-called microbe hunters had firmly established that bacteria are the cause of numerous diseases that are transmitted from person to person. Some illnesses, however, were shown to be completely unrelated to bacteria but rather attributable to dietary deficiencies. Among these disorders are beriberi, rickets, anemia, and scurvy. They have been almost totally eradicated as people have learned that a healthy diet must include fruits, vegetables, whole grain foods, and vitamin supplements.

—*Hans G. Graetzer, Ph.D.*

See also Malnutrition; Nutrition; Vitamins and minerals.

For Further Information:

Consumer Guide, editors of. *Complete Book of Vitamins and Minerals*. Lincolnwood, Ill.: Publications International, 1996.
Kasper, Dennis L., et al., eds. *Harrison's Principles of Internal Medicine*. 16th ed. New York: McGraw-Hill, 2005.
"Medicine and Surgery, History: Nutrition." In *The New Encyclopaedia Britannica*. 15th ed. Chicago: Encyclopædia Britannica, 2002.

Seasonal affective disorder

Disease/Disorder

Also known as: Recurrent major depression with seasonal pattern
Anatomy or system affected: Nervous system, psychic-emotional system
Specialties and related fields: Psychiatry
Definition: A subtype of depression characterized by seasonal fluctuation.

Key terms:

hypersomnia: a condition in which sleep periods are excessively long

major depressive episode: a group of symptoms that include depressed mood and a loss of interest or pleasure that must be identified before a psychiatric disorder of depression can be diagnosed

phototherapy: light therapy first introduced in 1984 to treat seasonal affective disorder

Causes and Symptoms

In order for a person to be diagnosed with seasonal affective disorder, the criteria for a major depressive episode as defined in the *Diagnostic and Statistical Manual of Mental Disorders: DSM-IV-TR* (4th ed., 2000) must be met. These criteria include having a depressed mood for most of the day, nearly every day, for a two-week period. Signs of a depressed mood can include reports of feeling sad, empty, or tearful. In addition, loss of interest or pleasure in almost all activities for most of the day, nearly every day, for at least two weeks can be part of a major depressive episode. If either of these two criteria is identified, then the patient must show four or more of the following symptoms: significant weight loss when not dieting or weight gain of more then 5 percent of body weight within a month, insomnia or hypersomnia nearly every day, psychomotor agitation or retardation nearly every day, fatigue or loss of energy nearly every day, feelings of worthlessness or inappropriate guilt, diminished ability to think or concentrate, and recurrent thoughts of death or suicide ideation. If the patient has experienced two recurrent major depressive episodes in the last two years that demonstrate temporal relationship to season, then a diagnosis of seasonal affective disorder can be made.

In addition to the DSM-IV-TR criteria for major depressive episode, a person with seasonal affective disorder may experience a number of other symptoms. Anxiety is a common symptom of depression and affects as many as 90 percent of all persons with depression. The depressed person often loses interest in sexual activities, and female patients

Information on Seasonal Affective Disorder

Causes: Unknown; probably hormone and neurotransmitter dysfunction

Symptoms: Seasonal pattern of depression, which may include anxiety, loss of interest in sex, abnormal menstruation, suicidal thoughts, withdrawal, reduced energy

Duration: Chronic during winter months

Treatments: Phototherapy, serotoninergic antidepressants

may experience abnormal menstruation. About two-thirds of all depressed patients contemplate suicide, and approximately 10 to 15 percent complete suicide. It should be noted that some depressed persons do not complain of mood disturbance even as they are withdrawing from family, friends, and activities. The majority of depressed persons complain about reduced energy and difficulty finishing tasks. Thus, they become impaired at school or work and lack the motivation to begin new projects.

Seasonal patterns of depression can also be identified among patients who have bipolar disorder. In this disorder, the patient experiences both major depressive episodes and elated moods. When a patient shows an elevated, expansive, or irritable mood that is excessive and impairs daily functioning, then a manic episode can be diagnosed. The elevated mood is euphoric and leads the person to engage in excessive behaviors that demonstrate poor judgment. These patients have an unlimited amount of energy and continue their activities without the need for sleep or rest. If a person experiences both manic episodes and recurrent major depressive episodes during certain seasons of the year, then the patient has a bipolar disorder with a seasonal pattern.

The causes of seasonal affective disorder are not well understood, but they probably involve dysfunction in a number of hormones and neurotransmitters, genetic influences, and personality. The seasonal mood changes have led to particular interest in studying the circadian rhythms of these individuals. Many studies have found that the circadian rhythms of persons with seasonal affective disorder are phase-delayed relative to the sleep-wake cycle. Seasonal affective disorder is considered an abnormal response to seasonal changes in length of the day and appears related to the photoperiod between sunrise and sunset. The hormone melatonin, which helps to regulate sleep-wake cycles, has been implicated. Melatonin is secreted by the pineal gland in response to darkness and is suppressed by bright light that enters through the retinal-central nervous system pathway. Genetic studies have shown that between 35 and 69 percent of persons with seasonal affective disorder have a family history of depression, and 7 to 37 percent have a family member who had seasonal depression.

Seasonal affective disorder is diagnosed following a clinical interview with the patient in order to identify the DSM-IV-TR criteria. The patient provides self-reports of possible symptoms, and the interviewer observes the person for any signs of depression that could fulfill the diagnostic requirements. In addition, seasonal affective disorder may not occur in isolation. Individuals may also suffer from other mental health problems, such as substance use disorders. Therefore, in addition to diagnosing seasonal affective disorder, the diagnostic process should also focus on ruling out other conditions that may demand additional or specialized treatment.

Treatment and Therapy

Phototherapy or light therapy involves exposing the patient to a bright light. The individual sits in front of a specific type of therapeutic light source for approximately one to two hours, usually in the morning each day. Light visors with a light source built into the brim also may be used for treatment. Antidepressant medication is often used in conjunction with phototherapy. Serotoninergic antidepressants are most often used to augment light therapy.

Perspective and Prospects

Prevalence rates point to the fact that winter seasonal affective disorder is more common than any other seasonal pattern. Evidence exists that people living in northern climates have a higher incidence of the disorder than do those living at other latitudes. Individuals with seasonal affective disorder typically experience depression as the amount of daylight decreases with advancing winter. Women have been found to represent at least 75 percent of patients with seasonal depression, being two to four times as likely than men to develop this problem. Most individuals who will develop this problem do so in their twenties and thirties. The rates of newly diagnosed seasonal affective disorder tend to decrease during the fifties and markedly decrease after age sixty-five. Understanding these age-related trends is likely to be a focus of future research that may perhaps uncover new understandings of the etiology of and treatment for the disorder.

Light therapy, the dominant treatment for this disorder, can be challenging for some because individuals must build time into their schedules to be exposed to the light. Future treatments in this area are likely to seek ways of better integrating exposure to light into the environment and activities of those affected. Light visors were a step in this direction, and other convenient methods can be expected.

—Frank J. Prerost, Ph.D.;
updated by Nancy A. Piotrowski, Ph.D.

See also Antianxiety drugs; Antidepressants; Anxiety; Bipolar disorders; Depression; Emotions: Biochemical causes and effects; Light therapy; Pharmacology; Psychiatric disorders; Psychiatry; Sleep; Sleep disorders; Suicide.

For Further Information:

Lee, T. "Seasonal Affective Disorder." *Clinical Psychology: Science and Practice* 5 (1998): 275-290.

Partonen, Timo, and Andres Magnusson, eds. *Seasonal Affective Disorder: Practice and Research.* 2d ed. New York: Oxford University Press, 2010.

Rosenthal, Norman E. *Winter Blues: Everything You Need to Know to Beat Seasonal Affective Disorder.* New York: Guilford Press, 2006.

Young, M., and P. Meaden. "Which Environmental Variables Are Related to the Onset of Seasonal Affective Disorder?" *Journal of Abnormal Psychology* 106 (1997): 554-562.

Seizures
Disease/Disorder

Anatomy or system affected: Brain, head, muscles, musculoskeletal system, nerves, nervous system

Specialties and related fields: Neurology, pediatrics

Definition: Asynchronous, paroxysmal discharges of neurons in the brain that result in body movements, unusual sensations, altered perceptions, and/or hallucinations that interfere with normal function and behavior.

Key terms:

aura: the initial event signaling the beginning of a seizure

clonic: referring to the alternate contraction and relaxation of muscles

convulsion: an involuntary contraction of the body musculature, tonic or clonic, that can be of either cerebral or spinal origin

epilepsy: a chronic brain disorder of various causes, characterized by recurrent seizures resulting from the excessive discharge of cerebral neurons

seizure: an unsynchronized, paroxysmal discharge of neurons in the brain that results in body movements, unusual sensations, altered perceptions, hallucinations, or various mixtures of such symptoms; also called an ictus

tonic: characterized by tension or contraction, especially muscular tension

Causes and Symptoms

Seizures can be divided into two fundamental groups-partial and generalized. In partial seizures, the abnormal discharge of neurons usually arises in a portion of one hemisphere and may spread to other parts of the brain during a seizure. Generalized seizures, however, have no evidence of localized onset; the clinical manifestations and abnormal electrical discharge give no indication of the locus of onset of the abnormality, if such a locus exists.

Partial seizures are divided into three groups: simple partial seizures, complex partial seizures, and partial seizures secondarily generalized. Simple partial seizures are associated with the preservation of consciousness and unilateral hemispheric involvement. The area of seizure may spread until the entire side is involved. This type of seizure, with motor, sensory, or autonomic signs, was originally called Jacksonian epilepsy. Complex partial seizures are associated with alteration or loss of consciousness and bilateral hemispheric involvement. A partial seizure secondarily generalized is a generalized tonic-clonic seizure that proceeds directly from either a simple partial seizure or a complex partial seizure. The distinction between simple partial seizures and complex partial seizures is clarified by the observation that neurologic problems that are confined to one hemisphere, such as a unilateral cerebral stroke, generally spare consciousness, whereas bilateral cerebral (or brain stem) involvement causes alteration of consciousness.

Information on Seizures

Causes: Often unknown; may include hypoglycemia, cardiovascular disorders, TIAs, movement disorders, toxic substances, metabolic disorders, sleep disorders, headaches, brain tumors, progressive neurological disease, fever, infection

Symptoms: Uncontrolled body movements, unusual sensations, altered perceptions, hallucinations that interfere with normal function and behavior

Duration: Acute to chronic

Treatments: Drug therapy, neurosurgery

If there is no evidence of localized onset, then the attack is a generalized seizure. Generalized seizures are more heterogeneous than partial seizures. The generalized seizures include generalized tonic-clonic (grand mal), absence (petit mal), atonic, myoclonic, clonic, and tonic seizures.

Tonic-clonic seizure is a common seizure pattern with sudden loss of consciousness, tonic contraction of muscles, loss of postural control, and a cry caused by contraction of respiratory muscles forcing exhalation. This is followed by a generalized contraction of the muscles of the four extremities. After two to five minutes of unconsciousness and the cessation of clonic contractions, the individual gradually regains consciousness. Fecal and urinary incontinence, as well as biting of the tongue, may occur. The individual does not remember the event and may not be completely functional for several days.

The absence seizure usually begins in childhood or early adolescence, and in many cases individuals outgrow the condition. Although unresponsiveness is the rule, motionlessness occurs in less than 10 percent of absence attacks; in fact, phenomena such as mild clonic motion and increased or decreased postural tone may accompany such attacks. Absence seizures are generally brief, usually lasting less than ten seconds and very rarely longer than forty-five seconds. The attacks are not associated with auras, hallucinations, or other symptoms characteristic of partial seizures, generalized tonic-clonic seizures, or infantile spasms. Individuals exhibiting these seizures are normal except for the seizures, but the seizures may occur as frequently as one hundred times a day.

Atonic seizures are characterized by a sudden loss of muscle tone. Myoclonic seizures are sudden and brief contractions of a single group of muscles or of the entire body. The patients fall but do not lose consciousness. Clonic and tonic seizures are characterized by alternation of contraction and relaxation and by contraction, respectively.

Infantile spasms are generalized seizures occurring in the first year of life. These are synchronous contractions of the muscles of the neck, trunk, and arms. About 90 percent of infants experiencing these attacks are mentally deficient.

Seizures may be further subdivided into epileptic (those involving recurrent seizures) and nonepileptic. The term "nonepileptic seizure," however, is somewhat problematic. For example, a seizure caused by hypoglycemia (low blood sugar) may not be considered an epileptic attack by some because it is a transient event easily corrected by metabolic manipulation. Of the organic nonepileptic seizures, the most common are of cardiovascular origin; others are caused by transient cerebral ischemia, movement disorders, toxic or metabolic problems, sleep disorders, and even headaches. Nonepileptic attacks may also be of nonorganic or psychiatric origin, such as with hysteria and schizophrenia, in which case they are called psychogenic seizures or pseudoseizures.

Attempts to find a cause for the sudden abnormal discharge of cerebral neurons has not been possible in all types of seizure activity. In some cases, a brain tumor, scar tissue remaining from trauma to the brain, or a progressive neurological disease may be responsible. In the great majority of cases, however, no pathologic basis for the seizures is evident, either during life or at autopsy. The latter type of seizure has been classified as "idiopathic." In certain circumstances, for example, fever, infection, or hyperglycemia, the response may include seizure. In many instances, these events are isolated and do not recur, and for this reason they are not categorized as epilepsy.

The cause of a seizure is related to the age of onset of the first attack. When seizures begin in the neonatal and infant period, the most likely causes are perinatal anoxia (a deficiency of oxygen), congenital brain defects, meningitis, birth injuries, or other metabolic problems, such as hypoglycemia or hypercalcemia (excessive calcium). Less common causes of seizures in young children include toxins such as lead poisoning, as well as rare degenerative diseases. In older children or adults, although metabolic or degenerative processes must be considered, other causes become more probable.

Head trauma accounts for the origin of many partial epileptic seizures in young adults, whereas brain tumors and vascular diseases are the major cause of such seizures in later life. Brain tumor is not a common cause of epilepsy in children, since 60 to 70 percent of brain tumors in children are located in the posterior fossa. Arteriosclerotic cerebrovascular disease is the most common cause of seizures in patients over the age of fifty. In about 4 percent of patients with brain infarction and 10 percent of those with intracerebral hemorrhage, seizures accompany the stroke; an additional 3 percent of patients who experience a stroke have recurrent seizures in later life, presumably generated by the cerebral scar.

Most idiopathic seizure activity appears to have its origin in an inherited propensity to cerebral dysrhythmia. Although there is a high incidence of electroencephalographic (EEG) abnormalities in close relatives of persons with recurrent seizures, not all family members have clinical seizures. In general, genetic factors are particularly important when recurrent seizures begin in childhood and decrease in importance with age.

In most studies of early seizures predicting future epilepsy, the conditions that are associated with high risk include a depressed skull fracture, an acute intracerebral hematoma, post-traumatic amnesia lasting more than twenty-four hours, and the presence of tears in the dura mater of the brain or focal neurologic signs.

Generalized tonic-clonic seizures sometimes develop during the course of chronic intoxication with alcohol or barbiturates, almost always in association with withdrawal or reduction of the drugs. How long a period of chronic drug intoxication or abuse must last to produce seizures upon withdrawal is uncertain, but such patients often give a history of many years (sometimes decades) of drug dependence. Usually, the patients experience one or more seizures or short bursts of two to six seizures over a period of hours. An episode of alcohol withdrawal rarely precipitates more than a single burst of convulsions, while convulsions may recur for several days after barbiturate withdrawal. Studies have shown that among those who have had withdrawal seizures without other evidence of neurological damage, seizures almost always occurred during the seven-hour to forty-eight-hour period following cessation of drinking. With alcohol withdrawal seizures, tremor, anorexia, and insomnia follow the seizure in perhaps 20 to 30 percent of cases. Delirium tremens is a less frequent event.

Treatment and Therapy

Prior to treatment, it is necessary for the physician to conduct a thorough investigation of the patient to identify any remediable cause of the seizures. This investigation would include metabolic diseases, endocrine system disturbances, cerebral tumors, abscess of the brain, or meningitis.

Persons who have recurrent convulsions controlled by medications can participate in sports and lead a relatively normal life; most countries will permit a person to drive an automobile if he or she has experienced no seizures for six months to one year. If seizures are uncontrolled, however, then automobile driving, swimming, the operation of unguarded machinery, and ladder climbing are not advised.

Drug therapy varies with the type of seizure presented. In the case of recurrent seizures, it generally consists of at least two to four years of daily medication. Careful neurologic examinations every four to six months, monitoring of seizure frequency correlated with drug blood level, and serial EEGs about once a year are also required. If there is a change in seizure frequency despite adequate drug blood levels, if there are focal neurologic signs or signs of increased intracranial pressure, or if evidence of focal changes on EEGs develop, further evaluation, including a computed tomography (CT) scan, is necessary. A small brain tumor may not be apparent even on a CT scan at the time of the initial evaluation, particularly in a patient with adult-onset epilepsy or in an older child or adolescent with partial seizures without a documented specific cause.

Absence seizures present less urgency. The patient rarely seeks medical advice until repeated episodes have occurred. Early treatment and prevention or reduction of repeated seizures can be beneficial. The drugs of choice for absence epilepsy are ethosuximide or valproate sodium. Medication is generally discontinued after two to four seizure-free years, depending on the presence or absence of generalized tonic-clonic seizures and the results of the

EEGs. After the medication is discontinued, and after follow-up for fifteen to twenty-three years, there is about a 12 percent incidence of recurrence.

If the seizure process is strong enough to require more than one drug, multiple drug administration needs to be maintained. The aim of the treatment is to achieve the best possible seizure control with the least amount of side effects. This goal may necessitate a compromise in patients with resistant seizures; such patients may prefer having an occasional seizure to being continuously sedated or unsteady. This is particularly true with patients who experience partial seizures that are not excessively disruptive.

The side effects of drugs may cause impairment of liver function in susceptible individuals. Thus, periodic monitoring of the patient's complete blood count and platelet count is necessary, as are liver function tests. This monitoring is done more frequently at the onset of therapy or after an upward adjustment of dosage.

The selection of specific drugs to be used for the prevention and control of seizures depends on the type of seizure. The most commonly used drugs include phenytoin, carbamazepine, phenobarbital, primidone, ethosuximide, methsuximide, clonazepam, valproate sodium, and trimethadione.

The pharmacokinetics and side effects of these drugs in infants and children differ somewhat from those observed in older children and adults. Absorption, plasma-protein binding, and metabolism are subject to age-specific variations. Younger children usually require a higher dose per kilogram to maintain a therapeutic blood level than do adults. Some of the classic signs of toxicity to the medications that are seen in adults may not be obvious in children.

If the seizures are related to a lesion in the brain, neurosurgical treatment is indicated. Surgery is the obvious form of treatment for demonstrable structural lesions such as cysts lying in accessible areas of the cerebral hemispheres. In a more restricted sense, surgical therapy is considered in patients without a mass lesion when the seizures are unresponsive to drug treatment and the patient has a consistent, electrophysiologically demonstrable focus emanating from, for example, a scar. Specific surgical treatments vary from case to case.

Up to 80 percent of properly selected patients have been found to benefit to some extent from surgical removal of the focal lesion. In some cases of intractable seizures associated with behavior disorders and hemiplegia of childhood, removal of a damaged cerebral hemisphere has been found to control the intractable seizures and improve the behavior disorder without causing further neurological deficit.

Perspective and Prospects

In the twentieth century, major developments were made in diagnosis and therapy. In 1929, Hans Berger recorded the first human electroencephalogram. Descriptions of EEG patterns and their correlation with clinical absences, partial seizures, and generalized tonic-clonic seizures led to important developments in classification and treatment.

Special EEG recordings with activation techniques, depth recordings, and long-term recordings for patients with intractable seizures became available to aid in the diagnosis and medical management of patients and in the selection of candidates for possible neurosurgical treatment.

Prolonged EEG recording by telemetry (the transmission of data electronically to a distant location) and ambulatory monitoring became helpful in making a diagnosis in patients who have brief spells of uncertain type. Electrical activity at the time of the attack can be documented. Videotaping with split-screen EEG recording and patient observation allows excellent correlation between the clinical and EEG manifestations, which aids in the classification and determination of appropriate therapy in difficult clinical problems. In those patients with intractable epilepsy, prolonged recording can document the frequency of seizures and correlation with anticonvulsive drug blood levels.

Radiological advances and CT scans in the 1970s, and later positron emission tomography (PET) scans, improved diagnostic skill in delineating potentially remediable lesions in patients with seizures.

During the twentieth century, many other medications became available for patients with seizures. The use of the operating microscope and technical advances in microsurgical techniques refined surgical treatments and improved the outlook for patients with structural lesions such as brain tumors, vascular malformations, and scars.

—*Genevieve Slomski, Ph.D.*

See also Addiction; Alcoholism; Arteriosclerosis; Batten's disease; Bites and stings; Brain; Brain damage; Brain disorders; Brain tumors; Electroencephalography (EEG); Epilepsy; Hallucinations; Head and neck disorders; Headaches; Hypoglycemia; Ischemia; Lead poisoning; Neuralgia, neuritis, and neuropathy; Neuroimaging; Neurology; Neurology, pediatric; Preeclampsia and eclampsia; Rabies; Schizophrenia; Sleep disorders; Snakebites; Strokes; Tetanus; Transient ischemic attacks (TIAs); Tumors.

For Further Information:

Bloom, Floyd E., M. Flint Beal, and David J. Kupfer, eds. *The Dana Guide to Brain Health*. New York: Dana Press, 2006. An easy-to-understand health guide to the brain from neuroscience, neurology, and psychiatry perspectives. More than seventy psychiatric and neurological disorders, their diagnoses, and their treatments are covered.

Delanty, Norman, ed. *Seizures: Medical Causes and Management*. Totowa, N.J.: Humana Press, 2002. Designed for health care personnel. Reviews seizures caused by fever and systemic infection, medications, alcohol or drugs, and environmental toxins.

Freeman, John M., Eileen P. G. Vining, and Diana J. Pillas. *Seizures and Epilepsy in Childhood: A Guide*. 3d ed. Baltimore: Johns Hopkins University Press, 2002. Designed for parents, an overall guide to the symptoms, diagnosis, and treatment of children with epilepsy. Third edition includes new chapters on alternative therapies and medicines, routine health care, insurance issues, and research resources.

Levy, René H., et al., eds. *Antiepileptic Drugs*. 5th ed. Philadelphia: Lippincott Williams & Wilkins, 2002. This useful work offers a quantitative analysis and interpretation of the drugs most often used in the treatment of recurrent seizures.

Rowan, A. James, and John R. Gates, eds. *Non-epileptic Seizures.* 2d ed. Boston: Butterworth-Heinemann, 2000. This book draws together a multidisciplinary perspective on knowledge of paroxysmal events that suggest a diagnosis of epilepsy but that are not of epileptic origin.

Solomon, Gail, Henn Kutt, and Fred Plum. *Clinical Management of Seizures.* 2d ed. Philadelphia: W. B. Saunders, 1983. Offers comprehensive treatment of seizures. After a brief historical perspective, the authors discuss the physiology, chemistry, and pharmacology of seizures; their classification; epidemiology and predisposing factors; treatment; and special management problems. Contains numerous charts, graphs, and illustrations.

Weaver, Donald F. *Epilepsy and Seizures: Everything You Need to Know.* Toronto, Ont.: Firefly Books, 2001. A lay guide covering research advances, history of the disease, different types, the mechanisms, diagnosis and treatment, and special situations, such as epilepsy in pregnant women, children, and the elderly.

Self-medication

Treatment

Also known as: Self-treatment, medications management

Anatomy or system affected: All

Specialties and related fields: All

Definition: Self-administration of drugs without the direction or supervision of a physician.

Key terms:

compliance: taking drugs as directed by a physician; completing therapeutic activities in proper fashion, as directed by a health care provider

drug interactions: the chemical effects of taking drugs in combination, where the effects will reduce, magnify, or alter the desired effects of the drug

illicit drugs: drugs that are illegal to possess, have addiction potential, and lack approved medical uses

over-the-counter drugs: pharmaceutical products, vitamins, herbal remedies, and other medicines that can be purchased by anyone, without a doctor's prescription

palliative care: care that decreases the suffering associated with health conditions by reducing the severity of symptoms, but does not provide a cure

prescription drugs: medicines that can be obtained only with the prescription of a doctor

Indications and Procedures

Every day, millions of people take medicinal drugs. Usually this is because they are experiencing symptoms, want to experience a particular feeling, or want to prevent a problem from developing and have information leading them to believe that the drug is the answer. For some, this occurs under the direction of a physician through the use of prescription medications. For others, this occurs through self-medication as a form of treatment. Most popularly, there are those who, through advertisements or personal experience, have learned that certain over-the-counter medications or popular legal drugs (such as cigarettes or alcohol) can be used to alleviate symptoms, provide palliative care, or cause certain symptoms or feelings. Others, via self-knowledge or guidance from alternative medicine specialists, will use teas, herbal remedies, and vitamins to achieve these same goals. Similarly, others may use illicit drugs to self-medicate in order to adjust their mood, physical feelings, or other abilities. For these individuals, it may

be that they have didactic knowledge about drug properties or have learned about drug effects through their experience with drugs. Relatedly, even those receiving prescribed drugs may abuse those drugs by using them in ways unapproved by their doctor. This may be due to judgments that they need more or less of the drug or need to mix it with something else to get the desired effect(s). Together, access to drugs, knowledge of dosages and drug effects, and having a culture that encourages use of medicinal remedies and drugs all contribute to self-medication.

Uses and Complications

Drug interactions can be a danger of self-medication. When individuals mix different medicines, legal drugs, or illegal drugs, there is a risk that they may cause themselves harm. Some drug interactions can cause medicinal drugs to be less effective for treating the condition needing attention. Others can lead to substantial discomfort or more serious conditions such as seizures or death. Similar problems can come from mixing certain medicinal substances and herbal remedies with each other or with certain foods. As such, anyone using self-medication as a treatment strategy should learn as much as possible about the drug(s) they are taking. Persons who self-medicate in addition to taking prescription drugs should inform their physicians of the nonprescription drugs they are taking.

Another problem of self-medication as a style of treatment is that unsupervised medical problems can often worsen without proper care. Using alcohol, cigarettes, or marijuana to alleviate conditions such as anxiety or depression may provide relief in the short term, but in the long term such use may worsen the mood problems and lead to substance abuse or dependence. Similarly, taking an antacid or laxative can be helpful for minor gastrointestinal problems, but prolonged use of such drugs can result in dangerous physical conditions not getting much-needed medical attention. Therefore, the limits of self-medication as a strategy must be known.

Perspective and Prospects

More than 30 percent of individuals living in the United States use an over-the-counter drug in any two-day period. It is estimated that 54 percent of three-year-olds receive over-the-counter drugs in any thirty-day period. Elderly adults use 25 percent of all over-the-counter drugs. Research also shows that 70 to 95 percent of all illnesses are managed without physician assistance. Additionally, over-the-counter drugs, herbal remedies, legal drugs, and illicit drugs constitute multibillion-dollar industries. Given these trends, self-medication as a treatment strategy is likely to continue. Increases can be expected as well because it is becoming easier to gain knowledge about how to use drugs safely. Furthermore, the practice of self-medication has the potential to decrease health care costs substantially by reducing the need for health care services, conserving valuable physician time.

The presence of self-medication as a positive force, however, must be balanced against problems such as a lack of compliance with medication regimens and the use of illicit and legal drugs to manage untreated mental and physical illnesses. When people do not take medicines as directed or fail to get proper medical treatment, problems can worsen. Work in the health care field therefore will need to address the longer-term problems that can develop as a result of these types of practices. Such investments may require increased time from service providers for purposes such as assessment and diagnosis, so as to uncover the hidden illnesses causing individuals to look for medicinal help in the first place. Additionally, barriers to treatment will have to be brought down so as to allow individuals who need medical and other health care to get the help they deserve.

—*Nancy A. Piotrowski, Ph.D.*

See also Addiction; Alcoholism; Alternative medicine; Antioxidants; Ergogenic aids; Herbal medicine; Internet medicine; Marijuana; Over-the-counter medications; Pain management; Palliative medicine; Pharmacology; Pharmacy; Prescription drug abuse; Side effects; Smoking; Substance abuse; Supplements; Vitamins and minerals; Weight loss medications.

For Further Information:

Chamberlain, Logan V. *What the Labels Won't Tell You: A Consumer's Guide to Herbal Supplements.* Loveland, Colo.: Interweave Press, 1998.

Gorman, Jack M. *The Essential Guide to Psychiatric Drugs.* 4th ed. New York: St. Martin's Press, 2007.

Graedon, Joe, and Teresa Graedon. *Dangerous Drug Interactions: How to Protect Yourself from Harmful Drug/Drug, Drug/Food, Drug/Vitamin Combinations.* Rev. ed. New York: St. Martin's Press, 1999.

Griffith, H. Winter. *Complete Guide to Prescription and Nonprescription Drugs.* Revised and updated by Stephen Moore. New York: Penguin Group, 2010.

Silverman, Harold M. *The Pill Book.* 13th ed. New York: Bantam Books, 2008.

Vandeputte, Charles. *Alcohol, Medications, and Older Adults: A Guide for Families and Other Caregivers.* St. Paul, Minn.: Johnson Institute, 1991.

Semen

Biology

Also known as: Ejaculate

Anatomy or system affected: Genitals, glands, reproductive system

Specialties and related fields: Urology

Definition: The fluid ejaculated by the male at orgasm, consisting of sperm and secretions from accessory glands.

Structure and Functions

Semen is released from the male reproductive system during ejaculation. It is a milky white, sticky fluid of 2 to 5 milliliters with an alkaline pH (7.2-7.8). It consists of spermatozoa (sperm) produced in the testes plus secretions of accessory glands: paired seminal vesicles that lie on the posterior surface of the bladder, the singular prostate gland that surrounds the urethra, and paired bulbourethral glands that lie just inferior to the prostate.

Sperm comprises only 5 percent of the semen, with 20 to 150 million sperm per milliliter. Seminal fluid contributes about 60 percent of the volume and contains high levels of fructose used by the sperm as an energy source. Seminal fluid also contains prostaglandins that stimulate smooth muscle contraction. This helps propel the semen through the urethra for release and aids in movement of sperm upward in the female reproductive tract. Two proteins, semenogelin I and II, inhibit sperm motility and protect the semen in the male urethra. The semenogelins cause the semen to form a temporary coagulate when deposited in the vagina. After fifteen to thirty minutes, the coagulum dissolves.

The prostate contributes about 30 percent of semen volume as a milky, slightly acidic fluid. It is high in citrate used as a nutrient by the sperm, plus several enzymes, including a protease called prostate-specific antigen (PSA). PSA hydrolyzes the semenogelins and helps to activate the motility of sperm. Prostatic fluid also contains seminalplasmin, an antibiotic active against *Escherichia coli (E. coli)* and several other bacteria that can cause urinary tract infections. The bulbourethral glands produce a thick, alkaline mucus that contributes only about 5 percent of semen volume. It is secreted in advance of ejaculation in order to neutralize any residual acidity from urine in the urethra. It also acts as a lubricant on the head of the penis to aid in vaginal penetration.

Disorders and Diseases

Disorders relating to semen involve pathologies of the individual glands. Infertility occurs in approximately 15 percent of males when there is a sperm count less than 20 million per milliliter, low sperm motility, or high levels of abnormal sperm. Decreased counts may be a result of testicular tumors, trauma, radiation, or infection with mumps virus. Infertility can also occur with autoimmunity when antibodies that bind to sperm are produced. Testicular cancer usually requires surgical removal of the testis. Semen can also transmit sexually transmitted infections, including human immunodeficiency virus (HIV).

Prostate hypertrophy, noncancerous enlargement of the prostate, occurs frequently in men over the age of fifty. It causes partial urethral obstruction, resulting in urinary hesitation, frequent urination, and possible painful urination. It may be treated with medication or corrected surgically. Prostate cancer occurs in one of every six men in their lifetime. Treatments include surgery, radiation, or hormonal therapy. Serum PSA increases in prostate cancer, and monitoring of PSA levels is important.

—*Ralph R. Meyer, Ph.D.*

See also Conception; Contraception; Erectile dysfunction; Genital disorders, male; Glands; Infertility, male; Masturbation; Men's health; Orchitis; Penile implant surgery; Prostate cancer; Prostate enlargement; Prostate gland; Prostate gland removal; Puberty and adolescence; Reproductive system; Sexual dysfunction; Sexuality; Sexually transmitted diseases (STDs); Sterilization; Testicles, undescended; Testicular cancer; Testicular surgery; Testicular torsion; Vas deferens; Vasectomy.

For Further Information:

Lilja, Hans, David Ulmert, and Andrew J. Vickers, "Prostate-Specific Antigen and Prostate Cancer: Prediction, Detection, and Monitoring." *Nature Reviews Cancer* 8 (2008): 268-278.

Marieb, Elaine N., and Katja Hoehn. *Human Anatomy and Physiology*. 8th ed. San Francisco: Pearson-Benjamin Cummings, 2009.
Poiani, Aldo. "Complexity of Seminal Fluid: A Review." *Behaviorial Ecology and Sociobiology* 60, no. 3 (2006): 289-310.

Sense organs

Anatomy

Anatomy or system affected: Ears, eyes, gastrointestinal system, mouth, nerves, nervous system, nose, skin

Specialties and related fields: Audiology, dentistry, dermatology, neurology, ophthalmology, optometry, otorhinolaryngology

Definition: Specialized structures anatomically suited to a particular sense-the eyes for vision, the nose for smell (olfaction), the taste buds for taste, the ears for hearing and balance, and the skin for such cutaneous sensations as warmth, cold, light touch, deep pressure, and pain.

Key terms:

chemoreception: sensitivity to chemical stimuli

cochlear: referring to the parts of the ear concerned with hearing

cutaneous: occurring within the skin

photoreception: sensitivity to light

retina: the light-sensitive part of the eye

stimulus: anything capable of producing a response

vestibular: referring to the parts of the ear concerned with balance

Structure and Functions

The sense organs of the body include the cutaneous sense organs, the organs of chemical reception, the organs of vision or sight, and the organs of hearing and balance. The skin is the major organ of sensation for touch, pressure, cold, warmth, and pain; the nasal epithelium and taste buds are the major organs of chemoreception; the eyes are the major organs of vision or sight; and the ears are the major organs of both hearing and balance.

There are five types of cutaneous receptors within the skin, each with a different type of sensory nerve ending and each with a different spatial pattern of distribution. Free (naked) nerve endings are sensitive to pain and are widely distributed over the body's skin surface, especially at the base of each hair. Overstimulation of any type of nerve ending also results in a sensation of pain, but these nerve endings are so exposed that any stimulation at all is felt as an overstimulation. All the remaining cutaneous receptors are encapsulated in one of several types of end organs. Of these, the end bulbs of Krause are sensitive to cold; they are most numerous around the conjunctiva of the eye and along the glans of the penis and the glans of the clitoris.

The Pacinian corpuscles each contain a single central nerve fiber, enclosed in many concentric layers of semitransparent tissue resembling the bulb of an onion. These structures, which are about 2 to 4 millimeters in diameter, are sensitive to deep pressure and are distributed throughout the skin, principally within the dermal papillae. They are most numerous on the palm of the hand, the sole of the foot, and the insides of many joints such as the front of the elbow or the back of the knee. The tactile (Meiss-

ner's) corpuscles each consist of an oval, bulblike swelling in which the nerve endings run around in spiral patterns at right angles to the long axis. Meissner's corpuscles are sensitive to light touch and are most numerous along the fingertips (and the hand in general), the tongue and lips, parts of the eye, and the skin of the mammary nipple or papilla. The corpuscles of Ruffini are enclosed in connective tissue sheaths perpendicular to the nerve that serves them. The axons of this nerve branch repeatedly within the corpuscle and these branches intertwine, each ending in a tiny knob. Corpuscles of Ruffini are sensitive to warmth and are very numerous over the fingertips, the forearm, and the skin of the face. The evidence to associate particular nerve endings with particular sensations (such as the Meissner's corpuscles with light touch) comes largely from patterns of spatial distribution: The areas of the body most sensitive to touch are also those with the highest densities of Meissner's corpuscles.

Neuromuscular spindles occur in most voluntary muscles and are sensitive to the state of contraction or relaxation of the muscle fibers. The spindle consists of a muscle fiber or small bundle of such fibers, around which are wrapped several turns of infrequently branching sensory nerve endings. The tendons of many muscles also frequently contain neurotendinous spindles, encapsulated structures in which a bundle of tendon fibers receive branched nerve endings. These nerve endings branch slightly just before reaching the tendon fibers but then lose their sheaths and branch profusely within the tendon. These neurotendinous spindles act as stretch receptors, sensitive to the state of stretching of the tendon.

Chemoreceptors of the body include those tissues sensitive to certain chemicals. The carotid body, a swelling within the carotid artery of the neck, contains tissue sensitive to the carbon dioxide or acid content of the blood; it stimulates the breathing reflex when the carbon dioxide level is too high. The taste buds of the tongue are sensitive to the taste of a variety of chemical substances present in moderate concentrations. Each taste bud contains gustatory cells along with nonsensitive supporting (sustentacular) cells. Experimental evidence points to four basic types of taste sensations: sweet (like sugar), bitter (like quinine), sour (like vinegar or citric acid), and salty (like sodium chloride). Sensitivity to each of these four basic tastes has its own characteristic pattern of distribution over the tongue and palate.

The nasal epithelium is responsible for olfaction, or smell, which is a sensitivity to chemical substances in much smaller concentrations. Most of the nasal epithelium is associated with the nose and the nasal passages, but a small part of this epithelium has become attached instead to the roof of the mouth, where it forms the vomeronasal (Jacobsohn's) organ, which "smells" the contents of the mouth (mostly food). The nasal epithelium is structurally unusual in that the cell bodies of the sensory cells originate within the epithelium and their nerve endings (axons) migrate inwardly to the brain, through the cribriform plate, forming the first cranial nerve or olfactory nerve. All other sensory nerves in the body grow outward from the central nervous system, and their cell bodies are located where their growth began.

Attempts have been made to classify smells according to a scheme similar to the bitter-sweet-sour-salty system used for tastes, but there are many more basic smells than there are tastes-lists vary from seven to twenty to more than ninety-and there is no general agreement on any of these schemes.

The eyes are the body's principal visual receptors. (Some evidence also exists of the brain's own ability to sense daily changes in the level of light intensity, especially in the pineal body.) The primary parts of the eye include the eyelids, cornea, lens, ciliary body, iris diaphragm, pupil, aqueous humor, vitreous humor, retina, choroid coat, scleroid coat, and optic nerve. The eyelids protect the front of the eye and prevent injury to the eye by closing. The cornea is the transparent covering of the front of the eye; the lens is the transparent, almost spherical body that focuses rays of incoming light onto the retina; and the ciliary body is a largely connective tissue structure (also containing some muscle tissue) that supports the lens. The colored part of the ciliary body is the iris diaphragm; muscle fibers within the iris diaphragm adjust the size of the pupil for different brightness levels of light. The opening in the middle of the iris diaphragm is called the pupil. The aqueous humor is the watery fluid in front of the lens, while the vitreous humor is the thick, jellylike fluid behind the lens.

The light-sensitive portion of the eye is the retina. It is almost spherical in shape and consists of two layers: a sensory layer on the inside (closer to the front) and a pigment layer surrounding and behind the sensory layer. Within the sensory layer are contained both the rods, which are sensitive to finer details, and the cones, which are sensitive to colors. The eye's most sensitive area is called the area centralis; it is centered upon a depression called the fovea. The choroid coat is the connective tissue layer immediately surrounding the retina, which is continuous with the pia mater that surrounds the brain. The scleroid coat is the stronger connective tissue layer that surrounds the choroid coat; it is continuous with the dura mater surrounding the brain. The optic nerve fibers originate from the sensory layer of the retina, where they converge toward a spot called the blind spot, marking the place where the nerve fibers turn inward toward the brain. A majority of the optic nerve fibers cross over to the opposite side of the brain via the optic chiasma, but a small proportion of the fibers remains on the same side without crossing over. Experiments on the physiology of vision have led researchers to conclude that there are three separate types of color receptors (cones) in the retina, sensitive principally to red, green, and blue regions of the spectrum. All other color sensations can be simulated experimentally in people with normal vision by a suitable combination of red, green, and blue stimuli.

The ears are special sense organs devoted to the two distinct functions of hearing and balance. The ear may be divided anatomically into outer, middle, and inner portions or functionally into a cochlear portion for hearing and a ves-

tibular portion for balance. The outer (external) ear consists of a flap called the pinna (or external ear flap) and a tube-like cavity called the external acoustic meatus. Within the external ear, sound impulses exist as waves of compressed or decompressed (rarefied) air, forming a series of longitudinal waves that vibrate in the same direction in which they are transmitted. The tympanic membrane (eardrum) is a vibrating membrane that marks the boundary between the outer and middle ears.

The middle ear consists of a cavity containing three tiny bones, the auditory ossicles. Within the middle ear, the vibrations of the tympanic membrane set up a series of vibrations within these tiny bones. The three auditory ossicles are called the malleus (hammer), incus (anvil), and stapes (stirrup). The malleus gets its name from its hammerlike shape, which includes a long handle (the manubrium) extending across the tympanic membrane. The incus, the second of the auditory ossicles, rests against the malleus at one end and the stapes at the other. The stapes is shaped like a stirrup, in which the foot is placed when riding a horse. The flat base of the stapes is called the footplate, in analogy to the corresponding part of a stirrup; this footplate rests against the fenestra ovalis of the inner ear. The opening in the stapes is penetrated by an artery called the stapedial artery. The cavity of the middle ear connects to the pharynx by means of a tube, the pharyngotympanic or Eustachian tube.

The inner ear is entirely housed within the petrosal bone. It can be divided into cochlear (hearing) and vestibular (balance) portions. The cochlear portion of the inner ear begins with two windows, the fenestra ovalis (oval window) and fenestra rotundum (round window), communicating between the middle ear and the inner ear. Behind the fenestra ovalis lies a vestibule, filled with a fluid called perilymph and extending into a long scala vestibuli. Behind the fenestra rotundum lies another long tube, the scala tympani, also filled with perilymph and running parallel to the scala vestibuli. Between these two tubes lies a third, the scala media or cochlear duct, filled with a different fluid called endolymph. Together, the three are prolonged into a spiral coil called the cochlea (Latin for "snail"), which has a bit more than three complete turns. At the end of this coil, the scala media ends, and the scala vestibuli and scala tympani join with one another by means of an intervening loop called the helicotrema. The basilar membrane separates the scala tympani and the cochlear duct. The spiral organ (organ of Corti) runs within the cochlear duct along the basilar membrane, not far beneath a tectorial membrane that is suspended within the cochlear duct.

The outer ear receives vibrations that travel through the air and transmits these vibrations to the tympanic membrane. In the middle ear, the vibrations of the tympanic membrane are transmitted through the malleus, incus, and stapes to the oval window. These vibrations are transmitted through the perilymph of the inner ear (vestibular portion), where they cause vibrations of the basilar membrane. The vibrating basilar membrane causes vibrations within the endolymph and also in the tectorial membrane, but the tectorial membrane is less flexible than the basilar membrane, creating regions of greater and lesser pressure within the endolymph. The hair cells of the spiral organ are sensitive to these pressure differences and send out nerve impulses to the brain, where they are interpreted as sounds.

The vestibular portion of the inner ear includes two interconnected chambers called the sacculus and the utriculus, both filled with endolymph. The sacculus has a downward extension called the lagena, and it also connects into the scala media of the cochlear portion of the ear. From the utriculus emerge three semicircular ducts, approximately at right angles to one another, all filled with endolymph: an anterior vertical duct, a posterior vertical duct, and a horizontal duct. Each semicircular duct runs through a bony semicircular canal, filled with perilymph. Each duct has a bulblike swelling, the ampulla, at one end. Each ampulla has a patch, or macula, of sensory structures called neuromasts, which are sensitive to movements in fluids such as endolymph. Other maculae, or patches of neuromasts, are located in the sacculus, the utriculus, and the lagena.

The vestibular portion of the inner ear is sensitive to movements and especially to acceleration. Normally, this acceleration is caused by gravity, but nonlinear movements (such as the swerving of a fast-moving vehicle around a curve) may also result in accelerations that cause fluid movements within the semicircular canals. These movements are perceived by the sensitive hair cells (neuromasts) within each ampulla. Spinning around or other sudden acceleration causes temporary dizziness (vertigo) and a consequent loss of balance.

Disorders and Diseases

Several types of medical specialists deal with problems of the various sense organs: Ophthalmologists deal with diseases of the eye; otorhinolaryngologists deal with diseases of the ears (oto-), nose (rhino-), and throat (larynx); and neurologists deal with all the senses. All these specialists first conduct diagnostic tests in order to detect any sensory malfunction and to determine the probable cause; they then provide whatever treatment may be available for each condition.

The ability to distinguish tastes diminishes gradually with age in older persons as the number of gustatory cells declines, but complete loss of taste is rare. Persons with diminished taste are at greater risk for accidental poisoning. Except for the decline of taste among the elderly, other defects of smell or taste are rare and are usually indicative of more serious neurological problems such as brain damage or nerve damage. The inability to smell is a rare condition known as anosmia. Loss of cutaneous sensations, even over a small portion of the body, is usually indicative of nerve damage.

Disorders of the eye range from easily correctable vision problems to total blindness. Impaired function of one or more of the three types of color receptors results in one of the several types of color blindness. The most common type, red-green color blindness, is inherited as a sex-linked recessive trait and is thus more common in men than in women. Blindness may result from various defects or injuries: A defective lens or cornea may limit vision to large objects, and a defective retina may limit perception to light and darkness only. Total blindness results if the optic nerve is damaged or missing. More common visual defects include myopia (nearsightedness), hyperopia (farsightedness), and astigmatism (differences in vision along different axes), all of which can be corrected with glasses or contact lenses or by surgical procedures. A failure of the mechanism that drains fluid from the interior of the eyeball may result in a buildup of ocular pressure, a condition known as glaucoma. In times past, when treatment for glaucoma was not readily available, most cases resulted in permanent blindness. Glaucoma can now be treated, however, either surgically or with drugs. Several changes occur to the lens of the eye in older individuals. As the lens becomes more rigid with advancing age, reading and other near-vision tasks become more difficult, a condition known as presbyopia. Also frequent among older people are cataracts, tiny opaque grains that cloud up the lens and reduce the ability to see clearly. Untreated cataracts may eventually result in blindness, but various forms of treatment are available to prevent this from occurring.

Diseases of the ear should always be treated as serious. Tinnitus, or ringing in the ears, can result from damage to the hair cells of the organ of Corti. Damage to the auditory nerve can result in deafness. Upper respiratory infections can travel up the Eustachian tube and cause a common childhood infection of the middle ear known as otitis media. Infections of the vestibular portion of the inner ear can result in recurrent or permanent dizziness (vertigo) because the inflamed cells transmit impulses that the body wrongly interprets as resulting from accelerations in unusual directions. Some plant poisons (or the drugs derived from them, such as ipecac) can also impair the function of the inner ear and result in sensations of dizziness, often followed by nausea and by the vomiting of the plant containing the poison. This reaction may have evolved as an adaptive response to possible poisons; the same reaction also results in vomiting in other situations that cause unusual accelerations in the vestibular portion of the inner ear, as in the case of seasickness or other motion sickness.

Perspective and Prospects

The many biblical references to deafness and blindness show that ancient civilizations were concerned about the proper functioning of the sense organs. The Greek philosopher Aristotle, also considered the greatest biologist of antiquity, enumerated five senses: touch, hearing, taste, smell, and sight. Detailed anatomical descriptions of the sense organs were made during the Renaissance by Bartolommeo Eustachio (or Eustachius) (1520-1574), after whom the Eustachian tube is named; by Giulio Casserio (1552?-1616); and by Andreas Vesalius (1514-1564), whose superbly illustrated texts set new standards for art as well as science. Further discoveries were made by such anatomists as Alfonso Corti (1822-1876), who first described the detailed internal structure of the inner ear. The detailed cellular structure of the retina was first elucidated by the Nobel Prize-winning anatomist and histologist Santiago Ramón y Cajal (1852-1934). Other anatomists who expanded the understanding of the microscopic anatomy of sensory structures include Abraham Vater (1684-1751), Filippo Pacini (1812-1883), Georg Meissner (1829-1905), and Jan Evangelista Purkinje (1787-1869).

—*Eli C. Minkoff, Ph.D.*

See also Appetite loss; Aromatherapy; Astigmatism; Audiology; Cataract surgery; Cataracts; Deafness; Dermatology; Ear surgery; Ears; Earwax; Eye surgery; Eyes; Hearing; Hearing loss; Microscopy, slitlamp; Myopia; Nasal polyp removal; Nasopharyngeal disorders; Nervous system; Numbness and tingling; Ophthalmology; Optometry; Otorhinolaryngology; Skin; Skin disorders; Smell; Synesthia; Systems and organs; Taste; Tinnitus; Touch; Vision; Vision disorders.

For Further Information:

Agur, Anne M. R., and Arthur F. Dalley. *Grant's Atlas of Anatomy.* 12th ed. Philadelphia: Wolters Kluwer Health/Lippincott Williams & Wilkins, 2009. This text contains many excellent, detailed illustrations.

Ferrari, Mario. *PDxMD Ear, Nose, and Throat Disorders.* Philadelphia: PDxMD, 2003. A clinical yet accessible reference text that provides a comprehensive list of disorders, with a summary of the condition, background, diagnosis, treatment, outcomes, prevention, and resources.

Møller, Aage R. *Sensory Systems: Anatomy, Physiology, and Pathophysiology.* Boston: Academic Press, 2003. An excellent text that describes how human sensory systems function, with comparisons of the five senses and detailed descriptions of the functions of each of them. Also covers how sensory information is processed in the brain to provide the basis for communication and for the perception of one's surroundings.

Riordan-Eva, Paul, and John P. Whitcher. *Vaughan and Asbury's General Ophthalmology.* 17th ed. New York: Lange Medical Books/McGraw-Hill, 2007. A clinical text that provides a range of information about the eye.

Rosse, Cornelius, and Penelope Gaddum-Rosse. *Hollinshead's Textbook of Anatomy.* 5th ed. Philadelphia: Lippincott-Raven, 1997. A very thorough, modern, detailed reference with good descriptions and illustrations.

Standring, Susan, et al., eds. *Gray's Anatomy.* 40th ed. New York: Churchill Livingstone/Elsevier, 2008. A great classic with the most thorough descriptions. The excellent color illustrations offer realistic detail in most cases and well-selected highlights in a few cases.

Sutton, Amy L., ed. *Eye Care Sourcebook: Basic Consumer Health Information About Eye Care and Eye Disorders.* 3d ed. Detroit, Mich.: Omnigraphics, 2008. A complete guide to eye care that includes such topics as eye anatomy, preventive vision care, refractive disorders and eye diseases, current research and clinical trials, and a list of organizations.

Wertenbaker, Lael T. *The Eye: Window to the World.* Reprint. New York: Scribner, 1984. Easy to read and understand, with good illustrations. Written for a popular audience.

Separation anxiety

Development

Anatomy or system affected: Psychic-emotional system

Specialties and related fields: Psychiatry, psychology

Definition: Common distress shown at the departure of a caregiver when a child is between ten to eighteen months of age and which may extend throughout the preschool years.

Physical and Psychological Factors

Infants are often wary or even fearful when someone other than the usual caregiver approaches them or tries to touch or carry them. This may be partly attributable to anticipation of separation. Furthermore, in the second year of life, negative reactions to strangers may compound toddlers' concerns about separation from the caregiver.

Self-initiated separations and those that are brief, in familiar settings, and explained by the departing caregiver are less likely to elicit distress. Factors that do not seem to be related to separation distress are gender, birth order, and experience within the normal range for a given culture and economic class. Usually, separation anxiety subsides by about three years of age.

Disorders and Effects

Researchers used to think that the intensity of separation distress was an index of the strength of the attachment bond. However, the child's reaction during reunion with the caregiver is a better indicator of the security of attachment.

Child psychiatrists have described an uncommon disorder (with a prevalence of 4 percent) called separation anxiety disorder. This disorder must be distinguished from many other types of disorders that children may have. Because a child is anxious does not mean that separation anxiety disorder is present. The disorder may develop in early childhood for no apparent reason or may develop after a life stress such as the death of a relative or a change in school or neighborhood. Children with this disorder show excessive anxiety about separation from the caregiver or home that is more characteristic of younger children and therefore developmentally inappropriate. Separation anxiety disorder is typically long-lasting and causes significant disruption to functioning, such as school avoidance, excessive worry about losing caregivers, and fear of being left alone.

A relationship may exist between very strong and long-lasting separation anxiety as an infant and separation anxiety disorder in later life, but infant distress about separation is very common, almost universal, and is usually relatively short-lived. Thus, there is usually little reason to be concerned about separation anxiety in infancy.

—*George A. Morgan, Ph.D.,*
and Robert J. Harmon, M.D.;
updated by Nancy A. Piotrowski, Ph.D.

See also Anxiety; Bonding; Developmental stages; Emotions: Biomedical causes and effects; Phobias; Psychiatry, child and adolescent.

For Further Information:

Berk, Laura E. *Child Development.* 8th ed. Boston: Pearson/Allyn & Bacon, 2009.

Caplan, Theresa. *The First Twelve Months of Life: Your Baby's Growth Month by Month.* New York: Bantam, 1995.

Craig, Grace J., Marguerite D. Kermis, and Nancy Digdon. *Children Today.* 2d ed. Toronto, Ont.: Prentice Hall, 2002.

Leach, Penelope. *Your Baby and Child: From Birth to Age Five.* London: Dorling Kindersley, 2003.

Mooney, Carol Garhart. *Theories of Childhood: An Introduction to Dewey, Montessori, Erikson, Piaget, and Vygotsky.* St. Paul, Minn.: Redleaf Press, 2000.

Septicemia

Disease/Disorder
Also known as: Blood poisoning, bacteremia
Anatomy or system affected: Blood, circulatory system
Specialties and related fields: Hematology, internal medicine, serology
Definition: Serious, systemic infection of the blood with pathogens that have spread from an infection in a part of the body, characteristically causing fever, chills, prostration, pain, headache, nausea, and/or diarrhea.

Key terms:

antibacterial therapy: treatment for patients with septicemia, best initiated with a combination of antibiotics when the infecting organism is unknown; when cultures define the causative microbe(s) or other data point to a specific organism, therapy can be tailored to the most appropriate, most specific, least toxic, and least expensive single antibiotic

bacteremia: also known as blood poisoning or septicemia; the rapid multiplication of bacteria and the presence of their toxins in the blood, a serious, life-threatening condition

bacteria: microorganisms with a wide variety of biochemical, often pathogenic, properties

septic shock: a dangerous condition in which there is tissue damage and a dramatic drop in blood pressure as a result of septicemia

shock treatment: the immediate treatment of septic shock, including the use of antibiotics and surgery and rapid fluid replacement by infusion

Causes and Symptoms

The rapid multiplication of bacteria and the presence of their toxins in the blood is a condition commonly known as blood poisoning, septicemia, or bacteremia. It is always a serious condition and represents a medical emergency that requires the prompt institution of therapy. A person in whom septicemia develops suddenly becomes seriously ill, with a high fever, chills, rapid breathing, headache, and often clouding of consciousness. Skin rashes or jaundice may occur, and sometimes the hands are unusually warm. In many cases, especially when large amounts of toxins are produced by the circulating bacteria, the person passes into a state of septic shock, which is life-threatening.

Bacteria in the bloodstream can produce two different types of complications: microbiologic and inflammatory. The microbiologic complications result from the local and systemic proliferation and seeding of the bacterial causative organism, which causes direct tissue or organ damage. The inflammatory complications are produced locally and can result in tissue or organ destruction independent of the toxic factors produced by the causative organism. Bacteremia triggers intravascular activation of the same inflammatory systems that are protective within tissues. These systems, which combine with stress-generated endocrine responses, produce a sequence of metabolic events, the end stage of which is the systemic vascular collapse traditionally called septic shock.

Shock symptoms vary with the extent and site of major

Information on Septicemia

Causes: Systemic bacterial infection
Symptoms: Fever, chills, pain, headache, nausea, rapid breathing, clouding of consciousness, rashes, jaundice, diarrhea
Duration: Acute
Treatments: Antibiotics (penicillin, chloramphenicol, ampicillin, neomycin); surgery (debridement, drainage); fluid replacement; oxygen therapy

tissue damage. They are similar to those for septicemia, with additional symptoms including cold hands and feet, often with blue-purple coloration caused by poor blood flow; a weak, rapid pulse; and markedly reduced blood pressure. There may be vomiting and diarrhea, and a poor output of urine may indicate that damage to the kidneys is occurring and that there is risk of renal failure. Heart failure and abnormal bleeding may also occur.

Septic shock is a dangerous condition in which there is tissue damage and a dramatic drop in blood pressure as a result of septicemia. Septic shock is usually preceded by signs of severe infection, often of the genitourinary or gastrointestinal systems. Fever, tachycardia, increased respiration, and confusion or coma may occur during shock. The classic septic shock syndrome results primarily from the sequence of events triggered by bacteremia, during which the bacterial toxins activate compounds that impair the functioning of surrounding cells in several ways. In many cases, the bacterial toxins are the main cause of trouble because they can cause damage to cells and tissues throughout the body and promote clotting of blood in the smallest blood vessels, seriously interfering with circulation. Consequently, damage occurs especially to tissues in the kidneys, heart, and lungs. The bacterial toxins may cause leakage of fluid from blood vessels and a reduction of the ability of the vessels to constrict, leading to a severe drop in blood pressure. Therefore, septic shock is a systematic vascular collapse, in which the systolic blood pressure of the patient is less than 90 millimeters of mercury. In septic shock, the low blood pressure has become unresponsive to adequate volume replacement. Morbidity and mortality associated with septic shock are high: About two-thirds of patients die.

Septicemia and septic shock can precipitate multiple organ failure. As the patient becomes hypermetabolic and febrile with progressive failure of one or more organs, the mortality rate can be as high as 90 percent. Septicemia is most common in people hospitalized with major disorders such as diabetes mellitus, cancer, or cirrhosis and who have a focus of infection somewhere in the body (often the intestines or urinary tract). Progression to septic shock is especially likely for people who have immunodeficiency disorders or are taking immunosuppressant drugs for cancer or an inappropriate antibiotic treatment. Newborn infants are also particularly at risk if septicemia develops.

Treatment and Therapy

A presumptive diagnosis of septicemia is often made on the basis of historical, physical, and laboratory data even in the absence of proof. The setting in which the episode is occurring should be evaluated promptly. Crucial to appropriate initial decision making are the background history, which may help to define the type of host-defense defect present, and prior blood culture data, which might predict the infecting organism. The physical examination should be quick and thorough, searching for the septic source as well as signs that might indicate progression to shock.

A diagnosis can be confirmed and the infective bacteria identified by growing a culture of the organisms from a blood sample. Several laboratory tests are often helpful in the evaluation of a potentially septic patient. In general, patients with fever should be considered septic until proved otherwise, and therapy should always be initiated for high-risk febrile patients in advance of a microbiologic confirmation of septicemia.

Common microorganisms that enter the bloodstream when the body's defenses break down include staphylococci from boils, abscesses, and wounds; streptococci from the tonsils, throat, or cuts; and pneumococci from the lungs. Other invaders of the bloodstream include the gonococci, the typhoid bacilli in typhoid fever, and *Escherichia coli (E. coli)* in bowel infections. All these bacteria may be detected by taking a blood culture.

Antibacterial therapy should be started as soon as septicemia is suspected. It is normally started by intravenous infusion of antibiotic drugs and glucose and/or saline solution. The focal site of infection is sought immediately and may be surgically removed. Surgical debridement (removal) and drainage of septic foci are especially important, and all severe localized infections should be widely debrided and drained. If the infection is recognized and treated promptly, there is usually a full recovery.

Broad antibacterial coverage is required in patients with severe septicemia. It is best to initiate therapy with a combination of antibiotics when the infecting organism is unknown. When cultures define the causative microbe(s) or other data point to a specific organism, therapy can then be tailored to the most appropriate, most specific, least toxic, and least expensive single antibiotic. Penicillin is usually used to combat staphylococcic, streptococcic, pneumococcic, and gonococcic infections; chloramphenicol and ampicillin are used against typhoid and paratyphoid infections; and neomycin is used against *E. coli* infections. Extreme care must be taken with the administration of chloramphenicol and neomycin because of their toxic side effects.

Antibiotics limit the microbiological complications of bacteremia, but other metabolic events, whether initiated by or independent of bacterial proliferation, may still produce substantial morbidity and mortality. Therefore, therapy in addition to antibiotics is recommended to counter this metabolic sequence.

Septic shock requires immediate treatment, including the use of antibiotics and surgery, rapid fluid replacement by infusion, and the maintenance of urine flow to prevent the effects of renal failure. Other measures must also be taken to raise the blood pressure and to promote a better supply of important nutrients to tissues, such as through intravenous infusion and oxygen therapy. The use of anti-inflammatory drugs is under active investigation.

Perspective and Prospects

Most febrile patients lacking other signs of severe septicemia will usually do well. Such patients usually respond quickly to fluid administration, antibacterial therapy, and drainage of the primary focus of infection. The presence of septic shock, however, dramatically increases morbidity and mortality. Even when the inciting infection is localized, shock is associated with at least 50 percent mortality. Full-blown septic shock has greater than 70 percent mortality. A favorable outcome in a patient in severe shock depends on the skill of management in the intensive care unit. Early diagnosis and therapy of severely septic patients will greatly decrease the morbidity and mortality of these individuals. The best means of preventing bacteremia is the proper care of burns and wounds and prompt application of antiseptic tinctures or preparations to ordinary cuts and tears.

Infections most commonly occur in the hospital setting, where many infected patients become bacteremic. About 5 percent of all hospital patients either are admitted with or develop an infection during hospitalization. This means that the number of patients at risk of developing septic shock is large. The clinician must be familiar with the manifestations and differential diagnosis of the patient who appears to suffer from septic shock and must have in mind rapid, comprehensive diagnostic and therapeutic plans of action. It is important to develop the concept of a preshock phase of septic shock predicated on identifying a subgroup of infected patients more likely than others to develop shock. In such patients, fluids should be administered and broad antibiotic coverage started early. Treatment before shock develops undoubtedly prevents some of the morbidity and mortality associated with septicemia.

—*Maria Pacheco, Ph.D.*

See also Antibiotics; Bacterial infections; Bacteriology; *E. coli* infection; Infection; Poisoning; Shock; Staphylococcal infections; Streptococcal infections; Typhoid fever; Toxicology.

For Further Information:

Goldman, Lee, and Dennis Ausiello, eds. *Cecil Textbook of Medicine*. 23d ed. Philadelphia: Saunders/Elsevier, 2007. An excellent, concise presentation of the topic. It is recommended that the reader have a good science background, especially in biology.

Litin, Scott C., ed. *Mayo Clinic Family Health Book*. 4th ed. New York: HarperResource, 2009. Good presentation of blood; concentrates on illnesses, both causes and treatments.

Mosby's Medical Dictionary. 8th ed. St. Louis, Mo.: Mosby/Elsevier, 2009. Offers a basic presentation of medical terms and concepts.

Rodak, Bernadette, ed. *Hematology: Clinical Principles and Applications*. 3d ed. St. Louis, Mo.: Saunders/Elsevier, 2007. A comprehensive textbook covering all aspects of hematology and hemostasis.

Strand, Calvin L., and Jonas A. Shulman. *Bloodstream Infections: Laboratory Detection and Clinical Considerations*. Chicago: American Society of Clinical Pathologists, 1988. A technical monograph reviewing the concepts and factors important in the selection and development of optimal blood culture systems for the detection of septicemia.

Wilson, Michael, Brian Henderson, and Rod McNab. *Bacterial Disease Mechanisms: An Introduction to Cellular Microbiology*. New York: Cambridge University Press, 2002. Basing their discussion on research advances in microbiology, molecular biology, and cell biology, the authors describe the interactions that exist between bacteria and human cells both in health and during infection.

Zucker-Franklin, D., et al. *Atlas of Blood Cells: Function and Pathology*. 3d ed. Philadelphia: Lea & Febiger, 2003. Great pictorial presentation of blood components in different stages of function and disease.

Serology

Specialty

Anatomy or system affected: Blood, immune system

Specialties and related fields: Bacteriology, cytology, hematology, immunology, microbiology, oncology, pathology, preventive medicine, public health, virology

Definition: The study of serum, the liquid portion of blood, the testing of which is used in blood typing, vaccination, diagnosis, and therapy.

Key terms:

antibody: a protein substance produced by lymphocytes in response to an antigen in order to combat bacterial, viral, chemical, or other invasive agents in the body

antigen: a chemical substance often on a bacterial or viral surface, containing antigenic determinants that initiate the body's immune response

antigenic determinant: a molecule on the surface of a cell or microorganism that is specific for evoking an immune response

bacteria: microscopic single-celled organisms that exist throughout the environment

host: the body of the person or animal infected

immunoglobulin: antibody; the globulin fraction of serum protein

microorganism: any bacterium, virus, or other minute organism; some are harmless in the body or are involved in essential body processes, while others are harmful and cause disease

pathogen: any disease-causing microorganism, such as bacteria, viruses, yeasts, fungi, and spirochetes

seronegative: the test result seen when blood does not contain the specific antibody or antigen being sought and the particular antigen-antibody reaction is not present

seropositive: the test result seen when blood contains the specific antibody or antigen being sought and the particular antigen-antibody reaction is present

Science and Profession

The term "serology" comes from the Latin *sero* (serum, a blood liquid) and *ology* (the study of). Many serologic testing procedures have been developed to determine the amounts of specific antibodies the individual has circulating in his or her bloodstream. These tests can help the physician diagnose disease conditions and develop appropriate treatment regimens. To understand serological testing in relation to blood typing and immunity-two major uses of serology-it is necessary to understand the structure and nature of blood cells and the workings of the human immune system.

The surface of red blood cells contains antigenic determinants that define the individual's blood group. There are more than twenty blood grouping systems; the most common, the ABO system, identifies individuals as being in A, B, AB, or O groups, depending on the antigenic determinant present on their red blood cells. The red blood cells of people in the A group are covered with A antigen, in the B group with B antigen, and in the AB group with both antigens. Red blood cells in the O group have neither A nor B antigens. The antigenic determinant causes the body to produce antibodies against other blood types. For example, if an individual's red blood cells are coated with A antigen, the body will produce antibodies against B antigen. Therefore, if a person with A blood is given B blood cells, these cells will be regarded as foreign, and the body's anti-B antibodies will dissolve them, leading to a severe, life-threatening hemolytic reaction.

All the blood groups in the ABO system are also classified as either negative or positive for Rh factor, another antigen found on the red blood cells, and so named because a similar antigen was first found in rhesus monkeys. About 85 percent of the population is Rh positive; that is, these individuals have Rh antigens on their red blood cells. If an Rh-negative person is given Rh-positive blood, he or she may tolerate the first transfusion, but a severe, even fatal, reaction can occur if a second is given. Furthermore, if an Rh-negative woman becomes pregnant with an Rh-positive baby, she may be exposed to Rh-positive red blood cells and may develop anti-Rh antibodies. This reaction may be of no significance for the first baby, but if a subsequent baby is also Rh-positive, the mother's antibodies will attack and dissolve the red blood cells of the fetus and may cause intrauterine anemia, heart failure, or miscarriage.

As on the red blood cells, there are antigenic determinants on the surfaces of invading microorganisms that trigger the body's immune process: When a virus, bacterium, or other infective agent enters the body, the immune system recognizes the invader as foreign. Once the organism is recognized as an enemy, the body begins to respond with the host-defense mechanism, an intricate process that not only destroys the offending pathogen but also protects against future infection by it.

Two factors determine whether an organism is antigenic and thus will trigger the immune response. First, there must be antigenic determinants present on the organism's surface that the body identifies as foreign, or nonself. Second, the organism must be large enough to carry antigenic determinants on its surface. Antigenic determinants are large molecules; the more there are on the organism's surface, the greater the antigenicity.

Antigens induce the production of certain white blood cells called lymphocytes. There are two basic types of lymphocytes involved in the immune process. One is the T cell, which originates in the bone marrow and travels to the thymus gland, where it becomes specialized for its immune function. The other lymphocyte is the B cell, which originates in the bone marrow and develops fully in the lymph system. T cells and B cells each develop into cells specialized for specific tasks in the immune process.

About 70 percent of T cells become helper-inducer cells, which have various functions. They promote the production of B cells, support B-cell activity, and increase the production of macrophages (cells that destroy foreign substances and dead cells). They also become "memory cells" capable of recognizing a pathogen to which the body has been exposed. If the particular pathogen reenters the body, the memory cells trigger the immune system to synthesize antibodies against it. T cells also become "killer" T cells that attack pathogens directly.

B cells produce the antibodies that are detected in seropositive blood tests. Antibodies, also called immunoglobulins, are rings, chains, or Y-shaped proteins that are carried in blood plasma. There are five groups of immunoglobulins involved in the immune system: IgG, IgA, IgM, IgD, and IgE. IgG makes up about 80 percent of all immunoglobulins and is found in tissue fluid and plasma. Its major function is to combat bacteria and viruses and to neutralize poisonous substances. IgA (13 percent) is found in the secretions of seromucous glands in the nose, gastrointestinal tract, eyes, and lungs. It also combats bacteria and viruses. IgM (6 percent) is found in blood plasma. It reacts with antigens during the first exposure to the disease organism. IgD (less than 1 percent) is found on the surface of most B cells. Its activities are not fully understood, but it is thought to be involved in the production of antibodies. IgE (less than 1 percent) is bound to mast cells found in connective tissue. It promotes allergic reactions.

Antibodies work in two ways-by direct attack on an antigen and by activating a protein complex called a complement. In direct attack, there are four ways in which antibodies destroy antigens: agglutination, which causes antigens to clump together; precipitation, which causes antigens to form insoluble substances; neutralization, which prevents antigens from producing toxic substances; and lysis, which causes the cell walls of antigens to rupture.

The activation of a complement causes three main activities: chemotaxis, which attracts macrophages and other white blood cells to the area, where they can eliminate the pathogens that are present; opsonization, which alters the structure of the antigen cell wall, making it easier for macrophages to engulf and destroy it; and inflammation, a process that helps to prevent the spread of pathogens.

Like T cells, some B cells become memory cells that help prevent reinfection by recognizing and destroying a pathogen that they have previously encountered.

Diagnostic and Treatment Techniques

The major use for seronegative-seropositive testing is in blood typing. The patient's blood type is recorded as part of his or her medical history and is required for a blood transfusion to ensure that the patient receives blood from a compatible donor. Blood typing is an activity conducted in, or

readily available to, virtually every medical facility. A major example is the Coomb's test, which detects antibodies on red blood cells in the bloodstream and establishes whether the patient has sensitized cells. This information is helpful in cross-matching donor and patient blood and in the diagnosis of hemolytic anemia.

Another important aspect of serologic testing is to determine the immune status of an individual-that is, whether a person or a local population is immune to a specific disease or is susceptible and therefore should be vaccinated. Such tests are geared to the identification of antibodies that protect against certain diseases. These antibodies are created by exposure to the disease-causing microorganism as a result of infection by the organism itself; vaccination, in which a modified form of the microorganism is used to trigger the body's immune response; or immunity that is acquired by a newborn baby from a mother, an immune state that lasts only a few months. A test that comes back seronegative or with very low antibody levels indicates that the patient is not immune to a given disease. A test that comes back seropositive indicates that the patient has circulating antibodies characteristic of a specific disease and that, if the amount of antibodies is high enough, the patient is immune to the disease.

A good example of immune status determination is the testing for hepatitis B surface antigen among health care workers. Hepatitis B is a blood-borne disease that can be transmitted when infected blood or other body fluids enter the bloodstream of another person. Transmission often occurs among health care workers because they are often exposed to the blood and body fluids of patients during operating procedures, dental procedures, or even when the nurse or other health care worker draws blood and is inadvertently stuck with the needle. Tests show that health care workers are seropositive for hepatitis B surface antigen at rates far above the general population. For example, 25 percent of surgeons and dentists become seropositive after five to ten years in practice. These tests prove that some health care workers are at high risk for contracting hepatitis B from their patients. Therefore, routine vaccination is recommended for those health care workers who are likely to be exposed to the blood and body fluids of patients carrying the hepatitis B virus.

Seronegative-seropositive testing can also reveal whether a person who has been vaccinated against a certain disease has achieved immunity (has "seroconverted" and developed antibodies in response to the antigen), whether the individual has not achieved immunity, or whether the individual has achieved immunity and then lost it.

No vaccine is 100 percent effective, but the better ones induce an immune response in 90 to 98 percent of individuals. For example, measles vaccine is about 95 percent effective. This means that most of the children who have received it are immune to measles, but 5 percent or so remain susceptible.

A few vaccines produce lifelong immunity. With most, however, the amount of antibody diminishes after time, and the vaccination must be repeated to maintain immunity. In other words, the patient is given a "booster" shot. In the late 1980s, many children who had received measles vaccine and who had seroconverted were found to be seronegative: They had lost their immunity to measles. This finding suggested that the measles vaccine conveyed an immunity that could diminish with time. Therefore, medical authorities and public health organizations revised their recommendations for mass vaccination against measles. Instead of only one vaccination of the infant at twelve to fifteen months of age, the protocol now recommends repeating the vaccination at a later date.

Serologic tests are used in virtually all branches of medicine. One group of seronegative-seropositive tests is used to detect fetal abnormalities. Another group, autoantibody tests, detects such diseases as autoimmune hepatitis, thyroiditis, and systemic lupus erythematosus (SLE). One example is testing for rheumatoid factor, an antibody that appears in the blood of adult patients with rheumatoid arthritis. Its presence will help the physician make a diagnosis and determine a course of treatment for a patient with joint inflammation. Similarly, specific antibodies will indicate specific disease conditions. A patient with lupus has antinuclear antibody (ANA). Rheumatic fever diagnosis requires evidence of the bacteria *Streptococcus pyogenes*. Syphilis patients have antibodies to the spirochete *Treponema pallidum*. Patients with mononucleosis are seropositive for heterophile antibodies.

Viral, bacterial, and fungal tests detect antibodies or antigens developed in response to infection. These include the antistreptolysin-O test for streptococcal antibodies, the febrile agglutination test to detect diseases caused by salmonella, and the latex particle agglutination (LPA) tests for antigens of other bacteria. Also in this group are the hepatitis-B surface and core antigen tests, which are used to screen blood donors as well as to identify persons who have been exposed to hepatitis B. Fungal serology tests are used to detect various fungal infections. The fluorescent treponemal antibody absorption test is used to diagnose syphilis.

Serologic tests called general humoral tests are used to detect and diagnose various bodily dysfunctions. Another group called the general cellular tests includes the lymphocyte transformation test to determine whether transplant donors and recipients are compatible. In this group, the terminal deoxynucleotidyl transferase test is used to diagnose leukemias and lymphomas, as well as to monitor the progress of treatment. In cancer therapy, the carcinoembryonic antigen test (CEA) is used to gauge the response of certain cancers to treatment or to detect the recurrence of certain cancers.

A major new field for serology is emerging with monoclonal antibody research. In this science, antibodies can be manufactured in the laboratory. Instead of injecting a patient with modified antigen and inducing the body to create antibodies to it (as in vaccination), physicians can provide the patient with the antibodies themselves. Because these antibodies are absolutely identical to their parent protein or cell and to one another, they are not subject to the variables present in antibodies produced by other methods. They have properties that make them ideal for treating certain diseases.

Once the analysis of tissue identifies a specific antigen, it may be possible to program monoclonal antibodies to search out and destroy them. It is also possible to link the antibodies to chemotherapeutic agents. Thus, monoclonal antibodies can not only target specific antigens but also bring medication to the specific tissues where it is required. In cancer therapy, these qualities promise to improve the efficiency of treatment greatly. With monoclonal antibodies, cancer-destroying drugs can be brought directly to the cancer cell and can destroy it without harming other body tissues, thus reducing the severity of side effects from chemotherapy.

Perspective and Prospects

The science of serology and serological testing for antibodies and antigens in the body have become mainstays of modern medical diagnosis and treatment for a wide range of diseases. Virtually every individual in the industrialized world and most members of the developing world urban populations undergo serologic testing as part of their regular medical routine.

Serological testing is part of every hospital workup, almost every routine medical examination, every blood transfusion, all transplant procedures, many diagnostic procedures, and many treatment regimens. It is the basis for most epidemiological studies that enumerate the extent of susceptibility to individual diseases in various populations and hence directs the development of immunization programs. It is an integral part of vaccine production and is critical in the development of new vaccines. With the development of monoclonal antibody research, serology enters a new era where the possibilities of improved serologic testing and therapeutic modalities seem almost unlimited.

Serological testing and therapy, so far, have been based on the manipulation and modification of living organisms. It is theoretically possible to develop vaccines and therapeutic agents that are completely synthetic in structure. This science promises greater specificity and efficacy, both for vaccines and for disease treatment.

—*C. Richard Falcon*

See also Anemia; Antibodies; Blood and blood disorders; Blood testing; Cholesterol; Cytology; Cytopathology; Diagnosis; Dialysis; Fluids and electrolytes; Forensic pathology; Hematology; Hematology, pediatric; Hemophilia; Hodgkin's disease; Host-defense mechanisms; Hypercholesterolemia; Hyperlipidemia; Hypoglycemia; Immune system; Immunization and vaccination; Immunology; Immunopathology; Jaundice; Laboratory tests; Leukemia; Malaria; Pathology; Phlebotomy; Plasma; Rh factor; Septicemia; Sickle cell anemia; Thalassemia; Transfusion.

For Further Information:

Bryant, Neville J. *An Introduction to Immunohematology.* 3d ed. Philadelphia: W. B. Saunders, 1994. *This book was written as a background text for laboratory personnel and students. Somewhat technical, but the writing is clear and the author covers the subject well.*

Chase, Allan. *Magic Shots*. New York: William Morrow, 1982. An excellent history of immunization that covers ancient medical practice and describes the work of such early pioneers as Edward Jenner and Louis Pasteur. Details the major discoveries that have taken place in the twentieth century, such as the development of the polio vaccine and the eradication of smallpox.

Griffith, H. Winter. *Complete Guide to Medical Tests*. Tucson, Ariz.: Fisher Books, 1988. A complete compendium of all tests used in hospitals and other medical facilities. All current seronegative-seropositive tests are described and categorized according to their diagnostic and therapeutic uses.

_____. *Complete Guide to Symptoms, Illness, and Surgery*. Revised and updated by Stephen Moore and Kenneth Yoder. Rev. 4th ed. New York: Perigee, 2000. Covers more than five hundred diseases and disorders and includes information about diagnostic tests that involve serology.

Litin, Scott C., ed. *Mayo Clinic Family Health Book*. 4th ed. New York: HarperResource, 2009. A superior medical reference for the general reader which gives a good presentation of blood.

Turgeon, Mary Louise. *Immunology and Serology in Laboratory Medicine*. 4th ed. St. Louis, Mo.: Mosby/Elsevier, 2009. A good introductory clinical text that details methodologies, clinical applications, and interpretations of basic serology.

Widmann, Frances K., and Carol Ann Itatani. *An Introduction to Clinical Immunology and Serology*. 2d ed. Philadelphia: F. A. Davis, 1998. Discusses immunology, immunopathology, and serologic testing methods. Includes bibliographical references and an index.

Serotonin

Biology

Also known as: 5-hydroxytryptamine (5-HT)
Anatomy or system affected: Nervous, muscular
Specialties and related fields: Neurology, biochemistry, psychology
Definition: A neurotransmitter synthesized in the brain and gastrointestinal tract that seems to be involved with various functions including appetite, digestion, memory, mood and social behavior, sexual desire, and sleep

Key terms:

5-HT receptor agonists: substances that bind to 5-HT receptors preventing the action of serotonin
enteramine: the original name used for serotonin
neurotransmitter: a substance in the body that carries the nerve signal from one nerve cell to another or to a muscle
sudden infantdeath syndrome (SIDS): the death of child less than one year of age due to unknown factors

Structure and Functions

Serotonin, scientifically known as 5-hydroxytryptamine (5-HT), is a neurotransmitter, which is a substance in the body that carries the nerve signal from one nerve cell to another or to a muscle. Serotonin, when released by an axon, travels across the synapse or neuromuscular junction, binds to its receptor in its target cell and stimulates a nerve impulse in the target cell. Along with adrenaline and dopamine, serotonin is one of several monoamine neurotransmitters. Serotonin is synthesized in the brain and gastrointestinal tract.

Serotonin or 5-HT is synthesized when a hydroxyl group (OH) is transferred to tryptophan, an amino acid, by the enzyme tryptophan hydroxylase. Between 80 and 90 percent of the body's serotonin is synthesized in the gastrointesti-

nal tract, but it is also found throughout the body in the central nervous system and in platelets.

Serotonin is believed to be involved in various functions including appetite, digestion, memory, mood and social behavior, sexual desire, and sleep. Research has found a relationship between mood and serotonin. Serotonin can also stimulate blood clot formation as it is synthesized by the platelets. Scientists believed that low levels of serotonin caused depression; however, studies have not been able to confirm serotonin's relationship to depression. Researchers working with mice that cannot synthesize serotonin have found no signs of depression in the animals, though the mice did display compulsive and aggressive behavior. It is possible that depression causes a reduction in serotonin production. Other possible reasons for the apparent connection between mood and serotonin include low tryptophan levels, a failure or lack of receptor sites, failure of serotonin to reach receptor sites, and reduced brain cell regeneration.

Men and women appear to react differently to changes in serotonin levels. A 2007 study in the journal *Biological Psychiatry* indicated that men with reduced levels of serotonin in the brain became impulsive while women developed a poorer mood and increased caution. Other studies seem to indicate that the interaction of serotonin and hormones may affect women during menopause, the postpartum period, and the premenstrual period-times when hormone levels fluctuate.

Disorders and Diseases

It is thought that a deficiency in serotonin may play a role in sudden infant death syndrome (SIDS). Mutant mice that synthesize lower levels of serotonin exhibit many SIDS characteristics including low heart rate and early death.

Humans with depression and mouse models of depression show a low level of a protein that assists in serotonin's function in the brain. Various drugs can alter the level of serotonin. Medications known as selective serotonin reuptake inhibitors (SSRIs) also known as serotonin-specific reuptake inhibitors or serotonergic antidepressants are prescribed to treat depression and anxiety because they have been found to increase extracellular serotonin levels. Like other neurotransmitters, serotonin is reabsorbed by the body after it has relayed a neural impulse. SSRIs hinder this reabsorption process, boosting serotonin levels. Some research suggests that high levels of serotonin improve transmission between brain cells, which improves one's mood. Other drugs that increase serotonin levels have been used clinically to treat migraine headaches and nausea.

Some substances, including dietary supplements such as St. John's wort, various medications and illicit drugs can overstimulate serotonin receptors. Carcinoid tumors which are often found in the gastrointestinal tract may cause high levels of serotonin. High serotonin may lead to a potentially life-threatening condition known as serotonin syndrome. Symptoms of this condition include agitation, confusion, diarrhea, headaches, increased heart rate and blood pressure, loss of muscle coordination, muscle rigidity, pupil dilation, shivering, and sweating.

Some research indicates that serotonin levels may be increased without medications. Possible methods include eating high protein foods that increase one's level of tryptophan, exercising, light, such as that used in treating seasonal affective disorder, and psychotherapy.

Drugs that bind to serotonin receptors, the 5-HT receptor agonists, can decrease the effects of serotonin. These drugs are often prescribed to reduce nausea from chemotherapy and radiation therapy. They are also used to treat migraine headaches.

Perspective and Prospects

Serotonin was first discovered during the 1930s by Vittorio Erspamer who first isolated the molecule from stomach cells while studying intestinal smooth muscles cells. When incubated with intestines, the molecule stimulated intestinal smooth muscle contraction. Since the compound was an amine, Erspamer named the compound enteramine. In 1948, Irvine Page, Maurice Rapport, and Arda Green at the Cleveland Clinic discovered a blood derived compound that was a vasoconstrictor. Hence, they called it serotonin. By 1952, serotonin and enteramine were shown to be the same compound.

While studying neurotransmitters in mussels, Betty Mack Twarog was unable to identify the neurotransmitter that regulated muscle relaxation in the mollusks. After she read the Cleveland Clinic researchers' paper on serotonin, she became intrigued, but the paper only addressed serotonin in mammals. About that time, Erspamer found enteramine in octopus salivary glands, and soon after this discovery, enteramine was identified as serotonin. Twarog obtained a sample of serotonin and soon confirmed her suspicions that the neurotransmitter in the mussels was serotonin. She later worked at the Cleveland Clinic and confirmed her theory that serotonin was also found in the brain. The work of these researchers was instrumental in the development of the field of neuroscience, which is the study of the nervous system.

—*Josephine Campbell;*
updated by Charles L. Vigue, PhD

For Further Information:
Bouchez, Colette. "Serotonin: 9 Questions and Answers." *WebMD.* WebMD, LLC. 19 Mar. 2015. http://www.webmd.com/depression/features/serotonin
McIntosh, James. "What Is Serotonin? What Does Serotonin Do?" *MNT.* MediLexicon International Ltd. Web. 19 Mar. 2015. http://www.medicalnewstoday.com/articles/232248.php
McIntosh, James. Serotonin: Facts, What Does Serotonin Do? Medical News Today, April 29, 2016. http://www.medicalnewstoday.com/kc/serotonin-facts-232248
Nauert, Rick. "Mice Study Suggests Lack of Serotonin Not Behind Depression." *Psych Central.* Psych Central. 28 Aug. 2014. Web. 20 Mar. 2015. http://psychcentral.com/news/2014/08/28/mice-study-suggests-lack-of-serotonin-not-behind-depression/74206.html
Whitaker-Azmitia, Patricia Mack. "The Discovery of Serotonin and Its Role in Neuroscience." *Nature.* Nature Publishing Group. 1999. Web. 20 Mar. 2015. http://www.nature.com/npp/journal/v21/n1s/full/1395355a.html

Severe acute respiratory syndrome (SARS)
Disease/Disorder
Anatomy or system affected: Immune system, lungs, respiratory system
Specialties and related fields: Critical care, emergency medicine, epidemiology, internal medicine, microbiology, public health, pulmonary medicine, virology
Definition: A newly recognized type of pneumonia, caused by a novel coronavirus, that may progress to respiratory failure and death.
Key terms:
coronavirus: a single-stranded ribonucleic acid (RNA) virus with a spherical shape and helical nucleocapsid surrounded by an envelope with a crown of glycoprotein spikes
electron microscopy: an imaging technique in which magnetically directed electrons in a vacuum tube are absorbed and deflected by structures, thus forming an image on a screen with very high resolution
Koch's postulates: criteria for judging whether given bacteria cause a given disease, including that the bacteria must be present in every case, that they must be isolated from the host and grown in pure culture, that the disease must be reproduced when the culture is inoculated into a healthy susceptible host, and that the bacteria must be recoverable from the experimentally infected host
tissue culture: a diagnostic method in which cells from plant or animal tissues bathed in sustaining liquid solution form a monolayer on a container that can be inoculated and observed for deterioration or destruction by replicating viruses

Causes and Symptoms

SARS first received worldwide attention in February, 2003, after a Chinese physician from Guangdong Province and twelve other guests at a hotel in Hong Kong became ill. Subsequent investigation of cases traced the illness back to November, 2002, when a businessman from Guangdong Province developed the new disease and soon died. Using electron microscopy, molecular techniques, and tissue cultures, researchers have identified a coronavirus in a variety of specimens from patients with SARS. Glycoprotein spikes on the outside of the envelope surrounding the viral capsid give the appearance of a crown, or corona, and make possible the identification by electron microscopy. The virus was cultured from lung and kidney specimens obtained at autopsy of the Chinese physician using African green monkey kidney cells. Pure cultures of the coronavirus have been inoculated into monkeys, producing pneumonia. With Koch's postulates fulfilled, researchers are confident that the coronavirus is the causative agent.

Human studies have revealed antibodies to this coronavirus only in SARS patients, suggesting that this is a new type of infection. Similar studies in animals have shown that SARS antibodies are present in wild animals, including the masked palm civet, raccoon dog, and ferret badger. While these animals have been found to host the SARS coronavirus, a 2006 study suggested that the natural reservoir host of SARS is likely the horseshoe bat. The crowded, unclean markets of Guangdong Province, which sell wild animals for human consumption, may have provided the opportunity for the virus to infect humans.

After an incubation period of two to sixteen days after exposure, patients develop fever, chills and rigors, myalgia (muscle pain), cough, headache, and dizziness. Less common symptoms are sputum production, sore throat, nausea and vomiting, and diarrhea. Radiographs and high-resolution computed tomography (CT) scans of the chest show ground-glass opacities and unilateral or bilateral air-space consolidation. Laboratory findings early in the illness often include lymphopenia, thrombocytopenia, and a variety of serum enzyme (lactate dehydrogenase, creatinine kinase, and alanine aminotransferase) elevations distinguishing SARS from pneumonia caused by usual bacterial pathogens.

SARS is often progressive in severity and is highly infective, especially for family members and health care workers. During the 2003 outbreak, the disease spread to many countries, with more than eight thousand cases and nine hundred deaths worldwide. The overall mortality rate was about 5 percent. Researchers wondered whether this respiratory illness would follow the seasonal pattern of similar viral illnesses, such as influenza. A SARS case diagnosed in Guangdong Province in January, 2004, led the Chinese government to order the mass slaughter of civets and rats in the hope of containing the disease.

Besides the livestock and human tolls, SARS inflicted economic and political damage. During the outbreak months in 2003, Asian countries saw a financial loss of roughly $28 billion. For the first time, the World Health Organization (WHO) issued an advisory suggesting that travelers avoid parts of the world infected with SARS. North American-based airlines cut 10 percent of their flights to Asia, resulting in a 60 percent drop in tourism. In Canada, China, and the United States, sporting events, public gatherings, film productions, religious services, and parades were canceled because of fears concerning SARS. An interesting footnote to the SARS legacy occurred in June, 2006, when Chinese researchers revealed that at least one of the reported SARS deaths in China during April, 2003, was actually the result of H5N1 avian influenza; raising the possibility that other cases and deaths attributed to SARS may have actually been human cases of H5N1 bird flu and that the Chinese government covered up the possibility that two pathogens were creating simultaneous outbreaks in order to avoid further economic disruption.

Treatment and Therapy

No specific diagnostic test for SARS is available, hampering early diagnosis and treatment. SARS cases can be suspected but not reliably distinguished from other types of pneumonia. Thus far, no antiviral agent has been found to be active against the SARS virus, and initial empiric therapy with antibacterial and antiviral agents has been directed at other pathogens that cause pneumonia that is indistinguishable from SARS.

Supportive measures directed toward respiratory failure,

> ## Information on
> ## Severe Acute Respiratory Syndrome (SARS)
>
> **Causes:** Coronavirus infection transmitted through contact with infected humans or animals
> **Symptoms:** Severe pneumonia, with respiratory failure, fever, chills and rigors, muscle pain, coughing, headache, dizziness
> **Duration:** Acute, sometimes fatal
> **Treatments:** Supportive measures, corticosteroids, isolation

often provided in an intensive care unit, are the mainstays of SARS therapy. In some cases of progressive pneumonia with respiratory failure, corticosteroid therapy has been used. Because of the alarming infectivity and spread of SARS, precautions against airborne droplets (respirators) and direct contact (gowns and gloves) are recommended. Despite such measures, spread has occurred, probably because of improper techniques used by inadequately trained personnel.

Perspective and Prospects

A coronavirus was first cultured from an adult patient with a common cold in 1965. It is now recognized that coronaviruses may cause up to 30 percent of common colds, but before SARS coronaviruses rarely produced pneumonia. These viruses also cause disease in a wide variety of animals, but usually in only one species. It is unclear how the SARS agent jumped from animals to humans. Furthermore, while some wild animals have been identified as having prior infection by the virus, the natural host remains uncertain. A more complete understanding of these issues will improve the chances of eliminating the disease from humans. Fortunately, only a few cases of SARS have been reported in the first few years of the twenty-first century, and these cases have been in laboratory workers or individuals directly exposed to civet cats. Since the 2002-2003 epidemic, human-to-human spread has ceased.

Extraordinarily rapid research has already produced sequencing of the SARS coronavirus genome. With this knowledge, molecular diagnostic techniques have been developed and should produce rapid and accurate diagnostic tests that will be widely available. Thousands of antiviral agents are being tested for activity against the virus, and new antivirals are being developed. Vaccines are available for some animal coronaviruses, and a SARS vaccine may be developed. In the meantime, there is hope that infection control and quarantine measures will be able to limit the spread of SARS.

—H. Bradford Hawley, M.D.;
updated by Randall L. Milstein, Ph.D.

See also Coronaviruses; Emerging infectious diseases; Environmental diseases; Environmental health; Epidemics and pandemics; Epidemiology; Microbiology; Pneumonia; Pulmonary diseases; Pulmonary medicine; Viral infections; Zoonoses.

For Further Information:

Kleinman, Arthur, and James L. Watson, eds. *SARS in China: Prelude to Pandemic?* Stanford, Calif.: Stanford University Press, 2006.

Ksiazek, Thomas G., et al. "A Novel Coronavirus Associated with Severe Acute Respiratory Syndrome." *New England Journal of Medicine* 348 (May 15, 2003): 1953-1966.

Lee, Nelson, et al. "A Major Outbreak of Severe Acute Respiratory Syndrome in Hong Kong." *New England Journal of Medicine* 348 (May 15, 2003): 1986-1994.

McIntosh, Kenneth, and Stanley Perlman. "Coronaviruses, Including Severe Acute Respiratory Syndrome (SARS)-Associated Coronavirus." In *Mandell, Douglas, and Bennett's Principles and Practice of Infectious Diseases*, 7th ed., edited by Gerald L. Mandell, John F. Bennett, and Raphael Dolin. New York: Churchill Livingstone/Elsevier, 2010.

Wang, Lin-Fa, et al. "Review of Bats and SARS." *Emerging Infectious Diseases* 12 (December, 2006): 1834-1840.

Severe combined immunodeficiency syndrome (SCID)

Disease/Disorder

Also known as: Bubble boy disease

Anatomy or system affected: Immune system

Specialties and related fields: Biotechnology, genetics, immunology, pediatrics

Definition: A syndrome in which the immune system is unable to produce T and B cells, resulting in catastrophic failure of the immune system. The underlying cause is a mutation in one of several key genes, and without specialized treatment, often with cells from a donor, death typically occurs before the age of one.

Key terms:

B cell: a lymphocyte that synthesizes immunoglobulins (antibodies)

graft-versus-host disease: a condition that occurs when transplanted organs or cells are recognized by the host's immune system as invaders, resulting in the donor cells being attacked by the host's immune system

leukemia: any of a variety of types of cancer involving the blood or bone marrow

reservoir: the host species in which a parasite is maintained in a given area and from which it may infect other species, initiating an epidemic

T cell: a lymphocyte responsible for cell-mediated immune responses, including graft rejection

X-linked gene: a gene located on the X chromosome

Causes and Symptoms

Severe combined immunodeficiency syndrome (SCID) is a genetic defect in which one of several genes involved in the immune system has a mutation that either prevents gene expression or causes the production of faulty products. The most common cause of SCID, accounting for about half of cases, is mutations in the X-linked gene IL2RG, which codes for the third chain of the interleukin-2 (IL-2) receptor, and also a part of several other interleukin receptors. Interleukin receptors are proteins embedded in the plasma membrane of cells in the immune system that interact with interleukin molecules, which carry important immune system signals. This type of SCID is called X-linked combined immunodeficiency (XCID), and the faulty interleukin

> ## Information on Severe Combined Immunodeficiency Syndrome (SCID)
>
> **Causes:** Various genetic defects
>
> **Symptoms:** Repeated, persistent infections that are unresponsive to standard treatments; may include meningitis, septic arthritis, opportunistic infections, graft-versus-host disease
>
> **Duration:** Chronic
>
> **Treatments:** Bone marrow transplantation, hormonal therapy, gene therapy

receptors prevent the development of Tdf cells and natural killer (NK) cells, both of which are required to prevent infections successfully. Because XCID is an X-linked defect, it is much more common in males.

The remaining cases of SCID are attributable to mutations in many different genes, with new defects being discovered every year. The types of genes involved range from those that code for proteins that interact with interleukin receptors and enzymes involved in purine metabolism, to genes that code for enzymes involved in antigen receptor production. In addition, a variety of lesser known defects and some genetic disorders show some, but not all, of the symptoms of SCID.

The most common of the remaining defects, accounting for about 20 percent of cases, is deficiency in the enzyme adenosine deaminase (ADA), which is involved in purine metabolism. This form of SCID, called ADA SCID, results in the accumulation of a toxic form of adenosine that especially affects lymphatic tissue. No T or B cells are produced. Deficiency in another enzyme, purine nucleoside phosphorylase (PNP), although much rarer, acts in a similar fashion.

Regardless of the underlying causes, symptoms are similar for most types of SCID. The overwhelming clinical symptom is problems with repeated, persistent infections that do not respond to standard treatment. Severe infections such as meningitis or septic arthritis may occur. Infections with opportunistic pathogens such as *Pneumocystis carinii* also frequently occur. Symptoms of graft-versus-host disease (GVHD) may occur in infants because of lymphocytes received from the mother or in patients following blood transfusion. A chest X ray typically shows lack of a thymic shadow, indicating that the thymus has not developed properly. There is often also a family history of immunodeficiency and infant deaths caused by serious infection.

Treatment and Therapy

Left untreated, most infants die within the first year, so rapid identification of the symptoms is extremely important. Prenatal diagnosis is possible and is recommended in families with a history of SCID or similar problems. If SCID is detected early enough, then several treatment options are available, even potential prenatal treatment.

For the majority of SCID cases, bone marrow transplantation is the standard treatment. To prevent GVHD, either the marrow must come from an identical twin or it must be depleted of T cells prior to transplantation. Although a close genetic match has the highest success rate, unmatched and T cell-depleted marrow can be used if matched marrow is unavailable. A survival rate of more than 90 percent has been accomplished when the marrow is from a parent or full sibling. It has typically been routine to use chemotherapy to kill the recipient's bone marrow before transplanting donor marrow, but in the case of SCID patients this has been found unnecessary (and seems to lower the survival rate) because the recipient has no T cells to cause rejection.

When transplantation is successful, donor stem cells present in the marrow populate the recipient's marrow and establish a functioning immune system. Unfortunately, some residual GVHD may occur, and over time T cell function seems to diminish in many cases, in spite of apparent initial success. The reasons for the latter problem are unknown.

Although transplantation may also work for ADA SCID, an alternative is polyethylene glycol (PEG)-bovine ADA replacement therapy. This treatment must be administered on an ongoing basis by frequent intravenous injections of PEG-ADA to maintain appropriate enzyme levels. Unfortunately, PEG-ADA is not always available and is extremely expensive, leaving transplantation the only option in some cases.

Still in the experimental stage is gene therapy to replace the defective genes. Experiments on this approach began in the early 1990s, and although the first attempts at curing ADA SCID showed partial success, the patients still required continued treatment with PEG-ADA. Since then, efforts have focused on better ways to insert the correct genes into the patient's own stem cells. Stem cells from the bone marrow must be isolated, treated, and then returned to the patient.

The most promising results came from experiments begun in 1999 involving gene therapy for XCID. Following the procedure, the infants developed apparently normal immune systems. Unfortunately, by the summer of 2002 one of the boys developed leukemia, and another developed it by the end of the same year. Some trials were stopped as a result. The apparent cause of the leukemia was insertion of the gene at an inappropriate location, a concern expressed early in the discussion of gene therapy for this disease. Gene therapy still holds great promise, but more work needs to be done to ensure its long-term safety and effectiveness.

—*Bryan Ness, Ph.D.*

See also Bone marrow transplantation; Congenital disorders; Gene therapy; Genetic diseases; Host-defense mechanisms; Immune system; Immunodeficiency disorders; Immunology; Immunopathology; Transplantation.

For Further Information:
Blaese, Michael R., et al. "T Lymphocyte-Directed Gene Therapy for ADA SCID: Initial Trial Results After Four Years." *Science* 270 (October 20, 1995): 475-480. A research report on the long-term results of the first gene therapy trials involving SCID.
Cohen, Philip. "Fresh Blow for Gene Treatments as Safety of a Second Virus Is Questioned." *New Scientist* 178 (June 7, 2003): 17. A brief article about the concerns over some children treated for SCID using gene therapy having developed leukemia.
Cooper, Max D., et al. "Immunodeficiency Disorders." *Hematology* 2003, no. 1 (January 1, 2003): 314-330. A thorough presentation on the cell biology behind immunodeficiency disorders with a detailed section on SCID.
Hawley, Robert G., and Donna A. Sobieski. "Of Mice and Men: The Tale of Two Therapies." *Stem Cells* 20 (2002): 275-278. Discusses the experimental gene therapy trials for both XCID and ADA SCID.
Schwarz, Klaus, et al. "Human Severe Combined Immune Deficiency and DNA Repair." *Bioessays* 25, no. 11 (November, 2003): 1061-1070. A current overview of the underlying causes of the various types of SCID and a discussion of the potential of gene therapy to cure it.
Scollay, Roland. "Gene Therapy: A Brief Overview of the Past, Present, and Future." *Annals of the New York Academy of Sciences* 953 (2001): 26-30. Discusses the potential of gene therapy in curing single-gene diseases, with some mention of SCID.

Sexual differentiation

Biology

Anatomy or system affected: Endocrine system, genitals, glands, reproductive system, uterus

Specialties and related fields: Embryology, endocrinology, genetics, gynecology, urology

Definition: The process by which an embryo becomes male or female under the influence of genetic and hormonal factors.

Key terms:

differentiation: the process of gradual remodeling of tissues in the embryo or fetus; in this context, the process of formation of the male or female reproductive organs

external genitalia: in the male, the penis and scrotum; in the female, the clitoris, the vaginal opening, and the folds (labia) around it

gender identity: the mental view of oneself as a girl or woman or as a boy or man

gonad: the internal organ in either sex that produces the reproductive cells (ova and sperm): the ovary in the female and the testis in the male

hormone: a chemical that is produced by a gland in the body and secreted into the blood; hormones act as coordinating signals

hormone receptor: a molecule contained in or on a cell that allows it to respond to a hormone; if receptors are not present, the hormone will have no effect

Müllerian ducts: the pair of tubes in the early embryo that will develop into the internal female organs (uterus, oviducts, and upper vagina)

urethra: the tube that drains the bladder; in the male, the urethra passes through the penis and carries sperm during ejaculation, while in the female, the urethra opens in front of the vagina but does not have a reproductive function

Wolffian ducts: the pair of tubes in the early embryo that will develop into the internal male organs (the epididymis, vas deferens, and seminal vesicles)

X and Y chromosomes: the chromosomes that determine genetic sex; females carry an XX pair, and males carry an XY pair

Fundamentals

The chromosomal sex of a human is determined at the time of conception, when the ovum from the mother is fertilized by a single sperm from the father. All ova (eggs) produced by a female contain one chromosome, denoted X. Sperm from the male can carry either an X or a Y chromosome. The Y chromosome is smaller than the X and contains fewer genetic codes. Men normally produce equal numbers of X- and Y-bearing sperm. The type of chromosome carried by the one sperm that fertilizes the ovum will determine the sex of the embryo. A Y-bearing sperm joining with the ovum will result in an embryo with one X and one Y; this embryo will develop as a male. If the ovum is fertilized with an X-bearing sperm, the embryo will have two X's and will develop as a female.

Although the genetic sex is determined at conception, male and female embryos initially look alike, both internally and externally. For the first seven weeks of development, each human embryo has the anatomical potential to develop in either a male or a female direction: This period is referred to as the sexually indifferent stage. Internally, the gonads, which lie in the kidney region, cannot yet be identified as ovaries or testes. The other internal reproductive organs are represented in every embryo by two pairs of ducts: the Müllerian ducts, which will later develop in the female but will be lost in the male; and the Wolffian ducts, which will later develop in the male but will regress in the female. Externally, male and female embryos possess the same rudimentary genital organs, which will later be remodeled to become either male or female genitalia.

The first organ to differentiate in the embryo is the gonad. Starting at about seven weeks of development in a male embryo, the cells within the gonad are reorganized to form a testis. This reorganization is brought about by the presence of the Y chromosome, which contains the codes for the production of a substance called testis-determining factor (TDF). The chemical nature of TDF has not yet been determined, but its existence is clear from experimental evidence. TDF acts on the gonad to cause it to become a testis. In the absence of a Y chromosome and TDF in a female embryo, the gonad develops into an ovary at about twelve weeks of development. If an individual has only one X chromosome (a condition known as Turner syndrome), the gonads will develop into ovaries, but these ovaries will not contain ova and so the person will be infertile.

The development of the other reproductive organs is not directly determined by the X and Y chromosomes, but rather by hormones secreted by the gonads. In the male, the fetal testes begin to produce testosterone by the tenth week of development, and this testosterone acts on the Wolffian duct system to cause it to develop into the epididymis, vas deferens, and seminal vesicles. The Müllerian duct system in the male regresses under the influence of another hormone from the testes, called Müllerian-inhibiting hormone (MIH). In the female, MIH is not produced, and the Müllerian ducts develop into the oviducts, uterus, and upper part of the vagina. The Wolffian ducts in the female regress in the absence of testosterone. Normal female development does not, at this stage, require any hormone produced by the ovaries, but instead occurs spontaneously in the absence of testicular hormones. Thus, the presence or absence of the Y chromosome determines which type of gonad develops, and the presence or absence of gonadal hormones determines which type of internal reproductive organs develop.

Similarly, the development of the external genitalia is hormonally directed. In the male, testosterone is converted by the action of the enzyme 5-alpha-reductase to 5-alpha-dihydrotestosterone (DHT). DHT acts on the undifferentiated external genital tissue, causing it to take on a male appearance: A pea-shaped structure (the genital tubercle) at the front of the crotch area grows to become the penis, a slitlike opening (the urethral groove) is enclosed within the penis to become the urethra when two folds behind the genital tubercle fuse together, and two swellings on the sides of the urethral groove become enlarged as the scrotum. In the female, it is the absence of DHT that causes development in the female direction: The genital tubercle remains as the relatively small clitoris; the folds do not fuse, allowing the urethral groove to remain as an open area where the vagina and urethral openings are located; and the swellings that become the scrotum in the male remain separated as the labia in the female.

Hormones also cause sexual differentiation of the brain, but the mechanism is not fully understood in humans. The most obvious result of brain differentiation is the difference in adult hormone production patterns. In the adult male, hormone production is relatively constant from day to day, and this results in constant production of sperm in the testes. In the female, hormone production changes in a monthly cycle that is associated with ovum maturation and ovulation. The difference in the pattern of hormone release in adult males and females appears to be attributable to hormonal programming of the fetal brain. Animal studies indicate that the development of the male pattern results from exposure of the fetal brain to testosterone or one of its derivatives. The female pattern of development is prevalent when testosterone is absent. In humans, testosterone also affects brain differentiation, but the effect appears to be less permanent than in animals.

It is not known for sure if there is any direct influence of the chromosomes or prenatal hormones on male and female behavior. Most researchers agree that human behavior is heavily influenced by social and cultural factors, so the importance of prenatal programming is difficult to assess. Indeed, it appears that gender identity, the internal view of oneself as male or female, is so heavily influenced by learning that a child with a disorder of sexual differentiation can be successfully reared in the gender that is opposite to that of the chromosomes. For example, a child born with female-appearing genitalia, but with XY chromosomes and internal testes, can be reared as a girl and will firmly adhere to this identity even if some masculinization occurs at the time of puberty.

Disorders and Diseases

Disorders of sexual differentiation result from errors in the signaling systems that normally direct male and female anatomical development. There are several different classes of these disorders, some of which result in a mixture of male and female reproductive organs. These disorders are rare, with the number of documented cases numbering only in the hundreds for most types.

True hermaphrodites are defined as individuals who possess both ovarian and testicular gonadal tissue. There may be one ovary and one testis, two gonads in which ovarian and testicular tissue are combined (ovotestes), or an ovotestis on one side and a normal ovary or testis on the other. True hermaphroditism can result from several distinct genetic anomalies. Some hermaphrodites have been shown to be chimeras: individuals that develop from the fusion of two separate embryos at an early stage. These individuals possess two distinct cell populations, one with an XX pair of chromosomes and one with XY. It is thought that expression of both of these chromosome pairs leads to the mixture of ovarian and testicular tissue seen in true hermaphrodites. A similar condition is mosaicism, in which the mixture of XX and XY cells is caused by errors of chromosome replication in a single early embryo. Other true hermaphrodites are neither chimeras nor mosaics; they appear to have a normal pair of XX or XY chromosomes, but on closer examination, one of the chromosomes is found to have a defect. For example, a Y chromosome may be missing a tiny piece, or an X chromosome may contain a portion of a Y.

There is much variation in the anatomical features of true hermaphrodites. One basic guideline is that the effects of the presence of testicular tissue are local. Thus, a true hermaphrodite with a testis on the left side and an ovary on the right will have Wolffian duct-derived (male) organs on the left side but Müllerian duct-derived (female) organs on the right. The external appearance depends on the relative levels of estrogen and testosterone but might include a typical male penis along with enlarged breasts. There are documented cases of ovulation and even pregnancy in true hermaphrodites. Successful sperm production appears to be less frequent than ovulation, and sperm production and ovulation are not seen in the same individual.

Pseudohermaphrodites are individuals whose external reproductive organs do not match their gonadal sex. Male pseudohermaphrodites have testes but external organs that appear to be female; female pseudohermaphrodites have ovaries and varying degrees of external male development.

Female pseudohermaphroditism has only one basic cause: the exposure of an XX fetus to masculinizing hormones. These hormones might come from the fetus itself, as in certain disorders involving the adrenal gland, or synthetic hormones given to a pregnant woman may have a masculinizing effect on a female fetus. The extent of masculinization depends on the timing of the hormone exposure, with earlier exposure leading to more extensive malelike appearance of the external genitalia, including fusion of the urethral folds and enlargement of the clitoris.

The internal organs are normal female.

Male pseudohermaphroditism arises from a wide variety of causes. There may be failure of testosterone production, or the reproductive organs may lack testosterone receptors, causing them to fail to respond to the hormone. Because of the hormonal abnormalities, the Wolffian duct organs may fail to develop, and the external genitalia will appear female to some extent. If MIH production is normal, internal female organs will not be present. The appearance at puberty is variable, depending on the exact hormonal deficiency. Some individuals undergo the typical male responses of increased muscle mass, deepening of the voice, and growth of beard and chest hair; others do not. Most male pseudohermaphrodites are infertile because of the hormonal problems.

Treatment of disorders of sexual development depends on the exact symptoms and their cause, but the prevailing overall philosophy is to attempt to produce an individual who will be able to function sexually as an adult, even if that means sacrificing fertility and rearing the child in the sex opposite to that of the chromosomes. Early diagnosis is a key, since most authorities agree that gender identity is irrevocably set by the age of eighteen to twenty-four months. After that time, few physicians would be willing to try to alter the individual's gender identity from that which has already been established.

For true hermaphrodites, the choice of sex for rearing usually depends on the predominant appearance of the external genitalia. If the genital tubercle has remained small, like a clitoris, the decision is usually for a female sex assignment; if the tubercle appears more penislike, the individual can be reared as a male. Usually, the gonadal tissue that does not correspond to the sex of rearing will be removed, to prevent the production of hormones that would interfere with the desired appearance. Appropriate hormone treatment and surgery can enhance the body form of the chosen sex. For example, testosterone treatment will cause beard growth, and estrogen treatment will cause breast development.

In the case of female pseudohermaphrodites, most can successfully be reared as girls. Surgical alteration of the external genitalia and hormone treatment to correct the original problem may be necessary. Assuming early diagnosis and treatment, most female pseudohermaphrodites will be fertile as adults.

Similarly, hormonal treatment of male pseudohermaphrodites who do not produce testosterone can allow these individuals to be reared as boys, even if they are not fertile later. There is no treatment, however, that will allow a male pseudohermaphrodite who is unresponsive to testosterone to develop a male appearance; these individuals are usually reared as girls, with female pubertal development induced by estrogen treatment.

A fascinating form of male pseudohermaphroditism is seen in the *guevedoces* (meaning "penis at twelve") of the Dominican Republic. In this island nation, the extensive intermarriage of related individuals has produced a population in which a certain genetic defect is seen in relatively high numbers. This genetic defect results in absence of the 5-alpha-reductase enzyme necessary to convert testosterone to DHT. Affected individuals are born with external genitalia that appear more female than male. The internal reproductive organs, which are stimulated by testosterone rather than by DHT, are normal for a male, although the testes may remain in the body cavity instead of descending into a scrotum. Female internal organs are absent, since MIH production is normal. Traditionally, these individuals were reared as girls until the time of puberty, when growth of the penis occurred under the influence of increasing levels of testosterone. (Although the penis would enlarge, the opening of the urethra would remain misplaced for a male, being on the bottom of or behind the penis, a condition known as hypospadias.) At this time, these individuals would make a transition to a male gender identity and sex role. Although initially reared as female, the *guevedoces* were typically heterosexual as adult males, participating in sexual activity with females. Physicians and psychologists have been puzzled by the fact that the *guevedoces* could switch their gender identity at such an advanced age, in the face of evidence suggesting that this should be impossible. This traditional switch of sex role at puberty is no longer seen, since most *guevedoces* are now diagnosed at birth and reared as males from the start.

Perspective and Prospects

Anatomical descriptions of people with disorders of sexual development are found in writings beginning in the pre-Christian era. The word "hermaphrodite" itself derives from the Greek myth about Hermaphroditos, the son of Hermes and Aphrodite, whose body was permanently merged with that of a nymph in a loving embrace. The myth probably arose from a desire to explain the existence of hermaphrodites.

Although the existence of hermaphrodites was known long ago, there was no understanding of the mechanism of sexual differentiation until modern times. During the nineteenth century, embryological studies firmly established the concept that the early human embryo is sexually indifferent anatomically. In the twentieth century, genetic and hormonal studies revealed the controlling factors in male and female development.

It was in the 1920s that the X and Y chromosomes were first discovered and recognized to be important in sex determination. Since the 1960s, researchers have had the ability to pinpoint the exact chromosome sites associated with many disorders of sexual differentiation. Ongoing efforts deal with the identification of the TDF coded by the Y chromosome and the mechanism by which TDF causes testicular development.

The nature of the hormonal control of sexual differentiation was determined by experiments such as those performed on rabbit embryos by A. Jost in the 1940s and 1950s. Jost systematically removed or transplanted embryonic testes and ovaries, and treated the embryos with estrogen and testosterone, in order to demonstrate the importance of hormones from the testis on the development of the internal and external reproductive organs.

Jost's conclusions for rabbits were confirmed in humans by studying individuals with disorders of sexual differentiation caused by genetic factors. Additional confirmation came from observations of the offspring of pregnant women treated with synthetic hormones as a possible preventive for miscarriage. Such treatment was later found to be ineffective in preventing miscarriage, but worse, the treated women often gave birth to masculinized female fetuses. It is now recognized that synthetic hormones in oral birth control pills can also masculinize female fetuses.

Discovery of the causes of true hermaphroditism and pseudohermaphroditism have allowed physicians to make important distinctions between these disorders, with a clear physical cause and manifestation, and the psychological disorders of sexuality that were previously confused with them. For example, until the middle of the twentieth century, the term "hermaphrodite" was used to refer not only to people with a mixture of male and female reproductive organs but also to those with a psychological confusion of gender identity. The latter individuals are now called transsexuals; they identify themselves by the gender that does not conform to the gender indicated by their reproductive organs. Transsexuals possess a complete set of normal reproductive organs and have no known chromosomal or hormonal abnormality. Another behavior is transvestism, which refers to the wearing of clothing of the opposite gender. Many transvestites are male heterosexuals who engage in this behavior to achieve sexual arousal; like transsexuals, transvestites have normal anatomy, chromosomes, and hormones. Finally, homosexual orientation is now considered to be a personality trait, rather than a disorder. Homosexuals are sexually and romantically attracted to individuals of the same gender; their reproductive organs, chromosomes, and hormone levels are the same as those of heterosexuals.

—*Marcia Watson-Whitmyre, Ph.D.*

See also Embryology; Gender identity disorder; Gender reassignment surgery; Genetics and inheritance; Hermaphroditism and pseudohermaphroditism; Hormones; Men's health; Reproductive system; Sexual dysfunction; Sexuality; Women's health.

For Further Information:

Henry, Helen L., and Anthony W. Norman, eds. *Encyclopedia of Hormones.* 3 vols. Boston: Academic Press, 2003. A comprehensive overview of the role of hormones, the major physiological systems in which they operate, and the biological consequences of an excess or deficiency of a particular hormone.

Kronenberg, Henry M., et al., eds. *Williams Textbook of Endocrinology.* 11th ed. Philadelphia: Saunders/Elsevier, 2008. Discusses normal sexual differentiation and then covers all the known disorders, including appearance, chromosomes, hormone levels, fertility, and treatment.

Moore, Keith L., and T. V. N. Persaud. *The Developing Human.* 8th ed. Philadelphia: Saunders/Elsevier, 2008. An outstanding textbook on human embryonic development, with specific information about the causes of congenital malformations and common defects occurring in each of the body's systems.

Morland, Iain, ed. *Intersex and After*. Durham, N.C.: Duke University Press, 2009. Scholars explore what it means for people born with ambiguous genitalia-intersexed persons-for theories of gender. Examines "the ethics of medical treatment and the repercussions of intersex surgery," showing "how biology, activism, law, morality, and ethics have a shared interest in the relationship between intersexuality and the meaning of sex, gender, and sexuality."

Simpson, Joe Leigh, and Sherman Elias. *Genetics in Obstetrics and Gynecology*. 3d ed. Philadelphia: W. B. Saunders, 2003. Deals with the genetic basis of disorders of sexual differentiation and provides a detailed, technical account of the results of various genetic defects.

Sexual dysfunction

Disease/Disorder

Anatomy or system affected: Genitals, psychic-emotional system, reproductive system

Specialties and related fields: Endocrinology, gynecology, psychiatry, psychology, urology

Definition: Impotence is the persistent inability of a man to achieve and maintain an erection adequate for penetration and sexual intercourse; frigidity is the disinterest in sex, usually applied to women, because of inadequate or unpleasurable sensation during intercourse.

Key terms:

corpora cavernosa: two passageways in the penis containing spongy reservoirs of tissue and blood vessels

etiology: the science of causes or origins, especially of diseases

neuropathy: malfunction of the nerves

organic disease: a disease caused or accompanied by an alteration in the structure of the tissues or organs

psychogenic: psychologic in origin

Causes and Symptoms

It is evident from the term "performance anxiety" that sexual anxiety is more easily recognized when it involves performance (that is, erections and orgasms) than when it involves subjective arousal. The most extreme example of this way of thinking is the familiar notion that women do not experience performance anxiety because it is only men who have to perform. When researchers searched for a corresponding term that refers not to performance but to subjectively felt arousal, they devised the oxymoronic-sounding term "pleasure anxiety." Performance anxiety refers to the fear of not being able to perform, while pleasure anxiety refers to the fear of feeling pleasure. Sex therapists have traditionally been much more concerned with the fear of not being able to perform.

To explain this blind spot in the field, it is clear that, historically, lack of desire has been considered a female disorder, whereas lack of performance has been considered a male disorder. From the male-identified point of view, the failure to perform is relatively understandable; it is often treated with humor, sympathy, or indulgence. Traditionally, however, the same indulgence has not been extended toward a woman when she cannot fulfill the role expected of her.

If there are any doubts that "frigidity" is a more accusatory term than "impotence," "impotence" as a diagnostic term retains its currency, whereas "frigidity" has largely been dropped. Researchers William H. Masters and Virginia E. Johnson were the first authorities to drop the term, and as a result of their influence it is rarely used in the field of sex therapy and research. It is still used, however, in the psychoanalytic literature.

The category of "inhibited sexual desire" in the American Psychiatric Association's *Diagnostic and Statistical Manual of Mental Disorders: DSM-III* (3d ed., 1980) indicated the difficulty in finding a nonjudgmental means of referring to the lack of erotic arousal: The term "inhibition" implies that the conditions for desire are present but that desire is being withheld. One of the implied accusations in the term "frigidity" is that the woman who does not experience erotic arousal is a cold, unfeeling, or withholding person. The work group on psychosexual disorders for the revision of the DSM-III-R published in 1987 first recognized this difficulty and recommended that "inhibited sexual desire" be renamed "hypoactive sexual desire disorder," arguing that this more awkward term is necessary because it reflects greater neutrality in terms of etiology.

In the 1970s researchers noted that the diagnosis of low sexual desire among couples seeking help with sexual dysfunction increased from approximately one-third of couples in the early 1970s to more than one-half of couples by the early 1980s. Men as well as women were identified with low sexual desire, or frigidity. Most of the knowledge of the causes of low sexual desire is based on clinical experience, rather than on more empirical and objective research. It has become clear that there is no single cause for low sexual desire. Rather, many cases involve several causal factors working simultaneously.

Virtually every standard work on sexual dysfunction lists religious orthodoxy as a major cause of sexual dysfunction. Some patients suffer from low sexual desire because they essentially lack the capacity for play (the obsessive-compulsive personality). Specific sexual phobias or aversions also may cause low sexual desire. Low-desire men almost uniformly have some degree of aversion to the vagina and female genitals. Women who have been sexually molested as children, or raped as adults, often have specific aversion reactions.

Some patients fear that if they allow themselves to feel any sexual desire at all, they will lose all control over themselves and begin acting out sexually in ways that would have disastrous consequences. Fear of pregnancy is often a "masked" cause of low sexual desire among women. Depression, hormonal issues, the side effects of medication, relationship problems, lack of attraction to one's partner, fear of closeness, and an inability to fuse feelings of love and sexual desire are among the many causes of low sexual desire in both men and women.

With regard to impotence, although the exact number is not known, it has been estimated that there are approximately ten million men in the United States suffering from impotence. In the past, it was thought that psychogenic causes accounted for 90 percent of impotence, with only 10 percent attributable to medical or postsurgical diseases, so-called physical or organic impotence. As medical knowledge increased, in the early 1990s it was estimated that medical or organic causes accounted for 50 to 70 percent of all patients suffering from impotence.

Until the 1980s, it was difficult to determine whether any given patient was impotent as a result of psychogenic causes or physical, organic ones. The availability of blood tests to measure hormone levels and of penile tumescence sleep laboratory testing now allows for accurate determination of the true cause of impotence in patients. Yet even when it is attributable to organic causes, impotence has significant psychological implications.

Impotence can be defined as the persistent inability to attain and maintain a rigid penis adequate for penetration and successful completion of intercourse. There are two types of impotence: primary and secondary. Primary impotence is the term used to describe the male who has never been able to achieve an erection adequate for sexual intercourse. This is a relatively rare condition. Except in very unusual circumstances that might have involved a surgical procedure on the penis during childhood, primary impotence is not caused by any physical defect but instead has a psychologic basis. Men with primary impotence are most often found to have had a severely repressive childhood. These patients generally exhibit considerable conflict in their relationships with women and have hostile or fearful attitudes toward females.

The majority of men with impotence have secondary impotence; that is, at one time in their lives they were capable of full erections and intercourse but have subsequently lost that ability. In the 1980s, other medical terms for impotence came into common use, such as "erectile dysfunction." As in the case of "frigidity," the word "impotence" has had negative connotations.

Diabetes mellitus is a rather common organic medical problem accounting for impotence in many men. It has been estimated that 50 percent of men who have had diabetes for twenty years become impotent. It is thought that diabetes results in impotence by causing neuropathy or malfunction of the nerves, as well as narrowing of the blood vessels. Arteriosclerosis, or hardening of the arteries, causes a narrowing of the blood vessels. Many patients who have arteriosclerosis involving the aorta or smaller blood vessels that supply blood to the penis will experience impotence.

Chronic kidney failure, cirrhosis (chronic liver disease), neurological diseases such as Parkinson's disease and multiple sclerosis, malfunction of the spinal cord (such as spina bifida or spinal cord injury), and low levels of testosterone are also frequent organic causes of impotence. Masters and Johnson have stated that alcoholism is the second most common cause of impotence. Pelvic fractures and trauma, radiation therapy, radical pelvic surgery (including removal of the prostate, bladder, or rectum), and aortic aneurysm repair can cause nerve and blood vessel injuries that can result in impotence and/or problems with ejaculation. Penile cancer, Peyronie's disease (curvature of the penis as a result of scar tissue formation), and priapism (prolonged

---

Information on Sexual Dysfunction

Causes: Stress, psychological factors, injury, hormonal disorders, disease, substance abuse, chronic kidney failure, spinal cord malfunction, history of sexual abuse

Symptoms: Impotence, inhibited sexual desire

Duration: Acute to chronic

Treatments: Behavior therapy, psychotherapy, medications, vacuum tumescence devices, surgical reconstruction

---

erection of the penis) are also causes of organic impotence. It has been reported that prescription drugs may account for 25 percent of patients with impotence. By far the most common group of drugs resulting in impotence are those taken for treatment of hypertension, or high blood pressure.

Treatment and Therapy

There are several difficulties inherent in devising a treatment program for low sexual desire. While most of the behavioral exercises devised by Masters and Johnson may enhance arousal and orgasm, they often fail in increasing sexual desire or motivation, since they were not designed to deal specifically with low sexual desire. A second problem is that many cases of low sexual desire not only are quite complex but are diverse in apparent etiology and maintenance factors as well. Each case of low desire must be examined on its own terms, and treatment must be tailored to the specific needs of the individual.

Behavior therapy and social learning theory contributed most of the effective techniques that constituted sex therapy in the 1980s. Other therapeutic approaches, however, have been used as adjunct techniques or proposed alternatives. One broad-spectrum approach attempts to integrate interventions from many theoretical orientations into a comprehensive treatment program, while remaining sensitive to the need to fine-tune the program to the individual.

The first step in this broad-spectrum approach is experiential/sensory awareness. Many patients with low sexual desire are unable to verbalize their feelings and are often unaware of their responses to situations involving sexual stimulation. The goal of this phase of therapy is to help patients recognize, using bodily cues, when they are experiencing feelings of anxiety, pleasure, anger, or disgust.

The second stage is the insight phase of therapy, in which patients, with the help of the therapist, attempt to learn and understand what is causing and maintaining their low desire. Frequently, patients with low sexual desire have misconceptions and self-defeating attitudes about the cause of the problem. Patients are helped to reformulate attitudes about the cause of the problem in a way that is conducive to therapeutic change.

The third stage, the cognitive phase of therapy, is designed to alter irrational thoughts that inhibit sexual desire. Patients are helped to identify self-statements that interfere with sexual desire. They are helped to accept the general assumption that their emotional reactions can be directly influenced by their expectations, labels, and self-statements. Patients are taught that unrealistic or irrational beliefs may be the main cause of their emotional reactions and that they can change these unrealistic attitudes. With change, patients can reevaluate specific situations more realistically and can reduce negative emotional reactions that cause low desire.

The final element of this treatment program consists of behavioral interventions. Behavioral assignments are used throughout the therapy process and include basic sex therapy as well as other sexual and nonsexual behavior procedures. Behavioral interventions are used to help patients change nonsexual behaviors that may be helping to cause or maintain the sexual difficulty. Assertiveness training, communication training, and skill training in negotiation are examples of such behavioral interventions.

The treatment of psychogenic impotence includes supportive psychotherapy and behavior-oriented tasks. If, during the course of evaluation, symptoms of depression such as loss of libido and appetite or sleep difficulties are present without a physical basis, the patient is often treated with an antidepressant medication. As mental depression lessens, sexual interest and potency will often return. Depression is the most common mental disorder detected when impotent patients undergo psychological studies.

There are certain causes of organic impotence that may be reversible with appropriate therapy. The alcoholic patient, for example, may regain his potency if his drinking problem can be resolved. The heavy cigarette smoker may similarly experience improvement in his general health and regain erections following cessation of smoking. Patients with newly discovered diabetes mellitus and high blood sugars may regain their erections following control of their diabetes with insulin, diet, or oral medications. This improvement will not be seen, however, in those individuals with long-standing diabetes who lose their erections.

Treatment programs for organic impotence are geared toward the problems of each individual and are often age-dependent. From 1980 to 1990, there were major advances not only in the diagnosis but also in the treatment of erectile insufficiency; moreover, many of those major treatment advances were nonsurgical. As a result of these nonsurgical advances and their positive rate of success, men often are encouraged to begin their treatment program with the most conservative technique possible. It has been estimated that approximately 90 percent of patients with erectile insufficiency are adequately treated with one of the following (conservative) medical programs: oral medication, self-injection, and vacuum tumescence devices.

Often the first step to medical management of erectile dysfunction is oral medication. Generally, these medications cause smooth muscle relaxation, thereby enhancing the blood flow into the penis. The drug Viagra (sildenafil), introduced in 1998, allows sufficient blood flow for an erection over a four- to five-hour period. Viagra boasted a success rate of almost 80 percent and was immediately in great demand. Dangerous side effects were noted, however, when sildenafil is used in conjunction with nitroglyc-

erin or long-acting nitrates in any form. These nitrate medications in combination with sildenafil produce significant blood pressure drops and are dangerous, especially to patients with compromised cardiac status. Soon after its introduction, concerns arose over the misuse of Viagra to enhance sexual performance instead of to treat impotence. Drugs similar to sildenafil, which are classified as phosphodiesterase V (PDE V) inhibitors, are new to the market. These drugs facilitate erectile function by stimulating the relaxation of smooth muscle tissue in the erectile bodies of the penis. This relaxation allows rapid blood flow into the penis and facilitates erectile function in men with erectile dysfunction. Additional drugs, including tadalafil (Cialis) and vardenafil (Levitra), have been approved for the treatment of erectile dysfunction in certain markets. Other agents, including apomorphine (Uprima), will stimulate central nervous system functions, providing improved erectile function. Uprima, which has been approved by the FDA Advisory Panel, is the first agent to act on the central nervous system to improve erectile dysfunction. Medications to increase sexual desire are also being investigated by various pharmaceutical companies in conjunction with the Food and Drug Administration (FDA).

Penile injection with drugs is a treatment for male impotence that was popularized in 1982 by Ronald Virag of Paris. Penile injection with vasoactive compounds to effect an erection, however, had not yet been approved by the FDA in the United States by the late 1990s. Thus patients were required to sign a legal release of liability if this method of treatment was chosen.

In the 1990s, there were approximately eighty thousand males using self-injection therapy (for the treatment of erectile impotence) in the United States. This method of treatment has gained much international acceptance and continues to be the focus of much clinical and laboratory research. This technique is relatively painless and quick, producing results in ten to twenty minutes. Treatment is initiated by administering a test dose of the medication. During this initial stage of treatment, the medication dosage level is adjusted. The patient is then taught the injection technique, given instructions on how to care for the medication and equipment, and given an assessment of erectile response. This method is considered simple, safe, and highly successful (with a success rate of approximately 75 to 80 percent). The major complications are priapism and penile scarring, which occurs in 1 to 2 percent of cases.

Another nonsurgical option available is vacuum tumescence therapy. This device enables the patient to attain penile enlargement and rigidity by inducing blood flow into the penile shaft. Once the blood flow is induced by the creation of a vacuum, it is trapped by the use of an occlusive device applied at the base of the penis. Although it produces a successful erection in approximately 75 percent of cases, the vacuum tumescence device and the accompanying obstructing rubber occlusive device prevent the ejaculate from being expelled in most cases.

Many men with erectile dysfunction are best treated by

surgical reconstruction. This group represents approximately 10 percent of the entire impotent population. Penile revascularization is one option. The patients who are best treated with penile revascularization are typically men under fifty years of age. Generally, these men are nonsmoking, healthy individuals whose potency problems are caused by a single lesion or injury. The purpose of penile revascularization is to channel more blood into the corpora cavernosa and thereby increase the corpora cavernosa pressure. Pressure can be increased by a variety of methods, including bypass artery-to-artery, bypass artery-to-vein, or closure of specific leaking areas in the corpora cavernosa.

Although available since the mid-1930s, penile prosthetics made their greatest strides after the introduction of synthetic materials (plastics) in the 1950s. Since then, major changes in design, function, and surgical technique have evolved. The prosthetics available by the late twentieth century were of three basic varieties: simple rods, flexible rods, and hydraulic devices (one-piece, two-piece, and multicomponent). Once implanted, prosthetics give the patient a return to "normal erectile dynamics." Although the tumescence-detumescence cycle is a result of the patient's prosthesis, sensation, satisfaction, and often even ejaculation remain as they were prior to surgery.

Perspective and Prospects

Anthropologists have found that impotence (erectile dysfunction) and frigidity (inhibited or low sexual desire) have been observed in both primitive and highly developed societies. During most of human history, it was taken for granted that women attain sexual gratification in the same manner as men. Little attention was paid to the failures.

One of the most significant social changes affecting attitudes toward these sexual dysfunctions has been the altered status of women in contemporary society. During the Victorian era, whether they worked or not, women were legally the wards of men and had virtually no civil rights. Many of the Victorian attitudes toward sex-fears, prejudices, taboos, and superstitions-remained powerful influences into the late twentieth century.

Researchers, however, have learned that they cannot understand the problem of impotence in women by comparing it with impotence in men, since the dynamics as well as the treatments for each disorder differ greatly. With the women's movement and the Masters and Johnson research into human sexuality, the archaic terms "impotence" and "frigidity" were called into question. More gender-neutral terms were used, and, particularly in the case of erectile insufficiency, organic as opposed to psychogenic etiologies were acknowledged. By the late twentieth century, erectile insufficiency had become a disorder more often treated by urologists than by psychiatrists.

With this changing attitude toward these sexual dysfunctions among the medical community as well as the public at large, more research was devoted to treating the problems effectively and to reassuring the patients. Age-old stereotypes came under attack, such as the notion that performance anxiety affects only men and that frigidity or low sexual desire is a disorder that affects only women. As more organic etiologies for both erectile dysfunction and low sexual desire are acknowledged, patients feel increasingly comfortable seeking medical attention, and the stigma of sexual dysfunction being purely psychological is slowly beginning to vanish.

—*Genevieve Slomski, Ph.D.*

See also Alcoholism; Anxiety; Aphrodisiacs; Arteriosclerosis; Cirrhosis; Diabetes mellitus; Erectile dysfunction; Genital disorders, female; Genital disorders, male; Hormones; Hypertension; Menopause; Men's health; Multiple sclerosis; Parkinson's disease; Prostate cancer; Psychiatry; Psychiatry, geriatric; Psychosomatic disorders; Renal failure; Sexuality; Spina bifida; Stress; Urinary disorders; Women's health.

For Further Information:

Crooks, Robert, and Karla Baur. *Our Sexuality*. 10th ed. Belmont, Calif.: Wadsworth, 2010. A college textbook that covers the span of human sexuality, including topics such as sexual health, dysfunction, and recent research.

Daniluk, Judith C. *Women's Sexuality Across the Life Span: Challenging Myths, Creating Meanings*. New York: Guilford Press, 1998. Examines how women experience sexuality from childhood through old age, with a focus on the complex interaction of psychological, social, cultural, and biological influences on the creation of individual sexual meanings.

Ellsworth, Pamela, and Bob Stanley. *One Hundred Questions and Answers About Erectile Dysfunction*. 2d ed. Sudbury, Mass.: Jones and Bartlett, 2008. A patient-oriented guide that cover basic questions about the condition such as causes, symptoms, and diagnosis; available treatments and how to choose among them; and ways of coping with common emotional and physical difficulties associated with the diagnosis and treatment.

Kaplan, Helen Singer. *The Sexual Desire Disorders: Dysfunctional Regulation of Sexual Motivation*. New York: Brunner/Mazel, 1995. This book provides current thinking on disorders of sexual desire and directions for contemporary treatment.

Miller, Karl E. "Treatment of Antidepressant-Associated Sexual Dysfunction." *American Family Physician* 61, no. 12 (June 15, 2000): 3728. Many classes of antidepressants, including the selective serotonin reuptake inhibitors (SSRIs), can impair sexual function. Michelson and associates evaluated the effectiveness of buspirone and amantadine in the treatment of sexual dysfunction associated with fluoxetine use.

Parker, James N., and Philip M. Parker, eds. *The Official Patient's Sourcebook on Impotence*. San Diego, Calif.: Icon Health, 2002. Draws from public, academic, government, and peer-reviewed research to provide a wide-ranging handbook for patients with impotence.

Phillips, Nancy A. "Female Sexual Dysfunction: Evaluation and Treatment." *American Family Physician* 62, no. 1 (July 1, 2000): 127-136. Sexual dysfunction includes desire, arousal, orgasmic, and sex pain disorders. Basic treatment strategies, which may be successfully provided by primary care physicians for most sexual dysfunctions, are discussed.

Taguchi, Yosh, and Merrily Weisbord, eds. *Private Parts: An Owner's Guide to the Male Anatomy*. 3d ed. Toronto, Ont.: McClelland & Stewart, 2003. A guide to male genital and sexual health, covering topics such as prostate trouble, erectile dysfunction, infertility, cancer, sexually transmitted diseases, vasectomies, and artificial insemination.

Sexual reassignment

Procedure

Key terms:

cisgender: a person whose sense of gender   identity

r identitycorresponds to the designation given at birth

feminizing genitoplasty: male-to-female surgical procedures including penectomy, orchiectomy, and
vaginoplasty

gender: the properties of organisms based on their reproductive roles

genderdysphoria: discomfort or anxiety that arises with
discontent with one's biological sex, with desire for another sex's physical characteristics and role

intersex: genitalia that are not absolutely identifiable as either male or female

masculinizing vaginoplasty: female-to-male surgical procedures including metoidioplasty and phalloplasty

trans man: a person born female who has transitioned to
male

trans woman: a person born male who has transitioned to
female

transition: the process of assuming the sexual identity that
is congruent with one's own private and subjective experience; this process may or may not include medical assistance such as cross-gender hormone replacement or
surgery

transgender: an umbrella term for anyone whose sense of
gender identity does not correspond to the designation
given at birth (gender-variant people); includes transsexual people

transsexual: one who wishes to assume a sexual identity
different from that assigned at birth, or someone who has
undergone surgery to change the sexual organs; pertains
to sexual characteristics but not necessarily to sexual
activities

Indications

At or before birth a baby's sex is assigned based on the
child's external genitalia. When a child's genitals are ambiguous, sometimes called intersex, generally a sex is assigned based on the sex that appears to be predominant.
Even in the absence of ambiguity and even well before puberty, some people feel a gender identity that differs from
the sex that was biologically assigned. The unease that this
disparity evokes is called gender dysphoria.

People whose gender identity differs from their anatomic
sex are transgender people, sometimes known as
transgendered. When a woman feels that the sex she was
assigned at birth is not who she is, she may either dress and
act as a man or elect to undergo surgery known as female-
to-male reassignment to bring her body more into line with
her sexual identity; a man whose sexual identity is female
may identify as female or undergo male-to-female surgical
procedures. When people transition from one sex to another, they are considered transsexual. The process of sexual reassignment is known as gender-confirmation surgery
or sex-reconstruction surgery.

Although many transgendered people report that they
felt gender dysphoria in childhood, one study found that
most do not disclose these feelings to their families until
later in their teens. Living with such unspoken disparity is
hard, and mental illness rates are higher in the
transgendered than in the cisgendered. In addition,
transgendered people are often targets of violence—which

may be self-inflicted. According to a 2010 study,
transgender people attempt suicide at a rate 25 times higher
than do the cisgendered. Childhood can be a time of trial for
anyone. For the transgendered, support from the family is
particularly important yet is available only for the fortunate. It is noteworthy that mental health has been shown to
improve in young transgendered people who transition
surgically.

Procedures

People who experience gender dysphoria may elect to undergo sex-reassignment surgery (SRS, also called by a variety of terms including gender-reassignment surgery, gen-
der-affirming surgery, sex-realignment surgery, sex-
reconstruction surgery, or gender-confirmation surgery).
The procedure (singular or several) seeks to alter physical
appearance and existing sexual organs to more closely resemble those of the gender with which the transgendered
person identifies.

In 1931 Berlin Dora Richter had the first known
vaginoplasty, which consisted simply of removing the penis; other such surgeries followed suit. The limits of this
disfigurement soon became apparent, and surgeons began
to develop more complex and, for the patient, satisfying
SRS procedures. The process was technically complex, but
also hampered by reluctance on the part of many medical
practitioners, in effect, to fix that which wasn't broken.
Over time, however, the medical community and families
of the transgendered began to be convinced that, to the afflicted, gender dysphoria is all too real and, in fact, might
be capable of being 'fixed'.

As demand for the surgeries continued, a 1992 study
found that 98.5% of those undergoing male-to-female surgeries, and 99% of those who underwent female-to-male
surgeries, did not regret their decisions. It may be prefera-
ble, when possible, to transit earlier in life, prior to puberty,
as trans people may experience considerable distress as
their bodies begin to show characteristics that they feel are
alien. Transgender surgery in people past puberty is also
complicated by the difference in pubic bones between the
sexes, as to accommodate childbirth a biological woman's
pelvis is wider and larger and set at a more obtuse angle
than a man's. Many variations in surgical procedures have
been tried and are as yet being devised. Although most
transgender surgeries go as planned, surgeons are human
and surgical mishaps do occasionally occur. Even when all
goes as planned SRS is in almost every case a lifetime commitment that before being undertaken must be thoroughly
considered and understood. With or without surgery,
hormone-replacement therapy has its own impacts, some
of which are noted below.

Male-to-Female SRS

Any procedure to construct a vagina is called vaginoplasty
(including surgical reconstruction following removal of
growths or to correct prolapse or congenital defects). Genital reconstruction for trans women often involves surgical
inversion of the penis to construct a vagina. Inversion

techniques using segments of the sigmoid colon or small intestine rather than the penis may produce a better semblance to genitals of cisgender women. Skin flaps from the penis and scrotum, sometimes in combination with a urethral flap, or nongenital skin grafts from other body parts may also be used. The neovagina may be lined with skin from the inferior pedicle or abdomen. The urethra is shortened and reoriented.

Ancillary procedures to more closely align with cisgender women include removal of testes (orchiectomy) and, if not inverted, penis (penectomy).

Trans women may choose aesthetic procedures such as breast augmentation and hair implants, and surgeries to feminize their facial contours.

Complications. Sex differences in pubic architecture, noted above, can make it difficult to allow sufficient septal thickness between the rectal wall and the neovagina; resultant weakness can cause fistula (tearing). When a vagina has been constructed, without sufficient post-surgical dilation the inner skin graft can shrink or collapse. In shortening the urethra, stricture (narrowing) may occur but is usually reparable.

Female-to-Male SRS

Genital reconstruction for trans men entails formation of a penis through phalloplasty or metoidioplasty. Phalloplasty involves extending the urethra with a tubed flap of tissue from another part of the body. During a second surgery, an erectile prosthesis may be implanted.

For metoidioplasty (sometimes known as metaoidioplasty), provision of testosterone gradually enlarges the clitoris to the point where it can be removed from the labia minora and lowered to the position occupied by the penis. Erectile tissue in the enlarged clitoris functions normally, as the clitoris develops from the same embryonic tissue as does the penis. The urethra need not be extended for metoidioplasty and thus is less expensive and has fewer complications, but then standing urination is no longer an option.

Technically, metoidioplasty is less complex and less expensive than phalloplasty. But, once recovered from surgery, people who have undergone phalloplasty are often more able to complete sexual penetration. This may be in part because the enlarged clitoris may not be capable of attaining the rigidity of a penis.

Medically assisted transition for trans men may include mastectomy and further surgical shaping of a male-contoured chest. Trans men may also undergo hysterectomy and removal of ovaries and Fallopian tubes (salpingo-oophorectomy).

Complications. Because the urethra of a trans man must be lengthened significantly, complications are more likely to occur. Postoperatively, about a quarter of patients in one study who had had their urethrae elongated had transient swelling that caused some urine dribbling, but this subsided without medical intervention. Trans men who had had the urethra extended had small changes of strictures, or narrowing of the urethra, or of a fistula, or hole in the ure-

thra, needing minor repair. Chest surgery to remove breasts will leave scarring. The nipples may have reduced sensation, and their placement may be asymmetrical.

HRT Effects

For transitions accompanied by hormones (hormone-replacement therapy), trans men will probably use testosterone in one of its forms, be it injectable, topically as a cream or gel, applied via patch, or by a pellet subcutaneously inserted; trans women may block their testosterone with an antiandrogen, commonly called a "t-blocker", while receiving estrogen and progesterone.

Although hormones have effects in everyone, often we overlook or minimize them. Sex hormones are the same for men and women, but their ratios differ across genders as well as being affected by time. Receiving hormones from the identified sex can ease the path of transition, but the unaccustomed influx can also rock one's psychic boat.

Some generalities apply. For trans men, previously unexperienced testosterone levels can affect the emotions, pushing anger up the roster of options. For trans women, as breasts develop they may not only be tender, but may leak milky fluid as well. Testosterone may cause hair to sprout in unexpected and perhaps inconvenient places, or familial baldness may wreak havoc on the hairline. For anyone receiving cross-gender HRT, acne may be worse this second time around and may even appear in places never before afflicted. Finally, when produced by hormones from a whole new quadrant, sexual desire may feel bafflingly unfamiliar.

Perspective and Prospects

Regardless of age, most people feel that they belong to a particular gender. Is that feeling of gender determined by the shape of our sex organs or by chemicals such as enzymes and hormones? If not, what causes it?

Because despite individual variations the structure of male and female brains varies slightly, some have questioned whether the brains of transgender people are more like their gender identities than their assigned gender. When Spanish investigators in one small study made MRI investigations of brains of a small number of female-to-male and male-to-female people, both before and after cross-sex hormonal treatment, results indicated that even before being treated the brains of transgendered people were in some ways more resembled the brains of their identified gender than those of their assigned gender. Subcortical areas, which tend to be thinner in men, were relatively thin in female-to-male subjects, while male-to-female subjects showed thinner right-hemisphere cortices, more characteristic of female brains. After hormonal treatment, these effects became more evident. But these researchers believe it an oversimplification to say that one sex is improperly housed in a body of the wrong sex. Instead, they propose that transgender people have transsexual brains.

The idea that being transgendered arises from hormonal imbalance has been debunked. A recent study in young people who do not identify with their assigned sex showed congruence between natally assigned sex and hormonal status; in other words, their sex hormones were in alignment with their anatomical sex. So if someone assigned to be female at birth because of possessing female genitalia has the same mix of estrogen, progesterone, and testosterone as did her mother, yet feels and has always felt male, it is not because of hormones.

Has a transgender gene been found? The short answer at this time is no. As embryos we all start as both genders with two sets of undeveloped (or ambiguous) gonads. Around the sixth week of development one of two things happens. Either a gene turns on and the female organs fade away, or that gene is silent and the female organs flourish; in either case the male organs do the converse. In most cases, that is. Mutations in engaged genes or chromosomes may subvert the process. Other mishaps may occur; receptors may not bind the sex hormones that should dock there, enzymes that ignite sex characteristics may misfire, a hormonal cascade may be torrential or constrained. From without, drugs and chemicals not intended for fetal acquaintance may find their way in and wreak changes. How these and other potentialities are timed and interact cannot but introduce uncertainties.

Not everyone considers sexuality a polarity of male or female; black to white encompasses an infinity of shades. The term transgender includes not only people whose gender identity differs from their assigned sex, but also those occupying various places along the spectrum of one sex to its opposite; bigender, pangender, agender. To be transgendered (the sex that one is) is not the same as sexual orientation (the sex that one prefers sexually); it differs as well from intersexed, which describes people born with ambiguous sex organs. Being transgendered may be more congruent with one's identity as heterosexual, homosexual, bisexual, asexual, or any variant. Or maybe it deserves a category of its own. But there is nothing physiologically wrong; there is nothing to 'cure'. (It is well to be mindful that, while transitioning to one's gender identity may solve one big problem, others may stubbornly persist.) All the same, the courage and openness of people like Caitlin Jenner, Chaz Bono, and Chelsea Manning has helped to bring awareness of the gender-atypical experience to the gender-typical population.

Although the mysteries behind our differences are yet to be unraveled, in the end only we can decide who we are.

—*Jackie Dial, PhD*

See also: Gender; Gender dysphoria; Gender reassignment; Genitoplasty; Orchiectomy; Penectomy; Sex realignment; Transgender; Vaginoplasty

For Further Information:

Lewis, Ricki. "Is Transgender Identity Inherited?" *DNAScience Blog*, March 2, 2017. Web August 27, 2017. http://blogs.plos.org/dnascience/2017/03/02/is-transgender-identity-inherited/

Olson, Johanna et al. "Baseline Physiologic and Psychosocial Characteristics of Transgender Youth Seeking Care for Gender Dysphoria." *Journal of Adolescent Health*, October 2015, 57:4: 374-380. Web August 10, 2017. http://www.jahonline.org/article/S1054-139X(15)00216-5/fulltext

Rogers, Ashley Lauren. "Eight Things That Really Happen When Transgender People Start Hormone Therapy." *Cosmopolitan*, September 29, 2015. Web August 14, 2017. http://www.cosmopolitan.com/sex-love/news/a46391/things-that-really-happen-when-trans-people-start-hormone-therapy/

Russo, Francine. "Is There Something Unique about the Transgender Brain?" *Scientific American*, January 1, 2016. Web August 10, 2017. https://www.scientificamerican.com/article/is-there-something-unique-about-the-transgender-brain/

Wanjek, Christopher. "Being Transgender Has Nothing to Do with Hormonal Imbalance." *LiveScience*, July 23, 2015. Web August10, 2017. https://www.livescience.com/51652-transgender-youth-dont-have-hormonal-imbalance.html

Sexuality

Biology

Anatomy or system affected: Genitals, psychic-emotional system, reproductive system

Specialties and related fields: Family medicine, genetics, gynecology, internal medicine, obstetrics, pediatrics, psychiatry, psychology

Definition: A complex, multidimensional, umbrella term referring to the identification of masculine and feminine gender, qualities associated with each gender, capacities for erotic stimulation, behaviors causing erotic stimulation, the biology of reproduction, and fundamental elements of individual personality and personal identity that relate to these; sexuality has procreative, recreational, and relational dimensions.

Key terms:

bisexuality: the capacity to be sexually attracted to and aroused by both genders; the term also implies a significant and consistent capacity for such arousal and does not refer to occasional attraction to or activity with both genders

celibacy: originally meaning "unmarried," it also refers to the willful or circumstantial refraining from sexual intercourse and, by implication, erotic behavior; though sometimes misconstrued as asexual, celibates are no less sexual than noncelibates

erogenous zones: bodily areas that are especially sensitive to touch, leading to sexual arousal; although a dozen or so such zones are common (for example, the clitoral glans and labia, penile glans and shaft, breasts, buttocks, inner thighs), these zones can differ from person to person

erotic: referring to sensory perceptions that are sensual (gratifying or pleasurable) and sexual; the context in which they occur will determine whether the perceptions become erotic (for example, breast and testicle examinations are typically not erotic, while caressing these same body parts in romantic settings typically is)

gender: strictly speaking, the behavioral and social aspects of being either a girl/woman or a boy/man; the term is more loosely used to refer to the biological and physical aspects of being male or female as well

gender identity: a person's inner sense and feeling of maleness/masculinity or femaleness/femininity, or both; it implies that one clearly identifies with one gender more than the other, although some people identify with both genders equally or near equally

gender role: behaviors and self-presentations that are

associated with being a boy/man or a girl/woman and that one uses to identify or recognize others as a boy/man or a girl/woman; the term also implies the sociocultural expectations of boys/men and girls/women

heterosexual: being principally attracted to and aroused by a person of the opposite gender; a synonymous term, "straight," refers to persons of either gender who are primarily heterosexual

homophobia: obsessive fear of and anxiety about homosexuals and their social and sexual activities; while several causes of homophobia are known, the most common is a homophobe's private, often unconscious fear and doubt about his or her own sexuality and sense of sexual adequacy

homosexual: being principally attracted to and aroused by persons of one's own gender; two synonymous terms are "gay," which can refer to all homosexuals or to homosexual boys/men exclusively, and "lesbian," which refers only to homosexual girls/women

Historical Overview

Sexuality is usually manifested and experienced as orientation toward and attraction to people of the same gender, the opposite gender, or both. Sexual orientation is also referred to as "sexual preference." The term "preference," however, can imply that sexual attraction and orientation are chosen and voluntary, that one can will oneself to find another person sexually appealing. In fact, most research suggests the opposite: People find themselves attracted to an individual or a particular gender without having thought about that attraction or having consciously willed it. The attraction and orientation are not chosen. People can wish not to be attracted in the ways that they are, and they may choose not to act on these feelings, but the attraction felt and experienced is outside voluntary control.

A female athlete may wish not to have the sexual feelings she does for her teammates. A male chemistry major may want himself not to find a female classmate as distracting as she is. A female attorney who is happily married may want the sexual feelings she experiences for her male client to cease. A celibate priest may desire the sexual feelings that he has toward some male and female members of his congregation to go away. As much as these individuals may want to will such feelings away, success in this endeavor is unlikely. Each, instead, must choose how to cope with the feelings, from acting on them directly, to carrying on in spite of them, to pretending that the feelings are not there.

The historical evidence suggests that the prevailing belief in most societies was that people had either a homosexual or a heterosexual orientation; regardless of what made people attracted to their own or to the opposite gender, sexual orientation was "either-or." In the twentieth century, most social scientists and sex researchers came to think about sexual orientation as lying on a continuum marked by degrees of likelihood of finding one's own or the opposite gender attractive. Sexologist Alfred C. Kinsey and his associates published their landmark works, *Sexual Behavior in the Human Male* in 1948 and *Sexual Behavior in the Human Female* in 1953, in which they used a continuum of sexual orientation to quantify a range of attraction, from those who found only members of the opposite gender attractive (whom they defined as "heterosexual") to those who found only members of the same gender attractive (whom they defined as "homosexual"). Between the two extremes were the majority of people, who find both genders attractive and arousing in varying degrees-and thus are defined as "bisexual."

In determining sexual orientation, researchers once focused on the gender of sex partners, which also was the criterion on which laypersons generally focused. If a male usually had female partners, they would consider him heterosexual; if a female usually had female partners, they would consider her homosexual. Yet sexual orientation, how one is attracted by and toward others, is more accurately considered to be primarily the subjective experience of how one feels inside, not the overt behavior that one demonstrates outside.

Research has shown that, in any given individual, there can be a large discrepancy between the gender of one's actual partners and the gender to which one is more attracted and drawn. Social and cultural circumstances often affect, even determine, whether one will behave the way one feels. People who are primarily attracted to opposite-gender persons may be influenced to have, and even pursue, same-gender partners by particular religious beliefs, certain restricted environments (such as prison), or the sense that this behavior is or is not permissible. Orientation is better understood in the minds and feelings of persons themselves: which gender attracts, how often, and how much. Personal histories that include procreating children, marriage, homosexual activities, and bisexual experimentation should not be used to identify sexual orientation.

Although many studies followed the early work of Kinsey, most experts believe that Kinsey and his colleagues produced the most valid observations about sexuality and sexual orientation. Conducting research in this field is difficult. Different studies use different survey tools, and not all are equally reliable. In addition, many people will not candidly or honestly discuss their sexual attitudes, attractions, or behaviors. Nevertheless, the best estimates that rely and build on the Kinsey group's earlier work suggest that about 10 percent of the population in Western countries is primarily gay or lesbian and that an additional 10 percent of the population is primarily bisexual. (There is less research available on non-Western nations, and much of what is available is methodologically less reliable.) In the United States, 60 million people are likely to be homosexual or bisexual. Far more important than the numbers, however, is the reality that gay, lesbian, and bisexual orientations are neither unusual nor peculiar. This remains true even though heterosexuality is the more common pattern of most people, most of the time-a finding true for all societies ever studied. Yet a minority pattern of attraction cannot, simply on the basis of numbers, be considered abnormal.

Expert and lay opinions about how sexual orientation develops differ, often considerably. Yet expert, if not lay, opinions do converge about when it develops: at about age four or five, which is a year to two earlier than when experts believe an individual's personal traits and characteristics emerge intact as an identifiable personality. Because erotic behavior and erogenous stimuli do not usually become an important part of one's personal world until puberty begins (the developmental marker used to interpret when childhood ends and adolescence begins), many do not learn what their orientation is until late adolescence or even well into adulthood. People who eventually come to have nearly exclusive heterosexual fantasies, attractions, and sexual affiliations often have had earlier, adolescent homosexual experiences. Likewise, people who eventually come to discover that their orientation is strongly homosexual have often married, borne children, and had long periods of gratifying heterosexual dating experiences.

Most people eventually come to identify their orientation, at least implicitly, in terms of direction and strength. Direction refers to the direction of sexual orientation, toward one's own or one's opposite gender. Strength refers to the degree of exclusivity associated with the direction of one's orientation: attracted only by the same or opposite gender, sometimes attracted by each, always attracted to each.

Bidirectional orientation is the least researched and least understood of sexual orientations. As with homosexual and heterosexual behavior, bisexual encounters, even if gratifying, do not in themselves mean that someone is bisexually oriented, and therefore bisexual. All sexual orientation is internal, not behavioral.

Some people, while learning about their sexual selves and their accompanying orientation, engage in experimental bisexual behavior. Some, with limited access to the gender toward which they are more predominantly or exclusively oriented, become sexually active with the gender toward which they are not oriented but which is more available. Some are sexually active with both genders for money. Some are sexually stimulated and aroused regardless of gender. (William H. Masters and Virginia E. Johnson, perhaps the leading sex researchers and sex educators of all time, label this group "ambisexual.") Some indicate that they have a definite orientation toward sexual activity with both genders. Among this last group, there are those who report having long-term, one-gender relationships that followed long-term, other-gender relationships, and there are others who report having concurrent sexual relationships with partners of both genders.

Although descriptions of active bisexuality are readily available in the research, the sheer variety of patterns substantially challenges research-based understandings of how sexual orientation originates and develops. What is known is that people with bisexual orientations are neither poorer nor better psychologically adjusted than heterosexuals or homosexuals, and that bisexuality, while poorly understood, reflects a comfortable and fulfilling sexual life and identity for a significant percentage of the general population.

Theories of Sexual Orientation

No other area of sexuality has generated more interest, theory, or research than orientation and how it originates. No one theory stands alone as proven, and not-yet-explained data shake the foundations of even the most useful theories. Nevertheless, scientific inquiry has disproven many earlier theories. The most promising theories fall into several categories, some of which can overlap to a degree: genetic, hormonal, psychodynamic, parental, familial, behavioral, societal, and cultural.

The first significant study of genetic causality for sexual orientation was published in 1952. The research compared one group of male identical twins with one group of male fraternal twins. In both groups, one twin was known to be homosexually oriented. Reasonably assuming that both twins of a pair would be exposed to essentially the same environments, the study counted how many second twins, whose sexual orientations were unknown at the start of the study, were also gay. If the rate of homosexuality for twins was higher among the group of identical twins than in the group of fraternal twins, it would be evidence that genetic makeup, which is virtually the same between identical twins, the main cause of sexual orientation.

Twelve percent of fraternal twins who were homosexual had a homosexual twin. Because male fraternal twins are genetically as similar and dissimilar as any pair of brothers, and the rate of homosexuality among the fraternal set was close to the rates that the Kinsey group found in the general population, the results were initially considered a breakthrough. The study also showed, however, that the twin of every known homosexual in the identical set was also homosexual. One hundred percent concordance rates are rare in studies of identical twins (even studies which might compare heights or weights between identical twins would not achieve 100 percent concordance) and are almost nonexistent in all other social groups on any variable ever studied. This particular study and its unique finding needed replication to be believed. Two later studies, published in 1968 and 1976, had quite different results, and the view that sexual orientation was principally a product of genetic conditions and variability was abandoned, though most researchers still believe genetics provides contributory influence.

Investigation into the role that hormonal factors play in sexual orientation divides between research on animals and research on humans. Studies clearly show that altering prenatal hormone exposure leads to male or female homosexual behavior in at least several animal species. Among humans, a number of studies have had findings that link prenatal exposure to specific sexual orientation outcomes. For example, females who were exposed to male hormones (androgens), especially testosterone, were more likely to develop lesbian orientations; males with Kleinfelter's syndrome, a chromosomal abnormality marked by a deficiency in androgens, are known to develop gay orientations at a greater frequency than the population average.

Other research on humans has shown that there are different hormone levels between adult homosexuals and heterosexuals. Some studies have found lower testosterone in homosexual males, some have found higher levels of estrogens (though present in both sexes, they are usually considered female hormones) in homosexual males, and other studies have found both. At least one study found higher blood testosterone in homosexual females than heterosexual females.

While this evidence seems illuminating on the surface, it is far from conclusive. First, although many studies show different hormone levels between heterosexual and homosexual persons, several studies have also found hormone levels to be the same in both groups. Second, administering sex hormones to adults does not affect their orientation in any way. Third, prenatal overexposure or underexposure to sex hormones is relatively rare. It would not account for the differences in orientation that are observed in the general adult population, nor is it beyond reason to view cases of abnormal hormonal prenatal environments as extraordinary and unrepresentative of how sexual orientation usually develops. Fourth, while animal studies often describe processes in particular species that are readily analogous to processes in humans, this does not seem to be the case with human sexuality in general or human sexual orientation in particular.

What seems clear is that there is no one-to-one link between sex hormones and sexual orientation. Prenatal hormones, which are known to influence brain development in many ways, may play an indirect role in predisposing individuals toward adapting certain adult sexual behavioral patterns of greater or lesser bisexuality.

Psychodynamic explanations focus on the nature of parent-child relationships and how parents encourage or discourage the growth of their children. Several studies showed homosexual males to have been reared in homes where mothers were dominant and overprotective and fathers were weak, passive, or emotionally uninvolved, a family constellation seen with less statistical frequency among heterosexual males. Other studies, however, showed strained, distant relationships between homosexual men and their fathers but could not find evidence of maternal dominance and overprotectiveness. One study even described the fathers of homosexual males as underprotective, generous, good, and dominant, while the mothers were not found to be overly protective or bossy. Another study simply found no differences in family constellation and dynamics between psychologically well-adjusted heterosexual and homosexual males and females. Given the varied results, the research outcomes from psychodynamic, parental, and familial studies lack cohesive evidence that homosexuality or any orientation results from poor parent-child relationships or dysfunctional family environments.

Behavioral, societal, and cultural theories assume that orientation is primarily learned as people become culturally assimilated and psychologically conditioned (rewarded and punished) for specific sexual feelings, thoughts, and behaviors. Therefore, in an environment where homoerotic feelings were accepted and valued, people would be more likely to develop homosexual, and perhaps bisexual, orientations. In an environment where homophobic attitudes were considered the norm, homoerotic feelings would more likely be abandoned. While these theories have utility in explaining certain sociological phenomena such as atypical gender role behavior (for example, tomboys) and observed shifts toward lesbian sexuality among some female rape victims, they seem to have less utility in explaining how orientation develops in the majority of the population.

Perspective and Prospects

Although answers to the question of how orientation develops are complex, researchers Alan P. Bell, Martin S. Weinberg, and S. K. Hammersmith published the two-volume work *Sexual Preference: Its Development in Men and Women* (1981) in an attempt to reveal the causal chain of sexual orientation development in more than thirteen hundred adult homosexual, heterosexual, and bisexual men and women. They based their findings both on lengthy face-to-face interviews with every person in their study and on a sophisticated and reliable statistical technique called path analysis.

Bell, Weinberg, and Hammersmith's research represents the most extensive collection of data on a large number of people in existence, and most experts are taking at least some of their findings to be conclusive. These results show that sexual orientation is strongly established in most people by late adolescence and that sexual feelings rarely undergo directional changes in adulthood. Atypical gender role behavior in childhood, such as boys preferring to play with dolls and not having an interest in more competitive activities, was found to be more likely than not to proceed homosexual orientations in adolescence and adulthood. Adult homosexuals and bisexuals had, on average, the same amount of heterosexual experience as heterosexual adolescents, though their heterosexual experiences were less rewarding and enjoyable than either their own homosexual experiences or the heterosexual experiences of heterosexuals. The study found that girls choosing their fathers as role models does not cause these girls to become lesbian (as several theories had maintained) and that the parental combination of a domineering, powerful mother and a weak, inadequate father does not cause homosexuality in males (as was once believed).

Although their study was methodologically well planned and statistically sound, Bell, Weinberg, and Hammersmith could not find solid support for any of the prevailing theories about the causality of sexual orientation. Some theories explain some of the observed data, and some theories seem to enhance understanding of the origins of sexual orientation in some elements of the population, but no theory or combination of theories explains all the data.

If this research has moved medical science along to some degree, it also serves to remind everyone, professional and nonprofessional alike, that the very complexity of human experience and how humans develop their identity warrants caution if it is ever to be accurately understood. The evidence is not complete. It is known that some aspects of the theories of the origins of sexual orientation are true and that others are false.

Learning one's own sexual orientation is a complex process requiring self-observation, self-reflection, and self-recollection. People discover what they like and who they like; the content and orientation of their sexual fantasies; and which gender feels closer to their sexual identity as persons (rather than the gender role that they feel a societal obligation to play). It is their own experiences of what is, and is not, sexually gratifying that teaches people how they are oriented sexually.

—*Paul Moglia, Ph.D.*

See also Aphrodisiacs; Erectile dysfunction; Gender identity disorder; Gender reassignment surgery; Hormones; Masturbation; Men's health; Precocious puberty; Psychiatry; Psychiatry, child and adolescent; Psychiatry, geriatric; Psychoanalysis; Puberty and adolescence; Reproductive system; Sexual differentiation; Sexual dysfunction; Sexually transmitted diseases (STDs); Women's health.

For Further Information:

Berzon, Betty. *Permanent Partners: Building Gay and Lesbian Relationships That Last*. Rev. ed. New York: Plume, 2004. A practical, realistic guide for same-gender partners in primary relationships. Berzon addresses the main conflict and confusing areas of relationships typically experienced by gay and lesbian couples.

Byer, Curtis O., Louis W. Shainberg, and Grace Galliano. *Dimensions of Human Sexuality*. 6th ed. Revised by Sharon P. Shriver. Boston: McGraw-Hill, 2002. An excellent, thorough, well-organized textbook on all areas of sexuality, with highlighted topics of special interest.

Corinna, Heather. *S.E.X.: The All-You-Need-to-Know Progressive Sexuality Guide to Get You Through High School and College*. New York: Marlowe, 2007. A candid discussion of sex and sexuality for teenagers and young adults. Topics include anatomy, sexual orientation and sexual identity, relationships, safer-sex practices, sexual abuse and rape, pregnancy and contraception, and sexually transmitted diseases, including HIV.

Dibble, Suzanne L., and Patricia A. Robertson. *Lesbian Health 101: A Clinician's Guide*. San Francisco: UCSF Nursing Press, 2010. The first comprehensive textbook on lesbian health for clinicians and students. Helpful to general readers as well. Also provides insight into women's health in general.

Fairchild, Betty, and Nancy Hayward. *Now That You Know: A Parent's Guide to Understanding Their Gay and Lesbian Children*. 3d ed. San Diego, Calif.: Harcourt Brace, 1998. A standard and compassionate reference for families with gay sons or lesbian daughters. Discusses the nature of homosexuality, counsels parents on how to respond supportively to gay and lesbian children, and informs parents on the pressing health and emotional issues that affect gays and lesbians.

Katz, Jonathan Ned. *The Invention of Heterosexuality*. Chicago: University of Chicago Press, 2007. Using the now-well-known premise of homosexuality as socially constructed, Katz, in this classic work, explores heterosexuality as a social construct as well.

Masters, William H., Virginia E. Johnson, and Robert C. Kolodny. *Human Sexuality*. 5th ed. New York: HarperCollins College, 1995. A well-organized, highly readable textbook covering biological, psychological, social, cultural, ethical, and religious perspectives on human sexuality.

Strong, Bryan, et al. *Human Sexuality: Diversity in Contemporary America*. 6th ed. Boston: McGraw-Hill, 2008. Excellent coverage of human sexuality and the differences and similarities across ethnicities, cultures, genders, and sexual orientations.

Sexually transmitted diseases (STDs)

Disease/Disorder

Also known as: Venereal diseases

Anatomy or system affected: Genitals, reproductive system

Specialties and related fields: Epidemiology, gynecology, internal medicine, public health, urology, virology

Definition: Diseases acquired through sexual contact or passed from a pregnant woman to her fetus, including diseases such as syphilis, gonorrhea, chlamydia, genital herpes, genital warts, viral hepatitis, and acquired immunodeficiency syndrome (AIDS).

Key terms:

antibody: a protein found in the blood and produced by the immune system in response to contact of the body with a foreign substance

asymptomatic: an infection without any symptoms

bacteria: microscopic single-celled organisms that multiply by means of simple division; bacteria are found everywhere, and most are beneficial-only a few species cause disease

immunity: the capacity to resist a disease caused by an infectious agent

infertility: the inability to produce offspring by a person in the childbearing years who has been having sex without contraception for twelve months

inflammation: a response of the body to tissue damage caused by injury or infection and characterized by redness, pain, heat, and swelling

latent: lying hidden or undeveloped within a person; unrevealed

pelvic inflammatory disease (PID): an extensive bacterial infection of the pelvic organs, such as the uterus, cervix, Fallopian tubes, and ovaries

protozoan: a single-celled organism that is more closely related to animals than are bacteria; only a few drugs are available that will kill protozoa without harming their animal hosts

virus: a noncellular particle of protein and nucleic acid; viruses, which can reproduce only inside cells, usually cause damage to their hosts by killing the cells they enter

Causes and Symptoms

Sexually transmitted diseases, or STDs (formerly called venereal diseases), have plagued humankind for centuries. The most prevalent, serious STDs are syphilis, gonorrhea, nongonococcal urethritis, trichomoniasis, genital herpes, genital warts, viral hepatitis, and AIDS. Others, troublesome but not as serious, include lice, scabies, and vaginal yeast infections. They are passed on from one person to another mostly by sexual contact, although some of these diseases may be acquired indirectly through contaminated objects or blood. In addition, nearly all these diseases can be passed on from an infected mother to her fetus, which may cause birth defects, severe and damaging infections, or even death. A person can acquire several STDs at the same time, and since recovery from an STD does not confer immunity, a person can get them again and again. Many of these diseases are asymptomatic, which allows them to spread and cause serious complications before a victim is

---

**Information on
Sexually Transmitted Diseases (STDs)**

Causes: Infection through sexual contact; also from contaminated blood or from infected mother to fetus

Symptoms: Varies; may include skin lesions or rash in genital area, itching, abdominal pain, painful urination, vaginal or penile discharge, birth defects, infertility

Duration: Acute to chronic with recurrent episodes

Treatments: Antibiotics, antiviral agents

---

aware of being infected. Finally, some STDs are treatable and some are not.

Syphilis is caused by *Treponema pallidum*. This bacterium normally infects the penis in males and the vagina or cervix in females, but it can also enter through a cut on the mouth or other parts of the skin. Once inside, the bacteria grow at the site of entry, then spread throughout the body through the lymph and blood vessels. The symptoms of syphilis are caused by the efforts of the immune response of the patient to fight off the infection. The disease occurs in three stages: primary, secondary, and tertiary. In primary syphilis, a flat, firm, painless, red sore called a chancre appears at the site of entry two to ten weeks after infection. Secondary syphilis is characterized by a red rash that appears two to ten weeks after the disappearance of the primary lesion. The rash will disappear in a few weeks. Without treatment, 40 percent of patients will progress to the tertiary stage within three to ten years. Tertiary syphilis is characterized by the formation of severe lesions called gummas on the skin, bones, or internal organs. Gummas on the spinal cord, brain, or heart can lead to seizures, insanity, or death. Almost all pregnant women with untreated primary or secondary syphilis will transmit the bacteria through the placenta to the developing baby, who will develop congenital syphilis. Many babies with congenital syphilis are spontaneously aborted or stillborn. Many others are born with characteristic birth defects, secondary or tertiary syphilis, or neurological damage, and may die shortly after birth.

Gonorrhea is caused by the *Neisseria gonorrhoeae* bacterium (also known as gonococcus). The bacterium infects the urethra in males and the cervix, vagina, or urethra in females. Most infected males get urethritis (inflammation of the urethra) along with symptoms of a pus-containing discharge from the penis and painful urination. Untreated, 1 percent of these men will develop complications of urethral blockage, epididymitis (inflammation of the epididymis, a sac through which sperm passes as it leaves the testicles), prostatitis (inflammation of the prostate, a gland that secretes fluid for semen), and infertility. Between 20 and 80 percent of women infected with gonococcus are asymptomatic or show only mild symptoms. Symptoms include burning or high frequency of urination, vaginal discharge, fever, and abdominal pain. In 20 to 30 percent of untreated women, gonococcus will spread to the Fallopian tubes and cause pelvic inflammatory disease (PID), which can lead to

infertility. Infected mothers can transmit the bacteria to their babies as they pass through the birth canal, causing ophthalmia neonatorum, a type of conjunctivitis (inflammation of the eye) that can cause blindness if untreated.

Most cases of nongonococcal urethritis (NGU) are caused by *Chlamydia trachomatis* types *d* through *k*. This bacterium infects the urethra in males and the cervix or urethra in females. The symptoms of chlamydia infection are often mild and go unnoticed. Males experience mild urethritis with a watery discharge, frequent urination, and painful urination. Females are either asymptomatic or experience mild cervicitis (inflammation of the cervix) or urethritis. Complications include epididymitis in males and PID and infertility in females. Infants born to mothers with cervicitis can develop eye (inclusion conjunctivitis) or lung (infant pneumonia) infections.

Trichomoniasis is caused by the protozoan *Trichomonas vaginalis*. In both sexes, the disease is often mild or asymptomatic. In males, the organism infects the prostate, seminal vesicles, and urethra. About 10 percent of infected males show signs of mild urethritis, with a thin, white urethral discharge. Secondary bacterial infection can lead to more severe urethritis and inflammation of the prostate and seminal vesicles. In females, the organism can infect the vulva, vagina, and cervix. Females may suffer from severe vaginitis, which includes a tender, red, and itchy genital area, and a profuse, frothy, foul-smelling, greenish-yellow discharge. Newborns may acquire the infection from an infected mother during delivery.

Most genital herpes infections are caused by herpes simplex virus type 2, but some are caused by herpes simplex virus type 1. The virus infects the penis in males and the cervix, vulva, vagina, or perineum in females. Two to seven days after infection, painful blisters appear in the genital area that ulcerate, crust over, and disappear in a few weeks. Herpesviruses are unique in that they can remain latent in the nerves and cause a recurrent infection at any time in the future. Fever, stress, sunlight, or local trauma may trigger the virus to come out of hiding and cause a recurrent infection. The virus can be transmitted from an infected mother to her baby either congenitally, through the placenta, or neonatally, as the baby passes through the birth canal. In congenital or neonatal herpes, the virus can infect all parts of the body, the death rate is high, and survivors commonly

---

Cases of Sexually Transmitted Diseases in the United States

(as reported by State Health Departments)

Year	Syphilis (all stages)	Chlamydia	Gonorrhea
1985	67,563	25,848	911,419
1995	69,358	478,577	392,651
2005	33,278	976,445	339,593

Source: Centers for Disease Control and Prevention (CDC).

have long-term neurological damage and recurrent infections.

Viral hepatitis is also an STD. At least three variants of the virus-hepatitis A virus (HAV), HBV, and HCV-are known to be transmitted sexually. HBV is the form most commonly transmitted sexually. Vaccines are available to immunize persons at risk for HAV and for HBV.

Genital warts are caused by human papillomaviruses (HPVs). In males, the warts appear on the penis, anus, and perineum. They are found on the vagina, cervix, perineum, and anus in females. The warts themselves may be removed, but the infection remains for the life of the patient. HPV infection seems to increase a woman's risk for cervical cancer. Two vaccines for HPV, Gardasil and Cervarix, are now available.

AIDS is caused by the human immunodeficiency virus (HIV). This virus is acquired through sexual contact as well as through intravenous drug use and blood transfusions. HIV infects and inactivates the T helper cells that are needed by the immune system to respond to and fight off infections. Without T helper cells, the immune system eventually becomes nonfunctional, and the affected person becomes susceptible to every type of infection possible. Two-thirds of all AIDS patients get pneumonia caused by *Pneumocystis carinii*. Other common diseases associated with AIDS patients are tuberculosis and other mycobacterial infections, viral infections such as those caused by cytomegalovirus and herpesviruses, fungal infections, cancers such as Kaposi's sarcoma, and neurological disorders. HIV can also be transmitted from an infected mother to her baby through the placenta. Virtually every person infected with HIV will eventually die of AIDS.

Treatment and Therapy

Sexually transmitted diseases can be diagnosed in several ways. One way is by observing the symptoms and case history of the patient. Characteristic sores or symptoms can lead a doctor to suspect a particular disease, and a sample of a scraping from a lesion or an unusual discharge can be examined under a microscope to identify the infecting organism. The syphilis, gonorrhea, chlamydia, and trichomoniasis organisms all have unique shapes that a doctor can recognize. For those STDs with mild symptoms or no symptoms, a doctor can try to grow the organism in the laboratory from samples taken from appropriate sites on the body. All organisms that cause STDs can be grown in the laboratory, and since these organisms are not normally present in humans, isolation of the organism from the body is a sign that the body has been infected by that organism. Finally, there are many blood tests that have been developed to test whether a person has specific antibodies in his or her blood that bind to one of these organisms. The presence of antibodies to an organism implies that one has been or is currently infected with that organism. In many cases, doctors will use several of these methods to confirm a diagnosis of an STD.

Specific treatment recommendations for each sexually transmitted disease are subject to periodic revision. Cur-

rent recommendations are reviewed by the Centers for Disease Control and are published in the *Morbidity and Mortality Weekly Report* every three or four years. It is important for physicians to review these recommendations in order to prescribe the best method for treating STDs. All the bacterial and the protozoal STDs can be treated and cured with antibiotics. It is important to seek early diagnosis and treatment of these diseases for three reasons: First, to prevent the disease from spreading; second, to prevent the various complications associated with the diseases; and third, to prevent the infection of infants by pregnant mothers. There is no cure for STDs caused by viruses; there are only drugs that slow the progress of the infection.

Syphilis is commonly treated with penicillin, or alternatively with erythromycin, doxycycline, or ceftriaxone. In most patients receiving appropriate therapy during primary or secondary syphilis, the active disease is totally and permanently arrested. Treatment during the latent stage stops the development of symptoms of the tertiary stage. There is no successful treatment for patients in tertiary syphilis. Cephalosporin antibiotics, such as cefixime and ceftriaxone, have replaced penicillins as therapeutic agents for gonorrhea because of widespread resistance of gonococci to penicillins. Quinolones, such as ciprofloxacin, and azithromycin are other antibiotics that can be effective treatment for gonococcal infections. Doxycycline or azithromycin are used to treat NGU caused by chlamydia, and trichomoniasis is treated with metronidazole or tinidazole.

Genital herpes is treated with antiviral agents such as acyclovir. Topical application of acyclovir is helpful in reducing the duration of primary, but not recurrent, infections. The use of oral acyclovir to suppress recurrent infections may cause more severe and more frequent infections once the therapy has stopped. Neonatal herpes is treated with acyclovir or vidarabine, which can reduce the severity of the infection but cannot reverse any herpes-related neurological damage or prevent recurrent infections. Genital warts can be removed by chemicals, freezing, electrocautery, or laser therapy. Antiviral drugs are useful in treating some STDs: acyclovir for genital herpes, zidovudine for AIDS, and interferon for hepatitis virus. They slow the progress of the disease in some persons, but they do not cure it.

As with any disease, prevention is the most desirable means of controlling STDs. With the exception of viral hepatitis and HPV, there are no vaccines for STDs; although much research is being done and many potential vaccines have been developed and tested, none is yet satisfactory for general and routine use. Therefore, behaviors resulting in disease avoidance are the only means of preventing most STDs. The only 100 percent effective way to prevent a sexually transmitted disease is abstinence. Abstinence means to refrain voluntarily from engaging in sexual activity. Since many of these diseases can be spread through sexual activity other than intercourse, abstinence must include all sexual activity. Choosing to exercise one's sexuality within a monogamous relationship for life can also help prevent sexually transmitted disease. The use of a condom or any other barrier method is only somewhat helpful in the prevention of STDs. Prevention of transmission of STDs from infected mothers to their babies involves early diagnosis and treatment of the mothers before birth and preventive medication of the babies after birth. In the past, ophthalmia neonatorum was the cause of blindness for half of the children admitted to schools for the blind. Therefore, the government made it mandatory to treat all newborns' eyes with silver nitrate, tetracycline, or erythromycin, to prevent this disease. The instillation of silver nitrate in babies' eyes does not prevent chlamydia eye infections, so babies born to mothers with chlamydia need additional antibiotic treatment. Prevention of neonatal herpes may involve delivery by cesarean section to avoid infection of the child as it passes through the birth canal. Preventing the spread of AIDS includes screening blood supplies, organ donors, and semen donors and avoiding contact with infected body fluids through sexual contact, blood transfusions, or intravenous drug use.

Control of STDs in a population is complex, since it is both a medical and a social problem. First, it is important that persons who contract a sexually transmitted disease receive early diagnosis and adequate treatment that will prevent further spread of the disease, serious complications, and infection of infants. This is difficult because many STDs are asymptomatic; therefore, people do not know they have the disease and have no reason to seek treatment. Many persons contract STDs from asymptomatic carriers. In addition, social stigma or embarrassment reduces the motivation of a victim to seek prompt medical care. Adequate treatment of STD victims is difficult if they do not want to return for subsequent treatment or will not take all their medication. Finally, people often contract several STDs at the same time, so detection of one STD should routinely instigate testing for other STDs.

Not only does the person with an STD need to be treated, but all the sexual contacts of that person need to be contacted, tested, and treated as well. Public health officials interview victims of STDs to determine the names and addresses of contacts and then try to find and treat the contacts. This is difficult if a victim does not remember who those contacts are, if he or she does not want to discuss his or her sexual activity, or if the contacts do not want to be bothered by the health department. In addition, many private physicians do not report cases of STDs to the public health department; therefore, in many cases, the sources of STDs are never interviewed.

A reduction in risky sexual behavior, such as unprotected sex, would aid in the control of STDs. Effective education to change sexual behavior must be predicated upon the motivation and cognitive development of the student. One-third of all cases involve teenagers and young adults; sexual activity in this age group is on the rise, and members of this group are more likely to have multiple sex partners. Prostitution for money or drugs also increases the incidence of STDs. Other control measures include development of vaccines for these diseases, mandatory reporting of all STDs, and education of the population regarding the dangers and risks involved in acquiring these diseases.

Perspective and Prospects

Syphilis was first recognized at the end of the fifteenth century in Europe, where it rapidly reached epidemic proportions and was called the "great pox." Gonorrhea was described and given its present name by the Greek physician Galen in 150 CE. From the fifteenth century to the eighteenth century, there was much confusion as to the nature of syphilis and gonorrhea, and many persons thought they were different stages of the same disease. In 1767, an English physician named John Hunter inoculated himself with a urethral discharge from a patient with gonorrhea in order to determine once and for all whether they were one disease or two. Unfortunately, that patient also had syphilis, so when Hunter developed symptoms of both gonorrhea and syphilis he concluded they were a single disease. It was not until 1838 that it was clearly proved that they were two separate diseases. Traditionally, 95 percent of all cases of sexually transmitted disease were either syphilis or gonorrhea. Since the late twentieth century, however, there has been a dramatic increase in the incidence of several other sexually transmitted diseases, such as genital herpes, NGU, AIDS, genital warts, and trichomoniasis.

The rise in incidence of STDs is of epidemic proportions. Worldwide in the 1990s, about 250 million new cases of STDs occurred annually. In the United States, about 12 million new cases, including 3 million in teenagers, occurred annually. By 1997, chlamydia had become the most frequently diagnosed STD in the United States, estimated at more than 4 million annually. Other STDs with high incidence included gonorrhea (1.3 million new cases annually) and genital herpes (0.5 million annually). Because there is no cure for genital herpes, it may be present in 20 percent of Americans. As of 2002, about 1 million North Americans were HIV-positive; only a portion of these had AIDS. By the late twentieth century, the U.S. government announced that the incidence of new cases of AIDS, about 56,000 at that time, had begun to decline. A decline in the numbers of persons dying from AIDS was also announced. It is estimated that there are 3 to 5 million new cases of NGU per year. One in five couples in the United States is infertile, and much of that infertility is caused by the complications associated with STDs, with chlamydial infection being the primary preventable cause of sterility in women. In the United States, it is estimated that 25 percent of all women are infected with trichomoniasis and more than 20 million people are infected with herpes simplex virus type 2.

Despite the fact that most STDs can be controlled, the incidence of many of the diseases is still quite high; thus, STDs obviously present a social as well as a medical problem. An increase in education concerning the signs and risks of these diseases, a reduction in promiscuity, and development of vaccines would help in controlling these destructive and fast-spreading diseases.

—Vicki J. Isola, Ph.D.;
updated by Armand M. Karow, Ph.D.

See also Acquired immunodeficiency syndrome (AIDS); Antibiotics; Bacterial infections; Candidiasis; Chlamydia; Clinics; Contraception; Epidemiology; Genital disorders, female; Genital disorders, male; Gonorrhea; Gynecology; Hepatitis; Herpes; Human immunodeficiency virus (HIV); Human papillomavirus (HPV); Immunization and vaccination; Pelvic inflammatory disease (PID); Preventive medicine; Protozoan diseases; Sexuality; Syphilis; Trichomoniasis; Urethritis; Uterus; Viral infections; Warts.

For Further Information:

Berek, Jonathan S., ed. *Berek and Novak's Gynecology.* 14th ed. Philadelphia: Lippincott Williams & Wilkins, 2007. A standard text covering all aspects of gynecology with an emphasis on diagnosis and treatment. Topics include biology and physiology, sexuality, evaluation of pelvic infections, and malignant diseases of the reproductive tract.

Biddle, Wayne. *A Field Guide to Germs.* 2d ed. New York: Anchor Books, 2002. This comprehensive book is easily accessible to the nonspecialist and includes a discussion of nearly every virus, bacterium, and fungus known to cause human and nonhuman animal disease.

Eng, Thomas Rand, and William T. Butler, eds. *The Hidden Epidemic: Confronting Sexually Transmitted Diseases.* Washington, D.C.: National Academy Press, 1997. This collection of well-written essays is the recommendation of a sixteen-member expert committee for the prevention and control of STDs in the United States.

Larsen, Laura. *Sexually Transmitted Diseases Sourcebook.* Detroit, Mich.: Omnigraphics, 2009. A general resource on the symptoms and treatment of STDs such as chlamydia, gonorrhea, HIV, hepatitis, herpes, HPV, syphilis, and PID. Includes facts about prevalence, risk factors, diagnosis, treatment, and prevention. Also includes a glossary and a list of resources.

Little, Marjorie. *Sexually Transmitted Diseases.* Rev. ed. Philadelphia: Chelsea House, 2000. This work, designed for students in grades nine through twelve, provides some historical information on STDs. Little covers curable diseases, such as syphilis and gonorrhea, as well as AIDS. Symptoms, diagnoses, treatments, and prevention are discussed.

Morse, Stephen A., Ronald C. Ballard, and King K. Holmes. *Atlas of Sexually Transmitted Diseases and AIDS.* 3d ed. New York: Mosby, 2003. A clinical text that provides photographs and illustrations, details global demographics, epidemiology, and diagnostic tests, among other features.

Shaw, Michael, ed. *Everything You Need to Know About Diseases.* Springhouse, Pa.: Springhouse Press, 1996. This well-illustrated consumer reference, compiled by more than one hundred doctors and medical experts, describes five hundred illnesses and conditions, their causes, symptoms, diagnosis, treatment, and prevention. Of particular interest is chapter 11, "Sexual Disorders and Diseases."

Shaking. *See* Tremors.

Shigellosis

Diseases/Disorder

Anatomy or system affected: Gastrointestinal system

Specialties and related fields: Bacteriology, gastroenterology, public health, epidemiology

Definition: An intestinal infection caused by *Shigella* bacteria.

Causes and Symptoms

Dr. Kiyoshi Shiga studied 36 patients during the 1897 Japanese dysentery epidemic and was able to identify the causative bacterium later named in his honor. Shigellosis is a

---

Information on Shigellosis

Causes: Bacterial infection; often related to poverty, malnutrition, poor hygiene, and overcrowding in developing countries

Symptoms: Abdominal cramps, painful urge to defecate, bloody and mucus-filled diarrhea, fever, malaise

Duration: Acute

Treatments: Antibiotics

---

worldwide disease affecting millions of people, particularly children, in areas where crowding and poverty occur. There are four subgroups: A (*S. dysenteriae*), B (*S. flexneri*), C (*S. boydii*), and D (*S. sonnei).* All four species are capable of causing disease with *S. dysenteriae* causing the majority of severe illness as well as most cases in developing nations. *S. sonnei* is the most common species in the United States and other developed countries. It is estimated that nearly a half million cases of shigellosis occur annually in the United States although only a small fraction are reported to public health departments.

Shigella only infects humans and other primates and is spread by person-to-person (fecal-oral route) contact or indirectly through contaminated food and water or flies. It is highly infectious with as few as 10-100 organisms being able to cause infection. Abdominal pain and diarrhea follow a short (1-3 days) incubation period. Some patients will have fever and stools with blood or mucus. *Shigella* invade the intestinal mucosa causing inflammation, but only rarely penetrate the mucosa and enter the bloodstream. *S. dysenteriae*, and sometimes other *Shigella* species as well as some strains of *Escherichia coli,* secrete Shiga toxin which increases the severity of the illness. Hemolytic uremic syndrome and Reiter's chronic arthritis occasionally occur as complications of *Shigella* infection.

Treatment and Therapy

In patients with acute diarrheal illness shigellosis may be suspected when microscopic examination of stool reveals white blood cells and red blood cells which are not found in cases of viral gastroenteritis. Stool cultures will grow *Shigella* confirming the diagnosis. Treatment with an appropriate antibiotic will not only decrease the duration and severity of illness, but will also make transmission to others less likely. Patients may shed *Shigella* in the stool for a month, but antibiotic treatment will reduce the shedding to a week or less. Fluoroquinolone, cephalosporin, and azithromycin antibiotics have all been used successfully for treatment, but antibiotic resistance is increasing making culture of the *Shigella* and antibiotic susceptibility testing of greater importance. Despite continued research an effective vaccine has not been found. Prevention depends upon a safe water supply with adequate chlorination, proper food handling and cooking, improved sanitation, and hand washing.

—Louis B. Jacques, MD;
updated by H. Bradford Hawley, MD

For Further Information:

Dupont, Herbert. "Bacillary Dysentery: *Shigella* and Enteroinvasive *Escherichia coli.*" In *Mandell, Douglas, and Bennett's Principles and Practice of Infectious Diseases*, 8th ed., edited by John E. Bennett, Raphael Dolin, and Martin J. Blaser. Philadelphia, Elsevier Saunders, 2015.

Horsman, Thomas A., William J. Zekan, Charles W. Stratton, and H. Bradford Hawley. "An Outbreak or Shigellosis In Kanawha County, West Virginia." *West Virginia Medical Journal* 76 (May, 1980): 103-108.

Lamba, Katherine, et al. "Shiga Toxin 1-Producing *Shigella sonnei* Infections, California, United States, 2014-2015." *Emerging Infectious Diseases* 22 (April 2016): 679-686.

Nuesch-Inderbinen, Magdalena, et al. "*Shigella* Antimicrobial Drug Resistance Mechanisms, 2004-2014." *Emerging Infectious Diseases* 22 (June 2016): 1083-1085.

Trofa, Andrew F., et al. "Dr. Kiyoshi Shiga: Discoverer of the Dysentery Bacillus." *Clinical Infectious Diseases* 29 (November 1999): 1303-1306.

Shingles

Disease/Disorder

Also known as: Herpes zoster

Anatomy or system affected: Nervous system, skin

Specialties and related fields: Dermatology, family medicine, gerontology, internal medicine, neurology, virology

Definition: Reactivation of the viral infection within a nerve cell that causes pain and a characteristic skin rash.

Key terms:

dermatome: a section of skin that is supplied by nerves that come off a single spinal nerve root.

Causes and Symptoms

Shingles results from the same virus (*varicella zoster*) that causes chickenpox. All individuals who have had chickenpox are at risk for shingles. The disease most commonly affects those over age fifty but can develop at any age, especially in immunocompromised individuals. After the initial manifestations of chickenpox resolve, the virus remains dormant in sensory dorsal nerve roots or ganglia. Each dorsal root receives sensation from receptors in a strip of skin on only one side of the body that are arranged in a segmental distribution called dermatome (map of the skin). Common sites for shingles outbreaks include the back along the distribution of a single dermatome wrapping around one side to the chest or abdomen. They may travel from the upper back to the arm or from the lower back to the leg. Shingles can also occur on the face and rarely can involve the optic nerve of the eye.

Varicella zoster can stay inactive in the nerve root for decades. It appears to be reactivated by stress, illness, decrease in immune function, or aging. The first symptom is often a sensation of tingling, burning, or sharp pain over the skin area supplied by the affected nerve root. Within several days, a rash appears, characterized by a cluster of blisters with surrounding redness spreading along the dermatomal pattern. The rash typically occurs only on one side of the body. Clinical diagnosis usually can be made by the characteristic rash. Alternately, fluid within the shingles blister may be sampled for viral culture to obtain a

---

Information on Shingles

Causes: Viral infection with *varicella zoster*; triggered by stress, illness, decrease in immune function, aging

Symptoms: Tingly, burning, or sharp pain; rash with blisters

Duration: Three days to several weeks

Treatments: Antiviral medications (acyclovir, famciclovir, valacyclovir); pain relief (cool compresses, anti-inflammatory drugs, mild narcotics)

---

definitive diagnosis.

Shingles blisters scab over in about three days and clear within several weeks. Until the blisters are completely scabbed over, the fluid within the blisters can transmit chickenpox via contact. Unvaccinated individuals who have never had chickenpox can develop chickenpox following contact with the fluid in the shingles blisters (e.g., from a grandparent with shingles holding a young child). Even though the fluid from shingles blisters can transmit chickenpox, this same fluid cannot transmit shingles -shingles cannot be acquired from contact exposure. About 20 percent of people continue to have severe pain along the course of the nerve after the rash has cleared. This condition is called postherpetic neuralgia (PHN). It can last for weeks and be so severe as to interfere with activities of daily living.

Treatment and Therapy

If shingles is diagnosed within three days of appearance of the rash, antiviral medications (acyclovir, famciclovir, or valacyclovir) can be used to stop viral replication and help shorten the course of the illness. Treatment also involves pain control with local cool compresses, calamine lotion, anti-inflammatory medications, or even mild narcotics. Gabapentin, a drug similar in structure to an inhibitory neurotransmitter, gamma aminobutyric acid (GABA), is useful against pain experienced in PHN. Antiviral therapy has no effect on PHN.

In 2006, *Zostavax* (zoster vaccine live) was approved for use in the United States to reduce the risk of shingles in older adults. The vaccine is administered in a single dose, usually to individuals over age 60. It is only about 50 percent effective in preventing shingles but about 67 percent effective in preventing PHN in those who do develop the disease.

Perspective and Prospects

The association between chickenpox and shingles was first made in 1888. The virus belongs to a family of viruses called herpes, which is derived from the Greek word *herpein*, meaning "to creep."

Because more than 90 percent of adults in the United States harbor the varicella zoster virus, shingles remains a significant clinical problem, particularly in the elderly and those with compromised immune systems.

A second shingles vaccine (*Shingrix*) was under FDA review in 2017. *Shingrix* is a two-dose vaccine that in clinical trials stimulated adequate antibody production to prevent shingles in 90 percent of individuals, and antibody levels remained adequate for at least four years.

– Veronica N. Baptista, MD;
updated by Tish Davidson, AM

See also: Blisters; Chickenpox; Herpes; Nervous system; Neuralgia, neuritis, and neuropathy; Neurology; Neurology, pediatric; Rashes; Viral infections.

For Further Information:

Doerr, Steven. "Shingles." MedicineNet.com July 5, 2017. http://www.medicinenet.com/shingles_herpes_zoster/article.htm (accessed July 30, 2017).

Janniger, Camilla K. "Herpes Zoster." Medscape.com July 20, 2017. http://emedicine.medscape.com/article/1132465-overview (accessed July 30, 2017).

"Shingles" In: Davidson, Tish. *Vaccines: History, Issues, and Science.* Santa Barbara, CA: Greenwood, 2017; 116-18.

"Shingles (Herpes Zoster)" U.S. Centers for Disease Control and Prevention (August 19, 2016). https://www.cdc.gov/shingles/index.html (accessed July 30, 2017).

Watson, C. Peter, ed. *Herpes Zoster and Postherpetic Neuralgia: Focus on Treatment and Prevention.* New York, NY: Springer Berlin Heidelberg, 2017.

Shock

Disease/Disorder

Anatomy or system affected: All

Specialties and related fields: Critical care, emergency medicine, family medicine, internal medicine

Definition: Shock is a life-threatening condition that may occur in response to a variety of circumstances (allergic reaction, infection, injury, blood loss, heart attack, toxic substances in the blood) which causes the heart to be unable to pump enough blood to supply the vital organs, which are therefore deprived of oxygen and nutrients and lose normal function; symptoms include rapid and shallow breathing, clammy skin, low blood pressure, rapid and weak pulse, and dizziness and if untreated will progress to unconsciousness and death.

Key terms:

blood pressure: the amount of pressure on blood vessel walls when the heart contracts and relaxes

cardiovascular system: the organ system consisting of the heart and all blood vessels (vasculature)

vasculature: all the blood vessels, including the arteries (blood vessels carrying blood away from the heart), the capillaries (the smallest blood vessels, where fluid and nutrients are exchanged), and the veins (blood vessels that return blood to the heart)

vital organs: organs of the body essential to life; the brain, heart, lungs, and sometimes the kidneys

Causes and Symptoms

The primary goal of the cardiovascular system is to provide blood flow, carrying oxygen and other nutrients to all tissues to meet their requirements. The cardiovascular system performs this function by maintaining a blood pressure high enough to push sufficient blood flow throughout the body, especially the vital organs. To keep the blood pressure up, the heart must pump sufficient amounts of blood even when the demand for increased blood flow to some tissues occurs. The blood vessels also play an important role in maintaining blood pressure. The heart and the blood vessels work in a coordinated manner to maintain blood pressure and blood flow.

A healthy heart is capable of adjusting the strength of its beats and the rate of its beats (the heart rate) to produce enough flow to match the demands placed on it by the tissues of the body. For example, during exercise, the exercising muscles require greater blood flow. If the heart does not pump the increased amount of blood that is necessary, then the blood pressure will fall. Hormones such as adrenaline help the heart beat faster and harder to meet the increased demand for blood by the muscles.

The blood vessels (vasculature) have a special structure and function to help maintain blood pressure. The arteries and veins are elastic in nature and squeeze on the blood like an inflated balloon does to the air inside it. In addition, the walls of blood vessels have special muscle tissue, called smooth muscle, that can contract to make the vessels' internal diameter smaller, which helps keep pressure up. If the vessels' internal diameter becomes too small, however, then the blood flow through them will decrease. The concept of blood vessels getting narrow and making it more difficult to push blood through is termed resistance to flow or vascular resistance. The balance of blood flow produced by the heart (cardiac output) and vascular resistance keeps blood pressure at the proper level. When one or both of these components falter, cardiac output and blood pressure fall, which, if untreated, leads to shock.

When the cardiovascular system cannot supply blood flow to the essential organs that is adequate to sustain their function, the body is said to be in shock. A reduction in cardiac output is the primary problem in shock. There are two major ways in which cardiac output can decrease enough to cause shock. When the ability of the heart to pump falls to about 40 percent of its normal capacity, it is termed cardiogenic shock. Cardiogenic shock may occur after a heart attack, heart valve disease, lung collapse, and other disorders.

Cardiogenic shock may occur in several ways. The most common cause is a myocardial infarction (heart attack). During a heart attack, the heart is damaged, and like any other muscle when injured, does not have the strength to pump much blood. Thus, cardiac output goes down and a fall in blood pressure will follow. Cardiogenic shock will progress to death if medical treatment is not rapidly obtained. After a myocardial infarction, while the heart is still healing, it has a reduced ability to pump blood. Exercise, even light exercise such as walking, must be resumed gradually. If it is not, the heart may not be able to pump enough blood to supply muscles even though demand for more flow is only slightly increased. This inability to meet the oxygen demand of the heart will cause further damage to the heart.

In cardiac tamponade, a type of obstructive circulatory shock, the stiff but pliable sac surrounding the heart (pericardium) fills with fluid or swells. This takes up room in the sac, squeezing the heart and prohibiting it from filling adequately from beat to beat. Therefore, the amount of blood pumped decreases, and a drop in blood pressure occurs. Cardiac tamponade can occur for several reasons. It can occur rapidly after trauma or heart surgery if the heart is punctured and bleeds into the pericardial sac. Cardiac tamponade occurs much more slowly when excess fluid is produced by the pericardium or when the pericardium becomes swollen. Both of these conditions can be caused by an infection.

A less common form of cardiogenic shock is caused by an extremely high heart rate. Normally, the heart beats at a rate between sixty and one hundred beats per minute. When the heart rate exceeds one hundred, the resulting condition is called tachycardia. Occasionally, in some people, the heart rate can go rapidly up to near two hundred beats per minute. The time between beats becomes so short that the heart does not have enough time to refill and cardiac output falls. If this condition persists, the blood pressure may fall, causing shock. When this occurs, the combination of the rapid heart rate and low blood pressure may cause a myocardial infarction.

Shock caused by a problem in the vascular system, not by a primary decrease in heart function, is generally termed hypovolemic shock. It is characterized by a lack of sufficient blood volume returned to the heart by the vascular system. Hypovolemic shock can be caused by a decrease in the body's total blood volume.

Excessive bleeding (hemorrhage) is the most common form of hypovolemic shock. The blood vessels are elastic in nature, and they must remain filled with blood for arterial pressure to be maintained. In addition, enough blood must be in the veins to push it back to the heart, to be pumped through the lungs and back out into the arteries. When blood loss is slight, the body attempts to compensate by contracting the veins and arteries, thereby maintaining enough pressure and sufficient cardiac output. When enough circulating blood volume is lost, approximately 15 percent to 20 percent, hypovolemic shock occurs.

There are other ways in which blood volume may decrease. When a person is burned severely, plasma (the fluid in which blood cells are suspended) is lost through the burn sites. Enough can be lost to cause hypovolemic shock. Different forms of dehydration can also result in shock. Prolonged diarrhea, vomiting, and sweating can ultimately result in shock if the person does not drink enough liquids to replace fluid lost. All these conditions lead to a loss in the circulating blood volume and subnormal return of blood to the heart, and thus reduced cardiac output.

A virtual loss in blood volume may also occur, resulting in neurogenic shock. Sometimes anesthesia, hypoxia (inadequate oxygen), low blood sugar, spinal cord injuries, or damage to the brain stem can cause the vascular smooth muscle around the arteries and veins to relax. This results in a loss of arterial and venous pressure. Blood tends to accumulate in the veins and is not returned to the heart, and cardiac output falls. A systemic (entire body) allergic reaction can cause a similar response, called anaphylactic shock.

Information on Shock

Causes: Injury; blood loss; heart attack or heart disorders; toxic substances in blood; prolonged diarrhea, vomiting, or sweating; severe burns; allergies; infection

Symptoms: Rapid, shallow breathing, clammy skin, low blood pressure (weak pulse), dizziness, unconsciousness, intense thirst

Duration: Acute

Treatments: Emergency resuscitation, medications, surgery

Severe infections, usually bacterial, can cause septic shock, which has a death rate of approximately 40 percent. In this type of shock, the immune system of the body responds to the infection. However, this response can cause damage to blood vessels or cause a release of chemicals that cause the vessels to dilate (expand). All types of shock can be deadly if they are not promptly treated.

Applications

In spite of the different causes of circulatory shock, the symptoms are quite common in nearly all cases of shock. The pulse (heart rate) is usually rapid and feeble. Breathing is generally rapid and shallow. The skin is pale, cool, and sometimes moist. The mouth is dry, and thirst is intense. Blood pressure is decreased. Some of these signs are attributable to the body's attempt to alleviate the problem.

The body has several defense mechanisms to help avoid circulatory shock. Several reflex systems function to maintain cardiac output and blood pressure. The body has sensors in the cardiovascular system that tell the brain what the pressure is in the arteries and the veins. When the brain senses a change in either or both of these pressures, it calls on its defenses.

When the arterial pressure sensors tell the brain that blood pressure is falling, the brain produces several responses. Through the nerves, the brain can make the heart beat faster and with greater force. In addition, the nerves can cause vascular smooth muscle to contract, making the vessels squeeze against the blood and increasing pressure. When the smooth muscle contracts, the veins squeeze blood back to the heart to enable it to pump more. The brain can also cause the release of adrenaline into the blood. This hormone can also cause the heart to beat harder and faster. The combined actions of this reflex mechanism attempt to compensate for the decreased cardiac output and blood pressure; however, these responses are only temporary before the person progresses to decompensation and death.

The sensors in the large veins and atria of the heart can cause a different response. Since most (75 percent) of the blood in the body is in the veins at any point in time, a 10 percent to 15 percent decrease in volume triggers the release of a hormone called vasopressin into the blood, which constricts the blood vessels to increase both arterial and venous pressure. The increase in venous pressure squeezes more blood back to the heart to improve cardiac output.

The squeeze on the arteries raises blood pressure. Vasopressin also causes the kidneys to retain water. This fluid retained by the kidney is returned to the blood to keep up the vascular volume.

Specialized blood vessels in the kidneys can also initiate a reflex response to a decrease in blood pressure. The kidneys release a hormone called renin into the blood. Renin activates another hormone, angiotensin, which is a powerful constrictor of blood vessels. Angiotensin increases the release of yet another hormone, aldosterone, which helps the kidneys to reabsorb more fluid. All the above reflexes work together to increase blood volume, cardiac output, and blood pressure, in an attempt to alleviate shock. Despite these mechanisms to prevent shock, however, the by-products of these reflexes actually produce negative effects in the body that eventually lead to more damage.

When average arterial blood pressure falls below 60 millimeters of mercury (mmHg), the blood flow to the blood vessels supplying the heart (coronary vessels) cannot be maintained. When this occurs in shock, it happens at a time when the heart needs its critical supply of oxygen. In fact, the heart is trying to beat harder and faster, which increases its need for oxygen. As a result, the heart can weaken. When weakened, it pumps less and thus cannot bring the pressure back to normal. The heart becomes weaker and weaker. This condition is termed cardiac failure. In addition to cardiac failure caused by reduced coronary blood flow, the body can produce a hormone called myocardial depressant factor (MDF). This hormone directly causes a weakening of the heart that is independent of coronary blood flow. MDF also causes the body's bacterial defense system to function poorly. The maintenance of heart function is important to defend against shock.

Because the blood vessels contract in most of the body during shock, blood flow to nonessential tissues such as skin, muscle, bone, and the intestines is reduced, depriving these tissues of oxygen. These tissues can tolerate short periods of low oxygen supply, but if shock persists for more than a few minutes, these tissues revert to other energy sources. The end products of these alternative energy sources are acids, which can begin a process of tissue damage. If this process is not controlled or reversed, tissues can die. If a critical amount of tissue in an organ dies, the organ cannot function and may fail. Acid produced by other tissues gets into the blood and can directly decrease the function of the heart and its ability to respond to beneficial reflex signals. Acid production makes it more difficult for the body to fight shock.

Derangements in blood clotting can occur during shock. Blood clots can form in the early stages of shock, blocking small vessels. This causes a loss of oxygen that results in acid production. Increased acid in the blood can increase the rate of formation of blood clots. Thus, the clotting system can start a vicious cycle that increases the severity of shock.

Even when shock is not bacterial in origin, the body needs its bacteria-fighting systems. During shock, the bacterial defenses are weakened. Normally, bacteria from the intestines constantly enter the blood and are rapidly neutralized. If this does not occur, endotoxic shock can intensify the already existing shock. Therefore, a capable bacteria-fighting system is important in defending against shock.

In shock, the blood vessels of the heart and brain are spared the constriction experienced by all other tissue blood vessels. In fact, arteries in these organs relax to permit as much blood flow as possible, maintaining oxygen supply to these vital organs. Even so, when very low blood pressure persists (less than 50 mmHg), the brain's function decreases. At this point, the brain sends fewer of the beneficial reflex signals to the heart and blood vessels. The final result is a continuous decline in blood pressure and death. Maintenance of brain blood flow is a very important factor in surviving shock.

Treatment and Therapy

Emergency procedures in response to circulatory shock entail contacting emergency service providers such as paramedics and keeping the victim warm and flat on his or her back, with slightly elevated legs. The victim must get medical attention immediately.

Treatment of shock can vary depending on the cause. In many cases, shock can be effectively treated with intravenous (IV) fluids and medication. Some cases require surgical intervention. In all cases, the status of body fluids must be monitored and treated. The body's blood volume is one of the most important things to maintain.

It is particularly important to optimize blood volume in forms of hypovolemic shock. With hemorrhagic shock, whole blood is given intravenously to replace lost blood. In other forms of hypovolemic shock, different intravenous fluids are usually given. In burn shock, when the blood's plasma weeps from the burn sites, blood plasma is the medicine of choice to restore lost volume. IV fluids are immediately started to restore lost volume until the needed blood products can be acquired. When hypovolemia is caused by excessive diarrhea, vomiting, or sweating, IV fluids are given to replenish lost volume.

In other cases of shock, special drugs are needed to alleviate the symptoms. Shock caused rapidly by a myocardial infarction, with cardiac arrest, can be immediately supported by cardiopulmonary resuscitation (CPR), provided by a trained individual. After resumption of the heartbeat, the heart can be helped with several types of drugs. In the case of sustained tachycardia, a drug such as amiodarone can lower the very rapid heart rate to normal, allowing the heart to fill properly and pump adequate blood. Cardiac tamponade must be corrected to allow the heart to pump usual amounts. If the onset is rapid, as when it is caused by chest trauma, then the fluid in the pericardial sac may need to be removed immediately. A needle is placed into the sac, and the excess fluid is removed to alleviate the pressure around the heart. If fluid accumulates slowly as with an infection and is recognized early, appropriate drug treatment for the infection (antibiotics) may resolve the problem. In cases of shock in which acidosis is a complication or even a potential complication, sodium bicarbonate, a chemical that can reduce the acidity of the blood, may be given. There is no universal treatment for the complex process of shock. For example, hemorrhage may become complicated by heart failure and/or septic shock. Each case must be treated in accordance with the patient's existing conditions.

Perspective and Prospects

Chinese writings of more than three thousand years ago indicate that a connection existed between the heart and the blood. Until the second century, it was thought that arteries carried air, not blood. Through the Middle Ages, it was believed that "spirits" were the essence of life or "vitality." This belief encouraged "bloodletting" as a treatment for many ailments, including shock. Leeches were applied to remove the "evil spirit" causing the sickness. This was not a very successful mode of therapy.

It was not until the seventeenth century that blood transfusions were tried, with the first experiments conducted by Richard Lower. In the 1660s, Jean-Baptiste Denis administered lamb's blood to a sixteen-year-old boy who was very weak and who had a high fever. The condition of the boy, who had been bled several times, improved for a short period of time. Others continued to experiment with transfusion as the remedy for loss of blood, but until the discovery of blood typing at the turn of the twentieth century, most attempts were of limited success.

The practice of giving transfusions greatly increased after the discovery of blood types in 1901 by Karl Landsteiner, who won the 1930 Nobel Prize in Physiology or Medicine for his work. By 1920, blood could be transfused from a bottle, since Luis Agote had discovered that citrated blood would not clot after being removed from the body. Blood banking was established in the 1920s by Russian scientists who discovered that citrated blood could be stored at 40 degrees Fahrenheit.

All types of shock are treated by determining and correcting the underlying cause. Oxygen is given in shock to improve the amount of circulating oxygen to the tissues. In hypovolemic shock, the goal is to improve the amount of circulating volume. This volume is replaced by intravenous fluids until blood products are available. Potent intravenous cardiac drugs that improve the contractions of the heart, improve blood pressure, or cause vasoconstriction may be used in cardiogenic and other types of shock. Mechanical devices have been developed (an intra-aortic balloon pump and a ventricular assist device) to use in severe cardiogenic shock that has not responded to traditional therapy. Synthetic epinephrine (adrenalin) is the first-line treatment for anaphylactic (allergic reaction) shock. It causes the smooth muscle in the bronchioles (tubes into the lungs) to relax and constricts blood vessels. Other treatments may include oxygen, antihistamines and corticosteroids. Septic shock is treated with IV antibiotics and fluids. Shock is a dangerous process that can occur for a variety of reasons. Quick detection and medical treatment are required to prevent negative outcomes.

—J. Timothy O'Neill, Ph.D.;
updated by Amy Webb Bull, D.S.N., A.P.N.

See also Allergies; Bites and stings; Bleeding; Blood and blood disorders; Blood pressure; Blood vessels; Burns and scalds; Cardiac arrest; Cardiopulmonary resuscitation (CPR); Critical care; Critical care, pediatric; Electrical shock; Emergency medicine; First aid; Heart attack; Heart failure; Hemophilia; Hemorrhage; Hypotension; Necrotizing fasciitis; Resuscitation; Septicemia; Transfusion; Unconsciousness; Vascular system.

For Further Information:

American College of Emergency Physicians. *Pocket First Aid*. New York: DK, 2003. An excellent reference guide illustrated with photographs and written in a clear, step-by-step format. Covers many first aid methods, from resuscitation of conscious and unconscious choking victims, to how to deal with bleeding, shock, spinal injuries, poisoning, seizures, fractures, and bandages.

Avraham, Regina. *The Circulatory System*. Philadelphia: Chelsea House, 2000. This text explains the function of the circulatory system in reasonably simple terms. Provides historical development of knowledge about the heart and blood vessels.

Holcomb, Susan Simmons. "Helping Your Patient Conquer Cardiogenic Shock." *Nursing* 32, no. 9 (September, 2002). 32cc1-32cc6. Reference for nurses who work in the intensive care unit.

Klein, Deborah G. "Shock and Sepsis." In *Introduction to Critical Care Nursing*, edited by Mary Lou Sole, Deborah G. Klein, and Marthe J. Moseley. 5th ed. St. Louis, Mo.: Saunders/Elsevier, 2009. A chapter in a critical-care nursing textbook.

Marx, John A., et al., eds. *Rosen's Emergency Medicine: Concepts and Clinical Practice*. 7th ed. Philadelphia: Mosby/Elsevier, 2010. A logical and straightforward presentation of current standards of emergency medicine. Intended to be a reference in busy emergency rooms. The writing is clear and to the point.

Porth, Carol M., and Glenn Matfin. "Heart Failure and Circulatory Shock." In *Essentials of Pathophysiology*, edited by Carol M. Porth. 2d ed. Philadelphia: Lippincott Williams & Wilkins, 2007. A chapter in a textbook on pathophysiology. Offers a detailed explanation of various types of shock.

Shock therapy

Treatment

Also known as: Electroshock, shock treatment, electroconvulsive therapy (ECT)

Anatomy or system affected: Brain, nerves, nervous system, psychic-emotional system

Specialties and related fields: Neurology, psychiatry

Definition: A psychiatric treatment in which chemical, electrical, or other measures are used to induce a coma, convulsions, or seizure in the brain, altering its chemistry and relieving psychiatric distress.

Key terms:

anesthetic: any of a variety of drugs used to cause a patient to become unconscious and amnesiac for a brief period of time; very short-acting anesthetics, such as methohexital, thiamylal sodium, thiopental sodium, and etomidate, are often used in conjunction with electroconvulsive therapy

convulsion: an instance of high-frequency and amplitude-random electrical activity in the brain; electroconvulsive therapy causes a convulsion in the brain, which is believed to be related to its mechanism of action

electrocardiogram: a recording of the electrical activity of the heart; used during electroconvulsive therapy to monitor changes in heart rate, rhythm, and conduction, any or all of which may be temporarily affected by this procedure

electroencephalogram: a brain wave trace used to monitor

the onset, termination, and duration of the convulsion or seizure

mood disorders: any of a number of mental conditions characterized by a primary disturbance of mood as distinct from thinking or behavior

muscle relaxant: any of a number of medications used to paralyze the muscles of the patient temporarily before delivering the electrical stimulus; the main medication used for this purpose is succinylcholine

organic brain syndrome (organicity): changes in memory, orientation, and perception that occur as a side effect of electroconvulsive therapy

psychotic disorder: a psychiatric condition in which an individual's mental state is out of touch with reality, as displayed by abnormal and bizarre perceptions, thoughts, behavior, judgment, and reasoning

seizure: used interchangeably with the term "convulsion"

Indications and Procedures

Shock therapy, also known as shock treatment, is an intervention that has been used for many years to treat severe psychiatric conditions, such as life-threatening depression and psychotic disorders. Many methods of shock treatment exist, ranging from chemically induced shock (via substances such as insulin) to electrically induced shock (from an electrical current). What all the methods share is the purpose of inducing a temporary loss of consciousness, convulsions, and/or seizure in an effort to disrupt brain activity and reset it to a healthier state.

Insulin shock therapy was developed in 1933 by Manfred Sakel. He found that intramuscular administrations of insulin were able to induce a coma that appeared effective for treating severe cases of schizophrenia. By and large, this approach was replaced with other methods of shock therapy, predominantly electroconvulsive therapy (ECT); however, it is still used today when other methods of shock therapy or intervention are judged to be less appropriate. Modern-day procedures are superior to what was originally done. The impact of the shock on the body is better controlled, and the shock treatment itself is more refined in its application.

Historically shock therapy is equated with ECT. Formerly called electroshock therapy, it is a very powerful treatment for psychiatric conditions such as mood disorders and psychotic disorders. It is based on the idea that electrically induced convulsions change the chemistry of the brain in a way that relieves the symptoms of severe mental illness, in which depression, mania, or both become debilitating.

In most situations, electroconvulsive therapy involves the participation of the psychiatrist providing the treatment and an anesthesiologist, who anesthetizes the patient for the procedure. The patient is instructed to take nothing by mouth for eight hours prior to the treatment, so that the stomach is empty for the induction of general anesthesia. The danger of having food or liquid in the stomach is that it might be aspirated into the lungs, where it could cause pneumonia, respiratory obstruction, or death. An intravenous needle is placed in an arm vein. The patient is then connected to a number of monitors, including a blood pressure cuff, electrocardiogram, and pulse oximeter (to measure the level of tissue oxygenation). The patient is then anesthetized with a short-acting intravenous drug (usually methohexital, also known as Brevital). This is followed by the administration of a short-acting muscle relaxant (usually succinylcholine). Ventilation is controlled by mask, using 100 percent oxygen. As soon as it is determined that the muscles are paralyzed, a mild electrical current is administered to the patient's brain. The duration of the stimulus is two seconds or less. There is a brief contraction of the muscles of the face, followed by a generalized seizure, which is monitored on the electroencephalogram. Small amounts of physical movement may be seen in the face, feet, or hands. These movements are not nearly as severe as those that occurred before the advent of muscle relaxants. The anesthesiologist continues to ventilate the patient until the effects of the muscle relaxant have worn off and spontaneous respiration is reestablished (three to five minutes). There is a period of confusion and disorientation that rapidly follows the treatment; it clears quickly. With each successive treatment, the patient is left with an ongoing loss of memory which will gradually clear after the course of therapy is finished. The average patient requires between six and twelve treatments. They are administered two or three times per week.

The decision to conduct electroconvulsive therapy usually comes after there has been failure in other forms of treatment, including medication and psychotherapy. Since there are so many medications and combinations of medication that can be used, however, ECT arguably cannot be thought of as a treatment of last resort, as it was in earlier decades. The idea of administering ECT generally arises when it is critical that the patient improve as rapidly as possible. This consideration is often punctuated by frustration on the part of the patient, the family, and/or the psychiatrist with the slowness of response to current therapeutic modalities. In the 1980s, ECT began to be considered earlier rather than later in the course of treatment. It is realistic to say that if one or two medications are not successful, it is unlikely that others will be successful. Yet there are always those cases in which a sudden and complete remission in mood and psychotic disorders occurs without the use of ECT.

Mood and psychotic disorders tend to recur. When treating a patient for the first time, the doctor cannot know whether the effect of ECT will last for a week, months, or years. Some people need only one course of ECT in a lifetime; others will respond well and remain symptom-free for many years, requiring further ECT when symptoms recur. For many patients who develop devastating symptoms with their illnesses, the early initiation of a course of ECT is warranted. Those who have responded well to ECT in the past will forgo medication trials in favor of starting ECT as soon as the symptoms reappear. For those patients who respond well to ECT but who have recurrences within weeks or months, maintenance ECT may be a reasonable option. With this regimen, a single treatment is given every four to twelve weeks in order to prevent a recurrence of psychiatric distress. The actual frequency of treatment is based on each patient's particular clinical course and history. For many patients, maintenance ECT has been a way of preventing multiple and frequent hospitalizations. Very little cognitive impairment is associated with low-frequency maintenance ECT, and patients go on to live very productive lives while being maintained in this way.

The following case is an example of the uses of electroconvulsive therapy in clinical practice: A seventy-five-year-old white, widowed female was referred by her psychiatrist for evaluation for electroconvulsive therapy. She had been well until two years prior to this evaluation. At that time, a month following the death of her husband, she began to experience a variety of symptoms, including loss of appetite with a ten-pound weight loss, decreased interest in her friends and the ordinary activities of life which she had found enjoyable, and sleep disturbance characterized by difficulty falling asleep and early morning awakening. The sleep difficulty was responsive to the use of triazolam, a sleep-inducing drug. Additionally, she began to experience episodes of dizziness that were made worse by antidepressant medications. She was not actively suicidal, but she did experience a wish to die and join her husband, whom she believed was waiting for her. She had been treated with tricyclic antidepressants (nortriptyline and desipramine) with lithium augmentation, but the side effects of constipation and dizziness made these medications intolerable. Her depression did not improve, and she began to exhibit medical signs of dehydration and malnutrition. The treating psychiatrist believed that electroconvulsive therapy was indicated and that it should be instituted as rapidly as possible as a lifesaving measure.

The patient was given a course of seven unilateral ECT treatments over the period of a month. She responded to the treatments with an elevation in her mood, an improvement in sleep and appetite, and increasing engagement with hospital staff and family. When she was discharged from the hospital, she showed evidence of mild memory impairment. In the weeks following her treatment, her memory improved, and she became brighter and resumed her normal activities with vigor. She was started on a small dose of fluoxetine (Prozac), an antidepressant known to have a milder side effect profile than the medications she had taken previously. After one year of follow-up, she was still doing well.

Electroconvulsive therapy continues to be widely practiced in the United States and abroad. There is consensus within the field of psychiatry that it is a valuable tool in the psychiatric armamentarium. Patients, patient advocates, and clinicians alike, however, continue to be concerned about its ethical and appropriate use. Practitioners support efforts of the lay community to ensure the proper and ethical use of ECT as long as it does not obstruct access to the treatment for those who require it.

Uses and Complications

Electroconvulsive therapy is used for a variety of psychiatric conditions, including major depressive disorder, depressed bipolar disorder, manic bipolar disorder, mixed bipolar disorder, schizophrenia, manic excitement, and catatonia. Before starting electroconvulsive therapy, all patients are screened for medical illnesses, for two reasons. First, a variety of medical illnesses are associated with depression or mania; the list is long and includes occult cancer, hypothyroidism, vitamin deficiencies, endocrine abnormalities, and brain tumors or infections, among many others. If there is a treatable cause for depression, it must be found and treated before the decision to perform electroconvulsive therapy is made. Once it is clear that the psychiatric illness is not being caused by something else, ECT may be used. It is important to note that there are certain untreatable medical causes for depression or mania in which the disorder may respond to ECT. For example, depressed patients with Alzheimer's disease may respond to ECT, showing significant improvements in mood. Brain-injured patients with depression may, in some circumstances, respond to electroconvulsive therapy.

The second reason for screening the patient is to establish that it is safe to proceed with ECT. A routine evaluation should include a medical history and physical examination, psychiatric history, mental status examination, blood count, blood chemistries, urinalysis, and electrocardiogram. Other tests may be done if they seem important to rule out other possible illnesses. Such tests might include a computed tomography (CT) scan, a magnetic resonance imaging (MRI) scan, an electroencephalogram (EEG, or brain wave study), or tests for antidepressant drug levels.

There are no absolute reasons not to perform electroconvulsive therapy. There are certain conditions, however, that produce a significant increase in risk with ECT. Cerebral aneurysm may increase the danger of electroconvulsive therapy. An aneurysm is a balloonlike swelling of an artery, which may cause severe brain damage if it bursts. The high blood pressure associated with ECT may cause a cerebral aneurysm to burst. Patients who have recently experienced a heart attack are at increased risk of dying with ECT. Electroconvulsive therapy should be delayed for six months, if possible, following a heart attack. Other illnesses that increase risk include emphysema, multiple sclerosis, and muscular dystrophy.

Despite these risks, electroconvulsive therapy is considered by many to be the safest of the somatic treatments available in psychiatry. The death rate from ECT itself is one patient in ten thousand-much lower, for example, than the death rate for patients taking antidepressant medications; the death rate from suicide in depressed people is much higher. Electroconvulsive therapy may be done safely with patients representing a broad range of age and physical condition. For the elderly, malnourished patient, it is clearly safer and more effective than medication. Prior to the use of muscle relaxants, broken bones and vertebrae were a considerable problem with ECT. This is no longer the case. Complications such as uncontrolled hypertension, stroke, and heart attack rarely occur; they are extremely unlikely, because the patients are medically screened prior to beginning the treatment.

In each situation, the risk of doing ECT must be weighed against the risk of not doing the treatment. If the patient is imminently suicidal-so that he or she cannot be left alone-ECT may be indicated even though the risk is high. Similarly, patients who are starving to death as a result of their illness may require immediate treatment. Patients with manic excitement or delirium, who are completely out of control and require seclusion, may require ECT despite increased risk. For individuals who cannot tolerate or effectively process antidepressant medications, as a result of a compromised liver or other health conditions, ECT may the most effective choice to save their lives.

The most disturbing and severe side effect of ECT is memory loss. It is believed that this side effect is attributable to the electricity that is passed through the brain. The postseizure state may also have some effect. What seems to be clear is that this memory deficit is not the result of physical damage to the brain. Some memories, especially those of events that occur around the time of the treatment, may be permanently lost. Many patients will lose their memory of the periods of most severe depression or mania. The ability to learn new information may be temporarily lost. Most people return to reasonable function within the first month and to complete function after six months.

There are a number of ways to gauge the response of a patient to ECT. It is a complicated process that has to take into account and weigh three factors: the improvement of the mood of the patient, the number of treatments or total seizure seconds, and the amount of confusion and/or memory loss that is produced. Additionally, it is important to gauge the emotional response of the patient and the family to the changes being brought about by the treatment.

With each successive treatment, the patient's mood should get better. If the patient has been depressed, there should be a decrease of the depressive symptoms. Appetite and sleep patterns should improve. There should be an increased level of activity, and social engagement should get better. These changes may first be noticeable to the family and hospital staff. Very often, the improvement becomes apparent to the patient later. Occasionally, the improvement will not be obvious until there has been a chance for the confusion and memory loss to resolve. If the patient is manic, there should be an improvement in symptoms of hyperactivity, grandiosity, irritability, and inability to organize activity and behavior. The response of mania to ECT is often very rapid, and the results may be quite gratifying.

If confusion occurs too early in the course of ECT and it is clear that more treatment needs to be done, decreasing the frequency of treatment from three times a week to once or twice a week may be indicated. Ultimately the decision to stop ECT is based on balancing the above-mentioned factors in an optimal way. This determination is made by the clinician with the input of the patient and all the others (psychiatrist, family, and staff) who know the patient best. If the patient does not seem to be improving and is not having memory difficulty, ECT should be continued. Some patients may need as many as twenty treatments to achieve resolution of psychiatric distress.

Electroconvulsive therapy is the most effective treatment for major mood disorders and for psychotic disorders with a mood component. The likelihood of success depends on the specific diagnosis as well as the accuracy of the diagnostic assessment. Patients who have not responded to adequate trials of medication are less likely to respond to ECT than are those who have not been treated with medication. This would seem to reflect the idea that treatment-resistant psychiatric distress is less likely to respond to any form of treatment.

Perspective and Prospects

Electroconvulsive therapy was discovered as a therapy of mental illness in 1938. It was first used by Ugo Cerletti and Lucio Bini in Italy. The basis of its use was the observation that patients with epilepsy did not suffer from schizophrenia. It was believed that there was something about brain seizures that either prevented or was protective against schizophrenia. While that clinical observation was not accurate, it became the impetus for research into the curative effects of electrically induced seizures.

The first electrical convulsions were induced without the benefit of general anesthesia. Patients had violent seizures and often suffered broken bones and teeth. They were held down in order to keep the seizures from causing excessive physical harm. The responses to ECT in certain patients were quite dramatic. Symptoms such as depression and mania could often be eliminated. Agitated behavior associated with schizophrenia could be mitigated, and patients suffering from catatonia would often become animated as a result of a course of electroconvulsive therapy. The therapy was soon brought to the United States, where it enjoyed frequent use until the early 1950s.

At that time, antipsychotic and antidepressant medications for the treatment of psychiatric illnesses became available. The drugs chlorpromazine and imipramine were shown to be effective in managing the symptoms of schizophrenia and mood disorders. As a result, electroconvulsive therapy was used less frequently and then only in severe, treatment-refractory cases. The political climate of the 1960s and 1970s and films such as *One Flew over the Cuckoo's Nest* (1975) portrayed ECT as a tool of the repressive and oppressing psychiatric establishment to exert behavioral and mind control over an unwitting public. Laws were passed in many jurisdictions making it more difficult for patients to obtain ECT. There were efforts to outlaw ECT. Now, however, even the most powerful patient advocacy groups accept the appropriate use of this treatment.

Electroconvulsive therapy has been utilized with increasing frequency for a number of reasons: recognition of its efficacy, the safety of electroconvulsive therapy in medically ill patients, the increased safety of anesthetic techniques, improved diagnostic criteria, an improved process of informed consent, and disappointing efficacy and side effects of medication in certain patients.

During the 1990s, an alternative stimulatory procedure

to the use of ECT as a standard treatment for severe depression was developed. Transcranial magnetic stimulation (TMS) is able to provide a similar adjustment to brain activity without the use of electric current or chemically induced shock. The procedure uses a magnetic coil to deliver a pulse to specified areas of the brain, generally in the region of the prefrontal cortex above the temple. The stimulating coil is held close to the scalp so that the field is focused and can pass through the skull. Rapid-rate TMS can deliver up to fifty stimuli per second. When stimulation is delivered at regular intervals, it is termed repetitive TMS (rTMS). TMS therapy can be used on an outpatient basis, reducing the necessity to hospitalize the patient. Unlike ECT, no side effects such as vomiting, fatigue, or memory loss are typically seen with TMS. The use of TMS is also being studied in connection with movement disorders, epilepsy, bipolar disorders, anxiety disorders, developmental stuttering, Tourette's syndrome, and schizophrenia.

One of the reasons for the renewed interest in ECT is the improvement in informed consent procedures. Physicians no longer adopt as authoritative an attitude toward patients as they did in the past. In the early years of ECT, patients were not informed of all the potential side effects of the treatment. They were often not told that they had alternatives and what the risks and side effects of the alternatives were. The result was that they experienced complications and side effects for which they were not prepared. They became disappointed and angry. Modern informed consent procedures allow the patient to participate as fully as possible in the decision to take any particular form of therapy. The patient is cognizant of the fact that there are choices and alternatives. The patient is also aware that he or she may decide to discontinue treatment at any time if there is no benefit and the side effects are intolerable. Accurate descriptions of side effects and complications are given to the patient. The patient is apprised of the fact that the treatment may fail and that the treatment is being done this time because it is the one that is most likely to help at this juncture. The patient learns that the choice is simply the best choice, not the only one. Both patients and doctors have benefited from such an enlightened approach to informed consent.

—*Frank Guerra, M.D.;*
updated by Nancy A. Piotrowski, Ph.D.

See also Bipolar disorders; Brain; Depression; Emotions: Biomedical causes and effects; Epilepsy; Memory loss; Nervous system; Neurology; Psychiatric disorders; Psychiatry; Psychiatry, child and adolescent; Psychiatry, geriatric; Schizophrenia; Seizures; Sleep disorders.

For Further Information:
Abrams, Richard. *Electroconvulsive Therapy.* 4th ed. New York: Oxford University Press, 2002. A textbook on electroconvulsive therapy that presents a complete picture of all aspects of treatment, from the scientific to the clinical.

American Psychiatric Association. *The Practice of Electroconvulsive Therapy: Recommendations for Treatment, Training, and Privileging.* 2d ed. Washington, D.C.: American Psychiatric Press, 2001. This book is the result of the work of a task force on electroconvulsive therapy in the American Psychiatric Association. It shows how psychiatrists have worked to make the practice of ECT as ethical and safe as possible. Argues for the importance of this form of treatment to psychiatric patients.

Endler, Norman S. *Holiday of Darkness.* Rev. ed. New York: John Wiley & Sons, 1990. This book documents the clinical depression of the author, a psychologist, who responded well to electroconvulsive therapy. A very important work that many patients who are contemplating the possibility of ECT may find comforting and useful.

Endler, Norman S., and Emmanuel Persad. *Electroconvulsive Therapy: The Myths and the Realities.* Toronto, Ont.: Hans Huber, 1988. Another good text on electroconvulsive therapy, written by a psychologist who experienced the treatment for his own depression. He has gone on to become a much-honored and internationally recognized teacher and researcher in the field of psychology.

Fink, Max. *Convulsive Therapy: Theory and Practice.* New York: Raven Press, 1979. This book continues to be an excellent introduction to electroconvulsive therapy by the leading practitioner and researcher in the United States. A classic text.

George, Mark S., and Robert H. Belmaker, eds. *Transcranial Magnetic Stimulation in Neuropsychiatry.* Blackwood, N.J.: American Psychiatric Press, 2000. Compares the effects of transcranial magnetic stimulation (TMS) and ECT in animal models of depression, showing that their similarities may further support the potential role of TMS as an antidepressant treatment.

Kellner, Charles H., et al. *Handbook of ECT.* Washington, D.C.: American Psychiatric Press, 1997. This source describes the procedure, its pros and cons, and how it works and is used in contemporary medicine.

Manning, Martha. *Undercurrents: A Therapist's Reckoning with Depression.* New York: HarperCollins, 1995. A memoir written by a therapist about her experience with depression and shock therapy.

Shunts

Procedure

Anatomy or system affected: Abdomen, brain, circulatory system, gastrointestinal system, head, liver, nervous system

Specialties and related fields: General surgery, neonatology, perinatology, vascular medicine

Definition: Surgically inserted tubes that are used to bypass blocked vessels that normally allow fluid to move from one region of the body to another.

Key terms:

anesthesia: the use of drugs to inhibit pain and alter consciousness

catheter: a tube passed into the body for fluid transport

incision: a cut made with a scalpel

portacaval: referring to a type of shunt used to carry blood from the portal vein to the inferior vena cava, allowing blood to bypass the liver

ventriculoperitoneal: referring to a type of shunt used to carry cerebrospinal fluid from the brain to the abdominal cavity

Indications and Procedures

The surgical placement of shunts is performed to reduce fluid pressures when the vessel that normally carries the fluid is blocked. Two major types of shunts are ventriculoperitoneal and portacaval. Ventriculoperitoneal shunts are used to remove excess fluid from the brain in hydrocephalus. Shunts used to decrease blood pressure in the portal veins are known as portacaval shunts.

Hydrocephalus is a condition characterized by an excessive amount of cerebrospinal fluid in the brain caused either by too much cerebrospinal fluid production or by the blockage of its flow. Hydrocephalus can occur at birth or be caused by head trauma, infection, or brain hemorrhage. If it occurs at birth, the main signs are an enlarged head that continues to grow more rapidly than normal. An infant's skull bones have yet to fuse, and the fluid pressure causes them to expand. The infant may have seizures, vomiting, abnormal reflexes, and other neurological signs. If hydrocephalus occurs in an adult, when the skull bones cannot expand, the pressure on the brain causes headaches, mental deterioration, loss of consciousness, and, if not treated, death.

Physicians use computed tomography (CT) scanning or magnetic resonance imaging (MRI) to find the blockage. The patient is then prepared for surgery to have a shunt inserted to drain the accumulating fluid. After the individual is anesthetized, the head is prepared for the operation. An incision is made through the skin of the head and a hole drilled into the skull, a procedure called craniotomy. A catheter that is part of the ventriculoperitoneal shunt is inserted into the ventricles of the brain and passed under the skin into the abdominal cavity, which is lined by the peritoneum. The peritoneum is a large membrane capable of absorbing the excess cerebrospinal fluid.

Portacaval shunts are used to reduce the blood pressure in the veins carrying blood from the digestive tract to the liver. Patients with abnormally elevated blood pressure in these veins have portal hypertension. This pressure reduces blood flow from the esophagus, stomach, and intestines, which leads to a pooling of blood and an engorgement of these vessels that may lead to their rupturing. Fluid leaking from the portal vein accumulates in the abdominal cavity, a condition known as ascites.

The most common cause of portal hypertension is cirrhosis of the liver, in which the liver is diseased and scar tissue forms. This scar tissue can block blood entering the liver from the portal vein and lead to portal hypertension. Occasionally, a thrombus (blood clot) will form in the portal vein and cause portal hypertension when the liver is not diseased. The patient may have ruptured vessels that bleed into the digestive tract, causing the feces to appear black. If the physician suspects portal hypertension, he or she will perform an ultrasound and arteriography to view the vessels.

A portacaval shunt operation may be necessary to reduce the pressure in the portal vein if other treatments have failed. In this surgical procedure, the patient is anesthetized and prepared for a major abdominal surgery called a laparotomy. An incision is made into the abdominal cavity, and the portal vein is exposed. The surgeon must then carefully place a catheter between the portal vein and another large abdominal vein. The latter vein is the inferior vena cava, which helps return blood to the heart from the lower body and the abdominal cavity. Another surgical option is for the surgeon to connect part of the portal vein to the inferior vena cava directly without the use of a catheter. The portacaval shunt diverts some of the blood that normally goes to the liver directly into the inferior vena cava, thus reducing the pressure within the portal vein.

Uses and Complications

The major problem associated with the ventriculoperitoneal shunt is the fact that it will need to be replaced as the infant grows. It is also possible for this tube to become blocked or infected. If the shunt remains in place for a long period of time, it may spontaneously penetrate an abdominal organ.

Portacaval shunt operations reduce the high blood pressure in the portal vein and help prevent bleeding. Unfortunately, they do not significantly improve liver function in most patients and may even cause further liver damage.

Perspective and Prospects

Early detection and treatment of increased intracranial pressure (pressure on the brain) in hydrocephalus and increased blood pressure in portal hypertension are important to the long-term health and survival of the patient.

Early treatment of hydrocephalus with shunt placement prevents further neurological damage and, if the increase in brain pressure is rapid, may even be necessary to prevent death. Drugs such as acetazolamide that inhibit the formation of cerebrospinal fluid may, in certain cases, prevent the need for shunt operations. These agents will likely prove most effective in patients with mild disease.

Physicians may try to stop bleeding from ruptured vessels that is caused by portal hypertension by injecting a solution into the veins to seal them (sclerotherapy). Dietary restriction of salt (sodium) and diuretic drugs may be tried to reduce blood pressure, vessel engorgement, and ascites fluid accumulation.

—Matthew Berria, Ph.D.,
and Douglas Reinhart, M.D.

See also Abdomen; Blood vessels; Brain; Brain disorders; Bypass surgery; Catheterization; Cirrhosis; Craniotomy; Fluids and electrolytes; Hydrocephalus; Hypertension; Liver; Liver disorders; Vascular system.

For Further Information:

Brunicardi, F. Charles, et al., eds. *Schwartz's Principles of Surgery.* 9th ed. New York: McGraw-Hill, 2010. A standard textbook on the topic. Intended for practicing surgeons, but valuable to general readers for its details.

Leikin, Jerrold B., and Martin S. Lipsky, eds. *American Medical Association Complete Medical Encyclopedia.* New York: Random House Reference, 2003. A concise presentation of numerous medical terms and illnesses. A good general reference.

Parker, James N., and Philip M. Parker, eds. *The Official Parent's Sourcebook on Hydrocephalus.* San Diego, Calif.: Icon Health, 2002. Guides patients in using the Web to educate themselves about hydrocephalus and draws from public, academic, government, and peer-reviewed research to provide comprehensive information on a range of topics related to the condition.

Toporek, Chuck, and Kellie Robinson. *Hydrocephalus: A Guide for Patients, Families, and Friends.* Sebastopol, Calif.: O'Reilly, 1999. Covers a range of topics related to the condition, including detailed discussion of shunt revision surgery.

Sickle cell disease

Disease/Disorder

Anatomy or system affected: Blood, cells, kidneys, lungs, spleen

Specialties and related fields: Genetics, hematology
Definition: Genetic disorders of the hemoglobin molecule.
Key terms:
anemia: the pathologic state of decreased concentration of hemoglobin
aplastic crisis: a sudden decrease in the bone marrow release of red blood cells, associated with very severe anemia
hemoglobin: the substance within red blood cells that transports oxygen and carbon dioxide
infarction: death in a tissue or organ caused by the obstruction of blood flow

---

Information on Sickle Cell Disease

Causes: Genetic disorder
Symptoms: Severe anemia, episodes of acute pain; complications may include septicemia, meningitis, pneumonia, severe upper respiratory tract infections, bone infarctions, kidney infections
Duration: Chronic with acute recurrent episodes
Treatments: Prophylactic antibiotics, hospitalization, analgesics

---

Causes and Symptoms

Sickle cell disease is a genetic disorder of hemoglobin, which gives the red color to blood. The hemoglobin molecule is made up of two pairs of globin polypeptide chains (two α chains and two β chains) and four heme molecules containing iron. Normal hemoglobin (hemoglobin A) is a remarkable protein that changes the biophysical configuration of its amino acid chains so that it can deliver oxygen safely to the tissues without oxidizing iron. Oxygen removal occurs during each cycle of blood flow from the lungs to the tissues. Sickle hemoglobin has a single amino acid substitution of valine for glutamic acid at the sixth position from the end of the β chain. Sickle hemoglobin has the unfortunate propensity to condense as rods in red blood cells when the oxygen is removed during the normal circulation of the blood. These rods distort the cells, making them stiff and rigid and unable to transverse the smaller blood vessels rapidly. The result is vasocclusion (obstruction) of the small and medium-sized blood vessels, damaging the endothelial inner lining of the blood vessel and thereby resulting in tissue necrosis (ischemia).

The most common genotypes of sickle cell disease are sickle cell anemia-homozygous sickle cell disease (SS disease), sickle cell hemoglobin C disease (SC disease), sickle cell $\beta0$ thalassemia (S$\beta0$ thalassemia), and sickle cell $\beta+$ thalassemia (S$\beta+$ thalassemia). Less common genotypes include sickle cell hemoglobin E disease (SE disease), sickle cell hemoglobin D Los Angeles (SD Los Angeles), and sickle cell hemoglobin O Arab (SO Arab). In addition to these conditions, more than four hundred other abnormal human hemoglobins can combine with sickle hemoglobin. This genetic heterogeneity accounts for the wide spectrum of clinical severity in patients with sickle cell disease, with some forms essentially asymptomatic, such as Hb SE or S deer lodge.

Sickle cell anemia (SS disease) is the most common and the most severe form of sickle cell disease. It results from the inheritance of the sickle cell gene from both parents. Its hallmark clinical manifestations are anemia and severe episodes of pain; similar but less frequent manifestations are seen with other forms of sickle cell disease. In sickle cell anemia, anemia is caused by the rapid destruction of the red blood cells as they circulate because of a shortened peripheral survival time of less than 30 days (normal is 120 days).

Acute painful episodes-particularly in the older child, adolescent, or adult-are characteristic of sickle cell anemia.

Sickle cell crisis often begins with pain in the abdomen or extremities and joints. Painful sickle crisis in the young child is usually precipitated by an acute fever, with excruciatingly tender swelling of the hands and feet (dactylitis) caused by small infarctions of the small growing bones of the hands and feet. Approximately 25 percent of SS patients have endless and repeated painful episodes throughout life requiring frequent hospital care.

The clinical course of sickle cell anemia involves intermittent episodes of acute painful illnesses interspersed with periods of clinical quiescence and relative well-being. Commonly occurring acute complications necessitating intensive medical care are septicemia and meningitis during childhood, recurrent sickle cell pain crises, cerebral infarction with stroke, acute chest syndrome (often termed pneumonia), severe upper respiratory tract infections, gallbladder disease with gallstones, aplastic crisis, hypersplenism with splenic sequestration crisis, bone infarctions, priapism (a painful erection of the penis not associated with sexual desire), and pyelonephritis (infection of the kidney).

An increased incidence of invasive infections caused by the bacteria *Streptococcus pneumoniae* is found in children with SS disease who are between the ages of four months and five years; this is thirty to one hundred times that which would be expected in a healthy population of the same race and age. Blood infections in SS infants and young children are associated with a rapid elevation of temperature, often to 104 degrees Fahrenheit, and the patient becomes even more anemic. In the untreated patient, death occurs within eight to twelve hours.

Chronic major organ failure in SS disease is the direct consequence of irreversible and ongoing damage to the endothelial lining of the small blood vessels as a result of sickle cells (sickle vasculopathy). Vascular damage begins years before the overt clinical symptoms are apparent. The spleen is the first organ to be destroyed, usually by five years of age. During childhood (three to ten years of age), 10 percent of children with this disease will have strokes, with resulting severe brain damage. Strokes cause paralysis and weakness of the extremities and difficulties in learning. This devastating complication in young children often makes functioning in school or living as self-sustaining adults difficult. Brain infarction can be accurately identified using computed tomography (CT) brain scans, magnetic resonance imaging (MRI), positron emission tomography (PET), and other diagnostic procedures. Sickle vasculopathy eventually culminates in young adulthood as end-stage kidney failure (glomerulosclerosis), sickle chronic restrictive lung disease, intracranial hemorrhages and brain damage, retinopathy with blindness, disabling leg ulcers, and painful generalized osteonecrosis of many of the bones of the body. Specialized medical care is required for the diagnosis and management of these permanent incurable complications.

Treatment and Therapy

Most acute complications of SS disease can be treated successfully so that the patient can attend school, be involved in social activities, and have a pleasant childhood and adolescence. Intensive care units with sophisticated monitoring equipment that are dedicated to infants and young children can manage and maintain the vital function of patients during severe illness episodes.

The institution of appropriate immunization programs for children with sickle cell anemia has substantially decreased their mortality and morbidity throughout the world. The importance of preventing the usual childhood infectious diseases such as hepatitis, whooping cough (pertussis), red measles (rubeola), rubella (German measles), diphtheria, tetanus, mumps, poliomyelitis, and *Hemophilus influenzae* septicemia allows 90 percent of these children to reach adulthood. The use of prophylactic antibiotics such as penicillin during young childhood (four months to five years) decreases the incidence of invasive pneumococcal blood infections. However, a recent ominous increase has been seen in penicillin resistance to pneumococcal serotype-specific strains, making prophylactic antibiotic prevention less effective. Salmonella contamination of chicken is still a major source of septicemia and salmonella osteomyelitis (bone infection).

Over time, children with sickle cell disease and their families begin to recognize the things that may precipitate a painful sickle cell crisis. Severe episodes require hospitalization and analgesic treatment, often with narcotic agents in addition to intravenous fluids.

Perspective and Prospects

Sickle cell anemia is the prototypical molecular disease. The causative gene modifying the chemical structure of the hemoglobin β chain (βA to βS)—replacing the amino acid glutamic acid with valine-originated in Africa. The disorder was transmitted to the United States, Arabia, Europe, and South and Central America as part of the slave trade. At that time, healthy persons carrying the sickle gene, who are said to have sickle cell trait, survived the rigors of a slave ship. As persons carrying the sickle cell trait migrated throughout the North and South American continents and Europe, genetic drift occurred, accounting for the 15 percent of patients with the various forms of sickle cell disease who are not phenotypically African in appearance.

Improvements in acute medical care during childhood and in the social and environmental situation for patients, as factors taken together, have made it possible for most children with sickle cell anemia and other forms of sickle cell disease to survive childhood. In the United States,

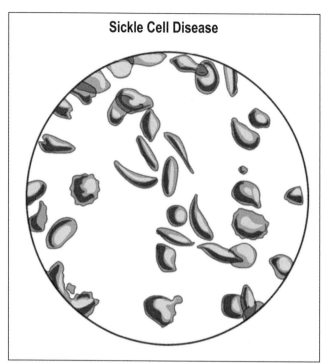

Sickle Cell Disease

The red blood cells are sickle-shaped rather than round, which causes blockage of capillaries.

Great Britain, and most European countries, umbilical cord blood diagnosis or peripheral blood sampling of newborns can diagnose the disorder at birth. This allows the children to be provided with responsive knowledgeable medical care and complete immunizations early in life.

The current focus of clinical investigations is prevention of the tissue destruction induced by the repeated endothelial damage caused when sickle cells obstruct blood vessels. Such prevention requires lifelong medical treatment. Drugs that can modify the rate of hemoglobin polymerization (precipitation) in the red blood cells include hydroxyurea, cytosine arabinoside, 5-azosididine, and other agents that increase the amount of fetal hemoglobin in red blood cells. By increasing the fetal hemoglobin, the rate of polymerization of hemoglobin S is modified so that there is less propensity for insoluble rods to be formed. The membranes of red blood cells become more flexible, allowing the cells to traverse the microvasculature and thereby decreasing the damage to blood vessels. Adhesion molecules (such as VCAM-1) act to provide the glue that binds the damaged sickle cell to the inner lining of the blood vessel, inducing permanent endothelial damage. Intensive search is underway to identify blocking agents for these adhesion molecules that can prevent the blood vessel occlusion.

Bone marrow transplantation with normal bone marrow (normal red blood cell precursors) from a donor with identical human leukocyte antigens (HLAs) is the only cure now available for sickle cell anemia. Bone marrow transplantation is limited by the paucity of HLA-compatible sibling donors who do not have sickle cell anemia.

Gene therapy holds the promise of a cure but has not been successfully developed for use in patients with sickle cell anemia. The advantage of gene therapy is that no HLA-compatible donor is required.

—*Darleen Powars, M.D.*

See also African American health; Anemia; Blood and blood disorders; Bone marrow transplantation; Fatigue; Genetic diseases; Hematology; Hematology, pediatric; Pain management; Thalassemia.

For Further Information:

Ballas, S. K. "Sickle Cell Anaemia: Progress in Pathogenesis and Treatment." *Drugs* 62 (2002): 1143-1172. A clearly presented review of sickle cell anemia, with available treatment options described.

Edelstein, Stuart J. *The Sickled Cell: From Myths to Molecules.* Cambridge, Mass.: Harvard University Press, 1986. A historical description of ancient African cultural beliefs and how they correlated to the modern molecular understanding of sickle hemoglobinopathies.

Embury, Stephen H., Robert P. Hebbel, Narla Mohandas, and Martin H. Steinberg, eds. *Sickle Cell Disease: Basic Principles and Clinical Practice.* New York: Raven Press, 1994. Chapters 26, 30, 35, 38, and 40 offer an in-depth description of the molecular and biochemical nature of sickle hemoglobin and clinical correlations.

O'Malley, Paul D., ed. *New Developments in Sickle Cell Disease Research.* New York: Nova Science, 2006. Covers a range of topics, from psychobiological reactivity to acute chest syndrome.

Pauling, Linus, H. Itano, S. J. Singer, and I. C. Wells. "Sickle Cell Anemia: A Molecular Disease." *Science* 110 (1949): 543-548. The discovery of the electrophoretic mobility of sickle Hb S as compared to normal Hb A defines the first molecular disease to be identified.

Powars, Darleen R. "Management of Cerebral Vasculopathy in Children with Sickle Cell Anaemia." *British Journal of Haematology* 108 (2000): 666-678. Explains that brain infarction (stroke) is the most devastating complication of sickle cell anemia.

Serjeant, Graham R., and Beryl E. Serjeant. *Sickle Cell Disease.* 3d ed. New York: Oxford University Press, 2001. Offers clinical observations of sickle cell disease based on long-term studies in Jamaica.

SIDS. *See* Sudden infant death syndrome (SIDS).

Signs and symptoms

Procedure

Anatomy or system affected: All

Specialties and related fields: All

Definition: Characteristics of a disease state perceived either by the affected individual (symptom) or by someone other than the affected individual (sign).

Key terms:

asymptomatic disease: a disease that has no obvious symptoms

diagnosis: the act of identifying a specific disease using signs and symptoms as evidence

prognosis: the predicted outcome of a disease

symptomatic disease: a disease or disorder that displays overt symptoms

Introduction

It is common practice to use the words "sign" and "symptom" interchangeably. There is, however, a subtle difference between the two terms; it concerns who is making the observation. Symptoms are subjective qualities that indicate an abnormality or disease. In other words, they are perceived by the affected individual. Examples of symptoms that a patient may describe are an itchy sensation in the skin, headache, joint pain, or nausea.

Signs are objective. They can be noticed by persons other than the affected individual, such as physicians, nurses, and relatives. Examples of outward signs of disease include hyperactivity in a child, forgetfulness in an elderly person, fever, rash, a swollen ankle, or vomiting. Sometimes, signs may not be immediately apparent and further testing may be necessary in order to reveal them. For example, a physician or nurse may check a patient's blood pressure, blood may be drawn for analysis, or a colonoscopy may be ordered.

Health care professionals use a combination of the signs that they observe and the symptoms described by the patient in order to determine the presence of a particular disorder. This process is called diagnosis. Once a diagnosis has been made, an appropriate course of treatment is evaluated.

Types of Signs and Symptoms

Signs and symptoms come in many different guises, and the way in which they present themselves gives health care professionals further clues as to the nature of the disorder-not only which disease is present but also how severe it is.

Blood pressure, pulse rate, body temperature, and breathing rate are known as vital signs. They are used as standard markers when monitoring an individual's state of health.

A sign or symptom is described as chronic if it is present for an extended period of time. For example, a chronic cough may be indicative of asthma, or a response to an environmental allergen. If a sign or symptom lessens in intensity or disappears, then it is a remitting symptom; conversely, if it worsens or reappears after a period of abatement, then it is relapsing. Some conditions are characterized by these types of signs. Relapsing-remitting multiple sclerosis is an example. In the relapse stage of this disease, the body's immune system attacks the sheath of myelin that surrounds nerves in the central nervous system. When the immune response has calmed down, special cells in the central nervous system, called glia, repair the myelin; the remission period is entered.

The presenting symptom is the symptom that first prompts the affected individual to consult a health care professional. If a symptom is general, involving the whole body-such as fatigue, weight loss, or fever-then it is called a constitutional symptom.

A condition that manifests in a tangible way is said to be a symptomatic disease or disorder. An asymptomatic condition, however, can be present without the affected individual being aware of it. Sometimes, routine screening methods such as a mammogram or prostate examination expose the presence of asymptomatic conditions before they become symptomatic, thereby increasing the chance for successful treatment. An asymptomatic infection is an infection by viruses or bacteria that does not result in obvious signs or symptoms. Often, sexually transmitted infections are asymptomatic: Examples include infection by the *Chlamydia trachomatis* bacterium (chlamydia) or the human papillomavirus (HPV). Some infections are asymptomatic while the bacteria or virus is incubating, which is the period of time between exposure to the infectious agent and the onset of symptoms. For example, the incubation period of the seasonal influenza virus is one to four days. Asymptomatic infections can be problematic because it is possible for the affected individual to transmit them to other people unknowingly.

Diseases can have primary and secondary symptoms. Alzheimer's disease is characterized primarily by symptoms such as memory loss and difficulty with concentration. As a result of the burden caused by these primary symptoms, an affected individual may develop depression. In the case of Alzheimer's disease, depression is a secondary symptom.

Prognostic signs or symptoms are those that give clues about the future course of the disease. The predicted outcome of the disease is called the prognosis. An example of a disease with an extremely poor prognosis is pancreatic cancer. Pancreatic cancer is rarely diagnosed in its early stages due to lack of symptoms; the chance of successful treatment becomes very low as the disease progresses. Less than 5 percent of pancreatic cancer patients survive for more than five years after diagnosis.

When an addictive substance is abruptly denied to an addicted body, withdrawal symptoms usually become apparent. In alcoholism, these symptoms range from headaches, nausea, and weakness to convulsions and delirium tremens (confusion and visual hallucination). Each addictive substance has a characteristic set of withdrawal symptoms.

Eponymous signs are named after the person who first described them. For example, Braxton Hicks' contractions (sometimes known as Hicks' sign), prelabor contractions occurring during pregnancy, were first described by John Braxton Hicks.

Perspective and Prospects

Many years ago, physicians could use only their limited powers of observation, along with patients' description of their symptoms, to make a diagnosis. The development of progressively sophisticated equipment and new methods for clinical testing has made the diagnostic procedure faster and more accurate. As a consequence, treatment is becoming increasingly effective.

A vast amount of medical information is now available to the layperson. Online discussion groups and "symptom checker" Web sites encourage the practice of self-diagnosis. In fact, the act of researching a disease using the Internet as a resource, and subsequently worrying that one is suffering from symptoms of that particular disease, is termed cyberchondria.

—*Claire L. Standen, Ph.D.*

See also Allied health; Alternative medicine; Biopsy; Blood pressure; Blood testing; Cancer; Cardiac rehabilitation; Death and dying; Diagnosis; Disease; Hospice; Imaging and radiology; Invasive tests; Laboratory tests; Noninvasive tests; Physical examination; Physical rehabiliation; Prognosis; Pulse rate; Screening; Syndrome.

For Further Information:
Kahan, Scott, Redona Miller, and Ellen Smith. *In a Page-Signs and Symptoms*. 2d ed. Philadelphia: Lippincott Williams & Wilkins, 2008.
Springhouse, ed. *Handbook of Signs and Symptoms*. 4th ed. Philadelphia: Lippincott Williams & Wilkins, 2009.
Tierney, Lawrence, and Mark Henderson. *The Patient History: Evidence-Based Approach*. New York: McGraw-Hill Medical, 2004.

Single photon emission computed tomography (SPECT)

Procedure

Also known as: Single photon emission tomography (SPET)

Anatomy or system affected: Blood, blood vessels, brain, circulatory system, head, heart

Specialties and related fields: Cardiology, nuclear medicine, psychiatry, pulmonary medicine, radiology

Definition: A nuclear imaging test used to provide three-dimensional information about the flow of blood through arteries and veins in order to diagnose a wide range of health conditions, including strokes, epilepsy, dementia, and tumors.

Key terms:

gamma rays: electromagnetic radiation emitted during radioactive decay with short wavelengths

ischemia: reduced blood flow

myocardial perfusion imaging (MPI): a type of cardiac stress test

neurotransmitter: a chemical that communicates nerve impulses from one nerve cell to another

photons: particles that travel at the speed of light

tracer: a substance that is injected into the body and releases energy which allows it to be followed along its path through the circulatory system and metabolism pathways

Indications and Procedures

Single photon emission computed tomography (SPECT) uses the radioisotopes xenon 133, technetium 99, and iodine 123 to acquire information about blood flow. A small amount of radioisotope is injected into a patient's vein to observe the flow of blood and metabolic pathways during the digestion of food. These radioisotopes are the radioactive forms of the naturally occurring elements of xenon, technetium, and iodine. These forms are referred to as radioactive because they emit gamma rays. These gamma rays can be measured directly by using a gamma ray detector containing a series of crystals that convert the gamma rays to photons of light. Photomultiplier tubes amplify the photons into electrical signals, which are then converted by a computer into detailed three-dimensional visual images on a screen.

SPECT is one of several nuclear imaging techniques used in medicine for diagnosis. Imaging is important as a noninvasive method of seeing inside the body, without requiring surgery. Other common techniques include X rays, magnetic resonance imaging (MRI) scans, computed to-

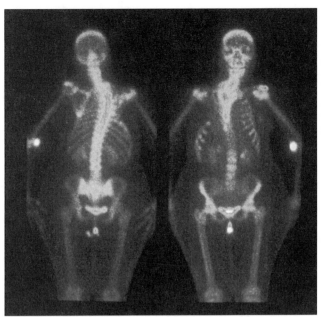

SPECT scan showing scoliosis, a curvature of the spine. (Oullette/Theroux/Publiphoto/Photo Researchers, Inc.)

mography (CT) scans, and ultrasound. The other nuclear imaging techniques include cardiovascular imaging, bone scanning, and positron emission tomography (PET). All these techniques assist in the detection of inadequate blood flow to tissues, aneurysms (weak locations in the walls of blood vessels), various blood cell disorders, and tumors.

Of these techniques, SPECT is the most similar to PET, but SPECT is less expensive and more readily available. SPECT radioisotopes emit single gamma rays with longer decay times than in PET, and thus have the disadvantage of producing less detailed images than PET.

Tomography refers to the technique of using rotating X rays to record an image within the body. With today's computers, the terminology of computed tomography (CT) is used. The imaging process of SPECT combines CT with the use of radioisotopes. These radioisotopes are often referred to as tracers because they allow physicians to follow the pathway traveled by the blood through the body. Tracers emit gamma rays that are collected by a computer, which then translates the data into two-dimensional cross sections that are added together to form a three-dimensional image. These radioactive tracers decay within minutes to hours and are eliminated in the urine, thus posing negligible harm to the body.

Uses and Complications

The sharp images that can be obtained using SPECT enable it to be a useful diagnostic tool for a variety of cardiovascular, cerebrovascular, and neurological disorders. SPECT is more sensitive than an electrocardiogram (ECG) for detecting ischemia. In order to diagnose ischemic heart disease, SPECT scanning enhances myocardial perfusion imaging (MPI) after a patient exerts stress in order to compare images from before and after stress to assess blood flow. SPECT has become an extensively used tool to diagnose

coronary artery disease (CAD). Because it is such a useful tool for detecting reduced blood flow, SPECT has also been widely used to detect tumors. For example, as part of the diagnosis of patients suspected of having aneurysms or tumors at the base of the skull, the internal carotid artery temporary balloon occlusion (TBO) test is enhanced by the use of SPECT to evaluate the cerebral blood flow. SPECT is also used to detect lymphoma tumors in the chest and abdomen, neuroendocrine tumors, stress fractures and stress reactions in the spine (known as spondylolysis), and liver lesions.

The high resolution of SPECT allows it to be a very useful tool for obtaining images of the striatum, a specific area of the brain containing the neurotransmitter dopamine. This dopamine activity can be monitored to help diagnose schizophrenia and various mood and movement disorders, including epilepsy, Alzheimer's disease, dementia, and obsessive-compulsive disorder.

Perspective and Prospects

Although a SPECT scan exposes the body to less radiation than does a CT scan or a chest X ray, pregnant or nursing women should not receive a SPECT scan. A nuclear medicine technologist will inject a patient with a small amount of radioactive tracer. After enough time is allowed for the

---

In the News:
Use of SPECT to Detect Pulmonary Embolism

Single photon emission computed tomography (SPECT) has been shown by researchers to be useful in the diagnosis of pulmonary embolism. According to the study titled "Detection of Pulmonary Embolism with Combined Ventilation-Perfusion SPECT and Low-Dose CT: Head-to-Head Comparison with Multidetector CT Angiography," SPECT plus low-dose CT had a sensitivity of 97 percent and specificity of 100 percent. This diagnostic effectiveness was much greater than that of the multidetector CT angiography alone, which had a sensitivity of 68 percent and specificity of 100 percent.

Pulmonary embolism is a blockage in an artery in the lung caused by a blood clot. Diagnosis can be problematic because a seemingly healthy individual can develop this condition quickly, often with no symptoms. Furthermore, the mortality rate is estimated to be a relatively high 30 percent.

The article published by researchers in Denmark in the December, 2009, issue of *The Journal of Nuclear Medicine* is one of several recent articles describing additional applications of SPECT to diagnose these types of blood flow abnormalities as well as coronary heart disease and even to diagnose brain damage and cancer. Researchers in Houston, Texas, have found that the combination of using SPECT along with the coronary artery calcium score (CACS) is more effective in diagnosing coronary heart disease than either method alone. These results were published in the November 10, 2009, issue of the *Journal of the American College of Cardiology.* ReGen Therapeutics has also reported that SPECT has shown the effectiveness of their drug zolpidem for treating brain damage.

—*Jeanne L. Kuhler, Ph.D.*

tracer to travel to the brain (usually ten to twenty minutes), a special camera called a gamma camera is used to acquire multiple images from multiple angles by rotating around the head. This gamma camera detects the gamma radiation emitted by the radioactive tracers. Thus, the patient needs to remain motionless during the scanning process so that clear images can be obtained. After the scanning process is finished, it is important for the patient to drink fluids to remove the radioactive tracers from the body.

—*Jeanne L. Kuhler, Ph.D.*

See also Angiography; Angioplasty; Computed tomography (CT) scanning; Echocardiography; Imaging and radiology; Magnetic resonance imaging (MRI); Mammography; Neuroimaging; Noninvasive tests; Nuclear medicine; Nuclear radiology; Positron emission tomography (PET) scanning; Radiation sickness; Radiation therapy; Radiopharmaceuticals; Ultrasonography.

For Further Information:

American Academy of Neurology, Therapeutics, and Technology Assessment Subcommittee. *Assessment: Brain SPECT*. Minneapolis: American Academy of Neurology, 1995.

Frankle, W. G., et al. "Neuroreceptor Imaging in Psychiatry: Theory and Applications." *International Review of Neurobiology* 67 (2005): 385-440.

Masdeu, J. C., et al. "Special Review: Brain Single Photon Emission Tomography." *Neurology* 44 (October, 1994): 1970-1977.

Van Heertum, R. "Single Photon Emission, CT, and Positron Emission Tomography in the Evaluation of Neurologic Disease." *Radiologic Clinics of North America* 39 (May, 2001).

Sinusitis

Disease/Disorder

Anatomy or system affected: Nose, respiratory system
Specialties and related fields: Family medicine, internal medicine, otorhinolaryngology
Definition: Irritation and swelling of the sinuses.
Key terms:

deviated septum: a condition that causes a shift of the bones and cartilage from the middle of the nose to either side, making one side of the nasal passages much smaller than the other

nasal polyps: noncancerous growths inside the nose; usually associated with allergies or asthma, which can block the sinus drainage tract

orbit: the bones and other tissues that surround the eye, commonly known as the eye socket

Causes and Symptoms

The sinuses are airspaces in the skull that exist in the forehead just above the eyes, on either side of the nose below the eyes, and in the area just above the nose and in between the eyes. The sinuses are lined with mucus and tiny hairs, called cilia, which trap inhaled particles and bacteria and move them back out through the nose. This action serves as a natural defense system to eliminate these potential irritants that are inhaled during normal breathing. The tracts through which the sinuses drain are relatively small and easily blocked by swelling of the area. This blockage can impair drainage and cause the buildup of normal sinus secretions.

The term "sinusitis" refers to irritation or swelling of the

> **Information on Sinusitis**
>
> **Causes:** Common cold; allergies; environmental exposure to smoke or air pollution; blockage from nasal polyps, deviated septum, or pregnancy
> **Symptoms:** Irritation or swelling of sinuses, congestion or pressure in nose or face, runny nose with secretions varying from clear to yellowish green to bloody, decreased sense of smell, productive cough, fever, tooth pain, bad breath
> **Duration:** Acute
> **Treatments:** Increased fluid intake, antihistamines, anti-inflammatory drugs, decongestants, humidified air, nasal irrigation, oral or nasal allergy medications, antibiotics if needed

---

sinuses and their membranes. Typical symptoms may include a feeling of congestion or pressure in the nose or face and runny nose with secretions that may vary in color from clear to yellowish green to bloody. The facial pressure is often worse when bending forward.

Most often, sinusitis is precipitated by the common cold. Another frequent cause is allergies, with typical symptoms of sneezing, runny nose, and itchy, watery eyes. An allergic patient who is sensitive to a particular airborne substance (pollen, ragweed, dust, animal dander) has a particularly vigorous response when these particles land in the nose and enter the sinuses. An increased production of mucus and the body's natural immune defenses combine to produce thick and copious nasal secretions that can fill the sinuses in an attempt to eliminate the offending agent.

Another factor that may predispose a patient to sinusitis is environmental exposure to smoke or air pollution, which are natural irritants to the sinuses. Problems that cause a blockage of the sinus drainage system by things such as nasal polyps, a deviated septum, or pregnancy (which leads to swelling of the nasal membranes as a result of hormonal changes) can interfere with mucus drainage from the sinuses. Finally, other genetic diseases such as cystic fibrosis or disorders of the immune system can predispose patients to sinusitis.

Although most cases of sinusitis are caused by viruses or allergies, these can often lead to infection by bacteria if they do not resolve promptly. Bacterial sinusitis requires treatment with antibiotics to avoid the rare but serious complications of infection of the orbit or infection of the brain and its surrounding tissues.

The distinction between bacterial and other causes of sinusitis is most accurately based on the patient's symptoms and a physical examination. A patient is more likely to have bacterial sinusitis if two or three of the following symptoms are present for at least seven days: facial pressure, nasal congestion, discolored nasal mucus, decreased sense of smell, productive or "wet" cough, fever, tooth pain on the upper jaw, or bad breath.

Sinus X rays, done frequently in the past, are not considered a reliable diagnostic test for sinusitis. Though sinus computed tomography (CT) scans allow intricate visual-

The Major Sinuses

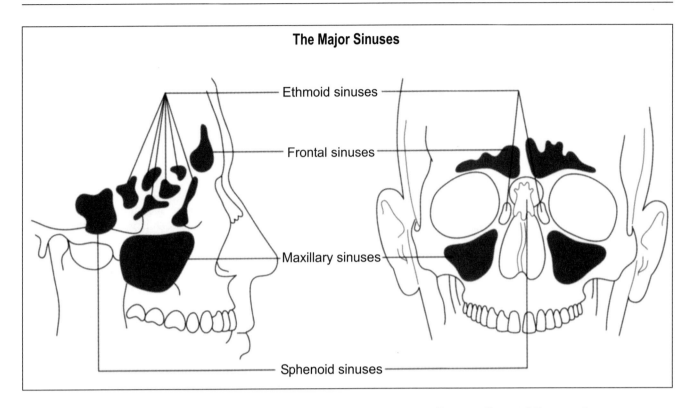

Ethmoid sinuses

Frontal sinuses

Maxillary sinuses

Sphenoid sinuses

ization of sinus anatomy, they do not reliably distinguish bacterial sinusitis from other forms and are useful only in cases of long-standing, refractory symptoms for which sinus surgery is being considered.

Treatment and Therapy

The initial treatment of sinusitis involves extra fluids, anti-inflammatory drugs such as ibuprofen, antihistamines, short-term use of nasal decongestant sprays (no longer than three days), and oral decongestants such as pseudoephedrine. Humidified air (for example, steam from a hot shower) and nasal irrigation with water or saline can offer short-term symptom relief.

If allergies are the cause of sinusitis, then oral or nasal allergy medications are appropriate. Examples are nonprescription antihistamines such as chlorpheniramine or diphenhydramine; they can cause drowsiness in some patients. Loratadine and other related, newer generation antihistamines are also available over the counter. They offer once-daily dosing and are significantly less sedating. Other nasal sprays such as topical steroids are available by prescription and offer significant relief.

If symptoms persist longer than seven to fourteen days, then antibiotic therapy may be necessary and evaluation by a health care provider is warranted. Many different types of antibiotics are effective for sinusitis, and prescription practices vary. Initial treatment is typically for two weeks.

Perspective and Prospects

Prior to the antibiotic era, the treatment of sinusitis involved drainage of the sinuses by extracting a tooth, puncturing the roof of the mouth, or entering the nose and creating a drainage tract through which secretions could be removed and the sinuses could be irrigated with fluid for cleansing. Given the invasiveness of these procedures, they

---

In the News: Balloon Sinuplasty

In late 2005, the Acclarent Company received permission from the Food and Drug Administration (FDA) to market a device to clear blocked sinuses similar to that used to clear blocked arteries in the heart. A flexible catheter tube inserted into the nostril guides a balloon into the targeted sinus. The balloon is inflated, spreading the bones of the passageway sufficiently to permit accumulated mucus or pus to drain. A minimally invasive outpatient procedure, balloon sinuplasty is performed under local anesthesia and takes one to two hours. Patients report little or no pain and can often return to normal activity within twenty-four hours. The sinuplasty devices cost from $1,200 to $1,500 and are not reusable. Total costs for the procedure run $4,000 to $6,800; the procedure is covered by some private insurance plans.

The procedure cannot be used if nasal polyps need to be removed. Nevertheless, it provides a possible alternative for sinusitis sufferers who do not need, or prefer not to undergo, surgical procedures involving cutting away bone or other tissue to open the blocked sinus. Surgeons using the devices praised them. The American Rhinologic Society was more cautious in its October, 2006, position statement, asserting that the technology had limited indication at the time. In November, 2006, the California Blue Cross labeled the procedure investigational and not medically necessary, noting that since the FDA's clearance was based on the devices' comparability to already approved procedures, it did not require submission of safety or effectiveness data. The most extensive 2006 clinical trial, which claimed that the procedure was safe and effective, followed 109 patients over twenty-four weeks. Longer-term efficacy remains unknown.

—Milton Berman, Ph.D.

have become uncommon with the development of effective antibiotic therapy.

The development of tiny, high-resolution cameras known as endoscopes in the 1950s created a revolution in the understanding of sinus disease. Direct visualization of the nasal passages and sinus drainage tracts allowed a better understanding of the sinus anatomy and thus led to the use of this equipment to facilitate surgical treatment.

Occasionally, patients with recurrent symptoms require surgical removal of infected sinus tissue and enlargement of the natural drainage tracts to minimize sinus obstruction. A specialist in otorhinolaryngology can perform such surgery using an endoscope, without the need for general anesthesia. Patients do not typically require hospitalization, and complications are rare.

—*Gregory B. Seymann, M.D.*

See also Allergies; Antihistamines; Bacterial infections; Common cold; Decongestants; Ear infections and disorders; Hay fever; Headaches; Multiple chemical sensitivity syndrome; Nasal polyp removal; Nasopharyngeal disorders; Otorhinolaryngology; Polyps.

For Further Information:

Beers, Mark H., et al., eds. *The Merck Manual of Diagnosis and Therapy.* 18th ed. Whitehouse Station, N.J.: Merck Research Laboratories, 2006.

Brook, Itzhak, ed. *Sinusitis: From Microbiology to Management.* New York: Taylor & Francis, 2006.

Kennedy, David W., and Marilyn Olsen. *Living with Chronic Sinusitis: A Patient's Guide to Sinusitis, Nasal Allergies, Polyps, and Their Treatment Options.* Long Island, N.Y.: Hatherleigh Press, 2007.

McCaffrey, Thomas. "Functional Endoscopic Sinus Surgery: An Overview." *Mayo Clinic Proceedings* 68 (June, 1993): 571-577.

Mickelson, Samuel, and Michael Benninger. "The Nose and Paranasal Sinuses." In *Textbook of Primary Care Medicine*, edited by John Noble. 3d ed. St. Louis, Mo.: Mosby, 2001.

Younis, Ramzi T., ed. *Pediatric Sinusitis and Sinus Surgery.* New York: Taylor & Francis, 2006.

Sjögren's syndrome

Disease/Disorder

Also known as: Dry eye/dry mouth or sicca syndrome

Anatomy or system affected: Eyes, immune system, mouth

Specialties and related fields: Dentistry, family medicine, rheumatology

Definition: An autoimmune disorder resulting in the loss of tears and saliva.

Causes and Symptoms

Sjögren's (pronounced SHOW-grins) syndrome is a chronic autoimmune disease in which the body's own immune cells attack and eliminate the glands that produce tears and saliva. This results in dryness of the eyes and mouth and is referred to as sicca syndrome. The causes of Sjögren's syndrome are not known, although evidence suggests that viral infection, heredity, and hormones may be involved. Sjögren's syndrome is one of the more prevalent autoimmune disorders, affecting as many as four million Americans. Nine of ten patients with Sjögren's syndrome are female.

Sjögren's syndrome can be difficult to diagnose because

Information on Sjögren's Syndrome

Causes: Unknown; possibly viral infection, heredity, hormones

Symptoms: Dry eyes, dry mouth, blurred vision, eye discomfort, recurrent mouth infections, swollen salivary glands, hoarseness, difficulty swallowing and eating, extreme fatigue

Duration: Chronic

Treatments: Moisture replacement (eyedrops, saliva-stimulating drugs, salivary packets); immunosuppressive drugs or NSAIDs

---

the symptoms are similar to those caused by other diseases. The symptoms can also mimic the side effects associated with a number of medications and may vary from individual to individual. Even when the symptoms are reported to a physician, dentist, or eye specialist, the proper diagnosis can be overlooked.

The classic symptoms are dry eyes (xerophthalmia) and dry mouth (xerostomia). Individuals with Sjögren's syndrome often have blurred vision, constant eye discomfort, recurrent mouth infections, swollen parotid (salivary) glands, hoarseness, and difficulty in swallowing and eating. Dryness of other mucous membranes of the body, such as the intestines, lungs, and reproductive system, may also occur. Extreme fatigue can also seriously alter the quality of life.

Sjögren's syndrome is most commonly diagnosed in people in their mid-forties. In some individuals, primary Sjögren's syndrome affects only the tear ducts and salivary glands. In other patients, it is present in conjunction with other diseases such as rheumatoid arthritis, systemic lupus erythematosus, systemic sclerosis (scleroderma), or polymyositis/dermatomyositis (secondary Sjögren's syndrome).

Treatment and Therapy

Once Sjögren's syndrome is suspected, blood tests for autoantibodies against nuclear or cytoplasmic proteins may be performed. Schirmer's test, which measures tear production, and salivary scintigraphy, which determines salivary gland function, may also be performed. A lower lip biopsy, to determine the extent of inflammation, may also be needed.

Moisture replacement therapies are designed to ease the symptoms of dryness. The routine use of eyedrops aids in controlling dryness of the eyes, and saliva-stimulating drugs and salivary packets help with difficulties in chewing and swallowing food. For individuals with more severe complications, immunosuppressive or nonsteroidal anti-inflammatory drugs (NSAIDs) may be prescribed.

Perspective and Prospects

Sjögren's syndrome is named after the Swedish eye doctor Henrik Sjögren, who first identified the syndrome in 1933. There is no known cure for Sjögren's syndrome, nor is there a current treatment to restore gland secretion. The outlook for individuals with this condition is usually good because Sjögren's syndrome is generally not life-threatening.

—Thomas L. Brown, Ph.D.

See also Autoimmune disorders; Eyes; Glands; Otorhinolaryngology; Rheumatoid arthritis; Scleroderma; Systemic lupus erythematosus (SLE); Tears and tear ducts; Vision disorders.

For Further Information:
Parker, James N., and Philip M. Parker, eds. *The Official Patient's Sourcebook on Sjögren's Syndrome.* San Diego, Calif.: Icon Health, 2002.

Rose, Noel R., and Ian R. Mackay, eds. *The Autoimmune Diseases.* 4th ed. St. Louis, Mo.: Academic Press/Elsevier, 2006.

Wallace, Daniel J., et al., eds. *The New Sjogren's Syndrome Handbook.* 3d ed. New York: Oxford University Press, 2005.

Skeletal disorders and diseases. *See* Bone disorders.

Skeleton. *See* Bones and the skeleton.

Skin

Anatomy

Anatomy or system affected: Nerves, nervous system

Specialties and related fields: Dermatology, neurology, oncology, plastic surgery

Definition: The largest organ of the body, which is vital to the survival of an organism for its protection against dehydration and abrasion, regulation of body temperature, and sensory reception.

Key terms:

basal cell carcinoma: the most common type of skin cancer; it grows slowly and seldom spreads beneath the skin

collagen: a fibrous protein found in the connective tissue, including skin, bone, ligaments, and cartilage

contact dermatitis: a common skin allergy characterized by inflamed skin; it occurs when skin comes in contact with substances such as poison ivy or allergenic cosmetics

dermatologist: a physician who treats the skin, including its structures, functions, and diseases

dermis: the layer of skin beneath the epidermis, consisting of dense connective tissue and blood vessels

epidermis: the outermost part of the skin, composed of four or five different layers called strata

keratin: an extremely tough protein that is the chief constituent of the epidermis, hair, nails, and tooth enamel

melanin: the dark pigment of the skin or hair that accounts for variations in skin color

melanoma: a cancer arising from a pigmented mole; it tends to spread to internal organs if left unchecked

psoriasis: a chronic skin disease characterized by red, scaly patches overlaid with thick, silvery gray scales

Structure and Functions

The anatomy of the skin consists of two major parts: the outer epidermis and the underlying dermis. The epidermis is composed of a particular kind of tissue called stratified squamous epithelium. Epithelium consists of cells that are packed together very tightly, a feature that is most important to an organ that must cover and protect the rest of the body. It is called squamous, which means "flat" in Latin, because its cells are flat and fit together like tiles. The word "stratified" describes the dozens of layers of cells that are piled up to create the epidermis. These cells form four or sometimes five strata, with their own characteristics and roles to perform.

The stratum basale, or basal layer, lies on a thin piece of tissue called the basement membrane, which is next to the dermis. The basal layer cells divide continuously throughout life, supplying new cells called keratinocytes for all the layers above the basal layer. About one-fourth of the stratum basale cells are called melanocytes because they produce the pigment melanin. As the keratinocytes are pushed up, they acquire a spiny shape; for this reason, the layer above the basal layer is called the stratum spinosum. While in the spiny layer, the upward-moving cells begin to produce the protein fibers that will eventually become waterproof keratin. As the spiny cells are moved further upward, they begin to flatten out. The layer that they form at this point is called the stratum granulosum because the keratin being formed is visible here, under the microscope, as large clumps or granules. Langerhans cells, which are very important in immunity and protection from disease, are also found in the granular layer. Only in thick skin, such as that found on the palms of the hands and the soles of the feet, do some of the migrating cells form a transparent layer of dead cells full of a shiny substance called eleidin. The shininess of this fourth layer earned it the name stratum lucidum.

The outermost part of the epidermis, the stratum corneum, is what most people think of as "the skin"-dead, dry cells that are completely waterproof because they are packed with keratin. The twenty-five layers of corneum cells form an efficient barrier to water loss and to the entrance of microorganisms. The epidermis has no blood vessels. The living, reproducing basal-layer cells must be nourished by nutrients passed from blood vessels in the dermis. Nerve endings that pick up the sensations of touch and pain extend upward into the epidermis, while those that sense pressure, heat, and cold extend only into the dermis.

Directly beneath the epidermis's basement membrane is the dermis. The dermis extends in a wavy or vertical tonguelike fashion into the epidermis to anchor it. The top of the dermis, which is called the papillary layer, thus forms ridges that account for one's fingerprints and toe prints. There are small blood vessels and fibers scattered throughout the papillary layer. The larger, lower part of the dermis is called the reticular layer. This thicker dermal layer has many more elastic and collagen fibers than does the papillary layer, and it is the location of oil glands, sweat glands, fat cells, hair follicles, and large blood vessels.

Directly under the skin, which is often called the cutis, is the jellylike, fat-filled subcutaneous layer. This packaging material provides heat insulation and energy storage, and it serves to attach the skin to the muscles and organs below.

The anatomy of the skin makes it able to perform a variety of functions. All these roles have one major purpose: to enable the skin to maintain homeostasis-that is, to keep the

The Structure of the Skin

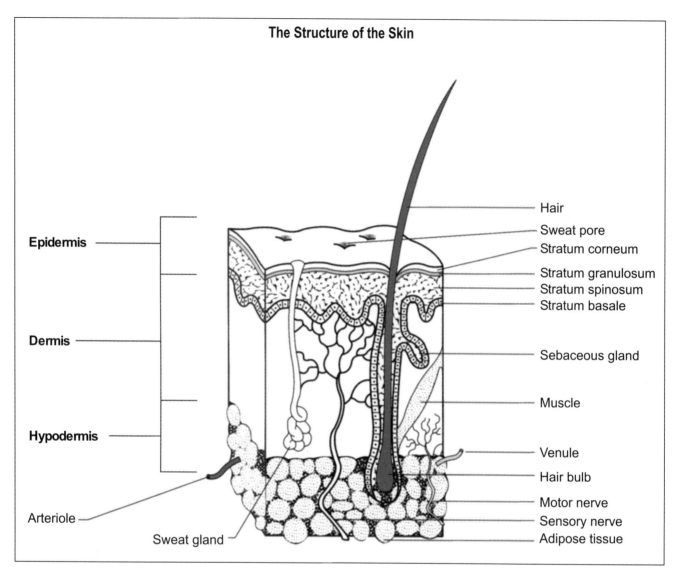

Epidermis

Dermis

Hypodermis

Arteriole

Sweat gland

Hair
Sweat pore
Stratum corneum
Stratum granulosum
Stratum spinosum
Stratum basale
Sebaceous gland
Muscle
Venule
Hair bulb
Motor nerve
Sensory nerve
Adipose tissue

body relatively stable inside, in spite of constantly changing conditions outside.

The intact skin acts as a barrier to invasion by the multitude of microorganisms that come into contact with its surface. The waterproof keratin in the epidermis prevents all substances that are able to dissolve in water from entering the body through the skin. The presence of the pigment melanin enables the skin to absorb harmful radiation from the sun safely, up to a point. Too much exposure to the sun causes sunburn, drying of the skin, a loss of elasticity, and wrinkling. More important, every sunburn increases the risk of skin cancer. Inheritance determines the amount of melanin possessed; although all races have the same number of melanocytes, people of different races differ greatly in the amount of melanin that their cells produce. The more melanin present, the darker the skin. The absence of a certain gene prevents melanin synthesis, causing those persons without the gene to be albinos. Skin color also varies because of the yellow pigment called carotene, which is found in the upper layers of the epidermis, and because of the red blood that is visible through the dermis of light-skinned people.

A very important function of skin is its role in temperature regulation. The body rids itself of excess heat by sweating. Excess heat passes from blood vessels into sweat glands, which conduct heat and perspiration to the surface. A large amount of heat can be lost as the sweat evaporates, thus maintaining normal body temperature. At other times, skin conserves heat by tightening blood vessels and reducing sweat secretion. Simultaneously, shivering, which is the involuntary contraction of skeletal muscles, releases internal heat to counteract excessive heat loss from the body. Only certain sweat glands-namely, those in the armpit and groin-produce the type of sweat that gives rise to an odor.

The waterproof quality of the skin prevents most substances from being absorbed through it into the body. Among the materials that can be absorbed are oxygen; vitamins A, D, E, and K; steroids such as cortisone cream; and, unfortunately, poisons such as insecticides.

The skin is able to produce a form of vitamin D that becomes active and useful to the body after passing through the kidneys. This synthesis requires a small amount of sunshine-far less than that necessary to cause a sunburn. If the skin does not produce enough vitamin D to enable the body to use calcium correctly, then vitamin D is needed in the diet.

Two very specialized accessory structures of the skin have their own particular functions. One of these skin derivatives is the pili, or hair. Except for the palms, soles, lips, and eyelids, the entire body contains hair. Each hair consists of a hair shaft that grows beyond the skin surface and a hair root lying inside a hair follicle. The follicle itself consists of epidermis that has grown downward into the dermis. Each hair follicle has an associated sebaceous gland that produces sebum, an oily substance, to lubricate the hair. Scalp hair protects the scalp from overexposure to the sun and from cold weather; eyelashes and tiny hairs inside the nose and ear canals help keep foreign material from entering.

The other important skin accessory is the nails. Each nail consists of a nail plate attached to a nail bed. Nails contain modified, highly keratinized cells from the stratum corneum. The basal cells that reproduce to make the nails grow lie under the cuticle at the base of the nail. Nails help to protect fingers and toes and enable humans to pick up tiny objects more efficiently.

Disorders and Diseases

The complex anatomy of the skin allows for the development of many possible defects and diseases. Three disorders that modern medical science attempts to understand and alleviate are psoriasis, cancer, and the many varieties of contact dermatitis.

Psoriasis, one of the most common of all skin conditions, is said to afflict about 3 percent of the American population. It commonly runs in families and affects both sexes equally. It may develop in childhood or old age but typically appears in the second or third decade of life. It most frequently occurs as scaly patches, or plaques, on the elbows, knees, and scalp but may appear on the back, belly, buttocks, and legs. Many people with psoriasis experience itching; surprisingly, some do not.

Human epidermis cells usually take about twenty-eight days to move from the stratum basale, where they are produced, to the top of the stratum corneum, where bathing removes them. This means that the cycle of normal epidermal cells in transit through the skin is accomplished in a month or more, allowing the cells time to mature. In psoriasis patients, this transit period is as short as four days. The reproducing basal cells divide five to ten times too rapidly, and the epidermis thickens enormously, but in patches. The skin cells of psoriasis patients are so abnormal that the patients' immune systems form antibodies that attack and destroy them, further damaging the ruptured, scaly surface. There is a notable tendency for psoriatic lesions or sores to form at sites of childhood injuries such as sunburns, scratches, scrapes, and areas where chickenpox was particularly widespread. These lesions often become pus-filled abscesses that contain enormous numbers of white blood cells. The epidermal cells no longer die at the stratum granulosum, and even the granules themselves are lost. The outermost corneum layer, which is usually dead, dry, and

protective, is full of living but abnormally functioning cells. In the dermis below, large, dilated, thin-walled blood vessels appear, and the epidermis directly above them is disproportionately thin. Scratching or picking at the plaques causes bleeding.

The exact cause of psoriasis is not yet known. Genetic factors play a role in its development, since one-third of all patients have a family member who is also afflicted. In addition to the physical discomfort and damage to self-esteem caused by this very obvious skin condition, it can lead to heat loss, fever, severe arthritis, heart failure, and even death.

The many forms of skin cancer can also cause great disfigurement and even death. Two frequently observed types are basal cell carcinoma and malignant melanoma. Basal cell cancers, which may begin in the hair follicle epithelium, are the most common skin cancers, accounting for almost 70 percent of all cases. Fortunately, they are also the most easily treated. They are most often found where sunlight strikes the hardest, on the neck, scalp, face, and shoulders. Basal cell cancers often start as small bumps but grow wider and more elevated, usually with a cavity in the center. Although their surface is shiny and filled with tiny blood vessels, their color may still be like that of normal skin. If left untreated, basal cell carcinomas may develop a crust or an ulcer that cannot heal. Although they seldom metastasize, shifting or spreading through the bloodstream to another part of the body, they often do great damage to the tissues and structures directly under them. Those that grow near ears and eyes can cause loss of function of those organs.

In almost all cases, the appearance of basal cell carcinomas is directly related to sun exposure. A few seem to be related to previous scars, burns, tattoos, or exposure to arsenic. It is important to be aware of the warning signs of basal cell carcinomas. Some can be felt as well as seen as reddish or dotted lumps; others look like open sores caused by scratches or insect bites that do not heal. Because these cancers, which often grow for two years before detection, have such varied appearances, they can be diagnosed accurately only by biopsy.

The most dangerous skin cancers are the malignant melanomas. They begin in the pigmented cells called melanocytes but usually and quite rapidly invade deeper tissue. Severe sunburns early in life seem to be their usual cause. Many start as small dark brown growths similar to moles, although they may become white, blue, or reddish and irregular in shape as they grow. Often they will bleed if rubbed. People who have acquired one hundred or more moles by young adulthood are considered genetically predisposed toward these dangerous melanomas; such people should use sunscreens every day all year long. It should be noted that half of all melanomas arise from apparently normal skin that has no moles. The malignant melanomas are much more dangerous than the basal cell carcinomas because they tend to release cancerous cells into the bloodstream that latch on to and grow into numerous internal organs.

Seldom life-threatening, contact dermatitis can still be very uncomfortable for a patient. Dermatitis is an inflammation of the skin that usually is a result of an allergic reaction and may include redness, swelling, blistering, crusting, and scaling among its symptoms. In all its many varieties, it probably forms the bulk of a dermatologist's practice. Contact dermatitis results from coming into contact with a causing substance, such as poison ivy, poison oak, or poison sumac. The sap from these plants contains urushiol, a substance to which 70 percent of all people are allergic.

Large numbers of persons are allergic to the metal nickel and can develop inflammations from wearing nickel rings, watches, earrings, or other jewelry. Nickel zippers and clothing snaps, eyeglass frames and sewing needles, and even coins can cause a reaction.

The chemicals in permanent hair dyes cause terrible swelling and itching of the face and neck in some people. Oddly, the scalp under the dyed hair is often unaffected. When dermatitis seems to result from hair dyes, it is often because the affected person has simultaneously been using certain sunscreens, the pain reliever benzocaine, or one of many other common medicines.

The chemical potassium dichromate is found in many detergents. People who experience dermatitis caused by detergent use should avoid other chromate-containing products as well. These include inks, paints, bleaches, and spackling, to name only a few.

Other people contract dermatitis caused by a formaldehyde allergy. Permanent-press clothing and sheets are made wrinkle-proof by the use of a formaldehyde-based substance. Individuals with a formaldehyde allergy must also avoid many paper products, cosmetics, and disinfectants that contain formaldehyde derivatives.

Susceptibility to contact dermatitis from rubber products is widespread. Surprisingly, it often appears long after the exposure and is most common in manufacturing workers.

In modern society, with its heavy reliance on over-the-counter drugs, cleaning products of all kinds, deodorants and cosmetics, insecticides and weed-killers, and innumerable other chemical products, the potential causes of contact dermatitis have been and will continue to be multiplied.

Perspective and Prospects

Research in dermatology both borrows from and sheds light upon many other branches of medical science. Immunology, endocrinology, biochemistry, surgery, and oncology are just a few of many.

Diseases of the skin can reveal the presence of many otherwise unseen internal disease conditions. Shiny, thin, reddish-yellow patches on the shins may be a sign of diabetes. Prediabetics are also susceptible to repeated yeast and fungal infections of the skin and have poor wound-healing ability.

Too little thyroid hormone causes coarse hair; thickened, dry, cool skin; and rough plaques on the shins. Too much thyroid hormone causes thin hair, excessive sweating, and, surprisingly, identical rough plaques on the shins.

Abnormally dark skin can be a sign of drug side effects, the presence of heavy metals, poor adrenal gland output, or pituitary tumors. Skin may also darken from excess iron intake or, very noticeably, from a widespread malignant melanoma.

Various bowel diseases may also cause skin conditions. The small intestine defect involving a flattened, malfunctioning lining can produce severely itchy blisters on the limbs and the back. Ulcers in the large intestine often produce deep, dirty-looking skin ulcers.

The presence of cancer in the breast, bowel, or lungs may precipitate thousands of external wartlike growths or flat, waxy-surfaced growths. Similarly, the gradual appearance, usually on the legs of the elderly, of fishlike skin may reveal the early presence of cancer of the lymph glands.

Alcoholism reveals itself in spider telangiectasia, webs of dilated capillaries on the skin surface. The presence of hepatitis, a serious viral infection of the liver, is indicated by the yellowing of the skin known as jaundice.

Two other links among dermatology, immunology, and oncology are the search for a vaccine against skin cancer and a new treatment called photopheresis. Since the late 1960s, there has been an ongoing attempt to develop a vaccine to prevent a recurrence of malignant melanoma. This is a particularly important pursuit because those who have survived one case of melanoma have a high risk of developing future ones.

Photopheresis patients take a drug called psoralen. Two hours later, their blood is drawn and exposed to ultraviolet light. The interaction between the psoralen and the light destroys abnormal white blood cells, after which the blood is returned to the body. Since 1987, photopheresis has been used to treat a cancer of the immune system that begins in the skin. Researchers hope eventually to use psoralen to treat arthritis and lupus, and to prevent the rejection of organ transplants.

For many years, drugs for internal conditions could be administered only orally or by injection. In both methods, the circulating amount may be too high to be safe immediately after it is given and too low to be effective as the hours go by. Dermatologists have greatly advanced medical science by developing transdermal patches. These patches enable a steady supply of a drug to enter the bloodstream by absorption through the skin. By the end of the twentieth century, patches had been developed to treat angina, high blood pressure, motion sickness, menopausal symptoms, and nicotine addiction.

One of the greatest traumas skin can suffer is a widespread burn. Although surgeons have had great success in transplanting many internal organs, they are unable to permanently transplant skin from another person. In 1981, they developed a marvelous technique to produce artificial skin. It uses animal skin protein seeded with a few skin cells taken from the patient. From this small patch, a large enough piece of skin can be grown to cover the wounds until the gradually healing skin replaces it.

From the earliest simple salves for skin rashes to the

great discoveries of transdermal patches and artificial skin, dermatologists have done and continue to do their share in advancing medical science.

—*Grace D. Matzen*

See also Abscess drainage; Abscesses; Acne; Acupressure; Acupuncture; Age spots; Albinos; Allergies; Athlete's foot; Bedsores; Biopsy; Birthmarks; Bites and stings; Blisters; Boils; Bruises; Burns and scalds; Candidiasis; Canker sores; Cells; Chickenpox; Cold sores; Collagen; Corns and calluses; Cradle cap; Cryosurgery; Cyst removal; Cysts; Dermatitis; Dermatology; Dermatology, pediatric; Dermatopathology; Diaper rash; Eczema; Edema; Electrical shock; Electrocauterization; Face lift and blepharoplasty; Fifth disease; Frostbite; Fungal infections; Glands; Grafts and grafting; Hair; Hair loss and baldness; Hair transplantation; Hand-foot-and-mouth disease; Heat exhaustion and heatstroke; Hives; Host-defense mechanisms; Human papillomavirus (HPV); Hyperhidrosis; Impetigo; Insect-borne diseases; Itching; Jaundice; Kawasaki disease; Laceration repair; Laser use in surgery; Leishmaniasis; Leprosy; Lesions; Lice, mites, and ticks; Lower extremities; Measles; Melanoma; Moles; Morgellons disease; Nails; Necrotizing fasciitis; Numbness and tingling; Pigmentation; Pityriasis alba; Pityriasis rosea; Plastic surgery; Poisonous plants; Porphyria; Psoriasis; Radiation sickness; Rashes; Ringworm; Rocky Mountain spotted fever; Rosacea; Roseola; Rubella; Scabies; Scarlet fever; Scleroderma; Sense organs; Shingles; Skin cancer; Skin disorders; Skin lesion removal; Smallpox; Stevens-Johnson syndrome; Stretch marks; Styes; Sunburn; Sweating; Systemic lupus erythematosus (SLE); Tattoos and body piercing; Touch; Upper extremities; Vitiligo; Warts; Wrinkles.

For Further Information:

Goodman, Thomas, and Stephanie Young. *Smart Face*. Englewood Cliffs, N.J.: Prentice Hall, 1988. An easy-to-read explanation of skin structure, problems, and care, with special emphasis on delicate facial skin. Contains an extensive appendix of consumer product information.

Jacknin, Jeanette. *Smart Medicine for Your Skin*. New York: Putnam, 2001. An accessible and comprehensive guide to skin problems and solutions that include traditional therapies and alternative medicine choices.

Lamberg, Lynne. *Skin Disorders*. Philadelphia: Chelsea House, 2001. This brief volume is an introduction to the study of skin problems. Contains a very helpful glossary, a bibliography, and a list of organizations to contact for more information.

Lees, Mark. *Skin Care: Beyond the Basics*. 3d ed. Clifton Park, N.Y.: Thomson/Delmar Learning, 2007. A text for estheticians and students in the field that provides practical information on treating many kinds of skin problems and discusses topics such as rosacea, sensitive skin, hormones and menopause, and postlaser skin care.

Mackie, Rona M. *Clinical Dermatology*. 5th ed. New York: Oxford University Press, 2003. A text written for dermatology students but useful for the general public for more precise and detailed information than that contained in popular works. Illustrated in color.

Siegel, Mary-Ellen. *Safe in the Sun*. New York: Walker, 1995. Presents information from research of leading dermatologists and ophthalmologists showing the relationship between sun exposure and damage to skin and eyes. Easily understood by the general public. Contains an extensive glossary and many pages of helpful further sources of information.

Turkington, Carol, and Jeffrey S. Dover. *The Encyclopedia of Skin and Skin Disorders*. 3d ed. New York: Facts On File, 2007. More than one thousand entries on skin-related topics, including diseases, treatments, resources and organizations, skin cancer, acne treatment, FDA approvals of new treatments, and remedies for wrinkled skin.

Weedon, David. *Skin Pathology*. 3d ed. New York: Churchill Livingstone/Elsevier, 2010. Text with extensive photographs, covering tissue reaction patterns; the epidermis, dermis, and subcutis; the skin in systemic and miscellaneous diseases; infections and infestations; and tumors, among other topics.

Skin cancer

Disease/Disorder

Anatomy or system affected: Lymphatic system, skin

Specialties and related fields: Dermatology, environmental health, immunology, oncology

Definition: Malignancies of the skin (and sometimes spreading to the internal organs) caused by the ultraviolet radiation in sunlight.

Cancer is the common term used to describe the large class of diseases called neoplasms. Neoplasms, which occur only in multicellular organisms, develop and function in an autonomous way that does not abide by the biological mechanisms that govern the growth and metabolism of the individual cells and the reactions that take place in a living organism. When such neoplasms grow at a rate faster than the tissues from which they arise, while at the same time invading those tissues, they are called malignant and are commonly described as cancerous. Benign neoplasms, which do not invade surrounding tissues, generally are not as dangerous as malignant ones.

Sun radiation is life-sustaining, but the higher-energy part of the sunlight spectrum brings the danger of skin cancer. When living tissue is irradiated, its molecular structure is disrupted, thus initiating a chain of reactions, many of which are not the usual ones associated with the living organism. Therefore, a change in the chromosomal composition and the development of unwanted cells is likely to occur. Such changes take place because of the formation of free radicals in the deoxyribonucleic acid (DNA) molecules that constitute the genetic code. The result is skin cancer, the most common form of cancer in both men and women in the United States.

Types of skin cancer. Skin neoplasms may be benign or malignant, acquired or congenital, although the majority are benign and acquired. The common mole (the medical term for which is melanocytic nevus) is a neoplasm of benign melanocytes that is often present at birth and which is known as a birthmark. Such moles are generally harmless unless they are large in size, in which case they may have up to a 10 percent chance of becoming malignant. Other melanocytic nevi are strawberry hemangiomas and portwine stains, which are of vascular origin.

The most common forms of skin cancer are the basal cell and squamous cell carcinomas, which arise from the corresponding part of the keratinocytes of the epidermis and are caused by the cumulative effects of ultraviolet radiation on the skin. They are generally localized, however, and rarely metastasize. These cancers are easily identified as persisting sores or crusting patches that grow mostly on sun-exposed parts of the body such as the hands, neck, arms, and nose. They can be treated with routine surgical procedures.

A malignant melanoma is formed from the pigment-forming melanocyte and almost certainly undergoes metastasis. It should therefore be removed surgically at the earliest possible stage. If the melanoma is detected at a later stage, chemotherapy and irradiation are the techniques usually applied. A malignant melanoma appears as a lesion that increases in size and turns several colors, such as black,

Information on Skin Cancer

Causes: Genetic factors, ultraviolet radiation from sun exposure

Symptoms: Lesion that increases in size and turns several colors (black, blue, white, brown); in later stages, itching, bleeding, and pain

Duration: Short-term to recurrent

Treatments: Surgical removal, chemotherapy, radiation therapy

blue, white, and brown. Symptoms such as itching, bleeding, and pain are not as common at first but are encountered at the later stages of development.

There are two additional skin malignancies that may be fatal: mycosis fungoides and Kaposi's sarcoma. Mycosis fungoides is a skin lymphoma that may be confined to one location for ten or more years before it metastasizes to internal organs, with death following. As a result, it is difficult to track this skin cancer, both clinically and histologically, and several biopsies (skin histological examinations) may be required to ascertain its presence. On the other hand, Kaposi's sarcoma occurs either as lesions (commonly among older Mediterranean men) or as skin abnormalities in HIV-infected people. The sarcoma is derived from skin blood vessels and appears as violet patches or lesions. As long as it is contained only in the skin, it is not fatal. Once the inner organs are affected, however, death is imminent, even though the lesions may be treated with irradiation and chemotherapy.

The effects of sunlight on skin. Extensive skin exposure to sunlight, such as at the beach, leads to the polymerization of skin chemicals (known as catecholamines) and the subsequent formation of different types of epidermal pigmentation (the melanins), which are responsible for tanning. Tanning occurs only if there is gradual exposure to sunlight; otherwise, a sunburn will arise. Photoprotection is believed to be one of the major biological functions of the melanin pigment. It appears that melanin formation can participate effectively in reducing the harmful effects of sunlight by an array of photoinduced chemical reactions, which result in the consumption of scavenging active oxygen species such as the superoxide anion and hydrogen peroxide. It has been determined that in biological systems, superoxide and hydrogen peroxide are formed in small quantities during normal processes. Both species are known to produce several biological effects, most of which are harmful to tissues. It should be pointed out, however, that although melanin may act as a free radical scavenger, it may also become energetically overloaded and may change to a toxic state. Evidence exists that melanin increases the radiative damage to cells, which leads to sunlight-induced skin cancer. In other words, melanin formation is good only when moderate exposure to sunlight occurs.

In the atmosphere 12 to 48 kilometers above the earth's surface lies a small layer of ozone. Although this layer does not contain much ozone-it is estimated to be about 3 millimeters thick under normal conditions of temperature and pressure-it has a profound effect on life. The ozone layer absorbs the harmful ultraviolet radiation from the sun, thus providing the mechanism for the heating of the stratosphere. A reduction in the ozone layer would lead to a large increase of ultraviolet rays intruding into the atmosphere, thus increasing the incidence of skin cancer. F. S. Rowland and M. J. Molina declared in 1974 that the presence of the volatile chlorofluorocarbons would eventually reduce the ozone layer. Some measurements done by scientists in 1979 showed a decrease in the layer, which led to the action taken by several governments to decrease and replace the chlorofluorocarbons commonly used in aerosols. As the average life span steadily increases, the incidence of skin cancer will increase as well. The use of effective sunscreens and sunglasses with high ultraviolet blocking is recommended for people who are exposed to large amounts of sunlight.

—*Soraya Ghayourmanesh, Ph.D.*

See also Cancer; Carcinogens; Carcinoma; Chemotherapy; Dermatology; Dermatopathology; Kaposi's sarcoma; Lesions; Lymphadenopathy and lymphoma; Malignancy and metastasis; Melanoma; Moles; Radiation therapy; Skin; Skin disorders; Skin lesion removal; Sunburn; Warts.

For Further Information:

Dollinger, Malin, et al. *Everyone's Guide to Cancer Therapy.* 5th ed. Kansas City, Mo.: Andrews McMeel, 2008. An excellent source of medical information about cancer, written for the general public. Describes various cancer sites in the body. Includes a helpful glossary of medical terminology.

James, William D., Timothy G. Berger, and Dirk M. Elston. *Andrews' Diseases of the Skin: Clinical Dermatology.* 10th ed. Philadelphia: Saunders/Elsevier, 2006. Includes discussions of skin cancer.

McClay, Edward F., and Jodie Smith. *One Hundred Questions and Answers About Melanoma and Other Skin Cancers.* Boston: Jones and Bartlett, 2004. Uses a reader-friendly format to survey a range of topics related to skin cancer.

Siegel, Mary-Ellen. *Safe in the Sun.* New York: Walker, 1995. This comprehensive book describes the benefits of sunlight, the risks of exposure and how to protect the skin, and how damage that has already occurred can be treated.

Skin Cancer Foundation. http://www.skincancer.org. Promotes public education about skin cancer through campaigns against sun exposure and in support of early detection and research into new diagnostic techniques and therapies.

Weedon, David. *Skin Pathology.* 3d ed. New York: Churchill Livingstone/Elsevier, 2010. Text with extensive photographs, covering tissue reaction patterns; the epidermis, dermis, and subcutis; the skin in systemic and miscellaneous diseases; infections and infestations; and tumors, among other topics.

Skin disorders

Disease/Disorder

Anatomy or system affected: Skin

Specialties and related fields: Dermatology, family medicine, occupational health

Definition: Diseases and conditions that affect the skin, ranging from harmless to life-threatening.

Key terms:

benign: in reference to a neoplasm, having a nonmalignant character

dermatology: the study of the skin, its chemistry, physiology, histopathology, cutaneous lesions, and the relationships of these lesions to systemic disease

malignant: in reference to a neoplasm, having the property of uncontrollable growth and dissemination, recurrence after removal, or both

melanin: dark brown or black molecules of pigment that normally occur in the skin, hair, pigmented coat of the retina, and pupil of the eye and in selected cells of the brain

metastasis: the shifting of a disease, or its local manifestations, from one portion of the body to another; in cancer, the appearance of neoplasms in parts of the body remote from the primary tumor

Anatomy of the Skin

The skin is the largest organ of the body. It provides a barrier between the external world and the internal world: It protects against external contamination and helps to maintain the sterility of the internal body. The skin also assists in temperature regulation; humans can survive only within a narrow temperature range. The skin has nerve receptors that supply the brain with information, providing an interface with the world. There are specialized receptors for touch, temperature, vibration, and position in space (proprioception).

Appendages to the skin are fingernails, toenails, and hair. They are mainly of psychological importance. Nails protect the tips of fingers and toes in humans but are not needed for protection as claws are in lower animals. Hair is analogous to feathers. In birds, tiny muscles attached to the base of each feather cause them to be ruffled; this creates air pockets and allows birds to conserve heat and keep warm. The same muscles persist in humans, causing "goose flesh," but they do not serve any other function. The main importance of these appendages is cosmetic. For example, people spend billions of dollars on hair care products each year. The motivation for this activity is psychological.

The two main layers in skin are the epidermis and dermis. The epidermis is the upper or outermost layer, and cells are continually formed at its base. As new cells are formed, existing cells are pushed toward the surface of the skin. These cells gradually lose their watery central contents, causing them to dry out (desiccate) and become flattened. This process normally spans approximately a month. Thus, the surface of the body is largely composed of dead cells that have become flattened. These cells are normally lost on a continual basis and create dandruff when shed from the scalp. On other parts of the body, sloughed cells provide excellent conditions for bacterial growth, accounting for the unpleasant odors that accompany poor hygiene habits.

Two other important types of cells are found in the epidermis: melanocytes and Langerhans cells. Melanocytes contain melanin and provide all the variations of pigmentation found in the human species. They multiply when stimulated by the ultraviolet radiation in sunlight. This causes the skin to become darker, a protective mechanism against damage from ultraviolet radiation. Langerhans cells contain surface receptors for immunoglobulins. They play a central role in allergic reactions of the skin, such as contact dermatitis or delayed hypersensitivity reaction.

The dermis is an inner layer of skin located beneath the epidermis. Its main function is protection. Within the dermis are highly specialized cells containing microscopic filaments. These cells impart tensile strength to the skin in much the same way that fibers strengthen fiberglass or reinforcing steel mesh strengthens concrete. Because they are so dense, they also serve as a barrier to the entry of most pathogens and many chemicals. Eccrine sweat glands are found in the dermis throughout the entire body. These produce a salty secretion (essentially salt water) that assists in thermoregulation through evaporative cooling. They are also sensitive to emotional stress. Apocrine sweat glands are primarily in the armpits (axilla) and groin and produce a milky secretion. When these secretions are broken down by bacteria on the surface of the skin, a characteristic odor is produced. The bases of hair follicles are also found in the dermis. The small sebaceous, or oil-secreting, gland associated with most hair follicles has the function of softening and moisturizing the hair.

Hair is found on most surfaces of the body; exceptions are the palms of the hands, the soles of the feet, and the glans penis in men. The texture and length of the hair vary with location on the body, gender, genetic heritage, and age. Dramatic increases in the growth and distribution of hair occur at puberty. With increasing age, hair is typically lost from the scalp and other body parts. It also changes color, assuming a gray or white color because of the loss of melanin at the base of the hair follicle.

Complications and Disorders

When normal skin anatomy and physiology are upset, several common diseases or disorders result. When the barrier provided by the skin is broken, bacteria, viruses, fungi, and other pathogens can invade the body, leading to infections. Locally, these infections can cause inflammation (redness and pain) of the skin; if widespread, they can lead to systemic infections. When the cells and other substances found in the skin become irregular or are abnormal, skin disorders or conditions result.

Skin disorders and conditions. Pigmentation of the skin results from the presence of melanocytes, cells that manufacture and contain melanin. Most humans have pigmentation over their entire bodies; the degree of pigmentation varies with different racial and ethnic groups. Local areas of increased color have a range of names depending on the size of the pigmented area. A freckle is small and discrete. A nevus is a larger area of hyperpigmentation. These conditions are attributable to underlying variations in the distribution of melanocytes. They are genetic in origin and permanent; they are also accentuated by exposure to sunlight. Melasmas are irregular, flat, light brown areas on the neck, cheeks, or forehead. They are caused by hormonal changes associated with pregnancy or contraceptive pills and by exposure to sunlight. Melasmas fade with the reduction of excess hormones. There are also color changes in the labia of females during pregnancy; these changes are both harmless and permanent.

Generalized increases in skin coloration can occur with some metabolic diseases. Addison's disease involves an increase in melanocyte-stimulating hormone. This leads to an overall bronzing of the body, with accentuation in creases of the palms and soles. The condition subsides with treatment of the underlying cause of the disease. Similar pigment increases are associated with some forms of lung cancer, hemochromatosis, and chronic arsenic exposure. The latter two conditions are caused by the deposition of iron (hemochromatosis) and arsenic in the skin.

Generalized decreases in skin coloration can also occur. If melanocytes fail to migrate to the skin during embryologic development, hair follicles will lack color, resulting in a condition called piebaldism. Characteristically, this is a white patch in the hair of the forehead. Vitiligo is caused by an immunologically mediated loss of melanocytes. Individuals with phenylketonuria (PKU) experience a generalized depigmentation of hair and eye color, in addition to mental retardation, if the condition is not adequately and promptly treated. An individual totally lacking melanocytes is called an albino; because melanin is also responsible for eye color, albinos have red eyes. The loss of hair is called alopecia. It can occur because of aging, sustained pulling on the hair with some hairstyles, and genetics. Women do not usually experience much alopecia until after the menopause. Conversely, some men start to lose their hair during their twenties.

Skin diseases. Eczema or dermatitis is a general term that describes a skin disease involving vesicles that ooze fluid. These conditions are usually characterized by a rash; they are inflammatory reactions, commonly caused by contact with a chemical or plant material. They can be caused by an adverse reaction to a drug or by sunlight. Bacteria, yeasts, or other fungi on the skin can cause eczema. Most rashes itch or burn; they can be spread by scratching. Athlete's foot is a common example of an eczematous dermatitis.

Maculopapular diseases encompass several common skin conditions, such as red measles (rubeola), German measles (rubella), and scarlet fever. Viruses that land on the skin cause these diseases. They are characterized by relatively large, localized areas of changed skin color (macules) that are also raised (papules) but not fluid-filled. After their clinical course is run, they disappear without leaving a scar. The more dangerous toxic shock syndrome also belongs to this group of diseases; it is caused by toxin from the bacteria *Staphylococcus aureus*.

Thickening of the skin and the formation of red to purple areas having sharply defined borders characterize papulosquamous skin diseases. The most common example is psoriasis. Other examples are pityriasis and ichthyosis. The pathology responsible for psoriasis is an alteration in the normal development of skin cells. In individuals with psoriasis, new skin cells develop and migrate to the surface in only five days instead of the usual thirty. This fact alone explains the flaking (rapid cell turnover), redness (thinner skin and a rich blood supply for new skin), and pain and itching (less protection for sensory nerve endings) experienced. Pityriasis includes a group of different conditions

---

Information on Skin Disorders

Causes: Infection, disease, allergies, environmental factors (e.g., ultraviolet radiation), hormonal changes, irritation, clogged sweat glands, eczema

Symptoms: May include inflammation, infection, flaking, pain, itching, redness, rashes, lesions, bleeding

Duration: Acute to chronic

Treatments: Topical ointments, antibiotics, corticosteroids, surgery, chemotherapy, radiation therapy

---

caused by different viruses. Patches or large spots develop on the skin. They usually resolve within a few weeks. Aside from being locally photosensitive, they usually are not serious. Ichthyosis describes a group of genetic conditions characterized by extreme scaling of the skin.

Vesiculobullous diseases have fluid-filled blisters that can vary in size from relatively small (vesicles) to relatively large (bullae). Insect bites, herpes, and some bacterial infections lead to the formation of vesicles or bullae. Such conditions are attributable to an immune reaction that leads to the formation of blisters at the junction between epidermis and dermis. They can be accompanied by intense pruritus (itching); scratching often leads to scarring.

Pustular diseases of the skin include acne, folliculitis, and candidiasis. They are characterized by the inflammation of hair follicles caused by surface bacteria or yeasts. Adequate personal hygiene is the most effective method of prevention. These diseases are usually not serious, but prolonged or repeated attacks can result in scarring and disfigurement. The sebaceous glands, which secrete oil at the base of hair follicles, can increase in size. The subsequent increase in oil output worsens the condition.

Clogged sweat glands can lead to acne. While this is primarily a problem for teenagers, it can affect individuals of any age. Exposure to cutting oils and other hydrocarbons such as gasoline and paint thinners can cause a similar condition called chloracne, which is inflammation in the base of hair follicles found on exposed skin in areas such as the nape of the neck, forearms, and face. The inability to sense temperature and regulate body heat through sweating is called anhidrosis, a condition that can cause shock and potentially death.

Other diseases that can affect the skin. Five such diseases are worthy of mention: leprosy, scleroderma, lupus, atherosclerosis, and diabetes mellitus. Leprosy, or Hansen's disease, is caused by infection by *Mycobacterium leprae*, a relative of the bacteria that cause tuberculosis. In leprosy, the causative organism accumulates in the skin and peripheral nerves. This causes disfigurement and loss of sensation, the latter being similar to that experienced by an uncontrolled diabetic. Disfigurement is responsible for the stigma associated with leprosy since ancient times: loss of fingers and toes, as well as mutilation of the nose and ears. Leprosy is caused by long-term association with the organism and can be adequately treated with appropriate antibiotics.

Scleroderma (literally, "hard skin") is an uncommon disease characterized by fibrosis of the skin and involvement of visceral organs. The skin involvement can range from an isolated, hardened patch to a life-threatening, generalized condition described as an ever-tightening case of steel. The skin becomes stretched tightly over the underlying skeleton. Skin tone is lost with restriction of movement.

Systemic lupus erythematosus is a disease of unknown etiology that is characterized by inflammation in many different organ systems. The skin is usually involved, as nearly all individuals with lupus develop a characteristic butterfly-shaped rash on their faces. This red coloration covers the cheeks and nose. Persons with lupus are also sensitive to sunlight, and many develop alopecia. Most of those affected are female. The disease waxes and wanes; treatment depends on the particular organs involved.

Atherosclerosis and diabetes can block the arteries supplying the nerves of the skin, leading to a loss of sensory input. When the patient is unable to experience pain, cuts and other abrasions on the skin are not noticed. Untreated, these lesions can lead to gangrene, sometimes requiring amputation of a body part.

Skin cancer. The most commonly diagnosed form of cancer is that involving the skin. It is not the most fatal form, but millions of cases are discovered annually. The origin of most skin cancers can be traced to excessive exposure to radiation from the sun. They can occur on any surface of the body, although they are more common on areas that are usually exposed to the sun, such as the face, the backs of the hand, and the neck. Skin cancers can arise in the epidermis or dermis. The majority are noncancerous, or benign. Epidermal nodules are characterized by local thickening of the epidermis, often accompanied by scaling of the skin in the affected area. Nodules in the dermis may appear as lumps with no alteration of the epidermis above them.

There are three malignant forms of skin cancer. Basal cell carcinoma arises from cells deep in the epidermis. This form of tumor rarely spreads (metastasizes), but it can be extensive and destructive locally. Squamous cell carcinoma is less common but can be invasive (involving adjacent tissues) and can metastasize. Melanoma is relatively uncommon but can grow extremely rapidly; it has the potential to be fatal in a matter of months. It involves the uncontrolled growth of melanocytes. Melanomas have irregular borders and color or pigmentation. Any pigmented lesion or suspicious change in the skin should be evaluated by a medical professional in a timely manner.

Prevention is the preferred method of dealing with skin cancer. When outside, loose-fitting clothing can provide protection from the sun, and a hat can protect the head. When exposure is unavoidable, a product with a sun-blocking agent will reduce exposure. Limiting the time of exposure to the sun until the body has reacted by producing additional melanocytes (tanned) is recommended.

Prolonged exposure to the sun also accelerates changes in the skin associated with aging. Collagen fibers provide the characteristic firm feel to the skin of a young person. With aging the skin becomes less firm, losing some of its tone, and begins to sag. Inadequate moisture also contributes to the loss of skin tone. Excessive exposure to the sun hastens both of these processes.

—*L. Fleming Fallon, Jr., M.D., Ph.D., M.P.H.*

See also Abscess drainage; Abscesses; Acne; Age spots; Aging; Albinos; Allergies; Bedsores; Birthmarks; Bites and stings; Blisters; Boils; Bruises; Canker sores; Carcinoma; Chickenpox; Cold sores; Corns and calluses; Cradle cap; Cyst removal; Cysts; Dermatitis; Dermatology; Dermatology, pediatric; Dermatopathlogy; Diaper rash; Eczema; Fifth disease; Grafts and grafting; Hair; Hair loss and baldness; Hand-foot-and-mouth disease; Herpes; Hives; Human papillomavirus (HPV); Hyperhidrosis; Impetigo; Inflammation; Insect-borne diseases; Itching; Kawasaki disease; Leprosy; Lesions; Measles; Melanoma; Moles; Morgellons disease; Necrotizing fasciitis; Neurofibromatosis; Pigmentation; Pityriasis alba; Pityriasis rosea; Poisonous plants; Psoriasis; Rashes; Ringworm; Rocky Mountain spotted fever; Rosacea; Scabies; Scleroderma; Skin; Skin cancer; Skin lesion removal; Stevens-Johnson syndrome; Stretch marks; Styes; Sunburn; Sweating; Systemic lupus erythematosus (SLE); Tattoo removal; Tattoos and body piercing; Vitiligo; Warts; Wrinkles.

For Further Information:

Burns, Tony, et al., eds. *Rook's Textbook of Dermatology.* 7th ed. Malden, Mass.: Blackwell Science, 2004. This is a core text in dermatology that will appeal to professionals and members of the general public who want a concise introduction to the subject. The aim of the book is to integrate basic science with clinical practice.

Frankel, David H., ed. *Field Guide to Clinical Dermatology.* 2d ed. Philadelphia: Lippincott Williams & Wilkins, 2006. Frankel, a noted internist and dermatologist, has enlisted widely respected and talented colleagues to help in the production of this book. It is a uniquely organized and easily readable field guide complete with 220 pages of excellent color illustrations.

Freinkel, Ruth K., and David T. Woodley, eds. *Biology of the Skin.* New York: Parthenon, 2001. Covers the basic biology of the skin, how the skin functions, effects of the environment, the molecules that direct cutaneous function, genetic influences, and methods in cutaneous research.

Goldsmith, Lowell A., Gerald S. Lazarus, and Michael D. Tharp. *Adult and Pediatric Dermatology: A Color Guide to Diagnosis and Treatment.* Philadelphia: F. A. Davis, 1997. This book provides excellent pictures to accompany good descriptions of dermatologic diseases.

Grob, J. J., et al., eds. *Epidemiology, Causes, and Prevention of Skin Diseases.* Cambridge, Mass.: Blackwell Science, 1997. This well-written book presents data on large groups of people. The sections on skin cancer are especially noteworthy.

Kenet, Barney, and Patricia Lawler. *Saving Your Skin: Prevention, Early Detection, and Treatment of Melanoma and Other Skin Cancers.* 2d ed. Chicago: Four Walls Eight Windows, 1998. Skin cancer is the focus of this title, which reviews the early symptoms of melanoma, its causes, and its treatment. Very few skin care titles do more than offer a chapter on the problem.

Sams, W. Mitchell, Jr., and Peter J. Lynch, eds. *Principles and Practice of Dermatology.* 2d ed. London: Churchill Livingstone, 1996. This is a new edition of a dermatology reference guide and text emphasizing accurate diagnosis by succinct discussions in eighty-five presentations featuring color photographs.

Weedon, David. *Skin Pathology.* 3d ed. New York: Churchill Livingstone/Elsevier, 2010. Text with extensive photographs, covering tissue reaction patterns; the epidermis, dermis, and subcutis; the skin in systemic and miscellaneous diseases; infections and infestations; and tumors, among other topics.

Skin grafting. *See* **Grafts and grafting.**

SALEM HEALTH

MAGILL'S
MEDICAL
GUIDE

Entries by Anatomy or System Affected

ALL
Abscesses
Accidents
Acupuncture
Adrenal glands
Aging
Aging: Extended care
Alternative medicine
Anatomy
Antibiotic resistance
Antibiotics
Antihypertensives
Anti-inflammatory drugs
Antioxidants
Autopsy
Biomarker
Bionics and biotechnology
Birth defects
Burkitt's lymphoma
Cancer
Carcinogens
Carcinoma
Chemotherapy
Chronic granulomatous disease
Clinical trials
Club drugs
Coccidioidomycosis
Cockayne disease
Collagen
Congenital disorders
Critical care
Cryosurgery
Cysts
Death and dying
Diagnosis
Dietary reference intakes (DRIs)
Disease
Embryology
Emergency medicine
Emergency rooms
Emerging infectious diseases
Environmental diseases
Enzyme therapy
Epidemics and pandemics
Epidemiology
Epidermal nevus syndromes
Essential nutrients
Family-centered care
Family medicine
Fascia
Fatigue
Fever
First aid
First responder
Food guide plate
Forensic pathology
Genetic diseases

Genetic engineering
Genetic imprinting
Genetics and inheritance
Genomics
Geriatric assessment
Geriatrics and gerontology
Grafts and grafting
Growth
Healing
Health
Herbal medicine
Histology
Homeopathy
Hospital readmission
Hydrotherapy
Hyperadiposis
Hyperthermia and hypothermia
Hypertrophy
Hypochondriasis
Iatrogenic disorders
Imaging and radiology
Immunopathology
Infection
Infection control
Inflammation
Insect-borne diseases
Internet medicine
Invasive tests
Leptin
Lesions
Longevity
Macronutrients
Magnetic resonance imaging (MRI)
Malignancy and metastasis
Malnutrition
Massage
Medical home
Meditation
Men's health
Mental hygiene
Metabolic disorders
Metabolic syndrome
Mucopolysaccharidosis (MPS)
Multiple births
Münchausen syndrome by proxy
Neonatology
Niacin
Noninvasive tests
Nursing
Nutrition
Occupational health
Oncology
Opportunistic infections
Orthorexia nervosa
Ovaries
Over-the-counter medications
Pain

Pain management
Palliative care
Palliative medicine
Paramedics
Parasitic diseases
Pathology
Pediatrics
Perinatology
Physical examination
Physician assistants
Physiology
Phytochemicals
Plastic surgery
Positron emission tomography (PET)
    scanning
Preventive medicine
Progeria
Prognosis
Prostheses
Protein
Proteomics
Psychiatry
Psychosomatic disorders
Puberty and adolescence
Radiation therapy
Radiopharmaceuticals
Reflexes
Retroviruses
Safety issues for children
Safety issues for the elderly
Screening
Self-medication
Shock
Signs and symptoms
Stem cells
Stress
Stress reduction
Substance abuse
Sudden infant death syndrome (SIDS)
Supplements
Surgery
Surgical procedures
Surgical technologists
Syndrome
Systemic lupus erythematosus (SLE)
Systemic sclerosis
Systems and organs
Teratogens
Terminally ill: Extended care
Tissue engineering
Toxic shock syndrome
Toxicology
Transitional care
Tumor removal
Tumors
Viral hemorrhagic fevers
Viral infections

Vitamin D deficiency
Vitamins and minerals
Well-baby examinations
Wounds
Xenotransplantation
Zoonoses

ABDOMEN
Abdominal disorders
Adrenalectomy
Amebiasis
Amniocentesis
Aneurysmectomy
Appendectomy
Appendicitis
Back pain
Bariatric surgery
Bladder removal
Bypass surgery
Campylobacter infections
Candidiasis
Cesarean section
Cholecystectomy
Cholecystitis
Colitis
Colon
Colon therapy
Colorectal cancer
Colorectal polyp removal
Colorectal surgery
Constipation
Culdocentesis
Cushing's syndrome
Diabetes mellitus
Dialysis
Diarrhea and dysentery
Digestion
Diverticulitis and diverticulosis
Eating disorders
Electrolysis
Endoscopic retrograde
    cholangiopancreatography (ERCP)
Endoscopy
Enemas
Fallopian tube
Fistula repair
Gallbladder
Gallbladder diseases
Gastrectomy
Gastroenteritis
Gastroenterology
Gastrointestinal disorders
Gastrointestinal system
Gastrostomy
Gaucher's disease
Gluten
Hernia
Hernia repair
Ileostomy and colostomy
Incontinence
Internal medicine

Intestinal disorders
Intestines
Irritable bowel syndrome (IBS)
Kidney transplantation
Kidneys
Laparoscopy
Liposuction
Lithotripsy
Liver
Liver transplantation
Mesothelioma
Nephrectomy
Nephrology
Obesity
Pancreas
Pancreatitis
Peristalsis
Peritonitis
Polyps
Pregnancy and gestation
Prostate cancer
Reproductive system
Roseola
Shunts
Small intestine
Splenectomy
Stents
Sterilization
Stevens-Johnson syndrome
Stomach
Stone removal
Stones
Tubal ligation
Tularemia
Ulcerative colitis
Ultrasonography
Urinary disorders
Urinary system
Urology
Vaginal birth after cesarean (VBAC)
Vasculitis
Virtual imaging

ANUS
Amebiasis
Anal cancer
Colon therapy
Colorectal polyp removal
Colorectal surgery
Endoscopy
Enemas
Episiotomy
Fistula repair
Hemorrhoid banding and removal
Hemorrhoids
Hirschsprung's disease
Human papillomavirus (HPV)
Intestinal disorders
Intestines
Irritable bowel syndrome (IBS)
Polyps

Rape and sexual assault
Rectum
Soiling
Sphincterectomy
Syphilis
Ulcerative colitis

ARMS
Amputation
Auras
Carpal tunnel syndrome
Casts and splints
Charcot-Marie-Tooth Disease
Cornelia de Lange syndrome
Cutis marmorata telangiectatica
    congenita
Diabetic neuropathy
Dyskinesia
Electrolysis
Fracture and dislocation
Fracture repair
Gigantism
Hand hygiene compliance
Hemiplegia
Liposuction
Muscles
Neonatal brachial plexus palsy
Phlebotomy
Pityriasis alba
Quadriplegia
Roseola
Rotator cuff surgery
Sarcoma
Skin lesion removal
Slipped disk
Spinocerebellar ataxia
Streptococcal infections
Tendinitis
Thalidomide
Tremors
Upper extremities

BACK
Ankylosing spondylitis
Back pain
Bone disorders
Bone marrow transplantation
Bones and the skeleton
Braces
Chiropractic
Cushing's syndrome
Disk removal
Dwarfism
Electrolysis
Juvenile rheumatoid arthritis
Kyphosis
Laminectomy and spinal fusion
Neuroimaging
Pityriasis alba
Pityriasis rosea
Sarcoma

Sciatica
Scoliosis
Slipped disk
Spine, vertebrae, and disks
Stevens-Johnson syndrome
Streptococcal infections
Sympathectomy
Tendon disorders

BLADDER
Abdomen
Abdominal disorders
Bed-wetting
Bladder cancer
Bladder removal
Candidiasis
Catheterization
Cystitis
Cystoscopy
Diabetic nephropathy
Diuretics
Endoscopy
Fetal surgery
Fistula repair
Hematuria
Incontinence
Internal medicine
Lithotripsy
Polyps
Pyelonephritis
Schistosomiasis
Smoking
Sphincterectomy
Stone removal
Stones
Toilet training
Ultrasonography
Uremia
Urethritis
Urinalysis
Urinary disorders
Urinary system
Urology
Williams syndrome

BLOOD
Acquired immunodeficiency syndrome
    (AIDS)
Anemia
Angiography
Antibodies
Aspergillosis
Avian influenza
Babesiosis
Biological therapies
Bleeding
Blood pressure
Blood testing
Blood vessels
Bone marrow transplantation
Bulimia

Candidiasis
Carbohydrates
Circulation
Cold agglutinin disease
Connective tissue
Cushing's syndrome
Cyanosis
Cytomegalovirus (CMV)
Deep vein thrombosis
Defibrillation
Dialysis
Dirofilaria immitis
Disseminated intravascular coagulation
    (DIC)
Diuretics
E. coli infection
Ebola virus
End-stage renal disease
Epstein-Barr virus
Ergogenic aids
Fetal surgery
Fetal tissue transplantation
Fistula repair
Fluids and electrolytes
Folate deficiency
Glycolysis
Gulf War syndrome
Heart
Hematocrit
Hematology
Hematomas
Hematuria
Hemoglobin
Hemolytic uremic syndrome
Hemophilia
Histiocytosis
Host-defense mechanisms
Hyperbaric oxygen therapy
Hypercholesterolemia
Hyperlipidemia
Hypoglycemia
Immune system
Immunization and vaccination
Jaundice
Laboratory tests
Leukemia
Liver
Lymph
Malaria
Menorrhagia
Methicillin-resistant staphylococcus
    aureus (MRSA) infection
Nephrology
Pharmacology
Phenylketonuria (PKU)
Phlebotomy
Plasma
Pulse rate
Rh factor
Salmonella infection
Schistosomiasis

Septicemia
Serology
Sickle cell disease
Single photon emission computed
    tomography (SPECT)
Snakebites
Staphylococcal infections
Sturge-Weber syndrome
Subdural hematoma
Thalassemia
Thrombocytopenia
Thrombolytic therapy and TPA
Thrombosis and thrombus
Thymus gland
Transfusion
Transplantation
Ultrasonography
Uremia
Von Willebrand's disease
Wiskott-Aldrich syndrome
Yellow fever

BLOOD VESSELS
Aneurysms
Angiography
Angioplasty
Anticoagulants
Arteriosclerosis
Avian influenza
Bedsores
Bile
Bleeding
Blood and blood disorders
Blood pressure
Blood testing
Blood vessels
Bruises
Bypass surgery
Carotid arteries
Catheterization
Cholesterol
Circulation
Claudication
Cluster headaches
Cold agglutinin disease
Cutis marmorata telangiectatica
    congenita
Deep vein thrombosis
Defibrillation
Diabetes mellitus
Disseminated intravascular coagulation
    (DIC)
Diuretics
Dizziness and fainting
Edema
Electrocauterization
Embolism
Embolization
End-stage renal disease
Endarterectomy
Erectile dysfunction

Eye infections and disorders
Facial transplantation
Hammertoe correction
Heart
Heart disease
Heat exhaustion and heatstroke
Hemangioma
Hematomas
Hemoglobin
Hemorrhoid banding and removal
Hemorrhoids
Hormone therapy
Hypercholesterolemia
Hypertension
Hypotension
Infarction
Intravenous (IV) therapy
Ischemia
Kawasaki disease
Klippel-Trenaunay syndrome
Leptospirosis
Methicillin-resistant staphylococcus
    aureus (MRSA) infection
Necrotizing fasciitis
Nephritis
Neuroimaging
Obesity
Phlebitis
Phlebotomy
Plaque
Plasma
Polycystic kidney disease
Polydactyly and syndactyly
Postural orthostatic tachycardia
    syndrome (POTS)
Pulse rate
Raynaud's Phenomenon
Rocky Mountain spotted fever
Roundworms
Schistosomiasis
Scleroderma
Scurvy
Single photon emission computed
    tomography (SPECT)
Stenosis
Stents
Strokes
Sturge-Weber syndrome
Temporal arteritis
Thalidomide
Thrombolytic therapy and TPA
Thrombosis and thrombus
Toxemia
Transient ischemic attacks (TIAs)
Umbilical cord
Varicose vein removal
Varicose veins
Vascular medicine
Vascular system
Vasculitis
Von Willebrand's disease

BONES

Amputation
Ankylosing spondylitis
Arthritis
Aspergillosis
Back pain
Bone cancer
Bone disorders
Bone grafting
Bone marrow transplantation
Bowlegs
Braces
Bunions
Casts and splints
Cells
Chiropractic
Cleft lip and palate
Cleft lip and palate repair
Connective tissue
Craniosynostosis
Cushing's syndrome
Cystic fibrosis
Dengue fever
Disk removal
Dwarfism
Ear surgery
Ears
Eating disorders
Ewing's sarcoma
Facial transplantation
Failure to thrive
Feet
Folate deficiency
Foot disorders
Fracture and dislocation
Fracture repair
Gaucher's disease
Gigantism
Hammertoe correction
Head and neck disorders
Hearing
Heel spur removal
Hip fracture repair
Hip replacement
Histiocytosis
Hormone therapy
Insulin-like growth factors
Jaw wiring
Joints
Kneecap removal
Knock-knees
Kyphosis
Leishmaniasis
Ligaments
Lower extremities
Marfan syndrome
Mesenchymal stem cells
Methicillin-resistant staphylococcus
    aureus (MRSA) infection
Motor skill development
Necrosis

Neurofibromatosis
Neurosurgery
Niemann-Pick disease
Nuclear medicine
Nuclear radiology
Orthopedic surgery
Orthopedics
Osteochondritis juvenilis
Osteoclast
Osteomyelitis
Osteonecrosis
Osteopathic medicine
Osteoporosis
Paget's disease
Periodontitis
Physical rehabilitation
Pigeon toes
Podiatry
Polydactyly and syndactyly
Prader-Willi syndrome
Rheumatology
Rickets
Rubinstein-Taybi syndrome
Sarcoma
Scoliosis
Spina bifida
Spinal cord disorders
Spine, vertebrae, and disks
Sports medicine
Syphilis
Teeth
Temporomandibular joint (TMJ)
    syndrome
Tendon disorders
Tendon repair
Upper extremities

BRAIN

Abscess drainage
Acidosis
Acquired immunodeficiency syndrome
    (AIDS)
Addiction
Adrenoleukodystrophy
Agnosia
Alcoholism
Altitude sickness
Alzheimer's disease
Amnesia
Anesthesia
Anesthesiology
Aneurysmectomy
Aneurysms
Angelman syndrome
Angiography
Anorexia nervosa
Anosmia
Antianxiety drugs
Anticoagulants
Antidepressants
Antipsychotic drugs

Gender reassignment surgery
Glands
Gynecology
Gynecomastia
Hormone therapy
Hypogonadism
Klinefelter syndrome
Mammography
Mastectomy and lumpectomy
Mastitis
Premenstrual syndrome (PMS)
Raynaud's Phenomenon
Stevens-Johnson syndrome
Tumor removal

CARDIOVASCULAR SYSTEM
Aortic stenosis
Atrial fibrillation
Diabetic nephropathy
Extracorporeal membrane oxygenation
  (ECMO)
Gluten
Hemoglobin
Hemolysis
Hyperbaric chamber
Hypokalemia
Osteogenesis imperfecta
Patent ductus arteriosus
Postural orthostatic tachycardia
  syndrome (POTS)
Statins

CELLS
Acid-base chemistry
Alzheimer's disease
Antibodies
Bacteriology
Batten's disease
Biological therapies
Biopsy
Breast cancer
Cholesterol
Cloning
Conception
Cytology
Cytomegalovirus (CMV)
Cytopathology
Defibrillation
Dehydration
Diuretics
Electrocauterization
Epstein-Barr virus
Erectile dysfunction
Ergogenic aids
Eye infections and disorders
Fatty acid
Fluids and electrolytes
Food biochemistry
Gaucher's disease
Gene therapy
Genetic counseling

Glycolysis
Gram staining
Gulf War syndrome
Hearing
Host-defense mechanisms
Hyperplasia
Immune system
Immunization and vaccination
In vitro fertilization
Karyotyping
Kinesiology
Laboratory tests
Lipids
Magnetic field therapy
Microbiology
Microscopy
Mutation
Necrosis
Osteoclast
Pharmacology
Phlebotomy
Plasma
Rhinoviruses
Sarcoma
Sickle cell disease
Sleep
Thymus gland
Turner syndrome

CENTRAL NERVOUS SYSTEM
Amphetamine
Antipsychotic drugs
Brain disorders
Caffeine
Deep brain stimulation
Delirium
Hippocampus
Minimally conscious state
Nicotine

CHEST
Achalasia
Aneurysmectomy
Antihistamines
Asthma
Bacillus Calmette-Guérin (BCG)
Bronchiolitis
Bronchitis
Bypass surgery
Cardiac rehabilitation
Cardiology
Choking
Cold agglutinin disease
Common cold
Congenital heart disease
Coughing
Defibrillation
Diaphragm
Electrocardiography (ECG or EKG)
Electrolysis
Emphysema

Gulf War syndrome
Gynecomastia
Heart
Heart transplantation
Heart valve replacement
Heimlich maneuver
Hiccups
Legionnaires' disease
Lung cancer
Lungs
Oxygen therapy
Pacemaker implantation
Palpitations
Pityriasis rosea
Pleurisy
Pneumocystis jirovecii
Pneumothorax
Pulmonary diseases
Pulmonary medicine
Respiration
Resuscitation
Rhinoviruses
Sarcoidosis
Streptococcal infections
Thoracic surgery
Trachea
Tuberculosis
Vasculitis
Virtual imaging
Whooping cough

CIRCULATORY SYSTEM
Acute respiratory distress syndrome
  (ARDS)
Aneurysms
Angina
Angiography
Angioplasty
Antibodies
Antihistamines
Apgar score
Arteriosclerosis
Autoimmune disorders
Avian influenza
Bilirubin
Biofeedback
Bleeding
Blood and blood disorders
Blood pressure
Blood testing
Blood vessels
Blue baby syndrome
Bypass surgery
Cardiac arrest
Cardiac rehabilitation
Cardiac surgery
Cardiology
Cardiopulmonary resuscitation (CPR)
Carotid arteries
Catheterization
Chest

Cholera
Cholesterol
Circulation
Claudication
Cold agglutinin disease
Computed tomography (CT) scanning
Congenital heart disease
Coronary artery bypass graft
Cutis marmorata telangiectatica
  congenita
Decongestants
Deep vein thrombosis
Defibrillation
Dehydration
Diabetes mellitus
Dialysis
Disseminated intravascular coagulation
  (DIC)
Diuretics
Dizziness and fainting
Drowning
Ebola virus
Echocardiography
Edema
Electrocardiography (ECG or EKG)
Electrocauterization
Embolism
Encephalitis
End-stage renal disease
Endarterectomy
Endocarditis
Ergogenic aids
Exercise physiology
Facial transplantation
Folate deficiency
Food allergies
Gigantism
Heart
Heart attack
Heart disease
Heart failure
Heart transplantation
Heart valve replacement
Heat exhaustion and heatstroke
Hematology
Hemolysis
Hemolytic disease of the newborn
Hemolytic uremic syndrome
Hemorrhoid banding and removal
Hemorrhoids
Hormone therapy
Hormones
Hyperbaric oxygen therapy
Hypercholesterolemia
Hypertension
Hypotension
Immune system
Intravenous (IV) therapy
Ischemia
Juvenile rheumatoid arthritis
Kawasaki disease

Kidneys
Kinesiology
Klippel-Trenaunay syndrome
Lead poisoning
Leukemia
Liver
Lymph
Lymphatic system
Marijuana
Methicillin-resistant staphylococcus
  aureus (MRSA) infection
Mitral valve prolapse
Motor skill development
Myoglobin
Neutrophil
Obesity
Osteochondritis juvenilis
Oxygen therapy
Pacemaker implantation
Palpitations
Patent ductus arteriosus
Phlebitis
Phlebotomy
Placenta
Plaque
Plasma
Postural orthostatic tachycardia
  syndrome (POTS)
Preeclampsia and eclampsia
Pulmonary heart disease
Pulmonary edema
Pulse rate
Resuscitation
Reye's syndrome
Rocky Mountain spotted fever
Roundworms
Sarcoidosis
Schistosomiasis
Scleroderma
Septicemia
Shunts
Single photon emission computed
  tomography (SPECT)
Smoking
Snakebites
Sports medicine
Staphylococcal infections
Stenosis
Stents
Steroid abuse
Streptococcal infections
Strokes
Sturge-Weber syndrome
Temporal arteritis
Testicular torsion
Thrombocytopenia
Thrombolytic therapy and TPA
Thrombosis and thrombus
Toxemia
Transfusion
Transient ischemic attacks (TIAs)

Transplantation
Typhoid fever
Typhus
Uremia
Varicose vein removal
Varicose veins
Vascular medicine
Vascular system
Vasculitis
Yellow fever

DIGESTIVE SYSTEM
Amylase
Bilirubin
Fecal bacteriotherapy
Pellagra

EARS
Adenoids
Adrenoleukodystrophy
Agnosia
Altitude sickness
Antihistamines
Aspergillosis
Audiology
Auras
Bell's palsy
Charcot-Marie-Tooth Disease
Cold agglutinin disease
Cornelia de Lange syndrome
Cytomegalovirus (CMV)
Deafness
Decongestants
Dyslexia
Ear infections and disorders
Ear surgery
Earwax
Facial transplantation
Fetal alcohol syndrome
Fragile X syndrome
Hearing
Hearing aids
Hearing loss
Hearing tests
Histiocytosis
Leukodystrophy
Lice, mites, and ticks
Measles
Motion sickness
Myringotomy
Nervous system
Neurology
Otoplasty
Otorhinolaryngology
Pharynx
Raynaud's Phenomenon
Rubinstein-Taybi syndrome
Sense organs
Speech disorders
Streptococcal infections
Tinnitus

Tonsillitis
Vasculitis
Vertigo
Williams syndrome
Wiskott-Aldrich syndrome

ELBOW
Arthroplasty
Hand hygiene compliance

ENDOCRINE SYSTEM
Addison's disease
Adrenalectomy
Adrenoleukodystrophy
Amenorrhea
Anorexia nervosa
Assisted reproductive technologies
Bariatric surgery
Biofeedback
Brain death
Breasts
Carbohydrates
Computed tomography (CT) scanning
Congenital adrenal hyperplasia
Congenital hypothyroidism
Corticosteroids
Cushing's syndrome
Diabetes mellitus
Dwarfism
End-stage renal disease
Endocrine disorders
Endocrine glands
Endocrinology
Ergogenic aids
Failure to thrive
Fibrocystic breast condition
Galactorrhea
Gender reassignment surgery
Gestational diabetes
Gigantism
Glands
Glucose tolerance test
Goiter
Gynecomastia
Hashimoto's thyroiditis
Health impact of sugar
Hormones
Hyperparathyroidism and
    hypoparathyroidism
Hypoglycemia
Hypothalamus
Insulin
Klinefelter syndrome
Lead poisoning
Liver
Melatonin
Nonalcoholic steatohepatitis (NASH)
Obesity
Overtraining syndrome
Pancreas
Pancreatitis

Parathyroidectomy
Pituitary gland
Placenta
Plasma
Polycystic ovary syndrome
Postpartum depression
Prader-Willi syndrome
Preeclampsia and eclampsia
Prostate gland
Prostate gland removal
Sexual differentiation
Small intestine
Steroid abuse
Steroids
Testicular cancer
Testicular surgery
Thymus gland
Thyroid disorders
Thyroid gland
Thyroidectomy
Turner syndrome
Weight loss medications
Williams syndrome

EYES
Acquired immunodeficiency syndrome
    (AIDS)
Adenoviruses
Adrenoleukodystrophy
Agnosia
Angelman syndrome
Ankylosing spondylitis
Antihistamines
Aspergillosis
Astigmatism
Auras
Batten's disease
Behçet's disease
Bell's palsy
Blindness
Blurred vision
Botox
Cataract surgery
Cataracts
Chlamydia
Color blindness
Conjunctivitis
Corneal transplantation
Cornelia de Lange syndrome
Cutis marmorata telangiectatica
    congenita
Cytomegalovirus (CMV)
Dengue fever
Diabetes mellitus
Diabetic nephropathy
Dyslexia
Electrolysis
Enteroviruses
Eye infections and disorders
Eye surgery
Face lift and blepharoplasty

Facial transplantation
Fetal alcohol syndrome
Fetal tissue transplantation
Galactosemia
Gigantism
Glaucoma
Gonorrhea
Gulf War syndrome
Hay fever
Juvenile rheumatoid arthritis
Keratitis
Kluver-Bucy syndrome
Laser use in surgery
Leptospirosis
Leukodystrophy
Lyme disease
Macular degeneration
Marfan syndrome
Marijuana
Microscopy
Motor skill development
Multiple chemical sensitivity syndrome
Myopia
Ophthalmology
Optometry
Pigmentation
Presbyopia
Pterygium/Pinguecula
Ptosis
Refractive eye surgery
Reiter's syndrome
Retina
Rubinstein-Taybi syndrome
Sarcoidosis
Scurvy
Sense organs
Sjögren's syndrome
Sphincterectomy
Spinocerebellar ataxia
Stevens-Johnson syndrome
Strabismus
Sturge-Weber syndrome
Styes
Syphilis
Tears and tear ducts
Trachoma
Transplantation
Vasculitis
Vision
Vision disorders
Williams syndrome

FEET
Athlete's foot
Bone disorders
Bones and the skeleton
Bowlegs
Bunions
Charcot-Marie-Tooth Disease
Cold agglutinin disease
Cornelia de Lange syndrome

Corns and calluses
Diabetic neuropathy
Dyskinesia
Flat feet
Foot disorders
Fragile X syndrome
Frostbite
Ganglion removal
Gout
Hammertoe correction
Hammertoes
Heel spur removal
Knock-knees
Lower extremities
Methicillin-resistant staphylococcus
    aureus (MRSA) infection
Nail removal
Nails
Orthopedic surgery
Orthopedics
Pigeon toes
Podiatry
Polydactyly and syndactyly
Raynaud's Phenomenon
Rubinstein-Taybi syndrome
Spinocerebellar ataxia
Sports medicine
Stevens-Johnson syndrome
Streptococcal infections
Tendinitis
Tendon repair
Thalidomide
Tremors

GALLBLADDER
Abscess drainage
Bariatric surgery
Bile
Cholecystectomy
Cholecystitis
Chyme
Endoscopic retrograde
    cholangiopancreatography (ERCP)
Fistula repair
Gallbladder cancer
Gallbladder diseases
Gastroenterology
Gastrointestinal system
Internal medicine
Laparoscopy
Liver transplantation
Malabsorption
Nuclear medicine
Polyps
Stone removal
Stones
Typhoid fever
Ultrasonography

GASTROINTESTINAL SYSTEM
Abdomen

Abdominal disorders
Achalasia
Acid reflux disease
Acidosis
Acquired immunodeficiency syndrome
    (AIDS)
Adenoviruses
Allergies
Amebiasis
Anal cancer
Angelman syndrome
Ankylosing spondylitis
Anorexia nervosa
Anthrax
Anus
Appendectomy
Appendicitis
Asbestos exposure
Avian influenza
Bacterial infections
Bariatric surgery
Beriberi
Bulimia
Bypass surgery
Campylobacter infections
Candidiasis
Carbohydrates
Childhood infectious diseases
Cholecystectomy
Cholecystitis
Cholera
Cholesterol
Chyme
Clostridium difficile (C. diff.)
Colic
Colitis
Colon
Colon therapy
Colonoscopy and sigmoidoscopy
Colorectal cancer
Colorectal polyp removal
Colorectal surgery
Computed tomography (CT) scanning
Constipation
Crohn's disease
Cystic fibrosis
Cytomegalovirus (CMV)
Diabetes mellitus
Diarrhea and dysentery
Digestion
Diverticulitis and diverticulosis
E. coli infection
Eating disorders
Ebola virus
Embolization
Endoscopic retrograde
    cholangiopancreatography (ERCP)
Endoscopy
Enemas
Enterocolitis
Esophagus

Fasting
Fecal bacteriotherapy
Fiber
Fistula repair
Folate deficiency
Food allergies
Food biochemistry
Food poisoning
Fructosemia
Fungal infections
Gallbladder
Gallbladder cancer
Gallbladder diseases
Gastrectomy
Gastroenteritis
Gastroenterology
Gastrointestinal disorders
Gastrostomy
Giardiasis
Glands
Glucose tolerance test
Gluten
Gluten intolerance
Gulf War syndrome
Hand-foot-and-mouth disease
Health impact of sugar
Hemolytic uremic syndrome
Hemorrhoid banding and removal
Hemorrhoids
Hernia
Hernia repair
Histiocytosis
Host-defense mechanisms
Hyperthyroidism and hypothyroidism
Ileostomy and colostomy
Incontinence
Insulin
Internal medicine
Intestinal disorders
Intestines
Irritable bowel syndrome (IBS)
Ketogenic diet
Klippel-Trenaunay syndrome
Kwashiorkor
Lactose intolerance
Laparoscopy
Leaky gut syndrome
Lipids
Liver
Malabsorption
Malnutrition
Marijuana
Meckel's diverticulum
Metabolism
Motion sickness
Muscles
Nausea and vomiting
Nonalcoholic steatohepatitis (NASH)
Noroviruses
Obesity
Pancreas

Pancreatitis
Peristalsis
Peritonitis
Pharynx
Pinworms
Poisoning
Polycystic kidney disease
Polyps
Proctology
Protozoan diseases
Pyloric stenosis
Radiation sickness
Rectum
Reiter's syndrome
Rotavirus
Roundworms
Salmonella infection
Scleroderma
Sense organs
Shigellosis
Shunts
Small intestine
Smallpox
Smoking
Soiling
Staphylococcal infections
Stenosis
Stevens-Johnson syndrome
Stomach
Tapeworms
Taste
Teeth
Toilet training
Toxoplasmosis
Trichinosis
Tumor removal
Typhoid fever
Ulcer surgery
Ulcerative colitis
Ulcers
Vagotomy
Vasculitis
Weaning
Weight loss and gain

GENITALS
Adrenoleukodystrophy
Aphrodisiacs
Assisted reproductive technologies
Behçet's disease
Candidiasis
Catheterization
Cervical, ovarian, and uterine cancers
Cervical procedures
Chlamydia
Circumcision, female and genital
  mutilation
Circumcision
Congenital adrenal hyperplasia
Contraception
Cyst removal

Embolization
Endometrial biopsy
Episiotomy
Erectile dysfunction
Ergogenic aids
Fragile X syndrome
Gender reassignment surgery
Genital disorders
Glands
Gonorrhea
Gynecology
Hemochromatosis
Hermaphroditism and
  pseudohermaphroditism
Herpes
Hormone therapy
Human papillomavirus (HPV)
Hydroceles
Hyperplasia
Hypospadias repair and urethroplasty
Infertility
Klinefelter syndrome
Kluver-Bucy syndrome
Lice, mites, and ticks
Masturbation
Mumps
Orchitis
Pap test
Pelvic inflammatory disease (PID)
Penile implant surgery
Prader-Willi syndrome
Rape and sexual assault
Reproductive system
Rubinstein-Taybi syndrome
Semen
Sexual differentiation
Sexual dysfunction
Sexuality
Sexually transmitted diseases (STDs)
Sperm banks
Sterilization
Stevens-Johnson syndrome
Streptococcal infections
Syphilis
Testicles
Testicular cancer
Testicular surgery
Testicular torsion
Toilet training
Trichomoniasis
Urethritis
Urology
Uterus
Vas deferens
Vasectomy

GLANDS
Abscess drainage
Addison's disease
Adrenalectomy
Adrenoleukodystrophy

Assisted reproductive technologies
Biofeedback
Breast cancer
Breast disorders
Breast-feeding
Breast surgery
Breasts
Cushing's syndrome
Cyst removal
Dengue fever
Diabetes mellitus
DiGeorge syndrome
Dwarfism
Endocrine disorders
Endocrine glands
Endocrinology
Epstein-Barr virus
Ergogenic aids
Eye infections and disorders
Gender reassignment surgery
Goiter
Gynecomastia
Hashimoto's thyroiditis
Hormones
Hyperhidrosis
Hyperparathyroidism and
  hypoparathyroidism
Hypoglycemia
Hypothalamus
Immune system
Internal medicine
Liver
Mastitis
Mumps
Neurosurgery
Nuclear medicine
Nuclear radiology
Pancreas
Parathyroidectomy
Pituitary gland
Prader-Willi syndrome
Prostate gland
Prostate gland removal
Quinsy
Semen
Sexual differentiation
Sleep
Steroids
Sweating
Testicular cancer
Testicular surgery
Thymus gland
Thyroid disorders
Thyroid gland
Thyroidectomy

GUMS
Abscess drainage
Bulimia
Cavities
Dengue fever

Dental diseases
Dentistry
Dentures
Fluoride treatments
Gingivitis
Gulf War syndrome
Gum disease
Jaw wiring
Mouth and throat cancer
Oral and maxillofacial surgery
Orthodontics
Periodontal surgery
Periodontitis
Root canal treatment
Scurvy
Teeth
Teething
Tooth extraction
Wisdom teeth

HAIR
Alopecia
Angelman syndrome
Anorexia nervosa
Collodion baby
Cornelia de Lange syndrome
Cushing's syndrome
Dermatitis
Dermatology
Gigantism
Gulf War syndrome
Hair
Hair transplantation
Hyperthyroidism and hypothyroidism
Klinefelter syndrome
Lice, mites, and ticks
Pigmentation
Radiation sickness

HANDS
Amputation
Arthritis
Arthroplasty
Bone disorders
Bursitis
Carpal tunnel syndrome
Casts and splints
Charcot-Marie-Tooth Disease
Cold agglutinin disease
Cornelia de Lange syndrome
Corns and calluses
Diabetic neuropathy
Dyskinesia
Fetal alcohol syndrome
Fracture and dislocation
Fragile X syndrome
Frostbite
Ganglion removal
Gigantism
Hand hygiene compliance
Methicillin-resistant staphylococcus

aureus (MRSA) infection
Nail removal
Nails
Neurology
Orthopedic surgery
Orthopedics
Polydactyly and syndactyly
Raynaud's Phenomenon
Rheumatology
Rubinstein-Taybi syndrome
Scleroderma
Skin lesion removal
Spinocerebellar ataxia
Sports medicine
Stevens-Johnson syndrome
Streptococcal infections
Tendinitis
Tendon repair
Thalidomide
Tremors
Upper extremities
Vasculitis

HEAD
Alopecia
Altitude sickness
Aneurysms
Angelman syndrome
Angiography
Antihistamines
Bell's palsy
Botox
Brain
Brain disorders
Brain tumors
Cluster headaches
Concussion
Cornelia de Lange syndrome
Craniosynostosis
Craniotomy
Deep brain stimulation
Dengue fever
Dizziness and fainting
Dyskinesia
Electroencephalography (EEG)
Epilepsy
Eye infections and disorders
Facial transplantation
Fetal alcohol syndrome
Fibromyalgia
Functional magnetic imaging (fMRI)
Hair transplantation
Head and neck disorders
Headaches
Hemiplegia
Hydrocephalus
Meningitis
Motion sickness
Nasal polyp removal
Neuroimaging
Neurology

Neurosurgery
Oral and maxillofacial surgery
Paget's disease
Pharynx
Phrenology
Rubinstein-Taybi syndrome
Seizures
Shunts
Single photon emission computed
   tomography (SPECT)
Spinocerebellar ataxia
Sports medicine
Stevens-Johnson syndrome
Strokes
Sturge-Weber syndrome
Tears and tear ducts
Temporomandibular joint (TMJ)
   syndrome
Thrombosis and thrombus
Tinnitus
Transcranial magnetic stimulation
   (TMS)
Tremors
Whiplash

HEART
Acidosis
Anemia
Aneurysmectomy
Aneurysms
Angina
Angiography
Angioplasty
Anorexia nervosa
Anticoagulants
Anxiety
Aortic stenosis
Apgar score
Arrhythmias
Arteriosclerosis
Aspergillosis
Atrial fibrillation
Avian influenza
Beriberi
Biofeedback
Bites and stings
Blood pressure
Blood vessels
Blue baby syndrome
Brucellosis
Bulimia
Bypass surgery
Cardiac arrest
Cardiac rehabilitation
Cardiac surgery
Cardiology
Cardiopulmonary resuscitation (CPR)
Carotid arteries
Catheterization
Congenital heart disease
Cornelia de Lange syndrome

Coronary artery bypass graft
Defibrillation
Depression
Diabetes mellitus
DiGeorge syndrome
Diphtheria
Dirofilaria immitis
Diuretics
Drowning
Echocardiography
Electrical shock
Electrocardiography (ECG or EKG)
End-stage renal disease
Endocarditis
Enteroviruses
Ergogenic aids
Exercise physiology
Fatty acid oxidation disorders
Fetal alcohol syndrome
Gangrene
Glycogen storage diseases
Heart attack
Heart disease
Heart failure
Heart transplantation
Heart valve replacement
Hemochromatosis
Hormone therapy
Hypercholesterolemia
Hypertension
Hyperthyroidism and hypothyroidism
Hypotension
Infarction
Internal medicine
Interstitial pulmonary fibrosis (IPF)
Intravenous (IV) therapy
Juvenile rheumatoid arthritis
Kawasaki disease
Kinesiology
Lyme disease
Marfan syndrome
Marijuana
Methicillin-resistant staphylococcus aureus (MRSA) infection
Mitral valve prolapse
Mononucleosis
Nuclear medicine
Obesity
Oxygen therapy
Pacemaker implantation
Palpitations
Patent ductus arteriosus
Plaque
Plasma
Postural orthostatic tachycardia syndrome (POTS)
Prader-Willi syndrome
Pulmonary heart disease
Pulmonary edema
Pulse rate
Renal failure

Respiratory distress syndrome
Resuscitation
Reye's syndrome
Rheumatic fever
Rheumatoid arthritis
Rubinstein-Taybi syndrome
Sarcoidosis
Scleroderma
Single photon emission computed tomography (SPECT)
Sleeping sickness
Sports medicine
Stenosis
Stents
Steroid abuse
Streptococcal infections
Strokes
Syphilis
Teeth
Thoracic surgery
Thrombolytic therapy and TPA
Thrombosis and thrombus
Transplantation
Ultrasonography
Uremia
Virtual imaging
Whooping cough
Williams syndrome

HIPS
Ankylosing spondylitis
Arthritis
Arthroplasty
Arthroscopy
Back pain
Bones and the skeleton
Bowlegs
Chiropractic
Dwarfism
Fracture and dislocation
Fracture repair
Hip fracture repair
Hip replacement
Knock-knees
Liposuction
Lower extremities
Orthopedic surgery
Orthopedics
Osteochondritis juvenilis
Osteonecrosis
Paget's disease
Physical rehabilitation
Pigeon toes
Rheumatology
Sciatica

IMMUNE SYSTEM
Acquired immunodeficiency syndrome (AIDS)
Adenoids
Adenoviruses

Allergies
Ankylosing spondylitis
Anorexia nervosa
Anthrax
Antibodies
Antihistamines
The Antivaccine Movement
Arthritis
Asthma
Bacillus Calmette-Guérin (BCG)
Bacterial infections
Bacteriology
Bedsores
Bile
Biological therapies
Bites and stings
Blood and blood disorders
Bone grafting
Bone marrow transplantation
Candidiasis
Cells
Chagas' disease
Childhood infectious diseases
Chronic fatigue syndrome
Clostridium difficile (C. diff.)
Cold agglutinin disease
Conjunctivitis
Cornelia de Lange syndrome
Coronaviruses
Corticosteroids
Coughing
Cytology
Cytomegalovirus (CMV)
Cytopathology
Dermatology
Dermatopathology
DiGeorge syndrome
Disseminated intravascular coagulation (DIC)
Ehrlichiosis
Endocrinology
Epstein-Barr virus
Facial transplantation
Fetal tissue transplantation
Food allergies
Fungal infections
Gluten intolerance
Gram staining
Guillain-Barré syndrome
Gulf War syndrome
Hashimoto's thyroiditis
Hay fever
Hematology
Hemolysis
Hemolytic disease of the newborn
Histiocytosis
Hives
Host-defense mechanisms
Human immunodeficiency virus (HIV)
Immunization and vaccination
Immunodeficiency disorders

Impetigo
Juvenile rheumatoid arthritis
Kawasaki disease
Leishmaniasis
Leprosy
Lymph
Lymphatic system
Magnetic field therapy
Malaria
Marburg virus
Mesenchymal stem cells
Microbiology
Mold and mildew
Monkeypox
Multiple chemical sensitivity syndrome
Mutation
Myasthenia gravis
Nephritis
Neutrophil
Noroviruses
Pancreas
Pharmacology
Pharynx
Plasma
Poisoning
Polymyalgia rheumatica
Pulmonary diseases
Pulmonary medicine
Renal failure
Rh factor
Rheumatoid arthritis
Rheumatology
Roseola
Sarcoidosis
Scarlet fever
Scleroderma
Serology
Severe acute respiratory syndrome
  (SARS)
Severe combined immunodeficiency
  syndrome (SCID)
Sjögren's syndrome
Small intestine
Stevens-Johnson syndrome
Temporal arteritis
Thalidomide
Thymus gland
Tonsils
Toxoplasmosis
Transfusion
Transplantation
Ulcerative colitis
Vasculitis
Vitiligo
Wiskott-Aldrich syndrome

INTESTINES
Abdomen
Abdominal disorders
Acidosis
Acquired immunodeficiency syndrome

(AIDS)
Adenoviruses
Amebiasis
Anus
Appendectomy
Appendicitis
Avian influenza
Bacterial infections
Bariatric surgery
Bulimia
Bypass surgery
Campylobacter infections
Carbohydrates
Celiac sprue
Cholera
Chyme
Colic
Colitis
Colon
Colon therapy
Colonoscopy and sigmoidoscopy
Colorectal cancer
Colorectal polyp removal
Colorectal surgery
Constipation
Crohn's disease
Cystic fibrosis
Diarrhea and dysentery
Digestion
Diverticulitis and diverticulosis
E. coli infection
Eating disorders
Endoscopy
Enemas
Enterocolitis
Fiber
Fistula repair
Food poisoning
Fructosemia
Gastroenteritis
Gastroenterology
Gastrointestinal disorders
Gastrointestinal system
Gluten
Hemorrhoid banding and removal
Hemorrhoids
Hernia
Hernia repair
Hirschsprung's disease
Ileostomy and colostomy
Infarction
Internal medicine
Intestinal disorders
Irritable bowel syndrome (IBS)
Kaposi's sarcoma
Lactose intolerance
Laparoscopy
Malabsorption
Malnutrition
Meckel's diverticulum
Metabolism

Obesity
Peristalsis
Peritonitis
Pinworms
Polyps
Proctology
Rectum
Roundworms
Small intestine
Soiling
Sphincterectomy
Stomach
Tapeworms
Toilet training
Trichinosis
Tumor removal
Typhoid fever
Ulcer surgery
Ulcerative colitis
Vasculitis

JOINTS
Amputation
Angelman syndrome
Ankylosing spondylitis
Arthritis
Arthroscopy
Back pain
Bowlegs
Braces
Brucellosis
Bursitis
Carpal tunnel syndrome
Casts and splints
Celiac sprue
Charcot-Marie-Tooth Disease
Cyst removal
Electrocauterization
Endoscopy
Ergogenic aids
Exercise physiology
Fracture and dislocation
Fragile X syndrome
Gout
Gulf War syndrome
Hemiplegia
Hip fracture repair
Hyaluronic acid injections
Juvenile rheumatoid arthritis
Klippel-Trenaunay syndrome
Kneecap removal
Knock-knees
Ligaments
Lyme disease
Methicillin-resistant staphylococcus
  aureus (MRSA) infection
Motor skill development
Obesity
Orthopedic surgery
Orthopedics
Osteoarthritis

Osteochondritis juvenilis
Osteomyelitis
Osteonecrosis
Physical rehabilitation
Pigeon toes
Polymyalgia rheumatica
Reiter's syndrome
Rheumatology
Rotator cuff surgery
Rubella
Sarcoidosis
Sarcoma
Scleroderma
Spondylitis
Sports medicine
Streptococcal infections
Syphilis
Temporomandibular joint (TMJ)
    syndrome
Tendinitis
Tendon repair
Tularemia
Von Willebrand's disease

KIDNEYS
Abdomen
Abdominal disorders
Abscess drainage
Addison's disease
Adrenalectomy
Anemia
Anorexia nervosa
Aspergillosis
Avian influenza
Babesiosis
Carbohydrates
Cholera
Cystic fibrosis
Diabetes mellitus
Diabetic nephropathy
Dialysis
Diuretics
Drowning
End-stage renal disease
Ergogenic aids
Fructosemia
Hantavirus
Hematuria
Hemolysis
Hemolytic uremic syndrome
Hypertension
Hypotension
Infarction
Insulin-like growth factors
Internal medicine
Intravenous (IV) therapy
Kidney cancer
Kidney disorders
Kidney transplantation
Laparoscopy
Leptospirosis

Lithotripsy
Metabolism
Methicillin-resistant staphylococcus
    aureus (MRSA) infection
Nephrectomy
Nephritis
Nephrology
Nuclear medicine
Nuclear radiology
Polycystic kidney disease
Polyps
Preeclampsia and eclampsia
Proteinuria
Pyelonephritis
Renal failure
Reye's syndrome
Rocky Mountain spotted fever
Sarcoidosis
Scleroderma
Scurvy
Sickle cell disease
Stone removal
Stones
Syphilis
Toilet training
Transplantation
Typhoid fever
Typhus
Ultrasonography
Uremia
Urinalysis
Urinary disorders
Urinary system
Urology
Vasculitis
Williams syndrome
Wilms tumor

KNEES
Amputation
Angelman syndrome
Arthritis
Arthroplasty
Arthroscopy
Bowlegs
Braces
Bursitis
Carticel®
Casts and splints
Endoscopy
Exercise physiology
Fracture and dislocation
Hyaluronic acid injections
Joints
Kneecap removal
Knock-knees
Liposuction
Lower extremities
Lyme disease
Orthopedic surgery
Orthopedics

Osgood-Schlatter disease
Osteonecrosis
Patellofemoral pain syndrome
Physical rehabilitation
Pigeon toes
Rheumatology
Sports medicine
Stevens-Johnson syndrome
Tendinitis
Tendon repair

LEGS
Amputation
Arthritis
Arthroscopy
Auras
Back pain
Bone disorders
Bones and the skeleton
Bowlegs
Bursitis
Bypass surgery
Casts and splints
Charcot-Marie-Tooth Disease
Claudication
Cornelia de Lange syndrome
Cutis marmorata telangiectatica
    congenita
Deep vein thrombosis
Diabetic neuropathy
Dwarfism
Dyskinesia
Electrolysis
Fracture and dislocation
Fracture repair
Gigantism
Hemiplegia
Hip fracture repair
Knee
Kneecap removal
Knock-knees
Liposuction
Lower extremities
Methicillin-resistant staphylococcus
    aureus (MRSA) infection
Muscle sprains, spasms, and disorders
Muscles
Muscular dystrophy
Numbness and tingling
Orthopedic surgery
Orthopedics
Paget's disease
Paralysis
Paraplegia
Physical rehabilitation
Pigeon toes
Poliomyelitis
Quadriplegia
Rheumatology
Roseola
Sarcoma

Sciatica
Slipped disk
Spinocerebellar ataxia
Sports medicine
Stevens-Johnson syndrome
Streptococcal infections
Tendinitis
Tendon disorders
Tendon repair
Thalidomide
Tremors
Varicose vein removal
Vascular system
Vasculitis
Venous insufficiency

LIGAMENTS
Ankylosing spondylitis
Astym® therapy
Back pain
Bowlegs
Casts and splints
Collagen
Connective tissue
Electrocauterization
Eye infections and disorders
Flat feet
Flexibility
Joints
Knock-knees
Muscle sprains, spasms, and disorders
Muscles
Orthopedic surgery
Orthopedics
Patent ductus arteriosus
Physical rehabilitation
Pigeon toes
Sports medicine
Tendon disorders
Tendon repair
Whiplash

LIVER
Abdomen
Abdominal disorders
Abscess drainage
Acquired immunodeficiency syndrome
   (AIDS)
Alcoholism
Amebiasis
Aspergillosis
Babesiosis
Bile
Bilirubin
Blood and blood disorders
Brucellosis
Cholecystitis
Chyme
Circulation
Cirrhosis
Cold agglutinin disease

Cystic fibrosis
Cytomegalovirus (CMV)
Edema
Embolization
Endoscopic retrograde
   cholangiopancreatography (ERCP)
Ergogenic aids
Fatty acid oxidation disorders
Fetal surgery
Fructosemia
Galactosemia
Gastroenterology
Gastrointestinal system
Gaucher's disease
Glucose tolerance test
Glycogen storage diseases
Hematology
Hemochromatosis
Hemoglobin
Hemolysis
Hepatitis
Histiocytosis
Hypercholesterolemia
Immune system
Insulin
Insulin-like growth factors
Internal medicine
Jaundice
Kaposi's sarcoma
Ketogenic diet
Leptospirosis
Liver cancer
Liver disorders
Liver transplantation
Malabsorption
Malaria
Mesenchymal stem cells
Metabolism
Methicillin-resistant staphylococcus
   aureus (MRSA) infection
Niemann-Pick disease
Nonalcoholic steatohepatitis (NASH)
Phenylketonuria (PKU)
Polycystic kidney disease
Reye's syndrome
Shunts
Thrombocytopenia
Transplantation
Typhoid fever
Wilson's disease
Yellow fever

LUNGS
Abscess drainage
Acquired immunodeficiency syndrome
   (AIDS)
Acute respiratory distress syndrome
   (ARDS)
Adenoviruses
Allergies
Altitude sickness

Antihistamines
Apgar score
Apnea
Asbestos exposure
Aspergillosis
Asphyxiation
Asthma
Avian influenza
Bacterial infections
Bronchi
Bronchiolitis
Bronchitis
Cardiopulmonary resuscitation (CPR)
Chest
Childhood infectious diseases
Chlamydia
Choking
Chronic obstructive pulmonary disease
   (COPD)
Cold agglutinin disease
Common cold
Coronaviruses
Coughing
Croup
Cystic fibrosis
Cytomegalovirus (CMV)
Diaphragm
Drowning
Edema
Embolism
Emphysema
Endoscopy
Exercise physiology
Fetal surgery
Hantavirus
Hay fever
Heart transplantation
Heimlich maneuver
Hiccups
Histiocytosis
H1N1 influenza
Human respiratory system
Hyperbaric oxygen therapy
Hyperventilation
Hypoxia
Infarction
Influenza
Internal medicine
Interstitial pulmonary fibrosis (IPF)
Intravenous (IV) therapy
Kaposi's sarcoma
Kinesiology
Legionnaires' disease
Leptospirosis
Lung cancer
Lung surgery
Marijuana
Measles
Mesothelioma
Mold and mildew
Multiple chemical sensitivity syndrome

Nicotine
Niemann-Pick disease
Oxygen therapy
Patent ductus arteriosus
Plague
Pleurisy
Pneumocystis jirovecii
Pneumonia
Pneumothorax
Pulmonary heart disease
Pulmonary diseases
Pulmonary edema
Pulmonary hypertension
Pulmonary medicine
Quinsy
Respiration
Respiratory distress syndrome
Resuscitation
Rhinoviruses
Roundworms
Sarcoidosis
Schistosomiasis
Scleroderma
Severe acute respiratory syndrome
  (SARS)
Sickle cell disease
Stevens-Johnson syndrome
Thoracic surgery
Thrombolytic therapy and TPA
Thrombosis and thrombus
Transplantation
Tuberculosis
Tumor removal
Vasculitis
Wiskott-Aldrich syndrome

LYMPHATIC SYSTEM
Acquired immunodeficiency syndrome
  (AIDS)
Adenoids
Antibodies
Autoimmune disorders
Bacillus Calmette-Guérin (BCG)
Bacterial infections
Biological therapies
Blood and blood disorders
Blood vessels
Breast cancer
Breast disorders
Bruises
Cervical, ovarian, and uterine cancers
Chlamydia
Cold agglutinin disease
Colorectal cancer
Coronaviruses
DiGeorge syndrome
Edema
Elephantiasis
Embolism
Epstein-Barr virus
Gaucher's disease

Hay fever
Hodgkin's disease
Immune system
Kawasaki disease
Klippel-Trenaunay syndrome
Leishmaniasis
Leptospirosis
Leukemia
Lower extremities
Lung cancer
Lymph
Lymphadenopathy and lymphoma
Mononucleosis
Overtraining syndrome
Prostate cancer
Roundworms
Rubella
Sarcoidosis
Skin cancer
Sleeping sickness
Small intestine
Splenectomy
Thymus gland
Tonsillectomy and adenoid removal
Tonsillitis
Tonsils
Tularemia
Upper extremities
Vascular medicine

MOUTH
Acid reflux disease
Acquired immunodeficiency syndrome
  (AIDS)
Adenoids
Angelman syndrome
Auras
Behçet's disease
Bell's palsy
Braces
Candidiasis
Canker sores
Chickenpox
Cold sores
Cornelia de Lange syndrome
Crowns and bridges
Dengue fever
Dental diseases
Dentistry
Dentures
DiGeorge syndrome
Dyskinesia
Eating disorders
Endodontic disease
Epstein-Barr virus
Esophagus
Facial transplantation
Fetal alcohol syndrome
Fluoride treatments
Gingivitis
Gum disease

Hand-foot-and-mouth disease
Heimlich maneuver
Herpes
Jaw wiring
Kawasaki disease
Lisping
Measles
Mouth and throat cancer
Oral and maxillofacial surgery
Orthodontics
Periodontal surgery
Pharynx
Plaque
Quinsy
Rape and sexual assault
Raynaud's Phenomenon
Reiter's syndrome
Root canal treatment
Rubinstein-Taybi syndrome
Sense organs
Sjögren's syndrome
Taste
Teething
Temporomandibular joint (TMJ)
  syndrome
Thumb sucking
Tooth extraction
Ulcers
Wisdom teeth

MUSCLES
Acidosis
Acupressure
Aerobics
Amputation
Anesthesia
Anesthesiology
Apgar score
Astym® therapy
Avian influenza
Back pain
Bed-wetting
Bedsores
Bell's palsy
Beriberi
Bile
Biofeedback
Botox
Bowlegs
Breasts
Carbohydrates
Charcot-Marie-Tooth Disease
Chest
Chiari malformations
Childhood infectious diseases
Chronic fatigue syndrome
Cushing's syndrome
Cystic fibrosis
Diaphragm
Ebola virus
Electrocauterization

Electromyography
Epstein-Barr virus
Exercise physiology
Eye infections and disorders
Facial transplantation
Fatty acid oxidation disorders
Fibromyalgia
Flat feet
Flexibility
Foot disorders
Gangrene
Glycogen storage diseases
Glycolysis
Guillain-Barré syndrome
Gulf War syndrome
Head and neck disorders
Hemiplegia
Hiccups
Hyperthyroidism and hypothyroidism
Insulin-like growth factors
Kinesiology
Knock-knees
Kwashiorkor
Leukodystrophy
Methicillin-resistant staphylococcus
   aureus (MRSA) infection
Motor neuron diseases
Motor skill development
Multiple chemical sensitivity syndrome
Multiple sclerosis
Muscle sprains, spasms, and disorders
Muscular dystrophy
Necrotizing fasciitis
Neurology
Numbness and tingling
Orthopedic surgery
Orthopedics
Osteopathic medicine
Overtraining syndrome
Palpitations
Palsy
Paralysis
Physical rehabilitation
Pigeon toes
Poisoning
Poliomyelitis
Ptosis
Rabies
Respiration
Restless legs syndrome
Rotator cuff surgery
Sarcoma
Scurvy
Seizures
Smallpox
Speech disorders
Sphincterectomy
Spinocerebellar ataxia
Sports medicine
Steroid abuse
Strabismus

Streptococcal infections
Tattoos and body piercing
Temporomandibular joint (TMJ)
   syndrome
Tendon disorders
Tendon repair
Tetanus
Tics
Torticollis
Tourette's syndrome
Tremors
Trichinosis
Tularemia
Upper extremities
Weight loss and gain
Williams syndrome
Yoga

MUSCULOSKELETAL SYSTEM

Acupressure
Amputation
Amyotrophic lateral sclerosis (ALS)
Anesthesia
Anesthesiology
Ankylosing spondylitis
Anorexia nervosa
Arthritis
Arthroplasty
Ataxia
Atrophy
Avian influenza
Back pain
Bed-wetting
Biofeedback
Bone cancer
Bone disorders
Bone grafting
Bone marrow transplantation
Bones and the skeleton
Braces
Breasts
Brucellosis
Bulimia
Casts and splints
Cartilage
Cells
Charcot-Marie-Tooth Disease
Chest
Childhood infectious diseases
Chiropractic
Chronic fatigue syndrome
Cleft lip and palate
Collagen
Computed tomography (CT) scanning
Congenital hypothyroidism
Connective tissue
Contracture
Dengue fever
Depression
Diaphragm
Dwarfism

Ear surgery
Ears
Ehrlichiosis
Ergogenic aids
Ewing's sarcoma
Exercise physiology
Feet
Fibromyalgia
Flat feet
Flexibility
Foot disorders
Fracture and dislocation
Fracture repair
Gigantism
Glycolysis
Guillain-Barré syndrome
Hammertoe correction
Head and neck disorders
Heel spur removal
Hematology
Hematomas
Hemiplegia
Hip fracture repair
Hyperparathyroidism and
   hypoparathyroidism
Jaw wiring
Joints
Juvenile rheumatoid arthritis
Kinesiology
Kneecap removal
Lead poisoning
Lower extremities
Marfan syndrome
Marijuana
Methicillin-resistant staphylococcus
   aureus (MRSA) infection
Motor neuron diseases
Motor skill development
Multiple sclerosis
Muscle sprains, spasms, and disorders
Muscles
Muscular dystrophy
Myasthenia gravis
Neurology
Nuclear medicine
Nuclear radiology
Numbness and tingling
Orthopedic surgery
Orthopedics
Osgood-Schlatter disease
Osteoarthritis
Osteochondritis juvenilis
Osteogenesis imperfecta
Osteomyelitis
Osteonecrosis
Osteopathic medicine
Osteopetrosis
Paget's disease
Palsy
Paralysis
Parkinson's Disease

Patellofemoral pain syndrome
Physical rehabilitation
Poisoning
Poliomyelitis
Prader-Willi syndrome
Precocious puberty
Rabies
Radiculopathy
Respiration
Restless legs syndrome
Rheumatoid arthritis
Rheumatology
Rickets
Rotator cuff surgery
Scoliosis
Seizures
Sleepwalking
Slipped disk
Speech disorders
Sphincterectomy
Spinal cord disorders
Spine, vertebrae, and disks
Spinocerebellar ataxia
Sports medicine
Staphylococcal infections
Strength training
Teeth
Tendinitis
Tendon disorders
Tendon repair
Tetanus
Tics
Tourette's syndrome
Trichinosis
Upper extremities
Walking
Weight loss and gain

NAILS
Anorexia nervosa
Athlete's foot
Collodion baby
Dermatology
Fungal infections
Malnutrition
Nail removal
Podiatry

NECK
Botox
Braces
Carotid arteries
Casts and splints
Chiari malformations
Choking
Congenital hypothyroidism
Dyskinesia
Encephalitis
Endarterectomy
Facial transplantation
Goiter

Hashimoto's thyroiditis
Head and neck disorders
Heimlich maneuver
Hyperparathyroidism and
    hypoparathyroidism
Laminectomy and spinal fusion
Mouth and throat cancer
Neuroimaging
Paralysis
Parathyroidectomy
Pharynx
Pityriasis alba
Slipped disk
Stevens-Johnson syndrome
Streptococcal infections
Sympathectomy
Thyroid disorders
Thyroid gland
Thyroidectomy
Torticollis
Trachea
Tracheostomy
Vagus nerve
Whiplash
Whooping cough

NERVES
Agnosia
Alzheimer's disease
Anesthesia
Anesthesiology
Angelman syndrome
Avian influenza
Back pain
Bell's palsy
Biofeedback
Brain
Bulimia
Carpal tunnel syndrome
Cells
Cluster headaches
Concussion
Dyskinesia
Electromyography
Encephalitis
Epilepsy
Eye infections and disorders
Facial transplantation
Fibromyalgia
Guillain-Barré syndrome
Hearing
Herpes
Hirschsprung's disease
Huntington's disease
Leprosy
Leukodystrophy
Listeria infections
Local anesthesia
Lower extremities
Lumbar puncture
Lyme disease

Marijuana
Motor neuron diseases
Motor skill development
Multiple chemical sensitivity syndrome
Multiple sclerosis
Neonatal brachial plexus palsy
Nervous system
Neuralgia, neuritis, and neuropathy
Neuroimaging
Neurology
Neurosis
Neurosurgery
Numbness and tingling
Palsy
Paralysis
Physical rehabilitation
Poliomyelitis
Postherpetic neuralgia
Ptosis
Radiculopathy
Sarcoidosis
Sciatica
Seizures
Sense organs
Shock therapy
Skin
Slipped disk
Spinal cord disorders
Spine, vertebrae, and disks
Spinocerebellar ataxia
Sturge-Weber syndrome
Sympathectomy
Tics
Tinnitus
Touch
Tourette's syndrome
Tremors
Upper extremities
Vagotomy
Vasculitis

NERVOUS SYSTEM
Abscess drainage
Acetaminophen
Acupressure
Addiction
Adenoviruses
Adrenoleukodystrophy
Agnosia
Alcoholism
Altitude sickness
Alzheimer's disease
Amnesia
Amputation
Amyotrophic lateral sclerosis (ALS)
Anesthesia
Anesthesiology
Aneurysms
Angelman syndrome
Anorexia nervosa
Anosmia

Anthrax
Antidepressants
Anxiety
Apgar score
Aphasia and dysphasia
Apnea
Aromatherapy
Aspirin
Ataxia
Atrophy
Attention-deficit disorder (ADD)
Auras
Autoimmune disorders
Avian influenza
Back pain
Balance disorders
Batten's disease
Behçet's disease
Beriberi
Biofeedback
Botulism
Brain
Brain damage
Brain death
Brain tumors
Brucellosis
Cells
Chagas' disease
Charcot-Marie-Tooth Disease
Chiari malformations
Chiropractic
Chronic wasting disease (CWD)
Cluster headaches
Cognitive development
Colon
Computed tomography (CT) scanning
Concussion
Congenital hypothyroidism
Creutzfeldt-Jakob disease (CJD)
Cutis marmorata telangiectatica
    congenita
Deafness
Defibrillation
Dementias
Developmental disorders
Developmental stages
Diabetes mellitus
Diabetic neuropathy
Diphtheria
Disk removal
Dizziness and fainting
Down syndrome
Drowning
Dwarfism
Dysarthria
Dyskinesia
Dyslexia
E. coli infection
Ear surgery
Ears
Ehrlichiosis

Electrical shock
Electroencephalography (EEG)
Electromyography
Encephalitis
Endocrinology
Enteroviruses
Epilepsy
Eyes
Facial transplantation
Fetal tissue transplantation
Fibromyalgia
Flexibility
Folate deficiency
Frontotemporal dementia (FTD)
Glands
Guillain-Barré syndrome
Hammertoe correction
Head and neck disorders
Headaches
Hearing tests
Heart transplantation
Hemiplegia
Hemolytic uremic syndrome
Histiocytosis
Huntington's disease
Hydrocephalus
Hyperthyroidism and hypothyroidism
Hypnosis
Hypothalamus
Intellectual disability
Intraventricular hemorrhage
Irritable bowel syndrome (IBS)
Kinesiology
Laminectomy and spinal fusion
Lead poisoning
Learning disabilities
Leprosy
Leptospirosis
Light therapy
Listeria infections
Local anesthesia
Lower extremities
Lumbar puncture
Lyme disease
Maple syrup urine disease (MSUD)
Marijuana
Measles
Memory erasure
Memory loss
Ménière's disease
Meningitis
Mental status exam
Mercury poisoning
Motion sickness
Motor neuron diseases
Motor skill development
Multiple chemical sensitivity syndrome
Multiple sclerosis
Mumps
Myasthenia gravis
Narcolepsy

Nausea and vomiting
Neuralgia, neuritis, and neuropathy
Neurofibromatosis
Neuroimaging
Neurology
Neurosis
Neurosurgery
Niemann-Pick disease
Nuclear radiology
Numbness and tingling
Orthopedic surgery
Orthopedics
Overtraining syndrome
Palsy
Paralysis
Paraplegia
Parkinson's Disease
Pellagra
Pharmacology
Phenylketonuria (PKU)
Physical rehabilitation
Pick's disease
Poisoning
Poliomyelitis
Porphyria
Precocious puberty
Preeclampsia and eclampsia
Prion diseases
Quadriplegia
Rabies
Radiculopathy
Restless legs syndrome
Reye's syndrome
Rocky Mountain spotted fever
Rubella
Sarcoidosis
Sciatica
Seasonal affective disorder
Seizures
Sense organs
Shingles
Shock therapy
Shunts
Skin
Sleep
Sleep disorders
Sleeping sickness
Sleepwalking
Slipped disk
Small intestine
Smell
Snakebites
Spina bifida
Spinal cord disorders
Spine, vertebrae, and disks
Spinocerebellar ataxia
Sports medicine
Staphylococcal infections
Strokes
Sturge-Weber syndrome
Stuttering

Sympathectomy
Synesthesia
Syphilis
Taste
Tay-Sachs disease
Teeth
Tetanus
Thrombolytic therapy and TPA
Tics
Tinnitus
Touch
Tourette's syndrome
Toxoplasmosis
Tremors
Typhus
Upper extremities
Vagotomy
Vertigo
Vision
Walking
West Nile virus
Wilson's disease
Yoga

NOSE
Adenoids
Allergies
Anosmia
Antihistamines
Aromatherapy
Auras
Avian influenza
Casts and splints
Chickenpox
Childhood infectious diseases
Cold agglutinin disease
Common cold
Cornelia de Lange syndrome
Decongestants
Dengue fever
Epstein-Barr virus
Facial transplantation
Fifth disease
Hay fever
H1N1 influenza
Influenza
Methicillin-resistant staphylococcus
   aureus (MRSA) infection
Mold and mildew
Nasal polyp removal
Nasopharyngeal disorders
Otorhinolaryngology
Pharynx
Polyps
Pulmonary medicine
Respiration
Rhinitis
Rhinoplasty and submucous resection
Rhinoviruses
Rosacea
Rubinstein-Taybi syndrome

Sense organs
Sinusitis
Skin lesion removal
Smell
Sore throat
Stevens-Johnson syndrome
Taste
Tears and tear ducts
Vasculitis

PANCREAS
Abscess drainage
Alcoholism
Carbohydrates
Cholecystitis
Chyme
Cystic fibrosis
Diabetes mellitus
Digestion
Endocrine glands
Endocrinology
Endoscopic retrograde
   cholangiopancreatography (ERCP)
Fetal tissue transplantation
Food biochemistry
Gastroenterology
Gastrointestinal system
Glands
Glucose tolerance test
Hemochromatosis
Insulin
Internal medicine
Malabsorption
Metabolism
Mumps
Pancreatitis
Polycystic kidney disease
Polycystic ovary syndrome
Stomach
Transplantation

PSYCHIC-EMOTIONAL SYSTEM
Acquired immunodeficiency syndrome
   (AIDS)
Addiction
Adrenoleukodystrophy
Alcoholism
Alzheimer's disease
Amnesia
Anesthesia
Anesthesiology
Angelman syndrome
Anorexia nervosa
Antianxiety drugs
Antidepressants
Antihistamines
Anxiety
Aphrodisiacs
Aromatherapy
Asperger syndrome
Attention-deficit disorder (ADD)

Auras
Autism
Bariatric surgery
Biofeedback
Bipolar disorders
Body dysmorphic disorder
Bonding
Brain
Bulimia
Chronic fatigue syndrome
Cognitive development
Colic
Death and dying
Dementias
Depression
Developmental disorders
Developmental stages
Dizziness and fainting
Down syndrome
Dyskinesia
Dyslexia
Eating disorders
Electroencephalography (EEG)
Encephalitis
Endocrinology
Factitious disorders
Failure to thrive
Fibromyalgia
Frontotemporal dementia (FTD)
Gulf War syndrome
Headaches
Hormone therapy
Hormones
Hydrocephalus
Hypnosis
Hypochondriasis
Hypothalamus
Interpartner violence
Kinesiology
Klinefelter syndrome
Learning disabilities
Light therapy
Marijuana
Memory loss
Menopause
Miscarriage
Morgellons disease
Motor skill development
Narcolepsy
Neurology
Neurosis
Neurosurgery
Obesity
Obsessive-compulsive disorder
Overtraining syndrome
Paranoia
Pharmacology
Phobias
Pick's disease
Postpartum depression
Post-traumatic stress disorder

Prader-Willi syndrome
Precocious puberty
Premenstrual syndrome (PMS)
Psychiatric disorders
Psychoanalysis
Psychosis
Rabies
Rape and sexual assault
Restless legs syndrome
Schizophrenia
Seasonal affective disorder
Separation anxiety
Sexual dysfunction
Sexuality
Shock therapy
Sleep
Sleep disorders
Sleeping sickness
Sleepwalking
Speech disorders
Sperm banks
Steroid abuse
Strokes
Suicide
Synesthesia
Tics
Tinnitus
Toilet training
Tourette's syndrome
Weight loss and gain
Wilson's disease

REPRODUCTIVE SYSTEM
Abdomen
Abortion
Acquired immunodeficiency syndrome
  (AIDS)
Adrenoleukodystrophy
Amenorrhea
Amniocentesis
Anorexia nervosa
Assisted reproductive technologies
Avian influenza
Breast-feeding
Breasts
Brucellosis
Candidiasis
Catheterization
Cervical, ovarian, and uterine cancers
Cervical procedures
Cesarean section
Childbirth
Childbirth complications
Chlamydia
Chorionic villus sampling
Circumcision, female and genital
  mutilation
Circumcision
Computed tomography (CT) scanning
Conception
Congenital adrenal hyperplasia

Contraception
Culdocentesis
Cyst removal
Cystic fibrosis
Cystoscopy
Dysmenorrhea
Eating disorders
Ectopic pregnancy
Endocrine glands
Endocrinology
Endometrial biopsy
Endometriosis
Episiotomy
Erectile dysfunction
Fallopian tube
Fetus
Fistula repair
Gamete intrafallopian transfer (GIFT)
Gender reassignment surgery
Genetic counseling
Genital disorders
Gestational diabetes
Gigantism
Glands
Gonorrhea
Gynecology
Hermaphroditism and
  pseudohermaphroditism
Hernia
Herpes
Hormone therapy
Human papillomavirus (HPV)
Hydroceles
Hypogonadism
Hypospadias repair and urethroplasty
Hysterectomy
In vitro fertilization
Infertility
Internal medicine
Klinefelter syndrome
Laparoscopy
Lead poisoning
Menopause
Menorrhagia
Menstruation
Miscarriage
Myomectomy
Obstetrics
Orchiectomy
Orchitis
Ovarian cysts
Pap test
Pelvic inflammatory disease (PID)
Penile implant surgery
Placenta
Polycystic ovary syndrome
Polyps
Precocious puberty
Preeclampsia and eclampsia
Pregnancy and gestation
Pregnancy test

Premature birth
Premenstrual syndrome (PMS)
Prostate cancer
Prostate enlargement
Prostate gland
Semen
Sexual differentiation
Sexual dysfunction
Sexuality
Sexually transmitted diseases (STDs)
Sperm banks
Sterilization
Steroid abuse
Stevens-Johnson syndrome
Stillbirth
Syphilis
Testicles
Testicular surgery
Testicular torsion
Toxemia
Trichomoniasis
Tubal ligation
Turner syndrome
Ultrasonography
Urology
Uterus
Vas deferens
Vasectomy
Von Willebrand's disease

RESPIRATORY SYSTEM
Abscess drainage
Acidosis
Acquired immunodeficiency syndrome
  (AIDS)
Acute respiratory distress syndrome
  (ARDS)
Adenoviruses
Adrenoleukodystrophy
Altitude sickness
Amyotrophic lateral sclerosis (ALS)
Anthrax
Antihistamines
Apgar score
Apnea
Asbestos exposure
Asphyxiation
Asthma
Avian influenza
Babesiosis
Bacterial infections
Bronchi
Bronchiolitis
Bronchitis
Cardiopulmonary resuscitation (CPR)
Cartilage
Chest
Childhood infectious diseases
Choking
Chronic obstructive pulmonary disease
  (COPD)

Cold agglutinin disease
Common cold
Computed tomography (CT) scanning
Coronaviruses
Coughing
Croup
Cystic fibrosis
Decongestants
Defibrillation
Diaphragm
Drowning
Dwarfism
Edema
Emphysema
Epiglottitis
Exercise physiology
Fetal surgery
Fluids and electrolytes
Food allergies
Fungal infections
Hantavirus
Hay fever
Head and neck disorders
Heart transplantation
Heimlich maneuver
Hiccups
H1N1 influenza
Human respiratory system
Hyperbaric chamber
Hyperbaric oxygen therapy
Hyperventilation
Hypoxia
Influenza
Internal medicine
Kinesiology
Laryngectomy
Legionnaires' disease
Lung cancer
Lung surgery
Lungs
Marijuana
Measles
Mesothelioma
Methicillin-resistant staphylococcus
  aureus (MRSA) infection
Mold and mildew
Monkeypox
Multiple chemical sensitivity syndrome
Nasopharyngeal disorders
Niemann-Pick disease
Obesity
Otorhinolaryngology
Oxygen therapy
Pharynx
Plague
Plasma
Pneumocystis jirovecii
Pneumonia
Pneumothorax
Poisoning
Pulmonary diseases

Pulmonary edema
Pulmonary heart disease
Pulmonary hypertension
Pulmonary medicine
Respiration
Resuscitation
Rheumatoid arthritis
Rhinitis
Rhinoviruses
Sarcoidosis
Severe acute respiratory syndrome
  (SARS)
Sinusitis
Sleep apnea
Smoking
Sore throat
Staphylococcal infections
Stevens-Johnson syndrome
Thoracic surgery
Thrombolytic therapy and TPA
Thrombosis and thrombus
Tonsillectomy and adenoid removal
Trachea
Tracheostomy
Transplantation
Tuberculosis
Tularemia
Typhus
Vasculitis
Voice and vocal cord disorders
Whooping cough

SKIN
Abscess drainage
Acne
Acquired immunodeficiency syndrome
  (AIDS)
Acupressure
Adenoviruses
Adrenoleukodystrophy
Allergies
Amputation
Anesthesia
Anesthesiology
Angelman syndrome
Anorexia nervosa
Anthrax
Antihistamines
Anxiety
Athlete's foot
Auras
Bacillus Calmette-Guérin (BCG)
Bariatric surgery
Batten's disease
Bedsores
Behçet's disease
Bites and stings
Blisters
Blood testing
Body dysmorphic disorder
Bruises

Burns and scalds
Candidiasis
Canker sores
Casts and splints
Cells
Chagas' disease
Chickenpox
Cleft lip and palate repair
Cold agglutinin disease
Cold sores
Collagen
Collodion baby
Corns and calluses
Cushing's syndrome
Cutis marmorata telangiectatica
  congenita
Cyanosis
Cyst removal
Dengue fever
Dermatitis
Dermatology
Dermatopathology
Diabetic neuropathy
Ebola virus
Eczema
Edema
Electrical shock
Electrocauterization
Electrolysis
Enteroviruses
Face lift and blepharoplasty
Facial transplantation
Fibrocystic breast condition
Fifth disease
Folate deficiency
Food allergies
Frostbite
Fungal infections
Gangrene
Glands
Gluten intolerance
Gulf War syndrome
Hair
Hair transplantation
Hand-foot-and-mouth disease
Hand hygiene compliance
Heat exhaustion and heatstroke
Hemangioma
Hematomas
Herpes
Histiocytosis
Hives
Hormone therapy
Host-defense mechanisms
Human papillomavirus (HPV)
Hyperbaric chamber
Hyperhidrosis
Hyperthyroidism and hypothyroidism
Impetigo
Intravenous (IV) therapy
Jaundice

Kaposi's sarcoma
Kawasaki disease
Kwashiorkor
Laceration repair
Laser use in surgery
Leishmaniasis
Leprosy
Lice, mites, and ticks
Light therapy
Lower extremities
Lyme disease
Measles
Melanoma
Mesenchymal stem cells
Methicillin-resistant staphylococcus
   aureus (MRSA) infection
Mold and mildew
Moles
Monkeypox
Morgellons disease
Multiple chemical sensitivity syndrome
Nails
Necrotizing fasciitis
Neurofibromatosis
Numbness and tingling
Otoplasty
Pellagra
Pigmentation
Pinworms
Pityriasis alba
Pityriasis rosea
Polycystic ovary syndrome
Polydactyly and syndactyly
Porphyria
Psoriasis
Radiation sickness
Reiter's syndrome
Ringworm
Rocky Mountain spotted fever
Rosacea
Roseola
Rubella
Sarcoidosis
Scabies
Scarlet fever
Sense organs
Shingles
Skin cancer
Skin disorders
Skin lesion removal
Smallpox
Streptococcal infections
Sturge-Weber syndrome
Styes
Sweating
Tattoo removal
Tattoos and body piercing
Touch
Toxoplasmosis
Tularemia
Typhoid fever

Typhus
Umbilical cord
Upper extremities
Vasculitis
Vitiligo
Von Willebrand's disease
Williams syndrome
Wiskott-Aldrich syndrome

SPINE
Anesthesia
Anesthesiology
Ankylosing spondylitis
Atrophy
Back pain
Brain tumors
Brucellosis
Charcot-Marie-Tooth Disease
Chiari malformations
Chiropractic
Diaphragm
Disk removal
Fetal tissue transplantation
Flexibility
Head and neck disorders
Kinesiology
Laminectomy and spinal fusion
Lumbar puncture
Marfan syndrome
Meningitis
Methicillin-resistant staphylococcus
   aureus (MRSA) infection
Motor neuron diseases
Multiple sclerosis
Narcotics
Nervous system
Neuralgia, neuritis, and neuropathy
Neuroimaging
Neurology
Neurosurgery
Orthopedic surgery
Orthopedics
Paget's disease
Paralysis
Paraplegia
Physical rehabilitation
Poliomyelitis
Quadriplegia
Radiculopathy
Sciatica
Scoliosis
Slipped disk
Spina bifida
Spinal cord disorders
Spondylitis
Sports medicine
Stenosis
Sympathectomy
Whiplash
Williams syndrome

SPLEEN
Abscess drainage
Aspergillosis
Brucellosis
Cold agglutinin disease
Gaucher's disease
Hematology
Hemoglobin
Hemolysis
Immune system
Internal medicine
Leptospirosis
Leukemia
Lymph
Lymphatic system
Malaria
Metabolism
Methicillin-resistant staphylococcus
   aureus (MRSA) infection
Mononucleosis
Niemann-Pick disease
Sarcoidosis
Sickle cell disease
Splenectomy
Thrombocytopenia
Transplantation
Typhoid fever

STOMACH
Abdomen
Abdominal disorders
Abscess drainage
Acid reflux disease
Adenoviruses
Allergies
Avian influenza
Bariatric surgery
Campylobacter infections
Chyme
Colitis
Digestion
Drowning
Eating disorders
Endoscopic retrograde
   cholangiopancreatography (ERCP)
Endoscopy
Esophagus
Food biochemistry
Food poisoning
Gastrectomy
Gastroenteritis
Gastroenterology
Gastrointestinal disorders
Gastrointestinal system
Gastrostomy
Hernia
Hernia repair
Internal medicine
Lactose intolerance
Malabsorption
Malnutrition

Metabolism
Motion sickness
Nausea and vomiting
Obesity
Peristalsis
Poisoning
Polyps
Pyloric stenosis
Radiation sickness
Stomach
Ulcer surgery
Ulcers
Vagotomy
Weaning
Weight loss and gain

TEETH
Angelman syndrome
Braces
Bulimia
Cavities
Cleft lip and palate repair
Cornelia de Lange syndrome
Crowns and bridges
Dental diseases
Dentistry
Dentures
Dysphagia
Eating disorders
Enamel
Endodontic disease
Fluoride treatments
Fracture repair
Gastrointestinal system
Gingivitis
Gum disease
Jaw wiring
Lisping
Mouth and throat cancer
Oral and maxillofacial surgery
Orthodontics
Periodontal surgery
Periodontitis
Plaque
Prader-Willi syndrome
Rickets
Root canal treatment
Rubinstein-Taybi syndrome
Scurvy
Teething
Temporomandibular joint (TMJ)
   syndrome
Thumb sucking
Tooth extraction
Wisdom teeth

TENDONS
Ankylosing spondylitis
Astym® therapy
Carpal tunnel syndrome
Casts and splints

Collagen
Connective tissue
Exercise physiology
Flexibility
Ganglion removal
Hammertoe correction
Hemiplegia
Joints
Kneecap removal
Orthopedic surgery
Orthopedics
Osgood-Schlatter disease
Physical rehabilitation
Rotator cuff surgery
Sports medicine
Tendinitis
Tendon disorders
Tendon repair

THROAT
Acid reflux disease
Acquired immunodeficiency syndrome
   (AIDS)
Adenoids
Antihistamines
Auras
Avian influenza
Catheterization
Choking
Croup
Decongestants
Diphtheria
Drowning
Eating disorders
Epiglottitis
Epstein-Barr virus
Esophagus
Fifth disease
Gastroenterology
Gastrointestinal system
Gonorrhea
Hay fever
Head and neck disorders
Heimlich maneuver
Hiccups
Histiocytosis
H1N1 influenza
Human papillomavirus (HPV)
Influenza
Laryngectomy
Laryngitis
Mononucleosis
Mouth and throat cancer
Nasopharyngeal disorders
Otorhinolaryngology
Pharyngitis
Pharynx
Polyps
Pulmonary medicine
Quinsy
Respiration

Rhinitis
Rhinoviruses
Smoking
Sore throat
Streptococcal infections
Tonsillectomy and adenoid removal
Tonsillitis
Tracheostomy
Tremors
Voice and vocal cord disorders
Whooping cough

TONGUE
Dysphagia
Folate deficiency
Taste
Vagus nerve

URINARY SYSTEM
Abdomen
Abdominal disorders
Abscess drainage
Adenoviruses
Adrenalectomy
Avian influenza
Bed-wetting
Bladder cancer
Bladder removal
Candidiasis
Catheterization
Chlamydia
Cold agglutinin disease
Cystic fibrosis
Cystitis
Cystoscopy
Dialysis
Diuretics
E. coli infection
End-stage renal disease
Endoscopy
Fetal surgery
Fistula repair
Gonorrhea
Hematuria
Hemolytic uremic syndrome
Hermaphroditism and
   pseudohermaphroditism
Hormone therapy
Host-defense mechanisms
Hyperplasia
Hypertension
Hypokalemia
Incontinence
Internal medicine
Kidney cancer
Kidney disorders
Kidney transplantation
Kidneys
Laparoscopy
Leptospirosis
Lithotripsy

Entries by Specialties and Related Fields

ALL
Abscesses
Accidents
Acupuncture
Adrenal glands
Aging
Aging: Extended care
Alternative medicine
Anatomy
Antibiotic resistance
Antibiotics
Antihypertensives
Anti-inflammatory drugs
Antioxidants
Autopsy
Biomarker
Bionics and biotechnology
Birth defects
Burkitt's lymphoma
Cancer
Carcinogens
Carcinoma
Chemotherapy
Chronic granulomatous disease
Clinical trials
Club drugs
Coccidioidomycosis
Cockayne disease
Collagen
Congenital disorders
Critical care
Cryosurgery
Cysts
Death and dying
Diagnosis
Dietary reference intakes (DRIs)
Disease
Embryology
Emergency medicine
Emergency rooms
Emerging infectious diseases
Environmental diseases
Enzyme therapy
Epidemics and pandemics
Epidemiology
Epidermal nevus syndromes
Essential nutrients
Family-centered care
Family medicine
Fascia
Fatigue
Fever
First aid
First responder
Food guide plate
Forensic pathology
Genetic diseases

Genetic engineering
Genetic imprinting
Genetics and inheritance
Genomics
Geriatric assessment
Geriatrics and gerontology
Grafts and grafting
Growth
Healing
Health
Herbal medicine
Histology
Homeopathy
Hospital readmission
Hydrotherapy
Hyperadiposis
Hyperthermia and hypothermia
Hypertrophy
Hypochondriasis
Iatrogenic disorders
Imaging and radiology
Immunopathology
Infection
Infection control
Inflammation
Insect-borne diseases
Internet medicine
Invasive tests
Leptin
Lesions
Longevity
Macronutrients
Magnetic resonance imaging (MRI)
Malignancy and metastasis
Malnutrition
Massage
Medical home
Meditation
Men's health
Mental hygiene
Metabolic disorders
Metabolic syndrome
Mucopolysaccharidosis (MPS)
Multiple births
Münchausen syndrome by proxy
Neonatology
Niacin
Noninvasive tests
Nursing
Nutrition
Occupational health
Oncology
Opportunistic infections
Orthorexia nervosa
Ovaries
Over-the-counter medications
Pain

Pain management
Palliative care
Palliative medicine
Paramedics
Parasitic diseases
Pathology
Pediatrics
Perinatology
Physical examination
Physician assistants
Physiology
Phytochemicals
Plastic surgery
Positron emission tomography (PET)
    scanning
Preventive medicine
Progeria
Prognosis
Prostheses
Protein
Proteomics
Psychiatry
Psychosomatic disorders
Puberty and adolescence
Radiation therapy
Radiopharmaceuticals
Reflexes
Retroviruses
Safety issues for children
Safety issues for the elderly
Screening
Self-medication
Shock
Signs and symptoms
Stem cells
Stress
Stress reduction
Substance abuse
Sudden infant death syndrome (SIDS)
Supplements
Surgery
Surgical procedures
Surgical technologists
Syndrome
Systemic lupus erythematosus (SLE)
Systemic sclerosis
Systems and organs
Teratogens
Terminally ill: Extended care
Tissue engineering
Toxic shock syndrome
Toxicology
Transitional care
Tumor removal
Tumors
Viral hemorrhagic fevers
Viral infections

Collagen
Colon
Connective tissue
Corticosteroids
CRISPR
Cystic fibrosis
Digestion
Endocrine glands
Endocrinology
Enzyme therapy
Ergogenic aids
Fatty acid
Fatty acid oxidation disorders
Fluids and electrolytes
Fluoride treatments
Food biochemistry
Food guide plate
Fructosemia
Galactosemia
Gaucher's disease
Genetic engineering
Genomics
Gigantism
Gingivitis
Glands
Glucagon
Glycerol
Glycogen storage diseases
Glycolysis
Gram staining
Gulf War syndrome
Hemoglobin
Histology
Hormones
Hyperadiposis
Hypothalamus
Insect-borne diseases
Insulin-like growth factors
Leptin
Leukodystrophy
Lipids
Lumbar puncture
Macronutrients
Malabsorption
Malaria
Melatonin
Mesenchymal stem cells
Metabolic disorders
Metabolism
Myoglobin
Nephrology
Neuroethics
Niemann-Pick disease
Nutrition
Ovaries
Pathology
Pharmacology
Phenylketonuria (PKU)
Pituitary gland
Plasma
Protein

Respiration
Retroviruses
Rhinoviruses
Serotonin
Sleep
Small intestine
Statins
Steroids
Thymus gland
Tourette's syndrome
Urinalysis
Wilson's disease

BIOTECHNOLOGY
Antibodies
Assisted reproductive technologies
Biological therapies
Bionics and biotechnology
Cloning
Computed tomography (CT) scanning
Defibrillation
Dialysis
Electrocardiography (ECG or EKG)
Electroencephalography (EEG)
Fatty acid oxidation disorders
Gene therapy
Genetic engineering
Genomics
Glycogen storage diseases
Huntington's disease
Hyperbaric oxygen therapy
Insect-borne diseases
Magnetic resonance imaging (MRI)
Malabsorption
Nephrology
Pacemaker implantation
Positron emission tomography (PET)
  scanning
Prostheses
Rhinoviruses
Severe combined immunodeficiency
  syndrome (SCID)
Sperm banks
Xenotransplantation

CARDIOLOGY
Acute respiratory distress syndrome
  (ARDS)
Aging: Extended care
Anemia
Aneurysms
Angina
Angiography
Angioplasty
Antihypertensives
Anxiety
Aortic aneurysm
Aortic stenosis
Arrhythmias
Arteriosclerosis
Aspergillosis

Atrial fibrillation
Biofeedback
Blood pressure
Blood vessels
Blue baby syndrome
Brucellosis
Bypass surgery
Cardiac arrest
Cardiac rehabilitation
Cardiac surgery
Cardiopulmonary resuscitation (CPR)
Carotid arteries
Catheterization
Chest
Circulation
Computed tomography (CT) scanning
Congenital heart disease
Coronary artery bypass graft
Critical care
Defibrillation
DiGeorge syndrome
Diphtheria
Dirofilaria immitis
Diuretics
Dizziness and fainting
Echocardiography
Electrocardiography (ECG or EKG)
Electrocauterization
Embolism
Emergency medicine
End-stage renal disease
Endocarditis
Enteroviruses
Exercise physiology
Extracorporeal membrane oxygenation
  (ECMO)
Fetal surgery
Gigantism
Heart
Heart attack
Heart disease
Heart failure
Heart transplantation
Heart valve replacement
Hematology
Hemochromatosis
Hemoglobin
Hormone therapy
Hypercholesterolemia
Hypertension
Hyperthyroidism and hypothyroidism
Hypokalemia
Hypotension
Infarction
Internal medicine
Ischemia
Kawasaki disease
Kinesiology
Leptin
Lesions
Lyme disease

Marfan syndrome
Mesenchymal stem cells
Metabolic syndrome
Methicillin-resistant staphylococcus
  aureus (MRSA) infection
Mitral valve prolapse
Mucopolysaccharidosis (MPS)
Muscles
Neonatology
Noninvasive tests
Nuclear medicine
Osteogenesis imperfecta
Oxygen therapy
Pacemaker implantation
Palliative care
Palpitations
Paramedics
Patent ductus arteriosus
Pellagra
Plaque
Plasma
Polycystic kidney disease
Postural orthostatic tachycardia
  syndrome (POTS)
Prader-Willi syndrome
Progeria
Prostheses
Pulmonary heart disease
Pulmonary edema
Pulmonary hypertension
Pulse pressure
Pulse rate
Rheumatic fever
Rubinstein-Taybi syndrome
Sarcoidosis
Single photon emission computed
  tomography (SPECT)
Spondylitis
Sports medicine
Staphylococcal infections
Stenosis
Stents
Systemic lupus erythematosus (SLE)
Thoracic surgery
Thrombolytic therapy and TPA
Thrombosis and thrombus
Tissue engineering
Transplantation
Ultrasonography
Uremia
Varicose veins
Vascular medicine
Vascular system
Vasculitis
Williams syndrome

CRITICAL CARE
Acidosis
Aging: Extended care
Amputation
Anesthesia

Anesthesiology
Aneurysmectomy
Anthrax
Apgar score
Botulism
Burns and scalds
Carotid arteries
Catheterization
Chronic granulomatous disease
Club drugs
Concussion
Craniotomy
Defibrillation
Diuretics
Drowning
Echocardiography
Electrical shock
Electrocardiography (ECG or EKG)
Electrocauterization
Electroencephalography (EEG)
Embolization
Emergency medicine
Epidemics and pandemics
Grafts and grafting
Hantavirus
Heart attack
Heart transplantation
Heat exhaustion and heatstroke
Hydrocephalus
Hyperbaric oxygen therapy
Hyperthermia and hypothermia
Hypotension
Hypoxia
Infarction
Insect-borne diseases
Intravenous (IV) therapy
Ischemia
Lumbar puncture
Methicillin-resistant staphylococcus
  aureus (MRSA) infection
Necrotizing fasciitis
Neonatology
Nursing
Oncology
Osteopathic medicine
Oxygen therapy
Pain management
Palliative care
Paramedics
Peritonitis
Psychiatry
Pulmonary medicine
Pulse rate
Radiation sickness
Resuscitation
Safety issues for children
Safety issues for the elderly
Severe acute respiratory syndrome
  (SARS)
Shock
Stevens-Johnson syndrome

Streptococcal infections
Thrombolytic therapy and TPA
Toxic shock syndrome
Tracheostomy
Transfusion
Whooping cough
Wounds

CYTOLOGY
Acid-base chemistry
Bionics and biotechnology
Biopsy
Blood testing
Breast disorders
Cancer
Carcinoma
Cells
Cholesterol
Cytopathology
Dermatology
Dermatopathology
Epstein-Barr virus
Eye infections and disorders
Fluids and electrolytes
Food biochemistry
Gaucher's disease
Gene therapy
Genetic counseling
Genomics
Glycolysis
Gram staining
Healing
Hematocrit
Hematology
Hirschsprung's disease
Histology
Hyperplasia
Immune system
Karyotyping
Laboratory tests
Lipids
Metabolism
Microscopy
Mutation
Neutrophil
Oncology
Pathology
Pharmacology
Plasma
Rhinoviruses
Sarcoma
Serology

DENTISTRY
Aging: Extended care
Anesthesia
Anesthesiology
Braces
Canker sores
Cavities
Cerebral palsy

Cockayne disease
Crowns and bridges
Dental diseases
Dentures
Eating disorders
Enamel
Endodontic disease
Fluoride treatments
Forensic pathology
Fracture repair
Gastrointestinal system
Gingivitis
Gum disease
Head and neck disorders
Jaw wiring
Lisping
Local anesthesia
Mouth and throat cancer
Oral and maxillofacial surgery
Orthodontics
Osteogenesis imperfecta
Periodontal surgery
Periodontitis
Plaque
Prader-Willi syndrome
Prostheses
Root canal treatment
Rubinstein-Taybi syndrome
Sense organs
Sjögren's syndrome
Teeth
Teething
Temporomandibular joint (TMJ)
     syndrome
Thumb sucking
Tooth extraction
Von Willebrand's disease
Wisdom teeth

DERMATOLOGY
Abscess drainage
Acne
Acquired immunodeficiency syndrome
     (AIDS)
Adrenoleukodystrophy
Allergies
Alopecia
Angelman syndrome
Anthrax
Anti-inflammatory drugs
Athlete's foot
Bedsores
Bile
Biopsy
Blisters
Body dysmorphic disorder
Burns and scalds
Carcinoma
Chickenpox
Chronic granulomatous disease
Coccidioidomycosis

Cockayne disease
Collodion baby
Corns and calluses
Cryosurgery
Cutis marmorata telangiectatica
     congenita
Cyst removal
Dermatitis
Dermatopathology
Dirofilaria immitis
Eczema
Electrocauterization
Electrolysis
Enteroviruses
Facial transplantation
Folate deficiency
Fungal infections
Ganglion removal
Gangrene
Gender dysphoria
Genetic engineering
Glands
Gluten intolerance
Grafts and grafting
Hair
Hair transplantation
Hand-foot-and-mouth disease
Healing
Hemangioma
Herpes
Histology
Hives
Hyaluronic acid injections
Hyperbaric chamber
Hyperhidrosis
Hyperthyroidism and hypothyroidism
Immunopathology
Impetigo
Laser use in surgery
Lesions
Lice, mites, and ticks
Light therapy
Local anesthesia
Lyme disease
Melanoma
Mesenchymal stem cells
Methicillin-resistant staphylococcus
     aureus (MRSA) infection
Moles
Monkeypox
Morgellons disease
Multiple chemical sensitivity syndrome
Nails
Necrotizing fasciitis
Neurofibromatosis
Pellagra
Pigmentation
Pinworms
Pityriasis alba
Pityriasis rosea
Plastic surgery

Podiatry
Polycystic ovary syndrome
Postherpetic neuralgia
Prostheses
Psoriasis
Puberty and adolescence
Reiter's syndrome
Ringworm
Rocky Mountain spotted fever
Rosacea
Sarcoidosis
Scabies
Scleroderma
Sense organs
Shingles
Skin
Skin cancer
Skin disorders
Skin lesion removal
Smallpox
Staphylococcal infections
Stevens-Johnson syndrome
Streptococcal infections
Stress
Sturge-Weber syndrome
Styes
Sweating
Systemic lupus erythematosus (SLE)
Tattoo removal
Tattoos and body piercing
Tissue engineering
Touch
Vasculitis
Vitiligo
Von Willebrand's disease
Wiskott-Aldrich syndrome

DIETETICS
Essential nutrients
Fasting
Folate deficiency
Glycerol
Health impact of sugar
Pellagra

EMBRYOLOGY
Amniocentesis
Assisted reproductive technologies
Birth defects
Blue baby syndrome
Chorionic villus sampling
Cloning
Conception
Down syndrome
Ectopic pregnancy
Fetal tissue transplantation
Fetus
Gamete intrafallopian transfer (GIFT)
Genetic counseling
Genetic diseases
Genetic engineering

Genetic imprinting
Genetics and inheritance
Genomics
Growth
Hermaphroditism and
    pseudohermaphroditism
In vitro fertilization
Karyotyping
Klinefelter syndrome
Meckel's diverticulum
Miscarriage
Mucopolysaccharidosis (MPS)
Multiple births
Neonatology
Obstetrics
Ovaries
Perinatology
Phenylketonuria (PKU)
Placenta
Pregnancy and gestation
Premature birth
Reproductive system
Rh factor
Sexual differentiation
Spina bifida
Syphilis
Teratogens
Ultrasonography
Uterus

EMERGENCY MEDICINE
Abdominal disorders
Abscess drainage
Acidosis
Adrenoleukodystrophy
Advance directives
Altitude sickness
Amputation
Anesthesia
Anesthesiology
Aneurysmectomy
Aneurysms
Angiography
Anthrax
Appendectomy
Appendicitis
Asphyxiation
Atrial fibrillation
Back pain
Bites and stings
Bleeding
Blurred vision
Botulism
Bruises
Burns and scalds
Cardiac arrest
Cardiology
Cardiopulmonary resuscitation (CPR)
Carotid arteries
Casts and splints
Catheterization

Cesarean section
Choking
Cholecystitis
Chronic granulomatous disease
Club drugs
Cold agglutinin disease
Computed tomography (CT) scanning
Concussion
Critical care
Croup
Defibrillation
Dizziness and fainting
Drowning
Echocardiography
Electrical shock
Electrocardiography (ECG or EKG)
Electrocauterization
Electroencephalography (EEG)
Embolization
Epiglottitis
First responder
Fracture and dislocation
Frostbite
Gangrene
Grafts and grafting
Head and neck disorders
Heart attack
Heart transplantation
Heat exhaustion and heatstroke
Heimlich maneuver
H1N1 influenza
Hyperbaric oxygen therapy
Hyperthermia and hypothermia
Hyperventilation
Hypotension
Hypoxia
Impetigo
Infarction
Influenza
Insulin
Interpartner violence
Interstitial pulmonary fibrosis (IPF)
Intravenous (IV) therapy
Jaw wiring
Laceration repair
Local anesthesia
Lung surgery
Meningitis
Mental status exam
Monkeypox
Nail removal
Necrotizing fasciitis
Noninvasive tests
Nursing
Osteopathic medicine
Oxygen therapy
Pain management
Palliative medicine
Paramedics
Peritonitis
Physician assistants

Plague
Plastic surgery
Pleurisy
Pneumonia
Pneumothorax
Poisoning
Pulmonary medicine
Pulse rate
Pyelonephritis
Radiation sickness
Rape and sexual assault
Resuscitation
Reye's syndrome
Rocky Mountain spotted fever
Safety issues for children
Safety issues for the elderly
Severe acute respiratory syndrome
    (SARS)
Shock
Snakebites
Spinal cord disorders
Splenectomy
Sports medicine
Stevens-Johnson syndrome
Streptococcal infections
Strokes
Surgical technologists
Thrombolytic therapy and TPA
Toxic shock syndrome
Tracheostomy
Transfusion
Transplantation
Tularemia
Wounds

ENDOCRINOLOGY
Addison's disease
Adolescent sexuality
Adrenalectomy
Adrenoleukodystrophy
Amenorrhea
Anorexia nervosa
Assisted reproductive technologies
Bariatric surgery
Biofeedback
Brain death
Breasts
Carbohydrates
Computed tomography (CT) scanning
Congenital adrenal hyperplasia
Congenital hypothyroidism
Corticosteroids
Cushing's syndrome
Diabetes mellitus
Dwarfism
End-stage renal disease
Endocrine disorders
Endocrine glands
Endocrinology
Ergogenic aids
Failure to thrive

Cloning
Defibrillation
Ergogenic aids
Facial transplantation
Fetal surgery
Fetal tissue transplantation
Gender dysphoria
Genetic engineering
Genomics
Gulf War syndrome
Longevity
Marijuana
Münchausen syndrome by proxy
Neurosis
Sperm banks
Xenotransplantation

EXERCISE
Walking

EXERCISE PHYSIOLOGY
Acidosis
Adipose tissue
Aerobics
Ataxia
Back pain
Biofeedback
Blood pressure
Bones and the skeleton
Cardiac rehabilitation
Carotid arteries
Defibrillation
Dehydration
Electrocardiography (ECG or EKG)
Ergogenic aids
Fascia
Glycolysis
Heart
Hemiplegia
Hypotension
Hypoxia
Juvenile rheumatoid arthritis
Kinesiology
Lungs
Massage
Metabolism
Motor skill development
Muscle sprains, spasms, and disorders
Muscles
Osteoarthritis
Overtraining syndrome
Physical rehabilitation
Pulmonary medicine
Pulse rate
Respiration
Slipped disk
Sports medicine
Stenosis
Steroid abuse
Sweating
Tendinitis

Vascular system

FAMILY MEDICINE
Abdominal disorders
Abscess drainage
Acne
Advance directives
Alcoholism
Allergies
Amenorrhea
Amyotrophic lateral sclerosis (ALS)
Anemia
Angina
Anorexia nervosa
Anosmia
Antianxiety drugs
Antidepressants
Antihistamines
Anti-inflammatory drugs
Antioxidants
Aspergillosis
Ataxia
Atrophy
Attention-deficit disorder (ADD)
Autism
Back pain
Bed-wetting
Bell's palsy
Beriberi
Biofeedback
Bleeding
Blisters
Blood pressure
Blurred vision
Body dysmorphic disorder
Bronchiolitis
Bronchitis
Bruises
Bulimia
Bunions
Burkitt's lymphoma
Candidiasis
Canker sores
Carotid arteries
Casts and splints
Cerebral palsy
Chagas' disease
Chickenpox
Childhood infectious diseases
Cholecystitis
Cholesterol
Chronic fatigue syndrome
Cirrhosis
Coccidioidomycosis
Cold sores
Common cold
Conjunctivitis
Constipation
Corticosteroids
Coughing
Cryosurgery

Cushing's syndrome
Cytomegalovirus (CMV)
Death and dying
Decongestants
Deep vein thrombosis
Defibrillation
Dehydration
Dengue fever
Depression
Diabetes mellitus
Diarrhea and dysentery
Digestion
Diphtheria
Dizziness and fainting
E. coli infection
Earwax
Eating disorders
Echocardiography
Ehrlichiosis
Electrocauterization
Enterocolitis
Epiglottitis
Ergogenic aids
Exercise physiology
Factitious disorders
Failure to thrive
Fatigue
Fever
Fifth disease
Fungal infections
Ganglion removal
Genital disorders
Geriatric assessment
Giardiasis
Gigantism
Gynecology
Headaches
Healing
Heart disease
Heat exhaustion and heatstroke
Hemiplegia
Hemolytic uremic syndrome
Hemorrhoid banding and removal
Hemorrhoids
Herpes
Hiccups
Hirschsprung's disease
Hives
H1N1 influenza
Hormone therapy
Hyperadiposis
Hyperlipidemia
Hypertension
Hypertrophy
Hypoglycemia
Hypoxia
Impetigo
Incontinence
Infarction
Infection
Inflammation

Esophagus
Essential nutrients
Failure to thrive
Fecal bacteriotherapy
Fiber
Fistula repair
Folate deficiency
Food allergies
Food biochemistry
Food poisoning
Gallbladder
Gallbladder cancer
Gallbladder diseases
Gastrectomy
Gastroenteritis
Gastrointestinal disorders
Gastrointestinal system
Gastrostomy
Giardiasis
Glands
Gluten
Gluten intolerance
Hemochromatosis
Hemolysis
Hemolytic uremic syndrome
Hemorrhoid banding and removal
Hemorrhoids
Hernia
Hernia repair
Hiccups
Ileostomy and colostomy
Infarction
Internal medicine
Intestinal disorders
Intestines
Irritable bowel syndrome (IBS)
Jaundice
Lactose intolerance
Laparoscopy
Leaky gut syndrome
Lesions
Liver
Liver cancer
Liver disorders
Liver transplantation
Malabsorption
Malnutrition
Meckel's diverticulum
Metabolism
Nausea and vomiting
Nonalcoholic steatohepatitis (NASH)
Noroviruses
Pancreas
Pancreatitis
Pellagra
Peristalsis
Peritonitis
Polycystic kidney disease
Polyps
Proctology
Pyloric stenosis

Rectum
Rotavirus
Salmonella infection
Scleroderma
Shigellosis
Small intestine
Soiling
Stenosis
Stevens-Johnson syndrome
Stomach
Stone removal
Stones
Systemic lupus erythematosus (SLE)
Tapeworms
Taste
Tissue engineering
Toilet training
Ulcer surgery
Ulcerative colitis
Ulcers
Vagotomy
Vagus nerve
Vasculitis
Von Willebrand's disease
Weight loss and gain
Wilson's disease

GENERAL SURGERY

Abscess drainage
Achalasia
Adenoids
Adrenalectomy
Amputation
Anesthesia
Anesthesiology
Aneurysms
Appendectomy
Arthroplasty
Back pain
Bariatric surgery
Biopsy
Bladder removal
Bone marrow transplantation
Brain tumors
Breast biopsy
Breast cancer
Breast disorders
Breast surgery
Bunions
Bypass surgery
Casts and splints
Catheterization
Cesarean section
Cholecystectomy
Chronic granulomatous disease
Circumcision, female, and genital
  mutilation
Circumcision
Coccidioidomycosis
Colon
Colonoscopy and sigmoidoscopy

Colorectal polyp removal
Colorectal surgery
Corneal transplantation
Cryosurgery
Culdocentesis
Cyst removal
Defibrillation
Disk removal
Ear surgery
Electrocauterization
Endarterectomy
Eye infections and disorders
Eye surgery
Face lift and blepharoplasty
Fistula repair
Gallbladder cancer
Ganglion removal
Gastrectomy
Gender dysphoria
Gender reassignment surgery
Gigantism
Grafts and grafting
Hair transplantation
Hammertoe correction
Heart transplantation
Heart valve replacement
Heel spur removal
Hemorrhoid banding and removal
Hernia repair
Hydroceles
Hydrocephalus
Hypospadias repair and urethroplasty
Hypoxia
Hysterectomy
Infarction
Intravenous (IV) therapy
Kidney transplantation
Kneecap removal
Laceration repair
Laparoscopy
Laryngectomy
Lesions
Liposuction
Liver transplantation
Lumbar puncture
Lung surgery
Mastectomy and lumpectomy
Meckel's diverticulum
Mesothelioma
Methicillin-resistant staphylococcus
  aureus (MRSA) infection
Mouth and throat cancer
Nasal polyp removal
Nephrectomy
Neurosurgery
Oncology
Ophthalmology
Orthopedic surgery
Otoplasty
Pain
Parathyroidectomy

Penile implant surgery
Periodontal surgery
Peritonitis
Phlebitis
Physician assistants
Plasma
Plastic surgery
Polydactyly and syndactyly
Polyps
Prostate gland removal
Prostheses
Pulse rate
Pyloric stenosis
Rhinoplasty and submucous resection
Rotator cuff surgery
Sarcoma
Shunts
Skin lesion removal
Small intestine
Sphincterectomy
Splenectomy
Staphylococcal infections
Sterilization
Stone removal
Streptococcal infections
Surgery
Surgical procedures
Surgical technologists
Sympathectomy
Tattoo removal
Tendon repair
Testicles
Testicular cancer
Testicular surgery
Thoracic surgery
Thyroidectomy
Tonsillectomy and adenoid removal
Tonsillitis
Toxic shock syndrome
Trachea
Tracheostomy
Transfusion
Transplantation
Tumor removal
Ulcer surgery
Ulcerative colitis
Vagotomy
Varicose vein removal
Vasectomy
Xenotransplantation

GENETICS
Adrenal glands
Adrenoleukodystrophy
Agnosia
Amniocentesis
Angelman syndrome
Antibiotic resistance
Assisted reproductive technologies
Attention-deficit disorder (ADD)
Autism

Batten's disease
Bioinformatics
Biological therapies
Biomarker
Bionics and biotechnology
Birth defects
Bone marrow transplantation
Breast cancer
Charcot-Marie-Tooth Disease
Chemotherapy
Chorionic villus sampling
Chronic granulomatous disease
Cloning
Cockayne disease
Cognitive development
Colorectal cancer
Congenital adrenal hyperplasia
Congenital disorders
Cornelia de Lange syndrome
CRISPR
Cystic fibrosis
Diabetes mellitus
DiGeorge syndrome
Down syndrome
Dwarfism
Embryology
Endocrinology
Enzyme therapy
Failure to thrive
Fetal surgery
Fetus
Fragile X syndrome
Fructosemia
Galactosemia
Gaucher's disease
Gender dysphoria
Gene therapy
Genetic counseling
Genetic diseases
Genetic engineering
Genetic imprinting
Genetics and inheritance
Genomics
Grafts and grafting
Hemangioma
Hematology
Hemoglobin
Hemophilia
Hermaphroditism and
    pseudohermaphroditism
Huntington's disease
Hyperadiposis
Immunodeficiency disorders
Immunopathology
In vitro fertilization
Intellectual disability
Karyotyping
Klinefelter syndrome
Klippel-Trenaunay syndrome
Laboratory tests
Leptin

Lesbian, gay, bisexual, transgender,
    and queer (LGBTQ)
Leukodystrophy
Malabsorption
Maple syrup urine disease (MSUD)
Marfan syndrome
Metabolic disorders
Motor skill development
Mucopolysaccharidosis (MPS)
Multiple births
Muscular dystrophy
Mutation
Neonatology
Nephrology
Neurofibromatosis
Neurology
Niemann-Pick disease
Obstetrics
Oncology
Ovaries
Paget's disease
Pain
Pediatrics
Phenylketonuria (PKU)
Polycystic kidney disease
Polydactyly and syndactyly
Polyps
Porphyria
Prader-Willi syndrome
Precocious puberty
Reproductive system
Retroviruses
Rh factor
Rhinoviruses
Rubinstein-Taybi syndrome
Sarcoidosis
Sarcoma
Severe combined immunodeficiency
    syndrome (SCID)
Sexual differentiation
Sexuality
Sickle cell disease
Sperm banks
Spinocerebellar ataxia
Synesthesia
Tay-Sachs disease
Tourette's syndrome
Transplantation
Tremors
Turner syndrome
Wilms tumor
Williams syndrome
Wiskott-Aldrich syndrome

GERIATRIC
Contracture
Psychiatry

**GERIATRICS AND
GERONTOLOGY**
Advance directives

Aging
Aging: Extended care
Alzheimer's disease
Arthroplasty
Assisted living facilities
Ataxia
Atrophy
Back pain
Blindness
Blood pressure
Blurred vision
Bone disorders
Brain disorders
Cartilage
Cataracts
Chronic obstructive pulmonary disease (COPD)
Critical care
Deafness
Death and dying
Dementias
Depression
Dyskinesia
Emergency medicine
End-stage renal disease
Eye infections and disorders
Eye surgery
Family-centered care
Family medicine
Fatigue
Fiber
Hip fracture repair
Hormone therapy
Hypotension
Incontinence
Interpartner violence
Joints
Massage
Memory loss
Neuroscience
Nursing
Osteoclast
Osteopathic medicine
Osteoporosis
Pain management
Palliative care
Paramedics
Parkinson's Disease
Physician assistants
Pick's disease
Psychiatry
Radiculopathy
Rheumatoid arthritis
Rheumatology
Safety issues for the elderly
Sleep disorders
Spine
Suicide
Temporal arteritis
Tremors
Vision disorders

GYNECOLOGY
Abdomen
Abortion
Acquired immunodeficiency syndrome (AIDS)
Amenorrhea
Assisted reproductive technologies
Biopsy
Bladder removal
Blurred vision
Breast biopsy
Breast cancer
Breast disorders
Breast-feeding
Breasts
Cervical, ovarian, and uterine cancers
Cervical procedures
Cesarean section
Childbirth
Childbirth complications
Chlamydia
Circumcision, female, and genital mutilation
Conception
Contraception
Cryosurgery
Culdocentesis
Cyst removal
Cystitis
Cystoscopy
Dysmenorrhea
Ectopic pregnancy
Electrocauterization
Embolization
Endocrinology
Endometrial biopsy
Endometriosis
Endoscopy
Episiotomy
Fibrocystic breast condition
Galactorrhea
Gender reassignment surgery
Genital disorders
Glands
Gonorrhea
Hermaphroditism and pseudohermaphroditism
Herpes
Hormone therapy
Human papillomavirus (HPV)
Hyperplasia
Hysterectomy
In vitro fertilization
Incontinence
Infertility
Internal medicine
Laparoscopy
Leptin
Lesions
Mammography
Mastitis

Menopause
Menorrhagia
Menstruation
Miscarriage
Myomectomy
Obstetrics
Ovarian cysts
Ovaries
Oxytocin
Pap test
Pelvic inflammatory disease (PID)
Polycystic ovary syndrome
Polyps
Postpartum depression
Preeclampsia and eclampsia
Pregnancy and gestation
Pregnancy test
Premenstrual syndrome (PMS)
Rape and sexual assault
Reiter's syndrome
Reproductive system
Sexual differentiation
Sexual dysfunction
Sexuality
Sexually transmitted diseases (STDs)
Sterilization
Syphilis
Toxic shock syndrome
Trichomoniasis
Tubal ligation
Turner syndrome
Ultrasonography
Urinary disorders
Urology
Uterus
Von Willebrand's disease

HEMATOLOGY
Acid-base chemistry
Acidosis
Acquired immunodeficiency syndrome (AIDS)
Anemia
Anticoagulants
Babesiosis
Biological therapies
Bleeding
Blood and blood disorders
Blood testing
Blood vessels
Bone grafting
Bone Marrow
Bone marrow transplantation
Bruises
Burkitt's lymphoma
Chronic fatigue syndrome
Circulation
Cold agglutinin disease
Connective tissue
Cyanosis
Cytology

Pancreas
Prostate cancer
Pulmonary diseases
Pulmonary medicine
Renal failure
Rheumatic fever
Rheumatoid arthritis
Rheumatology
Rhinitis
Rhinoviruses
Sarcoidosis
Scleroderma
Serology
Severe combined immunodeficiency
 syndrome (SCID)
Skin cancer
Small intestine
Smallpox
Stevens-Johnson syndrome
Stomach
Stress
Stress reduction
Systemic lupus erythematosus (SLE)
Thalidomide
Thymus gland
Transfusion
Transplantation
Tularemia
Wiskott-Aldrich syndrome
Xenotransplantation

INTERNAL MEDICINE
Abdomen
Abdominal disorders
Acidosis
Acquired immunodeficiency syndrome
 (AIDS)
Adenoids
Adrenal glands
Alcoholism
Allergies
Alzheimer's disease
Amebiasis
Amyotrophic lateral sclerosis (ALS)
Anemia
Angina
Anthrax
Antianxiety drugs
Antibodies
Anti-inflammatory drugs
Antioxidants
Anus
Anxiety
Aortic stenosis
Apnea
Arteriosclerosis
Arthritis
Ataxia
Auras
Babesiosis
Bacillus Calmette-Guérin (BCG)

Bacterial infections
Bariatric surgery
Bedsores
Behçet's disease
Bile
Biofeedback
Bleeding
Blood vessels
Blurred vision
Body dysmorphic disorder
Bronchiolitis
Bronchitis
Burkitt's lymphoma
Bursitis
Campylobacter infections
Candidiasis
Cardiac surgery
Carotid arteries
Casts and splints
Celiac sprue
Childhood infectious diseases
Cholecystitis
Cholera
Cholesterol
Chronic fatigue syndrome
Chronic granulomatous disease
Chyme
Cirrhosis
Coccidioidomycosis
Colitis
Colon
Common cold
Computed tomography (CT) scanning
Congenital hypothyroidism
Constipation
Coughing
Cushing's syndrome
Cyanosis
Cystic fibrosis
Defibrillation
Delirium
Dengue fever
Diabetes mellitus
Diabetic neuropathy
Dialysis
Diaphragm
Diarrhea and dysentery
Digestion
Disseminated intravascular coagulation
 (DIC)
Diuretics
Diverticulitis and diverticulosis
Dizziness and fainting
E. coli infection
Echocardiography
Edema
Electrocauterization
Embolism
Emphysema
Encephalitis
End-stage renal disease

Endocarditis
Endocrine glands
Endoscopic retrograde
 cholangiopancreatography (ERCP)
Enteroviruses
Epidemics and pandemics
Epiglottitis
Ergogenic aids
Factitious disorders
Family-centered care
Family medicine
Fatigue
Fever
Fiber
Fungal infections
Gallbladder
Gallbladder diseases
Gastroenteritis
Gastroenterology
Gastrointestinal disorders
Gastrointestinal system
Gaucher's disease
Genetic diseases
Geriatric assessment
Gigantism
Glucose tolerance test
Gluten
Gout
Guillain-Barré syndrome
Hantavirus
Headaches
Heart attack
Heart disease
Heart failure
Heat exhaustion and heatstroke
Hemangioma
Hematuria
Hemochromatosis
Hepatitis
Hernia
Histology
Hives
Hodgkin's disease
H1N1 influenza
Hormone therapy
Hyperbaric chamber
Hyperhidrosis
Hyperlipidemia
Hypertension
Hyperthermia and hypothermia
Hyperthyroidism and hypothyroidism
Hypertrophy
Hypoglycemia
Hypokalemia
Hypotension
Hypoxia
Impetigo
Incontinence
Infarction
Infection
Inflammation

Influenza
Insulin
Interpartner violence
Interstitial pulmonary fibrosis (IPF)
Intestinal disorders
Intestines
Jaundice
Kaposi's sarcoma
Kidney disorders
Klippel-Trenaunay syndrome
Legionnaires' disease
Leprosy
Leptospirosis
Lesions
Leukemia
Liver
Liver disorders
Lymph
Lymphadenopathy and lymphoma
Malaria
Malignancy and metastasis
Measles
Melanoma
Metabolic syndrome
Methicillin-resistant staphylococcus
  aureus (MRSA) infection
Mitral valve prolapse
Monkeypox
Multiple sclerosis
Nail removal
Nephritis
Nephrology
Niemann-Pick disease
Nonalcoholic steatohepatitis (NASH)
Non-steroidal anti-inflammatory drugs
  (NSAIDs)
Nuclear medicine
Obesity
Occupational health
Opportunistic infections
Osteopathic medicine
Pain
Palliative care
Palliative medicine
Pancreas
Pancreatitis
Parasitic diseases
Parkinson's Disease
Peristalsis
Peritonitis
Pharynx
Phlebitis
Physician assistants
Pick's disease
Plaque
Plasma
Pleurisy
Pneumonia
Polymyalgia rheumatica
Polyps
Postherpetic neuralgia

Proctology
Psoriasis
Puberty and adolescence
Pulmonary edema
Pulmonary medicine
Pulse rate
Pyelonephritis
Radiopharmaceuticals
Rectum
Renal failure
Reye's syndrome
Rocky Mountain spotted fever
Sarcoidosis
Scarlet fever
Schistosomiasis
Sciatica
Septicemia
Severe acute respiratory syndrome
  (SARS)
Sexuality
Sexually transmitted diseases (STDs)
Shingles
Shock
Sinusitis
Sleep
Sleeping sickness
Small intestine
Sports medicine
Staphylococcal infections
Stevens-Johnson syndrome
Stones
Streptococcal infections
Stress
Supplements
Syphilis
Systemic lupus erythematosus (SLE)
Tetanus
Thrombosis and thrombus
Toxic shock syndrome
Tremors
Tumors
Typhoid fever
Typhus
Ulcers
Ultrasonography
Urethritis
Viral infections
Vitamins and minerals
Weight loss medications
Wilson's disease
Wounds

MICROBIOLOGY
Acquired immunodeficiency syndrome
  (AIDS)
Amebiasis
Anthrax
Antibiotic resistance
Antibiotics
Antibodies
Autopsy

Bacillus Calmette-Guérin (BCG)
Bacterial infections
Bacteriology
Bionics and biotechnology
Brucellosis
Campylobacter infections
Chemotherapy
Chlamydia
Cholera
Chronic granulomatous disease
Coccidioidomycosis
Conjunctivitis
Creutzfeldt-Jakob disease (CJD)
Dengue fever
Diphtheria
E. coli infection
Enteroviruses
Epidemics and pandemics
Epstein-Barr virus
Fecal bacteriotherapy
Fluoride treatments
Fungal infections
Gastroenteritis
Gastroenterology
Gastrointestinal disorders
Genomics
Gonorrhea
Gram staining
Hematuria
Human immunodeficiency virus (HIV)
Immune system
Immunization and vaccination
Impetigo
Insect-borne diseases
Laboratory tests
Leptospirosis
Methicillin-resistant staphylococcus
  aureus (MRSA) infection
Microscopy
Mold and mildew
Opportunistic infections
Pathology
Pelvic inflammatory disease (PID)
Peritonitis
Pharmacology
Plasma
Pneumocystis jirovecii
Protozoan diseases
Serology
Severe acute respiratory syndrome
  (SARS)
Sleeping sickness
Staphylococcal infections
Streptococcal infections
Syphilis
Toxic shock syndrome
Trichinosis
Tuberculosis
Urinalysis
Urology

NEONATOLOGY
Amniotic fluid
Angelman syndrome
Apgar score
Apnea
Birth defects
Blue baby syndrome
Bonding
Breast disorders
Cesarean section
Childbirth
Childbirth complications
Cleft lip and palate
Cleft lip and palate repair
Collodion baby
Congenital disorders
Congenital heart disease
Cutis marmorata telangiectatica
  congenita
Disseminated intravascular coagulation
  (DIC)
E. coli infection
Embryology
Endocrinology
Extracorporeal membrane oxygenation
  (ECMO)
Failure to thrive
Fetal surgery
Genetic diseases
Hemolytic disease of the newborn
Hydrocephalus
Intraventricular hemorrhage
Karyotyping
Malabsorption
Maple syrup urine disease (MSUD)
Motor skill development
Multiple births
Neonatal brachial plexus palsy
Neurology
Nursing
Obstetrics
Patent ductus arteriosus
Pediatrics
Perinatology
Phenylketonuria (PKU)
Physician assistants
Premature birth
Pulse rate
Respiratory distress syndrome
Rh factor
Shunts
Spina bifida
Sudden infant death syndrome (SIDS)
Surgery
Syphilis
Tay-Sachs disease
Transfusion
Trichomoniasis
Umbilical cord
Well-baby examinations

NEPHROLOGY
Abdomen
Addison's disease
Anemia
Chronic granulomatous disease
Diabetes mellitus
Diabetic nephropathy
Dialysis
Diuretics
E. coli infection
Edema
End-stage renal disease
Ergogenic aids
Hematuria
Hemolysis
Hemolytic uremic syndrome
Hypokalemia
Internal medicine
Kidney cancer
Kidney disorders
Kidney transplantation
Kidneys
Leptospirosis
Lesions
Lithotripsy
Nephrectomy
Nephritis
Nuclear medicine
Palliative care
Polycystic kidney disease
Polyps
Preeclampsia and eclampsia
Proteinuria
Pyelonephritis
Renal failure
Sarcoidosis
Stenosis
Stone removal
Stones
Systemic lupus erythematosus (SLE)
Transplantation
Uremia
Urinalysis
Urinary disorders
Urinary system
Urology
Vasculitis
Wilms tumor
Williams syndrome

NEUROLOGY
Acquired immunodeficiency syndrome
  (AIDS)
Adrenoleukodystrophy
Aging: Extended care
Agnosia
Altitude sickness
Alzheimer's disease
Amnesia
Amyotrophic lateral sclerosis (ALS)
Anesthesia

Anesthesiology
Aneurysms
Angelman syndrome
Anorexia nervosa
Anosmia
Antidepressants
Antipsychotic drugs
Aphasia and dysphasia
Apnea
Asperger syndrome
Ataxia
Atrophy
Attention-deficit disorder (ADD)
Audiology
Auras
Back pain
Balance disorders
Batten's disease
Bell's palsy
Biofeedback
Blindsight
Botox
Brain
Brain damage
Brain death
Brain disorders
Brain tumors
Brucellosis
Capgras syndrome
Carotid arteries
Carpal tunnel syndrome
Cerebral palsy
Charcot-Marie-Tooth Disease
Chiari malformations
Chiropractic
Chronic wasting disease (CWD)
Cluster headaches
Cockayne disease
Cognitive enhancement
Concussion
Cornelia de Lange syndrome
Craniotomy
Creutzfeldt-Jakob disease (CJD)
Critical care
Cryosurgery
Cutis marmorata telangiectatica
  congenita
Deep brain stimulation
Delirium
Dementias
Depression
Developmental stages
Diabetes mellitus
Diabetic neuropathy
Disk removal
Dizziness and fainting
Dysarthria
Dyskinesia
Dyslexia
Dysphagia
Ear infections and disorders

Deep brain stimulation
Laminectomy and spinal fusion
Minimally conscious state
Osteopetrosis
Virtual imaging
Wernicke's aphasia

NUCLEAR MEDICINE
Chemotherapy
Imaging and radiology
Magnetic resonance imaging (MRI)
Noninvasive tests
Nuclear radiology
Pneumocystis jirovecii
Positron emission tomography (PET)
  scanning
Radiation therapy
Single photon emission computed
  tomography (SPECT)

NURSING
Abusive relationships
Acidosis
Adipose tissue
Aging: Extended care
Alzheimer's disease
Analgesic
Ataxia
Atrophy
Back pain
Bedsores
Cardiac rehabilitation
Carotid arteries
Casts and splints
Critical care
Defibrillation
Diuretics
Drowning
Emergency medicine
Epidemics and pandemics
Eye infections and disorders
Fiber
Home care
H1N1 influenza
Hypoxia
Infarction
Influenza
Intravenous (IV) therapy
Methicillin-resistant staphylococcus
  aureus (MRSA) infection
Minimally conscious state
Pediatrics
Physician assistants
Polycystic ovary syndrome
Pulse rate
Radiculopathy
Surgical procedures
Surgical technologists
Well-baby examinations

NUTRITION
Adipose tissue
Aging: Extended care
Anorexia nervosa
Antioxidants
Bariatric surgery
Bedsores
Bell's palsy
Bile
Breast-feeding
Bulimia
Carbohydrates
Cardiac rehabilitation
Celiac sprue
Cholesterol
Colon
Crohn's disease
Cushing's syndrome
Dietary reference intakes (DRIs)
Digestion
Essential nutrients
Exercise physiology
Eye infections and disorders
Fasting
Fatty acid oxidation disorders
Fiber
Food allergies
Food biochemistry
Food guide plate
Fructosemia
Galactosemia
Gastroenterology
Gastrointestinal system
Gestational diabetes
Gluten
Gluten intolerance
Glycerol
Glycogen storage diseases
Hemolytic uremic syndrome
Hyperadiposis
Hypercholesterolemia
Irritable bowel syndrome (IBS)
Jaw wiring
Ketogenic diet
Korsakoff's syndrome
Kwashiorkor
Lactose intolerance
Leptin
Leukodystrophy
Lipids
Macronutrients
Malabsorption
Malnutrition
Mastitis
Metabolic disorders
Metabolic syndrome
Metabolism
Niacin
Nursing
Obesity
Orthorexia nervosa

Osteoporosis
Pellagra
Phenylketonuria (PKU)
Phytochemicals
Pituitary gland
Plasma
Polycystic ovary syndrome
Protein
Rickets
Scurvy
Small intestine
Sports medicine
Supplements
Systemic lupus erythematosus (SLE)
Taste
Ulcer surgery
Ulcers
Vagotomy
Vitamin D deficiency
Vitamins and minerals
Weaning
Weight loss and gain
Weight loss medications

OBSTETRICS
Amniocentesis
Amniotic fluid
Apgar score
Assisted reproductive technologies
Back pain
Birth defects
Breast-feeding
Breasts
Cerebral palsy
Cervical, ovarian, and uterine cancers
Cesarean section
Childbirth
Childbirth complications
Chorionic villus sampling
Conception
Congenital disorders
Contraception
Critical care
Cytomegalovirus (CMV)
Disseminated intravascular coagulation
  (DIC)
Down syndrome
Embryology
Emergency medicine
Endometrial biopsy
Endoscopy
Episiotomy
Fallopian tube
Family-centered care
Family medicine
Fetal surgery
Fetus
Gamete intrafallopian transfer (GIFT)
Genetic counseling
Genetic diseases
Genital disorders

Gestational diabetes
Growth
Gynecology
Hirschsprung's disease
Incontinence
Intravenous (IV) therapy
Karyotyping
Listeria infections
Mastitis
Miscarriage
Multiple births
Neonatal brachial plexus palsy
Neonatology
Noninvasive tests
Ovaries
Perinatology
Pituitary gland
Placenta
Polycystic ovary syndrome
Postpartum depression
Preeclampsia and eclampsia
Pregnancy and gestation
Pregnancy test
Premature birth
Pyelonephritis
Reproductive system
Rh factor
Sexuality
Sperm banks
Stillbirth
Streptococcal infections
Teratogens
Toxemia
Trichomoniasis
Tubal ligation
Turner syndrome
Ultrasonography
Urology
Uterus
Vaginal birth after cesarean (VBAC)

OCCUPATIONAL HEALTH
Acidosis
Agnosia
Altitude sickness
Angelman syndrome
Asbestos exposure
Asphyxiation
Ataxia
Bacillus Calmette-Guérin (BCG)
Back pain
Biofeedback
Blurred vision
Brucellosis
Cardiac rehabilitation
Carpal tunnel syndrome
Charcot-Marie-Tooth Disease
Defibrillation
Gulf War syndrome
Hearing tests
Leptospirosis

Leukodystrophy
Lung cancer
Mercury poisoning
Mesothelioma
Multiple chemical sensitivity syndrome
Nasopharyngeal disorders
Pneumonia
Prostheses
Pulmonary diseases
Pulmonary medicine
Radiation sickness
Skin disorders
Slipped disk
Spinocerebellar ataxia
Stress reduction
Tendinitis
Tendon disorders
Tendon repair

OCCUPATIONAL THERAPY
Astym® therapy
Flexibility
Home care
Minimally conscious state
Williams syndrome

ONCOLOGY
Mesenchymal stem cells
Acquired immunodeficiency syndrome (AIDS)
Aging: Extended care
Amputation
Anal cancer
Analgesic
Anemia
Antibodies
Antioxidants
Anus
Asbestos exposure
Assisted suicide
Biological therapies
Biopsy
Bladder cancer
Bone cancer
Bone disorders
Bone Marrow
Bone marrow transplantation
Brain tumors
Breast cancer
Breasts
Burkitt's lymphoma
Cancer
Carcinoma
Cervical, ovarian, and uterine cancers
Chemotherapy
Cold agglutinin disease
Colon
Colorectal cancer
Computed tomography (CT) scanning
Cryosurgery
Cystoscopy

Cytology
Cytopathology
Dermatology
Dermatopathology
Disseminated intravascular coagulation (DIC)
Embolization
Epstein-Barr virus
Ewing's sarcoma
Family-centered care
Fibrocystic breast condition
Galactorrhea
Gallbladder cancer
Gastrectomy
Gastroenterology
Gastrointestinal system
Gastrostomy
Genetic imprinting
Genital disorders
Glioma
Gynecology
Hematology
Histology
Hodgkin's disease
Hormone therapy
Human papillomavirus (HPV)
Hyperbaric chamber
Hysterectomy
Intravenous (IV) therapy
Kaposi's sarcoma
Karyotyping
Kidney cancer
Laboratory tests
Laryngectomy
Laser use in surgery
Lesions
Leukemia
Light therapy
Liver cancer
Lumbar puncture
Lung cancer
Lungs
Lymph
Lymphadenopathy and lymphoma
Malignancy and metastasis
Mammography
Massage
Mastectomy and lumpectomy
Meckel's diverticulum
Mesothelioma
Mouth and throat cancer
Necrosis
Nephrectomy
Nuclear medicine
Nursing
Oral and maxillofacial surgery
Pain
Pain management
Palliative care
Pap test
Pathology

Pharmacology
Plastic surgery
Proctology
Prostate cancer
Prostate gland
Prostate gland removal
Prostheses
Pulmonary diseases
Radiation sickness
Radiation therapy
Radiopharmaceuticals
Rectum
Retroviruses
Sarcoma
Serology
Skin
Skin cancer
Skin lesion removal
Small intestine
Smoking
Stenosis
Stomach
Stress
Testicular cancer
Thalidomide
Thymus gland
Tonsils
Transplantation
Tumor removal
Tumors
Uterus
Wilms tumor
Wiskott-Aldrich syndrome

OPHTHALMOLOGY
Acquired immunodeficiency syndrome
   (AIDS)
Adenoviruses
Adrenoleukodystrophy
Aging: Extended care
Anesthesia
Anesthesiology
Anti-inflammatory drugs
Astigmatism
Batten's disease
Behçet's disease
Blindness
Blindsight
Blurred vision
Botox
Cataract surgery
Cataracts
Cockayne disease
Conjunctivitis
Corneal transplantation
Cutis marmorata telangiectatica
   congenita
Diabetic nephropathy
Dry eye
Eye infections and disorders
Eye surgery

Eyes
Glaucoma
Glycerol
Hyperbaric chamber
Juvenile rheumatoid arthritis
Keratitis
Kluver-Bucy syndrome
Laser use in surgery
Lesions
Light therapy
Lyme disease
Macular degeneration
Marfan syndrome
Microscopy
Myopia
Optometry
Osteogenesis imperfecta
Osteopetrosis
Presbyopia
Prostheses
Pterygium/Pinguecula
Ptosis
Refractive eye surgery
Reiter's syndrome
Retina
Rubinstein-Taybi syndrome
Sarcoidosis
Sense organs
Sphincterectomy
Spinocerebellar ataxia
Spondylitis
Stevens-Johnson syndrome
Strabismus
Sturge-Weber syndrome
Subdural hematoma
Tears and tear ducts
Trachoma
Vasculitis
Vision
Vision disorders

OPTOMETRY
Aging: Extended care
Astigmatism
Blindsight
Blurred vision
Cataract surgery
Cataracts
Cockayne disease
Color blindness
Conjunctivitis
Eye infections and disorders
Eye surgery
Eyes
Glaucoma
Keratitis
Myopia
Ophthalmology
Presbyopia
Pterygium/Pinguecula
Ptosis

Sarcoidosis
Sense organs
Spinocerebellar ataxia
Tears and tear ducts
Vision disorders
Williams syndrome

ORTHODONTICS
Bones and the skeleton
Braces
Cleft lip and palate repair
Dentistry
Jaw wiring
Periodontal surgery
Periodontitis
Teeth
Teething
Tooth extraction
Williams syndrome

ORTHOPEDICS
Amputation
Anti-inflammatory drugs
Arthritis
Arthroplasty
Arthroscopy
Ataxia
Atrophy
Back pain
Bariatric surgery
Bone cancer
Bone disorders
Bone grafting
Bones and the skeleton
Bowlegs
Braces
Bunions
Cancer
Carticel®
Cartilage
Casts and splints
Cerebral palsy
Charcot-Marie-Tooth Disease
Chiropractic
Connective tissue
Contracture
Craniosynostosis
Cutis marmorata telangiectatica
   congenita
Disk removal
Dwarfism
Endoscopy
Ergogenic aids
Ewing's sarcoma
Fascia
Feet
Flat feet
Flexibility
Foot disorders
Fracture and dislocation
Fracture repair

Astym® therapy
Ataxia
Atrophy
Back pain
Biofeedback
Bowlegs
Burns and scalds
Cardiac rehabilitation
Casts and splints
Cerebral palsy
Charcot-Marie-Tooth Disease
Cornelia de Lange syndrome
Disk removal
Dyskinesia
Electromyography
Exercise physiology
Facial transplantation
Fascia
Flexibility
Grafts and grafting
Hemiplegia
Home care
Hydrotherapy
Kinesiology
Knock-knees
Leukodystrophy
Lower extremities
Massage
Minimally conscious state
Motor skill development
Muscle sprains, spasms, and disorders
Muscles
Muscular dystrophy
Neonatal brachial plexus palsy
Neurology
Numbness and tingling
Orthopedic surgery
Orthopedics
Osteopathic medicine
Pain
Pain management
Palsy
Paralysis
Parkinson's Disease
Patellofemoral pain syndrome
Physical rehabilitation
Pigeon toes
Plastic surgery
Prostheses
Pulse rate
Radiculopathy
Rotator cuff surgery
Scoliosis
Slipped disk
Spinal cord disorders
Spine
Spinocerebellar ataxia
Sports medicine
Systemic lupus erythematosus (SLE)
Tendinitis
Tendon disorders

Torticollis
Upper extremities
Whiplash
Williams syndrome

PLASTIC SURGERY
Amputation
Bariatric surgery
Body dysmorphic disorder
Botox
Breast surgery
Breasts
Burns and scalds
Circumcision, female, and genital
  mutilation
Cleft lip and palate
Cleft lip and palate repair
Craniosynostosis
Cyst removal
DiGeorge syndrome
Face lift and blepharoplasty
Facial transplantation
Gender reassignment surgery
Grafts and grafting
Hair transplantation
Healing
Hyaluronic acid injections
Jaw wiring
Laceration repair
Liposuction
Malignancy and metastasis
Mastectomy and lumpectomy
Mesenchymal stem cells
Moles
Necrotizing fasciitis
Neonatal brachial plexus palsy
Neurofibromatosis
Oral and maxillofacial surgery
Otoplasty
Otorhinolaryngology
Prostheses
Ptosis
Rhinoplasty and submucous resection
Skin
Skin lesion removal
Spina bifida
Sturge-Weber syndrome
Surgical procedures
Tattoos and body piercing
Varicose vein removal
Varicose veins
Vision

PODIATRY
Athlete's foot
Bones and the skeleton
Bunions
Cerebral palsy
Corns and calluses
Diabetic neuropathy
Feet

Flat feet
Foot disorders
Gout
Hammertoe correction
Hammertoes
Heel spur removal
Joints
Lesions
Lower extremities
Methicillin-resistant staphylococcus
  aureus (MRSA) infection
Nail removal
Orthopedic surgery
Orthopedics
Polydactyly and syndactyly
Tendon disorders
Tendon repair
Acidosis
Acupressure
Acupuncture
Alternative medicine
Anemia
Aneurysmectomy
Antibodies
Antihistamines
Antihypertensives
Aromatherapy
Assisted living facilities
Bacillus Calmette-Guérin (BCG)
Back pain
Biofeedback
Blurred vision
Breast cancer
Brucellosis
Cardiac surgery
Cardiology
Cerebral palsy
Chemotherapy
Chiropractic
Cholesterol
Club drugs
Computed tomography (CT) scanning
Croup
Electrocardiography (ECG or EKG)
Endometrial biopsy
Exercise physiology
Family-centered care
Family medicine
Fiber
Food guide plate
Genetic counseling
Genetic engineering
Hormone therapy
Host-defense mechanisms
Immune system
Immunization and vaccination
Insect-borne diseases
Lead poisoning
Mammography
Massage
Meditation

Tardive dyskinesia
Tinnitus
Toilet training
Tourette's syndrome
Transcranial magnetic stimulation (TMS)
Traumatic brain injury
Tremors

PSYCHOLOGY
Abuse of the elderly
Abusive relationships
Addiction
Aging
Aging: Extended care
Alcoholism
Amnesia
Amyotrophic lateral sclerosis (ALS)
Angelman syndrome
Anorexia nervosa
Antidepressants
Antipsychotic drugs
Anxiety
Aromatherapy
Asperger syndrome
Attention-deficit disorder (ADD)
Auras
Bariatric surgery
Bed-wetting
Biofeedback
Bipolar disorders
Blindsight
Bonding
Brain
Brain damage
Bulimia
Capgras syndrome
Cardiac rehabilitation
Cerebral palsy
Cirrhosis
Club drugs
Cognitive development
Death and dying
Deep brain stimulation
Depression
Developmental disorders
Developmental stages
Dyslexia
Eating disorders
Electroencephalography (EEG)
Ergogenic aids
Facial transplantation
Factitious disorders
Failure to thrive
Family-centered care
Family medicine
Forensic pathology
Frontal lobe syndrome
Functional magnetic imaging (fMRI)
Gender dysphoria
Gender reassignment surgery

Genetic counseling
Gulf War syndrome
Gynecology
Hippocampus
Huntington's disease
Hypnosis
Hypochondriasis
Hypothalamus
Intellectual disability
Interpartner violence
Juvenile rheumatoid arthritis
Kinesiology
Klinefelter syndrome
Kluver-Bucy syndrome
Korsakoff's syndrome
Learning disabilities
Lesbian, gay, bisexual, transgender, and queer (LGBTQ)
Light therapy
Marijuana
Memory erasure
Memory loss
Mental status exam
Mirror neurons
Miscarriage
Motor skill development
Münchausen syndrome by proxy
Neonatal brachial plexus palsy
Neuropsychology
Neurorehabilitation
Neurosis
Obesity
Obsessive-compulsive disorder
Occupational health
Overtraining syndrome
Pain management
Palliative care
Paranoia
Phobias
Phrenology
Pick's disease
Plastic surgery
Polycystic ovary syndrome
Postpartum depression
Post-traumatic stress disorder
Premenstrual syndrome (PMS)
Psychosomatic disorders
Puberty and adolescence
Relaxation
Reminiscence therapy
Restless legs syndrome
Separation anxiety
Serotonin
Sexual dysfunction
Sexuality
Sleep
Sleep disorders
Sleepwalking
Speech disorders
Split-brain
Sports medicine

Steroid abuse
Stress
Stress reduction
Sturge-Weber syndrome
Sudden infant death syndrome (SIDS)
Suicide
Synesthesia
Systemic lupus erythematosus (SLE)
Temporomandibular joint (TMJ) syndrome
Tics
Toilet training
Tourette's syndrome
Transcranial magnetic stimulation (TMS)
Traumatic brain injury
Weight loss and gain
Wernicke's aphasia

PUBLIC HEALTH
Acquired immunodeficiency syndrome (AIDS)
Acute respiratory distress syndrome (ARDS)
Adenoviruses
Advance directives
Aging: Extended care
Amebiasis
Antibodies
Assisted living facilities
Babesiosis
Bacillus Calmette-Guérin (BCG)
Bacteriology
Blood testing
Brucellosis
Cerebral palsy
Chagas' disease
Chickenpox
Childhood infectious diseases
Cholera
Chronic obstructive pulmonary disease (COPD)
Club drugs
Common cold
Coronaviruses
Creutzfeldt-Jakob disease (CJD)
Dengue fever
Dermatology
Diarrhea and dysentery
E. coli infection
Ebola virus
Elephantiasis
Emergency medicine
Encephalitis
Epidemics and pandemics
Epidemiology
Food guide plate
Food poisoning
Forensic pathology
Gulf War syndrome
Hantavirus

H1N1 influenza
Human papillomavirus (HPV)
Immunization and vaccination
Influenza
Insect-borne diseases
Interpartner violence
Legionnaires' disease
Leishmaniasis
Leprosy
Leptospirosis
Lice, mites, and ticks
Macronutrients
Malaria
Malnutrition
Managed care
Marijuana
Measles
Meningitis
Methicillin-resistant staphylococcus
   aureus (MRSA) infection
Microbiology
Monkeypox
Multiple chemical sensitivity syndrome
Neurosis
Niemann-Pick disease
Nursing
Nutrition
Obesity
Occupational health
Osteopathic medicine
Parasitic diseases
Pharmacology
Physician assistants
Pinworms
Plague
Pneumonia
Poliomyelitis
Polycystic ovary syndrome
Prion diseases
Protozoan diseases
Psychiatry
Rabies
Radiation sickness
Rape and sexual assault
Retroviruses
Rhinoviruses
Roundworms
Salmonella infection
Schistosomiasis
Screening
Serology
Severe acute respiratory syndrome
   (SARS)
Sexually transmitted diseases (STDs)
Shigellosis
Sleeping sickness
Smallpox
Syphilis
Tapeworms
Tattoos and body piercing
Tetanus

Trichinosis
Trichomoniasis
Tuberculosis
Tularemia
Typhoid fever
Typhus
West Nile virus
Yellow fever
Zoonoses

PULMONARY MEDICINE
Acquired immunodeficiency syndrome
   (AIDS)
Acute respiratory distress syndrome
   (ARDS)
Adrenoleukodystrophy
Amyotrophic lateral sclerosis (ALS)
Antihistamines
Apnea
Asthma
Bronchi
Bronchiolitis
Bronchitis
Catheterization
Chest
Chronic granulomatous disease
Chronic obstructive pulmonary disease
   (COPD)
Coccidioidomycosis
Cold agglutinin disease
Coronaviruses
Coughing
Critical care
Cyanosis
Cystic fibrosis
Defibrillation
Diaphragm
Dirofilaria immitis
Drowning
Edema
Emergency medicine
Emphysema
Endoscopy
Epidemics and pandemics
Extracorporeal membrane oxygenation
   (ECMO)
Fluids and electrolytes
Forensic pathology
Fungal infections
Hantavirus
Hemoglobin
Human respiratory system
Hyperbaric chamber
Hyperbaric oxygen therapy
Hyperventilation
Hypoxia
Influenza
Internal medicine
Interstitial pulmonary fibrosis (IPF)
Leptospirosis
Lesions

Lung cancer
Lung surgery
Lungs
Mesothelioma
Methicillin-resistant staphylococcus
   aureus (MRSA) infection
Mold and mildew
Occupational health
Oxygen therapy
Paramedics
Patent ductus arteriosus
Pediatrics
Pharynx
Pleurisy
Pneumocystis jirovecii
Pneumonia
Pneumothorax
Polyps
Prader-Willi syndrome
Pulmonary diseases
Pulmonary edema
Pulmonary hypertension
Respiration
Respiratory distress syndrome
Sarcoidosis
Severe acute respiratory syndrome
   (SARS)
Single photon emission computed
   tomography (SPECT)
Sleep apnea
Smoking
Stevens-Johnson syndrome
Systemic lupus erythematosus (SLE)
Thoracic surgery
Thrombolytic therapy and TPA
Tissue engineering
Trachea
Tuberculosis
Tumors
Vasculitis

RADIOLOGY
Achalasia
Angiography
Atrophy
Back pain
Biopsy
Bone cancer
Brain tumors
Breast cancer
Cancer
Cartilage
Catheterization
Chronic granulomatous disease
Cold agglutinin disease
Computed tomography (CT) scanning
Critical care
Cushing's syndrome
Dysphagia
Embolization
Emergency medicine

Head and neck disorders
Heat exhaustion and heatstroke
Hematomas
Hydrotherapy
Hyperbaric chamber
Impetigo
Joints
Kinesiology
Macronutrients
Massage
Methicillin-resistant staphylococcus
  aureus (MRSA) infection
Motor skill development
Muscle sprains, spasms, and disorders
Muscles
Nail removal
Orthopedic surgery
Orthopedics
Overtraining syndrome
Pain
Patellofemoral pain syndrome
Physical rehabilitation
Pigeon toes
Pulse rate
Radiculopathy
Rotator cuff surgery
Safety issues for children
Slipped disk
Spine
Steroid abuse
Steroids
Tendinitis
Tendon disorders
Tendon repair

TOXICOLOGY
Acidosis
Bites and stings
Blood testing
Chemotherapy
Club drugs
Critical care
Cyanosis
Defibrillation
Diphtheria
Emergency medicine
Ergogenic aids
Food poisoning
Forensic pathology
Gaucher's disease
Hepatitis
Laboratory tests
Lead poisoning
Leukemia
Liver
Mold and mildew
Multiple chemical sensitivity syndrome
Neuroscience
Occupational health
Pharmacology
Poisoning

Sarcoidosis
Tremors
Urinalysis

UROLOGY
Abdomen
Adenoviruses
Bed-wetting
Bladder removal
Catheterization
Chronic granulomatous disease
Circumcision
Cold agglutinin disease
Congenital adrenal hyperplasia
Contraception
Cryosurgery
Cushing's syndrome
Cystic fibrosis
Cystitis
Cystoscopy
Diabetic nephropathy
Dialysis
Diuretics
E. coli infection
Endoscopy
Erectile dysfunction
Fetal surgery
Fluids and electrolytes
Gender reassignment surgery
Genital disorders
Hemolysis
Hemolytic uremic syndrome
Hermaphroditism and
  pseudohermaphroditism
Herpes
Hydroceles
Hyperplasia
Hypogonadism
Hypospadias repair and urethroplasty
Incontinence
Infertility
Kidney cancer
Kidney disorders
Kidneys
Laser use in surgery
Leptospirosis
Lesions
Lithotripsy
Nephrectomy
Nephrology
Nuclear medicine
Orchiectomy
Pediatrics
Penile implant surgery
Polycystic kidney disease
Polyps
Prostate cancer
Prostate enlargement
Prostate gland
Prostate gland removal
Proteinuria

Pyelonephritis
Reiter's syndrome
Reproductive system
Semen
Sexual differentiation
Sexual dysfunction
Sexually transmitted diseases (STDs)
Sperm banks
Staphylococcal infections
Sterilization
Stevens-Johnson syndrome
Stone removal
Stones
Testicles
Testicular cancer
Testicular surgery
Testicular torsion
Tissue engineering
Toilet training
Transplantation
Trichomoniasis
Ultrasonography
Uremia
Urethritis
Urinalysis
Urinary disorders
Urinary system
Vas deferens
Vasectomy
Wilms tumor

VASCULAR MEDICINE
Acidosis
Amputation
Aneurysms
Angiography
Angioplasty
Antihypertensives
Arteriosclerosis
Biofeedback
Bleeding
Blood pressure
Blood vessels
Bruises
Cardiac surgery
Cardiology
Carotid arteries
Cholesterol
Circulation
Claudication
Cold agglutinin disease
Computed tomography (CT) scanning
Congenital heart disease
Cutis marmorata telangiectatica
  congenita
Defibrillation
Dehydration
Diabetes mellitus
Electrocauterization
Embolism
Embolization

VIROLOGY